Calculations for dete... of local anesthetic a... tor in dental cartridg...

Typical local anesthetic concentrations

Strength		*mg/ml Equivalent*
0.5%	=	5 mg/ml
1.5%	=	15 mg/ml
2.0%	=	20 mg/ml
3.0%	=	30 mg/ml
4.0%	=	40 mg/ml

Typical vasoconstrictor concentrations

Strength		*mg/ml (or μg/ml) Equivalent*
1:20,000	=	0.05 mg/ml (50 μg/ml)
1:50,000	=	0.02 mg/ml (20 μg/ml)
1:100,000	=	0.01 mg/ml (10 μg/ml)
1:200,000	=	0.005 mg/ml (5 μg/ml)

General calculation guidelines

1. Convert % solution to mg/ml (or μg/ml) as shown above.
2. Multiply mg/ml (or μg/ml) × cartridge volume × number of cartridges = quantity of drug. *Note:* Cartridge volumes may vary between products.

Example: Two cartridges of a 2% lidocaine HCl and 1:100,000 epinephrine HCl solution were administered. The cartridge volume was 1.8 ml for each. What quantity of each drug was given?

Answer:

For lidocaine HCl: 20 mg/ml × 1.8 ml × 2 cartridges = 72 mg

For epinephrine HCl: 0.01 mg/ml × 1.8 ml × 2 cartridges = 0.036 mg or 10 μg/ml × 1.8 ml × 2 cartridges = 36 μg

Weights and Equivalents

Metric system

Weight

kilogram	=	kg	=	1000 grams
gram	=	g	=	1 gram
milligram	=	mg	=	0.001 gram
microgram	=	μg	=	0.001 milligram

Volume

liter	=	L	=	1000 milliliters
milliliter	=	ml	=	0.001 liter

Weight conversion pounds to kilograms

Kilograms (kg)	Pounds (lb)
1	2.2
10	22
15	33
20	44
40	88
60	132
80	176

Household equivalents - approximate

Utensil	Volume
1 teaspoonful	5 ml
1 tablespoonful	15 ml
1 teacupful	120 ml
1 tumbler glassful	240 ml
1 pint	480 ml

Mosby's
Dental Drug Reference 2005

Mosby's Dental Drug Reference 2005

Seventh Edition

Tommy W. Gage, RPh, DDS, PhD
Professor Emeritus
Department of Oral and Maxillofacial
Surgery and Pharmacology
Formerly Director of Curriculum
Academic Services
Baylor College of Dentistry
The Texas A&M University System Health Science Center
Dallas, Texas

Frieda Atherton Pickett, RDH, MS
Formerly, Associate Professor
Caruth School of Dental Hygiene
Baylor College of Dentistry
The Texas A&M University System Health Science Center
Dallas, Texas
Adjunct Associate Professor
Department of Dental Hygiene
East Tennessee State University
Johnson City, Tennessee

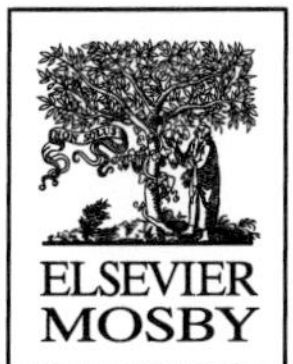

ELSEVIER
MOSBY

11830 Westline Industrial Drive
St. Louis, Missouri 63146

MOSBY'S DENTAL DRUG REFERENCE 2005 ISBN 0-323-04081-0

NOTICE

Pharmacology is constantly changing. As new research and experience broaden our knowledge, changes in practice, treatment and drug therapy may become necessary or appropriate. Readers are advised to check the most current information provided (i) on procedures featured or (ii) by the manufacturer of each product to be administered, to verify the recommended dose or formula, the method and duration of administration, and contraindications. It is the responsibility of the practitioner, relying on their own experience and knowledge of the patient, to make diagnoses, to determine dosages and the best treatment for each individual patient, and to take all appropriate safety precautions. To the fullest extent of the law, neither the Publisher nor the author assumes any liability for any injury and/or damage to persons or property arising out or related to any use of the material contained in this book.

Previous editions copyrighted 1994, 1996, 1997, 1999, 2001, 2003

International Standard Book Number 0-323-04081-0

Publishing Director: Linda Duncan
Executive Editor: Penny Rudolph
Developmental Editor: Courtney Sprehe
Publishing Services Manager: Julie Eddy
Designer: Andrea Lutes

Printed in the United States of America

Last digit is the print number: 9 8 7 6 5 4 3 2 1

Editorial Review Board

Authors' Comments

Our goal of creating a quick and concise drug reference resource remains steadfast. We are excited to present this seventh edition, trusting it will serve you even better than previous editions. We have revised the appendices and made them more user friendly. Your acceptance of this drug information resource has been extremely gratifying and has supported our vision for the need for such a volume. The book comes with a CD that provides color photographs of drug reactions in the oral cavity, plus over 950 patient information sheets that are taken from *Mosby's Drug Consult.* These patient handouts are available in English and Spanish.

In addition to updating each monograph, additional herbal and nonherbal remedies were added. We are continually working to keep the book as small as possible for convenience in handling, but the number of new drugs and drug products approved for marketing each year presents a considerable challenge. Our focus is on the most frequently prescribed medications, dental specialty products, and new products. Because of these reasons, not every drug that is available in the marketplace is listed. However, it does include the new drugs marketed through December 2004. The book is only as good as it is able to assist the practitioner to quickly locate drug facts. The authors are hopeful this edition will be equally acceptable and useful. Your comments for improvements are solicited. We receive many comments and suggestions from our readers, and we appreciate your input.

Preface

Mosby's Dental Drug Reference 2005 is designed to be used chairside in the dental office and by the student or resident as a quick, concise drug reference resource. Its *purpose is to assist in the rapid identification of drugs* patients may be taking as they present for dental care. The easy-to-use design provides rapid access to essential drug information to facilitate completion of the medical history review and patient evaluation.

This book is not intended to be a comprehensive drug compendium or to make specific recommendations about selecting and prescribing dental drugs. It contains concise and easy-to-read "micro" drug monographs with basic information about each drug.

Selected herbal and nonherbal remedies have been placed in a separate appendix to aid the dental practitioner in identifying dental implications of these products. Drugs are presented alphabetically by generic name in a succinctly ordered and standardized format with pertinent drug information for the dentist, dental hygienist, dental assistant, or student. A user-friendly cross index is the key to using the book for both brand and generic name identification. A second index, based on a therapeutic and pharmacologic classification, can also be used to identify the location of drug monographs. And in addition, it will aid in identifying drugs when the patient cannot recall the name or spelling of a drug being taken. This therapeutic index also groups drugs by classes or use, so the reader can easily identify other drugs within a given class or application. The seventh edition also contains an appendix with sample prescriptions suitable for use or as a guide in preparing prescriptions. Information is provided on more than 1600 drug products, including the most recently approved drugs and new drug products through 2004.

A special feature of this book is an emphasis on drug interactions of dental interest and the highlighting of oral side effects. The dental considerations section includes information that will be useful in developing patient management strategies. Useful fact tables are located on the front inside covers and in the appendix, with information about dose calculations. This volume also contains the 1997 AHA drug and dose recommendations for antibiotic prophylaxis for patients at risk for bacterial endocarditis and updated information prophylaxis for patients with prosthetic joints. We have also revised the tables listing drugs that can alter salivary flow and affect taste.

The accompanying CD features intraoral and extraoral color photographs of manifestations of oral reactions to drugs. This material was contributed by Drs. William Binnie and John Wright and is a must for every dental office. In addition, the CD features patient drug information sheets to accompany prescriptions. These sheets can be printed and customized for your particular need.

Each drug monograph is designed to include the following information:

GENERIC NAME of the drug

PRONUNCIATION of the generic name

COMMON BRAND NAMES for the generic drug as sold in the United States and Canada

DRUG CLASS to facilitate drug identification

CONTROLLED SUBSTANCES schedule as appropriate for the United States and Canada

ACTION, with a brief description of the mechanism of action of the drug

USES or indications for the drug, including those approved by the FDA. (Unapproved uses are identified as appropriate for selected drugs.)

DOSES AND ROUTES OF ADMINISTRATION to assist the dental professional in assessing the dose in relationship to the seriousness of the patient's disease and predicting potential side effects and drug interactions

SIDE EFFECTS/ADVERSE REACTIONS are grouped according to body systems; common side effects listed in italics, and life-threatening reactions listed in boldface type; information regarding oral manifestations of side effects listed separately

CONTRAINDICATIONS are identified for instances in which the medication should absolutely not be given or when risk benefit criteria must be established

PRECAUTIONS to be considered when prescribing and using the drug and identification of pregnancy categories

PHARMACOKINETICS, with brief descriptions for each drug

DRUG INTERACTIONS OF CONCERN TO DENTISTRY listed for the purpose of determining whether a given interaction is beneficial or harmful. This section is organized so that the response is given followed by a colon. This is followed by the drug(s) interacting with the monograph drug. For example, increased hypoglycemia: aspirin. When the monograph drug alters the effects of another drug the interaction is stated as the effect "with" or "of" another drug. For example: increased nausea: with codeine, hydrocodone. Another example is: increased blood levels of carbamazepine. Few drug interactions are absolute; therefore clinical judgment must always be applied for each interaction listed.

DENTAL CONSIDERATION includes general information related to dental concerns in treating a patient taking a given drug, suggestions for medical consultations, and recommendations for the patient/family in preventing dental complications or disease

Appendixes following the drug monograph section include the following:

APPENDIX A Abbreviations
APPENDIX B Drugs causing dry mouth
APPENDIX C Controlled substances chart
APPENDIX D FDA pregnancy categories
APPENDIX E Drugs that affect taste
APPENDIX F Combination products
APPENDIX G Dose calculations by weight
APPENDIX H Herbal and nonherbal remedies
APPENDIX I Drugs affecting the cytochrome P-450 isoenzymes
APPENDIX J Prescription examples
APPENDIX K Selected references
NEW DRUG UPDATES
In **Mosby's Dental Drug Reference 2005,** information on 13 recently approved drugs and six new combination products has been added. Also provided is information on 11 recently approved drugs not likely to be encountered in the dental office.

Located on the inside cover pages are useful tables, sample dose calculations, and drugs and doses for antibiotic prophylaxis.

Tommy W. Gage
Frieda Atherton Pickett

Acknowledgments

The authors wish to express their sincere gratitude for the contributions made by the Editorial Review Board who were selected on the basis of their extensive experience and knowledge. The authors also wish to offer a special thanks to Dr. Colvard for his aid in the preparation of Appendix H. A special word of appreciation goes to Mrs. Brigitte Wallaert-Sims for her assistance in data entry, in the laborious task of printing the completed manuscript, and in putting up with our demands.

Tommy W. Gage
Frieda Atherton Pickett

Contents

Mosby's
Dental Drug Reference 2005

Therapeutic/Pharmacologic Index

Drugs Classified by Usual Therapeutic/Pharmacologic Category

This section of the book features drugs classified by primary therapeutic or pharmacologic group, or both. Thus you can locate drugs by knowing their primary therapeutic use or general pharmacologic class. This arrangement makes it easy to find the matching drug monograph by using the generic name. The individual drug monographs are arranged by generic name in alphabetical order and can simply be found in the appropriate alphabet section. Colored tabs on the side of the book mark the alphabetical sections. An originator or common brand name is also listed for convenience and may help with identification. This arrangement allows the book user to see other drugs in the same classification that are included in this volume.

For example, take the case of a patient using a drug for depression and having difficulty recalling the drug name. Find the *Antidepressants* section. All of the antidepressants listed in this volume can be seen and may help stimulate the patient to recall the drug currently used. Or if you want to know which drugs are calcium channel antagonists, go to the *Antihypertensives* section and find the subtopic of calcium channel antagonists. The calcium channel antagonists included in this volume are listed. As you identify the drug, use the generic name to quickly tab to the appropriate alphabet section.

ADRENERGIC AGONISTS

albuterol sulfate (Proventil)
apraclonidine HCl (Iopidine)
brimonidine tartrate (Alphagan)
dipivefrin HCl (Propine C)
ephedrine sulfate
epinephrine HCl (Adrenalin)
isoetharine HCl (Isoethaine)
isoproterenol HCl (Isuprel)
levalbuterol HCl (Xopenex)
metaproterenol sulfate (Alupent)
pirbuterol acetate (Maxair)
terbutaline sulfate (Brethine)

ALZHEIMER'S

donepezil HCl (Aricept)
galantamine HBr (Reminyl)
memantine HCl (Namenda)
rivastigmine (Exelon)
tacrine HCl (Cognex)

AMINOGLYCOSIDES (TOPICALS)

gentamicin ophth. (Garamycin)
neomycin (Myciguent)
polymyxin B ophth. (Aerosporin)
tobramycin ophth. (Tobrex)

AMYOTROPHIC LATERAL SCLEROSIS

riluzole (Rilutek)

ANALGESICS (NONOPIOID)

acetaminophen (Tylenol)
aspirin
salsalate (Anaflex)

ANALGESICS (NSAIDS)

(see nonsteroidal antiinflammatory drugs)

ANALGESICS (OPIOIDS)

buprenorphine HCl (Buprenex)
codeine sulfate
dihydrocodeine bitartrate
fentanyl transdermal (Duragesic)
fentanyl transmucosal (Fentanyl Oralet, Actiq)
hydromorphone HCl (Dilaudid)
meperidine HCl (Demerol)
methadone HCl (Dolophine)
morphine sulfate (MS Contin)
oxycodone HCl (Roxicodone)
pentazocine HCl (Talwin Nx)
propoxyphene hydrochloride (Darvon)
propoxyphene napsylate (Darvon-N)
tramadol HCl (Ultram)

ANESTHETICS (LOCAL)

articaine HCl (Septocaine)
bupivacaine HCl (Marcaine)
lidocaine HCl (Xylocaine)
mepivacaine HCl (Carbocaine)
prilocaine HCl (Citanest)

ANESTHETICS (TOPICAL)

benzocaine (Hurricaine)
dyclonine HCl
lidocaine HCl (Xylocaine)
lidocaine transoral (DentiPatch)
tetracaine HCl (Pontocaine)

ANESTHETICS (GENERAL)

midazolam HCl (Versed)
propofol (Diprivan)

ANTACIDS

magaldrate (Riopan)

ANTAGONISTS

disulfiram (Antabuse)
flumazenil (Romazicon)
nalmefene HCl (Revex)
naloxone HCl (Narcan)
naltrexone HCl (ReVia, Trexan)

ANTIANGINALS

Nitrates

isosorbide dinitrate (Isordil)

isosorbide mononitrate (ISMO)
nitroglycerin (Transderm-Nitro)

Beta-adrenergic antagonists
atenolol (Tenormin)
metoprolol tartrate (Lopressor)
nadolol (Corgard)
propranolol HCl (Inderal)

Calcium channel antagonists
amlodipine (Norvasc)
bepridil (Vascor)
diltiazem HCl (Cardizem)
felodipine (Plendil)
nicardipine HCl (Cardene)
nifedipine (Procardia)
nislodipine (Sular)
verapamil (Calan)

ANTIANEMIC
darbepoetin alfa (Aranesp)
epoetin alfa (Procrit)

ANTIANXIETY/SEDATIVE-HYPNOTICS

Barbiturates
pentobarbital (Nembutal)
phenobarbital (Luminal)
secobarbital (Seconal)

Benzodiazepines
alprazolam (Xanax)
chlordiazepoxide HCl (Librium)
clorazepate dipotassium (Tranxene)
diazepam (Valium)
estazolam (ProSom)
flurazepam HCl (Dalmane)
lorazepam (Ativan)
midazolam (Versed)
oxazepam (Serax)
quazepam (Doral)
temazepam (Restoril)
triazolam (Halcion)

Antihistamines
diphenhydramine HCl (Benadryl)
hydroxyzine HCl (Atarax, Vistaril)
promethazine HCl (Phenergan)

Others
buspirone HCl (BuSpar)
chloral hydrate (Aquachloral)
doxepin HCl (Sinaquan)
meprobamate (Equanil, Miltown)
zaleplon (Sonata)
zolpidem (Ambien)

ANTIASTHMATICS
(see bronchodilators)

ANTICARIES
sodium fluoride

ANTICHOLELITHICS
ursodiol (Actigall)

ANTICHOLINERGICS
atropine sulfate (Sal-Tropine)
benztropine mesylate (Cogentin)
biperidin (Akineton)
dicyclomine HCl (Bentyl)
glycopyrrolate (Robinul)
hyoscyamine sulfate (Levsin)
mepenzolate (Cantil)
oxybutynin chloride (Ditropan)
propantheline bromide (Pro-Banthine)
scopolamine
tolterodine tartrate (Detrol)

ANTICOAGULANTS
dalteparin sodium (Fragmin)
danaparoid (Orgaran)
enoxaparin sodium (Lovenox)
fondaparinux sodium (Arixtra)
heparin
warfarin sodium (Coumadin)

ANTICONVULSANTS
acetazolamide (Diamox)
carbamazepine (Tegretol)
clonazepam (Klonopin)
diazepam (Valium)

divalproex (Depakote)
ethosuximide (Zarontin)
ethotoin (Peganone)
felbamate (Felbatol)
fosphenytoin sodium (Cerebyx)
gabapentin (Neurontin)
lamotrigine (Lamictal)
levetiracetam (Keppra)
mephobarbital (Mebaral)
methsuximide (Celontin)
oxcarbazepine (Trileptal)
phenobarbital (Luminal)
phenytoin sodium (Dilantin)
primidone (Mysoline)
tiagabine HCl (Gabitril)
topiramate (Topamax)
trimethadione (Tridione)
valproic acid (Depakene)
zonisamide (Zonegran)

ANTIDEPRESSANTS

Atypical

bupropion HCl (Wellbutrin)
nefazodone HCl (Serzone)
trazodone HCl (Desyrel)
venlafaxine HCl (Effexor)

Monoamine oxidase inhibitors

isocarboxazid (Marplan)
phenelzine sulfate (Nardil)
tranylcypromine sulfate (Parnate)

Serotonin-specific reuptake inhibitors

citalopram HCl (Celexa)
escitalopram oxalate (Lexapro)
fluoxetine (Prozac)
fluvoxamine maleate (Luvox)
paroxetine (Paxil)
sertraline (Zoloft)

Tetracyclics

maprotiline HCl (Ludiomil)
mirtazapine (Remeron)

Tricyclics

amitriptyline HCl(Elavil)
amoxapine (Asendin)
clomipramine (Anafranil)
desipramine HCl (Norpramin)
doxepin (Sinequan)
imipramine HCl (Tofranil)
nortriptyline HCl (Pamelor)
protriptyline HCl (Vivactil)
trimipramine maleate (Surmontil)

ANTIDIABETICS

acarbose (Precose)
acetohexamide (Dymelor)
chlorpropamide (Diabinese)
glimepiride (Amaryl)
glipizide (Glucotrol)
glyburide (DiaBeta)
insulin
metformin HCl (Glucophage)
miglitol (Glyset)
nateglinide (Starlix)
pioglitazone (Actos)
repaglinide (Prandin)
rosiglitazone maleate (Avandia)
tolazamide (Tolinase)
tolbutamide (Orinase)

ANTIDIARRHEALS

bismuth subsalicylate (Pepto-Bismol)
difenoxin/atropine (Motofen)
diphenoxylate/atropine (Lomotil)
loperamide HCl (Imodium-AD)
paregoric

ANTIDIURETIC HORMONE

desmopressin acetate (DDAVP)

ANTIDYSRHYTHMICS (ANTIARRHYTHMICS)

amiodarone HCl (Cordarone)
digoxin (Lanoxin)
diltiazem (Cardizem)
disopyramide (Norpace)
dofetilide (Tikosyn)
flecainide acetate (Tambocor)
lidocaine (Xylocaine Cardiac)
mexiletine HCl (Mexitil)
moricizine (Ethmozine)

procainamide HCl (Pronestyl)
propafenone (Rythmol)
propranolol HCl (Inderal)
quinidine (Quinaglute)
sotalol (Betapace)
tocainide HCl (Tonocard)

ANTIEMETICS

aprepitant (Emend)
chlorpromazine (Thorazine)
cyclizine HCl (Marezine)
dimenhydrinate (Dramamine)
dolasetron (Anzemet)
dronabinol (Marinol)
meclizine HCl (Bonine)
metoclopramide (Reglan)
ondansetron HCl (Zofran)
prochlorperazine (Compazine)
promethazine (Phenergan)
scopolamine (Transderm-Scop)
thiethylperazine maleate (Torecan)
trimethobenzamide (Tigan)

ANTIFUNGALS (TOPICAL)

amphotericin B (Fungizone)
butenafine (Mentax)
butoconazole nitrate (Femstat)
ciclopirox olamine (Loprox)
clotrimazole (Mycelex)
econazole nitrate (Spectazole)
itraconazole (Sporanox)
miconazole nitrate (Monistat)
naftifine HCl (Naftin)
nystatin (Mycostatin)
sulconazole nitrate (Exelderm)
terbinafine HCl (Lamisil)
terconazole (Terazol)

ANTIFUNGALS (SYSTEMIC)

fluconazole (Diflucan)
flucytosine (Ancobon)
itraconazole (Sporanox)
ketoconazole (Nizoral)
terbinafine HCl (Lamisil)

ANTIGOUTS

allopurinol (Zyloprim)
colchicine

ANTIHISTAMINES (H_2) ANTAGONISTS

cimetidine (Tagamet)
famotidine (Pepcid)
nizatidine (Axid)
ranitidine (Zantac)

ANTIHISTAMINES (H_1) ANTAGONISTS

azatadine maleate (Optimine)
azelastine HCl (Astelin, Optivar)
brompheniramine tannate (Brovex)
buclizine (Bucladin-S)
cetirizine HCl (Zyrtec)
chlorpheniramine maleate (Chlor-Trimeton)
clemastine fumarate (Tavist Allergy)
cyclizine (Marezine)
cyproheptadine HCl (Periactin)
desloratadine (Clarinex)
dexchlorpheniramine maleate (Polaramine)
dimenhydrinate (Dramamine)
diphenhydramine (Benadryl)
emedastine difumarate (Emadine)
fexofenadine HCl (Allegra)
hydroxyzine (Atarax, Vistaril)
ketotifen fumarate (Zaditor)
levocabastine (Livostin)
loratadine (Claritin)
meclizine (Bonine)
olopatadine HCl (Patanol)
promethazine (Phenergan)

ANTIHYPERCALCEMICS (OSTEOPOROSIS)

alendronate sodium (Fosamax)
etidronate disodium (Didronel)

calcitonin (Calcimar)
raloxifene (Evista)
risedronate sodium (Actonel)
teriparatide acetate (Forteo)
tiludronate disodium (Skelid)
zoledronic acid (Zometa)

ANTIHYPERLIPIDEMICS

atorvastatin calcium (Lipitor)
cholestyramine (Questran)
clofibrate (Atromid-S)
colesevelam HCl (Welchol)
colestipol HCl (Colestid)
ezetimibe (Zetia)
fenofibrate (Tricor)
fluvastatin sodium (Lescol)
gemfibrozil (Lopid)
lovastatin (Mevacor)
niacin (Nia-Bid)
pravastatin (Pravachol)
rosuvastatin calcium (Crestor)
simvastatin (Zocor)

ANTIHYPERTENSIVES

(also see diuretics)

Aldosterone antagonists
eplerenone (Inspra)
spironolactone (Aldactone)

Alpha-adrenergic antagonists
doxazosin mesylate (Cardura)
phentolamine mesylate (Regitine)
prazosin HCl (Minipress)
terazosin (Hytrin)

Alpha/beta-adrenergic antagonists
carvedilol (Coreg)
labetalol (Normodyne)

Angiotensin-converting enzyme inhibitors
benazepril (Lotensin)
captopril (Capoten)
enalapril maleate (Vasotec)
fosinopril (Monopril)
lisinopril (Prinivil, Zestril)
moexipril HCl (Univasc)
perindopril erbumine (Aceon)
quinapril (Accupril)
ramipril (Altace)
trandolapril (Mavik)

Angiotensin II receptor antagonists
candesartan cilexetil (Atacand)
eprosartan (Teveten)
irbesartan (Avapro)
losartan potassium (Cozaar)
olmesartan medoxomil (Benicar)
telmisartan (Micardis)
valsartan (Diovan)

Beta-adrenergic antagonists
Selective
atenolol (Tenormin)
betaxolol (Kerlone)
bisoprolol fumarate (Zebeta)
metoprolol tartrate (Lopressor)
nadolol (Corgard)
Nonselective
carteolol HCl (Cartrol)
carvedilol (Coreg)
penbutolol (Levatol)
pindolol (Visken)
propranolol HCl (Inderal)
timolol maleate (Blocadren)

Calcium channel antagonists
amlodipine besylate (Norvasc)
bepridil HCl (Vascor)
diltiazem (Cardizem)
felodipine (Plendil)
isradipine (DynaCirc)
nicardipine HCl (Cardene)
nifedipine (Procardia XL)
nislodipine (Sular)
verapamil (Calan)
Centrally acting
clonidine (Catapres)
clonidine transdermal (Catapres-TTS)
guanabenz acetate (Wytensin)
methyldopa (Aldomet)
Other
bosentan (Tracleer)
guanadrel sulfate (Hylorel)

guanethidine sulfate (Ismelin)
hydralazine HCl (Apresoline)
mecamylamine HCl (Inversine)
minoxidil (Loniten)
reserpine (Serpasil)

ANTIHYPOGLYCEMIC

glucagon (Glucagon Emergency Kit)

ANTIINFECTIVES (TOPICAL)

chlorhexidine gluconate (Peridex, PerioGard)
chlorhexidine gluconate (PerioChip)
erythromycin (Erytroderm)
mupirocin (Bactroban)
povidone-iodine (Betadine)

ANTIINFECTIVES (MISCELLANEOUS)

atovaquone (Mepron)
clofazimine (Lamprene)
daptomycin (Cubicin)
linezolid (Zyvox)
metronidazole (Flagyl)
pentamidine (NebuPent)
quinupristin/dalfopristin (Synercid IV)

ANTIINFECTIVES (SYSTEMIC)

(see specific class: penicillins, cephalosporins, etc.)

ANTIINFLAMMATORY ANTIARTHRITICS

allopurinol (Zyloprim)
aspirin
auranofin gold (Ridaura)
aurothioglucose (Solganal)
celecoxib (Celebrex)
choline salicylate (Arthropan)
colchicine
diflunisal (Dolobid)
etanercept (Enbrel)
etodolac (Lodine)
fenoprofen calcium (Nalfon)
gold sodium thiomalate (Myochrysine)
ibuprofen (Motrin)
indomethacin (Indocin)
infliximab (Remicade)
ketoprofen (Orudis)
leflunomide (Arava)
methotrexate (Rheumatrex)
nabumetone (Relafen)
naproxen sodium (Anaprox)
naproxen (Naprosyn)
oxaprozin (Daypro)
piroxicam (Feldene)
probenecid (Benemid)
rofecoxib (Vioxx)
salsalate (Anaflex)
sulindac (Clinoril)
tolmetin sodium (Tolectin)
valdecoxib (Bextra)

ANTIMALARIALS

chloroquine (Aralen)
hydroxychloroquine sulfate (Plaquenil)
primaquine phosphate
quinine sulfate

ANTIPARKINSONIANS

amantadine HCl (Symmetrel)
benztropine (Cogentin)
biperiden HCl (Akineton)
bromocriptine mesylate (Parlodel)
diphenhydramine (Benadryl)
entacapone (Comtan)
levodopa (Larodopa)
levodopa/carbidopa (Sinemet)
pergolide mesylate (Permax)
pramipexole dihydrochloride (Mirapex)
procyclidine HCl (Kemadrin)
ropinirole HCl (ReQuip)
selegiline HCl (Eldepryl)
tolcapone (Tasmar)
trihexyphenidyl HCl (Artane)

ANTIPSYCHOTICS

Phenothiazines

chlorpromazine HCl (Thorazine)
fluphenazine HCl (Prolixin)
mesoridazine besylate (Serentil)
perphenazine (Trilafon)
prochlorperazine (Compazine)
thioridazine HCl (Mellaril)
trifluoperazine HCl (Stelazine)

Butyrophenone

haloperidol (Haldol)

Thioxanthene

thiothixene (Navane)

Others

aripipraxole (Abilify)
clozapine (Clozaril)
loxapine HCl (Loxitane)
molindone HCl (Moban)
olanzapine (Zyprexa)
pimozide (Orap)
quetiapine fumarate (Seroquel)
risperidone (Risperdal)
ziprasidone HCl (Geodon)

Bipolar disease

lithium carbonate (Eskalith)
valproic acid (Depakene)

ANTISIALOGOGUES

atropine sulfate (SalTropine)
glycopyrrolate (Robinul)
propantheline bromide (Pro-Banthine)

ANTITHYROIDS

methimazole (Tapazole)

ANTITUBERCULARS

aminosalicylic acid (Paser)
cycloserine (Seromycin)
ethambutol HCl (Myambutol)
ethionamide (Trecator)
isoniazid (Nydrazid)
pyrazinamide
rifabutin (Mycobutin)
rifampin (Rifadin)
rifapentine (Priftin)

ANTITUSSIVES/ EXPECTORANTS

benzonatate (Tessalon)
codeine
dextromethorphan HBr (Benylin)
diphenhydramine (Benadryl)
guaifenesin (Humibid)
hydrocodone bitartrate (Hycodan)

ANTIVIRALS (SYSTEMIC)

Herpes viruses

acyclovir (Zovirax)
famciclovir (Famvir)
foscarnet sodium (Foscavir)
ganciclovir (Cytovene)
valacyclovir HCl (Valtrex)
valganciclovir HCl (Valcyte)

Hepatitis B virus

adefovir dipivoxil (Hepsera)
ribavirin (Copegus)

Influenza viruses

amantadine (Symmetrel)
oseltamivir phosphate (Tamiflu)
rimantadine HCl (Flumadine)
zanamivir (Relenza)

HIV-fusion inhibitors

enfuvirtide (Fuzeon)

HIV—nonnucleoside analogs

delavirdine mesylate (Rescriptor)
efavirenz (Sustiva)
nevirapine (Viramune)
tenofovir disoproxil fumarate (Viread)

HIV—nucleoside analogs

abacavir sulfate (Ziagen)
didanosine (ddl) (Videx)
emtricitabine (Emtriva)
lamivudine (3TC) (Epivir)
stavudine (d4T) (Zerit)
zalcitabine (Hivid)
zidovudine (AZT) (Retrovir)

HIV—protease inhibitors
- amprenavir (Agenerase)
- atazanavir sulfate (Reyataz)
- indinavir sulfate (Crixivan)
- nelfinavir mesylate (Viracept)
- ritonavir (Norvir)
- saquinavir mesylate (Invirase, Fortovase)

ANTIVIRALS (TOPICAL)
- acyclovir sodium (Zovirax)
- docosanol (Abreva)
- penciclovir (Denavir)
- vidarabine (Vira-A)

APHTHOUS STOMATITIS
- amlexanox (Aphthasol)
- chlorhexidine (Peridex)

APPETITE SUPPRESSANTS/ WEIGHT CONTROL
- diethylpropion HCl (Tenuate)
- methamphetamine (Desoxyn)
- orlistat (Xenical)
- phendimetrazine tartrate (Prelu-2)
- phentermine HCl (Ionamin)
- sibutramine (Meridia)

ASTHMA TREATMENT
(see bronchodilators)

ASTHMA PREVENTION
- montelukast (Singulair)
- salmeterol xinafoate (Serevent)
- zafirlukast (Accolate)
- zileuton (Zyflo)

ATTENTION DEFICIT HYPERACTIVITY DISORDER
- amphetamine (Adderall)
- atomoxetine HCl (Strattera)
- dexmethylphenidate HCl (Focalin)
- methylphenidate (Ritalin)

BARBITURATES
- pentobarbital (Nembutal)
- phenobarbital (Luminal)
- secobarbital (Seconal)

BRONCHODILATORS
- albuterol (Proventil, Ventolin)
- aminophylline (Truphylline)
- dyphylline (Dilor)
- ephedrine sulfate
- epinephrine HCl (Adrenalin)
- epinephrine HCl inhalation (Primatene Mist)
- formoterol fumarate (Foradil)
- ipratropium Br (Atrovent)
- isoproterenol HCl (Isuprel)
- levalbuterol (Xopenex)
- metaproterenol sulfate (Alupent)
- oxtriphylline (Choledyl)
- pirbuterol (Maxair)
- terbutaline sulfate (Brethine)
- theophylline (Theo-Dur)

CANCER CHEMOTHERAPY
- bicalutamide (Casodex)
- busulfan (Myleran)
- capecitabine (Xeloda)
- cyclophosphamide (Cytoxan)
- fluorouracil (Efudex)
- flutamide (Eulexin)
- hydroxyurea (Hydrea)
- interferon alfa-2a (Roferon-A)
- interferon alfa-2b (Intron-A)
- imatinib mesylate (Gleevec)
- letrozole (Femara)
- leucovorin calcium (Wellcovorin)
- lomustine (CeeNU)
- megestrol acetate (Megace)
- melphalan (Alkeran)
- mercaptopurine (Purinethol)
- methotrexate (Rheumatrex)
- mitotane (Lysodren)
- paclitaxel (Taxol)
- peginterferon alfa-2a (Pegasys)
- procarbazine HCl (Matulane)

tamoxifen citrate (Nolvadex)
toremifene citrate (Fareston)

CARDIAC GLYCOSIDES
digoxin (Lanoxin)

CENTRAL NERVOUS SYSTEM STIMULANTS
dextroamphetamine sulfate (Dexedrine)
methylphenidate (Ritalin)
methamphetamine (Desoxyn)
modafinil (Provigil)
pemoline (Cylert)

CEPHALOSPORINS
cefaclor (Ceclor)
cefadroxil (Duricef)
cefditoren pivoxil (Spectracef)
cefazolin sodium (Ancef)
cefdinir (Omnicef)
cefepime (Maxipime)
cefixime (Suprax)
cefpodoxime proxetil (Vantin)
cefprozil monohydrate (Cefzil)
ceftibuten (Cedax)
cefuroxime axetil (Ceftin)
cefditoren (Spectracef)
cephalexin (Keflex)
cephradine (Velosef)
loracarbef (Lorabid)

CHOLESTEROL LOWERING AGENTS
atorvastatin calcium (Lipitor)
fluvastatin sodium (Lescol)
lovastatin (Mevacor)
pravastatin sodium (Pravachol)
rosuvastatin calcium (Crestor)

CHOLINERGIC AGONISTS
bethanechol chloride (Urecholine)
pyridostigmine (Mestinon)

CHOLINESTRASE INHIBITORS
ambenonium (Mytelase)
neostigmine Br (Prostigmin)
pyridostigmine (Mestinon)

DECONGESTANTS
oxymetazoline HCl (Afrin)
phenylephrine HCl (Neo-Synephrine)
pseudoephedrine (Sudafed)

DEMENTIA/ALZHEIMER'S
donepezil (Aricept)
ergoloid mesylate (Hydergine)
galantamine (Reminyl)
rivastigmine tartrate (Exelon)
tacrine (Cognex)

DERMATOLOGICS
acitretin (Soriatane)
alefacept (Amevive)
alitretinoin (Panretin)
azelaic acid (Azelex)
capsaicin (Zostrix)
doxepin HCl (Zonalon)
isotretinoin (Accutane)
methotrexate (Folex)
minoxidil (Rogaine)
pimecrolimus (Elidel)
tacrolimus (Protopic)
tazarotene (Tazorac)
tretinoin (Retin-A)

DIURETICS
Loop diuretics
bumetanide (Bumex)
ethacrynate (Edecrin)
furosemide (Lasix)
torsemide (Demadex)

Potassium sparing
amiloride HCl (Midamor)
spironolactone (Aldactone)
triamterene (Dyrenium)

Thiazides
chlorothiazide (Diuril)
hydrochlorothiazide (HydroDIURIL)
polythiazide (Renese)

Thiazide-like
chlorthalidone (Hygroton)
indapamide (Lozol)
metolazone (Zaroxolyn)

Others
acetazolamide (Diamox)
dorzolamide HCl (Trusopt)
methazolamide (Neptazane)

ENDOCRINE

clomiphene citrate (Clomid)
conjugated estrogens (Premarin)
conjugated estrogens, synthetic (Cenestin)
danazol (Danocrine)
desmopressin (DDAVP)
dutasteride (Avodart)
esterified estrogens (Estrab)
estradiol transdermal (Estraderm)
estradiol valerate (Estrace)
estropipate (Ogen)
estrogen synthetic conjugated (Cenestin)
estrogen substances conjugated (Premarin)
finasteride (Proscar)
fluoxymesterone (Halotestin)
glucagon (Glucagon Emergency Kit)
levothyroxine (Synthroid)
liothyronine sodium (Cytomel)
liotrix (Euthroid)
medroxyprogesterone acetate (Provera)
norethindrone (Aygestin)
norgestrel (Ovrette)
oral contraceptives (many brands)
oxandrolone (Oxandrin)
oxymetholone (Anadrol)
raloxifene HCl (Evista)
stanozolol (Winstrol)
testosterone (Depo-Testosterone)
thyroid (Armour Thyroid)

ERECTILE DYSFUNCTION

alprostadil (Caverject)
sildenafil citrate (Viagra)
tadalafil (Cialis)
vardenafil HCl (Levitra)

ERGOT ALKALOIDS

(see migraine)
ergotamine tartrate (Ergomart)

EXPECTORANT

guaifenesin (Humibid)

FLUOROQUINOLONES

alatrofloxacin mesylate (Trovan IV)
ciprofloxacin HCl (Cipro)
enoxacin (Penetrex)
gatifloxacin (Tequin)
gemifloxacin mesylate (Factive)
levofloxacin HCl (Levaquin)
lomefloxacin (Maxaquin)
moxifloxacin HCl (Avelox)
norfloxacin (Noroxin)
ofloxacin (Floxin)
sparfloxacin (Zagam)
trovafloxacin mesylate (Trovan)

FOLATE ANTAGONIST

trimetrexate glucuronate (Neutrexin)

FREE RADICAL SCAVENGER

amifostine (Ethyol)

GASTROESOPHAGEAL REFLUX DISEASE

esomeprazole magnesium (Nexium)
lansoprazole (Prevacid)

omeprazole (Prilosec)
pantoprazole sodium (Protonix)
rabeprazole (Aciphex)

GASTROINTESTINAL DRUGS

balsalazide sodium (Colazal)
infliximab (Remicade)
lansoprazole (Prevacid)
mesalamine (Asacol)
metoclopramide HCl (Reglan)
misoprostol (Cytotec)
olsalazine sodium (Dipentum)
pancrelipase (Cotazym)
rabeprazole (Aciphex)
sucralfate (Carafate)
sulfasalazine (Azulfidine)
tegaserod maleate (Zelnorm)

GLAUCOMA TREATMENT

acetazolamide (Diamox)
apraclonidine (Iopidine)
betaxolol HCl (Betoptic)
bimatoprost (Lumigan)
brinzolamide (Azopt)
carteolol (Ocupress)
dipivefrin HCl (Propine)
dorzolamide (Trusopt)
emedastine (Emadine)
latanoprost (Xalatan)
levobunolol HCl (Betagan)
methazolamide (Neptazane)
pilocarpine (Isopto-Carpine)
timolol maleate (Timoptic)
travoprost (Travatan)
unoprostone isopropyl (Rescula)

GLUCOCORTICOIDS

Inhalant sprays

beclomethasone (Vanceril Inh)
budesonide (Rhinocort Inh)
flunisolide (Aerobid Inh)
fluticasone propionate (Flonase)
mometasone furoate monohydrate (Nasonex)
triamcinolone acetonide (Azmacort)

Systemic

betamethasone (Celestone)
cortisone acetate (Cortone)
dexamethasone (Dexadron)
fludrocortisone acetate (Florinef)
hydrocortisone (Cortef)
methylprednisolone (Medrol)
prednisolone (Delta-Cortef)
prednisone (Meticorten)
triamcinolone acetonide (Aristocort)

Topical

betamethasone (Diprolene)
clobetasol propionate (Temovate)
clobetasol propionate (Olux)
clocortolone pivalate (Cloderm)
desonide (DesOwen)
desoximetasone (Topicort)
dexamethasone (Decaderm)
diflorasone diacetate (Florone)
fluocinonide (Lidex)
flurandrenolide (Cordran)
fluticasone propionate (Cutivate)
halcinonide (Halog)
halobetasol propionate (Ultravate)
hydrocortisone (Allercort)
hydrocortisone buteprate (Pandel)
loteprednol etabonate (Lotemax)
prednicarbate (Dermatop)
rimexolone (Vexol)
triamcinolone acetonide (Kenalog)

HEMOSTATICS

absorbable gelatin sponge (Gelfoam)
aminocaproic acid (Amicar)
oxidized cellulose (Surgicel)
tranexamic acid (Cyklokapron)

IMMUNOMODULATORS
imiquimod (Aldara)
interferon alfa-2a (Roferon-A, Pegasys)
interferon alfa-2b (Intron-A)
interferon alfa-n_1 (Wellferon)
interferon alfa-n_3 (Alferon-N)
interferon beta-1A (Avonex)
interferon gamma-1B (Actimmune)
levamisole HCl (Ergamisol)
peginterferon alfa-2a (Pegasys)
peginterferon alfa-2B (PEG-Intron)

IMMUNOSUPPRESSANTS
azathioprine (Imuran)
cyclosporine (Sandimmune, Neoral)
daclizumab (Zenapax)
mycophenolate mofetil (CellCept)
prednisone (Meticorten)
tacrolimus (Prograf)
tacrolimus (Protopic)

IRRITABLE BOWEL SYNDROME
alosetron (Lotronex)

LEUKOTRIENE RECEPTOR ANTAGONIST
montelukast sodium (Singulair)
zafirlukast (Accolate)

LEUKOTRIENE PATHWAY INHIBITOR
zileuton (Zyflo)

LINCOSAMIDES
clindamycin HCl (Cleocin)
lincomycin (Lincocin)

MACROLIDES
azithromycin (Zithromax)
clarithromycin (Biaxin)
dirithromycin (DynaBac)
erythromycin (Erythrocin)

MALE PATTERN BALDNESS
finasteride (Propecia)
minoxidil (Rogaine)

MAST CELL STABILIZERS
cromolyn sodium (Intal)
lodoxamide tromethamine (Alomide)
nedocromil sodium (Tilade)
pemirolast (Alamast)

MIGRAINE
(see ergot alkaloids)
almotriptan maleate (Axert)
divalproex (Depakote)
eletriptan HBr (Replax)
frovatriptan succinate (Frova)
naratriptan HCl (Amerge)
propranolol HCl (Inderal)
rizatriptan benzoate (Maxalt)
sumatriptan succinate (Imitrex)
timolol (Blocadren)
zolmitriptan (Zomig)

MINERALS
ferrous gluconate (Fergon)
ferrous sulfate (Feosol)
ferrous fumarate (Feostat)
potassium chloride (Micro-K)
sodium fluoride

MONOCLONAL ANTIBODIES
adalimumab (Humira)
efalizumab (Raptiva)
omalizumab (Xolair)

MUCOLYTIC
dornase alfa (Pulmozyme)

MULTIPLE SCLEROSIS
tizanidine HCl (Zanaflex)

MYASTHENIA GRAVIS
ambenonium (Mytelase)
neostigmine (Prostigmin)
pyridostigmine bromide (Mestinon)

MYDRIATIC
atropine sulfate (optic) (Isopto Atropine)
homatropine HBr (optic) (Isopto Homatropine)

NARCOTICS
(see analgesics [opioid])

NITROIMIDAZOLE
metronidazole (Flagyl)

NONSTEROIDAL ANTIINFLAMMATORY DRUGS
aspirin
celecoxib (Celebrex)
diclofenac (Voltaren)
diflunisal (Dolobid)
etodolac (Lodine)
fenoprofen (Nalfon)
flurbiprofen (Ansaid)
ibuprofen (Motrin)
indomethacin (Indocin)
ketoprofen (Orudis)
ketorolac (Toradol)
meclofenamate sodium (Meclomen)
mefenamic acid (Ponstel)
meloxicam (Mobic)
nabumetone (Relafen)
naproxen (Naprosyn)
naproxen sodium (Anaprox)
oxaprozin (Daypro)
piroxicam (Feldene)
rofecoxib (Vioxx)
sulindac (Clinoril)
tolmetin (Tolectin)
valdecoxib (Bextra)

OBESITY MANAGEMENT
diethylpropion (Tenuate)
methamphetamine (Desoxyn)
orlistat (Xenical)
phendimetrazine (Prelu-2)
phentermine (Ionamin)
sibutramine (Merida)

OPHTHALMICS
atropine sulfate (optic) (Isopto Atropine)
azelastine HCl (Optivar)
betaxolol HCl (Betoptic)
bimatoprost (Lumigan)
brimonidine tartrate (Alphagan)
carteolol (Occupres)
ciprofloxacin (Ciloxan)
cyclosporine (Restasis)
dipivefrin (Propine)
epinastine HCl (Elestat)
erythromycin (Ilotycin)
flurbiprofen sodium (Ocufen)
gentamicin (Garamycin)
homatropine hydrobromide (optic) (Isopto Homatropine)
ketotifen (Zaditor)
levocabastine HCl (Livostin)
levofloxacin HCl (Quixin)
loteprednol (Lotemax, Alrex)
moxifloxacin HCl (Vigamox)
naphazoline HCl (Naphcon)
ofloxacin (Ocuflox)
olopatadine (Patanol)
permirolast (Alamast)
pilocarpine (Isopto Carpine)
polymyxin (Aerosporin)
sulfacetamide sodium (Sulamyd)
timolol (Timoptic)
tobramycin (Tobrex)
travoprost (Travatan)
trifluridine (Viroptic)
unoprostone isopropyl (Rescula)
vidarabine (Vira-A)

ORPHAN DRUGS
miglustat (Zavesca)

OTIC DRUGS
gatifloxacin (Zymar)
ofloxacin (Floxin Otic)

PENICILLINS
amoxicillin trihydrate (Amoxil)
amoxicillin/clavulanate (Augmentin)
ampicillin sodium (Omnipen)
dicloxacillin sodium (Dynapen)
oxacillin (Prostaphlin)
penicillin G benzathine (Bicillin)
penicillin V potassium (V-Cillin K)

PEPTIDE ANTIINFECTIVE
vancomycin HCl (Vancocin)

PERIODONTAL SPECIALTY PRODUCTS
chlorhexidine (PerioChip)
doxycycline hyclate (Atridox)
doxycycline hyclate (Periostat)
minocycline HCl (Arestin)

PERIPHERAL VASCULAR DISEASE
cilostazol (Pletal)
isoxsuprine HCl (Vasodilan)
papaverine HCl (Pavabid)
pentoxifylline (Trental)

PLATELET AGGREGATION INHIBITORS
aspirin
clopidogrel bisulfate (Plavix)
dipyridamole (Persantine)
ticlopidine (Ticlid)

PLATELET REDUCING AGENT
anagrelide HCl (Agrylin)

PNEUMOCYSTIC PNEUMONITIS
atovaquone (Mepron)
pentamidine (Pentam 300)
sulfamethoxazole/trimethoprim (Bactrim, Septra)
trimetrexate (Neutrexin)

PROSTAGLANDIN
alprostadil (Caverject)
bimatoprost (Lumigan)
latanoprost (Xalatan)
misoprostol (Cytotec)
travoprost (Travatan)

PROSTATE HYPERPLASIA
alfuzosin HCl (Uroxatral)
dutasteride (Avodart)
finasteride (Proscar)
tamsulosin HCl (Flomax)
terazosin HCl (Hytrin)

SALIVARY STIMULANTS (SIALOGOGUES)
amifostine (Ethyol)
cevimeline (Evoxac)
pilocarpine HCl (Salagen)

SELECTIVE SEROTONIN ANTAGONIST
alosetron HCl (Lotronex)
dolasetron mesylate (Anzemet)

SKELETAL MUSCLE RELAXANTS
baclofen (Lioresal)
carisoprodol (Soma)
chlorphenesin carbamate (Maolate)
chlorzoxazone (Paraflex)
cyclobenzaprine HCl (Flexeril)
dantrolene sodium (Dantrium)
metaxalone (Skelexan)
methocarbamol (Robaxin)
orphenadrine citrate (Norflex)

SMOKING CESSATION

bupropion HCl (Zyban)
nicotine polacrylex (Nicorette)
nicotine transdermal (Habitrol, ProStep)

STATINS- CHOLESTEROL-LOWERING

atorvastatin calcium (Lipitor)
fluvastatin sodium (Lescol)
lovastatin (Mevacor)
pravastatin sodium (Pravachol)
rosuvastatin sodium (Crestor)
simvastatin (Zocor)

SULFONAMIDES

sulfacetamide sodium (Sulamyd Sodium)
sulfamethoxazole (Gantanol)
sulfamethoxazole/trimethoprim (Septra, Bactrim)
sulfisoxazole (Gantrisin)

TETRACYCLINES

demeclocycline HCl (Declomycin)
doxycycline calcium (Vibramycin)
doxycycline hyclate (Atridox)
doxycycline hyclate (Periostat)
minocycline HCl (Minocin, Arestin)
tetracycline (Achromycin)
tetracycline fiber (Actisite)

URICOSURIC

probenecid (Benemid)
sulfinpyrazone (Anturane)

URINARY TRACT INFECTIONS

cinoxacin (Cinobac)
flavoxate HCl (Urispas)
fosfomycin tromethamine (Monurol)
methenamine (Hiprex)
nitrofurantoin (Furadantin)
phenazopyridine HCl (Pyridium)
sulfamethoxazole (Gantanol)
sulfamethoxazole/trimethoprim (Bactrim, Septra)

VASOCONSTRICTOR

epinephrine (Adrenalin)
phenylephrine (Neo-Synephrine)

VITAMINS

ascorbic acid
calcipotriene (Dovonex, D_3)
cyanocobalamin (Rubramin)
dihydrotachysterol (Hytakerol)
doxercalciferol (Hectorol)
folic acid (Folvite, B_9)
niacin (Nicolid)
phytonadione (Aqua MEPHYTON)
pyridoxine (B_6)
riboflavin (B_2)
thiamin HCl (B_1)
vitamin A (Aquasol A)
vitamin D (Calciferol)
vitamin E (Aquasol E)

WOUND REPAIR

becaplermin (Regranex)

XANTHINES AND XANTHINE DERIVATIVES

aminophylline (Somophyllin)
dyphylline (Dilor)
oxtriphylline (Choledyl)
pentoxifylline (Trental)
theophylline (Theo-Dur)

Individual Drugs

abacavir sulfate

(a-bak'a-veer)
Ziagen

Drug class.: Antiviral, nucleoside analog

Action: Converted to an active metabolite, carbovir triphosphate, that inhibits reverse transcriptase enzymes in human immunodeficiency virus type 1 (HIV-1), thereby inhibiting viral DNA growth

Uses: Used in combination with other antiviral drugs for treatment of HIV-1 infection

Dosage and routes:

• *Adult:* PO 300 mg bid in combination with other antiretroviral drugs

• *Child 3 mo–16 yr:* PO 8 mg/kg bid not to exceed adult dose; in combination with other antiviral drugs for HIV-1

Available forms include: Tabs 300 mg, oral sol 20 mg/ml in 240 ml vol

Side effects/adverse reactions:

▼ *ORAL:* Mucous membrane lesions

CNS: Insomnia, fatigue, headache, asthenia, lethargy, paresthesia, anorexia

CV: Edema

GI: Nausea, vomiting, diarrhea, anorexia, abdominal pain, ***lactic acidosis, pancreatitis, hepatotoxicity***

RESP: Shortness of breath, pharyngitis

INTEG: Rash, urticaria

META: Elevation of blood glucose, triglyceride elevation, alteration of liver enzymes

HEMA: Decreased lymphocytes

MS: Myalgia, arthralgia

MISC: ***Severe or fatal hypersensitivity reactions***

Contraindications: Hypersensitivity

Precautions: Do not breast-feed, pregnancy category C, bone marrow depression, renal or hepatic impairment, use with other antivirals to avoid emergence of resistant viruses, avoid alcohol use

Pharmacokinetics:

PO: Bioavailability (83%), plasma protein binding (50%), hepatic metabolism (alcohol dehydrogenase), primarily renal excretion, fecal excretion (16%)

Drug interactions of concern to dentistry:

• None reported

DENTAL CONSIDERATIONS

General:

• Examine for oral manifestation of opportunistic infection.

• Patient on chronic drug therapy may rarely have symptoms of blood dyscrasias, which include infection, bleeding, and poor healing.

• Avoid dental light in patient's eyes; offer dark glasses for patient comfort.

• Place on frequent recall because of oral side effects.

• Consider semisupine chair position for patient comfort if GI side effects occur.

Consultations:

• In a patient with symptoms of blood dyscrasias, request a medical consultation for blood studies and postpone treatment until normal values are reestablished.

• Medical consultation may be required to assess disease control.

Teach patient/family:

• Importance of good oral hygiene to prevent soft tissue inflammation

• To prevent trauma when using oral hygiene aids
• To be alert for the possibility of secondary oral infection and the need to see dentist immediately if signs of infection occur

absorbable gelatin sponge

Gelfoam

Drug class.: Hemostatic, purified gelatin sponge

Action: Absorbs blood, provides area for clot formation
Uses: Hemostasis adjunct in dental surgery
Dosage and routes:
Dental use
• *Adult:* TOP can be applied dry or moistened with normal saline solution; blot on sterile gauze to remove excess solution, shape to fit with light finger compression; hold pressure on dry foam for 1-2 min
Available forms include: Dental packs, size 4 (2 × 2 cm)
Side effects/adverse reactions:
• *None reported*
Contraindications: Hypersensitivity, frank infection
Precautions: Avoid use in presence of infection, potential nidus of infection, do not resterilize product
Pharmacokinetics:
IMPLANT: Absorbed in 4-6 wk
DENTAL CONSIDERATIONS
Teach patient/family:
• To immediately report any sign of infection to the dentist

acarbose

(ay′car-bose)
Precose
♣ Prandase

Drug class.: Oral antidiabetic

Action: Competitive and reversible inhibitor of membrane-bound α-glucosidase, hydrolase, and pancreatic α-amylase in the GI tract to delay the breakdown of carbohydrates to glucose, resulting in lower postprandial plasma glucose levels
Uses: Use as single drug or in combination with insulin or oral hypoglycemics (sulfonylureas, metformin) in type 2 diabetes (non–insulin-dependent diabetes mellitus [NIDDM]) when diet control is ineffective in controlling blood glucose levels
Dosage and routes:
• *Adult:* PO initial dose 25 mg tid at start of main meal; after testing may be increased to 50 mg tid at start of each meal; max dose >60 kg is 100 mg tid; max dose <60 kg is 50 mg tid
Caution: Doses must be individualized for each patient
Available forms include: Tabs 25, 50, 100 mg
Side effects/adverse reactions:
GI: Bloating, diarrhea, abdominal pain, flatulence
META: Elevations of AST/ALT
INTEG: Rash
MS: Edema, small reduction in hematocrit
Contraindications: Hypersensitivity, diabetic ketoacidosis, cirrhosis, inflammatory or obstructive GI disease, severe renal impairment
Precautions: Use glucose for hypoglycemia, monitor blood glucose

levels, pregnancy category B, avoid use in lactation, children

Pharmacokinetics:

PO: Limited oral absorption, absorbed dose excreted in urine, metabolized in the GI tract and major portion of dose excreted in feces

Drug interactions of concern to dentistry:

- None reported

DENTAL CONSIDERATIONS

General:

- Ensure that patient is following prescribed diet and takes medication regularly.
- Type 2 patients may also be using insulin. If symptomatic hypoglycemia occurs while taking this drug, use dextrose rather than sucrose because of interference with sucrose metabolism.
- Place on frequent recall to evaluate healing response.
- Patients with diabetes may be more susceptible to infection and have delayed wound healing.
- Question the patient about self-monitoring the drug's antidiabetic effect.
- Consider semisupine chair position for patient comfort when GI side effects occur.

Consultations:

- Medical consultation may be required to assess disease control and patient's ability to tolerate stress.

Teach patient/family:

- Importance of good oral hygiene to prevent soft tissue inflammation

acetaminophen

(a-seet-a-min'oh-fen)

Aceta, Acephen, Apacet, Aspirin Free Anacin Maximum Strength, Dapacin, Dynafed Feverall, Genepap, Genebs, Liquiprin, Mapap, Meda, Maranox, Neopap, Oraphen-PD, Panadol, Silapap, Tapanol, Tempra, Tylenol, Tylenol Extra Strength, Uni-ACE, and many others

Actimol, Apo-Acetaminophen, Atasol, Robigesic, Rounax

Drug class.: Nonnarcotic analgesic

Action: Analgesic action not fully determined; presumed to block the initiation of pain impulses by inhibition of prostaglandin synthesis; acts mainly in the CNS and to a lesser degree in peripheral nerves; antipyretic action results from inhibition of prostaglandin synthesis in the hypothalamic heat-regulating center

Uses: Mild-to-moderate pain, fever; also used in combination with other ingredients, including opioids

Dosage and routes:

- *Adult and child >12 yr:* PO 325-650 mg q4h prn or 1 g q6h, not to exceed 4 g/day; REC: 325-650 mg q4-6h prn, not to exceed 4 g/day
- *Adult:* PO for osteoarthritis, 1300 mg tid
- *Child 0-3 mo:* PO 40 mg/dose q4h
- *Child 4-12 mo:* PO 80 mg/dose q4h
- *Child 1-2 yr:* PO 120 mg/dose q4h
- *Child 2-3 yr:* PO/REC 160 mg/dose q4h
- *Child 4-5 yr:* PO/REC 240 mg/dose q4h

• *Child 6-8 yr:* PO/REC 320 mg/dose q4h
• *Child 9-10 yr:* PO/REC 320-400 mg/dose q4h
• *Child 11 yr:* PO/REC 480 mg/dose q4h
• *Child 12-14 yr:* PO/REC 640 mg/dose q4h
• *Child >14 yr:* PO/REC 650 mg/dose q4h

Available forms include: Rec supp 80, 120, 125, 300, 325, 650 mg; chew tab 80 mg; tabs 160, 325, 500, 650 mg; caps 325, 500 mg; elix 80, 120, 160, 325 mg/5 ml; liq 160 mg/5 ml, 500 mg/15 ml; sol (infant drops) 100 mg/1.66 ml, 100 mg/15 ml; gelcaps 500 mg; sprinkle cap 80, 160 mg; drops 80 mg/0.8 ml

Side effects/adverse reactions:
CNS: Stimulation, drowsiness
GI: ***Hepatotoxicity,*** nausea, vomiting, abdominal pain
HEMA: ***Leukopenia, neutropenia, hemolytic anemia*** (long-term use), ***thrombocytopenia, pancytopenia***
INTEG: ***Angioedema,*** rash, urticaria
TOXICITY: ***Cyanosis, anemia, neutropenia, jaundice, pancytopenia, CNS stimulation, delirium; then vascular collapse, convulsions, coma, death***

Contraindications: Hypersensitivity, chronic heavy alcohol use

Precautions: Anemia, hepatic disease, renal disease, chronic alcoholism, pregnancy category B

Pharmacokinetics:
PO: Onset 10-30 min, peak 0.5-2 hr, duration 4-6 hr, half-life 1-3 hr
REC: Slow, variable onset
For all routes, is metabolized in the liver, is excreted by the kidneys, crosses the placenta, and is found in breast milk

Drug interactions of concern to dentistry:
• Decreased effects: barbiturates, oral contraceptives, loop diuretics
• Nephrotoxicity: NSAIDs, salicylates (chronic, high-dose concurrent use)
• Liver toxicity: chronic use of hydantoins, chronic alcohol use, high-dose carbamazepine
• Possible increased effects of zidovudine
• Possible increased effects of acetaminophen: β-blockers, probenecid
• Increased bleeding: warfarin

DENTAL CONSIDERATIONS

General:
• Reports regarding the concomitant use of acetaminophen and warfarin seem to suggest a possible increase in anticoagulant effects, especially in patients with other diseases or contributing factors, diarrhea, age, debilitation, etc. Patients taking warfarin should be questioned about recent use of acetaminophen and current INR values. Acetaminophen has been shown to increase the INR depending on the amount of acetaminophen taken and duration of use. A new PT or INR value may be required if surgical procedures are planned. Data from one study (*JAMA* 279:657-662, 1998) indicated that use of four regular-strength acetaminophen tablets (325 mg) qd for 1 wk can increase the INR values. It is important to closely monitor INR values with use of acetaminophen over a long duration and in higher doses.

• Avoid prolonged use with aspirin-containing products or NSAIDs.
• Determine why the patient is taking the drug.
• Patients on chronic drug therapy may rarely have symptoms of blood dyscrasias, which can include infection, bleeding, and poor healing.
• Question patient about the use of other drug products, including OTC products, that also contain acetaminophen because of risk of acetaminophen overdose

Consultations:

• In a patient with symptoms of blood dyscrasias, request a medical consult for blood studies and postpone dental treatment until normal values are reestablished.

---

acetazolamide/ acetazolamide sodium

(a-set-a-zole'a-mide)

Ak-Zol, Dazamide, Diamox, Storzolamide

♣ Acetazolam, Apo-Acetazolamide

Drug class.: Diuretic, carbonic anhydrase inhibitor

Action: Inhibits carbonic anhydrase activity in proximal renal tubular cells to decrease reabsorption of water, sodium, potassium, bicarbonate; decreases carbonic anhydrase in CNS, increasing seizure threshold; able to decrease aqueous humor in eye, which lowers intraocular pressure

Uses: Open-angle glaucoma, narrow-angle glaucoma (preoperatively, if surgery delayed), epilepsy (petit mal, grand mal, mixed), edema in CHF, drug-induced edema, acute mountain sickness in climbers, drug-induced edema

Dosage and routes:

Closed-angle glaucoma (acute congestive glaucoma):

• *Adult:* PO/IM/IV 250 mg q4h, or 250 mg bid, to be used for short-term therapy; sus rel 500 mg bid

Open-angle glaucoma (chronic simple glaucoma):

• *Adult:* PO/IM/IV 250 mg–1 g/day; usually in divided doses for amounts over 250 mg

• *Child:* IM/IV 5 to 10 mg/kg/dose q6h; PO 10-15 mg/kg/day in equally divided doses q6-8h

Epilepsy:

• *Adults and children:* PO 8-30 mg/kg/day in divided doses; optimum dose range 375-1000 mg/day in combination with other anticonvulsants; initial dose is 250 mg/day

Acute mountain sickness:

• *Adults:* PO 500-1000 mg/day in divided doses; initiate doses 1-2 days before ascent

CHF:

• *Adults:* PO initial dose 5 mg/kg (250-375 mg) qd in AM; adjust dose to diuresis; best given on alternate days

Available forms include: Tabs 125, 250 mg; sus rel caps 500 mg; inj IM/IV 500 mg

Side effects/adverse reactions:

▼ *ORAL:* Dry/burning mouth, tongue, lips; paresthesia; metallic taste; thirst

CNS: Drowsiness, paresthesia, anxiety, depression, headache, dizziness, confusion, stimulation, fatigue, seizures, sedation, nervousness

GI: Nausea, vomiting, anorexia, ***hepatic insufficiency,*** constipation, diarrhea, melena, weight loss

HEMA: ***Aplastic anemia, hemolytic anemia, leukopenia, agranulocytosis, thrombocytopenia, purpura, pancytopenia***
GU: Frequency, hypokalemia, ***uremia,*** polyuria, glucosuria, hematuria, dysuria
EENT: Myopia, tinnitus
INTEG: Rash, ***Stevens-Johnson syndrome,*** photosensitivity, pruritus, urticaria, fever
ENDO: Hyperglycemia
Contraindications: Hypersensitivity to sulfonamides, severe renal disease, severe hepatic disease, electrolyte imbalances (hyponatremia, hypokalemia), hyperchloremic acidosis, Addison's disease, long-term use in narrow-angle glaucoma, COPD
Precautions: Hypercalciuria, pregnancy category C; chronic use of oral sulfonylureas has been associated with increased risk of CV mortality; risk is controversial
Pharmacokinetics:
PO: Onset 1-1.5 hr, peak 1-3 hr, duration 6-12 hr
PO (SUS REL): Onset 2 hr, peak 8-12 hr, duration 18-24 hr
IV: Onset 2 min, peak 15 min, duration 4-5 hr
65% absorbed if fasting (oral), 75% absorbed if given with food; half-life 2.5-5.5 hr; excreted unchanged by kidneys (80% within 24 hr); crosses placenta
Drug interactions of concern to dentistry:
- Toxicity: salicylates (large doses)
- Hypokalemia: corticosteroids (systemic use)
- Crystalluria: ciprofloxacin

DENTAL CONSIDERATIONS
General:
- Patients on chronic drug therapy may rarely have symptoms of blood dyscrasias, which can include infection, bleeding, and poor healing.
- Assess salivary flow as a factor in caries, periodontal disease, and candidiasis.
- Avoid drugs that may exacerbate glaucoma (e.g., anticholinergics).

Consultations:
- In a patient with symptoms of blood dyscrasias, request a medical consultation for blood studies and postpone dental treatment until normal values are reestablished.
- Consultation may be required to assess disease control.

Teach patient/family:
- Importance of good oral hygiene to prevent soft tissue inflammation
- Caution to prevent injury when using oral hygiene aids

When chronic dry mouth occurs, advise patient:
- To avoid mouth rinses with high alcohol content because of drying effects
- To use daily home fluoride products for anticaries effect
- To use sugarless gum, frequent sips of water, or saliva substitutes

acetohexamide

(a-set-oh-hex'a-mide)
Dymelor
Dimelor
Drug class.: Sulfonylurea (first generation), antidiabetic

Action: Causes functioning β cells in pancreas to release insulin, leading to drop in blood glucose levels; may improve binding between insulin and insulin receptors or increase number of insulin receptors; not effective if patient lacks functioning β cells

Uses: Stable adult-onset diabetes mellitus (type 2)

Dosage and routes:

• *Adult:* PO 250 mg–1.5 g/day; usually given before breakfast, unless large dose is required, then dose is divided in two

Available forms include: Tabs 250, 500 mg scored

Side effects/adverse reactions:

CNS: Headache, weakness, tinnitus, fatigue, dizziness, vertigo

GI: ***Hepatotoxicity, jaundice,*** heartburn, nausea, vomiting, diarrhea

HEMA: ***Leukopenia, thrombocytopenia, agranulocytosis, aplastic anemia, hemolytic anemia,*** increased AST/ALT, alk phosphatase

INTEG: Rash, allergic reactions, pruritus, urticaria, eczema, photosensitivity, erythema

ENDO: ***Hypoglycemia***

Contraindications: Hypersensitivity to sulfonylureas, juvenile or brittle diabetes

Precautions: Pregnancy category C, elderly, cardiac disease, renal disease, hepatic disease, thyroid disease, severe hypoglycemic reactions

Pharmacokinetics:

PO: Onset 1 hr, peak 2-4 hr, duration 12-24 hr, half-life 6-8 hr; completely absorbed by GI route; metabolized in liver; excreted in urine (active metabolites, unchanged drug)

Drug interactions of concern to dentistry:

• Increased hypoglycemic effects: salicylates (large doses)

• Decreased action: corticosteroids

• Disulfiram-like reaction: alcohol

DENTAL CONSIDERATIONS

General:

• Monitor vital signs at every appointment because of cardiovascular effects of diabetes.

• Patients on chronic drug therapy may rarely have symptoms of blood dyscrasias, which can include infection, bleeding, and poor healing.

• Place on frequent recall to evaluate healing response.

• Ensure that patient is following prescribed diet and takes medication regularly.

• Question patient about self-monitoring of drug's antidiabetic effect, including blood glucose values (SMBG) or finger-stick records.

• Avoid prescribing aspirin-containing products.

• Early morning appointments and a stress reduction protocol may be required for anxious patients.

• Patients with diabetes may be more susceptible to infection and have delayed wound healing.

Consultations:

• In a patient with symptoms of blood dyscrasias, request a medical consultation for blood studies and postpone dental treatment until normal values are reestablished.

• Medical consultation may include data from patient's blood glucose monitoring, including glycosylated hemoglobin (GHb) or HbA_{1c} testing.

Teach patient/family:

• Importance of good oral hygiene to prevent soft tissue inflammation

• Caution to prevent injury when using oral hygiene aids

• To avoid mouth rinses with high alcohol content

acitretin

(a-si-tre′tin)

Soriatane

Drug class.: Systemic retinoid

Action: Unclear; may enhance the inflammatory response and accelerate reappearance of the stratum corneum; binds to nuclear retinoic acid receptors (RARs) and may alter gene expression

Uses: Severe psoriasis; unlabeled uses: nonpsoritic dermatoses, keratinization disorders, palmoplantar keratoses, lichen planus, Darier's disease, Sjögren-Larrson syndrome; should be prescribed only by physicians knowledgeable in the use of systemic retinoids

Dosage and routes:

• *Adult:* PO initial dose 25-50 mg qd taken with the main meal, adjust dose by patient response; a negative pregnancy report is required before prescribing

Available forms include: Caps 10, 25 mg

Side effects/adverse reactions:

▼ *ORAL: Xerostomia (30%), ulcerative and nonulcerative stomatitis, taste perversion, cheilitis, gingival bleeding,* gingival hyperplasia

CNS: Fatigue, headache, dizziness, dysesthesia

CV: Flushing, ***pseudotumor cerebri***

GI: Abdominal pain, diarrhea, nausea, ***hepatitis, pancreatitis, hepatotoxicity***

RESP: Sinusitis

HEMA: Thrombocytosis

EENT: Rhinitis, xerophthalmia, earache, tinnitus, dry eyes, dry nose, conjunctivitis, epistaxis, blurred vision, eye pain, photophobia

INTEG: Abnormal skin color, dry skin, alopecia, bulbous eruption, dermatitis, rash, purpura, skin fissures and ulcerations, photosensitivity

META: Elevation in serum transaminase, lipid disturbances, hyperglyceridemia

MS: Arthralgia, myalgia, spinal hyperostosis

MISC: Joint pains, asthenia, chills, diaphoresis

Contraindications: Hypersensitivity, hypersensitivity to etretinate, pregnancy, ethanol use, concurrent use with vitamin A, hepatic disease, tetracyclines

Precautions: Women are advised to use effective contraception during use and for 3 yr after use, renal impairment, lactation, pregnancy category X, hyperlipidemia, cardiovascular disease

Pharmacokinetics:

PO: Peak serum levels 2-5 hr; food enhances bioavailability, highly plasma protein bound (99.9%), hepatic metabolism, active metabolite; excreted in urine and bile

Drug interactions of concern to dentistry:

• Avoid vitamin preparations containing vitamin A

• Avoid tetracyclines and other drugs that cause photosensitivity

DENTAL CONSIDERATIONS

General:

• Determine why patient is taking the drug.

• Apply lubricant to dry lips for patient comfort before dental procedures.

• Assess salivary flow as factor in caries, periodontal disease, and candidiasis.
• Palliative medication may be required for management of oral side effects.
• Place on frequent recall because of oral side effects.
• Consider semisupine chair position for patient comfort if GI side effects occur.
• Avoid dental light in patient's eyes; offer dark glasses for patient comfort.

Consultations:
• Medical consultation may be required to assess disease control.

Teach patient/family:
• Importance of good oral hygiene to prevent soft tissue inflammation
• Caution patient to prevent trauma when using oral hygiene aids
• To report oral lesions, soreness, or bleeding to dentist

When chronic dry mouth occurs, advise patient:
• To avoid mouth rinses with high alcohol content because of drying effects
• To use daily home fluoride products for anticaries effect
• To use sugarless gum, frequent sips of water, or saliva substitutes

---

acyclovir (topical)

(ay-sye'kloe-ver)

Zovirax

Drug class.: Antiviral

Action: A nucleoside antiviral that is converted to acyclovir triphosphate by herpes simplex thymidine kinase; it causes inhibition of DNA polymerase, thereby inhibiting HSV DNA replication

Uses: Management of initial genital herpes and in limited non–life-threatening mucocutaneous herpes simplex infection in immunocompromised patients

Dosage and routes:
• *Adult and adolescents 12 yr or older:* TOP apply to all lesions q3h while awake, 6 × daily × 1 wk

Available forms include: TOP oint 5% (50 mg/g) in 3 g and 15 g tubes; top cream 5%

Side effects/adverse reactions:

▼ *ORAL:* Stinging sensation (lip application)

INTEG: Rash, urticaria, stinging, burning, pruritus, vulvitis

Contraindications: Hypersensitivity

Precautions: Pregnancy category C, lactation; cutaneous use only; safety and efficacy in children under age 12 not established

DENTAL CONSIDERATIONS

General:
• Postpone dental treatment when oral herpetic lesions are present.

Teach patient/family:
• To dispose of toothbrush or other contaminated oral hygiene devices used during period of infection to prevent reinoculation of herpetic infection
• To apply with a finger cot or latex glove to prevent herpes infection on fingers
• To avoid mouth rinses with high alcohol content because of irritating effects

acyclovir sodium

(ay-sye'kloe-ver)

Zovirax

✦ Avirax, Alti-Acyclovir, Zovirax Wellstat Pac, Zovirax Zestab Pac

Drug class.: Antiviral

Action: A synthetic nucleoside that is converted to acyclovir triphosphate by herpes simplex thymidine kinase; it causes inhibition of DNA polymerase, thereby inhibiting HSV DNA replication

Uses: Initial episodes of herpes genitalis (HSV-2), *herpes simplex* encephalitis, neonatal *herpes simplex* in immunocompromised patients, *herpes zoster* in all patients, varicella (chickenpox); unapproved: prophylaxis of *herpes simplex* or *herpes zoster*

Dosage and routes:

Herpes simplex (mucocutaneous):

• *Adult:* PO 200-400 mg 5 × daily for 10 days in immunocompromised patients

Genital herpes:

• *Adult:* PO initial dose 200 mg q4h 5 × daily while awake for 10 days; chronic suppressive therapy 400 mg bid or 200 mg 3-5 × day up to 12 mo

Herpes zoster:

• 800 mg q4h, 5 × daily for 7-10 days

Chickenpox:

• *Child >2 yr:* PO 20 mg/kg per dose (limit 800 mg), 4 × daily for 5 days; start at earliest sign of symptoms

• *Adult and child >40 kg:* PO 800 mg 4 × daily × 5 days

Available forms include: Caps 200 mg; tabs 400 mg and 800 mg; powder for inj IV 500 mg and 1000 mg vials; susp 200 mg/5 ml

Side effects/adverse reactions:

▼ *ORAL:* Glossitis, medication taste

CNS: Malaise, ***convulsions,*** confusion, lethargy, hallucinations, dizziness, headache

CV: Peripheral edema

GI: Nausea, vomiting, diarrhea, abdominal pain

HEMA: ***Thrombocytopenia, leukopenia,*** lymphadenopathy

GU: ***Renal failure,*** elevated creatinine, hematuria

EENT: Visual abnormalities

INTEG: ***Erythema multiforme, toxic epidermal necrolysis,*** rash, urticaria, pruritus, phlebitis at IV site

META: Increased ALT/AST, hyperbilirubinemia, jaundice

MISC: ***Anaphylaxis,*** fever, myalgia

Contraindications: Hypersensitivity to this drug or valacyclovir

Precautions: Modify dose with acute or chronic renal impairment, safety of oral doses in pediatric patients <2 yr old not established, lactation, hepatic disease, renal disease, electrolyte imbalance, dehydration, pregnancy category B

Pharmacokinetics:

IV: Peak 1 hr, half-life 20 min–3 hr (terminal); metabolized by liver; excreted by kidneys as unchanged drug (95%); crosses placenta

PO: Peak levels 1.5-2 hr, plasma half-life 2.5-3 hr; low protein binding

Drug interactions of concern to dentistry:

• No dental drug interactions reported

DENTAL CONSIDERATIONS

General:

• Patients on chronic drug therapy

may rarely have symptoms of blood dyscrasias, which can include infection, bleeding, and poor healing.

• Determine why the patient is taking the drug.

Consultations:

• In a patient with symptoms of blood dyscrasias, request a medical consultation for blood studies and postpone dental treatment until normal values are reestablished.

• Medical consultation may be required to assess disease control.

Teach patient/family:

• Importance of good oral hygiene to prevent soft tissue inflammation

• Caution to prevent injury when using oral hygiene aids

• To avoid mouth rinses with high alcohol content because of drying effects

• To dispose of toothbrush or other contaminated oral hygiene devices used during period of infection to prevent reinoculation of herpetic infection

---

adalimumab

(ay-da-lim'yoo-mab)

Humira

Drug class.: monoclonal antibody, antinflammatory, immunosuppressant

---

Action: A recombinant human Ig G1 monoclonal antibody that binds to TNF-α blocking its interaction with the p55 and p75 cell surface receptors; modulates biologic responses induced or regulated by TNF

Uses: Treatment of signs and symptoms and inhibition of structural damage in moderately to severely active rheumatoid arthritis in adults who have an inadequate response to one or more disease-modifying antirheumatic drugs (DMARDs)

Dosage and routes:

• *Adult:* SC 40 mg every other week; alone or in combination with other DMARDs, methotrexate, glucocorticoids, salicylates, or NSAIDs

Available forms include: Prefilled syringe: 40 mg

Side effects/adverse reactions:

CNS: Headache, confusion, paresthesia, tremor

CV: Hypertension, arrhythmias, palpitation, tachycardia, ***myocardial infarction,*** peripheral edema

GI: Nausea, abdominal pain

RESP: Pneumonia, URI, asthma, bronchospasm, dyspnea

HEMA: ***Granulocytopenia, agranulocytosis,*** immunosuppression, leukopenia

GU: Hematuria, UTI, cystitis, renal calculus, menstrual disorder

EENT: Sinusitis

INTEG: Injection site reactions, erythema, itching, swelling, rash, risk of lupus-like syndrome

META: Hypercholesterolemia, hyperlipidemia, ↑ alkaline phosphatase, dehydration

MS: Back pain, joint disorders, muscle cramps, myasthenia

MISC: Flulike syndrome, ***serious infection (TB or opportunistic fungal infections), malignancies,*** allergic reactions

Contraindications: Hypersensitivity, patients with active infections

Precautions: Predisposition to infections, appearance of new infection with use, risk of exacerbation of demyelinating diseases, risk of malignancies, risk of TB reactivation; pregnancy category B, safety and effectiveness in children not established, lactation, use with caution in elderly

Pharmacokinetics: SC: peak serum levels 131 ± 56 hr; absolute bioavailability 64%, elimination half-life 10-18 days

Drug interactions of concern to dentistry:

• None reported

DENTAL CONSIDERATIONS

General:

• Patient may need assistance in getting into and out of dental chair.

• Adjust chair position for patient comfort.

• Determine why patient is taking the drug.

• Question patient about other drugs being taken.

• Examine for oral manifestation of opportunistic infection.

• Report oral infections to patient's physician; treat infections aggressively.

• Consider semisupine chair position for patient comfort if GI side effects occur.

Consultations:

• Medical consultation may be required to assess disease control and patient's ability to tolerate stress.

Teach patient/family:

• Importance of good oral hygiene to prevent soft tissue inflammation

• To immediately report any signs/symptoms of oral infection

adefovir dipivoxil

a-def′o-veer

Hepsera

Drug class.: Antiviral

Action: Prodrug of adefovir; adefovir is phosphorylated by tissue kinases to adefovir diphosphate; it inhibits HBV DNA polymerase (reverse transcriptase) causing DNA chain termination after incorporation into viral DNA

Uses: Treatment of chronic hepatitis B in adults showing evidence of active viral replication and with persistent elevations of ALT or AST or histologically active disease

Dosage and routes:

• *Adult:* PO 10 mg qd; doses must be adjusted for renal impairment or end-stage renal disease patients

Available forms include: Tabs 10 mg

Side effects/adverse reactions:

CNS*: Asthenia, headache*

GI: Abdominal pain, flatulence, diarrhea, dyspepsia, ***hepatic failure (post–liver transplant), lactic acidosis, hepatomegaly with steatosis***

GU: *Glucosuria, hematuria,* ***renal impairment, renal failure, nephrotoxicity***

EENT: Pharyngitis, sinusitis, cough

INTEG: Pruritus, rash

META: Elevations in ALT, AST, creatine kinase, amylase; hypophosphatemia

MISC: Fever

Contraindications: Hypersensitivity

Precautions: Severe acute exacerbations of hepatitis in patients who have discontinued drug, renal dysfunction with chronic use, HIV resistance, lactic acidosis, severe hepatomegaly with steatosis, monitor renal and hepatic function, pregnancy category C, safety and effectiveness in children and lactation not established

Pharmacokinetics:

PO: Approximate bioavailability

59%; converted to adefovir with absorption, peak plasma levels 0.5-4 hr; plasma protein binding <4%; excreted by glomerular filtration and active tubular secretion

Drug interactions of concern to dentistry:

• None reported

DENTAL CONSIDERATIONS

General:

• Examine for oral manifestation of opportunistic infection.
• Determine why patient is taking the drug.
• Consider semisupine chair position for patient comfort if GI side effects occur.
• Do not provide treatment if clinician does not have seroconversion to protective antibodies to hepatitis B.

Consultations:

• Medical consultation may be required to assess disease control and patient's ability to tolerate stress.
• Patients who report feeling symptoms of lactic acidosis, such as weakness, malaise, with unusual muscle pain, difficulty breathing, stomach pain with nausea, cold feeling in arms or legs, dizziness or light-headedness, and irregular heartbeat, should be immediately referred to their physician.

Teach patient/family:

• Importance of good oral hygiene to prevent soft tissue inflammation
• To prevent trauma when using oral hygiene aids
• Importance of updating health and drug history if physician makes any changes in evaluation/drug regimens

albuterol and albuterol sulfate

(al-byoo'ter-ole)

Aerosol: Proventil, Proventil HFA, Ventolin, Ventolin HFA
✤ Apo-Salvent, Novo-Salmol
INH solution: AccuNeb, Proventil
✤ Ventolin PF, Gen-Sal butamol PF, Apo-Salvent
Tablets: Proventil, Proventil Repetabs, Volmax
Syrup: Proventil
✤ Ventolin

Drug class.: Adrenergic β_2-agonist

Action: Causes bronchodilation by agonist action on β_2-receptors stimulating adenyl cyclase, thereby increasing levels of cAMP that relax smooth muscle with very little effect on heart rate; may also inhibit the release of immediate hypersensitivity mediators

Uses: Prevention and relief of bronchospasm in reversible obstructive airway disease, exercise-induced bronchospasm; unlabeled use acute, serious hyperkalemia in hemodialysis patients

Dosage and routes:

Oral INH sulfate solution:

• *Adult and child >12 yr:* INH 2.5 mg by nebulization over 5-15 min tid or qid
• *Child 2-12 yr:* INH 1.25-2.5 mg by nebulization over 5-15 min tid or qid

Oral INH aerosol:

• *Adult and child >4 yr (Proventil age limit 12 yr old):* INH 2 inhalations (180-200 μg) q4-6h

Prophylaxis for exercise-induced bronchospasm:

• *Adult and child >4 yr (Proventil age limit 12 yr old):* INH 2 inhalations 15 min before exercise

Tablets (extended release):
• *Adult and child >12 yr:* PO 2-4 mg tid or qid; limit 32 mg/day
• *Child 6-12 yr:* PO 2 mg tid or qid; limit 24 mg/day
Syrup:
• *Adult and child >12 yr:* PO 2-4 mg tid or qid; limit 8 mg qid
• *Child 6-12 yr:* PO 2 mg tid or qid; limit 24 mg/day
• *Child 2-6 yr:* PO 0.1 mg/kg tid; limit 2 mg tid
• *Elderly and patients sensitive to β-adrenergic agonists:* PO 2 mg tid or qid
Available forms include: Aerosol 90 μg/actuation; tabs 2, 4 mg; ext rel tabs 4, 8 mg; syr 2 mg/5 ml; inhal sol 0.083%, 0.5% and 0.63 or 1.25 mg/ml
Side effects/adverse reactions:
▼ *ORAL:* Taste changes, dry mouth, teeth discoloration
CNS: Tremors, anxiety, insomnia, headache, dizziness, stimulation, restlessness, hallucinations, flushing, irritability, fatigue
CV: Palpitation, tachycardia, hypertension, angina, hypotension, dysrhythmias
GI: Heartburn, nausea, vomiting, diarrhea
RESP: ***Bronchospasm,*** bronchitis
GU: Difficulty urinating
EENT: Dry nose, irritation of nose and throat, nasal congestion, epistaxis
MS: Muscle cramps
Contraindications: Hypersensitivity to sympathomimetics, tachydysrhythmias, severe cardiac disease
Precautions: Lactation, pregnancy category C, cardiac disorders, hyperthyroidism, diabetes mellitus, hypertension, prostatic hypertrophy, narrow-angle glaucoma, seizures, paradoxic bronchospasm
Pharmacokinetics:
PO: Onset 0.5 hr, peak 2.5 hr, duration 4-6 hr, half-life 2.5 hr
INH: Onset 5-15 min, peak 0.5-2 hr, duration 3-6 hr, half-life 4 hr
Metabolized in the liver; excreted in urine; crosses placenta, breast milk, blood-brain barrier
Drug interactions of concern to dentistry:
• None reported

DENTAL CONSIDERATIONS

General:
• Monitor vital signs at every appointment because of cardiovascular and respiratory side effects.
• Assess salivary flow as a factor in caries, periodontal disease, and candidiasis.
• Consider semisupine chair position for patients with respiratory disease.
• Midday appointments and a stress reduction protocol may be required for anxious patients.
• Be aware that aspirin or sulfite preservatives in vasoconstrictor-containing products can exacerbate asthma.
• Acute asthmatic episodes may be precipitated in the dental office. Sympathomimetic inhalants should be available for emergency use.
Consultations:
• Medical consultation may be required to assess disease control.
• Medical consultation may be required to assess patient's ability to tolerate stress.
Teach patient/family:
• For inhalation dosage forms, rinse mouth with water after each dose to prevent dryness

When chronic dry mouth occurs, advise patient:

- To avoid mouth rinses with high alcohol content because of drying effects
- To use daily home fluoride products for anticaries effect
- To use sugarless gum, frequent sips of water, or saliva substitutes

alefacept

(a-le′fa-sept)

Amevive

Drug class.: Biologic response modifier, immunosuppressant

Action: Binds to lymphocyte antigen (CD_2) interfering with lymphocyte activation; also causes a reduction in subsets of CD2+ T lymphocytes; also reduces circulating total CH4+ and CD8+ T lymphocyte counts

Uses: Treatment of moderate to severe chronic plaque psoriasis in adults who are candidates for systemic therapy or phototherapy

Dosage and routes:

- *Adult:* IV 7.5 mg as an IV bolus or IM 15 mg once weekly × 12 wk; a second 12 wk treatment course may be used providing the CD4 T lymphocyte count is within normal ranges

Available forms include: Powder for IV injection 7.5 mg; powder for IM injection 15 mg

Side effects/adverse reactions:

CNS: Dizziness

CV: Nausea

RESP: Increased cough

HEMA: ***Lymphopenia,*** decreased CD4+, CD8+ and T lymphocytes

EENT: Pharyngitis

INTEG: Pruritus, injection site pain

MS: Myalgia

MISC: Chills, ***malignancies, serious infections, allergic reactions***

Contraindications: Hypersensitivity, concurrent therapy with other immunosuppressive drugs or phototherapy

Precautions: Live or live-attenuated vaccines require regular monitoring of lymphocyte counts; pregnancy category B, lactation data not available (caution), elderly, safety and efficacy in pediatric patients not known

Pharmacokinetics: IM bioavailability 63%; metabolism data not reported

Drug interactions of concern to dentistry:

- None reported

alendronate sodium

(a-len′droe-nate)

Fosamax

Drug class.: Amino biphosphonate

Action: Acts as a specific inhibitor of osteoclast-mediated bone resorption

Uses: Osteoporosis treatment and prevention in men and postmenopausal women, glucocorticoid-induced osteoporosis in men and women receiving glucocorticoids at daily dose of 7.5 mg prednisone, Paget's disease of bone

Dosage and routes:

Osteoporosis–treatment:

- *Postmenopause:* PO 10 mg/day; must be taken at least 30 min before first food, beverage, or other

medication of the day; take with full glass of water and avoid lying down for 30 min after dose; supplemental calcium and vitamin D required for all patients if dietary intake is inadequate; or 70 mg once weekly
• *Men:* PO 10 mg once daily, or 70 mg once weekly
Prevention of osteoporosis in postmenopause:
• *Adult:* PO 5 mg/day or 35 mg once weekly taken as described above
Glucocorticoid-induced osteoporosis:
• *Adult:* PO 5 mg/day as described above; in postmenopausal women not receiving estrogen, the dose is 10 mg/day as described above
Paget's disease:
• *Adult:* PO 40 mg/day × 6 mo; take as described above; supplemental calcium and vitamin D required for all patients if dietary intake is inadequate
Available forms include: Tabs 5, 10, 35, 40, 70 mg
Side effects/adverse reactions:
ORAL: Taste alteration
CNS: Headache, nervousness
GI: Abdominal pain, nausea, constipation, diarrhea, acid regurgitation, gastritis, esophagitis
INTEG: Rash, erythema
MS: Pain, cramps
Contraindications: Hypersensitivity, hypocalcemia, esophageal abnormalities, inability to sit upright for 30 min
Precautions: Renal insufficiency, active upper GI disease, may see decrease in serum calcium/phosphate, ensure adequate calcium and vitamin D intake, pregnancy category C, lactation

Pharmacokinetics:
PO: Food, coffee, or juice reduces bioavailability; rapidly distributed to bone; not metabolized; almost complete urinary excretion
Drug interactions of concern to dentistry:
• Increased risk of GI side effects in doses >10 mg/day: Use NSAIDs, ASA with caution
• After administration, must wait at least 30 min before taking any other drug

DENTAL CONSIDERATIONS
General:
• Be aware of oral manifestations of Paget's disease (macrognathia, alveolar pain).
• Consider semisupine chair position for patient comfort because of pain experienced in osteoporosis and possible GI side effects of drug.
• Consider short appointments for patient comfort.
Consultations:
• Medical consultation may be required to assess disease control and patient's ability to tolerate stress.

alfuzosin HCl

(al-fyoo′-zoe-sin)
Uroxatral
Drug class.: Adrenoreceptor antagonist

Action: Selectively inhibits α_1-adrenergic receptors in the lower urinary tract relaxing smooth muscle in bladder neck to improve urine flow
Uses: Signs and symptoms of benign prostatic hyperplasia (BPH)

Dosage and routes:
• *Adult:* PO 10 mg (ext rel tab) taken immediately after the same meal daily
Available forms include: Ext rel tab 10 mg
Side effects/adverse reactions:
CNS: Headache, fatigue, dizziness
CV: Syncope, postural hypotension, chest pain, tachycardia
GI: Abdominal pain, dyspepsia, nausea, constipation
RESP: URI, bronchitis
GU: Impotence, priapism
EENT: Sinusitis, pharyngitis
INTEG: Rash
MISC: Pain
Contraindications: Hypersensitivity, moderate to severe hepatic impairment, potent inhibitors of CYP3A4 isoenzyme, other α_1-adrenergic blockers
Precautions: Increase in angina pectoris symptoms, severe renal impairment, known history of QT-interval prolongation, caution in use of drugs that prolong the QT interval, pregnancy category B, not for use in women or children
Pharmacokinetics:
PO: absolute bioavailability 49%, maximum plasma levels 8 hr; maximum absorption occurs immediately after a meal, plasma protein binding 82% to 90%, hepatic metabolism involving CYP3A4 isoenzymes, metabolites excreted in feces 69% and in urine 24%
Drug interactions of concern to dentistry:
• Potential for hypotension: antihypertensives drugs, other adrenergic antagonists
• Contraindicated with ketoconazole, itraconazole
• Possible risk of orthostatic hypotension may be increased with conscious sedation techniques
• Opioids and anticholinergic drugs may enhance urinary retention in BPH; use alternative analgesics (NSAIDs)
• Erythromycin is an inhibitor of CYP3A4, but no data reported for possible interaction: use with caution

DENTAL CONSIDERATIONS
General:
• Monitor vital signs at every appointment because of cardiovascular side effects.
• Consider semisupine chair position for patient comfort if GI side effects occur.
• After supine positioning, have patient sit upright for at least 2 min before standing to avoid orthostatic hypotension.

---

alitretinoin gel

(a-li-tret′-i-noyn)
Panretin
Drug class.: Topical retinoid

Action: Binds to all known intracellular retinoid receptor subtypes to function as a transcription factor in the regulation of gene expression that controls the process of cellular differentiation and proliferation in both normal and neoplastic cells
Uses: Topical treatment of cutaneous lesions in patients with AIDS-related Kaposi's sarcoma
Dosage and routes:
• *Adult:* TOP apply bid; can increase to tid or qid if application toxicity is not severe; apply enough gel to cover the lesion

Available forms include: Gel 0.1%, 60 g tube

Side effects/adverse reactions:
INTEG: Rash, pain, pruritus, erythema, edema, exfoliative dermatitis, vesiculation

Contraindications: Hypersensitivity, avoid application to mucous membranes and normal skin, hypersensitivity to retinoids

Precautions: Avoid pregnancy, pregnancy category D, discontinue breast-feeding when used, safe use in children unknown, patients >65 yr, occlusive dressings; do not use products containing DEET

Pharmacokinetics: TOP: limited absorption occurs with concentrations similar to naturally occurring retinoids

Drug interactions of concern to dentistry:

• Risk of photosensitivity reaction: tetracyclines, fluoroquinolones, other photosensitizing drugs

DENTAL CONSIDERATIONS

General:

• Patients will be taking antiviral drugs; note which drugs are being used, because some have potential for significant drug interactions.

• Take a complete medical history, including a current drug history with doses and duration of therapy.

allopurinol/allopurinol sodium

(al-oh-pure'i-nole)

Zyloprim

Apo-Allopurinol, Purinol, Zyloprim

Drug class.: Antigout drug, antihyperuricemic

Action: Inhibits the enzyme xanthine oxidase, reducing uric acid synthesis

Uses: Chronic gout, hyperuricemia associated with malignancies, recurrent calcium oxalate calculi, uric acid nephropathy

Dosage and routes:

Gout/hyperuricemia:

• *Adult:* PO 100-600 mg qd depending on severity, not to exceed 800 mg/day; maintenance dose 200-300 mg daily

• *Child 6-10 yr:* 300 mg qd or 100 mg tid

• *Child <6 yr:* 50 mg tid

Prevention of uric acid nephropathy in chemotherapy:

• *Adult:* PO 600-800 mg qd × 2 or 3 days with forced fluids

• *Adult:* IV 200-400 mg/m^2 daily

• *Child:* IV 200 mg/m^2 daily

Available forms include: Tabs 100, 300 mg; powder for inj 500 mg/vial

NOTE: Zyloprim for injection (allopurinol sodium) used only for patients with certain cancers for control of uric acid levels

Side effects/adverse reactions:

▼ *ORAL:* Metallic taste, stomatitis, lichenoid drug reaction, salivary gland swelling

CNS: Headache, drowsiness, neuritis, paresthesia

GI: Nausea, vomiting, anorexia, malaise, cramps, peptic ulcer, diarrhea

HEMA: ***Agranulocytosis, thrombocytopenia, aplastic anemia, pancytopenia, leukopenia, bone marrow depression, eosinophilia***

EENT: Retinopathy, cataracts, epistaxis

INTEG: Fever, chills, dermatitis, pruritus, purpura, erythema, ecchymosis, alopecia

MISC: Myopathy, arthralgia, hepatomegaly, ***cholestatic jaundice, renal failure***

Contraindications: Hypersensitivity

Precautions: Pregnancy category C, lactation, renal disease, hepatic disease, children

Pharmacokinetics:

PO: Peak 2-4 hr, half-life 1-2 hr; excreted in feces, urine

Drug interactions of concern to dentistry:

• Increased risk of rash: ampicillin, amoxicillin, bacampicillin, hetacillin

DENTAL CONSIDERATIONS

General:

• Patients on chronic drug therapy may rarely have symptoms of blood dyscrasias, which can include infection, bleeding, and poor healing.

Consultations:

• In a patient with symptoms of blood dyscrasias, request a medical consult for blood studies and postpone dental treatment until normal values are reestablished.

• Medical consult may be required to assess disease control.

Teach patient/family:

• Importance of good oral hygiene to prevent soft tissue inflammation

• To avoid mouth rinses with high alcohol content because of drying effects

---

almotriptan malate

(al-moh-trip'tan)

Axert

Drug class.: Selective serotonin agonist

Action: A selective serotonin agonist for $5HT_{1/b.1/d}$ receptors with effects on intracranial blood vessels, trigeminal sensory nerves (cranial vessel constriction) and inhibition of proinflammatory vasoactive neuropeptide release

Uses: Acute treatment of migraine with or without aura in adults

Dosage and routes:

• *Adult:* PO single dose of 6.25-12.5 mg; can repeat in 2 hr if headache reoccurs; limit 2 doses in 24 hr

Available forms include: Tab 6.25, 12.5 mg

Side effects/adverse reactions:

▼ *ORAL: Dry mouth,* taste alteration

CNS: Headache, somnolence, dizziness, asthenia, paresthesia, anxiety

CV: Slight increase in BP, palpitation

GI: Nausea, abdominal pain, dyspepsia

EENT: Pharyngitis, rhinitis, ear pain, tinnitus, dry eyes

INTEG: Pruritus, rash, dermatitis

META: Hyperglycemia

MS: Myalgia, weakness

Contraindications: Hypersensitivity, heart disease, uncontrolled hypertension, hemiplegic or basilar migraine, use of another serotonin agonist, ergotamine-type drug in last 24 hr, MAOIs

Precautions: Hypertension, diabetes, hepatitis, renal impairment, elevated cholesterol, obesity, smoking, postmenopause, male >40 yr, preexisting heart disease, elderly, pregnancy category C, lactation, safety/efficacy for pediatric patients not evaluated

Pharmacokinetics:

PO: Bioavailability 80%, peak effect 2.5 hr, half-life 3.1 hr, plasma protein binding 35%, metabolized by CYP3A4 and monoamine oxidase A, most excreted in urine (70%), feces (13%)

Drug interactions of concern to dentistry:

• Avoid concurrent use of ketoconazole, itraconazole, erythromycin

DENTAL CONSIDERATIONS

General:

• This is an acute-use drug; it is doubtful that patients will undergo dental treatment during acute migraine attacks.

• Be aware of patient's disease, its severity, frequency when known.

Consultations:

• If treating chronic orofacial pain, consult with physician of record.

• Medical consultation may be required to assess disease control and patient's ability to tolerate stress.

Teach patient/family:

• That dryness of the mouth may occur when taking this drug; avoid mouth rinses with high alcohol content because of additional drying effects

• Importance of updating health and drug history if physician makes any changes in evaluation or drug regimens

---

alosetron HCl

(a-loe'se-tron)

Lotronex

Drug class.: Selective serotonin antagonist, neuroenteric modulator

Action: A selective 5-HT_3 (serotonin) receptor antagonist; especially those 5-HT_3 receptors in enteric neurons of the GI tract

Uses: Treatment of women with diarrhea-predominant irritable bowel syndrome (IBS) failing to respond to conventional therapy

NOTE: Available only through enrolled physicians in the Lotronex risk management program

Dosage and routes:

• *Adult:* PO initial 1 mg/day × 4 wk; can be increased to 1 mg bid if symptoms not controlled and patient tolerates initial dose; discontinue drug if symptoms continue with higher dose for 4 wk

Available forms include: Tabs 1.124 mg (equivalent to 1 mg base)

Side effects/adverse reactions:

▼ *ORAL:* Unusual taste (rare)

CNS: Sleep disorders, depression

CV: Hypertension, arrhythmias (infrequent)

GI: Nausea, GI discomfort, abdominal pain, gas symptoms, dyspepsia, hemorrhoids, constipation, ***serious complications of constipation, ischemic colitis***

EENT: Allergic rhinitis, throat pain, eye, ear and nose infections

META: Increase in ALT, abnormal bilirubin

MISC: Allergies (rare)

Contraindications: Hypersensitivity; patients with constipation, chronic or severe constipation, history of sequelae from constipation, intestinal obstruction, stricture, toxic megacolon, GI perforation, adhesions, ischemic colitis, Crohn's disease, ulcerative colitis, diverticulitis

Precautions: Food retards absorption, elderly, reduced hepatic or renal function, notify physician immediately if severe constipation or worse occurs, pregnancy category B, lactation, children; physicians prescribing this drug must be enrolled in Glaxo Smith Kline's Prescribing Program

Pharmacokinetics:
PO: Rapid absorption, bioavailability 50%-60%, peak plasma levels 1 hr, widely distributed, plasma protein binding 82%, extensively metabolized (cytochrome P450 enzymes), excreted mostly in urine (73%), feces (24%)

Drug interactions of concern to dentistry:

• Does not appear to induce CYP450 isoenzymes; no interactions are documented

• Avoid use of drugs (opioids) that could lead to increased risk of constipation

• Use NSAIDs or acetaminophen for mild to moderate dental pain

DENTAL CONSIDERATIONS

General:

• Short appointments and a stress reduction protocol may be required for anxious patients.

• Consider semisupine chair position for patient comfort because of GI side effects of disease.

• Avoid drugs with anticholinergic activity, such as antihistamines, opioids, benzodiazepines, propantheline, atropine, and scopolamine.

• Question patient about tolerance of NSAIDs or aspirin related to GI disease.

Consultations:

• Consider consulting with physician before prescribing drugs that can cause constipation (opioids).

• Consultation with physician may be needed if sedation or general anesthesia is required.

• Medical consultation may be required to assess disease control and patient's ability to tolerate stress.

Teach patient/family:

• Importance of updating health and drug history if physician makes any changes in evaluation or drug regimens

---

alprazolam

(al-pray′zoe-lam)
Xanax, Xanax XR
Alti-Alprazola, Apo-Alpraz, Gen-alprazolam, Novo-Alprazol, Nu-Alpraz, Xanax TS

Drug class.: Benzodiazepine

Controlled Substance Schedule IV

Action: Produces CNS depression by interacting with benzodiazepine receptors to facilitate the action of the inhibitory neurotransmitter γ-aminobutyric acid (GABA)

Uses: Generalized anxiety disorder, panic disorders, anxiety with depressive symptoms; unapproved: agoraphobia

Dosage and routes:

Anxiety disorder:

• *Adult:* PO 0.25-0.5 mg tid, not to exceed 4 mg in divided doses/day

Panic disorder:

• *Adult:* PO 0.5 mg tid; may increase dose by no more than 1 mg/day

• *Geriatric or debilitated:* PO 0.25 mg bid-tid

Available forms include: Tab 0.25, 0.5, 1, 2 mg; ext rel tab 0.5, 1, 2, and 3 mg; oral sol 0.5 mg/5 ml; intensol sol 1 mg/ml

Side effects/adverse reactions:

ORAL: Dry mouth

CNS: Dizziness, drowsiness, confusion, headache, anxiety, tremors, stimulation, fatigue, depression, insomnia, hallucinations

CV: Orthostatic hypotension, ***ECG changes, tachycardia,*** hypotension

GI: Constipation, nausea, vomiting, anorexia, diarrhea
EENT: *Blurred vision,* tinnitus, mydriasis
INTEG: Rash, dermatitis, itching
Contraindications: Hypersensitivity to benzodiazepines, acute narrow-angle glaucoma, psychosis, pregnancy category D, child <18 yr, ketoconazole, itraconazole, ritonavir, indinavir, saquinavir
Precautions: Elderly, debilitated, hepatic disease, renal disease; dependence, potential for abuse; pregnancy category D, avoid in lactation, safety and efficacy in patients <18 yr old not established
Pharmacokinetics:
PO: Onset 30 min, peak 1-2 hr, duration 4-6 hr, half-life 12-15 hr; therapeutic response 2-3 days; metabolized by liver; excreted by kidneys; crosses placenta, breast milk
Drug interactions of concern to dentistry:
• Increased CNS depression: alcohol, other CNS depressants, clarithromycin, erythromycin, fluconazole, miconazole, fluoxetine, isoniazid, fluvoxamine, nefazodone, rifamycin; St. John's wort (herb), kava (herb)
• Contraindicated with ketoconazole, itraconazole, ritonavir, indinavir, saquinavir

DENTAL CONSIDERATIONS
General:
• Monitor vital signs at every appointment because of cardiovascular side effects.
• After supine positioning, have patient sit upright for at least 2 min to avoid orthostatic hypotension.
• Assess salivary flow as a factor in caries, periodontal disease, and candidiasis.
• Psychologic and physical dependence may occur with chronic administration.
Consultations:
• Medical consultation may be required to assess disease control.
Teach patient/family:
When chronic dry mouth occurs, advise patient:
• To avoid mouth rinses with high alcohol content because of drying effects
• To use daily home fluoride products for anticaries effect
• To use sugarless gum, frequent sips of water, or saliva substitutes

alprostadil

(al-pros′ta-dil)
Caverject, Caverject Impulse, Edex, Muse

Drug class.: Naturally occurring prostaglandin (E_1, PGE_1)

Action: Induces erection by relaxation of trabecular smooth muscle and by dilation of cavernosal arteries
Uses: Treatment of erectile dysfunction due to neurogenic, vasculogenic, psychogenic, or mixed etiology
(NOTE: Another alprostadil-containing product, Prostin VR Pediatric, is used to maintain ductus arteriosus patency in neonates until surgery can be performed.)
Dosage and routes:
Male gender:
• *Adult:* Intracavernosal–initial dose must be determined in physician's office, individualized dose for each patient; initial doses range from 1.25-2.5 μg, titrate dose in increments of 5-10 μg until erection suitable for intercourse is ob-

tained; administer with supplied self-injection system by injecting into the corpora cavernosa; onset varies from 5-20 min, duration <60 min; do not give more than 2 doses in 24 hr; use more than 3 × wk is not recommended; alternate side and site of injection

- *Adult:* Intraurethral–the dose must be individualized in the physician's office; no more than 2 doses in 24 hr, follow package instructions for correct administration technique

Available forms include: Vial powder with diluent and self-injection system 5, 10, 20, 40 μg/ml, 10, 20 μg/0.5 ml ; pellets: 125, 250, 500, and 1000 μg; instructions for use and administration accompany package

Side effects/adverse reactions:

CNS: Headache, dizziness, fainting

CV: Hypotension, hypertension, abnormal ECG

RESP: Flulike syndrome, cough, URI

GU: Penile pain, priapism, fibrosis, hematoma, rash or edema at site of injection, prostatic disorder, penile trauma, urinary frequency

INTEG: Rash

EENT: Nasal congestion, sinusitis, rhinitis, blurred vision

META: Hypercholesterolemia, hypertriglyceridemia

MS: Pain, leg cramps

Contraindications: Hypersensitivity, conditions predisposing to priapism (sickle cell anemia, sickle trait, multiple myeloma, or leukemia), penile deformation, penile implants, or Peyronie's disease; intercourse with a pregnant woman (unless condom used)

Precautions: Patients on anticoagulant therapy, use of sterile technique, care of syringe, physician instruction in use required, sexually transmitted disease

Pharmacokinetics: Rapidly metabolized and cleared from body by urinary excretion

Drug interactions of concern to dentistry:

- None reported

DENTAL CONSIDERATIONS

- None

amantadine HCl

(a-man'ta-deen)

Symmetrel

Endantadine, Gen-Amantadine, Symmetrel

Drug class.: Antiviral, antiparkinsonian agent

Action: Prevents uncoating of nucleic acid in viral cell, preventing penetration of virus to host; causes release of dopamine and norepinephrine from neurons; may block reuptake of dopamine and norepinephrine into presynaptic neurons

Uses: Prophylaxis or treatment of respiratory tract illness caused by influenza type A; drug-induced extrapyramidal reactions; parkinsonism

Dosage and routes:

Influenza type A:

- *Adult and child >12 yr:* PO 200 mg/day in single dose or divided bid
- *Adult >65 yr:* PO 100 mg daily
- *Child 9-12 yr:* PO 100 mg q12h
- *Child 1-9 yr:* PO 2.2-4.4 mg/kg/day q12h, not to exceed 150 mg/day

Extrapyramidal reaction/parkinsonism:

- *Adult:* PO 100 mg bid, up to 400 mg/day in EPS; give for 1 wk, then

100 mg as needed in parkinsonism
Available forms include: Caps 100 mg; syr 50 mg/5 ml; tab 100 mg
Side effects/adverse reactions:
▼ *ORAL: Dry mouth,* glossitis
CNS: ***Convulsions,*** headache, dizziness, drowsiness, fatigue, anxiety, psychosis, impaired concentration, insomnia, depression, hallucinations, tremors
CV: ***CHF,*** orthostatic hypotension
GI: Nausea, vomiting, constipation
HEMA: ***Leukopenia***
GU: *Frequency, retention*
EENT: Blurred vision
INTEG: Photosensitivity, dermatitis
Contraindications: Hypersensitivity, lactation, child <1 yr
Precautions: Epilepsy, CHF, orthostatic hypotension, psychiatric disorders, hepatic disease, renal disease (necessitates dose adjustment); pregnancy category C
Pharmacokinetics:
PO: Onset 48 hr, half-life 24 hr; not metabolized; excreted in urine (90%) unchanged; crosses placenta; excreted in breast milk
Drug interactions of concern to dentistry:
• Increased anticholinergic response: anticholinergic drugs
• Increased CNS depression: alcohol, other CNS depressants
DENTAL CONSIDERATIONS
General:
• Monitor vital signs at every appointment because of cardiovascular side effects.
• Assess salivary flow as a factor in caries, periodontal disease, and candidiasis.
• After supine positioning, have patient sit upright for at least 2 min to avoid orthostatic hypotension.
• Avoid dental light in patient's eyes; offer dark glasses for patient comfort.
• Short appointments and stress reduction protocol may be required for anxious patients.
• Consider semisupine chair position for patients with respiratory distress.
Teach patient/family:
• To avoid mouth rinses with high alcohol content because of drying effects
• To use electric toothbrush if patient has difficulty holding conventional devices

ambenonium chloride

(am-be-noe'nee-um)
Mytelase
Drug class.: Cholinesterase inhibitor

Action: An acetylcholinesterase inhibitor; inhibits destruction of acetylcholine, which increases concentration at sites in which acetylcholine is released; this facilitates transmission of impulses across the myoneural junction
Uses: Myasthenia gravis, when other drugs cannot be used
Dosage and routes:
• *Adult:* PO 5 mg tid or qid, then gradually increased q1-2d; 5-75 mg/dose is usually sufficient
Caution: doses more than 200 mg per day
Available forms include: Tabs 10 mg
Side effects/adverse reactions:
▼ *ORAL: Increased salivary secretions*
CNS: ***Paralysis, loss of consciousness, convulsions,*** drowsiness, diz-

ziness, headache, weakness, incoordination

CV: ***Cardiac arrest,*** tachycardia, dysrhythmias, bradycardia, hypotension, AV block, ECG changes, syncope

GI: Nausea, diarrhea, vomiting, cramps, gastric secretions, dysphagia, increased peristalsis

RESP: ***Respiratory depression, bronchospasm, constriction, laryngospasm, respiratory arrest,*** increased secretions, dyspnea

GU: Frequency, incontinence, urgency

EENT: Miosis, blurred vision, lacrimation, visual changes

INTEG: Rashes, urticaria, sweating

Contraindications: Obstruction of intestine or renal system, hypersensitivity

Precautions: Seizure disorders, bronchial asthma, coronary occlusion, hyperthyroidism, dysrhythmias, peptic ulcer, megacolon, poor GI motility, pregnancy category C, bradycardia, hypotension, lactation, children

Pharmacokinetics:

PO: Onset 20-30 min, duration 3-8 hr

Drug interactions of concern to dentistry:

- Avoid drugs with anticholinergic activity and neuromuscular blocking agents
- Avoid systemic use of ester-type local anesthetics because of reduced plasma cholinesterase activity
- Use glucocorticoids with caution

DENTAL CONSIDERATIONS

General:

- Control excessive salivary flow with rubber dam and suction.
- Avoid drugs that reduce salivary flow, because they will antagonize this drug.
- Patient may be unable to keep mouth open for long periods because of disease; short appointments may be necessary.
- Monitor vital signs at every appointment because of cardiovascular side effects. Evaluate respiration characteristics and rate.
- Consider semisupine chair position for patient comfort because of GI side effects of the drug.
- After supine positioning, have patient sit upright for at least 2 min to avoid orthostatic hypotension.

Consultations:

- Consultation with physician may be needed if sedation or general anesthesia is required.
- Medical consultation may be required to assess disease control and patient's ability to tolerate stress.
- **Teach patient/family:**
- Use of electric toothbrush if patient has difficulty holding conventional devices
- Importance of updating health and drug history, reporting changes in health status, drug regimen changes, or disease/treatment status

amifostine

(am-i-fos′teen)

Ethyol

Drug class.: Cytoprotective, radioprotective

Action: Amifostine is converted to an active free-thiol metabolite that reduces cytotoxicity by binding to and detoxifying cisplatin metabolites or other alkylating agents; acts as a free-radical scavenger

Uses: (1) Incidence reduction in moderate to severe xerostomia in patients undergoing postoperative head and neck radiation for cancer where the radiation port includes a substantial part of the parotid gland; (2) reduction in cumulative renal toxicity associated with repeated cisplatin use in patients with advanced ovarian or non–small cell lung cancers

Dosage and routes:

Xerostomia reduction:

• *Adult:* IV infusion 200 mg/m^2 given once daily in a 3 min IV infusion starting 15-30 min before standard radiation therapy (1.8-2.0 Gy)

Cisplatin toxicity reduction:

• *Adult:* IV infusion 910 mg/m^2 given once daily in a 15 min IV infusion 30 min before beginning cisplatin use

Available forms include: Vial 500 mg powder

Side effects/adverse reactions:

CNS: Somnolence, dizziness

CV: Hypotension

GI: Nausea, vomiting, hiccups

INTEG: Skin rash, flushing

META: Hypocalcemia

MISC: Hypersensitivity reactions (rare)

Contraindications: Hypersensitivity to aminothiol compounds

Precautions: Patients should be well hydrated, monitor blood pressure, safety not established in CV disease; elderly, cerebrovascular disease, pregnancy category C, lactation, children

Pharmacokinetics: *IV infusion:* Rapidly cleared from plasma ~6 min, rapidly metabolized to an active free thiol metabolite, dephosphorylated by alk phosphatase, eliminated by rapid tissue distribution and metabolism, small amounts excreted in urine

Drug interactions of concern to dentistry:

• None reported

DENTAL CONSIDERATIONS

General:

• This is an in-hospital or outpatient chemotherapy-administered drug. Confirm the patient's disease and treatment status.

• Dental treatment may be provided if necessary during treatment.

• Monitor vital signs at every appointment because of cardiovascular side effects.

• Consider semisupine chair position for patient comfort if GI side effects occur.

• Patients taking opioids for acute or chronic pain should be given alternative analgesics for dental pain.

• Short appointments and a stress reduction protocol may be required for anxious patients.

• Palliative medication may be required for management of oral side effects caused by chemotherapeutic drugs.

• Assess salivary flow as a factor in caries, periodontal disease, and candidiasis.

• Chlorhexidine mouth rinse before and during chemotherapy may reduce severity of mucositis.

• Apply lubricant to dry lips for patient comfort before dental procedures.

• Examine for oral manifestation of opportunistic infection.

Consultations:

• Medical consultation may be required to assess immunologic status during cancer therapy and determine safety risks posed by dental treatment.

• Consultation with physician may be needed if sedation or general anesthesia is required.

Teach patient/family:

• To prevent trauma when using oral hygiene aids

• Importance of good oral hygiene to prevent soft tissue inflammation, infection

• To report oral lesions, soreness, or bleeding to dentist

When chronic dry mouth occurs, advise patient:

• To avoid mouth rinses with high alcohol content because of drying effects

• To use daily home fluoride products for anticaries effect

• To use sugarless gum, frequent sips of water, or saliva substitutes

• Importance of updating health and drug history, reporting changes in health status, drug regimen changes, or disease/treatment status

---

amiloride HCl

(a-mil'oh-ride)

Midamor

Drug class.: Potassium-sparing diuretic

Action: Acts primarily on distal tubule and secondarily by inhibiting reabsorption of sodium and increasing potassium retention

Uses: Edema in CHF in combination with other diuretics, for hypertension as an adjunct with other diuretics to maintain potassium-

Dosage and routes:

• *Adult:* PO 5 mg qd, added to the usual antihypertensive or diuretic, can increase dose to 5 mg bid (with persistent hypokalemia 15-20 mg/day with monitoring)

Available forms include: Tab 5 mg

Side effects/adverse reactions:

▼ *ORAL: Dry mouth, increased thirst*

CNS: Headache, dizziness, fatigue, weakness, paresthesias, tremor, depression, anxiety

CV: Orthostatic hypotension

GI: Nausea, diarrhea, vomiting, anorexia, cramps, constipation, abdominal pain, jaundice, bleeding

HEMA: ***Aplastic anemia, neutropenia*** (rare)

GU: Polyuria, dysuria, frequency, impotence

EENT: Loss of hearing, tinnitus, blurred vision, nasal congestion, increased intraocular pressure

INTEG: Rash, pruritus, alopecia, urticaria

META: Acidosis, hyponatremia, ***hyperkalemia,*** hypochloremia, abnormal liver function

MS: Cramps, joint pain

Contraindications: Anuria, hypersensitivity, hyperkalemia, impaired renal function

Precautions: Dehydration, pregnancy category B, diabetes, acidosis, lactation

Pharmacokinetics:

PO: Onset 2 hr, peak 6-10 hr, duration 24 hr, half-life 6-9 hr; excreted in urine, feces

Drug interactions of concern to dentistry:

• Decreased effects: corticosteroids, NSAIDs, indomethacin

DENTAL CONSIDERATIONS

General:

• Monitor vital signs at every appointment because of cardiovascular side effects.

• Assess salivary flow as a factor in caries, periodontal disease, and candidiasis.
• After supine positioning, have patient sit upright for at least 2 min to avoid orthostatic hypotension.
• Patients on chronic drug therapy may rarely have symptoms of blood dyscrasias, which can include infection, bleeding, and poor healing.
• Limit use of sodium-containing products such as saline IV fluids for those patients with a dietary salt restriction.

Consultations:

• Medical consultation may be required to assess patient's ability to tolerate stress.
• Medical consultation may be required to assess disease control.
• In a patient with symptoms of blood dyscrasias, request a medical consultation for blood studies and postpone dental treatment until normal values are reestablished.

Teach patient/family:

• Importance of good oral hygiene to prevent soft tissue inflammation
• Caution to prevent injury when using oral hygiene aids

When chronic dry mouth occurs, advise patient:

• To avoid mouth rinses with high alcohol content because of drying effects
• To use daily home fluoride products for anticaries effect
• To use sugarless gum, frequent sips of water, or saliva substitutes

aminocaproic acid

(a-mee-noe-ka-proe'ik)
Amicar
Drug class.: Hemostatic

Action: Inhibits fibrinolysis by inhibiting plasminogen activator substances

Uses: Hemorrhage from hyperfibrinolysis; adjunctive therapy in hemophilia, postsurgical hemorrhage

Dosage and routes:

• *Adult:* PO/IV infusion 5 g loading dose, then 1-1.25 g qh if needed, not to exceed 30 g/day

Dental extractions:

• *Adult:* PO/IV: 50-100 mg/kg IV q6h for 2-3 days starting 4 hr before procedure; then 50-100 mg/kg PO q6h for 5-7 days (Benitz WE, Tatro DS: *The pediatric drug handbook,* ed 2, Chicago, 1988, Year Book).

NOTE: TOP: Oral rinse 1.25g/5 ml swished for 30 sec qid for 7-10 days has also been used. Reports indicate that this may be effective for gingival bleeding, but not bleeding from sockets (Casdorph DL: Topical aminocaproic acid in hemophiliac patients undergoing dental extractions, *DICP* 24:160-161, 1990).

Available forms include: Inj IV 5 g/20 ml vial; tab 500 mg; syr 250 mg/ml

Side effects/adverse reactions:

CNS: Headache, dizziness, ***convulsions,*** malaise, fatigue, hallucinations, delirium, psychosis, weakness

CV: Edema, ***dysrhythmias,*** orthostatic hypotension, bradycardia, peripheral ischemia

GI: Nausea, vomiting, abdominal cramps, diarrhea
RESP: Dyspnea
HEMA: ***Thrombosis, leukopenia, agranulocytosis, thrombocytopenia***
GU: ***Renal failure,*** dysuria, frequency, oliguria, ejaculatory failure, menstrual irregularities
EENT: Tinnitus, nasal congestion, conjunctival suffusion, visual disorder
MS: Myalgia, weakness, fatigue, rhabdomyolysis, myoglobinuria
MISC: Rash, allergic reactions

Contraindications: Hypersensitivity, abnormal bleeding, postpartum bleeding, disseminated intravascular coagulation, upper urinary tract bleeding, new burns

Precautions: Neonates/infants, mild or moderate renal disease, hepatic disease, thrombophlebitis, cardiac disease, pregnancy category C, lactation

Pharmacokinetics:
PO: Peak 2 hr, excreted by kidneys as unmetabolized drug, rapidly absorbed

DENTAL CONSIDERATIONS

General:
• Monitor vital signs at every appointment because of cardiovascular side effects.
• After supine positioning, have patient sit upright for at least 2 min to avoid orthostatic hypotension.
• Consider additional local hemostasis measures to prevent excessive bleeding in patients with hemophilia.
• Determine why the patient is taking the drug.
• Avoid drugs such as aspirin; NSAIDs may have the potential to prolong bleeding.

Consultations:
• Medical consultation may be required to assess disease control.
• Medical consultation may be required to assess patient's ability to tolerate stress.

Teach patient/family:
• Importance of good oral hygiene to prevent soft tissue inflammation
• Caution to prevent injury when using oral hygiene aids

---

aminophylline (theophylline ethylenediamine)

(am-in-off'i-lin)
Phyllocontin, Truphylline
Drug class.: Xanthine

Action: Relaxes smooth muscle of respiratory system by blocking phosphodiesterase, which increases AMP

Uses: Bronchial asthma, bronchospasm, Cheyne-Stokes respirations

Dosage and routes:
• *Adult:* PO 5 mg/kg loading dose, then 2-3 mg/kg q8h as tolerated; IV dose must be individualized
• *Child:* PO 5 mg/kg loading dose, then 3-4 mg/kg q6-8h as tolerated; IV doses must be individualized

Available forms include: Inj IV 250 mg/10 ml; rec supp 250, 500 mg; oral liq 105 mg/5 ml; tabs 100, 200 mg; con rel tabs 225 mg

Side effects/adverse reactions:
▼ *ORAL:* Bitter taste
CNS: Anxiety, restlessness, insomnia, dizziness, ***convulsions,*** headache, light-headedness, muscle twitching
CV: Palpitation, sinus tachycardia, hypotension, flushing, dysrhythmias

GI: Nausea, vomiting, anorexia, diarrhea, dyspepsia, anal irritation (suppositories), epigastric pain
RESP: Increased rate
GU: Urinary frequency
INTEG: Flushing, urticaria
Contraindications: Hypersensitivity to xanthines, tachydysrhythmias
Precautions: Elderly, CHF, cor pulmonale, hepatic disease, active peptic ulcer disease, diabetes mellitus, hyperthyroidism, hypertension, children, pregnancy category C, glaucoma, prostatic hypertrophy
Pharmacokinetics:
IV: Peak 30 min; 16 mg of anhydrous aminophylline provides a dose equivalent to 100 mg anhydrous theophylline
Drug interactions of concern to dentistry:
• Increased action: erythromycin (macrolides), ciprofloxacin
• Cardiac dysrhythmia: CNS stimulants, hydrocarbon inhalation anesthetics
• Decreased effects: barbiturates, carbamazepine
• Decreased effects of benzodiazepines
DENTAL CONSIDERATIONS
General:
• Monitor vital signs at every appointment because of cardiovascular and respiratory side effects.
• Consider semisupine chair position for patient comfort because of respiratory disease and GI side effects of the drug.
• Midday appointments and a stress reduction protocol may be required for anxious patients.
• Be aware that aspirin or sulfite preservatives in vasoconstrictor-containing products can exacerbate asthma.
• Acute asthmatic episodes may be precipitated in the dental office. Sympathomimetic inhalants should be available for emergency use.
Consultations:
• Medical consultation may be required to assess disease control.

aminosalicylic acid

(a-mee-noe-sal-i-sil′ik)
Paser
Drug class.: Antitubercular antiinfective

Action: Bacteriostatic for *M. tuberculosis;* postulated mechanisms are related to inhibition of folic acid synthesis or inhibition of the cell wall component, mycobactin
Uses: Tuberculosis, in combination with other *M. tuberculosis* antiinfectives
Dosage and routes:
Multidrug-resistant TB cases:
• *Adult:* PO 4 g tid
Available forms include: Packets 4 g; carton of 30 packets
Side effects/adverse reactions:
CV: Pericarditis
GI: Nausea, vomiting, diarrhea, abdominal pain, jaundice, hepatitis
HEMA: ***Agranulocytosis, thrombocytopenia,*** leukopenia, anemia, reduction in prothrombin
GU: Crystalluria
EENT: Optic neuritis
INTEG: ***Exfoliative dermatitis,*** rash, eruptions
MISC: Fever, infectious mononucleosis–like and lymphoma-like symptoms
Contraindications: Hypersensitivity, severe renal impairment
Precautions: Hepatic dysfunction, refrigeration required for storage, malabsorption of vitamin B_{12},

pregnancy category C, no data on safe use in children or lactation
Pharmacokinetics:
PO: Protect granules by giving with acidic foods, mean peak serum levels 6 hr, 50%-60% protein bound; acetylated form excreted mostly in urine
Drug interactions of concern to dentistry:
• None reported
DENTAL CONSIDERATIONS
General:
• Determine that noninfectious status exists by ensuring that (1) anti-TB drugs have been taken for more than 3 wk, (2) culture confirmed TB susceptibility to antiinfectives, (3) patient has had three consecutive negative sputum smears, and (4) patient is not in the coughing stage.
• Determine why patient is taking drug (i.e., for prophylaxis or active therapy).
• Explain importance of taking medication for full length of regimen to ensure effectiveness of treatment and to prevent the emergence of resistant strains.
• Patients on chronic drug therapy may rarely have symptoms of blood dyscrasias, which can include infection, bleeding, and poor healing.
• Consider semisupine chair position for patient comfort if GI side effects occur.
Consultations:
• Medical consultation may be required to assess disease control and patient's ability to tolerate stress.
• In a patient with symptoms of blood dyscrasias, request a medical consultation for blood studies and postpone treatment until normal values are reestablished.
Teach patient/family:
• Importance of updating health and drug history if physician makes any changes in evaluation or drug regimens
• To prevent trauma when using oral hygiene aids

amiodarone HCl

(a-mee'oh-da-rone)
Cordarone, Cordarone IV, Pacerone
✱ Cordarone Intravenous
Drug class.: Antidysrhythmic (class III)

Action: Prolongs action potential duration and effective refractory period, slows conduction, noncompetitive α- and β-adrenergic receptor inhibition, blocks sodium channels, prolongs nodal conduction
Uses: Documented life-threatening ventricular tachycardia; unapproved: ventricular fibrillation not controlled by first-line agents
Dosage and routes:
• *Adult:* PO loading dose 800-1600 mg/day 1-3 wk, then 600-800 mg/day 1 mo; maintenance 200-600 mg/day; usually given by IV infusion, must follow package insert (oral doses follow IV infusion and suppression of arrhythmias)
Available forms include: Tabs 200, 400 mg; INJ 50 mg/ml
Side effects/adverse reactions:
▼ *ORAL:* Bitter taste sensation, dry mouth
CNS: Headache, dizziness, involuntary movement, tremors, peripheral neuropathy, malaise, fatigue, ataxia, paresthesias, insomnia
*CV: Hypotension, bradycardia, **sinus arrest, CHF, dysrhythmias,***

SA node dysfunction prolonged QT interval

GI: ***Hepatotoxicity,*** nausea, vomiting, diarrhea, abdominal pain, anorexia, constipation

RESP: ***Pulmonary fibrosis,*** pulmonary inflammation

EENT: ***Corneal microdeposits,*** blurred vision, halos, photophobia, dry eyes

INTEG: Rash, photosensitivity, bluish-gray skin discoloration, alopecia, spontaneous ecchymosis

ENDO: Hyperthyroidism or hypothyroidism

MS: Weakness, pain in extremities

MISC: Flushing, abnormal smell, edema, coagulation abnormalities

Contraindications: Hypersensitivity, cardiogenic shock, marked sinus bradycardia, second- or third-degree heart block

Precautions: Goiter, Hashimoto's thyroiditis, SN dysfunction, second- or third-degree AV block, electrolyte imbalances, bradycardia; pregnancy category D, lactation, not recommended for children

Pharmacokinetics:

PO: Onset 1-3 wk, peak 3-7 hr, half-life 15-100 days; metabolized by liver (CYP 3A4); excreted in bile; *IV:* rapid onset, peak levels 10 min

Drug interactions of concern to dentistry:

- Bradycardia, hypotension: inhalation anesthetics, lidocaine, anticholinergics, vasoconstrictors
- Increased photosensitization: tetracyclines
- Do not use with grapefruit juice, gatifloxacin, moxifloxacin, or sparfloxacin
- Amiodarone is both a substrate and an inhibitor of CYP 3A4; potential interactions with strong inhibitors of CYP 3A4 isoenzymes (see Appendix I)

DENTAL CONSIDERATIONS

General:

- Monitor vital signs at every appointment because of cardiovascular and respiratory side effects.
- Assess salivary flow as a factor in caries, periodontal disease, and candidiasis.
- Avoid dental light in patient's eyes; offer dark glasses for patient comfort.
- After supine positioning, have patient sit upright for at least 2 min before standing to avoid orthostatic hypotension.
- Use vasoconstrictors with caution, in low doses, and with careful aspiration. Avoid gingival retraction cord with epinephrine.
- Stress from dental procedures may compromise cardiovascular function; determine patient risk.
- Delay or avoid dental treatment if patient shows signs of cardiac symptoms or respiratory distress.

Consultations:

- Medical consultation may be required to assess patient's ability to tolerate stress.
- Medical consultation may be required to assess disease control.

Teach patient/family:

- Importance of updating health and drug history, reporting changes in health status, drug regimen changes, or disease/treatment status

When chronic dry mouth occurs, advise patient:

- To avoid mouth rinses with high alcohol content because of drying effects
- To use daily home fluoride products for anticaries effect

• To use sugarless gum, frequent sips of water, or saliva substitutes

amitriptyline HCl

(a-mee-trip'ti-leen)
Elavil
Apo-Amitriptyline, Levate, Novotriptyn
Drug class.: Antidepressant-tricyclic

Action: Inhibits both norepinephrine and serotonin (5-HT) uptake in the brain, although the precise antidepressant mechanism remains unclear

Uses: Major depression; unapproved: enuresis and neurogenic pain

Dosage and routes:

• *Adult:* PO 75 mg/day in divided doses or 50-100 mg hs, may increase to 150 mg qd; IM 20-30 mg qid or 80-120 mg hs; hospitalized patients may use doses in the range of 200-300 mg/day

• *Adolescent/geriatric:* PO 30 mg/day in divided doses, with 20 mg hs; may be increased to 150 mg/day

Enuresis

• *Child up to 6 yr:* PO 10 mg/day hs

• *Child >6 yr:* PO 10 mg/day hs, can increase up to 25 mg maximum

Available forms include: Tabs 10, 25, 50, 75, 100, 150 mg; inj IM 10 mg/ml

Side effects/adverse reactions:

ORAL: Dry mouth, unpleasant taste, stomatitis, salivary gland pain

CNS: Dizziness, drowsiness, confusion, headache, anxiety, tremors, stimulation, weakness, insomnia, nightmares, EPS (elderly), increased psychiatric symptoms, seizures, ataxia, paresthesias

CV: Orthostatic hypotension, ***ECG changes, tachycardia, hypertension,*** palpitation, syncope, prolonged QT interval

GI: Diarrhea, ***paralytic ileus, hepatitis,*** increased appetite, cramps, epigastric distress, jaundice, nausea, vomiting

HEMA: ***Agranulocytosis, thrombocytopenia, eosinophilia, leukopenia***

GU: Retention

EENT: Blurred vision, tinnitus, mydriasis, ophthalmoplegia

INTEG: Rash, urticaria, sweating, pruritus, photosensitivity

Contraindications: Hypersensitivity to tricyclic antidepressants, recovery phase of MI; concurrent use with or 14 days after use of an MAOI, sparfloxacin, grepafloxacin

Precautions: Suicidal patients, convulsive disorders, prostatic hypertrophy, asthma, schizophrenia, psychotic disorders, severe depression, increased intraocular pressure, narrow-angle glaucoma, urinary retention, cardiac disease, hepatic disease, renal disease, hyperthyroidism, electroshock therapy, elective surgery, child <12 yr, pregnancy category C, elderly, MAOIs, St. John's wort

Pharmacokinetics:

PO/IM: Onset 45 min, peak 2-12 hr, therapeutic response 2-3 wk, half-life 10-50 hr; metabolized by liver; excreted in urine, feces, breast milk; crosses placenta

Drug interactions of concern to dentistry:

• Increased anticholinergic effects: muscarinic blockers, antihistamines, phenothiazines

• Increased effects of direct-acting sympathomimetics (epinephrine, levonordefrin)

• Possible risk of increased CNS depression: alcohol, barbiturates, benzodiazepines, CNS depressants, antidepressants
• Possible increase in serum levels: fluconazole, ketoconazole, bupropion, fluvoxamine, paroxatine, sertraline
• Decreased antihypertensive effect: clonidine, guanadrel, guanethidine
• Possible decrease in serum levels: barbiturates, St. John's wort (herb)

DENTAL CONSIDERATIONS

General:

• Take vital signs every appointment because of cardiovascular side effects.
• Assess salivary flow as a factor in caries, periodontal disease, and candidiasis.
• Patients on chronic drug therapy may rarely have symptoms of blood dyscrasias, which can include infection, bleeding, and poor healing.
• After supine positioning, have patient sit upright for at least 2 min to avoid orthostatic hypotension.
• Use vasoconstrictors with caution, in low doses, and with careful aspiration. Avoid use of gingival retraction cord with epinephrine.
• Place on frequent recall because of oral side effects.

Consultations:

• In a patient with symptoms of blood dyscrasias, request a medical consultation for blood studies and postpone dental treatment until normal values are reestablished.
• Medical consultation may be required to assess disease control.
• Physician should be informed if significant xerostomic side effects occur (e.g., increased caries, sore tongue, problems eating or swallowing, difficulty wearing prosthesis) so a medication change can be considered.

Teach patient/family:

• Importance of good oral hygiene to prevent soft tissue inflammation
• Caution to prevent injury when using oral hygiene aids

When chronic dry mouth occurs, advise patient:

• To avoid mouth rinses with high alcohol content because of drying effects
• To use daily home fluoride products for anticaries effect
• To use sugarless gum, frequent sips of water, or saliva substitutes

amlexanox

(am-lex'an-ox)

Aphthasol

Drug class.: Topical antiinflammatory

Action: Mechanism of action is unknown; has antiinflammatory and antiallergic activities; accelerates the resolution of pain and healing of aphthous ulcers

Uses: Aphthous ulcers in patients with normal immune systems

Dosage and routes:

• *Adult:* TOP squeeze dab (0.5 cm) of paste onto fingertip and dab each ulcer qid, after oral hygiene, after each meal, and hs; use until ulcer heals; initiate treatment with onset of early symptoms

Available forms include: Oral paste 5%, 5 g tube

Side effects/adverse reactions:

▼ *ORAL:* Transient stinging and burning on application, contact mucositis

GI: Nausea, diarrhea

Contraindications: Hypersensitivity

Precautions: Wash hands immediately before and after each use; discontinue if mucositis appears, pregnancy category B, lactation, children

Pharmacokinetics: ***TOP:*** Systemic absorption from GI tract if swallowed, drug and metabolites excreted in urine

Drug interactions of concern to dentistry:

- None reported

DENTAL CONSIDERATIONS

General:

- Recurrent aphthous ulcers may be associated with systemic conditions; evaluate as needed if healing has not occurred after 10 days.

Teach patient/family:

- To apply paste as directed and wash hands immediately before and after each use
- To report oral lesions or soreness to dentist

---

amlodipine besylate

(am-loe'di-peen)

Norvasc

Drug class.: Calcium channel blocker

Action: Inhibits calcium ion influx across cell membrane during cardiac depolarization; produces relaxation of coronary vascular smooth muscle; dilates coronary arteries; decreases SA/AV node conduction; dilates peripheral arteries

Uses: Hypertension as a single agent or in combination with other antihypertensives, chronic stable angina pectoris, vasospastic angina

Dosage and routes:

Hypertension:

- *Adult:* PO 5 mg/day; max daily dose 10 mg
- *Geriatric or small, fragile adult, hepatic impairment:* PO 2.5 mg/day

Angina (stable or vasospastic):

- *Adult:* PO 5-10mg qd

Available forms include: Tabs 2.5, 5, 10 mg

Side effects/adverse reactions:

▼ *ORAL:* Dry mouth, altered taste; gingival overgrowth has been reported with other calcium channel blockers

CNS: Headache, fatigue, lethargy, somnolence, dizziness, light-headedness, asthenia, depression

CV: Flushing, peripheral edema, palpitation, syncope, CHF, tachycardia, arrhythmia, chest pain

GI: Nausea, dyspepsia, discomfort, diarrhea, flatulence

RESP: Pulmonary edema, dyspnea

GU: Sexual difficulties

HEMA: ***Leukopenia, thrombocytopenia***

EENT: Diplopia, eye pain

INTEG: Pruritus, rash, purpura, erythema multiforme

MS: Muscle cramps, joint stiffness

Contraindications: Sick sinus syndrome, second- or third-degree heart block, hypotension less than 90 mm Hg systolic, cardiogenic shock, severe CHF

Precautions: Pregnancy category C, CHF, hypotension, hepatic impairment, lactation, children, renal disease

Pharmacokinetics:

PO: Peak plasma levels 6-12 hr, half-life 30-50 hr; highly protein bound; metabolized in liver; excreted in urine

Drug interactions of concern to dentistry:
- None reported

DENTAL CONSIDERATIONS

General:
- Monitor cardiac status; take vital signs at each appointment because of CV side effects. Consider a stress reduction protocol to prevent stress-induced angina during the dental appointment.
- Determine why patient is taking the drug (hypertension or angina).
- After supine positioning, have patient sit upright for at least 2 min to avoid orthostatic hypotension.
- Limit use of sodium-containing products such as saline IV fluids for those patients with a dietary salt restriction.
- Assess salivary flow as a factor in caries, periodontal disease, and candidiasis.
- Short appointments and a stress reduction protocol may be required for anxious patients.
- Ensure that patient's prescription nitroglycerin tablets are easily available if angina occurs. Check expiration date (shelf life is 3 months after opening).

Consultations:
- Medical consultation may be required to assess disease control and patient's ability to tolerate stress.

Teach patient/family:
- Need for frequent oral prophylaxis if gingival overgrowth occurs

When chronic dry mouth occurs, advise patient:
- To avoid mouth rinses with high alcohol content because of drying effects
- To use daily home fluoride products for anticaries effect
- To use sugarless gum, frequent sips of water, or artificial saliva

amoxapine

(a-mox′a-peen)

Asendin

Drug class.: Antidepressant—tricyclic

Action: Inhibits both norepinephrine and serotonin (5-HT) uptake in the brain, although the precise antidepressant mechanism remains unclear

Uses: Depression

Dosage and routes:
- *Adult:* PO 50 mg bid-tid, may increase to 100 mg tid on third day of therapy, not to exceed 300 mg/day unless lower doses have been given for at least 2 wk; may be given daily dose hs, not to exceed 600 mg/day in divided doses in hospitalized patients

Available forms include: Tabs 25, 50, 100, 150 mg

Side effects/adverse reactions:

▼ *ORAL: Dry mouth,* stomatitis

CNS: Dizziness, drowsiness, confusion, headache, anxiety, tremors, tardive dyskinesia, stimulation, weakness, insomnia, nightmares, EPS (elderly), increased psychiatric symptoms, paresthesia

CV: Orthostatic hypotension, ECG changes, tachycardia, ***hypertension,*** palpitation

GI: Diarrhea, constipation, ***paralytic ileus, hepatitis,*** nausea, vomiting, increased appetite, cramps, epigastric distress, jaundice

HEMA: ***Agranulocytosis, thrombocytopenia, eosinophilia, leukopenia***

GU: ***Acute renal failure,*** urinary retention

EENT: Blurred vision, tinnitus, mydriasis, ophthalmoplegia

INTEG: Rash, urticaria, sweating, pruritus, photosensitivity

Contraindications: Hypersensitivity to tricyclic antidepressants, recovery phase of MI, convulsive disorders, prostatic hypertrophy

Precautions: Suicidal patients, severe depression, increased intraocular pressure, narrow-angle glaucoma, urinary retention, cardiac disease, hepatic disease, hyperthyroidism, electroshock therapy, elective surgery, elderly, pregnancy category C, MAOIs

Pharmacokinetics:

PO: Peak blood levels 90 min, steady state 7 days, half-life 8 hr; metabolized by liver; excreted by kidneys; crosses placenta

Drug interactions of concern to dentistry:

• Increased anticholinergic effects: muscarinic blockers, antihistamines, phenothiazines

• Increased effects of direct-acting sympathomimetics (epinephrine, levonordefrin)

• Potential risk of increased CNS depression: alcohol, barbiturates, benzodiazepines, CNS depressants

• Decreased antihypertensive effect: clonidine, guanadrel, guanethidine

• Avoid concurrent use with St. John's wort

DENTAL CONSIDERATIONS

General:

• Take vital signs every appointment because of cardiovascular side effects.

• Assess salivary flow as a factor in caries, periodontal disease, and candidiasis.

• Patients on chronic drug therapy may rarely have symptoms of blood dyscrasias, which can include infection, bleeding, and poor healing.

• After supine positioning, have patient sit upright for at least 2 min to avoid orthostatic hypotension.

• Use vasoconstrictors with caution, in low doses, and with careful aspiration. Avoid use of gingival retraction cord with epinephrine.

• Place on frequent recall because of oral side effects.

Consultations:

• In a patient with symptoms of blood dyscrasias, request a medical consultation for blood studies and postpone dental treatment until normal values are reestablished.

• Medical consultation may be required to assess disease control.

• Physician should be informed if significant xerostomic side effects occur (e.g., increased caries, sore tongue, problems eating or swallowing, difficulty wearing prosthesis) so a medication change can be considered.

Teach patient/family:

• Importance of good oral hygiene to prevent soft tissue inflammation

• Caution to prevent injury when using oral hygiene aids

When chronic dry mouth occurs, advise patient:

• To avoid mouth rinses with high alcohol content because of drying effects

• To use daily home fluoride products for anticaries effect

• To use sugarless gum, frequent sips of water, or saliva substitutes

amoxicillin/clavulanate potassium

(a-mox-i-sil'in)/(klav'yoo-la-nate)

Augmentin, Augmentin ES-600, Augmentin SR

✦ Clavulin-125 F, Clavulin-250 F, Clavulin-500 F

Drug class.: Aminopenicillin with a β-lactamase inhibitor

Action: Aminopenicillins bind to specific receptors, penicillin-binding proteins, thereby interfering with cell wall synthesis that ultimately results in cell lysis; β-lactamase inhibitors bind to β-lactamase enzymes thereby preventing the hydrolysis of the β-lactam ring of penicillin

Uses: For treatment of infections caused by susceptible β-lactamase–producing strains of microorganisms as listed: lower respiratory tract infections, otitis media, and sinusitis caused by *H. influenzae, M. catarrhalis;* skin and skin structure infections caused by *S. aureus, E. coli, Klebsiella* species; urinary tract infections caused by *E. coli, Klebsiella, Enterobacter* species; Augmentin ES-600: treatment of recurrent or persistent otitis media, *S. pneumoniae,* and β-lactamase–producing strains of *H. influenzae* or *M. catarrhalis*

Dosage and routes:

• *Adult:* PO one 500 mg tab q12h or one 250 mg tab q8h depending on severity of infection

• *Child:* PO 20-40 mg/kg/day in divided doses q8h

NOTE: Do not use the 250/125 mg tab until child weighs at least 40 kg or more.

Severe and respiratory tract infections:

• *Adult:* PO one 875 mg tab q12h or one 500 mg tab q8h

Recurrent or persistent otitis media (for Augmentin ES-600 only):

• *Child 3 mo and older and less than 40 kg:* PO (amoxicillin) 90 mg/kg/day in two equal doses

Available forms include:

Amoxicillin/clavulanate K amounts: Tabs 250/125, 500/125, 875/125, 1000/62.5 mg; chew tabs 125/31.25, 200/28.5, 250/62.5, 400/57 mg; powder for oral susp 125/31.25, 200/28.5, 250/62.5, 400/57 mg/5 ml when reconstituted; note that the single dose of clavulanate K should not exceed 125 mg. Augmentin 250 mg tab and Augmentin 250 mg chewable tab do not contain the same amount of clavulanic acid. They are not interchangeable; ES-600 oral suspension (amoxicillin 600 mg and clavulanic acid 42.9 mg/5 ml), ext rel tab 1000 mg amoxicillin and 62.5 mg clavulanic acid.

NOTE: Oral suspensions are not interchangeable because of differences in clavulanic acid content.

Side effects/adverse reactions:

▼ *ORAL:* Discolored tongue, glossitis, increased thirst, candidiasis, stomatitis

CNS: Headache

GI: Nausea, diarrhea, vomiting, increased AST/ALT, abdominal pain, colitis, antibiotic-associated pseudomembranous colitis

HEMA: ***Bone marrow depression, granulocytopenia, leukopenia, eosinophilia,*** thrombocytopenic purpura, anemia

GU: Vaginitis, moniliasis, ***glomer-***

ulonephritis, oliguria, proteinuria, hematuria
INTEG: Pemphigus-like reaction
META: Hyperkalemia, hypokalemia, alkalosis, hypernatremia
SYST: ***Anaphylaxis,*** pruritus, urticaria, angioedema, bronchospasm (allergy symptoms)
Contraindications: Hypersensitivity to penicillins; neonates, clavulanate K–associated cholestatic/hepatic dysfunction
Precautions: Pregnancy category B, hypersensitivity to cephalosporins, hepatic function impairment
Pharmacokinetics:
PO: Good oral absorption with or without food; peak 2 hr, duration 6-8 hr, half-life 1-1.33 hr; metabolized in liver; excreted in urine; crosses placenta; enters breast milk
Drug interactions of concern to dentistry:
• Decreased antimicrobial effectiveness: tetracyclines, erythromycins, lincomycins
• Increased amoxicillin concentrations: probenecid
• Increased risk of skin rashes: allopurinol
When used for dental infection:
• Oral contraceptives: advise patient of a potential risk for decreased contraceptive action, to maintain compliance with oral contraceptive use while using antibiotics, and to consider the use of additional nonhormonal contraception

DENTAL CONSIDERATIONS
General:
• Take precautions regarding allergy to medication.
• Determine why the patient is taking the drug.
Consultations:
• Medical consultation may be required to assess disease control.
Teach patient/family:
• Importance of good oral hygiene to prevent soft tissue inflammation
• Caution to prevent injury when using oral hygiene aids
When used for dental infection, advise patient:
• To report sore throat, oral burning sensation, fever, and fatigue, any of which could indicate superinfection
• To take at prescribed intervals and complete dosage regimen
• To immediately notify the dentist if signs or symptoms of infection increase

amoxicillin trihydrate

(a-mox-i-sil′in)
Amoxil, Trimox
Apo-Amoxi, Novamoxin, Nu-Amox
Drug class.: Aminopenicillin

Action: Aminopenicillins bind to specific receptors, penicillin binding proteins, thereby interfering with cell wall synthesis that ultimately results in cell lysis
Uses: Nose, throat, sinus infections; pneumonia, otitis media, skin infections, urinary tract infections; effective for susceptible strains (β-lactamase negative) of *E. coli, P. mirabilis, H. influenzae, S. faecalis, S. pneumoniae, H. pylori, N. gonorrhoeae,* selected staphylococci
Dosage and routes:
Systemic infections:
• *Adult and child ≥40 kg:* PO 250 mg q8h or 500 mg q12h or 875 mg

q12h depending on severity/type of infection

• *Child 3 mo to 40 kg:* PO 20-45 mg/kg/day in divided doses q8h; optional dose 200 mg q12h (in place of 125 mg q8h) or 400 mg q12h (in place of 250 mg q8h)

Acute gonorrhea:

• *Adult:* PO 3 g as single dose

Bacterial endocarditis prophylaxis:

• *Adult:* PO 2 g 1 hr before dental procedure

• *Child:* PO 50 mg/kg of body weight, not to exceed the adult dose, 1 hr before dental procedure

Prosthetic joint prophylaxis (when indicated):

• *Adult:* PO 2 g 1 hr before dental procedure

Anthrax exposure (B. anthracis):

• *Adult:* PO 500 mg tid

• *Child <9 yr:* PO 80 mg/kg/day divided equally into 2-3 doses

Available forms include: Caps 250, 500 mg; tabs 500, 875 mg; chew tabs 125, 250 mg; powder for oral susp 125, 200, 250, 400 mg/5 ml in 80, 100, 150 ml bottles, pediatric powder for oral susp 50 mg/ml in 15, 30 ml

Side effects/adverse reactions:

▼ *ORAL:* Discolored tongue, glossitis, increased thirst, candidiasis, stomatitis

CNS: Headache

GI: Nausea, vomiting, diarrhea, increased AST/ALT, abdominal pain, colitis

HEMA: ***Bone marrow depression, granulocytopenia,*** anemia, increased bleeding time

INTEG: Pemphigus-like reaction

SYST: ***Anaphylaxis*** (allergy symptoms), pruritus, urticaria, angioedema, bronchospasm

Contraindications: Hypersensitivity to penicillins

Precautions: Pregnancy category B, hypersensitivity to cephalosporins, serious allergic reactions are reported, superinfections, chewable tablets contain phenylalamine (phenylketonurics), neonates

Pharmacokinetics:

PO: Rapid oral absorption, serum protein binding 20%, peak 1-2 hr, duration 6-8 hr, half-life 1-1.33 hr; metabolized in liver; excreted in urine; crosses placenta; enters breast milk

Drug interactions of concern to dentistry:

• Decreased antimicrobial effectiveness: tetracyclines, erythromycins, lincomycins

• Increased amoxicillin concentrations: probenecid

• Suspected increase in methotrexate toxicity

When used for dental infection:

• Oral contraceptives: advise patient of a potential risk for decreased contraceptive action, to maintain compliance with oral contraceptive use while using antibiotics, and to consider the use of additional nonhormonal contraception

DENTAL CONSIDERATIONS

General:

• Take precautions regarding allergy to medication.

• Determine why the patient is taking the drug.

Consultations:

• Medical consultation may be required to assess disease control

Teach patient/family:

• Importance of good oral hygiene to prevent soft tissue inflammation

• Caution to prevent injury when using oral hygiene aids

When used for dental infection, advise patient:

- To report sore throat, oral burning sensation, fever, and fatigue, any of which could indicate superinfection
- To take at prescribed intervals and complete dosage regimen
- To immediately notify the dentist if signs or symptoms of infection increase

---

amphetamine sulfate

(am-fet′a-meen)

amphetamine sulfate (generic)

amphetamine mixtures

See Appendix F, combination products

Controlled Substance Schedule II

Drug class.: Amphetamine

Action: Precise mechanism of action of amphetamines in ADHD or narcolepsy is not clear; amphetamines facilitate the release of norepinephrine and dopamine from CNS adrenergic neurons; effects on specific noradrenergic/dopaminergic pathways may influence patient response; peripheral adrenergic effects include elevation of blood pressure; heart rate may be slowed by reflex response in usual doses

Uses: Narcolepsy, attention deficit disorder with hyperactivity (ADHD)

Dosage and routes:

Narcolepsy:

- *Adult:* PO 5-60 mg qd in divided doses
- *Child >12 yr:* PO 10 mg qd increasing by 10 mg/day at weekly intervals
- *Child 6-12 yr:* PO 5 mg qd increasing by 5 mg/wk, max 60 mg

ADHD:

- *Child >6 yr:* PO 5 mg qd-bid increasing by 5 mg/day at weekly intervals
- *Child 3-6 yr:* PO 2.5 mg qd increasing by 2.5 mg/day at weekly intervals

Available forms include: Tab 5, 10 mg, immediate-release tab 5, 7.5, 10, 12.5, 15, 20, 30 mg, ext rel cap 10, 20, 30 mg

Side effects/adverse reactions:

▼ *ORAL:* Dry mouth, metallic taste

CNS: Hyperactivity, insomnia, restlessness, talkativeness, dizziness, headache, chills, dysphoria, irritability, aggressiveness, tremor, dependence, addiction

CV: palpitation, tachycardia, hypertension, bradycardia, dysrhythmias

GI: Anorexia, diarrhea, constipation, weight loss, nausea, cramps

GU: Impotence, change in libido

INTEG: Urticaria

Contraindications: Hypersensitivity to sympathomimetics, amines, hyperthyroidism, hypertension, glaucoma, severe arteriosclerosis, drug abuse, cardiovascular disease, anxiety

Precautions: Gilles de la Tourette's syndrome, pregnancy category C, lactation, child <3 yr

Pharmacokinetics:

PO: Onset 30 min, peak 1-3 hr, duration 4-20 hr, half-life 10-30 hr; metabolized by liver, urinary excretion pH dependent; crosses placenta, excreted in breast milk

Drug interactions of concern to dentistry:

- Increased sensitivity to effects of

sympathomimetics; increased risk of serotonin syndrome with SSRIs
• Increased pressor response: tricyclic antidepressants

DENTAL CONSIDERATIONS

General:
• Monitor vital signs at every appointment because of cardiovascular side effects.
• Assess salivary flow as a factor in caries, periodontal disease, and candidiasis.
• Psychologic and physical dependence may occur with chronic use.
• Consider short appointments, frequent recall if patient becomes restless during a dental appointment.

Consultations:
• Medical consultation may be required to assess disease control and patient's ability to tolerate stress.

Teach patient/family:
• Importance of updating health and drug history, reporting changes in health status, drug regimen changes, or disease/treatment status
• Importance of good oral hygiene to prevent soft tissue inflammation/infection
• To prevent trauma when using oral hygiene aids

When chronic dry mouth occurs, advise patient:
• To avoid mouth rinses with high alcohol content because of drying effects
• To use daily home fluoride products for anticaries effect
• To use sugarless gum, frequent sips of water, or saliva substitutes

amphotericin B (topical)

(am-foe-ter′i-sin)

Fungizone Oral Suspension

Drug class.: Polyene antifungal

Action: Increases cell membrane permeability in susceptible organisms by binding to cell membrane sterols

Uses: Oral mucocutaneous infections caused by *Candida* species

Dosage and routes:
• *Adult and child:* SOL oral suspension rinse with 1 ml (100 mg) qid; shake well before using, place dose on tongue using the dropper, swish as long as reasonable, can swallow.

Available forms include: Oral suspension 100 mg/ml in 24 ml dropper bottle

Side effects/adverse reactions:

GI: Nausea, vomiting, diarrhea

INTEG: Urticaria, angioedema (rare), ***Stevens-Johnson syndrome***

Contraindications: Hypersensitivity

Precautions: Pregnancy category C, lactation; not for systemic fungal infections

Pharmacokinetics: Topical rinse only, poorly absorbed if swallowed

Drug interactions of concern to dentistry:
• None reported

DENTAL CONSIDERATIONS

General:
• Determine why the patient is taking the drug.
• Broad-spectrum antibiotics may contribute to oral *Candida* infections.

Teach patient/family:
• That long-term therapy may be

needed to clear infection; complete entire course of medication
• Not to use commercial mouthwashes for mouth infection unless prescribed by dentist
• That patient with removable dental appliance should soak appliance in antifungal agent overnight
• To prevent reinoculation of *Candida* infection by disposing of toothbrush or other contaminated oral hygiene devices used during period of infection

ampicillin/ampicillin sodium/ampicillin trihydrate

(am-pi-sil′in)

Ampicillin sodium (parenteral): Ampicin, Penbritin

Ampicillin (oral) Principen,

🍁 Apo-Ampi, Novo-Ampicillin, Nu-Ampi, Penbritin

Drug class.: Aminopenicillin

Action: Aminopenicillins bind to specific receptors, penicillin binding proteins, thereby interfering with cell wall synthesis that ultimately results in cell lysis

Uses: Sinus infections, pneumonia, otitis media, skin infections, UTIs; effective for susceptible strains of β-lactamase negative) *E. coli, P. mirabilis, H. influenzae, S. faecalis, S. pneumoniae, S. typhosa, N. gonorrhoeae, N. meningitidis, L. monocytogenes,* shigella, enterococci

Dosage and routes:

Systemic infections:

• *Adult and adolescent:* PO 250-500 mg q6h depending on severity of infection; IV/IM 2-8 g qd in divided doses q4-6h
• *Child up to 20 kg:* PO (oral susp only) 12.5-25 mg/kg q6h, or 16.7-33.3 mg/kg q8h; *IV/IM:* 12.5 mg/kg q6h

Bacterial endocarditis prophylaxis:

• *Adult:* IV or IM for patients unable to take oral medications and who are not allergic to penicillin 2 g within 30 min of dental procedure
• *Child:* IV or IM for patients unable to take oral medications and who are not allergic to penicillin 50 mg/kg of body weight not to exceed the adult dose

Prosthetic joint prophylaxis (when indicated):

• *Adult:* IV or IM for patients unable to take oral medications and who are not allergic to penicillin 2 g 1 hr before dental procedure

Available forms include: Powder for inj IV/IM 125, 250, 500 mg and 1, 2, 10 g; caps 250, 500 mg; powder for oral susp 125, 250 mg/5 ml in 100, 150, 200 ml

Side effects/adverse reactions:

▼ *ORAL:* Discolored tongue, glossitis, increased thirst, candidiasis, stomatitis

CNS: ***Coma, convulsions,*** lethargy, hallucinations, anxiety, depression, twitching

GI: Nausea, vomiting, diarrhea

HEMA: ***Bone marrow depression, granulocytopenia,*** anemia, increased bleeding time

GU: Vaginitis, moniliasis, ***glomerulonephritis,*** oliguria, proteinuria, hematuria

INTEG: Rash, urticaria

SYST: ***Anaphylaxis,*** pruritus, urticaria, angioedema, bronchospasm (allergy symptoms)

Contraindications: Hypersensitivity to penicillins

Precautions: Pregnancy category B, hypersensitivity to cephalosporins, neonates

Pharmacokinetics:

PO: Peak 2 hr

IV: Peak 5 min

IM: Peak 1 hr, half-life 50-110 min; metabolized in liver; excreted in urine, bile, breast milk; crosses placenta, protein binding 20%

Drug interactions of concern to dentistry:

- Decreased antimicrobial effectiveness: tetracyclines, erythromycins, lincomycins
- Increased ampicillin concentrations: probenecid
- Increased skin rash: allopurinol
- Decreased effects of atenolol
- Suspected increased risk of methotrexate toxicity

When used for dental infection:

- Oral contraceptives: advise patient of a potential risk for decreased contraceptive action, to maintain compliance with oral contraceptive use while using antibiotics, and to consider the use of additional nonhormonal contraception

DENTAL CONSIDERATIONS

General:

- Take precautions regarding allergy to medication.
- Determine why the patient is taking the drug.

Consultations:

- Medical consultation may be required to assess disease control.

Teach patient/family:

- Importance of good oral hygiene to prevent soft tissue inflammation
- Caution to prevent injury when using oral hygiene aids

When used for dental infection, advise patient:

- To report sore throat, oral burning sensation, fever, and fatigue, any of which could indicate superinfection
- To take at prescribed intervals and complete dosage regimen
- To immediately notify the dentist if signs or symptoms of infection increase

amprenavir

(am-pren'a-veer)

Agenerase

Drug class.: Antiviral

Action: Inhibits human immunodeficiency virus (HIV) protease enzymes resulting in the formation of immature, noninfectious viral particles

Uses: HIV-1 infection, in combination with other antiretroviral agents

Dosage and routes:

- *Adult:* PO 1200 mg bid in combination with other antiretroviral drugs
- *Child 13-16 yr:* PO 1200 mg bid in combination with other antiretroviral drugs
- *Child 4-12 yr or 13-16 yr weighing less than 50 kg:* PO 20 mg/kg bid or 15 mg/kg tid (max 2400 mg/day) in combination with other antiretroviral drugs

Oral solution:

- *Child 4-12 yr or 13-16 yr weighing less than 50 kg:* PO 22.5 mg/kg (1.5 ml/kg) bid or 17 mg/kg (1.1 ml/kg) tid in combination with other antiretroviral drugs; max daily limit 2800 mg; contraindicated in child <4 yr and in infants

• *Child 13-16 yr weighing more than 50 kg:* PO 1400 mg bid

Available forms include: Caps 50, 150 mg; oral sol 15 mg/ml in 240 ml

(NOTE: Capsules and oral solution are not interchangeable on an mg per mg basis.)

Side effects/adverse reactions:

▼ *ORAL: Perioral paresthesia, taste disorders*

CNS: Headache, peripheral paresthesia, depression, mood disorder

GI: Nausea, vomiting, diarrhea, abdominal pain

HEMA: ***Acute hemolytic anemia***

INTEG: Rash, ***Stevens-Johnson syndrome***

META: Hyperglycemia, hyperlipidemia, hypercholesterolemia

MISC: Fatigue

Contraindications: Concurrent use with midazolam, triazolam, bepridil, disulfiram, metronidazole, pimozide, and ergotlike drugs; hypersensitivity; serious reactions could occur with lidocaine (systemic) or other antiarrhythmics and tricyclic antidepressants; avoid use of drugs metabolized by CYP3A4 enzymes; lactation

Precautions: Exacerbation of diabetes, hyperglycemia, use of additional vitamin E, hemophilia, viral resistance, risk of cross allergy with sulfonamides, fat redistribution, pregnancy category C, hepatic disease, patients on oral contraceptives, sildenafil; oral solution contains propylene glycol with risk of toxicity to children <4 yr old

Pharmacokinetics:

PO: Rapid oral absorption (except with fatty meal), bioavailability of oral solutions is less than capsules, peak plasma concentration 1-2 hr, plasma protein binding 90%, hepatic metabolism (CYP3A4), excreted in feces (75%) and urine

Drug interactions of concern to dentistry:

• Contraindicated with midazolam, triazolam, tricyclic antidepressants

• Increased plasma levels of erythromycin, clarithromycin, itraconazole, alprazolam, chlorazepate, diazepam, carbamazepine, loratadine, flurazepam, ketoconazole, itraconzole; lidocaine (systemic use for cardiac arrhythmias)

• Decreased effectiveness: dexamethasone, St. John's wort (herb)

• Use with caution: sildenafil

DENTAL CONSIDERATIONS

General:

• Palliative medication may be required for management of oral side effects.

• Examine for oral manifestation of opportunistic infection.

• Patients on chronic drug therapy may rarely have symptoms of blood dyscrasias, which can include infection, bleeding, and poor healing.

• Consider semisupine chair position for patient comfort if GI side effects occur.

Consultations:

• In a patient with symptoms of blood dyscrasias, request a medical consultation for blood studies and postpone treatment until normal values are reestablished.

• Medical consultation may be required to assess disease control and patient's ability to tolerate stress.

Teach patient/family:

• Importance of good oral hygiene to prevent soft tissue inflammation

• To prevent trauma when using oral hygiene aids

• Importance of updating health and drug history if physician makes any changes in evaluation or drug regimens
• That secondary oral infection may occur; must see dentist immediately if infection occurs

anagrelide hydrochloride

(an-ag′gre-lide)
Agrylin

Drug class.: Platelet-reducing agent

Action: Unclear; may involve a reduction in megakaryocyte hypermaturation without affecting WBC count or coagulation, insignificant reduction in RBC count; platelet aggregation may be inhibited in larger doses

Uses: Treatment of essential thrombocythemia secondary to myeloproliferative disorders, to reduce elevated platelet counts and risk of thrombosis

Dosage and routes:

• *Adult:* PO (requires close medical supervision)–initial dose 0.5 mg qid or 1.0 mg bid; after 1 wk adjust dose to maintain platelet count below 600,000/µl; limit dose increases to 0.5 mg/day; dose limit 10 mg/day and 2.5 mg per single dose

Available forms include: Tabs 0.5 mg and 1.0 mg

Side effects/adverse reactions:

▼ *ORAL:* Aphthous stomatitis
CNS: Headache, dizziness, paresthesia, seizures
CV: Palpitation, edema, tachycardia
GI: Diarrhea, abdominal pain, nausea, dyspepsia, flatulence, vomiting, anorexia, ***pancreatitis,*** ulceration
RESP: ***Pulmonary infiltrate, pulmonary hypertension***
EENT: Rash, urticaria
MS: Back pain, arthralgia
MISC: Asthenia, malaise

Precautions: Cardiac disease, renal impairment, hepatic impairment, monitor reduction in platelets, risk of thrombocytopenia especially while correct dose is being found, sudden discontinuance of use, pregnancy category C, lactation, children <16 yr

Pharmacokinetics:

PO: Extensive hepatic metabolism, urinary excretion, half-life 1.3 hr

Drug interactions of concern to dentistry:

• Possible risk of hemorrhage: NSAIDs, aspirin

DENTAL CONSIDERATIONS

General:

• Laboratory studies should include routine CBCs.
• Patients have risk of thrombohemorrhagic complications; prolonged bleeding time, anemia, or splenomegaly may occur in some patients with this disease. However, thrombosis may also occur in some patients.
• Mucosal bleeding can be a symptom of disease.
• Patients with severe symptoms may be taking chemotherapy.
• Monitor vital signs at every appointment because of cardiovascular side effects.
• Consider semisupine chair position for patient comfort when GI side effects occur.

Consultations:

• Medical consultation with hematologist or physician directing therapy is essential before dental treatment.

Teach patient/family:

• To inform dentist of unusual bleeding episodes following dental treatment

• Importance of updating health and drug history if physician makes any changes in evaluation or drug regimens

apraclonidine

(a-pra-kloe′ni-deen)

Iopidine

Drug class.: Selective α_2-adrenergic agonist

Action: Reduces elevated or normal intraocular pressure

Uses: Control or prevention of increases in intraocular pressure related to laser surgery of eye; short-term control of increased intraocular pressure as an adjunctive drug

Dosage and routes:

• *Adult:* TOP INSTILL 1 or 2 gtt (0.5% sol) tid; allow a 5 min interval between other required ophthalmic drops

• *Adult:* TOP prelaser surgery use 1 gtt (1% sol) 1 hr before surgery and 1 gtt when surgery is completed

Available forms include: Sterile ophthalmic sol 0.5% and 1.0%

Side effects/adverse reactions:

▼ *ORAL:* Dry mouth, taste alterations (both 1%)

CNS: Insomnia, paresthesia, headache, dizziness

CV: Bradycardia, vasovagal syncope, palpitation

GI: Abdominal pain, diarrhea, emesis, nausea

RESP: Dyspnea, asthma

EENT: Hyperemia, discomfort, edema, tearing, mydriasis, blurred vision

INTEG: Pruritus

MISC: Facial edema

Contraindications: Hypersensitivity to this drug or clonidine; concurrent use of monoamine oxidase inhibitors

Precautions: Tachyphylaxis, impaired renal or liver function, depression, pregnancy category A, lactation, children, cardiovascular disease, cardiovascular drugs

Pharmacokinetics: *TOP:* Onset 1 hr, maximum effect 3-5 hr; some systemic absorption

Drug interactions of concern to dentistry:

• No drug interactions have been reported; this is a new drug and data are lacking

• Avoid using drugs that can exacerbate glaucoma: anticholinergic drugs

DENTAL CONSIDERATIONS

General:

• Protect patient's eyes from accidental spatter during dental treatment.

• Avoid dental light in patient's eyes; offer dark glasses for patient comfort.

• Determine why the patient is taking the drug.

• Assess salivary flow as a factor in caries, periodontal disease, and candidiasis.

Consultations:

• Medical consultation may be required to assess disease control.

Teach patient/family:

When chronic dry mouth occurs, advise patient:

- To avoid mouth rinses with high alcohol content because of drying effects
- Of need for daily home fluoride to prevent caries
- To use sugarless gum, frequent sips of water, or saliva substitutes

---

aprepitant

(ap-re′pi-tant)

Emend

Drug class.: Antiemetic

Action: A selective antagonist for human substance P/neurokinin (NK_1) receptors in the CNS

Uses: Prevention of acute and delayed nausea/vomiting associated with cancer chemotherapy including high-dose cisplatin; for acute use only

Dosage and routes:

- *Adult:* PO 125 mg 1 hr before chemotherapy; then 80 mg qd on days 2 and 3 after chemotherapy; used in combination with a glucocorticoid and a 5-HT_3 receptor antagonist

Available forms include: Caps 80, 125 mg

Side effects/adverse reactions:

▼ *ORAL:* Salivation, taste alteration

CNS: Dizziness, anorexia, headache, insomnia

CV: Edema, deep vein thrombosis, tachycardia

GI: Abdominal pain, constipation, diarrhea, gastritis, nausea, vomiting, acid reflux

RESP: Hiccups, URI, cough

HEMA: Neutropenia, anemia, ***thrombocytopenia***

GU: Dysuria, renal insufficiency, pelvic pain

EENT: Tinnitus, pharyngitis

INTEG: Alopecia, rash, rarely angioedema, urticaria, Stevens-Johnson syndrome

META: Dehydration, diabetes mellitus, hypokalemia, weight loss, abnormal metabolic enzyme levels

MS: Asthenia, myalgia, weakness

MISC: Fatigue, fever, mucous membrane disorder, sweating, peripheral neuropathy, septic shock

Contraindications: Hypersensitivity, contraindicated with pimozide

Precautions: Use with caution in patients taking drugs metabolized by CYP3A4 enzymes; not for chronic use; acts as a moderate inhibitor of CYP3A4 and an inducer of CYP3A4 and CYP2C9; pregnancy category B, use with caution in lactation, safety and efficacy in pediatric patients not established

Pharmacokinetics:

PO: Absolute bioavailability 60%-65%, peak plasma levels ~4 hr; plasma protein binding >95%, extensive metabolism mainly by CYP3A4, to lesser extent by CYP1A2 and CYP2C19; eliminated primarily by metabolism

Drug interactions of concern to dentistry:

- Increased plasma concentrations of midazolam and other benzodiazepines metabolized by CYP3A4 (see Appendix I)
- Increased plasma levels: concurrent use of drugs that inhibit CYP3A4 enzymes (fluconazole,

itraconazole, ketoconazole, erythromycin, and clarithromycin) (see Appendix I)
• Decreased plasma levels: concurrent use of drugs that induce CYP3A4 enzymes (carbamazepine) (see Appendix I)

DENTAL CONSIDERATIONS

General:

• Patients using this drug are also undergoing or have recently undergone cancer chemotherapy. Take a complete health history.
• Chemotherapy patients may show stomatitis and ulceration; palliative therapy may be required.
• Consider semisupine chair position for patient comfort if GI side effects occur.
• Examine for oral manifestation of opportunistic infection.
• Short appointments and a stress reduction protocol may be required for anxious patients.
• Patients taking opioids for acute or chronic pain should be given alternative analgesics for dental pain.
• Patients on chronic drug therapy may rarely have symptoms of blood dyscrasias, which can include infection, bleeding, and poor healing.
• Consult physician; prophylactic or therapeutic antibiotics may be indicated to prevent or treat infection if surgery or periodontal debridement is required for patients undergoing chemotherapy.

Consultations:

• Medical consultation may be required to assess immunologic status during cancer therapy and determine safety risks posed by dental treatment.
• Consultation with physician may be needed if sedation or general anesthesia is required.
• Medical consultation may be required to assess disease control and patient's ability to tolerate stress.

Teach patient/family:

• Importance of good oral hygiene to prevent soft tissue inflammation
• To prevent trauma when using oral hygiene aids
• Importance of updating health and drug history if physician makes any changes in evaluation/drug regimens

---

aripiprazole

ay-ri-pip′ ray-zole

Abilify

Drug class.: Antipsychotic

Action: Antipsychotic mechanism unknown; it has partial agonist activity at D_2 and 5-HT_{2A} receptors, also has antagonist activity for α_1-receptors

Uses: Treatment of schizophrenia

Dosage and routes:

• *Adult:* PO 10-15 mg qd; doses may be adjusted after 2 wk; dose range 10-30 mg daily

With CYP3A4 inhibitors:

• Reduce dose by 50%

With CYP2D6 inhibitors:

• Reduce dose by 50%

With CYP3A4 inducers:

• Dose should be doubled

Available forms include: Tabs 2, 5, 10, 15, 20, and 30 mg

Side effects/adverse reactions:

▼ *ORAL:* Face edema, jaw pain; infrequent stomatitis, candidiasis, tongue edema, dry mouth

CNS: Somnolence, headache, asthenia, anxiety, insomnia, akathesia, tremor, ***neuroleptic malignant syndrome,*** dyskinesia, depression, nervousness
CV: Hypotension, palpitation, bradycardia
GI: Nausea, vomiting, constipation, anorexia, dysphagia
RESP: Coughing, dyspnea, pneumonia
HEMA: Anemia, ecchymosis
GU: Incontinence
EENT: Rhinitis, blurred vision, rhinitis, ear pain
INTEG: Rash, dry skin
META: ↑ creatine phosphokinase, ↑ liver enzymes
MS: Arthralgia, cramps
MISC: Fever, flulike symptoms

Contraindications: Hypersensitivity

Precautions: Known cardiovascular diseases, cerebrovascular disease, or other conditions predisposing the patient to hypotension; seizures, may impair judgement or motor skills, elevated body temperature, suicide, dysphagia, dehydration, severe renal or hepatic impairment, pregnancy category C, avoid breast-feeding and use in children

Pharmacokinetics:
PO: Absolute bioavailability 87%, peak plasma levels 3-5 hr, plasma protein binding >99%, metabolized by CYP3A4, CYP2D6 enzymes, active metabolite dehydro-aripiprazole, excreted mostly in feces and a lesser amount in urine

Drug interactions of concern to dentistry:

- Possible lowering of blood levels: carbamazepine and other inducers of CYP3A4 isoenzymes (see Appendix I)
- Increased blood levels: ketoconazole and other inhibitors of CYP3A4 or CYP2D6 isoenzymes (see Appendix I)
- Caution with CNS depressants and alcohol

DENTAL CONSIDERATIONS

General:

- Assess for presence of extrapyramidal motor symptoms, such as tardive dyskinesia and akathisia. Extrapyramidal motor activity may complicate dental treatment.
- Consider semisupine chair position for patient comfort if GI side effects occur.

Consultations:

- Consultation with physician may be needed if sedation or general anesthesia is required.
- Medical consultation may be required to assess disease control and patient's ability to tolerate stress.

Teach patient/family:

- To consult physician if signs of tardive dyskinesia or akathisia are present
- Importance of good oral hygiene to prevent soft tissue inflammation
- Use of electric toothbrush if patient has difficulty holding conventional devices
- Importance of updating health and drug history if physician makes any changes in evaluation/drug regimens

articaine HCl (local)

(ar-te'kane)

Septocaine

♣ Ultracaine-DS, Astracaine, Astracaine Forte

Drug class.: Amide local anesthetic with vasoconstrictor (epinephrine)

Action: Inhibits ion fluxes across membranes, particularly sodium transport across cell membrane; decreases rise of depolarization phase of action potential; blocks nerve action potential

Uses: Local, infiltrative, or conductive anesthesia in both simple and complex dental and periodontal procedures

Dosage and routes:

Infiltration:

• *Adult:* INJ 0.5-2.5 ml (20-100 mg)

Nerve block:

• *Adult:* INJ 0.5-3.4 ml (20-136 mg)

Oral surgery:

• *Adult:* INJ 1.0-5.1 ml (40-204 mg)

Maximum recommended doses should not exceed 7 mg/kg or 3.2 mg/lb. Reduce doses for pediatric patients, elderly patients, and patients with cardiac or liver disease.

• *Child:* Use not recommended for child <4 yr. Do not exceed maximum recommended dose and adjust for age, body weight, and physical condition (7.0 mg/kg or 3.2 mg/lb).

Example calculations illustrating amount of drug administered per dental cartridge(s):

# cartridges (1.7 ml)	mg of articaine (4%)	mg (μg) of vasoconstrictor (1:100,000)
1	68	0.017 (17)
2	136	0.034 (34)
3	204	0.051 (51)

Available forms include: Inj 4% with epinephrine 1:100,000 in 1.7 ml vol (50 per carton)

Side effects/adverse reactions:

▼ *ORAL: Facial edema, gingivitis,* glossitis, tongue edema, mouth ulcer, taste perversion, dry mouth

CNS: Headache, paresthesia, migraine

CV: Syncope, tachycardia (infrequent)

GI: Nausea, vomiting, diarrhea

RESP: Pharyngitis

HEMA: Ecchymosis

GU: Dysmenorrhea

EENT: Rhinitis, ear pain

INTEG: Pruritus, rash

META: Edema, thirst

MS: Arthralgia, myalgia

MISC: Infection, localized pain

Contraindications: Hypersensitivity to amides or sodium metabisulfite

Precautions: Accidental intravascular injections may be associated with convulsions, CNS depression, or cardiorespiratory depression; reduce dose for elderly, debilitated, or pediatric patients; exaggerated response to intravascular epinephrine, severe hepatic impairment, pregnancy category C, lactation

Pharmacokinetics: Onset 1-6 min; duration about 1 hr; p Ka 7.8, p H of sol is 5.0; peak blood levels in 25 min, plasma level after 68 mg is 385 ng/ml, after 204 mg is 900 ng/ml, 60%-80% plasma protein bound, metabolized by plasma carboxylesterase; liver P450 enzymes metabolize 5%-10% of available articaine; urinary excretion mainly

Drug interactions of concern to dentistry:

• CNS depressants: increased risk of CNS depression with all CNS depressants, especially in children and when larger doses are used

• Avoid placing dental cartridges in disinfectant solutions with heavy metals or surface-active agents; may see release of metal ions into local anesthetic solutions with tissue irritation following injection

• Risk of cardiovascular side effects; rapid intravascular administration of local anesthetic containing vasoconstrictor, either alone or in patients taking tricyclic antidepressants, MAOIs, digitalis drugs, cocaine, phenothiazines, β-blockers, and in presence of halogenated hydrocarbon general anesthetics; use smallest effective vasoconstrictor dose and careful aspiration technique

• Avoid use of vasoconstrictors in patients with uncontrolled hyperthyroidism, diabetes, angina, or hypertension; refer these patients for medical treatment before elective dental procedures

DENTAL CONSIDERATIONS

General:

• Monitor vital signs at every appointment because of cardiovascular side effects.

• Apply lubricant to dry lips for patient comfort before dental procedures.

• Use vasoconstrictor with caution, in low doses, and with careful aspiration.

Teach patient/family:

• To use care to prevent injury while numbness exists and to not chew gum or eat following dental anesthesia

• To report any signs of infection, muscle pain, or fever to dentist when feeling returns

• To report any unusual soft tissue reactions

ascorbic acid (vitamin C)

(a-skor′bic)

Cevi-Bid, Dull-C, Vita-C

♣ Apo-C

Drug class.: Vitamin C, water-soluble vitamin

Action: Needed for wound healing, collagen synthesis, antioxidant, carbohydrate metabolism, absorption of iron, and other metabolic processes

Uses: Vitamin C deficiency, scurvy, urine acidification, and supplemental use in a variety of debilitated patients with poor vitamin C intake

Dosage and routes:

Recommended daily allowance (RDA):

• *Adult nonsmoker:* PO 60 mg/day

• *Adult smoker:* PO 100 mg/day

Scurvy:

• *Adult:* PO/SC/IM/IV 200-1000 mg qd, then 50 mg or more qd

• *Child:* PO/SC/IM/IV 100-300 mg qd, then 35 mg or more qd

Wound healing/chronic disease/fracture:

• *Adult:* SC/IM/IV/PO 300-500 mg qd

• *Child:* SC/IM/IV/PO 100-200 mg added doses

Urine acidification:

• *Adult:* SC/IM/IV/PO 4-12 g qd in divided doses

Available forms include: Tabs 250, 500, 1000, 1500 mg; caps 500 mg; timed rel tabs 500, 1000 mg; crys 4 g/tsp; powd 4 g/tsp; sol 100 mg/ml; inj SC/IM/IV 500 mg/ml; loz 60 mg

Side effects/adverse reactions:

▼ *ORAL:* Enamel erosion, caries (chewable form, chronic use)

CNS: Headache, insomnia, dizziness, fatigue, flushing

GI: Nausea, vomiting, diarrhea, anorexia, heartburn, cramps

HEMA: ***Hemolytic anemia in patients with G6PD***

GU: Polyuria, urine acidification, oxalate or urate renal stones

Contraindications: None significant

Precautions: Gout, pregnancy category A

Pharmacokinetics:

PO/INJ: Metabolized in liver; unused amounts excreted in urine (unchanged) and metabolites; crosses placenta and excreted in breast milk

Drug interactions of concern to dentistry:

• Increased urinary excretion: salicylates, barbiturates

DENTAL CONSIDERATIONS

General:

• An increased incidence of caries and soft tissue injury has been reported with excessive use of chewable ascorbic acid tablets.

aspirin (acetylsalicylic acid)

(as'pir-in)

Arthritis Foundation Pain Reliever, ASA, Ascriptin, Aspergum, Aspirin, Bayer Children's Aspirin, Ecotrin, Empirin, Genuine Bayer, Maximum Bayer, Norwich Extra-Strength, St. Joseph Adult Chewable Aspirin, ZORprin, others

Combinations: Often combined with other analgesic drugs

🍁 Entrophen, Novasen, Apo-ASA, Apo-Asen, Coryphen, Arthrisin, Atria SR, PMS-ASA

Drug class.: Nonnarcotic analgesic salicylate

Action: Inhibits prostaglandin synthesis by interfering with cyclooxygenase needed for biosynthesis; possesses analgesic, antiinflammatory, antipyretic properties

Uses: Mild-to-moderate pain or fever, including arthritis, thromboembolic disorders, transient ischemic attacks in men, rheumatic fever, post–myocardial infarction

Dosage and routes:

Arthritis:

• *Adult:* PO 3.2-6 g/day in divided doses q4-6h

Juvenile rheumatoid arthritis:

• *Child:* PO 60-110 mg/kg/day in divided doses q6-8h

Pain/fever:

• *Adult:* PO/REC 500 mg q3h, 325-650 mg q4h or 1000 mg q6h

• *Child 2-3 yr:* PO/REC 160 mg q4h

• *Child 4-5 yr:* PO/REC 240 mg q4h

• *Child 6-8 yr:* PO/REC 325 mg q4h

• *Child 9-10 yr:* PO/REC 400 mg q4h
• *Child 11 yr:* PO/REC 480 mg q4h
• *Child 12 yr:* PO/REC 650 mg q4h

Platelet aggregation inhibitor:
• *Adult:* PO 80-325 mg/day

Transient ischemic attacks in men:
• *Adult:* PO 325 mg-1.0 g/day

Available forms include: Tabs 81, 165, 325, 500, 650, 975 mg; chew tabs 81 mg; caps 325, 500 mg; con rel tabs 800 mg; time rel tabs 650 mg; supp 120, 200, 300, 600 mg, and 1.2 g; gum 227.5 mg

Side effects/adverse reactions:
▼ *ORAL:* Increased bleeding (chronic, high doses)
CNS: ***Coma, convulsion,*** stimulation, drowsiness, dizziness, confusion, headache, flushing, hallucinations
CV: Rapid pulse, pulmonary edema
GI: Nausea, vomiting, ***GI bleeding, hepatitis,*** diarrhea, heartburn, anorexia
RESP: Wheezing, hyperpnea
HEMA: ***Thrombocytopenia, agranulocytosis, leukopenia, neutropenia, hemolytic anemia,*** increased pro-time, bleeding time
EENT: Tinnitus, hearing loss
INTEG: Rash, urticaria, bruising
ENDO: Hypoglycemia, hyponatremia, hypokalemia

Contraindications: Hypersensitivity to salicylates, GI bleeding, bleeding disorders, children <3 yr, children with flulike symptoms, pregnancy category C, lactation, vitamin K deficiency, peptic ulcer

Precautions: Anemia, hepatic disease, renal disease, Hodgkin's disease, preoperative, postoperative

Pharmacokinetics:
PO: Onset 15-30 min, peak 1-2 hr, duration 4-6 hr
REC: Onset slow, duration 4-6 hr, half-life 1-3.5 hr; metabolized by liver; excreted by kidneys; crosses placenta; excreted in breast milk

Drug interactions of concern to dentistry:
• Increased risk of GI complaints and occult blood loss: alcohol, NSAIDs, corticosteroids
• *Buffered aspirin:* Decreased absorption of tetracycline
• Recent report indicated ibuprofen may block clot-preventing effects of aspirin

Interactions when used as a dental drug:
• Increased risk of bleeding: oral anticoagulants, valproic acid, dipyridamole
• Increased risk of hypoglycemia: sulfonylureas
• Increased risk of toxicity: methotrexate, lithium, zidovudine
• Decreased effects of probenecid, sulfinpyrazone
• Avoid prolonged or concurrent use with NSAIDs, corticosteroids, acetaminophen
• Suspected reduction in antihypertensives and vasodilator effects of ACE inhibitors; monitor blood pressure if used concurently

DENTAL CONSIDERATIONS

General:
• Patients on chronic drug therapy may rarely have symptoms of blood dyscrasias, which can include infection, bleeding, and poor healing.
• Avoid prescribing buffered aspirin-containing products if patient is on a sodium-restricted diet.
• Chewable forms of aspirin should

not be used for 7 days following oral surgery because of possible soft tissue injury.

• Evaluate allergic reactions: rash, urticaria; patients with allergy to salicylates may not be able to take NSAIDs; drug may need to be discontinued.

Consultations:

• In a patient with symptoms of blood dyscrasias, request a medical consultation for blood studies and postpone dental treatment until normal values are reestablished.

• Take precautions if dental surgery is anticipated because of risk of increased bleeding; avoid prescribing aspirin before dental surgery.

• Tinnitus, ringing, roaring in ears after high-dose and long-term therapy necessitates referral for salicylism.

Teach patient/family:

• That aspirin or buffered aspirin tablets should not be placed directly on a tooth or mucosal surface because of the risk of chemical burn

• To read label on other OTC drugs; may contain aspirin

• To avoid alcohol ingestion; GI bleeding may occur

---

atazanavir sulfate

(at-a-za-na'-veer)

Reyataz

Drug class.: Antiviral, HIV-1 protease inhibitor

Action: Selectively inhibits virus-specific processing of viral Gag and Gag-pol polymerase in HIV-1 infected cells, thereby preventing formation of mature virus

Uses: HIV-1 infection in combination with other antiretroviral medications

Dosage and routes:

• *Adult:* PO 400 mg/day; with efavirenz 600 mg and ritonavir 100 mg

Available forms include: Caps 100, 150, 200 mg

Side effects/adverse reactions:

▼ *ORAL:* Oral ulcers, taste perversion

CNS: Headache, fever, fatigue, depression, insomnia, dizziness

CV: ***Asymptomatic AV block,*** chest pain, palpitation, hypotension

GI: Nausea, abdominal pain, vomiting, diarrhea, ***lactic acidosis,*** symptomatic hyperlactemia

RESP: Increased cough

HEMA: ↓ hemoglobin, ↓ neutrophils

GU: Decreased male fertility, UTI, urinary frequency

EENT: Otitis tinnitus

INTEG: Rash, photosensitivity, dry skin, eczema, pruritus

META: Jaundice, ↑ *bilirubin levels,* ↑ *ALT, AST;* lipodystrophy

MS: Back pain, arthralgia, myalgia

MISC: ***Angioedema,*** pain

Contraindications: Hypersensitivity, midazolam, triazolam, sildenafil, ergot derivatives, pimozide, and many other drugs metabolized by CYP3A4 isoenzymes (see Appendix I), St. John's wort

Precautions: Prolongs PR interval, use with caution in preexisting conduction disorders; diabetes mellitus, hyperglycemia, hepatic impairment, monitor liver function, HBV infection, redistribution of body fat, pregnancy category B, do not breast-feed infants, safety and efficacy in children not established

Pharmacokinetics:
PO: Rapidly absorbed, plasma protein binding 86%, hepatic metabolism by CYP3A isoenzymes, extensively metabolized, excreted in feces (79%) and urine (13%)

Drug interactions of concern to dentistry:
• Avoid drugs metabolized by CYP3A4 isoenzymes; however, the package insert notes that significant drug interactions are not expected with azithromycin, erythromycin, itraconazole, or ketoconazole; use with caution and monitor

DENTAL CONSIDERATIONS
General:
• Short appointments and a stress reduction protocol may be required for anxious patients.
• Use precaution if sedation or general anesthesia is required; risk of hypotensive episode exists.
• Consider semisupine chair position for patient comfort if GI side effects occur.
• Patient history should include all medications and herbal or nonherbal remedies taken by the patient.
• Assess salivary flow as a factor in caries, periodontal disease, and candidiasis.
• Examine for oral manifestation of opportunistic infection.
• Palliative medication may be required for management of oral side effects.
• Advise patient if dental drugs prescribed have a potential for photosensitivity.
• Precaution if dental surgery is anticipated, general anesthesia required.
• Patients on chronic drug therapy may rarely have symptoms of blood dyscrasias, which can include infection, bleeding, and poor healing.

Consultations:
• Consultation with physician may be needed if sedation or general anesthesia is required.
• Medical consultation may be required to assess disease control and patient's ability to tolerate stress.

Teach patient/family:
• To be aware of oral side effects and potential sequelae
• Importance of updating health and drug history, reporting changes in health status, drug regimen changes, or disease/treatment status
• Importance of good oral hygiene to prevent soft tissue inflammation/infection
• To prevent trauma when using oral hygiene aids

atenolol

(a-ten'oh-lole)
Tenormin
✤ Apo-Atenol, Novo-Atenolol
Drug class.: Antihypertensive, selective β_1-blocker

Action: This is a selective β_1-adrenergic antagonist. At higher doses selectivity may be lost with antagonism of β_2-receptors as well. The antihypertensive mechanism of action is unclear, but may include a reduction in cardiac output and inhibition of renin release by the renal juxtaglomerular apparatus. Peripheral resistance decreases with long-term use. The antianginal action (when indicated for this use) may be related to a decrease in myocardial oxygen demand and negative chronotropic and inotropic effects. The antiarrhythmic action (when indicated for this use) has been related to a reduction in spontaneous pacemaker firing and slowing of AV nodal conduction.

Uses: Mild-to-moderate hypertension, treatment and prophylaxis of angina pectoris, arrhythmia, adjunct therapy in hypertrophic cardiomyopathy, MI therapy and prophylaxis, adjunct therapy in pheochromocytoma, prophylaxis for vascular headache, adjunct therapy in thyrotoxicosis, mitral valve prolapse syndrome

Dosage and routes:

Hypertension:

• *Adult:* PO 50 mg qd, increasing q1-2wk to 100 mg qd used alone or in combination with other antihypertensive drugs

Angina pectoris:

• *Adult:* PO 50 mg/day, can increase to 100 mg/day in 1 wk; max dose 200 mg/day

Available forms include: Tabs 25, 50, 100 mg; inj 5 mg/10 ml ampules

Side effects/adverse reactions:

▼ *ORAL:* Dry mouth

CNS: Insomnia, fatigue, dizziness, mental changes, memory loss, hallucinations, depression, lethargy, drowsiness, strange dreams, catatonia

CV: Profound hypotension, bradycardia, CHF, cold extremities, postural hypotension, second- or third-degree heart block

GI: Nausea, diarrhea, mesenteric arterial thrombosis, ischemic colitis, vomiting

RESP: Bronchospasm, dyspnea, wheezing

HEMA: Agranulocytosis, thrombocytopenia, purpura

GU: Impotence

EENT: Sore throat, dry burning eyes

INTEG: Rash, fever, alopecia

ENDO: Hypoglycemia

Contraindications: Hypersensitivity to β-blockers, cardiogenic shock, second- or third-degree heart block, sinus bradycardia, CHF, cardiac failure

Precautions: Major surgery, pregnancy category D, lactation, diabetes mellitus, severe renal disease, thyroid disease, COPD, asthma, well-compensated heart failure

Pharmacokinetics:

PO: Peak 2-4 hr; half-life 6-7 hr; excreted unchanged in urine; protein binding 5%-15%; up to 50% excreted unchanged in feces as unabsorbed drug

Drug interactions of concern to dentistry:

• Decreased antihypertensive effects: NSAIDs, indomethacin, salicylates

• May slow metabolism of lidocaine

• Decreased β-blocking effects (or decreased β-adrenergic effects) of epinephrine, levonordefrin, isoproterenol, and other sympathomimetics

• Reduced bioavailability suspected with ampicillin

DENTAL CONSIDERATIONS

General:

• Monitor vital signs at every appointment because of cardiovascular and respiratory side effects.

• After supine positioning, have patient sit upright for at least 2 min before standing to avoid orthostatic hypotension.

• Patients on chronic drug therapy may rarely have symptoms of

blood dyscrasias, which can include infection, bleeding, and poor healing.
• Assess salivary flow as a factor in caries, periodontal disease, and candidiasis.
• Stress from dental procedures may compromise cardiovascular function; determine patient risk.
• Short appointments and a stress reduction protocol may be required for anxious patients.
• Use vasoconstrictors with caution, in low doses, and with careful aspiration. Avoid use of gingival retraction cord with epinephrine.

Consultations:
• In a patient with symptoms of blood dyscrasias, request a medical consultation for blood studies and postpone dental treatment until normal values are reestablished.
• Medical consultation may be required to assess disease control and stress tolerance of patient.
• Use precautions if general anesthesia is required for dental surgery.

Teach patient/family:
• Importance of good oral hygiene to prevent soft tissue inflammation
• Caution to prevent injury when using oral hygiene aids

When chronic dry mouth occurs, advise patient:
• To avoid mouth rinses with high alcohol content because of drying effects
• To use daily home fluoride products for anticaries effect
• To use sugarless gum, frequent sips of water, or saliva substitutes

atomoxetine HCl

(at-oh-mox' e-teen)

Strattera

Drug class.: Selective norepinephrine reuptake inhibitor

Action: Proposed to enhance noradrenergic function by selective inhibition of the presynaptic norepinephrine transporter; it has little or no affinity for other neuronal transporters or receptor sites; mechanism of action in ADHD is unknown

Uses: Treatment of attention deficit hyperactivity disorder

Dosage and routes:
• *Child and adolescent up to 70 kg:* PO initial dose 0.5 mg/kg/day and increased after 3 days to target daily dose of ~1.2 mg/kg either as a single AM dose or in two equally divided doses AM and PM; daily dose limit 1.4 mg/kg or 100 mg.
• *Adult and child or adolescent >70 kg:* PO initial dose 40 mg/day, increase after 3 days to total daily dose of ~80 mg either as a single AM dose or in two equally divided doses AM and PM; after 2-4 wk more, dose may be increased to 100 mg; daily dose limit 100 mg

Available forms include: Caps 10, 18, 25, 40, 60 mg

Side effects/adverse reactions:

▼ *ORAL:* Dry mouth

CNS: Aggression, irritability, somnolence, mood swings, anorexia, dizziness, headache, crying

CV: Increased blood pressure, tachycardia, palpitation, chest pain

GI: Vomiting, dyspepsia, nausea, abdominal pain, constipation

RESP: Cough, UTI, rhinorrhea, nasal congestion

GU: Urinary retention, impotence, dysmenorrhea, prostatitis
EENT: Ear infection, mydriasis
INTEG: Dermatitis, pruritus
MS: Arthralgia
MISC: Fatigue, decreased appetite, flu, weight loss

Contraindications: Hypersensitivity, MAOI used concurrently or within 2 weeks of taking MAOI, narrow-angle glaucoma

Precautions: Hypertension, tachycardia, CV disease, monitor weight and growth changes, urinary retention, pregnancy category C, nursing, use in geriatric patients not established, use of herbs, poor metabolizers of CYP2D6 drugs, hepatic impairment

Pharmacokinetics:
PO: Absolute bioavailability 63%-94%, peak plasma levels in 1-2 hr, half-life 5 hr; plasma protein binding 98%, metabolized primarily by CYP2D6 to active metabolite (4-hydroxyatomoxetine); excreted as glucuronide mainly in urine (80%) and some in feces (17%)

Drug interactions of concern to dentistry:

- No dental drug interactions reported; however, drugs that inhibit CYP2D6 enzymes (paroxetine, fluoxetine) can increase plasma levels (see Appendix I)
- Albuterol and other β_2-agonists should be used with caution because of potential effects on the cardiovascular system

DENTAL CONSIDERATIONS

General:

- Assess salivary flow as a factor in caries, periodontal disease, and candidiasis.
- Monitor vital signs at every appointment because of cardiovascular side effects.
- Consider semisupine chair position for patient comfort if GI side effects occur.
- Use vasoconstrictor with caution, in low doses, and with careful aspiration.

Consultations:

- Medical consultation may be required to assess disease control and patient's ability to tolerate stress.

Teach patient/family:

- Importance of good oral hygiene to prevent soft tissue inflammation/infection

When chronic dry mouth occurs, advise patient:

- To avoid mouth rinses with high alcohol content because of drying effects
- To use daily home fluoride products for anticaries effect
- To use sugarless gum, frequent sips of water, or saliva substitutes

---

atorvastatin calcium

(a-tore′va-sta-tin)

Lipitor

Drug class.: Cholesterol-lowering agent

Action: Inhibits HMG-Co A reductase enzyme, which reduces cholesterol synthesis; reduced synthesis of LDL and VLDL; plasma triglyceride levels may also be decreased

Uses: As an adjunct in homozygous familial hypercholesterolemia, mixed lipidemia, elevated serum triglyceride levels and type IV hyperproteinemia, also reduces total cholesterol, LDL-C, apo B, and triglyceride levels; patient should first be placed on cholesterol-lowering diet; familial hypercholesterolemia age 10-17 yr

Dosage and routes:
• *Adult:* PO initial 10-40 mg daily; dose can be modified according to lipid lab values at 2-4 wk; dose range 10-80 mg daily
Available forms include: Tabs 10, 20, 40, 80 mg
Side effects/adverse reactions:
▼ *ORAL: Angioneurotic edema, lichenoid reaction*
CNS: Headache, insomnia
CV: Chest pain
GI: Flatulence, dyspepsia, abdominal pain, nausea
RESP: Bronchitis, rhinitis, sinusitis
INTEG: Rash, pruritus
META: Elevated liver enzymes
GU: UTI, ***renal failure secondary to rhabdomyolysis***
MS: Myalgia, arthralgia, back pain, ***rhabdomyolysis***
MISC: Allergy, peripheral edema, flulike syndrome
Contraindications: Hypersensitivity, active liver disease, pregnancy, lactation
Precautions: Chronic alcohol liver disease, pregnancy X, monitor liver function and lipid levels
Pharmacokinetics:
PO: Absolute bioavailability 14%, first-pass metabolism, half-life 14 hr, 98% protein bound, peak plasma levels 1-2 hr; metabolized by CYP3A4 isoenzymes, excretion in the bile
Drug interactions of concern to dentistry:
• Severe myopathy or rhabdomyolysis: erythromycin, niacin, itraconazole, ketoconazole
• Increase in plasma levels: erythromycin, itraconazole, alcohol, ketoconazole (see Appendix I)
• Suspected increase in midazolam effects when used in general anesthesia (***Anesthesia*** 58:899-904. 2003)

DENTAL CONSIDERATIONS
General:
• Consider semisupine chair position for patient comfort if GI side effects occur.

---

atovaquone
(a-toe'va-kwone)
Mepron
Drug class.: Antipneumocystic (antiprotozoal)

Action: Mechanism of action unknown; may act through ubiquinone to inhibit synthesis of ATP and nucleic acids
Uses: Treatment and prevention of mild to moderate *P. carinii* pneumonia in patients who are intolerant to trimethoprim-sulfamethoxazole
Dosage and routes:
Treatment:
• *Adult and child 13-16 yr:* PO 750 mg bid with a meal × 21 days
Prevention:
• *Adult and child 13-16 yr:* PO 1500 mg qd at mealtime
Available forms include: Oral susp 750 mg/5 ml
Side effects/adverse reactions:
▼ *ORAL: Candidiasis,* taste alteration
CNS: Headache, insomnia, dizziness, anxiety
CV: Hypotension, hyponatremia
GI: Nausea, vomiting, abdominal pain, diarrhea, constipation
RESP: Cough
HEMA: ***Neutropenia,*** anemia
INTEG: Rash, sweating
MISC: Fever, hypoglycemia, asthenia

Contraindications: Hypersensitivity

Precautions: Pregnancy category C, lactation, children, elderly, GI diseases with malabsorption complications, hepatic disease; must do CBC, ALT, and AST values

Pharmacokinetics: Fatty meals enhance absorption; highly protein bound (99%); two peak plasma periods (first 1-8 hr, second 24-96 hr); metabolites excreted in urine

Drug interactions of concern to dentistry:

• Aspirin: there are no data on drug interactions related to specific dental medications; however, because of its high protein binding there is always a risk of displacement when other highly protein bound drugs are administered.

DENTAL CONSIDERATIONS

General:

• Examine patient for signs of oral manifestations of opportunistic infections.

• Place on frequent recall because of drug and disease oral side effects.

• Consider semisupine chair position because of GI side effects.

• Consider semisupine chair position for patients with respiratory disease.

• Patients on chronic drug therapy may rarely have symptoms of blood dyscrasias, which can include infection, bleeding, and poor healing.

Consultations:

• Medical consultation may be required to assess disease control and stress tolerance.

• In a patient with symptoms of blood dyscrasias, request a medical consultation for blood studies and postpone dental treatment until normal values are reestablished.

• Acute oral infection may require physician consultation for coordination of antiinfective therapy.

Teach patient/family:

• Importance of good oral hygiene to prevent soft tissue inflammation

• Caution to prevent injury when using oral hygiene aids

• Importance of dietary suggestions to maintain oral and systemic health

• That secondary oral infections may occur; must see dentist immediately if infection occurs

atropine sulfate

(a'troe-peen)

Sal-Tropine

Drug class.: Anticholinergic

Action: Inhibits muscarinic actions of acetylcholine at postganglionic parasympathetic neuroeffector sites; dries secretions by antagonism of muscarinic cholinergic receptors

Uses: Reduction of salivary and bronchial secretions

Dosage and routes:

• *Adult:* PO 0.4 mg given 30-60 min before drying effect is required for dental procedure

• *Child:* PO >90 lb, 0.4 mg; 65-90 lb, 0.4 mg; 40-65 lb, 0.3 mg

Available forms include: Tabs 0.4 mg

Side effects/adverse reactions:

▼ *ORAL: Dry mouth,* burning sensation

CNS: Headache, dizziness, ***coma (toxic dose),*** involuntary movement, confusion, anxiety, flushing, drowsiness, insomnia

CV: Hypotension, paradoxic bradycardia, angina, PVCs, hypertension, tachycardia, ectopic ventricular beats
GI: Nausea, vomiting, abdominal pain, anorexia, constipation, ***paralytic ileus,*** abdominal distention
GU: Retention, hesitancy, impotence, dysuria
EENT: Blurred vision, photophobia, glaucoma, eye pain, pupil dilation, nasal congestion
INTEG: Rash, urticaria, contact dermatitis, dry skin, flushing
MISC: Suppression of lactation, decreased sweating

Contraindications: Hypersensitivity to belladonna alkaloids, angle-closure glaucoma, GI obstructions, myasthenia gravis, thyrotoxicosis, ulcerative colitis, prostatic hypertrophy, tachycardia/tachydysrhythmias, asthma

Precautions: Pregnancy category C, lactation, renal disease, CHF, hyperthyroidism, COPD, hepatic disease, child <6 yr, hypertension, geriatric

Pharmacokinetics:
PO: Onset 0.5-1 hr, moderate protein binding, duration of action 4-6 hr, renal excretion

Drug interactions of concern to dentistry:
- Increased anticholinergic effects: tricyclic antidepressants, antihistamines, opioid analgesics, antipsychotic medications, or other drugs with anticholinergic activity
- Decreased absorption of ketoconazole

DENTAL CONSIDERATIONS

General:
- Give PO dose 30-60 min before drying effects are required for dental procedures.
- Request that patient remove contact lenses before using because of possible drying effects in the eyes.
- Caution patients that they may feel a dry, burning sensation in the throat and experience blurred vision.
- This drug is intended for acute use, usually in single doses only; therefore chronic dry mouth should not be a concern.
- Avoid dental light in patient's eyes; offer dark glasses for patient comfort.

Consultations:
- Medical consultation is advisable before using this drug in patients with a history of GI disease, cardiac disease, or glaucoma.

atropine sulfate (optic)

(a'troe-peen)

Atropine-1, Atropine Care, Atropisol, Isopto Atropine

♣ Mims Atropine, Atropisol

Drug class.: Mydriatic (anticholinergic)

Action: Blocks response of iris sphincter muscle and muscle of accommodation of ciliary body to cholinergic stimulation, resulting in dilation and paralysis of accommodation

Uses: Iritis, cycloplegic refraction

Dosage and routes:
- *Adult:* INSTILL SOL 1-2 gtt of a 1% sol qd-tid for iritis or 1 hr before refracting (cycloplegic refraction); INSTILL OINT bid-tid
- *Child:* INSTILL SOL 1-2 gtt of a 0.5% sol qd-tid for iritis or bid × 1-3 days before exam (cycloplegic refraction); INSTILL OINT qd-bid 2-3 days before exam

Uveitis:
• *Adult:* INSTILL SOL 1-2 gtt into eye(s) up to 4 × daily
• *Child:* INSTILL SOL 1 or 2 gtt of 0.5% sol into eye(s) up to 3 × daily
Available forms include: Oint 1%; sol 0.5%, 1%, 2%
Side effects/adverse reactions:
▼ *ORAL: Dry mouth*
SYST: Tachycardia, confusion, fever, flushing, dry skin, abdominal discomfort (infants: bladder distention, irregular pulse, respiratory depression)
Contraindications: Hypersensitivity, infants <3 mo, open- or narrow-angle glaucoma, conjunctivitis, Down syndrome
Pharmacokinetics:
INSTILL: Peak 30-40 min (mydriasis), 60-180 min (cycloplegia); duration of dilation up to 6-12 days
DENTAL CONSIDERATIONS
General:
• Avoid dental light in patient's eyes; offer dark glasses for patient comfort.

---

auranofin

(au-rane′oh-fin)
Ridaura
Drug class.: Gold salt, antirheumatic

Action: Specific antiinflammatory action unknown; may decrease phagocytosis, lysosomal activity, inhibit prostaglandin synthesis or inhibit various enzyme systems, clinically there appears to be some suppression of synovitis during the active stage of rheumatoid disease
Uses: Rheumatoid arthritis, unapproved: juvenile arthritis
Dosage and routes:
• *Adult:* PO 6 mg qd or 3 mg bid, may increase to 9 mg/day after 3 mo, if tolerated
Available forms include: Caps 3 mg
Side effects/adverse reactions:
▼ *ORAL: Stomatitis, lichenoid drug reaction,* metallic taste, glossitis, gingivitis
CNS: Dizziness, syncope
GI: Diarrhea, abdominal cramping, stomatitis, nausea, vomiting, enterocolitis, anorexia, flatulence, dyspepsia, jaundice, increased AST/ALT, melena, constipation
RESP: ***Interstitial pneumonitis, fibrosis,*** cough, dyspnea
HEMA: ***Thrombocytopenia, agranulocytosis, aplastic anemia, leukopenia, eosinophilia***
GU: Proteinuria, hematuria, increased BUN, creatinine, vaginitis
INTEG: Rash, pruritus, dermatitis, ***exfoliative dermatitis,*** urticaria, alopecia, photosensitivity
Contraindications: Hypersensitivity to gold, necrotizing enterocolitis, bone marrow aplasia, child <6 yr, lactation, pulmonary fibrosis, exfoliative dermatitis, blood dyscrasias, recent radiation therapy
Precautions: Elderly, CHF, diabetes mellitus, allergic conditions, ulcerative colitis, renal disease, liver disease, pregnancy category C
Pharmacokinetics:
PO: Peak 2 hr; steady state 8-16 wk; 20%-25% absorbed by GI tract; excreted in urine and feces
DENTAL CONSIDERATIONS
General:
• Patients on chronic drug therapy may rarely have symptoms of blood dyscrasias, which can include infection, bleeding, and poor healing.

• Consider semisupine chair position for patients with arthritic disease.

Consultations:

• In a patient with symptoms of blood dyscrasias, request a medical consultation for blood studies and postpone dental treatment until normal values are reestablished.

Teach patient/family:

• Importance of good oral hygiene to prevent soft tissue inflammation

• To avoid mouth rinses with high alcohol content because of drying and irritating effects

---

aurothioglucose/gold sodium thiomalate

(aur-oh-thye-oh-gloo'kose)

Aurolate (gold sodium thiomalate), Solganal (aurothioglucose)

Drug class.: Antiinflammatory gold compound

Action: Specific antiinflammatory action unknown; may decrease phagocytosis, lysosomal activity, inhibit prostaglandin synthesis or inhibit various enzyme systems, clinically there appears to be some suppression of synovitis during the active stage of rheumatoid disease

Uses: Rheumatoid arthritis; juvenile arthritis; unapproved: psoriatic arthritis, Felty's syndrome

Dosage and routes:

Aurothioglucose:

• *Adult:* IM 10 mg, then 25 mg qwk × 2-3 wk, then 25-50 mg/wk until total of 800 mg-1 g is administered, then 25-50 mg q3-4wk if there is improvement without toxicity; limit 50 mg/wk

• *Child 6-12 yr:* IM 2.5 mg × 1 wk, 6.25 mg qwk × 2-3 wk, then 12.5 mg/wk until total dose of 200-250 mg, then 6.25-12.5 mg q2-3wk

Gold sodium thiomalate:

• *Adult:* IM 10 mg, then 25 mg after 1 wk, then 25-50 mg qwk for total of 1 g, then 25-50 mg q2wk × 20 wk, then 25-50 mg q3-4wk for maintenance

• *Child:* IM 10 mg × 1 wk, 1 mg/kg 2nd wk (limit 50 mg), then maintenance dose

Available forms include: IM inj 50 mg/ml

Side effects/adverse reactions:

▼ *ORAL:* Stomatitis, metallic taste

CNS: Dizziness, ***encephalitis,*** EEG abnormalities, confusion, hallucinations

CV: Bradycardia, rapid pulse

GI: ***Hepatitis,*** vomiting, nausea, jaundice, diarrhea, cramping, flatulence

RESP: ***Pulmonary fibrosis,*** interstitial pneumonitis, pharyngitis

HEMA: ***Thrombocytopenia, agranulocytosis, aplastic anemia, leukopenia, eosinophilia, neutropenia***

GU: Proteinuria, ***nephrosis, tubular necrosis,*** hematuria

EENT: Iritis, corneal ulcers

INTEG: Rash, pruritus, dermatitis, ***exfoliative dermatitis, angioedema,*** urticaria, alopecia, photosensitivity

MISC: ***Anaphylaxis***

Contraindications: Hypersensitivity to gold, SLE, uncontrolled diabetes mellitus, marked hypertension, recent radiation therapy, CHF, lactation, renal disease, liver disease

Precautions: Decreased tolerance in elderly, children, blood dyscrasias, pregnancy category C

Pharmacokinetics: *IM:* Peak 4-6

hr; half-life 3-27 days; half-life increases up to 168 days with eleventh dose; excreted in urine and feces

Drug interactions of concern to dentistry:

• None reported

DENTAL CONSIDERATIONS

General:

• Patients on chronic drug therapy may rarely have symptoms of blood dyscrasias, which can include infection, bleeding, and poor healing.

• Palliative medication may be required for management of oral side effects.

• Consider semisupine chair position for patient comfort because of arthritic disease.

Consultations:

• Medical consultation may be required to assess disease control and patient's ability to tolerate stress.

• In a patient with symptoms of blood dyscrasias, request a medical consultation for blood studies and postpone dental treatment until normal values are reestablished.

Teach patient/family:

• Importance of good oral hygiene to prevent soft tissue inflammation

• To be aware of the possibility of secondary oral infection and the need to see dentist immediately if infection occurs

• To report oral lesions, soreness, or bleeding to dentist

• To avoid mouth rinses with high alcohol content because of drying effects

azatadine maleate

(a-za'ta-deen)

Optimine

Drug class.: Antihistamine, H_1-receptor antagonist

Action: Acts on blood vessels, GI system, and respiratory system by competing with histamine for H_1-receptor site; decreases allergic response by blocking histamine

Uses: Allergy symptoms, rhinitis, chronic urticaria, pruritus

Dosage and routes:

• *Adult and child >12 yr:* PO 1-2 mg bid, not to exceed 4 mg/day

Available forms include: Tabs 1 mg

Side effects/adverse reactions:

▼ *ORAL:* Dry mouth

CNS: Dizziness, drowsiness, poor coordination, fatigue, anxiety, euphoria, confusion, paresthesia, neuritis, sweating, chills

CV: Hypotension, palpitation, tachycardia

GI: Constipation, nausea, vomiting, anorexia, diarrhea

RESP: Increased thick secretions, wheezing, chest tightness

HEMA: ***Thrombocytopenia, agranulocytosis, hemolytic anemia***

GU: Retention, dysuria, frequency, impotence

EENT: Blurred vision, dilated pupils, tinnitus, nasal stuffiness, dry nose/throat

INTEG: Rash, urticaria, photosensitivity

Contraindications: Hypersensitivity to H_1-receptor antagonist, acute asthma attack, lower respiratory tract disease, child <12 yr

Precautions: Increased intraocular pressure, renal disease, cardiac disease, bronchial asthma, seizure disorder, stenosed peptic ulcers, hyperthyroidism, prostatic hypertrophy, bladder neck obstruction, pregnancy category B, elderly, lactation

Pharmacokinetics:

PO: Peak 4 hr, half-life 9-12 hr; minimally bound to plasma proteins; metabolized in liver; excreted by kidneys; crosses placenta, blood-brain barrier

Drug interactions of concern to dentistry:

- Increased CNS depression: all CNS depressants, alcohol
- Increased anticholinergic effect: anticholinergics

DENTAL CONSIDERATIONS

General:

- Assess salivary flow as a factor in caries, periodontal disease, and candidiasis.
- Patients on chronic drug therapy may rarely have symptoms of blood dyscrasias, which can include infection, bleeding, and poor healing.
- Consider semisupine chair position for patient comfort because of respiratory disease.
- Monitor vital signs at every appointment because of cardiovascular side effects.

Consultations:

- In a patient with symptoms of blood dyscrasia, request a medical consultation for blood studies and postpone dental treatment until normal values are reestablished.

Teach patient/family:

- Importance of good oral hygiene to prevent soft tissue inflammation
- Caution to prevent injury when using oral hygiene aids
- *When chronic dry mouth occurs, advise patient:*
- To avoid mouth rinses with high alcohol content because of drying effects
- To use daily home fluoride products for anticaries effect
- To use sugarless gum, frequent sips of water, or saliva substitutes

---

azathioprine

(ay-za-thye′oh-preen)

Imuran

Drug class.: Immunosuppressant

Action: Produces immunosuppression by inhibiting purine synthesis in cells, thereby preventing RNA and DNA synthesis

Uses: Renal transplants to prevent graft rejection, refractory rheumatoid arthritis; unapproved use in refractory ITP, glomerulonephritis, nephrotic syndrome, bone marrow transplant; unapproved: pemphigoid and pemphigus, chronic ulcerative colitis, Behçet's syndrome, Crohn's disease

Dosage and routes:

Prevention of rejection:

- *Adult and child:* PO/IV 3-5 mg/kg/day, then maintenance of at least 1-2 mg/kg/day

Refractory rheumatoid arthritis:

- *Adult:* PO 1 mg/kg/day, may increase dose after 2 mo by 0.5 mg/kg/day, not to exceed 2.5 mg/kg/day

Unlabeled use in pemphigoid, pemphigus:

- *Adult:* PO 1 mg/kg of body weight per day; can titrate dose after 6-8 wk at 0.5 mg/kg of body weight per day; max dose 2.5 mg/kg of body weight per day; maintenance dose: determine the

minimum effective dose by reducing dose at 0.5 mg/kg of body weight per day q4-8wk
Available forms include: Tabs 50 mg; inj IV 100 mg
Side effects/adverse reactions:
▼ *ORAL: Stomatitis, oral ulceration*
GI: ***Pancreatitis, hepatotoxicity, jaundice,*** nausea, vomiting, esophagitis
HEMA: ***Leukopenia, thrombocytopenia, anemia, pancytopenia***
INTEG: Rash
MS: Arthralgia, muscle wasting
Contraindications: Hypersensitivity, pregnancy category D
Precautions: Severe renal disease, severe hepatic disease, chronic use increases risk of neoplasia
Pharmacokinetics: Metabolized in liver; excreted in urine (active metabolite); crosses placenta
Drug interactions of concern to dentistry:
- Increased blood dyscrasias: NSAIDs, especially phenylbutazone, dapsone, phenothiazines
- Increased immunosuppression, risk of infection: corticosteroids

DENTAL CONSIDERATIONS
General:
- Patients on chronic drug therapy may rarely have symptoms of blood dyscrasias, which can include infection, bleeding, and poor healing.
- To prevent infection if surgery or deep scaling is planned, prophylactic antibiotics may be indicated in patients who develop neutropenia.
- Determine why the patient is taking the drug.
- Alert the patient to the possibility of secondary oral infection; must see dentist immediately if infection occurs.

Consultations:
- In a patient with symptoms of blood dyscrasias, request a medical consultation for blood studies and postpone dental treatment until normal values are reestablished.
- Medical consultation may be required to assess disease control.
- Medical consultation may be required to assess patient's ability to tolerate stress.

Teach patient/family:
- Importance of good oral hygiene to prevent soft tissue inflammation
- Caution to prevent injury when using oral hygiene aids
- To avoid mouth rinses with high alcohol content because of drying effects and irritation of mucous membranes

---

azelaic acid
(a-zel'ay-ik)
Azelex, Finevin
Drug class.: Topical antimicrobial, antiacne

Action: Exact mechanism unknown; may inhibit synthesis of cellular protein; has antimicrobial activity against *P. acnes* and *S. epidermidis,* it may also normalize keratinization and decrease comedone formation
Uses: Topical therapy of mild-to-moderate inflammatory acne vulgaris; unapproved: melasma
Dosage and routes:
- *Adult and child <12 yr:* TOP wash skin and pat skin dry, apply thin film to affected area bid

Available forms include: Cream 20% in 30, 50 g tube
Side effects/adverse reactions:
INTEG: Irritation, pruritus, burning, hypopigmentation

Contraindications: Hypersensitivity

Precautions: Prevent contact with eyes, pregnancy category B, child <12 yr, lactation, severe skin irritation

Pharmacokinetics:

TOP: Less than 4% systemic absorption

Drug interactions of concern to dentistry:

• None reported

DENTAL CONSIDERATIONS

General:

• Topical use rarely causes exacerbation of recurrent herpes labialis.

• Keep away from mouth and other mucous membranes; wash eyes if cream comes in contact; irritation can occur.

---

azelastine HCl (otic)

(a-zel′as-teen)

Optivar Ophthalmic

Drug class.: Antihistamine

Action: Selective H_1-antagonist; may inhibit release of other mediators from mast cells

Uses: Temporary relief of signs and symptoms of allergic conjunctivitis

Dosage and routes:

• *Adult:* TOP 1 drop in affected eye(s) bid

Available forms include: Sol 0.05% in 6 ml

Side effects/adverse reactions:

CNS: Headache

EENT: Transient burning, stinging

Contraindications: Hypersensitivity

Precautions: Pregnancy category C, lactation; safety/effectiveness in children <3 yr unknown, renal impairment

Pharmacokinetics:

TOP: Low systemic absorption, low plasma levels, plasma protein binding 88%; metabolized to active metabolite by CYP450 isoenzymes (*N*-desmethylazelastine); excreted primarily in feces

Drug interactions of concern to dentistry:

• None reported

DENTAL CONSIDERATIONS

General:

• Protect patient's eyes from accidental spatter during dental treatment.

---

azelastine HCl

(a-zel′as-teen)

Astelin Nasal Spray

Drug class.: Antihistamine

Action: Acts by competitive antagonism of H_1-receptors to antagonize the wheal and flare responses and nasal hypersecretion; may also inhibit the release of other inflammatory mediators, including kinins and leukotrienes

Uses: Control of symptoms associated with seasonal allergic rhinitis, nonallergic vasomotor rhinitis, nasal pruritus

Dosage and routes:

• *Adult and child >12 yr:* Nasal spray 2 sprays per nostril bid

• *Child 5-11 yr:* Nasal spray 1 spray per nostril bid

Available forms include: Nasal spray unit, 137 μg per actuation

Side effects/adverse reactions:

ORAL: Bitter taste, dry mouth

CNS: Somnolence, headache

GI: Nausea

RESP: Paroxysmal sneezing

EENT: Nasal burning

MISC: Fatigue

Contraindications: Hypersensitivity

Precautions: Child <5 yr, pregnancy category C, lactation, renal impairment

Pharmacokinetics:

INH: Low absorption, metabolism to active metabolite, desmethylazelastine; excretion mostly in feces (75%), urine (25%)

Drug interactions of concern to dentistry:

• Increased risk of anticholinergic effects: anticholinergics

• Possible additive sedation: alcohol, anxiolytics, opioid analgesics

DENTAL CONSIDERATIONS

General:

• Assess salivary flow as factor in caries, periodontal disease, and candidiasis.

Teach patient/family:

• ***When chronic dry mouth occurs, advise patient:***

• To avoid mouth rinses with high alcohol content because of drying effects

• To use daily home fluoride products for anticaries effect

• To use sugarless gum, frequent sips of water, or saliva substitutes

---

azithromycin/ azithromycin dihydrate

(az-ith-roe-mye'sin)

Zithromax

Drug class.: Macrolide antibiotic

Action: Binds to50S ribosomal subunits of susceptible bacteria and suppresses protein synthesis

Uses: Mild-to-moderate infections of the upper/lower respiratory tract; COPD exacerbations caused by *H. influenzae, M. catarrhalis,* or *S. pneumoniae;* gonorrhea, chancroid, uncomplicated skin and skin structure infections caused by *M. catarrhalis, S. pneumoniae, S. pyogenes, S. aureus, S. agalactiae, H. influenzae, Clostridium, L. pneumophila;* nongonococcal urethritis; cervicitis caused by *C. trachomatis;* otitis media caused by *H. influenzae, S. pneumoniae, M. catarrhalis;* chlamydia; *M. avium* complex in HIV infection

Dosage and routes:

• *Adult and child =16 yr:* PO 500 mg on day 1, then 250 mg qd on days 2-5 for a total dose of 1.5 g, or 500 mg/day × 3 days; do not take oral suspension with meals; take 1 hr before or 2 hr after eating; patients with bacterial exacerbation of COPD may take 500 mg qd for 3 days or 500 mg on day 1 and 250 mg on days 2-5

Community-acquired pneumonia:

• *Adult:* IV 500 mg by infusion × 2 days, then begin oral doses of 500 mg/day to complete a 7-10 day course of treatment

Chlamydia/chancroid/urinary infections:

• *Adult:* PO 1 g in a single dose

Gonorrhea:

• *Adult:* PO 2 g in a single dose

Otitis media (acute):

• *Child age 6 mo and older:* PO 10 mg/kg/day, then 5 mg/kg daily on days 2-5 or 30 mg/kg in single dose; do not exceed adult dose

Mycobacterium avium complex:

• *Adult:* PO 1200 mg qwk (prevention); disseminated MAC infections 600 mg/day with ethambutol

Bacterial endocarditis prophylaxis:

• *Adult:* PO for patients allergic to amoxicillin, 500 mg 1 hr before dental procedure

• *Child:* PO for patients allergic to

amoxicillin, 15 mg/kg of body weight not to exceed the adult dose 1 hr before dental procedure

Available forms include: Tab 250 (Z-Pak 6 tabs), 500, 600 mg; powder for oral susp 100/5 ml (in 300 mg bottle), 200 mg/5 ml (in 600, 900 mg bottles); 1 g packet; powder for inj 500 mg in 10 ml vial

Side effects/adverse reactions:

▼ *ORAL:* Stomatitis, candidiasis, angioedema (allergy)

CNS: Dizziness, headache, vertigo, somnolence, fatigue

CV: Palpitation, chest pain

GI: Nausea, vomiting, diarrhea, abdominal pain, ***hepatotoxicity,*** heartburn, dyspepsia, flatulence, melena

GU: Vaginitis, nephritis

INTEG: ***Cholestatic jaundice,*** rash, urticaria, pruritus (allergy), photosensitivity

Contraindications: Hypersensitivity to azithromycin or erythromycin, pimozide therapy

Precautions: Pregnancy category C; lactation; hepatic, renal, cardiac disease; elderly; child <16 yr IV use

Pharmacokinetics:

PO: Peak 12 hr, duration 24 hr, half-life 11-57 hr; excreted in bile, feces, urine primarily as unchanged drug

Drug interactions of concern to dentistry:

- Increased serum levels: carbamazepine, cyclosporine, pimozide
- Risk of severe myopathy, rhabdomyolysis: HMG-CoA reductase inhibitors (statins)
- Decreased action of clindamycin, penicillin, lincomycin
- Oral contraceptives: advise patient of a potential risk for decreased contraceptive action, to maintain compliance with oral contraceptive use while using antibiotics, and to consider the use of additional nonhormonal contraception
- Possible increase in anticoagulant effect: warfarin
- Increased serum levels of theophylline

DENTAL CONSIDERATIONS

General:

- An alternative drug of choice for mild infection caused by susceptible organisms in patients allergic to penicillin.
- Determine why the patient is taking the drug.
- Consider semisupine chair position for patient comfort if GI side effects occur.

Teach patient/family:

When used for dental infection, advise patient:

- To report sore throat, oral burning sensation, fever, fatigue, any of which could indicate superinfection
- To take at prescribed intervals and complete dosage regimen
- To immediately notify the dentist if signs or symptoms of infection increase

---

baclofen

(bak'loe-fen)

Lioresal, Lioresal Intrathecal

🍁 Alpha-Baclofen, PMS-Baclofen, Novo-Baclofen, Nu-Baclofen, Lioresal

Drug class.: Skeletal muscle relaxant, central acting

Action: Precise mechanism of action is unknown; inhibits both monosynaptic and polysynaptic reflexes in the spinal cord and may act as an agonist for $GABA_B$ receptors; also causes some CNS depression

Uses: Skeletal muscle spasticity in multiple sclerosis, spinal cord injury, children with cerebral palsy; intrathecal dose form for severe spasticity in spinal cord injury or those not responsive to oral dose form; unapproved: trigeminal neuralgia

Dosage and routes:

• *Adult:* PO 5 mg tid × 3 days, then 10 mg tid × 3 days, then 15 mg tid × 3 days, then 20 mg tid × 3 days, then titrated to response, not to exceed 80 mg/day

Trigeminal neuralgia:

• *Adult:* PO 50-60 mg/day

Intrathecal dose form:

• *Adult:* INJ necessitates use of implantable pumps and titration of doses for each individual

Available forms include: Tabs 10, 20 mg; intrathecal 0.5 mg/ml, 10 mg/20 ml, 10 mg/5 ml

Side effects/adverse reactions:

ORAL: Dry mouth, taste alteration

CNS: Dizziness, weakness, fatigue, drowsiness, headache, disorientation, insomnia, paresthesias, tremors, convulsions, anxiety

CV: Hypotension, chest pain, palpitation, edema

GI: Nausea, vomiting, constipation, increased AST, alk phosphatase, abdominal pain, anorexia

GU: Urinary frequency, incontinence

EENT: Nasal congestion, blurred vision, mydriasis, tinnitus

INTEG: Rash, pruritus, urticaria

MS: Hypotonia

META: Elevated AST, alk phosphatase, blood sugar

Contraindications: Hypersensitivity

Precautions: Peptic ulcer disease, renal disease, hepatic disease, stroke, seizure disorder, diabetes mellitus, pregnancy category C, lactation, elderly, psychotic disorders, ovarian cysts, MAOIs

Pharmacokinetics:

PO: Peak 2-3 hr, duration <8 hr, half-life 2.5-4 hr; partially metabolized in liver; excreted in urine (unchanged)

Drug interactions of concern to dentistry:

• Increased CNS depression: alcohol, all CNS depressants

• Muscle hypertonia: tricyclic antidepressants

When used in dentistry:

• Warn patient of sedative effects while taking medication

DENTAL CONSIDERATIONS

General:

• Monitor vital signs at every appointment because of cardiovascular side effects.

• Assess salivary flow as a factor in caries, periodontal disease, and candidiasis.

• After supine positioning, have patient sit upright for at least 2 min to avoid orthostatic hypotension.

Teach patient/family:

When chronic dry mouth occurs, advise patient:

• To avoid mouth rinses with high alcohol content because of drying effects

• To use daily home fluoride products for anticaries effect

• To use sugarless gum, frequent sips of water, or saliva substitutes

B

balsalazide disodium

(bal-sal'a-zide)
Colazal
Drug class.: Antiinflammatory

Action: Converted by colon bacteria to mesalamine (5-aminosalicylic acid), mechanism of action unknown, may act topically in bowel by blocking synthesis of arachidonic acid metabolites
Uses: Mild to moderately active ulcerative colitis
Dosage and routes:
• *Adult:* PO 2.25 g (three capsules) taken tid for total daily dose of 6.75 g × 8-12 wk
Available forms include: Cap 750 mg
Side effects/adverse reactions:
▼ *ORAL: Dry mouth (1%)*
CNS: Headache, insomnia, fatigue, anorexia, dizziness
CV: Hot flushes
GI: Abdominal pain, diarrhea, nausea, vomiting, flatulence, rectal bleeding
RESP: Respiratory infection, pharyngitis, coughing
HEMA: Anemia
EENT: Rhinitis, sinusitis
INTEG: Rash, pruritus
MS: Back pain, myalgia
MISC: Arthralgia, fever
Contraindications: Hypersensitivity, including hypersensitivity to mesalamine or salicylates
Precautions: Hepatic or renal impairment, pyloric stenosis, pregnancy category B, lactation, pediatric patients not evaluated
Pharmacokinetics:
PO: Drug reaches colon intact; bacterial azoreductases release 5-aminobenzyl-B-analine and mesalamine (active metabolite); low, variable systemic absorption; peak concentration 1-2 hr, protein binding ≈99%; less than 1% renal excretion; most excreted in feces (65%)
Drug interactions of concern to dentistry:
• None reported
DENTAL CONSIDERATIONS
General:
• Consider semisupine chair position for patient comfort because of GI side effects of disease.
Consultations:
• To reduce any potential risk of antibiotic-associated pseudomembranous colitis, a consultation is recommended before selecting an antibiotic for a dental infection.

becaplermin

(bee-kap'ler-min)
Regranex Gel
Drug class.: Topical wound repair

Action: A recombinant human platelet–derived growth factor (rhPDGF-BB) that promotes chemotactic recruitment and proliferation of cells involved in wound repair and formation of granulation tissue
Uses: As an adjunct to good ulcer care practices in lower extremity diabetic, neuropathic ulcers that extend into subcutaneous tissues or beyond and have adequate blood supply
Dosage and routes:
• *Adult and child >16 yr:* TOP Calculate the amount of gel to apply by the area (l × w) of the ulcer according to manufacturer's formula in gel package insert; apply the gel once daily in a 1/16-

inch-thick layer spread evenly on the ulcerated area; as the ulcer heals, the dose must be recalculated at weekly or biweekly intervals

Available forms include: Gel 0.01% in 2, 7.5, and 15 g tubes

Side effects/adverse reactions:

INTEG: Erythematous rashes, pain, infection

Contraindications: Hypersensitivity, neoplasms at the site of application, ulcers caused by vascular insufficiency

Precautions: Nonsterile, low-bioburden product that is not for use in ulcers that heal by primary intention, external use only, do not apply with fingers, pregnancy category C, lactation, children <16 yr

Drug interactions of concern to dentistry:

- Unknown

DENTAL CONSIDERATIONS

General:

- Patients requiring use of this medication will probably be limited in activities or bedridden.
- Determine why patient is taking the drug.
- Diabetes: question patient about self-monitoring of blood glucose values or finger-stick records.
- Diabetics may be more susceptible to infection and have delayed wound healing.
- Examine for oral manifestation of opportunistic infection.
- Patients with advanced diabetes should be questioned about any limitations in activities or stress tolerance. Some will also be receiving dialysis treatment if renal function is compromised. Dental treatment can usually be performed the day after dialysis.

Consultations:

- Medical consultation may be required to assess disease control and patient's ability to tolerate stress.
- Medical consultation may include data from patient's blood glucose monitoring, including glycosylated hemoglobin (GHb) or Hb
- A_{1c} testing.
- Patients in dialysis may require antibiotic prophylaxis; determine need.

Teach patient/family:

- Importance of good oral hygiene to prevent soft tissue inflammation
- To prevent trauma when using oral hygiene aids
- Importance of updating health and drug history if physician makes any changes in evaluation or drug regimens

---

beclomethasone dipropionate/ beclomethasone dipropionate HFA

(be-kloe-meth'a-sone)

Oral inhalation: Qvar

Nasal inhalation: Beconase, Beconase AQ Nasal, Vancenase AQ 84 mcg, Vancenase Pockethaler

Drug class.: Corticosteroid, synthetic

Action: Glucocorticoids have multiple actions that include anti-inflammatory and immunosuppressant effects. They inhibit phospholipase A_2, interfering with or reducing the synthesis of prostaglandins and leukotrienes. They also bind to cytoplasmic glucocorticoid receptors (GRs) and enter the cell nucleus to bind with DNA. This results in the synthesis of various enzymes such as collagenase, elastase, and cytokines that play important roles in inflammation control and immunosuppression. They also suppress the production of lymphocytes, monocytes, and eosinophils.

Uses: Chronic asthma, prevent recurrent nasal polyps, allergic and nonallergic rhinitis

Dosage and routes:

Oral inhalation (QVAR only):

• *Adults and adolescents:* INH 40-160 μg bid; limit to 320 μg bid

• *Child 5-11 yr:* INH 40 μg bid; limit 80 μg bid

Nasal inhalation:

• *Adult and child >12 yr:* INSTILL 1-2 sprays in each nostril bid-qid; 84 μg double strength: use once daily

• *Child 6-12 yr:* INSTILL 1 spray in each nostril once daily

Pockethaler:

• *Adult and child >12 yr:* INH 1 spray in each nostril bid-qid

Available forms include: Aerosol 42, 84 μg/actuation in canisters, and pockethaler containing 200 metered actuations; QVAR 40, 80 μg/actuations

Side effects/adverse reactions:

▼ *ORAL: Dry mouth, candidiasis (rare)*

RESP: ***Bronchospasm***

EENT: Hoarseness, sore throat

Contraindications: Hypersensitivity; status asthmaticus (primary treatment); nonasthmatic bronchial disease; bacterial, fungal, or viral infections of mouth, throat, or lungs; child <3 yr

Precautions: Nasal disease/surgery, pregnancy category C

Pharmacokinetics:

INH: Onset 10 min, half-life 3-15 hr; crosses placenta; metabolized in lungs, liver, GI system; excreted in feces (metabolites)

DENTAL CONSIDERATIONS

General:

• Evaluate respiration characteristics and rate.

• Assess salivary flow as a factor in caries, periodontal disease, and candidiasis.

• Place on frequent recall because of oral side effects.

• Be aware that aspirin or sulfite preservatives in vasoconstrictor-containing products can exacerbate asthma.

• Acute asthmatic episodes may be precipitated in the dental office. Sympathomimetic inhalants should be available for emergency use.

• Midday appointments and a stress reduction protocol may be required for anxious patients.

Consultations:

• Medical consultation may be required to assess patient's ability to tolerate stress.

Teach patient/family:

• That gargling and rinsing with water after each dose helps prevent candidiasis

When chronic dry mouth occurs, advise patient:

• To avoid mouth rinses with high alcohol content because of drying effects

• To use daily home fluoride products for anticaries effect

• To use sugarless gum, frequent sips of water, or saliva substitutes

benazepril

(ben-a'ze-pril)
Lotensin

Drug class.: Angiotensin-converting enzyme (ACE) inhibitor

Action: Selectively suppresses renin-angiotensin-aldosterone system; inhibits ACE; prevents conversion of angiotensin I to angiotensin II; results in dilation of arterial, venous vessels

Uses: Hypertension, alone or in combination with thiazide diuretics

Dosage and routes:

• *Adult:* PO 10 mg qd initially, then 20-40 mg/day divided bid or qd as a single drug

Renal impairment and with diuretics: PO 5 mg qd with creatine clearance <30 ml/min/1.73 m^2, increase as needed to max of 40 mg/day

Available forms include: Tabs 5, 10, 20, 40 mg

Side effects/adverse reactions:

▼ *ORAL: Angioedema, dry mouth (rare)*

CNS: Anxiety, hypertonia, insomnia, paresthesia, headache, dizziness, fatigue

CV: Hypotension, postural hypotension, syncope, palpitation, angina

GI: Nausea, constipation, vomiting, gastritis, melena

RESP: Cough, asthma, bronchitis, dyspnea, sinusitis

HEMA: ***Neutropenia, agranulocytosis***

GU: Increased BUN, creatinine, decreased libido, impotence, UTI

INTEG: Rash, flushing, sweating

MS: Arthralgia, arthritis, myalgia

META: Hyperkalemia, hyponatremia

Contraindications: Hypersensitivity to ACE inhibitors, pregnancy category D, lactation, children

Precautions: Impaired renal or liver function, dialysis patients, hypovolemia, blood dyscrasias, CHF, COPD, asthma, elderly

Pharmacokinetics:

PO: Peak 0.5-1 hr, half-life 10-11 hr; serum protein binding 97%; metabolized by liver, metabolites excreted in urine

Drug interactions of concern to dentistry:

• Increased hypotension: alcohol, phenothiazines

• Decreased hypotensive effects: indomethacin and possibly other NSAIDs, sympathomimetics

• Suspected reduction in the antihypertensive and vasodilator effects by salicylates; monitor blood pressure if used concurrently

DENTAL CONSIDERATIONS

General:

• Monitor vital signs at every appointment because of cardiovascular and respiratory side effects.

• After supine positioning, have patient sit upright for at least 2 min to avoid orthostatic hypotension.

• Patients on chronic drug therapy may rarely have symptoms of blood dyscrasias, which can include infection, bleeding, and poor healing.

• Assess salivary flow as a factor in caries, periodontal disease, and candidiasis.

• Limit use of sodium-containing products such as saline IV fluids for those patients with a dietary salt restriction.

• Use vasoconstrictors with caution, in low doses, and with careful aspiration.
• Stress from dental procedures may compromise cardiovascular function; determine patient risk.
• Short appointments and a stress reduction protocol may be required for anxious patients.

Consultations:

• Medical consultation may be required to assess disease control and patient's ability to tolerate stress.
• In a patient with symptoms of blood dyscrasias, request a medical consultation for blood studies and postpone dental treatment until normal values are reestablished.
• Take precautions if dental surgery is anticipated and sedation or general anesthesia is required; there is risk of a hypotensive episode.

Teach patient/family:

• Importance of good oral hygiene to prevent soft tissue inflammation
• Caution to prevent injury when using oral hygiene aids

When chronic dry mouth occurs, advise patient:

• To avoid mouth rinses with high alcohol content because of drying effects
• To use daily home fluoride products for anticaries effect
• To use sugarless gum, frequent sips of water, or saliva substitutes

benzocaine (topical)

(ben'zoe-kane)

Benzocaine liquid 20%: Maximum Strength Anbesol, Maximum Strength Orajel, Orajel Mouth Aid
Benzocaine gel 20%: Americaine Anesthetic Lubricant, Hurricaine, Maximum Strength Orojel, Maximum Strength Anbesol, Orajel Mouth-Aid, Orajel Brace-Aid, Senso Gard
Benzocaine gel 15%: Orabase Gel
Benzocaine gel 10%: Numzident, Zilactin-B Medicated, Rid-A-Pain, Oraljel/d, Denture Orajel, Baby Orajel Nighttime
Benzocaine gel 7.5%: Baby Anbesol, Baby Orajet
Benzocaine gel 2%: Baby Orajel Tooth and Gum Cleanser
Benzocaine cream 6%: Bicozene, Lanacaine, Orabase Lip 5%
Benzocaine lotion 8%: Dermoplast
Benzocaine lotion 2.5%: Babee Teething
Benzocaine lotion 0.2%: Numzit Teething
Benzocaine spray 20%: Americaine, Dermoplast, Hurricaine, Lanacaine, Solarcaine

Drug class.: Topical ester, local anesthetic Action: Inhibits conduction of nerve impulses from sensory nerves

Uses: Oral irritation, toothache, cold sore, canker sore, pain, teething pain, pain caused by dental prostheses or orthodontic appliances

Dosage and routes:

• *Adult and child >6 yr:* TOP apply

to affected area according to manufacturer's labeled instructions
Available forms include: Cream 5%, 6%; gel 2%, 20%, 15%, 10%, 7.5%, 6%; spray 20%; lotion 2.5%, 8%
Side effects/adverse reactions:
▼ *ORAL: Numbness, tingling*
EENT: Itching, irritation
INTEG: Rash, urticaria
Contraindications: Hypersensitivity
Precautions: Pregnancy category C
Pharmacokinetics:
TOP: Onset 1 min, duration 0.5-1 hr; esters metabolized by plasma esterases; excreted as urinary metabolites

DENTAL CONSIDERATIONS
General:
- Do not use for topical anesthesia if medical history reveals allergy to procaine, PABA, parabens, or other ester-type local anesthetics.
- Use smallest effective amount in infants and children.
- Avoid applying to large denuded areas of mucosa to prevent excessive systemic absorption and potential toxicity.

---

benzonatate

(ben-zoe'na-tate)
Tessalon

Drug class.: Antitussive, nonnarcotic

Action: Inhibits cough reflex by anesthetizing stretch receptors in respiratory system, lungs, and pleura
Uses: Nonproductive cough relief
Dosage and routes:
- *Adult and child ≥10 yr:* PO 100 mg tid, not to exceed 600 mg/day

Available forms include: Perles 100 mg; caps 200 mg
Side effects/adverse reactions:
CNS: Dizziness, drowsiness, headache
CV: Increased BP, chest tightness, numbness
GI: Nausea, constipation, upset stomach
EENT: Nasal congestion, burning eyes
INTEG: Urticaria, rash, pruritus
Contraindications: Hypersensitivity
Precautions: Pregnancy category C, lactation
Pharmacokinetics:
PO: Onset 15-20 min, duration 3-8 hr; metabolized by liver; excreted in urine

Drug interactions of concern to dentistry:
- Increased CNS depression: slight risk of increased sedation with other CNS depressants

DENTAL CONSIDERATIONS
General:
- Elective dental treatment may not be possible with significant coughing episodes.

---

benztropine mesylate

(benz'troe-peen)
Cogentin
✦ Apo-Benzotropine, PMS Benztropine

Drug class.: Anticholinergic, antidyskinetic

Action: Blockade of central acetylcholine receptors

Uses: Parkinson symptoms, extrapyramidal symptoms associated with neuroleptic drugs

Dosage and routes:

Drug-induced extrapyramidal symptoms:

• *Adult:* IM/IV 1-2 ml 1-2 × daily; give PO dose as soon as possible; PO 1-4 mg qd-bid, increase by 0.5 mg q5-6d

Parkinson symptoms:

• *Adult:* PO 0.5-1 mg qd, increased 0.5 mg q5-6d titrated to patient response

Available forms include: Tabs 0.5, 1, 2 mg; inj IM/IV 1 mg/ml

Side effects/adverse reactions:

ORAL: Dry mouth, glossitis

CNS: Confusion, anxiety, restlessness, irritability, delusions, hallucinations, headache, sedation, depression, incoherence, dizziness, memory loss

CV: Palpitation, tachycardia, hypotension, bradycardia

GI: Constipation, ***paralytic ileus,*** nausea, vomiting, abdominal distress, epigastric distress

GU: Hesitancy, retention

EENT: Blurred vision, photophobia, dilated pupils, difficulty swallowing, dry eyes, mydriasis

INTEG: Rash, urticaria, dermatosis

MS: Muscular weakness, cramping

MISC: Increased temperature, flushing, decreased sweating, hyperthermia, heatstroke, numbness of fingers

Contraindications: Hypersensitivity, narrow-angle glaucoma, myasthenia gravis, GI/GU obstruction, child <3 yr, peptic ulcer, megacolon

Precautions: Pregnancy category C, elderly, lactation, tachycardia, prostatic hypertrophy, liver or kidney disease, drug abuse history, dysrhythmias, hypotension, hypertension, psychiatric patients

Pharmacokinetics:

IM/IV: Onset 15 min, duration 6-10 hr

PO: Onset 1 hr, duration 6-10 hr

Drug interactions of concern to dentistry:

• Increased anticholinergic effect: antihistamines, anticholinergics, and meperidine

• Decreased effects of phenothiazines

DENTAL CONSIDERATIONS

General:

• Monitor vital signs at every appointment because of cardiovascular side effects.

• Assess salivary flow as a factor in caries, periodontal disease, and candidiasis.

• After supine positioning, have patient sit upright for at least 2 min to avoid orthostatic hypotension.

• Avoid dental light in patient's eyes; offer dark glasses for patient comfort.

• Do not use ingestible sodium bicarbonate products, such as the air polishing system (Prophy Jet), within 1 hr of taking benztropine.

• Place on frequent recall because of oral side effects.

Consultations:

• Medical consultation may be required to assess disease control.

• Medical consultation may be required to assess patient's ability to tolerate stress.

Teach patient/family:

• Importance of good oral hygiene to prevent soft tissue inflammation

• Use of electric toothbrush if patient has difficulty holding conventional devices

When chronic dry mouth occurs, advise patient:
• To avoid mouth rinses with high alcohol content because of drying effects
• To use daily home fluoride products for anticaries effect
• To use sugarless gum, frequent sips of water, or saliva substitutes

bepridil HCl

(be'pri-dil)
Vascor

Drug class.: Calcium channel blocker

Action: Inhibits calcium ion influx across cell membrane during cardiac depolarization; produces relaxation of coronary vascular smooth muscle; dilates coronary arteries; decreases SA/AV node conduction; dilates peripheral arteries; this drug also inhibits fast sodium inward current

Uses: Stable angina, used alone or in combination with propranolol

Dosage and routes:

Angina:

• *Adult:* PO 200 mg qd, can titrate to 300 mg or 400 mg qd; usual dose 200 mg/day

Available forms include: Film-coated tabs 200, 300 mg

Side effects/adverse reactions:

ORAL: Dry mouth, taste changes (gingival overgrowth has been reported with other calcium channel blockers)

CNS: Headache, asthenia, tremor, vertigo, anorexia, drowsiness, insomnia, dizziness, light-headedness, nervousness, fatigue, anxiety, depression, weakness, confusion

*CV: Edema, **ventricular fibrillation, torsades de pointes,*** dysrhythmia, CHF, bradycardia, hypertension, palpitation, AV block, ventricular tachycardia

GI: Nausea, dyspepsia, diarrhea, constipation, gastric upset, increased liver function studies

RESP: Dyspnea, cough, URI

EENT: Rhinitis, blurred vision

GU: Nocturia, polyuria, impotence

INTEG: Rash

Contraindications: Sick sinus syndrome, second- or third-degree heart block, Wolff-Parkinson-White syndrome, hypotension <90 mm Hg (systolic), cardiogenic shock, serious ventricular arrhythmias

Precautions: CHF, hypotension, hepatic injury, pregnancy category C, lactation, children, renal disease, may induce new arrhythmias, prolongs QT interval with risk of torsades de pointes

Pharmacokinetics:

PO: Onset 60 min, absolute bioavailability 60%, peak 2-3 hr, half-life 42 hr; 99% plasma protein bound; completely metabolized in liver; excreted in urine and feces

Drug interactions of concern to dentistry:

• Decreased effect: indomethacin, possibly other NSAIDs, phenobarbital
• Increased effect: parenteral and inhalational general anesthetics or other drugs with hypotensive actions
• Increased effects of carbamazepine

DENTAL CONSIDERATIONS

General:

• Monitor cardiac status; take vital signs at every appointment because of cardiovascular side effects. Con-

sider a stress reduction protocol to prevent stress-induced angina during the dental appointment.
• After supine positioning, have patient sit upright for at least 2 min to avoid orthostatic hypotension.
• Limit use of sodium-containing products such as saline IV fluids for those patients with a dietary salt restriction.
• Assess salivary flow as a factor in caries, periodontal disease, and candidiasis.

Consultations:

• Medical consultation may be required to assess disease control and stress tolerance of patient.

Teach patient/family:

• Need for frequent oral prophylaxis if gingival overgrowth occurs

When chronic dry mouth occurs, advise patient:

• To avoid mouth rinses with high alcohol content because of drying effects
• To use daily home fluoride products for anticaries effect
• To use sugarless gum, frequent sips of water, or saliva substitutes

betamethasone valerate/ betamethasone dipropionate

(bay-ta-meth'a-sone)

Betamethasone dipropionate augmented cream 0.05%: Diprolene, Diprolene AF
Betamethasone dipropionate augmented ointment 0.05%: Diprolene
Betamethasone dipropionate augmented gel 0.05%: Diprolene
Betamethasone dipropionate augmented lotion 0.05%: Diprolene
Betamethasone dipropionate cream 0.05%: Alphatrex, Diprosone, Maxivate, Teldar
♣ Topilene, Topisone
Betamethasone dipropionate oint 0.05%: Alphatrex, Diprolene, Diprosone, Maxivate
♣ Topilene, Topisone
Betamethasone dipropionate lotion 0.05%: Alphatrex, Diprosone, Maxivate
♣ Topisone, Occlucort
Betamethasone valerate cream 0.1 or 0.01%: ♣ Betatrex, Psorion, Valisone, Valisone Reduced Strength, Bentovate-1/2, Celestoderm-V/2, Ectosone Mild, Metaderm Mild, Metaderm Regular, NovoBetament, Prevex B, Betaderm
Betamethasone valerate foam: Luxiq

Action: Glucocorticoids have multiple actions that include anti-inflammatory and immunosuppressant effects. They inhibit phospholipase A_2, interfering with or reducing the synthesis of prostaglandins and leukotrienes. They also bind to cytoplasmic GRs and enter the cell nucleus to bind with DNA. This results in the synthesis of various enzymes such as collagenase, elastase, betamethasone, and cytokines that play important roles in inflammation and immunosuppression. They also suppress the production of lymphocytes, monocytes, and eosinophils.

Uses: Psoriasis, eczema, contact dermatitis, pruritus, oral ulcerative inflammatory lesions

Dosage and routes

• *Adult and child:* TOP apply to affected area qid

Available forms include: Oint 0.05%; cream 0.05%; lotion 0.01%, 0.05%, 0.1%; gel 0.05% (gel available in 15 and 45 g tubes); foam 1.2 mg/g in 100 g

Side effects/adverse reactions:

▼ *ORAL: Thinning of mucosa, stinging sensation (oral application)*

INTEG: Burning, dryness, itching, irritation, acne, folliculitis, hypertrichosis, perioral dermatitis, hypopigmentation, atrophy, striae, miliaria, allergic contact dermatitis, secondary infection

Contraindications: Hypersensitivity to corticosteroids, fungal infections

Precautions: Pregnancy category C, lactation, viral infections, bacterial infections

DENTAL CONSIDERATIONS

General:

• Place on frequent recall to evaluate healing response.

Teach patient/family:

• That, when used for oral lesions, patient should return for oral evaluation if response of oral tissues has not occurred in 7-14 days

• Importance of good oral hygiene to prevent soft tissue inflammation

• To apply at bedtime or after meals for maximum effect

• To apply with cotton-tipped applicator by pressing, not rubbing, paste on lesion

• That use on oral herpetic ulcerations is contraindicated

betamethasone/ betamethasone sodium phosphate/ betamethasone sodium phosphate and betamethasone acetate

(bay-ta-meth'a-sone)

Betamethasone oral: Celestone ♣ Betnesol

Betamethasone sodium phosphate injection USP: Celestone Phosphate, Cel-U-Jec

Betamethasone sodium phosphate and betamethasone acetate USP: Celestone Soluspan

Drug class.: Glucocorticoid, long acting

Action: Glucocorticoids have multiple actions that include anti-inflammatory and immunosuppressant effects. They inhibit phospholipase A_2, interfering with or reducing the synthesis of prostaglandins and leukotrienes. They also bind to cytoplasmic GRs and enter the cell nucleus to bind with DNA. This results in the synthesis of various enzymes such as collagenase, elastase, and cytokines that play important roles in inflammation and immunosuppression. They also suppress the production of lymphocytes, monocytes, and eosinophils.

Uses: Severe inflammation, shock, adrenal insufficiency, collagen disorders

Dosage and routes:

Betamethasone tablets or syrup:

- *Adult:* PO 0.6-7.2 mg/day as a single dose or in divided doses; all doses must be individualized for the patient depending on the disease and patient response
- *Child:* 62.5-250 μg/kg of body weight in 3 or 4 divided doses daily for most indications; for adrenal cortical insufficiency: 17.5 μg/kg of body weight

Betamethasone sodium phosphate injection:

- *Adult:* IM or IV up to 9 mg/day; intraarticular, intralesional, or soft tissue injection up to 9 mg as needed

Betamethasone sodium phosphate and betamethasone acetate suspension:

- *Adult:* IM can be mixed with paraben-free 1% or 2% lidocaine for injection, 0.5-9 mg/day; intrabursal INJ 1.0 ml/0.6 mg; intraarticular INJ 0.5-2.0 mg (1.5-12 mg) depending on joint size; intradermal or intralesional INJ 1.2 mg/cm^2 of affected skin up to 6 mg at weekly intervals

Available forms include: Tabs 0.6 mg, effervescent tabs 0.5 mg; syrup 0.6 mg/5 ml; inj 4 mg betamethasone phosphate/ml in 5 ml vials; 3 mg betamethasone acetate with 3 mg betamethasone sodium phosphate in 5 ml vials

Side effects/adverse reactions:

▼ *ORAL: Candidiasis, dry mouth*

CNS: Depression, flushing, sweating, headache, mood changes

CV: Hypertension, ***circulatory collapse, thrombophlebitis, embolism,*** tachycardia, edema

GI: Diarrhea, nausea, abdominal distention, ***GI hemorrhage, pancreatitis,*** increased appetite

HEMA: ***Thrombocytopenia***

EENT: Fungal infections, increased intraocular pressure, blurred vision

INTEG: Acne, poor wound healing, ecchymosis, petechiae

MS: Fractures, osteoporosis, weakness

Contraindications: Psychosis, hypersensitivity, idiopathic thrombocytopenia, acute glomerulonephritis, amebiasis, fungal infections, nonasthmatic bronchial disease, child <2 yr, AIDS, TB

Precautions: Pregnancy category C, diabetes mellitus, glaucoma, osteoporosis, seizure disorders, ulcerative colitis, CHF, myasthenia gravis, renal disease, peptic ulcer, esophagitis

Pharmacokinetics:

PO: Peak 1-2 hr, duration 2.33 days

IM: Peak 8 hr, duration 6 days; half-life 3-4.5 hr

Drug interactions of concern to dentistry:

- Decreased action: barbiturates
- Increased GI side effects: alcohol, salicylates, and other NSAIDs
- Increased action: ketoconazole, macrolide antibiotics

DENTAL CONSIDERATIONS

General:

- Monitor vital signs at every appointment because of cardiovascular side effects.
- Patients on chronic drug therapy

may rarely have symptoms of blood dyscrasias, which can include infection, bleeding, and poor healing.

• Symptoms of oral infections may be masked.

• Determine dose and duration of steroid therapy for each patient to assess risk for stress tolerance and immunosuppression.

• Avoid prescribing aspirin-containing products.

• Place on frequent recall to evaluate healing response.

• Prophylactic antibiotics may be indicated to prevent infection if surgery or deep scaling is planned.

• Patients who have been or are currently on chronic steroid therapy (>2 wk) may require supplemental steroids for dental treatment.

Consultations:

• In a patient with symptoms of blood dyscrasias, request a medical consultation for blood studies and postpone dental treatment until normal values are reestablished.

• Medical consultation may be required to assess disease control.

• Consultation may be required to confirm steroid dose and duration of use.

Teach patient/family:

• Importance of good oral hygiene to prevent soft tissue inflammation

• Caution to prevent injury when using oral hygiene aids

---

betaxolol HCl

(be-tax'oh-lol)

Kerlone

Drug class.: Antihypertensive, selective β_1-blocker

Action: This is a selective β_1-adrenergic antagonist. At higher doses selectivity may be lost with antagonism of β_2-receptors as well. The antihypertensive mechanism of action is unclear, but may include a reduction in cardiac output and inhibition of renin release by the renal juxtaglomerular apparatus. Peripheral resistance decreases with long-term use. The antianginal action (when indicated for this use) may be related to a decrease in myocardial oxygen demand and negative chronotropic and inotropic effects. The antiarrhythmic action (when indicated for this use) has been related to a reduction in spontaneous pacemaker firing and slowing of AV nodal conduction.

Uses: Hypertension, alone or in combination with other antihypertensive drugs, especially thiazide diuretics

Dosage and routes:

• *Adult:* PO 10 mg qd, increasing to 20 mg qd if response is inadequate after 14 days

Available forms include: Tabs 10, 20 mg

Side effects/adverse reactions:

▼ *ORAL: Dry mouth (less than 2%)*

CNS: Dizziness, fatigue, lethargy, depression, headache

CV: Bradycardia, hypotension, dysrhythmias

GI: Nausea, dyspepsia, diarrhea

RESP: ***Bronchospasm,*** dyspnea, pharyngitis

GU: Impotence

EENT: Eye irritation, conjunctivitis, keratitis

INTEG: Rash, urticaria

Contraindications: Hypersensitivity to β-blockers, cardiogenic shock, second- or third-degree heart block, sinus bradycardia, CHF, cardiac failure

Precautions: Major surgery, pregnancy category C, lactation, diabetes mellitus, renal disease, thyroid disease, COPD, asthma, well-compensated heart failure, aortic or mitral valve disease

Pharmacokinetics:

PO: Peak 3-4 hr, half-life 14-22 hr; protein binding 50%; some hepatic metabolism; excreted in urine mostly unchanged

Drug interactions of concern to dentistry:

• Decreased antihypertensive effects: NSAIDs, indomethacin

• May slow metabolism of lidocaine

• Decreased β-blocking effects (or decreased β-adrenergic effects) of epinephrine, levonordefrin, isoproterenol, and other sympathomimetics

DENTAL CONSIDERATIONS

General:

• Monitor vital signs at every appointment because of cardiovascular and respiratory side effects.

• After supine positioning, have patient sit upright for at least 2 min to avoid orthostatic hypotension.

• Assess salivary flow as a factor in caries, periodontal disease, and candidiasis.

• Stress from dental procedures may compromise cardiovascular function; determine patient risk.

• Short appointments and a stress reduction protocol may be required for anxious patients.

• Use vasoconstrictors with caution, in low doses, and with careful aspiration. Avoid use of gingival retraction cord with epinephrine.

Consultations:

• Medical consultation may be required to assess disease control and stress tolerance of patient.

• Use precautions if general anesthesia is required for dental surgery.

Teach patient/family:

• Importance of good oral hygiene to prevent soft tissue inflammation

• Caution to prevent injury when using oral hygiene aids

When chronic dry mouth occurs, advise patient:

• To avoid mouth rinses with high alcohol content because of drying effects

• To use daily home fluoride products for anticaries effect

• To use sugarless gum, frequent sips of water, or saliva substitutes

betaxolol HCl (optic)

(be-tax'oh-lol)

Betoptic Solution, Betoptic S-Suspension

Drug class.: Selective β_1-blocker

Action: Reduces intraocular pressure by reducing production of aqueous humor

Uses: Chronic open-angle glaucoma, ocular hypertension

Dosage and routes:

• *Adult:* INSTILL 1-2 drops bid

Available forms include: Susp 0.25%; sol 0.5%

Side effects/adverse reactions:

CNS: Insomnia, dizziness, headache, depression (all rarely occur)

CV: Bradycardia (rare)

RESP: ***Bronchospasm*** (rare)

EENT: Eye irritation, conjunctivitis, keratitis

Contraindications: Hypersensitivity, asthma, second- or third-degree heart block, right ventricular failure, congenital glaucoma (infants), COPD

Precautions: Pregnancy category C

Pharmacokinetics: Onset 30 min, max effect 2 hr, duration 12 hr

Drug interactions of concern to dentistry:

• Avoid use of anticholinergic drugs, atropine-like drugs, propantheline, and diazepam (benzodiazepines)

DENTAL CONSIDERATIONS

General:

• Monitor vital signs at every appointment because of cardiovascular side effects.

• Check compliance of patient with prescribed drug regimen for glaucoma.

• Avoid dental light in patient's eyes; offer dark glasses for patient comfort.

Consultations:

• Consultation with physician may be needed if sedation or anesthesia is required.

bethanechol chloride

(be-than'e-kole)

Drug class.: Cholinergic stimulant

Action: Stimulates muscarinic ACh receptors directly; mimics effects of parasympathetic nervous system stimulation; stimulates gastric motility, stimulates ganglia

Uses: Urinary retention (postoperative, postpartum), neurogenic atony of bladder with retention; unapproved: gastric atony

Dosage and routes:

• *Adult:* PO 10-50 mg tid-qid

Available forms include: Tabs 5, 10, 25, 50 mg

Side effects/adverse reactions:

▼ *ORAL: Increased salivation*

CNS: ***Convulsions,*** dizziness, headache, confusion, weakness

CV: ***Cardiac arrest, circulatory collapse,*** hypotension, bradycardia, orthostatic hypotension, reflex tachycardia

GI: Nausea, bloody diarrhea, vomiting, cramps, fecal incontinence

RESP: ***Acute asthma, dyspnea***

GU: Frequency, incontinence

EENT: Miosis, lacrimation, blurred vision

INTEG: Rash, urticaria, flushing, increased sweating, hypothermia

Contraindications: Hypersensitivity, severe bradycardia, asthma, severe hypotension, hyperthyroidism, peptic ulcer, parkinsonism, seizure disorders, CAD, coronary occlusion, mechanical obstruction

Precautions: Hypertension, pregnancy category C, lactation, child <8 yr, urinary retention

Pharmacokinetics:

PO: Onset 30-90 min, duration 6 hr

SC: Onset 5-15 min, duration 2 hr; excreted by kidneys

Drug interactions of concern to dentistry:

• Decreased effects: anticholinergics

DENTAL CONSIDERATIONS

General:

• Monitor vital signs at every appointment because of cardiovascular and respiratory side effects.

• After supine positioning, have patient sit upright for at least 2 min to avoid orthostatic hypotension.

Consultations:

• For excessive, troublesome salivation, reassure patient that treatment duration is usually limited to a few days; otherwise consult to lower bethanechol dose.

bicalutamide

(bye-ka-loo'ta-mide)

Casodex

Drug class.: Nonsteroidal antiandrogen, antineoplastic

Action: Competitively inhibits the action of androgens by binding to androgen receptors in target tissues

Uses: Combination therapy with a luteinizing hormone–releasing hormone (LHRH) analog for advanced prostate cancer

Dosage and routes:

- *Adult:* PO 50 mg daily with or without food

Available forms include: Tabs 50 mg

Side effects/adverse reactions:

▼ *ORAL: Dry mouth (<5%)*

CNS: Headache, dizziness, paresthesia, insomnia

CV: Hot flashes, hypertension, peripheral edema

GI: Diarrhea, abdominal pain, constipation, flatulence, vomiting

RESP: Dyspnea, cough

HEMA: Anemia

GU: Nocturia, hematuria, UTI, incontinence, inhibition of spermatogenesis

INTEG: Rash, sweating

ENDO: Gynecomastia, hyperglycemia

MS: Back pain, asthenia, bone pain

MISC: Breast pain, weight loss

Contraindications: Hypersensitivity, women who may become pregnant, pregnancy category X

Precautions: Hepatic impairment, lactation, children

Pharmacokinetics:

PO: Rapid absorption; 96% plasma protein binding; hepatic metabolism; excretion in feces and urine

Drug interactions of concern to dentistry:

- Avoid drugs that could exacerbate urinary retention, such as anticholinergics

DENTAL CONSIDERATIONS

General:

- Patients taking opioids for acute or chronic pain should be given alternative analgesics for dental pain.
- Palliative medication may be required for management of oral side effects.
- Assess salivary flow as a factor in caries, periodontal disease, and candidiasis.
- Monitor vital signs at every appointment because of cardiovascular and respiratory side effects.
- Short appointments may be required for patient comfort.
- Consider semisupine chair position for patient comfort because of disease and drug side effects.
- Place on frequent recall because of oral side effects.

Consultations:

- Medical consultation may be required to assess disease control and patient's ability to tolerate stress.

Teach patient/family:

- Importance of updating medical/drug record if physician makes any changes in evaluations/drug regimens

When chronic dry mouth occurs, advise patient:

- To avoid mouth rinses with high alcohol content because of drying effects
- Of need for daily home fluoride to prevent caries
- To use sugarless gum, frequent sips of water, or saliva substitutes

bimatoprost ophthalmic solution

(bye'ma-to-prost)

Lumigan

Drug class.: A prostamide (synthetic structural analog of prostaglandin)

Action: Mimics the intraocular pressure–lowering activity of natural prostamides; believed to lower intraocular pressure (IOP) by increasing outflow of aqueous humor through both the trabecular meshwork and uveoscleral routes

Uses: Reduction of elevated IOP in patients with open-angle glaucoma or ocular hypertension who are intolerant of, or insufficiently responsive to, other IOP-lowering drugs

Dosage and routes:

• *Adult:* TOP 1 drop in affected eye(s) once daily in PM

Available forms include: Sterile sol 0.03% in 2.5, 5, 7.5 ml

Side effects/adverse reactions:

CNS: Headache

RESP: URI, colds

EENT: Conjunctival hyperemia, growth of eyelashes, dryness, burning, ocular pruritus, eye pain, pigmentation, eyelash darkening, foreign body sensation, visual disturbance

META: Abnormal liver function tests

MS: Asthenia

MISC: Hirsutism

Contraindications: Hypersensitivity

Precautions: Increased pigmentation in iris and eyelid, change in eye color, changes in eyelashes (color, length, shape); uveitis, macular edema; renal or hepatic impairment, remove contact lenses to apply, pregnancy category C, lactation, pediatric use

Pharmacokinetics:

TOP: Very low absorption, no systemic accumulation, some tissue distribution, 12% of absorbed dose seen in the plasma, metabolized to multiple metabolites, excreted mostly in urine (67%), feces (25%)

Drug interactions of concern to dentistry:

• None reported

DENTAL CONSIDERATIONS

General:

• Avoid drugs with anticholinergic activity, such as antihistamines, opioids, benzodiazepines, propantheline, atropine, and scopolamine.

• Protect patient's eyes from accidental spatter during dental treatment.

• Avoid dental light in patient's eyes; offer dark glasses for patient comfort.

Consultations:

• Medical consultation may be required to assess disease control.

Teach patient/family:

• Importance of updating health and drug history if physician makes any changes in evaluation or drug regimens

biperiden HCl/ biperiden lactate

(bye-per'i-den)

Akineton

Drug class.: Anticholinergic

Action: Centrally acting competitive anticholinergic

Uses: Parkinson symptoms, extrapyramidal symptoms secondary to neuroleptic drug therapy

Dosage and routes:

Extrapyramidal symptoms:

• *Adult:* PO 2 mg tid-qid; IM/IV 2 mg q30min, if needed, not to exceed 8 mg/24 hr

Parkinson symptoms:

• *Adult:* PO 2 mg tid-qid; max daily dose 16 mg/24 hr

Available forms include: Tabs 2 mg; inj IM/IV 5 mg/ml (lactate)

Side effects/adverse reactions:

▼ *ORAL: Dry mouth, glossitis*

CNS: Confusion, anxiety, restlessness, irritability, delusions, hallucinations, headache, sedation, depression, incoherence, dizziness, euphoria, tremors, memory loss

CV: Palpitation, tachycardia, postural hypotension, bradycardia

GI: Constipation, ***paralytic ileus,*** nausea, vomiting, abdominal distress

GU: Hesitancy, retention

EENT: Blurred vision, photophobia, dilated pupils, difficulty swallowing, mydriasis

INTEG: Rash, urticaria, dermatosis

MS: Weakness, cramping

MISC: Increased temperature, flushing, decreased sweating, hyperthermia, heatstroke, numbness of fingers

Contraindications: Hypersensitivity, narrow-angle glaucoma, myasthenia gravis, GI/GU obstruction, megacolon, stenosing peptic ulcers

Precautions: Pregnancy category C, elderly, lactation, tachycardia, prostatic hypertrophy, dysrhythmias, liver or kidney disease, drug abuse, hypotension, hypertension, psychiatric patients, children

Pharmacokinetics:

IM/IV: Onset 15 min, duration 6-10 hr

PO: Onset 1 hr, duration 6-10 hr

Drug interactions of concern to dentistry:

• Increased anticholinergic effect: antihistamines, anticholinergic-acting drugs, meperidine

• Increased CNS depression: alcohol, CNS depressants

• Decreased effects of phenothiazines

DENTAL CONSIDERATIONS

General:

• Monitor vital signs at every appointment because of cardiovascular side effects.

• After supine positioning, have patient sit upright for at least 2 min to avoid orthostatic hypotension.

• Assess salivary flow as a factor in caries, periodontal disease, and candidiasis.

• Avoid dental light in patient's eyes; offer dark glasses for patient comfort.

Consultations:

• Medical consultation may be required to assess disease control and patient's ability to tolerate stress.

Teach patient/family:

• To use electric toothbrush if patient has difficulty holding conventional devices

• Importance of good oral hygiene to prevent soft tissue inflammation

When chronic dry mouth occurs, advise patient:

• To avoid mouth rinses with high alcohol content because of drying effects

• To use daily home fluoride products for anticaries effect

• To use sugarless gum, frequent sips of water, or saliva substitutes

bismuth subsalicylate

(bis'meth)

Bismatrol, Bismatrol Extra Strength, Pepto-Bismol, Pepto-Bismol Maximum Strength, Pink-Bismuth

✤ PMS–bismuth subsalicylate

Drug class.: Antidiarrheal, also used in combination with antibiotics (amoxicillin, clarithromycin, metronidazole, tetracyclines), proton pump inhibitors (omeprazole or lansoprazole), or ranitidine for *H. pylori* infection

Action: Mechanism of action is not known; may act through antisecretory, antimicrobial, or antiinflammatory effects

Uses: Diarrhea (cause undetermined), prevention of diarrhea when traveling; unapproved: gastritis, duodenal ulcer associated with *H. pylori*

Dosage and routes:

- *Adult:* PO 30 ml or 2 tabs q30-60 min, not to exceed 8 doses for >2 days
- *Child 9-12 yr:* PO 15 ml or 1 tab
- *Child 6-9 yr:* PO 10 ml or 2/3 tab
- *Child 3-6 yr:* PO 5 ml or 1/3 tab

Available forms include: Caps 262 mg; Chew tabs 262 mg; susp 130 mg/15 ml, 262 mg/15 ml, 524 mg/15 ml

Side effects/adverse reactions:

▼ *ORAL: Metallic taste, gray discoloration of tongue*

CNS: Confusion, twitching

GI: Increased fecal impaction (high doses), dark stools

HEMA: Increased bleeding time

EENT: Hearing loss, tinnitus

Contraindications: Child <3 yr

Precautions: Anticoagulant therapy

Pharmacokinetics:

PO: Onset 1 hr, peak 2 hr, duration 4 hr

Drug interactions of concern to dentistry:

- Salicylate toxicity: other salicylates
- Decreased absorption of tetracyclines
- Suspected reduction in antihypertensives and vasodilator effects of ACE inhibitors; monitor blood pressure if used concurently

DENTAL CONSIDERATIONS

General:

- Avoid prescribing aspirin-containing products for analgesia.

bisoprolol fumarate

(bis-oh'proe-lol)

Zebeta

Drug class.: Antihypertensive, selective β_1-blocker

Action: Produces fall in BP without reflex tachycardia or significant reduction in heart rate; acts to block β_1-adrenergic receptors; elevated plasma renins are reduced; blocks β_1-adrenergic receptors in bronchial and vascular smooth muscle only at high doses

Uses: Hypertension as a single agent or in combination with other antihypertensives; unapproved: angina pectoris, PVCs, supraventricular tachydysrhythmias

Dosage and routes:

- *Adult:* PO 5 mg/day, limit 20 mg/day
- *Geriatric:* PO 2.5 mg/day

Available forms include: Tabs 5, 10 mg

Side effects/adverse reactions:
▼ *ORAL: Dry mouth*
CNS: Insomnia, dizziness, ***depression,*** mental changes, hallucinations, anxiety, headaches, nightmares, confusion, fatigue
CV: Bradycardia, palpitation, ***cardiac arrest, AV block,*** hypotension, dysrhythmias, CHF
GI: Hiccups, nausea, vomiting, colitis, cramps, diarrhea, constipation, flatulence
RESP: ***Bronchospasm,*** dyspnea, wheezing
HEMA: ***Agranulocytosis, eosinophilia, thrombocytopenic purpura***
GU: Impotence
EENT: Sore throat, dry burning eyes
INTEG: Rash, purpura, alopecia, dry skin, urticaria, pruritus

Contraindications: Hypersensitivity to β-blockers, cardiogenic shock, second- or third-degree heart block, sinus bradycardia, CHF, bronchial asthma

Precautions: Pregnancy category C, major surgery, lactation, diabetes mellitus, renal disease, thyroid disease, COPD, heart failure, CAD, nonallergic bronchospasm, hepatic disease

Pharmacokinetics:
PO: Half-life 9-12 hr; highly protein bound; 50% excreted unchanged in urine, rest as metabolites

Drug interactions of concern to dentistry:
- Decreased antihypertensive effects: NSAIDs, indomethacin, sympathomimetics
- May slow metabolism of lidocaine
- Decreased β-blocking effects (or decreased β-adrenergic effects) of epinephrine, levonordefrin, isoproterenol, and other sympathomimetics

DENTAL CONSIDERATIONS

General:
- Monitor vital signs at every appointment because of cardiovascular side effects.
- After supine positioning, have patient sit upright for at least 2 min to avoid orthostatic hypotension.
- Patients on chronic drug therapy may rarely have symptoms of blood dyscrasias, which can include infection, bleeding, and poor healing.
- Assess salivary flow as a factor in caries, periodontal disease, and candidiasis.
- Stress from dental procedures may compromise cardiovascular function; determine patient risk.
- Short appointments and a stress reduction protocol may be required for anxious patients.
- Use vasoconstrictors with caution, in low doses, and with careful aspiration. Avoid use of gingival retraction cord with epinephrine.

Consultations:
- In a patient with symptoms of blood dyscrasias, request a medical consultation for blood studies and postpone dental treatment until normal values are reestablished.
- Medical consultation may be required to assess disease control and patient's ability to tolerate stress.
- Take precautions if general anesthesia is required for dental surgery.

Teach patient/family:
When chronic dry mouth occurs, advise patient:
- To avoid mouth rinses with high

alcohol content because of drying effects
- To use daily home fluoride products for anticaries effect
- To use sugarless gum, frequent sips of water, or saliva substitutes

bosentan

(boe-sen'-tan)

Tracleer

Drug class.: Antihypertensive

Action: Acts as an antagonist for endothelin-1 receptors (endothelin A and B), thereby antagonizing the vasoconstrictor action of endothelin-1 endogenous peptide

Uses: Treatment of pulmonary arterial hypertension in patients with WHO class III and IV symptoms

Dosage and routes:
- *Adult:* PO initial dose is 62.5 mg bid × 4 wk; then increase to 125 mg bid as a maintenance dose; patients with low body weight should use the lower dose, 62.5 mg, as a maintenance dose

Available forms include: Tabs: 62.5 and 125 mg

Side effects/adverse reactions:

CNS: Headache, fatigue

CV: Flushing, hypotension, palpitation

GI: Dyspnea

HEMA: Decrease in hemoglobin, hematocrit

EENT: Nasopharyngitis

INTEG: Pruritus

ENDO: ***Potential liver injury,*** *abnormal liver function, altered liver enzymes*

MISC: Lower-limb edema

Contraindications: Hypersensitivity, pregnancy, concurrent use of cyclosporine or glyburide

Precautions: Potential for serious liver injury, risk of major birth defect, hepatic impairment, pregnancy category X, use during lactation or in children has not been determined, necessitates monthly tests for pregnancy during use

Pharmacokinetics:

PO: Bioavailability 50%, highly plasma protein bound (98%), hepatic metabolism (CYP 2C9 and CYP 3A4), active metabolites, biliary excretion

Drug interactions of concern to dentistry:
- Increased plasma concentrations: ketoconazole and possible other drugs that inhibit or induce CYP 450 enzymes involved with metabolism
- See contraindications for other drugs

DENTAL CONSIDERATIONS

General:
- Acute pulmonary arterial hypertension rarely occurs and is a major medical problem. Patients are at high risk.
- Chronic pulmonary arterial hypertension also occurs. Patients may be taking a variety of antihypertensive medications. It is advisable to consult with the physician of record to determine quality of disease control, patient's ability to tolerate stress, and, with this particular drug, liver function.

Teach patient/family:
- Importance of good oral hygiene to prevent tissue inflammation and dental caries
- Importance of updating health and drug history if physician makes any changes in evaluation or drug regimens

brimonidine tartrate

(bri-moe'ni-deen)

Alphagan, Alphagan-P

Drug class.: α-adrenergic receptor agonist

Action: Selective α_2-receptor adrenergic agonist that reduces aqueous humor production and increases uveoscleral outflow

Uses: Lowering of intraocular pressure in open-angle glaucoma or ocular hypertension; prevention of postoperative intraocular pressure elevation after argon laser trabeculoplasty

Dosage and routes:

• *Adult:* OPTH 1 drop in affected eye(s) tid q8h

Available forms include: Sol 0.2% and 0.5%; 5, 10, 15 ml; Alphagan-P : 0.15% in 5, 10 ml, 15 ml

Side effects/adverse reactions:

▼ *ORAL: Dry mouth, abnormal taste*

CNS: Headache, drowsiness, fatigue, insomnia, depression

CV: Hypertension, palpitation, syncope

EENT: Ocular hyperemia, burning, stinging, ocular allergy, blurring, foreign body reaction, photophobia

MS: Muscular pain

Contraindications: Hypersensitivity, MAOI

Precautions: Wait 15 min after using before inserting contact lens; tricyclic antidepressants, β-blockers, CNS depressants; severe CV disease, hepatic or renal impairment, depression, cerebral or coronary insufficiency, Raynaud's phenomenon, orthostatic hypotension, thromboangiitis obliterans, pregnancy category B, lactation, children <2 yr

Pharmacokinetics:

TOP: Peak plasma levels 1-4 hr; half-life 3 hr; hepatic metabolism, urinary excretion

Drug interactions of concern to dentistry:

Drug interactions have not been studied; however, the following possibilities exist:

• Increased CNS depression: opioids, sedatives, alcohol, and general anesthetics

• Possible risk of interference with lowering intraocular pressure: anticholinergic drugs or drugs with anticholinergic actions; tricyclic antidepressants

DENTAL CONSIDERATIONS

General:

• Assess salivary flow as factor in caries, periodontal disease, and candidiasis.

• Avoid dental light in patient's eyes; offer dark glasses for patient comfort.

• Question patient about compliance with prescribed drug regimen for glaucoma.

• Avoid drugs with anticholinergic activity, such as antihistamines, opioids, benzodiazepines, propantheline, atropine, and scopolamine.

• Monitor vital signs at every appointment because of cardiovascular side effects.

Consultations:

• Consultation with physician may be needed if sedation or general anesthesia is required.

Teach patient/family:

• Importance of updating health and drug history if physician makes any changes in evaluation or drug regimens

When chronic dry mouth occurs, advise patient:
• To avoid mouth rinses with high alcohol content because of drying effects
• To use daily home fluoride products for anticaries effect
• To use sugarless gum, frequent sips of water, or saliva substitutes

brinzolamide (optic)

(brin-zoh'la-mide)

Azopt

Drug class.: Carbonic anhydrase inhibitor

Action: Reduces intraocular pressure through inhibition of carbonic anhydrase enzyme

Uses: Ocular hypertension, open-angle glaucoma

Dosage and routes:
• *Adult:* OPTH 1 drop in affected eye tid

Available forms include: Ophthalmic suspension 1% in 2.5, 5, 10, 15 ml

Side effects/adverse reactions:

▼ *ORAL: Bitter taste, dry mouth (>1%)*

CNS: Headache, dizziness

GI: Diarrhea

EENT: Blurred vision, blepharitis, dry eye, ocular pain, foreign body sensation

MISC: Allergy

Contraindications: Hypersensitivity

Precautions: Pregnancy category C, lactation, no pediatric data for use

Pharmacokinetics:

TOP: Some systemic absorption, active metabolite, plasma protein binding 60%, urinary excretion

Drug interactions of concern to dentistry:
• Avoid drugs that can exacerbate glaucoma (e.g., anticholinergics)

DENTAL CONSIDERATIONS

General:
• Avoid dental light in patient's eyes; offer dark glasses for patient comfort.
• Question patient about compliance with prescribed drug regimen for glaucoma.

Consultations:
• Medical consult may be required to assess disease control.

bromocriptine mesylate

(broe-moe-krip'teen)

Parlodel, Parlodel SnapTabs

✤ Alti-Bromocriptine, Apo-Bromocriptine

Drug class.: Dopamine receptor agonist, ovulation stimulant

Action: Inhibits prolactin release by activating postsynaptic dopamine receptors; activation of striatal dopamine receptors could be reason for improvement in Parkinson's disease

Uses: Female infertility, Parkinson's disease, prevention of postpartum lactation, amenorrhea caused by hyperprolactinemia, acromegaly

Dosage and routes:

Hyperprolactinemic indications:
• *Adult:* PO 0.5-2.5 mg with meals; may increase by 2.5 mg q3-7d; usual range 5-7.5 mg

Acromegaly:
• *Adult:* PO 1.25-2.5 mg × 3 days hs, may increase by 1.25-2.5 mg q3-7d, usual range 20-30 mg/day

Postpartum lactation:
• *Adult:* PO 2.5 mg qd-tid with meal × 14 or 21 days
Parkinson's disease:
• *Adult:* PO 1.25 mg bid with meals, may increase q2-4wk by 2.5 mg/day, not to exceed 100 mg qd
Available forms include: Caps 5 mg; tabs 2.5 mg
Side effects/adverse reactions:
▼ *ORAL: Dry mouth*
CNS: Headache, ***convulsions,*** depression, restlessness, anxiety, nervousness, confusion, hallucinations, dizziness, fatigue, drowsiness, abnormal involuntary movements, psychosis
CV: ***Shock,*** orthostatic hypotension, decreased BP, palpitation, extrasystole, dysrhythmias, bradycardia
GI: Nausea, vomiting, anorexia, cramps, constipation, diarrhea, hemorrhage
GU: Frequency, retention, incontinence, diuresis
EENT: Blurred vision, diplopia, burning eyes, nasal congestion
INTEG: Rash on face/arms, alopecia
Contraindications: Hypersensitivity to ergot, severe ischemic disease, pregnancy category D, severe peripheral vascular disease
Precautions: Lactation, hepatic disease, renal disease, children
Pharmacokinetics:
PO: Peak 1-3 hr, duration 4-8 hr, half-life 3 hr; 90%-96% protein bound; metabolized by liver (inactive metabolites); excreted in urine, feces
Drug interactions of concern to dentistry:
• Decreased action: phenothiazines, loxapine, haloperidol, droperidol, amitriptyline
• Increased plasma levels: erythromycin
DENTAL CONSIDERATIONS
General:
• Monitor vital signs at every appointment because of cardiovascular side effects.
• After supine positioning, have patient sit upright for at least 2 min to avoid orthostatic hypotension.
• Assess salivary flow as a factor in caries, periodontal disease, and candidiasis.
• Short appointments may be required because of disease effects on musculature.
Consultations:
• Medical consultation may be required to assess disease control.
Teach patient/family:
• To avoid mouth rinses with high alcohol content because of drying effects

---

brompheniramine tannate

(brome-fen-ir'a-meen)
Brovex, Brovex CT
Drug class.: Antihistamine, H_1-receptor antagonist

Action: Acts on blood vessels, GI system, respiratory system by competing with histamine for H_1-receptor sites; decreases allergic response by blocking histamine
Uses: Allergy symptoms, rhinitis, hay fever
Dosage and routes:
• *Adult and child >12 yr:* PO 12-24 mg q12h; limit 48 mg/day
• *Child 6-12 yr:* PO 6-12 mg q12h; limit 24 mg/day

• *Child 2-6 yr:* PO 6 mg q12h; limit 12 mg/day

Available forms include: Chew tab 12 mg, oral susp 12 mg/5ml

Side effects/adverse reactions:

▼ *ORAL: Dry mouth*

CNS: Dizziness, drowsiness, poor coordination, fatigue, anxiety, euphoria, confusion, paresthesia, neuritis

CV: Hypotension, palpitation, tachycardia

GI: Nausea, vomiting, anorexia, constipation, diarrhea

RESP: Increased thick secretions, wheezing, chest tightness

HEMA: ***Thrombocytopenia, agranulocytosis, hemolytic anemia***

GU: Retention, dysuria, frequency, impotence

EENT: Blurred vision, dilated pupils, tinnitus, nasal stuffiness, dry nose/throat

INTEG: Photosensitivity

Contraindications: Hypersensitivity to H_1-receptor antagonists, acute asthma attack, lower respiratory tract disease, child <6 yr

Precautions: Increased intraocular pressure, renal disease, cardiac disease, hypertension, bronchial asthma, seizure disorder, stenosed peptic ulcers, hyperthyroidism, prostatic hypertrophy, bladder neck obstruction, pregnancy category C

Pharmacokinetics:

PO: Peak 2-5 hr, duration to 48 hr, half-life 12-34 hr; metabolized in liver; excreted by kidneys

Drug interactions of concern to dentistry:

• Increased CNS depression: alcohol, all CNS depressants

• Additive photosensitization: tetracyclines

• Increased drying effect: anticholinergics

• Hypotension: general anesthetics

DENTAL CONSIDERATIONS

General:

• Assess salivary flow as a factor in caries, periodontal disease, and candidiasis.

• Consider semisupine chair position for patients with respiratory disease.

• Determine why the patient is taking the drug.

Teach patient/family:

• Importance of good oral hygiene to prevent soft tissue inflammation

• To avoid mouth rinses with high alcohol content because of drying effects

budesonide

(byoo-des' oh-nide)

Entocortec

Drug class.: glucocorticoid, long acting

Action: Glucocorticoids have multiple actions that include anti-inflammatory and immunosuppressant effects. They inhibit phospholipase A_2 interfering with or reducing the synthesis of prostaglandins and leukotrienes. They also bind to cytoplasmic GRs and enter the cell nucleus to bind with DNA. This results in the synthesis of various enzymes such as collagenase, elastase, and cytokines that play important roles in inflammation and immunosuppression. They also suppress the production of lymphocytes, monocytes, and eosinophils.

Uses: Treatment of mild-to-moderate active Crohn's disease of the ileum or ascending colon

Dosage and routes:

• *Adult:* PO 9 mg/day in AM × 8 wk; a repeat 8 wk course can be given for recurring episodes; doses can be tapered to 6 mg/day × 2 wk before complete cessation.

Available forms include: Caps 3 mg

Side effects/adverse reactions:

▼ *ORAL:* Candidiasis

CNS: Headache, dizziness, fatigue, paresthesia, hyperkinesias, tremor, vertigo, agitation, confusion, insomnia

CV: Hypertension, palpitation

GI: Nausea, dyspepsia, abdominal pain, flatulence, vomiting

RESP: URI

HEMA: Leukocytosis

GU: Dysuria, nocturia

EENT: Ear infection

INTEG: Acne, alopecia, dermatitis, eczema

META: Hypokalemia

MS: Asthenia, myalgia

MISC: Symptoms of hypercorticism, back pain, pain (unspecified)

Contraindications: Hypersensitivity

Precautions: Tuberculosis, hypertension, diabetes mellitus, osteoporosis, peptic ulcer, glaucoma, cataracts, suppression of the hypothalamic-pituitary-adrenal (HPA) axis, pregnancy category C, discontinue use during nursing or discontinue drug, use in children has not been established, geriatric patients

Pharmacokinetics:

PO: Complete absorption, peak plasma levels 30 min to 10 hr; plasma protein binding 85%-90%, high first-pass metabolism (80%-90%), metabolized mainly by CYP3A4 isoenzymes, metabolites excreted in urine and feces

Drug interactions of concern to dentistry:

• Decreased action: barbiturates

• Increased GI side effects: alcohol, salicylates, NSAIDs

• Increased action: ketoconazole, macrolide antibiotics

• Potent inhibitors of CYP3A4 (see Appendix I) cause significant increases in plasma levels

DENTAL CONSIDERATIONS

General:

• Monitor vital signs at every appointment because of cardiovascular side effects.

• Patients on chronic drug therapy may rarely have symptoms of blood dyscrasias, which can include infection, bleeding, and poor healing.

• Symptoms of oral infection may be masked.

• Determine dose and duration of steroid therapy to assess for risk of stress tolerance and immunosuppression.

• Avoid prescribing aspirin-containing products.

• Place on frequent recall to evaluate healing response.

• Prophylactic antibiotics may be indicated to prevent infection if surgery or deep scaling is planned.

• Patients who have been or are currently on chronic steroid therapy (>2 wk) may require supplemental steroids for dental treatment.

• Consider semisupine chair position for patient comfort if GI side effects occur.

• Examine for oral manifestation of opportunistic infection.

Consultations:

• In a patient with symptoms of blood dyscrasias, request a medical consultation for blood studies and postpone treatment until normal values are reestablished.

• Medical consultation may be required to assess disease control and patient's ability to tolerate stress.

• Consultation may be required to confirm steroid dose and duration of use.

Teach patient/family:

• Importance of updating health and drug history, reporting changes in health status, drug regimen changes, or disease/treatment status

• Importance of good oral hygiene to prevent soft tissue inflammation/infection

• To prevent trauma when using oral hygiene aids

---

budesonide

(byoo-des'oh-nide)

Pulmacort Turbuhaler, Pulmicort Respules, Rhinocort Aqua, Rhinocort Nasal Inhaler

Drug class.: Corticosteroid, synthetic

Action: Glucocorticoids have multiple actions that include anti-inflammatory and immunosuppressant effects. They inhibit phospholipase A_2, interfering with or reducing the synthesis of prostaglandins and leukotrienes. They also bind to cytoplasmic GRs and enter the cell nucleus to bind with DNA. This results in the synthesis of various enzymes such as collagenase, elastase, and cytokines that play important roles in inflammation and immunosuppression. They also suppress the production of lymphocytes, monocytes, and eosinophils.

Uses: Management of symptoms of perennial allergic rhinitis in adults and children, perennial nonallergic rhinitis in adults

Dosage and routes:

For intranasal use only:

• *Adult and child ≥6 yr (Rhinocort):* INH 2 sprays in each nostril AM, PM, up to 4 sprays in each nostril in AM, then reduce to smallest amount for symptom control

Adult and child ≥6 yr (Rhinocort Aqua): INH 1 spray in each nostril qd; maximum dose 4 sprays/nostril per day

For oral inhalation (Turbohaler):

• *Adult:* INH 1-2 inhalations bid, limit to 2-4 inhalations/day

• *Child >6 yr:* INH 1 inhalation/day, limit to 2 inhalations/day

For oral inhalation (Respules):

• *Child >12 mo:* INH NEB 0.5 mg either qd or bid in divided doses

• *Child 12 mo-8 yr:* INH used only for maintenance therapy in chronic asthma

Available forms include: Metered inhaler: 7 g canister (contains 200 doses); each actuation provides 32 μg; nebulizer 0.25, 0.5 mg in 2 ml plastic amps; turbihaler 200 μg in each actuation (200 doses); INH susp 0.25 mg/2 ml

Side effects/adverse reactions:

▼ *ORAL: Dry mouth, alteration of taste*

CNS: Nervousness

GI: Nausea

RESP: Wheezing, dyspnea

EENT: Irritation of nasal membranes, sneezing, coughing, epistaxis, candidosis, altered smell, nasal septum injury

INTEG: Rash, pruritus, facial edema
MS: Myalgia, arthralgia
Contraindications: Hypersensitivity; bacterial, viral, or fungal infections of mouth, throat, or lungs
Precautions: Pregnancy category B, lactation, child age <6 yr with nonallergic rhinitis; larger doses may cause symptoms of hypercorticism and suppress HPA function
Pharmacokinetics: INH approximately 20% of inhaled dose is absorbed; highly protein bound; liver metabolism; urinary excretion
Drug interactions of concern to dentistry:
• None reported
DENTAL CONSIDERATIONS
General:
• Evaluate respiration characteristics and rate.
• Assess salivary flow as a factor in caries, periodontal disease, and candidiasis.
• Midday appointments are suggested with stress reduction protocol for anxious patients.
• Place on frequent recall because of oral side effects.
• Acute asthmatic episodes may be precipitated in the dental office. Rapid-acting sympathomimetic inhalants should be available for emergency use. Budesonide is not a rapid-acting drug and is not intended for use in acute asthmatic attacks.
Consultations:
• Medical consultation may be required to assess disease control.
Teach patient/family:
• Importance of good oral hygiene to prevent soft tissue inflammation
• That gargling and rinsing with water after each dose helps prevent fungal infection
When chronic dry mouth occurs, advise patient:
• To avoid mouth rinses with high alcohol content because of drying effects
• To use daily home fluoride products for anticaries effect
• To use sugarless gum, frequent sips of water, or artificial saliva substitutes

---

bumetanide

(byoo-met'a-nide)
Bumex
Drug class.: Loop diuretic

Action: Acts on loop of Henle to decrease the reabsorption of chloride and sodium with resultant diuresis
Uses: Edema in CHF, liver disease, renal disease (nephrotic syndrome), pulmonary edema, ascites (nephrotic syndrome), hypertension
Dosage and routes:
• *Adult:* PO 0.5-2.0 mg qd, may give second or third dose at 4-5 hr intervals, not to exceed 10 mg/day, may be given on alternate days or intermittently; IV/IM 0.5-1.0 mg/day, may give second or third dose at 2-3 hr intervals, not to exceed 10 mg/day
Available forms include: Tabs 0.5, 1, 2 mg; inj IV/IM 0.25 mg/ml
Side effects/adverse reactions:
▼ *ORAL: Dry mouth, increased thirst*
CNS: Headache, fatigue, weakness, vertigo
CV: ***Circulatory collapse,*** chest

pain, hypotension, ECG changes
GI: Nausea, ***acute pancreatitis, jaundice,*** diarrhea, vomiting, anorexia, cramps, upset stomach, abdominal pain
HEMA: ***Thrombocytopenia, agranulocytosis, neutropenia***
GU: Polyuria, ***renal failure,*** glycosuria
EENT: Loss of hearing, ear pain, tinnitus, blurred vision
INTEG: Rash, pruritus, ***Stevens-Johnson syndrome,*** purpura, sweating, photosensitivity
ENDO: Hyperglycemia
ELECT: Hypokalemia, hypochloremic alkalosis, hypomagnesemia, hyperuricemia, hypocalcemia, hyponatremia
MS: Cramps, arthritis, stiffness

Contraindications: Hypersensitivity to sulfonamides, anuria, hepatic coma, hypovolemia, lactation

Precautions: Dehydration, ascites, severe renal disease, pregnancy category C

Pharmacokinetics:
PO: Onset 0.5-1 hr, duration 4 hr
IM: Onset 40 min, duration 4 hr
IV: Onset 5 min, duration 2-3 hr; excreted by kidneys; crosses placenta; excreted by breast milk

Drug interactions of concern to dentistry:
- Decreased diuretic effect: NSAIDs, indomethacin
- Masked ototoxicity: phenothiazines
- Increased electrolyte imbalance: nondepolarizing skeletal muscle relaxants, corticosteroids

DENTAL CONSIDERATIONS

General:
- Monitor vital signs at every appointment because of cardiovascular side effects.
- Patients on chronic drug therapy may rarely have symptoms of blood dyscrasias, which can include infection, bleeding, and poor healing.
- After supine positioning, have patient sit upright for at least 2 min to avoid orthostatic hypotension.
- Assess salivary flow as a factor in caries, periodontal disease, and candidiasis.
- Limit use of sodium-containing products such as saline IV fluids for patients with a dietary salt restriction.
- Patients on high-potency diuretics should be monitored for serum K^+ levels.

Consultations:
- In a patient with symptoms of blood dyscrasias, request a medical consultation for blood studies and postpone dental treatment until normal values are reestablished.
- Medical consultation may be required to assess disease control.

Teach patient/family:
- Importance of good oral hygiene to prevent soft tissue inflammation
- Caution to prevent injury when using oral hygiene aids

When chronic dry mouth occurs, advise patient:
- To avoid mouth rinses with high alcohol content because of drying effects
- To use daily home fluoride products for anticaries effect
- To use sugarless gum, frequent sips of water, or saliva substitutes

bupivacaine HCl (local)

(byoo-piv'a-kane)

Marcaine, Sensorcaine, Sensorcaine-MPF

With vasoconstrictor: Marcaine Hydrochloride with Epinephrine, Sensorcaine with Epinephrine, Sensorcaine-MPF with Epinephrine

Drug class.: Amide local anesthetic

Action: Inhibits ion fluxes across membranes, particularly sodium transport across cell membrane; decreases rise of depolarization phase of action potential; blocks nerve action potential

Uses: Local dental anesthesia, epidural anesthesia, peripheral nerve block, caudal anesthesia

Dosage and routes:

Dental injection–infiltration or conduction block:

• *Bupivacaine 0.5% with epinephrine 1:200,000:* Max dose 1.3 mg/kg or 0.6 mg/lb; limit 90 mg* per dental appointment for healthy patients; doses must be adjusted downward for medically compromised, debilitated, or elderly patients and for each individual patient. **Always use the lowest effective dose, a slow injection rate, and careful aspiration technique.**

Example calculations illustrating amount of drug administered per dental cartridge

# of cartridges (1.8 ml)	mg of bupivacaine (0.5%)	mg (μg) of vasoconstrictor (1:200,000)
1	9	0.009 (9)
2	18	0.018 (18)
4	36	0.036 (36)
6	54	0.054 (54)
10	90	0.090 (90 g)

*Maximum dose is cited from the *USP-DI,* ed 23, 2003, US Pharmacopeial Convention, Inc. Doses may differ in other published reference resources.

• Package insert does not recommend bupivacaine for children <12 yr.

Available forms include: Inj 0.25%, 0.5%, 0.75%; inj with epinephrine 1:200,000 in 0.25%, 0.5%, 0.75%

Side effects/adverse reactions:

▼ *ORAL:* Numbness, tingling, *trismus*

CNS: ***Convulsions, loss of consciousness,*** drowsiness, disorientation, tremors, shivering, anxiety, restlessness

CV: ***Myocardial depression, cardiac arrest, dysrhythmias,*** bradycardia, hypotension, hypertension, fetal bradycardia

GI: Nausea, vomiting

RESP: ***Status asthmaticus, respiratory arrest, anaphylaxis***

EENT: Blurred vision, tinnitus, pupil constriction

INTEG: Rash, urticaria, allergic reactions, edema, burning, skin discoloration at injection site, tissue necrosis

Contraindications: Hypersensitivity, cross sensitivity between amides (rare), severe liver disease, 0.75% sol in dentistry

Precautions: Elderly, severe drug allergies, pregnancy category C, use in children (risk of local injury because of long duration of anesthesia)

Pharmacokinetics: INJ onset 4-17 min, duration 4-12 hr; excreted in urine (metabolites); metabolized by liver

Drug interactions of concern to dentistry:

• CNS depressants: may see increased risk of CNS depression with all CNS depressants, especially in children and when larger doses are used

• Avoid placing dental cartridges in disinfectant solutions with heavy metals or surface-active agents; may see release of metal ions into local anesthetic solutions, with tissue irritation following injection

• Avoid excessive exposure of dental cartridges to light or heat; it hastens deterioration of vasoconstrictor; color change in local anesthetic solution indicates breakdown of vasoconstrictor

• Risk of cardiovascular side effects: rapid intravascular administration of local anesthetic containing vasoconstrictor, either alone or in patients taking tricyclic antidepressants, MAOIs, digitalis drugs, cocaine, phenothiazines, β-blockers, and in the presence of halogenated hydrocarbon general anesthetics; always use the smallest effective vasoconstrictor dose and careful aspiration technique

• Avoid use of vasoconstrictors in patients with uncontrolled hyperthyroidism, diabetes, angina, or hypertension; refer these patients for medical treatment before elective dental procedures

DENTAL CONSIDERATIONS

General:

• Monitor vital signs at every appointment because of cardiovascular and respiratory side effects.

• Lubricate dry lips before injection or dental treatment as required.

Teach patient/family:

• To use care to prevent injury while numbness exists; do not chew gum or eat following dental anesthesia

• That numbness with this drug is expected to last for a considerable period

• To report any signs of infection, muscle pain, or fever to dentist when oral sensations return

• To report any unusual soft tissue reactions

---

buprenorphine HCl

(byoo-pre-nor′feen)

Buprenex, Subutex

Drug class.: Opioid agonist-antagonist

Controlled Substance Schedule III

Action: Binds to mu subclass opioid receptors to produce analgesia, also has narcotic antagonist activity usually demonstrated by higher doses

Uses: Relief of moderate to severe pain (injection) and for treatment of opioid dependence (tablets)

Dosage and routes:

Analgesia:

• *Adult and child 13 yr and older:* IM (deep) 0.3 mg or IV (slowly over 2 min) 0.3 mg at 6 hr intervals; a second dose (0.3 mg) if needed can be given in 30-60 min with caution depending on the patient's history/health; dose should be reduced in elderly patients, debilated patients, or patients taking other CNS depressants

• *Child 2-12 yr:* IM or IV 2-6 µg/kg q4-6h; fixed dose interval should not be used but established by patient response to the initial dose

Opioid dependence:

• *Adult:* SL 12-16 mg/day in a single dose; use is limited to physicians qualified and certified to treat opioid addiction; other dosing requirements apply to patients taking heroin or other short-acting opioids and to patients taking methadone or other long-acting opioids

Available forms include: Sublingual tabs 2, 8 mg; ampules 0.3 mg/ml

Side effects/adverse reactions:

▼ *ORAL:* Dry mouth

CNS: Sedation, dizziness, insomnia, vertigo, headache, confusion, depression

CV: Hypotension, vasodilation, hypertension, tachycardia, bradycardia, flushing

GI: Nausea, vomiting, constipation, abdominal pain

RESP: Hypoventilation, dyspnea, cyanosis

GU: Urinary retention

EENT: Miosis, rhinitis, visual abnormalities

INTEG: Sweating, pruritus

MS: Back pain

MISC: Withdrawal syndrome, ***allergic reactions,*** injection site pain, chills

Contraindications: Hypersensitivity

Precautions: Hepatic impairment, hepatitis, risk of allergic reaction, bile tract disease, impaired respiration (COPD, corpulmonale, decreased respiratory reserve, hypoxia, hypercapnia, preexisting respiratory depression); naloxone may not be effective as a narcotic reversal agent, head injury, impairment of reaction time, low abuse potential, opioid-dependent patients, debilitated patients, elderly, pregnancy category C, children <2 yr, use not advised during lactation

Pharmacokinetics:

IM: Onset 15-30 min, duration 4-6 hr; absorption 90%-100%; hepatic metabolism; excreted in feces (68%-71%); also renal excretion

Drug interactions of concern to dentistry:

• Increased risk of respiratory and cardiovascular collapse: benzodiazepines

• Increased CNS depression: all CNS depressants, concomitant use of other opioids

DENTAL CONSIDERATIONS

General:

• Patients taking this drug for opioid dependence; avoid the use of any drug with abuse potential.

• Consider aspirin, acetaminophen, or NSAIDs for the management of dental-related pain.

• Monitor vital signs at every appointment because of cardiovascular side effects.

• After supine positioning, have patient sit upright for two or more minutes to avoid orthostatic hypotension.

• Assess salivary flow as a factor in caries, periodontal disease, and candidiasis.
• Consider semisupine chair position for patient comfort if GI or respiratory side effects occur.
• Take precautions if dental surgery is anticipated and general anesthesia is required.
• If opioid or sedative drugs are required for patient management and comfort, advise current drug abuse care facility or aftercare program as appropriate.

Consultations:
• Consultations may be difficult to obtain where treatment confidentiality of drug dependence is followed.
• Medical consultation may be required to assess disease control in the patient.

Teach patient/family:
• Importance of good oral hygiene to prevent soft tissue inflammation.
When chronic dry mouth occurs, advise patient:
• To avoid mouth rinses with high alcohol content because of drying effects
• To use daily home fluoride products for anticaries effect
• To use sugarless gum, frequent sips of water, or saliva substitutes

---

bupropion hydrochloride

(byoo-proe'pee-on)
Wellbutrin, Wellbutrin SR, Zyban
Drug class.: Antidepressant

Action: Weak uptake inhibitor of the neuronal uptake of dopamine, serotonin, norepinephrine; antidepressant and smoking cessation mechanism unknown

Uses: Depression; smoking cessation treatment (Zyban)

Dosage and routes:
Depression:
• *Adult:* PO 100 mg bid initially, then increase after third day to 100 mg tid if needed; may increase after 1 mo to 150 mg tid; usual dose 300 mg/day in three equally divided doses; limit use of higher doses to 450 mg/day
Smoking cessation:
• *Adult:* PO initial dose 150 mg/day × 3 days, can increase to 150 mg bid if required; max daily dose 300 mg; initiate dose while patient is still smoking to allow for achievement of steady-state blood levels; set stop smoking date within 2 wk of administration; continue doses for 7-12 wk; if progress is not made by week 7 it is unlikely patient will stop smoking during the session; maintenance doses may be required through week 12; may be used in combination with nicotine transdermal system

Available forms include: Tabs 75, 100 mg; sus rel tabs 100, 150, 200 mg; Zyban sus rel tabs 100 and 150 mg

Side effects/adverse reactions:
▼ *ORAL: Dry mouth,* taste alteration
CNS: Headache, agitation, confusion, dizziness, insomnia, ***seizures,*** akathisia, delusions, sedation, tremors
CV: Dysrhythmias, hypertension, palpitation, tachycardia, hypotension, flushing
GI: Nausea, vomiting, constipation, increased appetite, abdominal pain
GU: Impotence, frequency, retention

EENT: Blurred vision, auditory disturbance, pharyngitis, sinusitis
INTEG: Rash, pruritus, sweating
MS: Arthralgia, myalgia

Contraindications: Hypersensitivity, seizure disorder, eating disorders (bulimia, anorexia), ritonavir, MAOIs; concurrent use of Wellbutrin and Zyban, abrupt discontinuation of alcohol or benzodiazepines

Precautions: Renal and hepatic disease, recent MI, cranial trauma, pregnancy category B, lactation, children, low abuse potential; increased CNS or psychiatric symptoms may occur with use

Pharmacokinetics:
PO: Onset 2-4 wk, half-life 12-14 hr, metabolized by liver, peak plasma levels 3-6 hr; time to steady state levels 8 days; plasma protein binding 84%, metabolized by CYP2D6 isoenzymes, urinary excretion 87%, fecal 10%

Drug interactions of concern to dentistry:
• Increased adverse reactions (seizures): tricyclic antidepressants, phenothiazines, benzodiazepines, alcohol, haloperidol, and trazodone
• Decreased serum levels with carbamazepine
• Inhibits CYP2D6 isoenzymes; use with caution; other drugs metabolized by this enzyme (see Appendix I)

DENTAL CONSIDERATIONS

General:
• Assess salivary flow as a factor in caries, periodontal disease, and candidiasis.
• Short appointments and a stress reduction protocol may be required for anxious patients.
• See nicotine doseforms for additional smoking cessation considerations.

Consultations:
• Medical consultation may be required to assess disease control and patient's ability to tolerate stress.
• Physician should be informed if significant xerostomic side effects occur (e.g., increased caries, sore tongue, problems eating or swallowing, difficulty wearing prosthesis) so a medication change can be considered.

Teach patient/family:
When chronic dry mouth occurs, advise patient:
• To avoid mouth rinses with high alcohol content because of drying effects
• To use daily home fluoride products for anticaries effect
• To use sugarless gum, frequent sips of water, or saliva substitutes

---

buspirone HCl

(byoo-spye'rone)
BuSpar
♣ Bustab

Drug class.: Antianxiety agent

Action: Unknown; may act by inhibiting 5-HT receptors or dopamine receptors

Uses: Management and short-term relief of anxiety disorders; unapproved: PMS

Dosage and routes:
• *Adult:* PO 5 mg tid, may increase by 5 mg/day q2-3d, not to exceed 60 mg/day

Available forms include: Tabs 5, 10, 15 mg

Side effects/adverse reactions:
▼ *ORAL: Dry mouth,* burning tongue, salivation

CNS: Dizziness, headache, depression, stimulation, insomnia, nervousness, light-headedness, numbness, paresthesia, incoordination, tremors, excitement, involuntary movements, confusion, akathisia
CV: Tachycardia, palpitation, CVA, CHF, MI, hypotension, hypertension
GI: Nausea, diarrhea, constipation, flatulence, increased appetite, rectal bleeding
RESP: Hyperventilation, chest congestion, shortness of breath
GU: Frequency, hesitancy, menstrual irregularity, change in libido
EENT: Sore throat, tinnitus, blurred vision, nasal congestion, red/itching eyes, change in smell
INTEG: Rash, edema, pruritus, alopecia, dry skin
MS: Pain, weakness, muscle cramps, spasms
META: Increase in AST and ALT
MISC: Sweating, fatigue, weight gain, fever

Contraindications: Hypersensitivity, child <18 yr, concurrent use or use within 14 days of discontinuing MAOI

Precautions: Pregnancy category B, lactation, elderly, impaired hepatic/renal function

Pharmacokinetics:
PO: Peak plasma levels 30-60 min, highly protein bound; metabolized in liver, first-pass metabolism by CYP3A4 isoenzymes; mainly renal excretion of metabolites, some fecal excretion; full antianxiety effects may not be seen until after 2 wk

Drug interactions of concern to dentistry:

• Increased sedation: alcohol, all CNS depressants
• Increased plasma levels: fluconazole, ketoconazole, itraconazole, miconazole, erythromycin, clarithromycin, troleandomycin

DENTAL CONSIDERATIONS

General:

• Monitor vital signs at every appointment because of cardiovascular side effects.
• Assess salivary flow as a factor in caries, periodontal disease, and candidiasis.
• Short appointments and a stress reduction protocol may be required for anxious patients.
• Determine why the patient is taking the drug.

Consultations:

• Medical consultation may be required to assess disease control.

Teach patient/family:

When chronic dry mouth occurs, advise patient:

• To avoid mouth rinses with high alcohol content because of drying effects
• To use daily home fluoride products for anticaries effect
• To use sugarless gum, frequent sips of water, or saliva substitutes

---

busulfan

(byoo-sul'fan)

Busulfex, Myleran

Drug class.: Antineoplastic

Action: Changes essential cellular ions to covalent bonding with resultant alkylation, which interferes with biologic function of DNA; activity is not phase specific; effect is due to myelosuppression

Uses: Chronic myelogenous leukemia, orphan drug in preparative therapy for malignancies treated with bone marrow transplant

Dosage and routes:

• *Adult:* PO 1.8 mg/m^2/day initially until WBC levels fall to 15,000/mm^3, then drug is stopped until WBC levels rise over 50,000/mm^3, then 1-12 mg/day

• *Child:* PO 0.06-0.12 mg/kg or 1.8-4.6 mg/m^2 day; dose is titrated to maintain WBC levels at 20,000/mm^3

Available forms include: Tabs 2 mg

Side effects/adverse reactions:

▼ *ORAL: Dry mouth, cheilosis, stomatitis*

CV: ***Endocardial fibrosis***

GI: Diarrhea, weight loss, nausea, vomiting, anorexia

RESP: ***Irreversible pulmonary fibrosis,*** pneumonitis

HEMA: ***Thrombocytopenia, leukopenia, pancytopenia, severe bone marrow depression,*** anemia

GU: ***Renal toxicity,*** impotence, sterility, amenorrhea, gynecomastia, hyperuricemia, adrenal insufficiency–like syndrome

EENT: Cataracts

INTEG: Hyperpigmentation, dermatitis, alopecia

META: Hyperglycemia, hypokalemia, ALT increase, hypophosphatemia

MISC: ***Chromosomal aberrations,*** weakness, fatigue

Contraindications: Radiation, chemotherapy, lactation, pregnancy category D, blastic phase of chronic myelocytic leukemia, hypersensitivity

Precautions: Childbearing-age men and women, leukopenia, thrombocytopenia, anemia, hepatotoxicity, renal toxicity

Pharmacokinetics:

PO: Well absorbed orally; hepatic metabolism, excreted in urine; crosses placenta; excreted in breast milk; long retention of metabolites in body

Drug interactions of concern to dentistry:

• Acetaminophen may reduce clearance if given 72 hr or less before busulfan is administered

DENTAL CONSIDERATIONS

General:

• Patients taking opioids for acute or chronic pain should be given alternative analgesics for dental pain.

• Consider semisupine chair position for patient comfort if GI side effects occur.

• Chlorhexidine mouth rinse (nonalcoholic) before and during chemotherapy may reduce severity of mucositis.

• Patients on chronic drug therapy may rarely have symptoms of blood dyscrasias, which can include infection, bleeding, and poor healing.

• Palliative medication may be required for management of oral side effects.

• Apply lubricant to dry lips for patient comfort before dental procedures.

• Assess salivary flow as factor in caries, periodontal disease, and candidiasis.

• Patients in active chemotherapy treatment should have adequate WBC count before completing dental procedures that may produce a wound. Consultation with the oncologist may be required to determine WBC values before treatment.

Consultations:

• Medical consultation may be required to assess disease control and patient's ability to tolerate stress.

• In a patient with symptoms of blood dyscrasias, request a medical consultation for blood studies and postpone dental treatment until normal values are reestablished.
• Consult oncologist; prophylactic or therapeutic antibiotics may be indicated to prevent/treat infection if surgery or deep scaling is planned.

Teach patient/family:
• Importance of good oral hygiene to prevent soft tissue inflammation
• To prevent trauma when using oral hygiene aids
• To report oral lesions, soreness, or bleeding to dentist
• That secondary oral infection may occur; must see dentist immediately if infection occurs
• Importance of updating medical/drug record if physician makes any changes in evaluation or drug regimen

When chronic dry mouth occurs, advise patient:
• To avoid mouth rinses with high alcohol content because of drying effects
• To use daily home fluoride products for anticaries effect
• To use sugarless gum, frequent sips of water, or artificial saliva substitutes

---

butenafine

(byoo'ten-a-feen)
Lotrimin Ultra (OTC), Mentax
Drug class.: Antifungal

Action: Inhibits epoxidation of squalene, thereby interfering with the synthesis of fungal cell membranes
Uses: Tinea pedis caused by *E. floccosum, T. mentagrophytes,* or *T. rubrum;* and tinea versicolor caused by *Malassezia furfur*
Dosage and routes:
• *Adult:* TOP apply to affected area and adjacent skin once daily for 4 wk; bid for 2 wk may be sufficient for some infections
Available forms include: Cream 1% in 15, 30 g sizes
Side effects/adverse reactions:
INTEG: Dermatitis, burning, stinging, erythema, itching
Contraindications: Hypersensitivity
Precautions: External use only, pregnancy category B, lactation, children <12 yr, not for oral use
Pharmacokinetics:
TOP: Some systemic absorption, hepatic metabolism

DENTAL CONSIDERATIONS
General:
• There are no dental drug interactions or relevant considerations to dentistry for this drug.

---

butoconazole nitrate

(byoo-toe-koe'na-zole)
Femstat 3, Gynazole-1, Mycelex-3
Drug class.: Antifungal

Action: Binds sterols in fungal cell membrane, which increases permeability
Uses: Vulvovaginal infections caused by *Candida*
Dosage and routes:
• *Adult:* INTRA VAG 1 applicator × 6 days (second/third trimester pregnancy)
• *Three-day treatment:* INTRAVAG insert 1 applicator for 3 days
Available forms include: Vaginal cream 2%

Side effects/adverse reactions:
GU: Rash, stinging, burning, vulvovaginal itching, soreness, swelling, discharge
Contraindications: Hypersensitivity
Precautions: Pregnancy category C, lactation
DENTAL CONSIDERATIONS
General:
• Examine oral mucous membranes for signs of yeast infection.
• Broad-spectrum antibiotics for dental infections may cause vaginal yeast infection.

calcipotriene

(kal-si-poe'try-een)
Dovonex
Drug class.: Vitamin D_3 analog (synthetic)

Action: Regulation of skin cell production and development
Uses: Chronic, mild-to-moderate plaque psoriasis
Dosage and routes:
• *Adult:* TOP Apply small amount to skin bid, rub in gently; do not exceed 100 g cream/ointment per wk
• *Adult:* TOP SCALP SOL After combing hair, apply small amount to lesions only, bid
Available forms include: Ointment, cream 0.005%; 60, 100 g; scalp sol in 60 ml
Side effects/adverse reactions:
INTEG: Local irritation, itching, burning, dry skin, dermatitis
Contraindications: Hypersensitivity, hypercalcemia, evidence of vitamin D toxicity
Precautions: Pregnancy category C, external use only, elderly >65 yr, lactation, children, hypercalcemia

Drug interactions of concern to dentistry:
• None reported
DENTAL CONSIDERATIONS
General:
• Be aware that psoriasis may have oral manifestations.

calcitonin (salmon)

(kal-si-toe'nin)
Calcimar, Miacalcin Nasal Spray, Miacalcin, Osteocalcin, Salmonine
Drug class.: Synthetic polypeptide calcitonins

Action: Inhibits bone resorption; reduces osteoclast function; reduces serum calcium levels in hypercalcemia
Uses: Paget's disease, postmenopausal osteoporosis, hypercalcemia, unlabeled use in intractable bone pain
Dosage and routes:
Paget's disease:
• *Adult:* SC/IM 50-100 IU daily; monitor disease symptoms, serum alk phosphatase, and urinary hydroxyproline; maintenance dose of 50 IU qd-qid may be sufficient
Postmenopausal osteoporosis:
• *Adult:* SC/IM 100 IU daily with supplemental calcium and vitamin D; NASAL spray 200 IU daily
Hypercalcemia:
• *Adult:* SC/IM 4 IU q12h for 1-2 days, increasing if required to 8 IU q12h; maximum dose 8 IU q6-12h
Available forms include: Inj 200 IU/ml; nasal spray 200 IU in 2 ml
Side effects/adverse reactions:
ORAL: Dry mouth, metallic taste (all infrequent)
CNS: Headache, dizziness, insomnia, anorexia, anxiety, depression

CV: Hypertension, angina pectoris, tachycardia, palpitation
GI: Nausea, vomiting, diarrhea, abdominal pain
RESP: URI, coughing, dyspnea, bronchospasm
HEMA: Lymphadenopathy, anemia
GU: Frequency of urination, cystitis, hematuria, renal calculus
EENT (NASAL SPRAY): Epistaxis, rhinitis, nasal irritation, dryness, sores, crusting, tinnitus
INTEG: Erythematous skin rashes, flushing face and hands, inflammation at injection site, pruritus
ENDO: Goiter, hyperthyroidism
MS: Myalgia, arthrosis
MISC: Fatigue, flulike symptoms, severe allergic reactions

Contraindications: Hypersensitivity (skin test before use)

Precautions: Allergy, hypocalcemic tetany, routine monitoring of urine sediment, osteogenic sarcoma in Paget's disease, pregnancy category C, lactation, children

Pharmacokinetics:
NASAL: Low bioavailability
IM/SC: Therapeutic response; see decrease in serum calcium in 2 hr, duration 6-8 hr; pain relief in bone may take 8-10 days; Paget's disease response may take several months; rapidly metabolized in kidney and other tissues; renal excretion

Drug interactions of concern to dentistry:
- Supplemental calcium and vitamin D may already be used; do not use additional amounts

DENTAL CONSIDERATIONS
General:
- Consider semisupine chair position for patient comfort because of effects of disease.
- Consider semisupine chair position for patient comfort if GI side effects occur.
- Assess salivary flow as factor in caries, periodontal disease, and candidiasis.

Teach patient/family:
- Importance of good oral hygiene to prevent soft tissue inflammation

When chronic dry mouth occurs, advise patient:
- To avoid mouth rinses with high alcohol content because of drying effects
- To use daily home fluoride products for anticaries effect
- To use sugarless gum, frequent sips of water, or saliva substitutes

---

candesartan cilexetil

(kan-de-sar'tan)
Atacand

Drug class.: Angiotensin II (AT_1) receptor antagonist, antihypertensive

Action: Blocks the vasoconstrictor and aldosterone-releasing effects of angiotensin II

Uses: Hypertension, as a single drug or in combination with other antihypertensives

Dosage and routes:
- *Adult:* Usual starting dose 16 mg once a day when used as monotherapy if not volume depleted; can be given qd or bid with total daily dose range 8-32 mg

Available forms include: Tabs 4, 8, 16, 32 mg

Side effects/adverse reactions:
CNS: Headache, dizziness, fatigue, anxiety
CV: Peripheral edema, chest pain, tachycardia, palpitation
GI: Dyspepsia

RESP: URI, bronchitis, cough
GU: Hematuria
EENT: Pharyngitis, rhinitis, sinusitis
INTEG: Rash, sweating
MS: Back pain, myalgia

Contraindications: Hypersensitivity

Precautions: Discontinue drug if pregnancy occurs, risk of fetal and neonatal injury, correct volume depletion if present, renal impairment, pregnancy category C (first trimester) and D (second and third trimesters), lactation

Pharmacokinetics:
PO: Pro-drug rapidly converted to candesartan on absorption, absolute bioavailability 15%, peak serum levels 3-4 hr, highly plasma protein bound (99%), minor hepatic metabolism, 67% excreted in feces, 33% in urine

Drug interactions of concern to dentistry:
• Potential for increased hypotensive effects with other hypotensive and sedative drugs

DENTAL CONSIDERATIONS
General:
• Monitor vital signs at every appointment in patients with history of hypertension.
• Evaluate respiration characteristics and rate because of respiratory side effects.
• Consider semisupine chair position for patient comfort if GI side effects occur.
• Limit use of sodium-containing products such as saline IV fluids for those patients with a dietary salt restriction.
• Stress from dental procedures may compromise cardiovascular function; determine patient risk.
• Short appointments and a stress reduction protocol may be required for anxious patients.
• Use precaution if sedation or general anesthesia is required; risk of hypotensive episode.

Consultations:
• Medical consultation may be required to assess disease control and patient's ability to tolerate stress.

Teach patient/family:
• Importance of updating health and drug history if physician makes any changes in evaluation or drug regimens

capecitabine

(ka-pe-site'a-been)
Xeloda

Drug class.: Antineoplastic

Action: A pro-drug that is enzymatically converted to 5-fluorouracil (5-FU). 5-FU is metabolized by both normal and tumor cells to other metabolites that prevent the synthesis of thymidylate (essential for DNA synthesis), thus inhibiting cell division, or by action as an antimetabolite that can interfere with RNA processing and protein synthesis

Uses: First-line treatment of patients with metastatic colorectal cancer and metastatic breast cancer resistant to both paclitaxel or an anthracycline-containing chemotherapy regimen; colorectal cancer when treatment with a fluoropyrimidine alone is preferred

Dosage and routes:
• *Adult:* PO 2500 mg/m^2/day in two divided doses AM and PM for 2 wk followed by a 1 wk rest period given in 3 wk cycles; take within 30 min of the end of a meal

Available forms include: Tabs 150, 500 mg

Side effects/adverse reactions:

▼ *ORAL: Stomatitis, taste alteration, candidiasis*

CNS: Fatigue, weakness, fever, headache, dizziness

CV: Edema, chest pain, ***cardiotoxicity, MI, dysrhythmias***

GI: Severe diarrhea, nausea, vomiting, abdominal pain, constipation, GI bleeding, ileus

RESP: Dyspnea, cough, URI

HEMA: ***Neutropenia, thrombocytopenia, lymphopenia,*** anemia

EENT: Eye irritation, abnormal vision, sore throat, epistaxis

INTEG: Dermatitis, hand and foot syndrome (tingling, swelling, desquamation, pain), alopecia, skin discoloration, photosensitivity, sweating

META: Hyperbilirubinemia, decreased appetite

MS: Back pain, arthralgia, pain in limbs, paresthesia

MISC: Peripheral neuropathy, viral infections

Contraindications: Hypersensitivity to 5-FU, pregnancy, severe renal impairment

Precautions: Food reduces absorption, renal insufficiency, altered coagulation when taken with Coumadin, patients >80 yr, pregnancy category D, hepatic dysfunction because of liver metastases, lactation, children <18 yr, avoid use of folic acid

Pharmacokinetics:

PO: Readily absorbed, peak blood levels 1.5 hr, plasma protein binding <60%, extensively metabolized in liver to 5-FU, renal excretion (95.5%)

Drug interactions of concern to dentistry:

- Dental drug interactions not reported; however, patients taking this drug with coumarin oral anticoagulants have altered coagulation parameters or bleeding (or both), INR or PT should be physician monitored

DENTAL CONSIDERATIONS

General:

- Monitor vital signs at every appointment because of cardiovascular side effects.
- Patients on chronic drug therapy may have symptoms of blood dyscrasias, which can include infection, bleeding, and poor healing.
- Patients taking opioids for acute or chronic pain should be given alternative analgesics for dental pain.
- Short appointments and a stress reduction protocol may be required for anxious patients.
- Consider semisupine chair position for patient comfort if GI side effects occur.
- Question patient about tolerance of NSAIDs or aspirin related to GI effects of drug.
- Consider local hemostasis measures to control and prevent excessive bleeding.
- Examine for oral manifestation of opportunistic infection.
- Be aware of oral side effects and potential sequelae.
- Palliative medication may be required for management of oral side effects.
- Avoid dental light in patient's eyes; offer dark glasses for patient comfort.
- Prophylactic or therapeutic antibiotics may be indicated to prevent

or treat infection if surgery or periodontal debridement is required.

Consultations:

• In a patient with symptoms of blood dyscrasias, request a medical consultation for blood studies and postpone treatment until normal values are reestablished.

• Medical consultation may be required to assess disease control and patient's ability to receive dental treatment.

• Consultation with physician may be needed if sedation or general anesthesia is required.

Teach patient/family:

• To prevent trauma when using oral hygiene aids

• That secondary oral infection may occur; need to see dentist immediately if infection occurs

• Importance of good oral hygiene to prevent soft tissue inflammation

• To report oral lesions, soreness, or bleeding to dentist

• Importance of updating health and drug history if physician makes any changes in evaluation or drug regimens

---

capsaicin

(kap'say-sin)

Capsin, Capzasin-P, Dolorac, No Pain-HP, Pain Doctor, Pain X, R-Gel, Zostrix, Zostrix-HP

Drug class.: Topical analgesic for selected pain syndromes

Action: Exact mechanism unknown; may deplete and prevent reaccumulation of substance P in peripheral sensory neurons

Uses: Neuralgia associated with herpes zoster or diabetic neuropathy; pain of osteoarthritis and rheumatoid arthritis; unapproved: postmastectomy pain, causalgia, and TMD pain

Dosage and routes:

• *Adult and child >2 yr:* TOP apply sparingly to affected area tid or qid; transient burning may occur

Available forms include: Cream 0.025% in 45, 90 g tubes; cream 0.075% in 30, 60 g tubes; lotion 0.025%, 0.075% in 60 ml; gel 0.025%, 0.05% in 15, 30, 42.5 g; roll-on 0.075% in 60 ml

Side effects/adverse reactions:

EENT: Coughing if inhaled

INTEG: Local burning sensation, stinging

Contraindications: Hypersensitivity, persons especially sensitive to hot peppers, children <2 yr

Precautions: Pregnancy category not reported, lactation, avoid use on broken skin

Drug interactions of concern to dentistry:

• None reported

DENTAL CONSIDERATIONS

General:

• Determine why the patient is taking the drug.

• Consider location of lesions and alter dental procedures accordingly.

Teach patient/family:

• To wash hands thoroughly after use and avoid contact with mouth or eyes

---

captopril

(kap'toe-pril)

Capoten

Drug class.: Angiotensin-converting enzyme (ACE) inhibitor

Action: Selectively suppresses renin-angiotensin-aldosterone system; inhibits ACE; prevents conversion of angiotensin I to angiotensin II

Uses: Hypertension, heart failure not responsive to conventional therapy, left ventricular dysfunction (LVD) after MI, diabetic nephropathy; unapproved: hypertension of scleroderma

Dosage and routes:

Hypertension (alone or with other antihypertensives, esp. thiazide diuretics):

• *Initial dose-Adult:* PO 25 mg bid/tid; may increase to 50 mg bid-tid at 1-2 wk intervals; usual range 25-150 mg bid-tid; max 450 mg

CHF:

• *Adult:* PO 6.25-12.5 mg tid, given with a diuretic, digitalis; may increase to 25-50 mg bid-tid, after 14 days; may increase to 150 mg tid if needed; use low starting dose if hypovolemic

LVD post-MI:

• *Adult:* PO single dose of 6.25 mg; then 12.5 mg tid increasing to 25 mg tid over several days, then to 50 mg tid over several wk

Diabetic nephropathy:

• *Adult:* PO 25 mg tid

Available forms include: Tabs 12.5, 25, 50, 100 mg

Side effects/adverse reactions:

▼ *ORAL:* Dry mouth, glossitis, oral ulceration (Stevens-Johnson syndrome), angioedema, bleeding, lichenoid drug reaction

CNS: Fever, chills, headache, dizziness, fatigue

CV: Hypotension, chest pain, palpitation, angina pectoris, syncope, ***MI***

GI: Abdominal pain, vomiting, nausea, diarrhea

RESP: ***Bronchospasm,*** dyspnea, cough

HEMA: ***Neutropenia***

GU: ***Nephrotic syndrome, acute reversible renal failure,*** polyuria, oliguria, frequency, impotence, dysuria, nocturia, proteinuria

INTEG: *Angioedema,* rash, pemphigus-like reaction, alopecia, pruritus, photosensitivity

META: Hyperkalemia

Contraindications: Hypersensitivity, pregnancy category D, lactation, heart block, children, K-sparing diuretics

Precautions: Dialysis patients, hypovolemia, leukemia, scleroderma, lupus erythematosus, blood dyscrasias, CHF, diabetes mellitus, renal disease, thyroid disease, COPD, asthma, discontinue drug if pregnancy is detected

Pharmacokinetics:

PO: Peak 1-1.5 hr, duration 2-6 hr, half-life 3 hr; metabolized by liver (metabolites); excreted in urine; crosses placenta; excreted in breast milk

Drug interactions of concern to dentistry:

• Increased hypotension: alcohol, phenothiazines

• Decreased hypotensive effects: indomethacin and possibly other NSAIDs, sympathomimetics

• Suspected reduction in the antihypertensive and vasodilator effects by salicylates; monitor blood pressure if used concurrently

DENTAL CONSIDERATIONS

General:

• Monitor vital signs at every appointment because of cardiovascular side effects.

• After supine positioning, have

patient sit upright for at least 2 min before standing to avoid orthostatic hypotension.

• Patients on chronic drug therapy may rarely have symptoms of blood dyscrasias, which can include infection, bleeding, and poor healing.

• Assess salivary flow as a factor in caries, periodontal disease, and candidiasis.

• Limit use of sodium-containing products such as saline IV fluids for patients with a dietary salt restriction.

• Stress from dental procedures may compromise cardiovascular function; determine patient risk.

• Short appointments and a stress reduction protocol may be required for anxious patients.

Consultations:

• Medical consultation may be required to assess patient's ability to tolerate stress.

• In a patient with symptoms of blood dyscrasias, request a medical consultation for blood studies and postpone dental treatment until normal values are reestablished.

• Take precautions if dental surgery is anticipated and sedation or general anesthesia is required; there is risk of a hypotensive episode.

Teach patient/family:

• Importance of good oral hygiene to prevent soft tissue inflammation

• Caution to prevent injury when using oral hygiene aids

When chronic dry mouth occurs, advise patient:

• To avoid mouth rinses with high alcohol content because of drying effects

• To use daily home fluoride products for anticaries effect

• To use sugarless gum, frequent sips of water, or saliva substitutes

---

carbamazepine

(kar-ba-maz'e-peen)

Atretol, Carbatrol, Epitol, Tegretol, Tegretol Chewtabs, Tegretol XR, Teril

♣ Taro-Carbamazepine, Tegretol CR

Drug class.: Anticonvulsant

Action: Exact mechanism unknown, inhibits nerve impulses by limiting influx of sodium ions across cell membrane in motor cortex, may also decrease polysynaptic transmission

Uses: Tonic-clonic, complex-partial, mixed seizures; trigeminal neuralgia; unapproved: neurogenic pain, some psychotic disorders, diabetes insipidus, alcohol withdrawal

Dosage and routes:

Seizures:

• *Adult and child >12 yr:* PO 200 mg bid, may be increased at weekly intervals by 200 mg/day in divided doses q6-8h or 2 × daily with ext rel tab; adjustment is needed to minimum dose to control seizures; up to 1.6 g/day; maintenance dose 800-1200 mg/day; dose limit in children 12-15 yr is 1200 mg; if oral suspension is used adjust to smaller doses at more frequent intervals

• *Child 6-12 yr:* PO 100 mg bid, can increase at weekly intervals by 100 mg/day q6-8h or 2 × daily for ext rel tab; maximum dose is 1000 mg/day; if oral suspension is used adjust to smaller doses at more frequent intervals

Trigeminal neuralgia:

• *Adult:* PO 100 mg bid, may increase 100 mg q12h until pain subsides, not to exceed 1.2 g/day; maintenance is 200-400 mg bid; adjust dose if oral suspension is used to smaller doses at more frequent intervals

Available forms include: Chew tabs 100 mg; tabs 200 mg; ext rel tabs 100, 200, 400 mg; ext rel caps 200, 300 mg; oral susp 100 mg/5 ml

Side effects/adverse reactions:

▼ *ORAL: Dry mouth, oral ulceration, glossitis, lichenoid reaction*

CNS: Drowsiness, ***paralysis,*** dizziness, confusion, fatigue, headache, hallucinations

CV: ***Hypertension, CHF,*** hypotension, aggravation of CAD

GI: Nausea, constipation, diarrhea, ***hepatitis,*** anorexia, vomiting, abdominal pain, increased liver enzymes

RESP: Pulmonary hypersensitivity (fever, dyspnea, pneumonitis)

HEMA: ***Thrombocytopenia, agranulocytosis, leukocytosis, neutropenia, aplastic anemia, eosinophilia,*** increased pro-time

GU: Frequency, retention, albuminuria, glycosuria, impotence

EENT: Tinnitus, blurred vision, diplopia, nystagmus, conjunctivitis

INTEG: Rash, ***Stevens-Johnson syndrome,*** urticaria

Contraindications: Hypersensitivity to carbamazepine or tricyclic antidepressants, bone marrow depression, concomitant use of MAOIs

Precautions: Glaucoma, hepatic disease, renal disease, cardiac disease, psychosis, pregnancy category D, lactation, child <6 yr

Pharmacokinetics:

PO: Onset slow, peak 4-8 hr, half-life 14-16 hr; metabolized in liver by CYP450 3A4 isoenzymes; excreted in urine, feces; crosses placenta; excreted in breast milk; trigeminal neuralgia pain relief 8-72 hr

Drug interactions of concern to dentistry:

• Decreased metabolism: erythromycin, clarithromycin, propoxyphene, troleandomycin, metronidazole, ketoconazole, fluconazole, itraconazole, or any drug that inhibits CYP450 3A4 enzymes (see Appendix I)

• Increased serum levels: tricyclic antidepressants, fluoxetine, fluvoxamine, nefazodone, ketoconazole, itraconazole

• Increased CNS depression: haloperidol, phenothiazines

• Decreased half-life: doxycycline

• Potential hepatotoxicity: chronic high doses of carbamazepine with acetaminophen

• Decreased effects of phenobarbital, corticosteroids, benzodiazepines, doxycycline, sertraline

DENTAL CONSIDERATIONS

General:

• Monitor vital signs at every appointment because of cardiovascular side effects.

• Patients on chronic drug therapy may rarely have symptoms of blood dyscrasias, which can include infection, bleeding, and poor healing.

• Assess salivary flow as a factor in caries, periodontal disease, and candidiasis.

• Short appointments and a stress reduction protocol may be required for anxious patients.

• Talk with patient about type of epilepsy, seizure frequency, and quality of seizure control.

Consultations:

• In a patient with symptoms of blood dyscrasias, request a medical consultation for blood studies and postpone dental treatment until normal values are reestablished.

• Medical consultation may be required to assess disease control and patient's ability to tolerate stress.

Teach patient/family:

• Importance of good oral hygiene to prevent soft tissue inflammation

• Caution to prevent injury when using oral hygiene aids

• Caution patients about driving or performing other tasks requiring alertness.

When chronic dry mouth occurs, advise patient:

• To avoid mouth rinses with high alcohol content because of drying effects

• To use daily home fluoride products for anticaries effect

• To use sugarless gum, frequent sips of water, or saliva substitutes

---

carisoprodol

(kar-eye-soe-proe'dole)
Soma

Drug class.: Skeletal muscle relaxant, central acting

Action: Mechanism unknown, may act by blocking interneuronal activity in spinal cord, produces nonspecific CNS sedation

Uses: Adjunct for relief of acute, painful musculoskeletal conditions

Dosage and routes:

• *Adult and child >12 yr:* PO 350 mg tid and hs

Available forms include: Tabs 350 mg

Side effects/adverse reactions:

▼ *ORAL: Glossitis, swelling of lips*

CNS: Dizziness, weakness, drowsiness, headache, tremor, depression, insomnia, ataxia, irritability

CV: Postural hypotension, tachycardia

GI: Nausea, vomiting, hiccups, epigastric discomfort

EENT: Diplopia, temporary loss of vision

INTEG: Rash, pruritus, fever, facial flushing

Contraindications: Hypersensitivity, intermittent porphyria

Precautions: Renal disease, hepatic disease, addictive personalities, pregnancy category C, elderly, children <12 yr

Pharmacokinetics:

PO: Onset 0.5 hr, duration 4-6 hr, half-life 8 hr; metabolized by liver; excreted in urine; crosses placenta; excreted in breast milk (large amounts)

Drug interactions of concern to dentistry:

• Increased CNS depression: alcohol, all CNS depressants

DENTAL CONSIDERATIONS

General:

• When used in dentistry, may be more effective when used in combination with aspirin or NSAIDs.

Teach patient/family:

• To use electric toothbrush if patient has difficulty holding conventional devices

carteolol HCl

(kar-tee'oh-lole)

Cartrol

Drug class.: Nonselective β-adrenergic blocker

Action: This is a nonselective β_1- and β_2-adrenergic antagonist. The antihypertensive mechanism of action is unclear but may include a reduction in cardiac output and inhibition of renin release by the renal juxtaglomerular apparatus. Peripheral resistance decreases with long-term use. The antianginal action (when indicated for this use) may be related to a decrease in myocardial oxygen demand and negative chronotropic and inotropic effects. The antiarrhythmic action (when indicated for this use) has been related to a reduction in spontaneous pacemaker firing and slowing of AV nodal conduction.

Uses: Mild-to-moderate hypertension, alone or with other antihypertensive drugs; unapproved: angina pectoris

Dosage and routes:

• *Adult:* PO 2.5 mg tid initially, may gradually increase to desired response up to 10 mg/day

Available forms include: Tabs 2.5, 5 mg

Side effects/adverse reactions:

▼ *ORAL: Dry mouth*

CNS: Dizziness, mental changes, drowsiness, fatigue, headache, catatonia, depression, anxiety, nightmares, paresthesia, lethargy, insomnia, decreased concentration

CV: ***Bradycardia, CHF, ventricular dysrhythmias, AV block, peripheral vascular insufficiency,*** palpitation, orthostatic hypotension

GI: Nausea, vomiting, diarrhea, flatulence, constipation, anorexia

RESP: ***Bronchospasm,*** dyspnea, wheezing, nasal stuffiness, pharyngitis

HEMA: ***Agranulocytosis, thrombocytopenic purpura*** (rare)

GU: Impotence, dysuria, ejaculatory failure, urinary retention

EENT: Tinnitus, visual changes, sore throat, double vision, dry/burning eyes

INTEG: Rash, alopecia, urticaria, pruritus, fever

MS: Joint pain, arthralgia, muscle cramps, pain

MISC: Facial swelling, decreased exercise tolerance, weight change, Raynaud's disease

Contraindications: Hypersensitivity to β-blockers, cardiogenic shock, second- or third-degree heart block, sinus bradycardia, CHF, bronchial asthma

Precautions: Major surgery, pregnancy category C, lactation, diabetes mellitus, renal disease, thyroid disease, COPD, well-compensated heart failure, CAD, nonallergic bronchospasm

Pharmacokinetics:

PO: Onset 1-2 hr, peak 2-4 hr, duration 8-12 hr, half-life 6-8 hr; metabolized by liver (metabolites inactive); crosses placenta; excreted in breast milk, urine, bile

Drug interactions of concern to dentistry:

• Hypertension, bradycardia: sympathomimetics (epinephrine, ephedrine)

• Slow metabolism of drug: lidocaine

• Increased hypotension, myocar-

dial depression: fentanyl derivatives, hydrocarbon inhalation anesthetics
• Decreased hypotensive effect: indomethacin and other NSAIDs

DENTAL CONSIDERATIONS

General:

• Monitor vital signs at every appointment because of cardiovascular side effects.
• Patients on chronic drug therapy may rarely have symptoms of blood dyscrasias, which can include infection, bleeding, and poor healing.
• After supine positioning, have patient sit upright for at least 2 min before standing to avoid orthostatic hypotension.
• Limit use of sodium-containing products such as saline IV fluids for patients with a dietary salt restriction.
• Assess salivary flow as a factor in caries, periodontal disease, and candidiasis.
• Stress from dental procedures may compromise cardiovascular function; determine patient risk.
• Short appointments and a stress reduction protocol may be required for anxious patients.

Consultations:

• In a patient with symptoms of blood dyscrasias, request a medical consultation for blood studies and postpone dental treatment until normal values are reestablished.
• Take precautions if dental surgery is anticipated and anesthesia is required.
• Medical consultation may be required to assess disease control and patient's ability to tolerate stress.

Teach patient/family:

• Importance of good oral hygiene to prevent soft tissue inflammation
• Caution to prevent injury when using oral hygiene aids

When chronic dry mouth occurs, advise patient:

• To avoid mouth rinses with high alcohol content because of drying effects
• To use daily home fluoride products for anticaries effect
• To use sugarless gum, frequent sips of water, or saliva substitutes

---

carteolol HCl

(kar-tee'oe-lole)

Ocupress

Drug class.: β-adrenergic blocker

Action: Nonselective β-adrenergic blocking agent, reduces production of aqueous humor by unknown mechanisms

Uses: Chronic open-angle glaucoma, ocular hypertension

Dosage and routes:

• *Adult:* INSTILL 1 drop in affected eye bid

Available forms include: Sol 1%

Side effects/adverse reactions:

CNS: Ataxia, dizziness, lethargy
CV: Bradycardia, hypotension, dysrhythmias
GI: Nausea
RESP: ***Bronchospasm***
EENT: Eye irritation, conjunctivitis

Contraindications: Hypersensitivity, asthma, second- and third-degree heart block, right ventricular failure, congenital glaucoma (infants), COPD

Precautions: Pregnancy category C, lactation, elderly, children

Pharmacokinetics:
INSTILL: Onset 1 hr, peak effects 2 hr, duration of action 6-8 hr

Drug interactions of concern to dentistry:
• Avoid use of anticholinergic drugs, including atropine-like drugs, propantheline, and diazepam (benzodiazepine)

DENTAL CONSIDERATIONS
General:
• Check compliance of patient with prescribed drug regimen for glaucoma.
• Avoid dental light in patient's eyes; offer dark glasses for comfort.

Consultations:
• Consultation with physician may be needed if sedation or anesthesia is required.

---

carvedilol

(kar've-di-lole)
Coreg

Drug class.: Nonselective β-adrenergic blocking agent with α_1-blocking activity

---

Action: This is a nonselective β_1- and β_2-adrenergic antagonist. The antihypertensive mechanism of action is unclear, but it may include a reduction in cardiac output and inhibition of renin release by the renal juxtaglomerular apparatus. Peripheral resistance decreases with long-term use. The antianginal action (when indicated for this use) may be related to a decrease in myocardial oxygen demand and negative chronotropic and inotropic effects. The antiarrhythmic action (when indicated for this use) has been related to a reduction in spontaneous pacemaker firing and slowing of AV nodal conduction.

Uses: Essential hypertension, alone or with other antihypertensives, CHF, treatment of heart attack patient with left ventricular dysfunction; unlabeled use in angina

Dosage and routes:
Essential hypertension:
• *Adult:* PO initially 6.25 mg bid for 7-14 days, then 12.5 mg bid if required for 7-14 days, then 25 mg bid; take with food

CHF:
• *Adult:* PO individualize doses, correct fluid retention, start with 3.125 mg bid for 2 wk, patients must be closely monitored by physician; if tolerated doses may be increased to 6.25, 12.5, and 25 mg bid in successive intervals of 2 wk

Available forms include: Tabs 3.125, 6.25, 12.5, 25 mg

Side effects/adverse reactions:
ORAL: Dry mouth (<1%)
CNS: Dizziness, insomnia, somnolence, headache
CV: ***Heart block,*** orthostatic hypotension, syncope, bradycardia, peripheral edema, fatigue
GI: *Diarrhea,* hepatocellular injury, abdominal pain
RESP: ***Status asthmaticus,*** rhinitis, pharyngitis, dyspnea
HEMA: ***Thrombocytopenia***
GU: UTI, impotence
INTEG: Pruritus, rash
EENT: Blurred vision
MS: Back pain
META: Hypertriglyceridemia
MISC: Infection

Contraindications: Class IV heart failure, bronchial asthma, bronchospastic diseases, second- or third-degree AV block, cardiogenic shock or severe bradycardia, hypersensitivity

Precautions: Elderly, hepatic impairment, renal impairment, pregnancy category C, lactation, child <18 yr

Pharmacokinetics:

PO: Rapid oral absorption, hepatic metabolism, metabolites excreted in feces, 98% plasma protein binding

Drug interactions of concern to dentistry:

- Decreased hypotensive effect: indomethacin, NSAIDs
- Increased hypotension, myocardial depression: hydrocarbon inhalation anesthetics
- Hypertension, bradycardia: sympathomimetics (epinephrine, ephedrine)
- Bradycardia: fluoxetine, paroxetine

DENTAL CONSIDERATIONS

General:

- Monitor vital signs at every appointment because of cardiovascular side effects.
- After supine positioning, have patient sit upright for at least 2 min before standing to avoid orthostatic hypotension.
- Assess salivary flow as a factor in caries, periodontal disease, and candidiasis.
- Patients on chronic drug therapy may rarely have symptoms of blood dyscrasias, which can include infection, bleeding, and poor healing.
- Limit use of sodium-containing products, such as saline IV fluids, for those patients with a dietary salt restriction.
- Stress from dental procedures may compromise cardiovascular function; determine patient risk.
- Short appointments and a stress reduction protocol may be required for anxious patients.

Consultations:

- In a patient with symptoms of blood dyscrasias, request a medical consultation for blood studies and postpone dental treatment until normal values are reestablished.
- Medical consultation may be required to assess disease control and patient's ability to tolerate stress.

Teach patient/family:

- To report oral lesions, soreness, or bleeding to dentist

When chronic dry mouth occurs, advise patient:

- To avoid mouth rinses with high alcohol content because of drying effects
- Of need for daily home fluoride to prevent caries
- To use sugarless gum, frequent sips of water, or saliva substitutes

cefaclor

(sef'a-klor)

Ceclor, Ceclor CD

Drug class.: Antibiotic, cephalosporin (second generation)

Action: Inhibits bacterial cell wall synthesis, rendering cell wall osmotically unstable

Uses: For use in the treatment of the following infections when caused by susceptible strains of named microorganisms: otitis media caused by *S. pneumoniae, H. influenzae,* staphylococci, and *S. pyogenes;* lower respiratory tract infections caused by *S. pneumoniae, H. influenzae,* and *S. pyo-*

genes; pharyngitis and tonsillitis caused by *S. pyogenes;* urinary tract infections caused by *E. coli, P. mirabilis, Klebsiella* species, and coagulase-negative staphylococci; skin and skin structure infections caused by *S. aureus* and *S. pyogenes;* and in vitro activity against *Peptococcus, Peptostreptococcus,* and *Propionibacterium* (clinical significance unknown)

Dosage and routes:

• *Adult:* PO 250-500 mg q8h, not to exceed 4 g/day

• *Child >1 mo:* PO 20-40 mg/kg/qd in divided doses q8h, not to exceed 1 g/day

Available forms include: Caps 250, 500 mg; powder for oral susp 125, 187, 250, 375 mg/5 ml; ext rel tabs 375, 500 mg

Side effects/adverse reactions:

▼ *ORAL: Candidiasis, glossitis*

CNS: Headache, dizziness, weakness, paresthesia, fever, chills

GI: Diarrhea, anorexia, nausea, vomiting, pain, bleeding, increased AST/ALT, bilirubin, LDH, alk phosphatase, abdominal pain

RESP: Dyspnea

HEMA: ***Leukopenia, thrombocytopenia, agranulocytosis, neutropenia, lymphocytosis, eosinophilia, pancytopenia, hemolytic anemia,*** anemia

GU: ***Nephrotoxicity, renal failure,*** proteinuria, vaginitis, pruritus, candidiasis, increased BUN

INTEG: ***Anaphylaxis,*** rash, urticaria, dermatitis

Contraindications: Hypersensitivity to cephalosporins, infants <1 mo

Precautions: Hypersensitivity to penicillins, pregnancy category B, lactation, renal disease

Pharmacokinetics:

PO: Peak 0.5-1 hr, half-life 36-54 min; 25% bound by plasma proteins; 60%-85% eliminated unchanged in urine in 8 hr; crosses placenta; excreted in breast milk

Drug interactions of concern to dentistry:

• Decreased bactericidal effects: tetracyclines, erythromycins

• Increased and prolonged serum levels: probenecid

• Oral contraceptives: advise patient of a potential risk for decreased contraceptive action, to maintain compliance with oral contraceptive use while using antibiotics, and to consider the use of additional nonhormonal contraception

DENTAL CONSIDERATIONS

General:

• Take precautions regarding allergy to medication.

• Determine why the patient is taking the drug.

Consultations:

• Medical consultation may be required to assess disease control.

Teach patient/family:

• Importance of good oral hygiene to prevent soft tissue inflammation

• To avoid mouth rinses with high alcohol content because of drying effects and possible drug-drug reaction

When used for dental infection, advise patient:

• To report sore throat, oral burning sensation, fever, fatigue, any of which could indicate superinfection

• To take at prescribed intervals and complete dosage regimen

• To immediately notify the dentist if signs or symptoms of infection increase

cefadroxil

(sef-a-drox'il)

Duricef

Drug class.: Cephalosporin (first generation)

Action: Inhibits bacterial cell wall synthesis, rendering cell wall osmotically unstable

Uses: Gram-negative bacilli: *E. coli, P. mirabilis, Klebsiella* (UTI only); gram-positive organisms: *S. pneumoniae, S. pyogenes, S. aureus;* upper/lower respiratory tract, urinary tract, skin infections; otitis media; tonsillitis; particularly for UTI

Dosage and routes:

• *Adult:* PO 500 mg-1 g q12h; dosage reduction indicated in renal impairment (CrCl <50 ml/min); limit 4 g/day

• *Child:* PO 30 mg/kg/day or 15 mg/kg q12h

Bacterial endocarditis prophylaxis

• *Adult:* PO 2 g 1 hr before dental procedure

• *Child:* PO 50 mg/kg 1 hr before dental procedure, not to exceed the adult dose

Available forms include: Caps 500 mg; tabs 1 g; oral susp 125, 250, 500 mg/5 ml

Side effects/adverse reactions:

▼ *ORAL:* Candidiasis, glossitis

CNS: Headache, dizziness, weakness, paresthesia, fever, chills

GI: Diarrhea, anorexia, ***pseudomembranous colitis,*** nausea, vomiting, pain, bleeding, increased AST/ALT, bilirubin, LDH, alk phosphatase, abdominal pain

RESP: Dyspnea

HEMA: ***Leukopenia, thrombocytopenia, agranulocytosis, neutropenia, lymphocytosis, eosinophilia, pancytopenia, hemolytic anemia***

GU: ***Nephrotoxicity, renal failure,*** proteinuria, vaginitis, pruritus, candidiasis, increased BUN

INTEG: ***Anaphylaxis,*** rash, urticaria, dermatitis

Contraindications: Hypersensitivity to cephalosporins, infants <1 mo

Precautions: Hypersensitivity to penicillins, pregnancy category B, lactation, renal disease

Pharmacokinetics:

PO: Peak 1-1.5 hr, half-life 1-2 hr; 20% bound by plasma proteins; crosses placenta; excreted in breast milk

Drug interactions of concern to dentistry:

• Decreased bactericidal effects: tetracyclines, erythromycins

• Increased and prolonged serum levels: probenecid

• Oral contraceptives: advise patient of a potential risk for decreased contraceptive action, to maintain compliance with oral contraceptive use while using antibiotics, and to consider the use of additional nonhormonal contraception

DENTAL CONSIDERATIONS

General:

• Take precautions regarding allergy to medication.

• Determine why the patient is taking the drug.

Consultations:

• Medical consultation may be required to assess disease control.

Teach patient/family:

• Importance of good oral hygiene to prevent soft tissue inflammation

• To avoid mouth rinses with high

alcohol content because of drying effects and possible drug-drug reaction

When used for dental infection, advise patient:

- To report sore throat, oral burning sensation, fever, fatigue, any of which could indicate superinfection
- To take at prescribed intervals and complete dosage regimen
- To immediately notify the dentist if signs or symptoms of infection increase

---

cefazolin sodium

(sef-a'zoe-lin)

Ancef, Zolicef

Drug class.: Cephalosporin (first generation)

Action: Inhibits bacterial cell wall synthesis, rendering cell wall osmotically unstable

Uses: Indicated for use when caused by susceptible microorganisms: respiratory tract infections caused by *S. pneumoniae, Klebsiella* species, *H. influenzae, S. aureus,* and group A β-hemolytic streptococci; UTI infections caused by *E. coli, P. mirabilis, Klebsiella* species, and some enterobacter and enterococci; skin and skin structure infections caused by *S. aureus,* group A β-hemolytic streptococci; biliary tract infections caused by *E. coli, P. mirabilis, S. aureus, Klebsiella* species, and various strains of streptococci; bone and joint infections caused by *S. aureus;* genital infections caused by *E. coli, P. mirabilis, Klebsiella* species, and some enterococci; septicemia caused by *S. aureus, S. viridans, P. mirabilis, E. coli,* and *Klebsiella* species, group A β-hemolytic streptococci

Dosage and routes:

Life-threatening infections:

- *Adult:* IM/IV 1-1.5 g q6h
- *Child >1 mo:* IM/IV 100 mg/kg/day

Mild-to-moderate infections:

- *Adult:* IM/IV 500 mg-1 g q4-6h
- *Child >1 mo:* IM/IV 25-50 mg/kg/day in 3-4 equal doses

Dosage reduction indicated in renal impairment (CrCl <54 ml/min)

Bacterial endocarditis prophylaxis:

- *Adult:* IM or IV patients unable to take oral medications (caution allergy to amoxicillin) 1 g 30 min before dental procedure
- *Child:* IM or IV 25 mg/kg of body weight not to exceed the adult dose 30 min before dental procedure

Prosthetic joint prophylaxis (when indicated):

- *Adult:* IM or IV 1 g 1 hr before dental procedure

Available forms include: Inj IM/IV 250, 500 mg; 1, 5, 10 g

Side effects/adverse reactions:

▼ *ORAL:* Candidiasis

CNS: Headache, dizziness, weakness, paresthesia, fever, chills

GI: Diarrhea, anorexia, nausea, vomiting, pain, glossitis, bleeding, increased AST/ALT, bilirubin, LDH, alk phosphatase, abdominal pain

HEMA: ***Leukopenia, thrombocytopenia, agranulocytosis, anemia, neutropenia, lymphocytosis, eosinophilia, pancytopenia, hemolytic anemia***

GU: ***Nephrotoxicity, renal failure,*** proteinuria, vaginitis, pruritus, increased BUN
INTEG: ***Anaphylaxis,*** rash, urticaria, dermatitis
Contraindications: Hypersensitivity to cephalosporins, infants <1 mo
Precautions: Hypersensitivity to penicillins, pregnancy category B, lactation, renal disease
Pharmacokinetics: *IM:* Peak 0.5-2 hr, half-life 1.5-2.25 hr
IV: Peak 10 min, eliminated unchanged in urine 70%-86% protein bound

Drug interactions of concern to dentistry:
• Decreased bactericidal effects: tetracyclines, erythromycins
• Increased and prolonged serum levels: probenecid
• Oral contraceptives: advise patient of a potential risk for decreased contraceptive action, to maintain compliance with oral contraceptive use while using antibiotics, and to consider the use of additional nonhormonal contraception

DENTAL CONSIDERATIONS
General:
• Take precautions regarding allergy to medication.
• Determine why the patient is taking the drug.
Consultations:
• Medical consultation may be required to assess disease control.
Teach patient/family:
• Importance of good oral hygiene to prevent soft tissue inflammation
• To avoid mouth rinses with high alcohol content because of drying effects and possible drug-drug reaction

When used for dental infection, advise patient:
• To report sore throat, oral burning sensation, fever, fatigue, any of which could indicate superinfection
• To take at prescribed intervals and complete dosage regimen
• To immediately notify the dentist if signs or symptoms of infection increase

cefdinir

(sef'di-ner)
Omnicef
Drug class.: Cephalosporin (third generation)

Action: Inhibits bacterial cell wall synthesis, rendering cell wall osmotically unstable
Uses: Infections caused by susceptible strains of organisms that cause community-acquired pneumonia, acute exacerbation of chronic bronchitis, pharyngitis, tonsillitis, uncomplicated skin and skin structure infections, acute maxillary sinusitis, and acute bacterial otitis media
Dosage and routes:
• *Adult and child <13 yr:* PO dose depends on type of infection and patient; range is from 300 mg q12h to 600 mg q24h for 5-10 days taken with or without food
• *Child <6 mo-12 yr:* PO dose depends on type of infection and patient: range is from 7 mg/kg of body weight q12h to 14 mg/kg of body weight q24h for 5-10 days with or without food
Available forms include: Caps 300 mg; powder for oral suspension 125 mg/5 ml

Side effects/adverse reactions:
▼ *ORAL:* None reported, but most antiinfectives carry a risk of opportunistic candidiasis
CNS: Dizziness, insomnia, somnolence
GI: Diarrhea, nausea, abdominal pain, ***antibiotic-associated pseudomembranous colitis***
RESP: Dyspnea
HEMA: Eosinophilia
GU: Vaginal candidiasis
INTEG: Rash, cutaneous candidiasis
META: Abnormal liver function tests, elevated AST/ALT, bilirubin, potassium, and urinary pH
MS: Asthenia, ***anaphylaxis***
Contraindications: Hypersensitivity
Precautions: Hypersensitivity to other cephalosporins, penicillins, or penicillamine; renal impairment (need dose reduction); ulcerative colitis, pseudomembranous colitis, bleeding disorders, renal impairment, hemodialysis, β-lactamase–resistant organisms, pregnancy category B, not detected in breast milk, child <6 mo
Pharmacokinetics:
PO: Slow absorption, peak serum levels 2-4 hr, bioavailability ranges from 16%-25%, depending on dose and dose form, plasma protein binding 60%-70%, little to no metabolism, renal excretion
Drug interactions of concern to dentistry:
• Absorption retarded by iron salts, magnesium, or aluminum antacids: take antiinfective dose at least 2 hr before antacids or iron preparations
• Increased plasma levels: probenecid
• Oral contraceptives: advise patient of a potential risk for decreased contraceptive action, to maintain compliance with oral contraceptive use while using antibiotics, and to consider the use of additional nonhormonal contraception

DENTAL CONSIDERATIONS
General:
• Use precaution regarding allergy to medication.
• Determine why patient is taking the drug.
• Examine for oral manifestation of opportunistic infection.
Consultations:
• Medical consultation may be required to assess disease control.
Teach patient/family:
• Importance of good oral hygiene to prevent soft tissue inflammation

cefditoren pivoxil

(sef'di-toe-reen)
Spectracef
Drug class.: Cephalosporin, third generation

Action: Inhibits bacterial cell wall synthesis, rendering cell wall osmotically unstable
Uses: Mild to moderate infections in adults and children >12 yr; for susceptible microorganisms causing (1) acute bacterial exacerbation of chronic bronchitis (*H. influenzae, H. parainfluenzae, S. pneumoniae* (penicillin susceptible only), or *M. catarrhalis;* (2) pharyngitis/tonsillitis (*S. pyogenes*); (3) uncomplicated skin and skin-structure infections (*S. aureus* and *S. pyogenes*)

Dosage and routes:
Acute bacterial exacerbation of chronic bronchitis:
• *Adult and child >12 yr:* PO 400 mg bid × 10 days
Pharyngitis, tonsillitis, uncomplicated skin and skin structure infections:
• *Adult and child >12 yr:* PO 200 mg bid × 10 days
Severe renal failure:
• *Adult and child >12 yr:* PO not to exceed 200 mg daily
Moderate renal impairment:
• *Adult and child >12 yr:* PO not to exceed 200 mg bid
Available forms include: Tab 200 mg
Side effects/adverse reactions:
▼ *ORAL:* Dry mouth, ulceration, candidiasis, stomatitis, taste perversion
CNS: Headache, abnormal dreams, anorexia, dizziness, insomnia
CV: Peripheral edema
GI: Diarrhea, nausea, abdominal pain, dyspepsia, vomiting, ***pseudomembranous colitis***
HEMA: Leukopenia, thrombocytopenia, ↑ coagulation time
GU: Vaginal candidiasis, urinary frequency
EENT: Pharyngitis, rhinitis, sinusitis
INTEG: ***Toxic epidermal necrosis,*** pruritus, rash, urticaria, Stevens-Johnson syndrome, erythema multiforme
META: Hyperglycemia, altered liver function tests
MS: Asthenia, myalgia
MISC: ***Anaphylaxis,*** fever
Contraindications: Known allergy to cephalosporins, carnitine deficiency, milk protein hypersensitivity (tablets contain sodium caseinate)
Precautions: Penicillin-allergic patients, diarrhea, not for prolonged treatment, risk of resistance emergence, alteration of normal GI flora, decrease in prothrombin activity (long-term use, renal or hepatic impairment, taking anticoagulants), take with meals, pregnancy category B, lactation, safety and efficiency has not been established in children <12 yr, elderly patients with impaired renal function, reduce dose in severe renal impairment
Pharmacokinetics:
PO: Absorption enhanced by a fatty meal, peak plasma levels (fasting) 1.5-3 hr, hydrolyzed by esterases on absorption, low plasma protein (serum albumin) binding, parent drug excreted by glomerular filtration and tubular secretion
Drug interactions of concern to dentistry:
• Reduced absorption: concurrent use with antacids, H_2-receptor antagonist
• Increased and prolonged serum levels: probenecid
• Does not alter pharmacokinetics of ethinyl estradiol
DENTAL CONSIDERATIONS
General:
• Precaution regarding allergy to medication.
• Assess salivary flow as a factor in caries, periodontal disease, and candidiasis.
• Determine why patient is taking the drug.
• Consider semisupine chair position for patient comfort if GI side effects occur.
• Consult with patient's physician

if an acute dental infection occurs and another antiinfective is required.

• Examine for oral manifestation of opportunistic infection.

• Patients on chronic drug therapy may rarely have symptoms of blood dyscrasias, which can include infection, bleeding, and poor healing.

Consultations:

• Medical consultation may be required to assess disease control

• In a patient with symptoms of blood dyscrasias, request a medical consultation for blood studies and postpone treatment until normal values are reestablished.

Teach patient/family:

• Importance of good oral hygiene to prevent soft tissue inflammation and infection

When chronic dry mouth occurs, advise patient:

• To avoid mouth rinses with high alcohol content because of drying effects

• To use daily home fluoride products for anticaries effect

• To use sugarless gum, frequent sips of water, or saliva substitutes

cefepime HCl

(sef′e-pim)

Maxipime

Drug class.: Cephalosporin (fourth generation)

Action: Inhibits bacterial cell wall synthesis, rendering cell wall osmotically unstable

Uses: Urinary tract infections (uncomplicated and complicated), uncomplicated skin and soft tissue infections, complicated intraabdominal infections (in combination with metronidazole), and pneumonia caused by susceptible strains of microorganisms, including *S. pneumoniae;* febrile neutropenia

Dosage and routes:

Mild to moderate infections:

• *Adult:* IV/IM 0.5-1.0 g q12h depending on severity of the infection for 7-10 days; IM doses for mild infections only

Moderate to severe infections:

• *Adult:* IV 1.0-2.0 g q12h for 10 days depending on severity of the infection; adjust all doses in patients with renal impairment

Available forms include: Powder for injection vials 500 mg, 1, 2 g

Side effects/adverse reactions:

▼ *ORAL:* Candidiasis

CNS: Headache, light-headedness

CV: ***Phlebitis***

GI: Diarrhea, pseudomembranous colitis, vomiting, dyspepsia

GU: Vaginitis

EENT: Blurred vision

INTEG: Urticaria, pruritus, rash

META: Elevation of liver function tests

MISC: Local reactions, fever

Contraindications: Hypersensitivity to cephalosporins or penicillins

Precautions: Renal impairment, overgrowth of resistant organisms, colitis, monitor prothrombin, pregnancy category B, lactation, child <12 yr; renal insufficiency patient at risk for encephalopathy, myoclonus, seizures, renal failure

Pharmacokinetics:

IV: Peak levels vary with dose and occur within 0.5-1 hr, protein binding 20%, urinary excretion (85% of dose), therapeutic serum levels up to 8 hr

IM: Peak levels 0.5-1.5 hr

Drug interactions of concern to dentistry:

- Increased risk of nephrotoxicity, ototoxicity: aminoglycosides in high doses, furosemide

DENTAL CONSIDERATIONS

General:

- Precaution regarding allergy to medication.
- Determine why patient is taking the drug.
- Oral contraceptives: advise patient of a potential risk for decreased contraceptive action, to maintain compliance with oral contraceptive use while using antibiotics, and to consider the use of additional nonhormonal contraception

Consultation:

- Medical consultation may be required to assess disease control.

Teach patient/family:

- Importance of good oral hygiene to prevent soft tissue inflammation
- To report sore throat, oral burning sensation, fever, fatigue, any of which could indicate presence of a superinfection

---

cefixime

(sef-ix'eem)

Suprax

Drug class.: Cephalosporin (third generation)

Action: Inhibits bacterial cell wall synthesis, rendering cell wall osmotically unstable

Uses: Uncomplicated UTI *(E. coli, P. mirabilis),* pharyngitis and tonsillitis *(S. pyogenes),* otitis media *(H. influenzae, M. catarrhalis),* acute bronchitis, and acute exacerbations of chronic bronchitis *(S. pneumoniae, H. influenzae)*

Dosage and routes:

- *Adult:* PO 400 mg qd as a single dose or 200 mg q12h
- *Child >50 kg or >12 yr:* PO use adult dosage
- *Child <50 kg or <12 yr:* PO (oral susp) 8 mg/kg/day as a single dose or 4 mg/kg q12h

Available forms include: Tabs 200, 400 g; powder for oral susp 100 mg/5 ml

Side effects/adverse reactions:

▼ *ORAL:* Candidiasis, glossitis

CNS: Headache, dizziness, paresthesia, fever, chills, lethargy, fatigue, confusion

GI: Nausea, vomiting, diarrhea, anorexia, pain, bleeding, increased AST/ALT, bilirubin, LDH, alk phosphatase, heartburn, dysgeusia, flatulence

RESP: ***Bronchospasm,*** dyspnea, tight chest

HEMA: ***Leukopenia, thrombocytopenia, agranulocytosis, neutropenia, lymphocytosis, eosinophilia, pancytopenia, hemolytic anemia***

GU: ***Proteinuria, nephrotoxicity, renal failure,*** pyuria, dysuria, vaginitis, pruritus, increased BUN

INTEG: ***Exfoliative dermatitis, anaphylaxis,*** rash, urticaria

Contraindications: Hypersensitivity to cephalosporins, infants <6 mo

Precautions: Hypersensitivity to penicillins, pregnancy category B, lactation, renal disease

Pharmacokinetics:

PO: Peak 1 hr, half-life 3-4 hr; 65% bound by plasma proteins, 50% eliminated unchanged in urine; crosses placenta; excreted in breast milk

Drug interactions of concern to dentistry:

• Decreased bactericidal effects: tetracyclines, erythromycins

• Increased and prolonged serum levels: probenecid

• Oral contraceptives: advise patient of a potential risk for decreased contraceptive action, to maintain compliance with oral contraceptive use while using antibiotics, and to consider the use of additional nonhormonal contraception

DENTAL CONSIDERATIONS

General:

• Take precautions regarding allergy to medication.

• Determine why the patient is taking the drug.

Consultations:

• Medical consultation may be required to assess disease control.

Teach patient/family:

• Importance of good oral hygiene to prevent soft tissue inflammation

• To avoid mouth rinses with high alcohol content because of drying effects and possible drug-drug reaction

When used for dental infection, advise patient:

• To report sore throat, oral burning sensation, fever, fatigue, any of which could indicate superinfection

• To take at prescribed intervals and complete dosage regimen

• To immediately notify the dentist if signs or symptoms of infection increase

cefpodoxime proxetil

(cef-pode-ox'eem)

Vantin, Vantin Oral Suspension

Drug class.: Cephalosporin (third generation)

Action: Inhibits bacterial cell wall synthesis, rendering cell wall osmotically unstable

Uses: Upper/lower respiratory tract infections, pharyngitis (tonsillitis), gonorrhea, UTI, uncomplicated skin and skin structure infections caused by susceptible organisms, acute otitis media, community-acquired pneumonia, acute bacterial exacerbation of chronic bronchitis, anorectal infections in women

Dosage and routes:

• *Adult:* PO 100-200 mg q12h for 5 days; more severe infections 400 mg q12h

Otitis media:

• *Child 5 mo–12 yr:* PO 10 mg/kg/day in one dose (max daily dose 400 mg) or 5 mg/kg (max 200 mg/dose) bid for 5-10 days

Available forms include: Tabs 100, 200 mg; oral susp 50, 100 mg/5 ml in 50, 75, 100 ml

Side effects/adverse reactions:

▼ *ORAL:* Candidiasis, glossitis

CNS: Headache, dizziness, weakness, paresthesia, fever, chills

GI: Diarrhea, anorexia, nausea, vomiting, abdominal pain, bleeding, increased AST/ALT, bilirubin, LDH, alk phosphatase

RESP: Dyspnea

HEMA: ***Leukopenia, thrombocytopenia, agranulocytosis, neutropenia, lymphocytosis, eosinophilia, pancytopenia, hemolytic anemia***

GU: ***Nephrotoxicity, renal failure,***

proteinuria, vaginitis, pruritus, candidiasis, increased BUN
INTEG: ***Anaphylaxis,*** rash, urticaria, dermatitis
Contraindications: Hypersensitivity to cephalosporins
Precautions: Hypersensitivity to penicillins, lactation, renal disease, pregnancy category B, safety and efficacy in infants <5 mo not established
Pharmacokinetics:
PO: Half-life 2-3 hr; excreted unchanged in urine; alter dose with renal impairment
Drug interactions of concern to dentistry:
• Decreased bactericidal effects: tetracyclines, erythromycins
• Increased and prolonged serum levels: probenecid
• Oral contraceptives: advise patient of a potential risk for decreased contraceptive action, to maintain compliance with oral contraceptive use while using antibiotics, and to consider the use of additional nonhormonal contraception

DENTAL CONSIDERATIONS
General:
• Take precautions regarding allergy to medication.
• Determine why the patient is taking the drug.
Consultations:
• Medical consultation may be required to assess disease control.
Teach patient/family:
• Importance of good oral hygiene to prevent soft tissue inflammation
• To avoid mouth rinses with high alcohol content because of drying effects and possible drug-drug reaction

When used for dental infection, advise patient:
• To report sore throat, oral burning sensation, fever, fatigue, any of which could indicate superinfection
• To take at prescribed intervals and complete dosage regimen
• To immediately notify the dentist if signs or symptoms of infection increase

---

cefprozil monohydrate

(sef-pro'zil)
Cefzil
Drug class.: Cephalosporin (second generation)

Action: Inhibits bacterial cell wall synthesis, rendering cell wall osmotically unstable
Uses: Pharyngitis/tonsillitis, otitis media, secondary bacterial infection of acute bronchitis, sinusitis; acute bacterial sinusitis; acute bacterial exacerbation of chronic bronchitis and uncomplicated skin and skin structure infections
Dosage and routes:
Upper respiratory infections:
• *Adult and child ≥13 yr:* PO 250 mg q12h or 500 mg qd × 10 days
Otitis media:
• *Child 6 mo-12 yr:* PO 15 mg/kg q12h × 10 days
Lower respiratory infections:
• *Adult:* PO 500 mg bid × 10 days
Skin/skin structure infections:
• *Adult:* PO 250-500 mg q12h × 10 days
Available forms include: Tabs 250, 500 mg; susp 125, 250 mg/5 ml
Side effects/adverse reactions:
ORAL: Candidiasis, glossitis
CNS: Dizziness, headache, weakness, paresthesia, fever, chills

GI: ***Pseudomembranous colitis,*** diarrhea, nausea, vomiting, pain, anorexia, bleeding, increased AST/ALT, bilirubin, LDH, alk phosphatase, abdominal pain, flatulence
RESP: ***Anaphylaxis,*** dyspnea
HEMA: ***Leukopenia, thrombocytopenia, agranulocytosis, anemia, neutropenia, lymphocytosis, eosinophilia, pancytopenia, hemolytic anemia***
GU: ***Nephrotoxicity, proteinuria, increased BUN, renal failure, hematuria,*** vaginitis, genitoanal pruritus, candidiasis
INTEG: Rash, urticaria, dermatitis
Contraindications: Hypersensitivity to cephalosporins
Precautions: Pregnancy category B, lactation, elderly, hypersensitivity to penicillins, renal disease
Pharmacokinetics:
PO: Peak 6-10 hr, elimination half-life 25 hr; plasma protein binding 99%; extensively metabolized to an active metabolite
Drug interactions of concern to dentistry:
• Decreased bactericidal effects: tetracyclines, erythromycins
• Increased and prolonged serum levels: probenecid
• Oral contraceptives: advise patient of a potential risk for decreased contraceptive action, to maintain compliance with oral contraceptive use while using antibiotics, and to consider the use of additional nonhormonal contraception
DENTAL CONSIDERATIONS
General:
• Take precautions regarding allergy to medication.
• Determine why the patient is taking the drug.
• Examine for evidence of oral manifestations of blood dyscrasia (infection, bleeding, poor healing) and superinfection.
Consultations:
• Medical consultation may be required to assess disease control.
Teach patient/family:
• Importance of good oral hygiene to prevent soft tissue inflammation
• To avoid mouth rinses with high alcohol content because of drying effects and possible drug-drug reaction
When used for dental infection, advise patient:
• To report sore throat, oral burning sensation, fever, fatigue, any of which could indicate superinfection
• To take at prescribed intervals and complete dosage regimen
• To immediately notify the dentist if signs or symptoms of infection increase

---

ceftibuten

(sef-tye'byoo-ten)
Cedax, Cedax Oral Suspensioin
Drug class.: Cephalosporin (third generation)

Action: Inhibits bacterial cell wall synthesis, rendering cell wall osmotically unstable
Uses: Acute exacerbations of chronic bronchitis caused by susceptible strains of *H. influenzae, M. catarrhalis, S. pneumoniae;* acute otitis media caused by susceptible strains of *H. influenzae, M. catarrhalis, S. pyogenes;* pharyngitis and tonsillitis caused by *S. pyogenes*
Dosage and routes:
• *Adult and child >12 yr:* PO 400 mg qd × 10 days

• *Child:* SUSP 9 mg/kg qd × 10 days, susp administered 2 hr before or 1 hr after a meal

Available forms include: Caps 400 mg; susp 90, 180 mg/5 ml in 30, 60, 120 ml volumes

Side effects/adverse reactions:

▼ *ORAL:* Candidiasis, dry mouth (<1%)

CNS: Headache, dizziness, weakness, paresthesia, fever, chills

GI: Diarrhea, dyspepsia, nausea, vomiting, abdominal pain, bleeding, anorexia, increased AST/ALT, bilirubin, LDH, alk phosphatase, antibiotic-associated pseudomembranous colitis

RESP: Dyspnea

HEMA: ***Leukopenia, thrombocytopenia, agranulocytosis, neutropenia, lymphocytosis, eosinophilia, pancytopenia, hemolytic anemia***

GU: ***Nephrotoxicity, renal failure,*** proteinuria, vaginitis, pruritus, candidiasis, increased BUN

INTEG: Rash, pruritus, ***anaphylaxis,*** urticaria, dermatitis

Contraindications: Hypersensitivity to cephalosporins

Precautions: Hypersensitivity to penicillins, lactation, renal impairment, pregnancy category B, lactation, infants <6 mo, pseudomembranous colitis, oral suspension contains 1 g sucrose/5 ml

Pharmacokinetics:

PO: Half-life 2-3 hr; protein binding 6%, excreted mostly unchanged in urine; alter dose with renal impairment

Drug interactions of concern to dentistry:

• Decreased bactericidal effects: tetracyclines, erythromycins

• Increased and prolonged serum levels: probenecid

• Aminoglycosides increase nephrotoxic potential

• Oral contraceptives: advise patient of a potential risk for decreased contraceptive action, to maintain compliance with oral contraceptive use while using antibiotics, and to consider the use of additional nonhormonal contraception

DENTAL CONSIDERATIONS

General:

• Take precautions regarding allergy to medication.

• Assess salivary flow as factor in caries, periodontal disease, and candidiasis.

• Oral suspension contains sucrose; patient should rinse mouth after use.

• Determine why the patient is taking the drug.

Consultations:

• Medical consultation may be required to assess disease control.

Teach patient/family:

• Importance of good oral hygiene to prevent soft tissue inflammation

When used for dental infection, advise patient:

• To report sore throat, oral burning sensation, fever, fatigue, any of which could indicate superinfection

• To take at prescribed intervals and complete dosage regimen

• To immediately notify the dentist if signs or symptoms of infection increase

cefuroxime axetil

(sef-fyoor-ox'eem)

Ceftin, Kefurox, Zinacef

Drug class.: Cephalosporin (second generation)

Action: Inhibits bacterial cell wall synthesis, rendering cell wall osmotically unstable

Uses: Gram-negative bacilli *(H. influenzae, E. coli, Neisseria, P. mirabilis, Klebsiella);* gram-positive organisms *(S. pneumoniae, S. pyogenes, S. aureus);* serious lower respiratory tract, urinary tract, skin, gonococcal infections; septicemia; meningitis; early Lyme disease; acute bronchitis, acute bacterial maxillary sinusitis, pharyngitis, tonsillitis, impetigo, bone and joint infections

Dosage and routes:

- *Adult and child ≥13 yr:* PO 250 mg q12h, may increase to 500 mg q12h in serious infections; for severe infections give IV/IM according to package insert directions; dose range 750 mg-1.5 g q8h for 5-10 days

Urinary tract infections:

- *Adult:* PO 125 mg q12h, may increase to 250 q12h if needed × 7-10 days

Pharyngitis or tonsillitis:

- *Child 3 mo-12 yr:* PO oral susp 20 mg/kg/day in two equal doses

Otitis media:

- *Child 3 mo-12 yr:* PO oral susp 30 mg/kg/day in two equal doses × 10 days

Available forms include: Tabs 125, 250, 500 mg; powder for inj 750 mg and 1.5, 7.5 g; oral susp 125 mg/5 ml, 250 mg/5 ml in 50 ml and 100 ml

Side effects/adverse reactions:

▼ *ORAL:* Candidiasis, glossitis

CNS: Headache, dizziness, weakness, paresthesia, fever, chills

GI: Nausea, vomiting, diarrhea, anorexia, pseudomembranous colitis, bleeding, increased AST/ALT, bilirubin, LDH, alk phosphatase, abdominal pain

RESP: ***Anaphylaxis***

HEMA: ***Leukopenia, thrombocytopenia, agranulocytosis, neutropenia, lymphocytosis, eosinophilia, pancytopenia, hemolytic anemia***

GU: ***Nephrotoxicity, renal failure,*** proteinuria, vaginitis, pruritus, candidiasis, increased BUN

INTEG: Rash, urticaria, dermatitis

Contraindications: Hypersensitivity to cephalosporins, infants <3 mo

Precautions: Hypersensitivity to penicillins, pregnancy category B, lactation, renal disease

Pharmacokinetics:

PO: Half-life 1-2 hr in normal renal function, 65% excreted unchanged in urine

Drug interactions of concern to dentistry:

- Decreased bactericidal effects: tetracyclines, erythromycins
- Increased and prolonged serum levels: probenecid
- Oral contraceptives: advise patient of a potential risk for decreased contraceptive action, to maintain compliance with oral contraceptive use while using antibiotics, and to consider the use of additional nonhormonal contraception

DENTAL CONSIDERATIONS

General:

• Take precautions regarding allergy to medication.

• Determine why the patient is taking the drug.

Consultations:

• Medical consultation may be required to assess disease control.

Teach patient/family:

• Importance of good oral hygiene to prevent soft tissue inflammation

• To avoid mouth rinses with high alcohol content because of drying effects and possible drug-drug reaction

When used for dental infection, advise patient:

• To report sore throat, oral burning sensation, fever, fatigue, any of which could indicate superinfection

• To take at prescribed intervals and complete dosage regimen

• To immediately notify the dentist if signs or symptoms of infection increase

---

celecoxib

(sel-e-cox'ib)

Celebrex

Drug class.: Nonsteroidal antiinflammatory, analgesic

Action: May be related to a selective inhibition of inducible cyclooxygenase 2 (COX 2) enzymes preventing the synthesis of prostaglandins

Uses: Relief of signs and symptoms of osteoarthritis and relief of signs and symptoms of rheumatoid arthritis in adults; also approved for reducing the number of intestinal polyps in patients with familial adenomatous polyposis; acute pain and primary dysmenorrhea

Dosage and routes:

Osteoarthritis:

• *Adult:* PO 200 mg/day as a single dose or 100 mg bid

Rheumatoid arthritis:

• *Adult:* PO 100-200 mg bid

Familial adenomatosis polyposis:

• *Adult:* PO 400 mg bid with food

Acute pain and primary dysmenorrhea:

• *Adult:* PO initial dose 400 mg; can be followed by 200 mg later in day if required, then 200 mg bid prn

Available forms include: Caps 100, 200 mg

Side effects/adverse reactions:

▼ *ORAL: Dry mouth, stomatitis, taste alteration*

CNS: Headache, dizziness, insomnia, anxiety

CV: May aggravate hypertension, palpitation, syncope, ***CHF***

GI: Abdominal pain, diarrhea, dyspepsia, flatulence, nausea, ***severe GI bleeding***

RESP: Pharyngitis, URI, aggravates bronchospasm

HEMA: Anemia, ecchymosis, ***thrombocytopenia***

GU: UTI, ***acute renal failure***

EENT: Rhinitis, sinusitis, tinnitus, deafness, blurred vision

INTEG: Skin rash, pruritus, urticaria, Sweet's syndrome (acute febrile neutrophilic dermatosis)

META: Hyperchloremia, hypophosphatemia, elevated BUN, elevated liver enzymes (AST, ALT)

MS: Myalgia, arthralgia

MISC: ***Anaphylaxis,*** back pain

Contraindications: Hypersensitivity, allergy to sulfonamides, patients who have experienced asthma, urticaria, or allergic-type reactions to ASA or NSAIDs

Precautions: Geriatric patients weighing <50 kg use lowest dose, children <18 yr, severe hepatic or renal impairment, upper active GI disease, GI bleeding, avoid in late pregnancy (category D after 34 wk), pregnancy category C, lactation, dehydrated patients, heart failure, hypertension, asthma, patients suspected or known to be poor CYP2C9 isoenzyme metabolizers

Pharmacokinetics:

PO: Fatty meal delays absorption, peak plasma levels 3 hr, half-life 11 hr, metabolism (CYP450 2C9 isoenzymes), metabolites excreted in feces (57%) and urine (27%)

Drug interactions of concern to dentistry:

- Increased plasma levels: fluconazole
- Increased risk of GI bleeding: long-duration NSAIDs, aspirin (except low doses), oral glucocorticoids, alcoholism, smoking, older age, and generally poor health
- Increased plasma levels of lithium
- Possible risk of increased INR in elderly patients taking warfarin
- Possible reduction in blood pressure control: ACE inhibitors
- First-time users of SSRIs also taking NSAIDs may have a higher risk of GI side effects; until more data are available, it may be advisable to avoid use of NSAIDs in these patients (*Br J Clin Pharmacol* 55:591-595, 2003)

DENTAL CONSIDERATIONS

General:

- Patients on chronic drug therapy may rarely have symptoms of blood dyscrasias, which can include infection, bleeding, and poor healing.
- Assess salivary flow as a factor in caries, periodontal disease, and candidiasis.
- Consider semisupine chair position for patient comfort because of disease and GI side effects of drug.

Teach patient/family:

- Importance of good oral hygiene to prevent soft tissue inflammation
- Importance of updating health and drug history if physician makes any changes in evaluation or drug regimens
- Use of electric toothbrush if patient has difficulty holding conventional devices

When chronic dry mouth occurs, advise patient:

- To avoid mouth rinses with high alcohol content because of drying effects
- To use daily home fluoride products for anticaries effect
- To use sugarless gum, frequent sips of water, or saliva substitutes

cephalexin/cephalexin HCl monohydrate

(sef-a-lex'in)

Cephalexin: *Biocef, Keflex*

Novo-Lexin, PMS-Cephalexin

Cephalexin HCl monohydrate: Keftab

Drug class.: Cephalosporin (first generation)

Action: Inhibits bacterial cell wall synthesis, rendering cell wall osmotically unstable

Uses: Use for the following infections when caused by susceptible microorganisms: respiratory tract infections caused by *S. pneumo-*

niae and group A β-hemolytic streptococci; otitis media caused by *S. pneumoniae, H. influenzae, M. catarrhalis,* staphylococci, and streptococci; skin and skin structure infections caused by staphylococci and streptococci; bone infections caused by staphylococci and *P. mirabilis;* and GU tract infections caused by *E. coli, P. mirabilis,* and *K. pneumoniae*

Dosage and routes:

• *Adult:* PO 250 mg q6h, or 500 mg q12h; up to 4 g/day

• *Child up to 40 kg:* PO 6.25-50 mg/kg/day in 4 equal doses; dose range varies with type of infection and severity

Moderate skin infections:

• *Adult:* PO 500 mg q12h

Severe infections:

• *Adult:* PO 500 mg-1 g q6h

• *Child:* PO 50-100 mg/kg/day in 4 equal doses

Otitis media:

• *Child up to 40 kg:* PO 75-100 mg/kg/day in 4 equal doses; dosage reduction indicated in renal impairment (CrCl <50 ml/min)

Bacterial endocarditis prophylaxis:

• *Adult:* PO 2 g 1 hr before dental procedure for those patients unable to take amoxicillin

• *Child:* PO 50 mg/kg of body weight 1 hr before dental procedure, not to exceed the adult dose for those patients unable to take amoxicillin

Available forms include: Caps 250, 500 mg; tabs 250, 500 mg, 1 g; oral susp 125, 250 mg/5 ml; monohydrate tabs 500 mg

Side effects/adverse reactions:

▼ *ORAL:* Candidiasis, glossitis

CNS: Headache, dizziness, weakness, paresthesia, fever, chills

GI: Nausea, vomiting, diarrhea, anorexia, ***pseudomembranous colitis,*** bleeding, increased AST/ALT, bilirubin, LDH, alk phosphatase, abdominal pain

RESP: ***Anaphylaxis,*** dyspnea

HEMA: ***Leukopenia, thrombocytopenia, agranulocytosis, neutropenia, lymphocytosis, eosinophilia, pancytopenia, hemolytic anemia***

GU: ***Nephrotoxicity, renal failure,*** proteinuria, vaginitis, pruritus, candidiasis, increased BUN

INTEG: Rash, urticaria, dermatitis

Contraindications: Hypersensitivity to cephalosporins, infants <1 mo

Precautions: Hypersensitivity to penicillins, pregnancy category B, lactation, renal disease

Pharmacokinetics:

PO: Peak 1 hr, duration 6-8 hr, half-life 30-72 min; 5%-15% bound by plasma proteins, 90%-100% eliminated unchanged in urine; crosses placenta; excreted in breast milk

Drug interactions of concern to dentistry:

• Decreased bactericidal effects: tetracyclines, erythromycins

• Increased and prolonged serum levels: probenecid

• Oral contraceptives: advise patient of a potential risk for decreased contraceptive action, to maintain compliance with oral contraceptive use while using antibiotics, and to consider the use of additional nonhormonal contraception

DENTAL CONSIDERATIONS

General:

• Take precautions regarding allergy to medication.

• Determine why the patient is taking the drug.

Consultations:

• Medical consultation may be required to assess disease control.

Teach patient/family:

• Importance of good oral hygiene to prevent soft tissue inflammation

• To avoid mouth rinses with high alcohol content because of drying effects and possible drug-drug reaction

When used for dental infection, advise patient:

• To report sore throat, oral burning sensation, fever, fatigue, any of which could indicate superinfection

• To take at prescribed intervals and complete dosage regimen

• To immediately notify the dentist if signs or symptoms of infection increase

---

cephradine

(sef′ra-deen)

Velosef

Drug class.: Cephalosporin (first generation)

Action: Inhibits bacterial cell wall synthesis, rendering cell wall osmotically unstable

Uses: Gram-negative bacilli: *H. influenzae, E. coli, P. mirabilis, Klebsiella;* gram-positive organisms: *S. pneumoniae, S. pyogenes, S. aureus;* serious respiratory tract, urinary tract, skin, and skin structure infections; otitis media

Dosage and routes:

• *Adult:* IM/IV 500 mg–1 g q4-6h, not to exceed 8 g/day; PO 250 mg q6h or 500 mg q12h; limit PO dose to 4 g/day

• *Child >9 mo:* PO 25-50 mg/kg/day, divided into equal doses q6-12h

• *Child >1 yr:* IV/IM 50-100 mg/kg/day in 4 equal doses

Available forms include: Powder for inj IM/IV 250, 500 mg and 1, 2 g; caps 250, 500 mg; oral susp 125, 250 mg/5 ml in 100 ml and 200 ml

Side effects/adverse reactions:

▼ *ORAL:* Candidiasis, glossitis

CNS: Headache, dizziness, weakness, paresthesia, fever, chills

GI: Nausea, vomiting, diarrhea, anorexia, ***pseudomembranous colitis,*** bleeding, increased AST/ALT, bilirubin, LDH, alk phosphatase, abdominal pain

RESP: ***Anaphylaxis,*** dyspnea

HEMA: ***Leukopenia, thrombocytopenia, agranulocytosis, neutropenia, lymphocytosis, eosinophilia, pancytopenia, hemolytic anemia***

GU: ***Nephrotoxicity, renal failure,*** proteinuria, vaginitis, pruritus, candidiasis, increased BUN

INTEG: Rash, urticaria, dermatitis

Contraindications: Hypersensitivity to cephalosporins, infants <9 mo

Precautions: Hypersensitivity to penicillins, pregnancy category B, lactation, renal disease

Pharmacokinetics:

PO: Peak 1 hr

IV: Peak 5 min

IM: Peak 1 hr

Half-life 0.75-1.5 hr; 20% bound by plasma proteins, 80%-90%

eliminated unchanged in urine; crosses placenta; excreted in breast milk

Drug interactions of concern to dentistry:

• Decreased bactericidal effects: tetracyclines, erythromycins

• Increased and prolonged serum levels: probenecid

• Oral contraceptives: advise patient of a potential risk for decreased contraceptive action, to maintain compliance with oral contraceptive use while using antibiotics, and to consider the use of additional nonhormonal contraception

DENTAL CONSIDERATIONS

General:

• Take precautions regarding allergy to medication.

• Determine why the patient is taking the drug.

Consultations:

• Medical consultation may be required to assess disease control.

Teach patient/family:

• Importance of good oral hygiene to prevent soft tissue inflammation

• To avoid mouth rinses with high alcohol content because of drying effects and possible drug-drug reaction

When used for dental infection, advise patient:

• To report sore throat, oral burning sensation, fever, fatigue, any of which could indicate superinfection

• To take at prescribed intervals and complete dosage regimen

• To immediately notify the dentist if signs or symptoms of infection increase

cetirizine hydrochloride

(se-ti'ra-zeen)

Zyrtec

Reactine

Drug class.: Antihistamine

Action: Competitive antagonist for peripheral H_1-receptors

Uses: Treatment of symptoms of seasonal allergic rhinitis, perennial allergic rhinitis, chronic urticaria

Dosage and routes:

• *Adult and child >12 yr:* PO 5-10 mg bid, limit 10 mg/day

• *Child 6-11 yr:* PO 5-10 mg once daily

• *Child 2-5 yr:* PO 2.5 mg once daily, can be increased to 5 mg once day or 2.5 mg bid if required

• *Infants 6 mo and older:* SYR if required

Available forms include: Tabs 5, 10 mg; syrup 5 mg/5 ml in 120 ml and pints

Side effects/adverse reactions:

ORAL: Dry mouth (5%), taste alteration, tongue edema, orofacial dyskinesia (all rare)

CNS: Sedation, drowsiness, dizziness, headache, somnolence, depression

CV: Palpitation, tachycardia, hypertension, cardiac failure

GI: Constipation, diarrhea

HEMA: ***Hemolytic anemia, thrombocytopenia***

GU: Difficult urination, urinary retention, dysmenorrhea

EENT: Pharyngitis, dry nose or throat, tinnitus, earache

INTEG: Pruritus, rash, dry skin

MS: Myalgia, arthralgia

MISC: Photosensitivity

Contraindications: Hypersensitivity to cetirizine or hypersensitivity to hydroxyzine

Precautions: Renal impairment (requires dose reduction), elderly, glaucoma, urinary obstruction, pregnancy category B, lactation

Pharmacokinetics:

PO: Peak plasma levels 1 hr, duration up to 24 hr, half-life 8-11 hr; highly protein bound; rapid oral absorption, minimal metabolism; excreted mostly unchanged in urine

Drug interactions of concern to dentistry:

• No drug interactions reported, but should be similar to other antihistamines; anticipate increased sedation with other CNS depressants and increased anticholinergic effects with anticholinergic drugs

DENTAL CONSIDERATIONS

General:

• Assess salivary flow as factor in caries, periodontal disease, and candidiasis.

Teach patient/family:

When chronic dry mouth occurs, advise patient:

• To avoid mouth rinses with high alcohol content because of drying effects

• To use daily home fluoride products for anticaries effect

• To use sugarless gum, frequent sips of water, or saliva substitutes

cevimeline HCl

(ce-vi-me'leen)

Evoxac

Drug class.: Cholinergic (muscarinic) agonist

Action: Acts directly on cholinergic (muscarinic) receptor sites in the CNS and in exocrine glands (i.e., salivary glands); also binds to cholinergic receptors in the GI and GU tracts; derivative of acetylcholine; peripheral effects may resemble pilocarpine

Uses: Treatment of symptoms of dry mouth associated with Sjögren's syndrome

Dosage and routes:

• *Adult:* PO 30 mg tid (higher doses have not been demonstrated to provide greater effects)

Available forms include: Caps 30 mg

Side effects/adverse reactions:

▼ *ORAL: Salivation,* facial edema (rare), salivary gland enlargement, ulcerative stomatitis

CNS: Confusion, headache, dizziness, fatigue, insomnia

CV: Palpitation, chest pain

GI: Diarrhea, nausea, abdominal pain, vomiting, dyspepsia

GU: Urinary frequency, sinusitis, UTI, polyuria

RESP: Rhinitis, coughing, bronchitis, URI

EENT: Pharyngitis, conjunctivitis, bronchitis, abnormal vision, eye pain, ear pain, visual blurring, lacrimation

INTEG: Diaphoresis, rash, allergy, erythematous rash

MS: Back pain, arthralgia

MISC: Asthenia, pain, skeletal pain

Contraindications: Hypersensitivity, uncontrolled asthma, acute iritis, narrow-angle glaucoma

Precautions: Has the potential to alter heart rate or cardiac conduction; use with care in cardiovascular disease, asthma, bronchitis, COPD, seizure disorders, Parkinson's disease, urinary tract/bladder obstruction, cholecystitis, cholangitis, biliary obstruction, GI ulcers, pregnancy category C, lactation, children (no data), history of adverse effects to other cholinergic agonists

Pharmacokinetics:

PO: Good oral absorption, peak concentration in 1.5-2 hr, <20% bound to plasma proteins, half-life 4-6 hr, hepatic metabolism by cytochrome P-450 (CYP2D6 and CYP3A3/4), renal excretion (97%)

Drug interactions of concern to dentistry:

• Use with caution in patients taking β-adrenergic blockers: possible conduction disturbances.

• There are no specific data on dental drug interactions; however, use caution with other cholinergic agonist.

• There is always the possibility that a cholinergic antagonist could interfere with this drug's action.

• Although there are no supporting data, use with caution in patients taking drugs that inhibit cytochrome P-450 (CYP3A3/4 and CYP2D6 isoenzymes); see Appendix I.

DENTAL CONSIDERATIONS

General:

• Assess salivary flow as a factor in caries, periodontal disease, and candidiasis.

• Place on frequent recall to assess effectiveness.

• Consider semisupine chair position for patient comfort if GI side effects occur.

Consultations:

• Medical consultation may be required to assess disease control.

• Medical consultation may be necessary before prescribing for those patients with cardiovascular or respiratory disease.

Teach patient/family:

• That this drug may cause visual disturbances, especially with night driving, which may impair driving safety

• That the patient should drink extra fluids (water) to compensate for excessive sweating

When chronic dry mouth occurs, advise patient:

• To avoid mouth rinses with high alcohol content because of drying effects

• Of need for daily home fluoride to prevent caries

• To use sugarless gum, frequent sips of water, or saliva substitutes

---

chloral hydrate

(klor-al hye'drate)

Aquachloral Supprettes

♣ Novo-Chlorhydrate, PMS-Chloral Hydrate

Drug class.: Sedative-hypnotic, chloral derivative

Controlled Substance Schedule IV, Schedule F

Action: Active metabolite, trichloroethanol, produces mild CNS depression

Uses: Sedation, insomnia

Dosage and routes:

Sedative-hypnotic:

• *Adult:* PO/REC 250 mg tid pc; preoperative 500 mg-1 g 30 min before surgery or bedtime

• *Child:* PO 25-50 mg/kg of body weight/day not to exceed 1 g/dose

Insomnia-hypnotic dose:

• *Adult:* PO/REC 500 mg-1g 0.5 hr hs

Available forms include: Caps 500 mg; syr 250, 500 mg/5 ml; supp 325, 500, 648 mg

Side effects/adverse reactions:

▼ *ORAL: Unpleasant taste, mucosal irritation*

CNS: Drowsiness, dizziness, stimulation, nightmares, ataxia, hangover (rare), light-headedness, headache, paranoia

CV: Hypotension, dysrhythmias

GI: Nausea, vomiting, flatulence, diarrhea, ***gastric necrosis***

RESP: ***Depression***

HEMA: ***Eosinophilia, leukopenia***

INTEG: Rash, urticaria, angioedema, fever, purpura, eczema

Contraindications: Hypersensitivity to this drug, severe renal disease, severe hepatic disease, GI disorders (oral forms), gastritis

Precautions: Severe cardiac disease, depression, suicidal individuals, asthma, intermittent porphyria, pregnancy category C, lactation, elderly; no specific reversal agent available, use extreme caution in dose calculation when used in pediatric patients for sedation

Pharmacokinetics:

PO: Onset 0.5-1 hr, duration 4-8 hr

REC: Onset slow, duration 4-6 hr; metabolized by liver; excreted by kidneys (inactive metabolite) and in feces; crosses placenta; excreted in breast milk; metabolite is highly protein bound

Drug interactions of concern to dentistry:

• Increased action of both drugs: alcohol, all CNS depressants, including nitrous oxide

DENTAL CONSIDERATIONS

General:

• Consider semisupine chair position for patient comfort because of GI effects of drug.

• Administer syrup in juice or beverage to mask taste and reduce GI upset.

• Contraindicated for use in patients with GI ulcerative disease.

• Have someone drive patient to and from dental office when used for conscious sedation.

• Geriatric patients are more susceptible to drug effects; use lower dose.

• Psychologic and physical dependence may occur with chronic administration.

---

chlordiazepoxide HCl

(klor-dye-az-e-pox'ide)

Libritabs, Librium, Mitran, Reposans-10

✤ Apo-Chlordiazepoxide, Novo-Poxide

Drug class.: Benzodiazepine antianxiety

Controlled Substance Schedule IV

Action: Produces CNS depression by interacting with a benzodiazepine receptor to facilitate the action of the inhibitory neurotransmitter γ-aminobutyric acid (GABA)

Uses: Short-term management of anxiety, acute alcohol withdrawal, preoperatively for relaxation

Dosage and routes:

Mild anxiety:

• *Adult:* PO 5-10 mg tid-qid

• *Child >6 yr:* PO 5 mg bid-qid, not to exceed 10 mg bid-tid

Severe anxiety:

• *Adult:* PO 20-25 mg tid-qid

Preoperatively:
• *Adult:* PO 5-10 mg tid-qid on day before surgery; IM 50-100 mg 1 hr before surgery
Alcohol withdrawal:
• *Adult:* PO/IM/IV 50-100 mg, not to exceed 300 mg/day
Available forms include: Caps 5, 10, 25 mg; tabs 10, 25 mg; powder for IM inj 100 mg
Side effects/adverse reactions:
▼ *ORAL:* Dry mouth
CNS: Dizziness, drowsiness, confusion, headache, anxiety, tremors, stimulation, fatigue, depression, insomnia, hallucinations
CV: Orthostatic hypotension, ***ECG changes, tachycardia,*** hypotension
GI: Constipation, nausea, vomiting, anorexia, diarrhea
EENT: Blurred vision, tinnitus, mydriasis
INTEG: Rash, dermatitis, itching
Contraindications: Hypersensitivity to benzodiazepines, narrow-angle glaucoma, psychosis, pregnancy category D, child <18 yr; ritonavir, indinavir, saquinavir
Precautions: Elderly, debilitated, hepatic disease, renal disease
Pharmacokinetics:
PO: Onset 30 min, peak plasma levels 0.5-4 hr, plasma protein binding 96%, duration 4-6 hr, half-life 5-30 hr; metabolized by liver; active metabolites excreted by kidneys; crosses placenta, breast milk
Drug interactions of concern to dentistry:
• Delayed elimination: erythromycin
• Increased CNS depression: CNS depressants, alcohol, disulfram, nefazodone
• Increased serum levels and prolonged effects of benzodiazepines: ketoconazole, itraconazole, fluconazole, miconazole (systemic), cimetidine, fluvoxamine, omeprazole, rifabutin, rifampin (see Appendix I)
• Contraindicated with ritonavir, indinavir, saquinavir (see Appendix I)
• Possible increase in CNS side effects: Kava (herb)
• Decreased plasma levels: St. John's wort (herb)

DENTAL CONSIDERATIONS
General:
• After supine positioning, have patient sit upright for at least 2 min to avoid orthostatic hypotension.
• Assess salivary flow as a factor in caries, periodontal disease, and candidiasis.
• Psychologic and physical dependence may occur with chronic administration.
• Geriatric patients are more susceptible to drug effects; use lower dose.
• Have someone drive patient to and from dental office if used for conscious sedation.
Consultations:
• Medical consultation may be required to assess disease control.
Teach patient/family:
• Importance of good oral hygiene to prevent soft tissue inflammation
• To avoid mouth rinses with high alcohol content because of drying effects

chlorhexidine gluconate

(klor-hex'i-deen)

Peridex, Perio

♣ GardOro-Clense

Drug class.: Antiinfective–oral rinse

Action: Adsorbed on tooth surfaces, dental plaque, and oral mucosa; a sustained reduction of plaque organisms occurs

Uses: Treatment of gingivitis; unlabeled use: acute aphthous ulcers and denture stomatitis

Dosage and routes:

Gingivitis:

• *Adult:* Rinse 15 ml for 30 sec bid after brushing and flossing teeth; expectorate after rinsing

Denture stomatitis: Soak dentures for 1-2 min bid, with patient following oral rinse instructions

Available forms include: Oral rinse, 0.12% in 16 oz bottles

Side effects/adverse reactions:

▼ *ORAL: Staining of teeth, tongue, and restorations; increased calculus formation; taste alteration;* mucosal desquamation and irritation; transient parotitis

Contraindications: Hypersensitivity

Precautions: Pregnancy category B, lactation, efficacy not established for children <18 yr, not intended for periodontitis

Pharmacokinetics: Approximately 30% of chlorhexidine is retained in the oral cavity and slowly released; poorly absorbed orally

Drug interactions of concern to dentistry:

• Disulfiram-like effects resulting from alcohol content: Antabuse, metronidazole

DENTAL CONSIDERATIONS

General:

• Perform dental examination and prophylaxis/scaling/root planing before starting rinse.

• Place on frequent recall because of oral side effects.

• Use discretion when prescribing to patients with anterior facial restorations with rough surfaces or margins.

Teach patient/family:

• Instruct patient to eat, brush, and floss before using rinse

• Do not rinse with water after using chlorhexidine

• Not to dilute solution; not to swallow solution

• Inform patient of oral side effects

chlorhexidine gluconate chip

(klor-hex'i-deen)

Perio Chip

Drug class.: Antiinfective

Action: Interferes with the integrity of the bacterial cell membrane, causing leakage of the intracellular components; penetrates into the cell, precipitates the cytoplasm, and the cell dies; effective against numerous supragingival and subgingival bacteria

Uses: Adjunct to scaling and root planing for reduction of the subgingival bacterial flora

Dosage and routes:

• *Adult:* Insert chip into a periodontal pocket with probing depth ≥5 mm; up to eight chips may be inserted per single visit; treatment recommended once every 3 mo in pockets ≥5 mm in depth; if chip dislodges within 48 hr of placement, replace with new chip; do not replace chips lost after 48 hr, but reevaluate in 3 mo; if chip is dislodged 7 days or more after placement, consider this a full course of treatment

Available forms include: CHIP 2.5 mg

Side effects/adverse reactions:

▼ *ORAL: Localized pain, tenderness, aching, throbbing, toothache*

NOTE: All other side effects reported did not differ from placebo chip

Contraindications: Hypersensitivity

Precautions: Not recommended for acutely abscessed periodontal pocket, pregnancy category C, use in children not established

Pharmacokinetics:

TOP: 40% of chlorhexidine released in first 24 hr, remainder released over 7-10 days; no detectable plasma levels

Drug interactions of concern to dentistry:

• None reported

DENTAL CONSIDERATIONS

General:

• Do not brush or use dental floss at site of chip placement.

Teach patient/family:

• To notify dentist immediately if chip is dislodged or if pain, swelling, or other symptoms occur

chloroquine HCl/ chloroquine phosphate

(klor'oh-kwin)

Aralen HCl, Aralen Phosphate

Drug class.: Antimalarial

Action: Inhibits parasite replications, transcription of DNA to RNA by forming complexes with DNA of parasite; unapproved: juvenile arthritis, rheumatoid arthritis, discoid or systemic lupus erythematosus, solar urticaria

Uses: Malaria caused by *P. vivax, P. malariae, P. ovale, P. falciparum* (some strains); rheumatoid arthritis; amebiasis

Dosage and routes:

Malaria suppression:

• *Adult:* IM 200-250 mg, may be repeated in 6 hr, limit 1 g/day; PO 500 mg on exactly the same day each week (500 mg phosphate = 300 mg base)

• *Child:* IM or SC 4.4 mg/kg, may be repeated in 6 hr; dose limit 12.5 mg/kg/day; PO 5 mg/kg weekly, calculated as base, on same day each week; not to exceed adult dose

Amebiasis:

• *Adult:* PO 1 g qd × 2 wk, then 500 mg qd × 2-3 wk

Rheumatoid arthritis:

• *Adult:* PO up to 4 mg/kg/day

Available forms include: Tabs 250, 500 mg; inj IM 50 mg/ml

Side effects/adverse reactions:

▼ *ORAL: Stomatitis, discolored mucosa, lichenoid drug reaction*

CNS: ***Convulsion,*** headache, stimulation, fatigue, irritability, bad dreams, dizziness, confusion, psychosis, decreased reflexes

CV: Hypotension, heart block, asystole with syncope, ECG changes
GI: Nausea, vomiting, anorexia, diarrhea, cramps, weight loss
HEMA: ***Thrombocytopenia, agranulocytosis, hemolytic anemia, leukopenia***
EENT: Blurred vision, corneal changes, retinal changes, difficulty focusing, tinnitus, vertigo, deafness, photophobia, corneal edema
INTEG: ***Exfoliative dermatitis,*** alopecia, pruritus, pigmentary changes, skin eruptions, lichenoid eruptions, eczema

Contraindications: Hypersensitivity, retinal field changes, porphyria, children (long-term use)

Precautions: Pregnancy category C, children, blood dyscrasias, severe GI disease, neurologic disease, alcoholism, hepatic disease, G6PD deficiency, psoriasis, eczema

Pharmacokinetics:
PO: Peak 1-2 hr, half-life 3-5 days; metabolized in the liver; excreted in urine, feces, breast milk; crosses placenta

Drug interactions of concern to dentistry:
• Hepatotoxicity: alcohol, hepatotoxic drugs

DENTAL CONSIDERATIONS

General:
• Patients on chronic drug therapy may rarely have symptoms of blood dyscrasias, which can include infection, bleeding, and poor healing.
• Avoid dental light in patient's eyes; offer dark glasses for patient comfort.
• Determine why the patient is taking the drug.

Consultations:
• In a patient with symptoms of blood dyscrasias, request a medical consultation for blood studies and postpone dental treatment until normal values are reestablished.

Teach patient/family:
• Importance of good oral hygiene to prevent soft tissue inflammation
• To avoid mouth rinses with high alcohol content because of drying effects

---

chlorothiazide

(klor-oh-thye'a-zide)
Diurigen, Diuril
Drug class.: Thiazide diuretic

Action: Acts on distal tubule by increasing excretion of water, sodium, chloride, potassium

Uses: Edema, hypertension, diuresis

Dosage and routes:
Edema, hypertension:
• *Adult:* PO/IV 500 mg-1 g qd in 2 divided doses
Diuresis:
• *Child >6 mo:* PO 22 mg/kg/day in 2 divided doses
• *Child <6 mo:* PO up to 33 mg/kg/day in 2 divided doses
Available forms include: Tabs 250, 500 mg; oral susp 250 mg/5 ml; inj 500 mg

Side effects/adverse reactions:
▼ *ORAL: Dry mouth, increased thirst,* lichenoid drug reaction
CNS: Dizziness, fatigue, weakness, drowsiness, paresthesia, anxiety, depression, headache
CV: Irregular pulse, orthostatic hypotension, palpitation, volume depletion
GI: Nausea, vomiting, anorexia,

hepatitis, constipation, diarrhea, cramps, pancreatitis, GI irritation
HEMA: ***Aplastic anemia, hemolytic anemia, leukopenia, agranulocytosis, thrombocytopenia, neutropenia***
GU: Frequency, **uremia,** polyuria, glucosuria
EENT: Blurred vision
INTEG: Rash, urticaria, purpura, photosensitivity, fever
META: Hyperglycemia, hyperuricemia, hypomagnesemia, increased creatinine, BUN
ELECT: Hypokalemia, hypercalcemia, hyponatremia, hypochloremia

Contraindications: Hypersensitivity to thiazides or sulfonamides, anuria, renal decompensation, pregnancy category D

Precautions: Hypokalemia, renal disease, hepatic disease, gout, COPD, lupus erythematosus, diabetes mellitus, elderly

Pharmacokinetics:
PO: Onset 2 hr, peak 4 hr, duration 6-12 hr; crosses placenta; excreted in breast milk

Drug interactions of concern to dentistry:

- Increased photosensitization: tetracyclines
- Decreased hypotensive response, nephrotoxicity: indomethacin and other NSAIDs

DENTAL CONSIDERATIONS

General:

- Monitor vital signs at every appointment because of cardiovascular side effects.
- After supine positioning, have patient sit upright for at least 2 min before standing to avoid orthostatic hypotension.
- Patients on chronic drug therapy may rarely have symptoms of blood dyscrasias, which can include infection, bleeding, and poor healing.
- Assess salivary flow as a factor in caries, periodontal disease, and candidiasis.
- Limit use of sodium-containing products such as saline IV fluids for patients with a dietary salt restriction.
- Stress from dental procedures may compromise cardiovascular function; determine patient risk.
- Short appointments and a stress reduction protocol may be required for anxious patients.
- Patients taking diuretics should be monitored for serum K^+ levels.

Consultations:

- In a patient with symptoms of blood dyscrasias, request a medical consultation for blood studies and postpone dental treatment until normal values are reestablished.
- Medical consultation may be required to assess disease control and patient's ability to tolerate stress.
- Physician should be informed if significant xerostomic side effects occur (increased caries, sore tongue, problems eating or swallowing, difficulty wearing prosthesis) so a medication change can be considered.

Teach patient/family:

- Importance of good oral hygiene to prevent soft tissue inflammation
- Caution to prevent injury when using oral hygiene aids

When chronic dry mouth occurs, advise patient:

- To avoid mouth rinses with high alcohol content because of drying effects
- To use daily home fluoride products for anticaries effect

• To use sugarless gum, frequent sips of water, or saliva substitutes

chlorphenesin carbamate

(klor-fen′e-sin)

Maolate

Drug class.: Skeletal muscle relaxant, central acting

Action: Unknown; may be related to sedative properties; does not directly relax muscle or depress nerve conduction

Uses: Adjunct for relieving pain in acute, painful musculoskeletal conditions

Dosage and routes:

• *Adult:* PO 800 mg tid, maintenance 400 mg qid, not to exceed 8 wk

Available forms include: Tabs 400 mg

Side effects/adverse reactions:

CNS: Dizziness, weakness, drowsiness, headache, tremor, depression, insomnia, confusion

CV: Postural hypotension, tachycardia

GI: Nausea, vomiting, hiccups

HEMA: ***Blood dyscrasias, leukopenia, thrombocytopenia, agranulocytosis***

EENT: Diplopia, temporary loss of vision

INTEG: Rash, pruritus, fever, facial flushing

SYST: ***Anaphylaxis,*** drug fever

Contraindications: Hypersensitivity, child <12 yr, intermittent porphyria, carbamate derivatives

Precautions: Renal disease, hepatic disease, addictive personality, pregnancy category unknown, elderly, lactation, using for >8 wk, impairment of mental alertness

Pharmacokinetics:

PO: Onset 0.5 hr, peak 1-2 hr, duration 4-6 hr, half-life 4 hr; metabolized by liver; excreted in urine; crosses placenta; excreted in breast milk (large amounts)

Drug interactions of concern to dentistry:

• Increased CNS depression: alcohol, tricyclic antidepressants, narcotics, barbiturates, sedatives, hypnotics

DENTAL CONSIDERATIONS

General:

• Patients on chronic drug therapy may rarely have symptoms of blood dyscrasias, which can include infection, bleeding, and poor healing.

• After supine positioning, have patient sit upright for at least 2 min to avoid orthostatic hypotension.

• Consider semisupine chair position for patient comfort if GI side effects occur.

Consultations:

• In a patient with symptoms of blood dyscrasias, request a medical consultation for blood studies and postpone dental treatment until normal values are reestablished.

Teach patient/family:

• Importance of good oral hygiene to prevent soft tissue inflammation

• Caution to prevent trauma when using oral hygiene aids

• To report oral lesions, soreness, or bleeding to dentist

chlorpheniramine maleate

(klor-fen-eer'a-meen)

Aller-Chlor, Allergy, Efidac 24, Chlo-Amine, Chlor-Trimeton

✤ Chlor-Tripolon, Novo-Pheniram

Drug class.: Antihistamine, H_1-receptor antagonist

Action: Acts on blood vessels, GI system, respiratory system by competing with histamine for H_1-receptor site; decreases allergic response by blocking histamine

Uses: Allergy symptoms, rhinitis

Dosage and routes:

- *Adult and child >12 yr:* PO 2 mg tid-qid, not to exceed 36 mg/day; time rel 8-12 mg bid-tid, not to exceed 36 mg/day; IM/IV/SC 5-40 mg/day
- *Child 6-11 yr:* PO 1 mg q4-6h, not to exceed 12 mg/day
- *Child 2-5 yr:* PO 0.5 mg q4-6h, not to exceed 4 mg/day

Available forms include: Chew tabs 2 mg; tabs 4 mg; time rel tabs 8, 12 mg; time rel caps 8, 12 mg; syr 2 mg/5 ml; inj IM/SC/IV 10, 100 mg/ml

Side effects/adverse reactions:

▼ *ORAL: Dry mouth*

CNS: Dizziness, drowsiness, poor coordination, fatigue, anxiety, euphoria, confusion, paresthesia, neuritis

GI: Nausea, anorexia, diarrhea

RESP: Increased thick secretions, wheezing, chest tightness

HEMA: ***Thrombocytopenia, agranulocytosis, hemolytic anemia***

GU: Retention, dysuria, frequency

EENT: Blurred vision, dilated pupils, tinnitus, nasal stuffiness, dry nose, throat

INTEG: Photosensitivity

Contraindications: Hypersensitivity to H_1-receptor antagonists, acute asthma attack, lower respiratory tract disease

Precautions: Increased intraocular pressure, renal disease, cardiac disease, hypertension, bronchial asthma, seizure disorder, stenosed peptic ulcers, hyperthyroidism, prostatic hypertrophy, bladder neck obstruction, pregnancy category B, elderly

Pharmacokinetics:

PO: Onset 20-60 min, duration 8-12 hr, half-life 20-24 hr; detoxified in liver; excreted by kidneys (metabolites/free drug)

Drug interactions of concern to dentistry:

- Increased CNS depression: alcohol, all CNS depressants
- Increased anticholinergic effect: other anticholinergics, phenothiazines, tricyclic antidepressants

DENTAL CONSIDERATIONS

General:

- Assess salivary flow as a factor in caries, periodontal disease, and candidiasis.
- Consider semisupine chair position for patients with respiratory disease.
- Determine why the patient is taking the drug.

Teach patient/family:

- Importance of good oral hygiene to prevent soft tissue inflammation
- Caution to prevent injury when using oral hygiene aids

When chronic dry mouth occurs, advise patient:

- To avoid mouth rinses with high alcohol content because of drying effects

• To use daily home fluoride products for anticaries effect
• To use sugarless gum, frequent sips of water, or saliva substitutes

chlorpromazine HCl

(klor-proe'ma-zeen)
Thorazine
♣ Chlorpromanyl, Novo-Chlorpromazine, Largactil Oral Drops, Largactil
Drug class.: Phenothiazine antipsychotic

Action: Blocks neurotransmission at dopaminergic synapses in the cerebral cortex, hypothalamus, and limbic system; exhibits strong peripheral α-adrenergic, anticholinergic blocking action; mechanism for antipsychotic effects is unclear
Uses: Psychotic disorders, mania, schizophrenia, anxiety, intractable hiccups, nausea, vomiting, preoperatively for relaxation, acute intermittent porphyria, behavioral problems in children
Dosage and routes:
Psychiatry:
• *Adult:* PO 10-50 mg q1-4h initially, then increase up to 2000 mg/day if necessary; IM 10-50 mg q1-4h
• *Child:* PO 0.25 mg/lb q4-6h or 0.5 mg/kg; IM 0.25 mg/lb q6-8h or 0.5 mg/kg; REC 0.5 mg/lb q6-8h or 1 mg/kg
Nausea and vomiting:
• *Adult:* PO 10-25 mg q4-6h prn; IM 25-50 mg q3h prn; REC 50-100 mg q6-8h prn, not to exceed 400 mg/day; IV 25-50 mg qd-qid
• *Child:* PO 0.25 mg/lb q4-6h prn; IM 0.25 mg/lb q6-8h prn not to exceed 40 mg/day (<5 yr) or 75 mg/day (5-12 yr); REC 0.5 mg/lb q6-8h prn; IV 0.55 mg/kg q6-8h
Intractable hiccups:
• *Adult:* PO 25-50 mg tid-qid; IM 25-50 mg (used only if PO dose does not work); IV 25-50 mg in 500-1000 ml saline (only for severe hiccups)
Available forms include: Tabs 10, 25, 50, 100, 200 mg; sus rel caps 30, 75, 150, 200, 300 mg; syr 10 mg/5 ml; conc 30, 100 mg/ml; supp 25, 100 mg; inj IM/IV 25 mg/ml
Side effects/adverse reactions:
▼ *ORAL: Dry mouth,* lichenoid reaction
CNS: Extrapyramidal symptoms: pseudoparkinsonism, akathisia, dystonia, tardive dyskinesia, seizures, headache
CV: Orthostatic hypotension, ***cardiac arrest, tachycardia,*** hypertension, ECG changes
GI: Nausea, vomiting, anorexia, constipation, diarrhea, jaundice, weight gain
RESP: ***Laryngospasm, respiratory depression,*** dyspnea
HEMA: ***Leukopenia, leukocytosis, agranulocytosis,*** anemia
GU: Urinary retention, urinary frequency, enuresis, impotence, amenorrhea, gynecomastia, breast engorgement
EENT: Blurred vision, glaucoma, dry eyes
INTEG: Rash, photosensitivity, dermatitis
Contraindications: Hypersensitivity, circulatory collapse, liver damage, cerebral arteriosclerosis, coronary disease, severe hypertension/hypotension, blood dyscrasias, coma, child <2 yr, brain damage, bone marrow depression, alcohol and barbiturate withdrawal states

Precautions: Pregnancy category C, lactation, seizure disorders, hypertension, hepatic disease, cardiac disease, elderly

Pharmacokinetics:

PO: Onset erratic, peak 2-4 hr, duration may be detected for up to 6 mo after last dose

IM: Onset 15-30 min, peak 15-20 min, duration may be detected for up to 6 mo after last dose

IV: Onset 5 min, peak 10 min, duration may be detected for up to 6 mo after last dose

REC: Onset erratic, peak 3 hr, elimination half-life 10-30 hr; 95% bound to plasma proteins; metabolized by liver; excreted in urine (metabolites); crosses placenta; enters breast milk

Drug interactions of concern to dentistry:

- Increased sedation: other CNS depressants, alcohol, barbiturate anesthetics, opioid analgesics
- Hypotension, tachycardia: epinephrine (systemic)
- Increased extrapyramidal effects: related drugs such as haloperidol, droperidol, and metoclopramide
- Additive photosensitization: tetracyclines
- Increased anticholinergic effects: anticholinergics

DENTAL CONSIDERATIONS

General:

- Monitor vital signs at every appointment because of cardiovascular side effects.
- Patients on chronic drug therapy may rarely have symptoms of blood dyscrasias, which can include infection, bleeding, and poor healing.
- After supine positioning, have patient sit upright for at least 2 min before standing to avoid orthostatic hypotension.
- Assess salivary flow as a factor in caries, periodontal disease, and candidiasis.
- Avoid dental light in patient's eyes; offer dark glasses for patient comfort.
- Assess for presence of extrapyramidal motor symptoms, such as tardive dyskinesia and akathisia. Extrapyramidal motor activity may complicate dental treatment.
- Geriatric patients are more susceptible to drug effects; use a lower dose.

Consultations:

- In a patient with symptoms of blood dyscrasias, request a medical consultation for blood studies and postpone dental treatment until normal values are reestablished.
- Take precautions if dental surgery is anticipated and anesthesia is required.
- If signs of tardive dyskinesia or akathisia are present, refer to physician.
- Physician should be informed if significant xerostomic side effects occur (increased caries, sore tongue, problems eating or swallowing, difficulty wearing prosthesis) so a medication change can be considered.

Teach patient/family:

- Importance of good oral hygiene to prevent soft tissue inflammation
- Caution to prevent injury when using oral hygiene aids
- To use electric toothbrush if patient has difficulty holding conventional devices

When chronic dry mouth occurs, advise patient:
- To avoid mouth rinses with high alcohol content because of drying effects
- To use daily home fluoride products for anticaries effect
- To use sugarless gum, frequent sips of water, or saliva substitutes

chlorpropamide

(klor-proe'pa-mide)
Diabinese
♣ Apo-Chlorpromaide, Novo-propamide

Drug class.: Antidiabetic, sulfonylurea (first generation)

Action: Causes functioning β-cells in pancreas to release insulin, leading to drop in blood glucose levels; may improve insulin binding to insulin receptors or increase the number of insulin receptors; not effective if patient lacks functioning β-cells

Uses: Stable adult-onset diabetes mellitus (type 2)

Dosage and routes:
- *Adult:* PO 100-250 mg qd, initially, then 100-500 mg maintenance according to response; not to exceed 750 mg/day

Available forms include: Tabs 100, 250 mg

Side effects/adverse reactions:

▼ *ORAL:* Lichenoid drug reaction

CNS: Headache, weakness, dizziness, drowsiness, tinnitus, fatigue, vertigo

GI: ***Hepatotoxicity, cholestatic jaundice,*** nausea, vomiting, diarrhea, heartburn

HEMA: ***Leukopenia, thrombocytopenia, agranulocytosis, aplastic anemia, pancytopenia, hemolytic anemia***

INTEG: Rash, allergic reactions, pruritus, urticaria, eczema, photosensitivity, erythema

ENDO: ***Hypoglycemia***

Contraindications: Hypersensitivity to sulfonylureas, juvenile or brittle diabetes

Precautions: Elderly, cardiac disease, thyroid disease, renal disease, hepatic disease, severe hypoglycemic reactions, pregnancy category C, avoid use in lactation, use in children not established

Pharmacokinetics:

PO: Completely absorbed by GI route, onset 1 hr, peak 3-6 hr, duration 60 hr, half-life 36 hr; 90%-95% is plasma protein bound; metabolized in liver; excreted in urine (metabolites and unchanged drug), breast milk

Drug interactions of concern to dentistry:
- Increased hypoglycemic effects: salicylates, NSAIDs, ketoconazole, miconazole
- Decreased action: corticosteroids, sympathomimetics
- Disulfiram-like reaction: alcohol

DENTAL CONSIDERATIONS

General:
- Patients on chronic drug therapy may rarely have symptoms of blood dyscrasias, which can include infection, bleeding, and poor healing.
- Short appointments and a stress reduction protocol may be required for anxious patients.
- Question patient about self-monitoring of drug's antidiabetic effect, including blood glucose values or finger-stick records.

• Ensure that patient is following prescribed diet and regularly takes medication.
• Determine if medication controls disease. Patients with diabetes may be more susceptible to infection and have delayed wound healing.
• Avoid prescribing aspirin-containing products.

Consultations:

• In a patient with symptoms of blood dyscrasias, request a medical consultation for blood studies and postpone dental treatment until normal values are reestablished.
• Medical consultation may be required to assess disease control.
• Medical consultation may include data from patient's blood glucose monitoring, including glycosylated hemoglobin or HbA_{1c} testing.

Teach patient/family:

• Importance of good oral hygiene to prevent soft tissue inflammation
• Caution to prevent injury when using oral hygiene aids
• To avoid mouth rinses with high alcohol content because of drying effects

chlorthalidone

(klor-thal′i-done)

Hygroton, Thalitone

🍁 Apo-Chlorthalidone, Novo-Thalidone, Uridon

Drug class.: Diuretic with thiazide-like effects

Action: Acts on distal tubule by increasing excretion of water, sodium, chloride, potassium

Uses: Edema, hypertension, diuresis, CHF

Dosage and routes:

• *Adult:* PO 25-100 mg/day or 100-200 mg qid; adjust dose to response
• *Child:* PO 2 mg/kg 3 × weekly

Available forms include: Tabs 15, 25, 50, 100 mg

Side effects/adverse reactions:

▼ *ORAL: Dry mouth, increased thirst*

CNS: Dizziness, fatigue, weakness, drowsiness, paresthesia, anxiety, depression, headache

CV: Irregular pulse, orthostatic hypotension, palpitation, volume depletion

GI: Nausea, vomiting, anorexia, ***hepatitis,*** constipation, diarrhea, cramps, pancreatitis, GI irritation

HEMA: ***Aplastic anemia, hemolytic anemia, leukopenia, agranulocytosis, thrombocytopenia, neutropenia***

GU: Frequency, ***uremia,*** glucosuria, polyuria

EENT: Blurred vision

INTEG: Rash, urticaria, purpura, photosensitivity, fever

META: Hyperglycemia, hyperuremia, increased creatinine, BUN

ELECT: Hypokalemia, hypomagnesemia, hypercalcemia, hyponatremia, hypochloremia

Contraindications: Hypersensitivity to thiazides or sulfonamides, anuria, renal decompensation

Precautions: Hypokalemia, renal disease, pregnancy category B, hepatic disease, gout, diabetes mellitus, elderly, lactation

Pharmacokinetics:

PO: Onset 2 hr, peak 6 hr, duration 24-72 hr, half-life 40 hr; excreted unchanged by kidneys; crosses placenta; enters breast milk

Drug interactions of concern to dentistry:
• Increased photosensitization: tetracyclines
• Decreased hypotensive response, nephrotoxicity: NSAIDs, indomethacin

DENTAL CONSIDERATIONS
General:
• Monitor vital signs at every appointment because of cardiovascular side effects.
• After supine positioning, have patient sit upright for at least 2 min before standing to avoid orthostatic hypotension.
• Patients on chronic drug therapy may rarely have symptoms of blood dyscrasias, which can include infection, bleeding, and poor healing.
• Assess salivary flow as a factor in caries, periodontal disease, and candidiasis.
• Limit use of sodium-containing products such as saline IV fluids for those patients with a dietary salt restriction.
• Short appointments and a stress reduction protocol may be required for anxious patients.
• Stress from dental procedures may compromise cardiovascular function; determine patient risk.

Consultations:
• In a patient with symptoms of blood dyscrasias, request a medical consultation for blood studies and postpone dental treatment until normal values are reestablished.
• Medical consultation may be required to assess disease control and patient's ability to tolerate stress.

Teach patient/family:
• Importance of good oral hygiene to prevent soft tissue inflammation
• Caution to prevent injury when using oral hygiene aids

When chronic dry mouth occurs, advise patient:
• To avoid mouth rinses with high alcohol content because of drying effects
• To use daily home fluoride products for anticaries effect
• To use sugarless gum, frequent sips of water, or saliva substitutes

chlorzoxazone

(klor-zox'a-zone)
Paraflex, Parafon Forte DSC, Remular-S

Drug class.: Skeletal muscle relaxant, centrally acting

Action: Depresses multisynaptic pathways in the spinal cord
Uses: Adjunct for relief of muscle spasm in musculoskeletal conditions
Dosage and routes:
• *Adult:* PO 250-750 mg tid-qid
Available forms include: Tabs 250, 500 mg; caplets 250, 500 mg
Side effects/adverse reactions:
CNS: Dizziness, drowsiness, headache, insomnia, stimulation, malaise
GI: Nausea, ***hepatotoxicity, jaundice,*** vomiting, anorexia, diarrhea, constipation
HEMA: ***Granulocytopenia, anemia***
GU: Urine discoloration
INTEG: ***Angioedema,*** rash, pruritus, petechiae, ecchymoses
SYST: ***Anaphylaxis***
Contraindications: Hypersensitivity, impaired hepatic function
Precautions: Safety in pregnancy not established, lactation, hepatic disease, elderly

Pharmacokinetics:
PO: Onset 1 hr, peak 3-4 hr, duration 6 hr, half-life 1 hr; metabolized in liver; excreted in urine (metabolites)

Drug interactions of concern to dentistry:
• Increased CNS depression: alcohol, narcotics, barbiturates, sedatives, hypnotics

DENTAL CONSIDERATIONS
General:
• Determine why the patient is taking the drug.
• Consider semisupine chair position if back is involved.
• When used for dental-related problems, consider aspirin or NSAIDs to improve response.

cholestyramine

(koe-less-teer'a-meen)
LoCholest Light, Prevalite, Questran, Questran Lite
Drug class.: Antihyperlipidemic

Action: Absorbs, combines with bile acids to form insoluble complex that is excreted through feces; loss of bile acids lowers cholesterol levels
Uses: Primary hypercholesterolemia, pruritus associated with biliary obstruction, diarrhea caused by excess bile acid, digitalis toxicity, xanthomas
Dosage and routes:
• *Adult:* PO 4 g qd or bid ac; maintenance dose 8-24 g in 2-6 divided doses
• *Child:* PO 4 g/day in 2 divided doses; administer with food or drink
Available forms include: 4 g cholestyramine in 5, 5.5, 5.7, 6.4, 9 g powder
Side effects/adverse reactions:
CNS: Headache, dizziness, drowsiness, vertigo, tinnitus
GI: Constipation, abdominal pain, nausea, fecal impaction, hemorrhoids, flatulence, vomiting, steatorrhea, peptic ulcer
HEMA: ***Hyperchloremic acidosis; bleeding;*** decreased pro-time, decreased vitamin A, D, K; red cell folate content
INTEG: Rash; irritation of perianal area, tongue, skin
MS: Muscle, joint pain
Contraindications: Hypersensitivity, biliary obstruction
Precautions: Pregnancy category C, lactation, children
Pharmacokinetics:
PO: Excreted in feces, max effect in 2 wk

Drug interactions of concern to dentistry:
• Decreased absorption of tetracyclines, cephalexin, phenobarbital, corticosteroids, clindamycin, penicillins; administer doses several hours apart

DENTAL CONSIDERATIONS
General:
• Consider semisupine chair position for patient comfort because of GI effects of disease.

choline salicylate

(koe'leen)
Arthropan
Drug class.: Salicylate analgesic

Action: Inhibits prostaglandin synthesis by interfering with cyclooxygenase need for biosynthesis; possesses analgesic, antipyretic, and antiinflammatory properties

Uses: Mild-to-moderate pain or fever, arthritis, juvenile rheumatoid arthritis

Dosage and routes:

Arthritis:

• *Adult:* PO 870-1740 mg qid

Pain/fever:

• *Adult and child >12 yr:* PO 870 mg q3-4h prn; maximum 6 doses/day

Available forms include: Liq 870 mg/5 ml (salicylate equivalent to 650 mg aspirin)

Side effects/adverse reactions:

CNS: ***Coma, convulsions,*** stimulation, drowsiness, dizziness, confusion, headache, flushing, hallucinations

CV: Rapid pulse, pulmonary edema

GI: Nausea, vomiting, GI bleeding, diarrhea, heartburn, ***hepatitis,*** anorexia

RESP: Wheezing, hyperpnea

HEMA: ***Thrombocytopenia, agranulocytosis, leukopenia, neutropenia, hemolytic anemia,*** increased pro-time

EENT: Tinnitus, hearing loss

INTEG: Rash, urticaria, bruising

ENDO: Hypoglycemia, hyponatremia, hypokalemia

Contraindications: Hypersensitivity to salicylates, GI bleeding, bleeding disorders, child <3 yr, vitamin K deficiency, child with flulike symptoms; avoid use in third trimester of pregnancy

Precautions: Anemia, hepatic disease, renal disease, Hodgkin's disease, pregnancy category C, lactation, geriatric patients

Pharmacokinetics:

PO: Onset 15-30 min; metabolized by liver; excreted by kidneys; crosses placenta; excreted in breast milk

Drug interactions of concern to dentistry:

• Increased risk of hypoglycemia: oral hypoglycemics

• Increased risk of GI complaints: alcohol, NSAIDs, steroids

• Avoid prolonged or concurrent use with ASA, NSAIDs, corticosteroids, acetaminophen

• Increased effects of anticoagulants, valproic acid, methotrexate, dipyridamole

• Decreased effects of probenecid, sulfinpyrazone

• Suspected reduction in antihypertensives and vasodilator effects of ACE inhibitors; monitor blood pressure if used concurrently

DENTAL CONSIDERATIONS

General:

• Patients on chronic drug therapy may rarely have symptoms of blood dyscrasias, which can include infection, bleeding, and poor healing.

• Consider semisupine chair position for patient comfort if GI side effects occur.

• Determine why the patient is taking the drug.

• Evaluate allergic reactions: rash, urticaria; patients with allergy to salicylates may not be able to take NSAIDs. Drug may need to be discontinued.

• Consider semisupine chair position for patient comfort because of arthritic disease.

Consultations:

• In a patient with symptoms of blood dyscrasias, request a medical consultation for blood studies and postpone dental treatment until normal values are reestablished.

• Medical consultation may be re-

quired to assess disease control and patient's ability to tolerate stress.
• Tinnitus, ringing, roaring in ears after high-dose and long-term therapy requires referral for evaluation for salicylism.

Teach patient/family:
• Importance of good oral hygiene to prevent soft tissue inflammation
• Caution to prevent trauma when using oral hygiene aids
• To read label on other OTC drugs; many contain aspirin
• To report oral lesions, soreness, or bleeding to dentist
• To avoid alcohol ingestion; GI bleeding may occur

---

ciclopirox olamine (topical)

(sye-kloe-peer'ox)
Loprox, Penlac Nail Lacquer
Drug class.: Topical antifungal

Action: Interferes with fungal cell membrane, increasing its permeability and causing leaking of cell nutrients

Uses: Tinea cruris, tinea corporis, tinea pedis, tinea versicolor, cutaneous candidiasis, nail solution for immunocompetent patients with mild to moderate onychomycosis of nails without lunula involvement; caused by *T. rubrum*

Dosage and routes:
• *Adult and child >10 yr:* TOP rub into affected area bid; nail polish apply at bedtime once daily; nail SOL apply solution once daily to all affected nails, used in a comprehensive care program for nails

Available forms include: Cream 1%, lotion 1%, nail lacquer 8%

Side effects/adverse reactions:
INTEG: Rash, urticaria, stinging, burning, pruritus, pain

Contraindications: Hypersensitivity, systemic antifungal treatment

Precautions: Pregnancy category B, lactation, child <10 yr

DENTAL CONSIDERATIONS

General:
• There are neither dental drug interactions nor relevant considerations to dentistry for this drug.

---

cilostazol

(sil-os'-ta-zol)
Pletal
Drug class.: Phosphodiesterase inhibitor

Action: Inhibits phosphodiesterase III enzymes, decreasing cAMP degradation to increase cAMP in platelets and blood vessels; reversibly inhibits platelet aggregation and causes vasodilation in vascular beds

Uses: Reduction of symptoms of intermittent claudication (leg pain on walking)

Dosage and routes:
• *Adult:* PO 100 mg bid at least 30 min before or 2 hr after breakfast and dinner

NOTE: With inhibitors of CYP3A4 isoenzymes, give 50 mg bid

Available forms include: Tabs 50, 100 mg

Side effects/adverse reactions:
▼ *ORAL: Glossitis, gingival bleeding*
CNS: Headache, palpitation, dizziness, vertigo, tachycardia
CV: Peripheral edema

GI: Diarrhea, abdominal pain, dyspepsia, nausea, flatulence, vomiting
RESP: Bronchitis
HEMA: Anemia, purpura, ecchymosis
GU: UTI
EENT: Pharyngitis, rhinitis
INTEG: Dry skin, urticaria
META: Increased creatinine, hyperlipidemia, hyperuricemia
MS: Arthralgia, leg cramps
MISC: Infection, malaise, asthenia

Contraindications: Hypersensitivity, CHF; use not recommended in lactation

Precautions: Pregnancy category C, lactation, children, smoking

Pharmacokinetics:
PO: High-fat meal enhances absorption; metabolized by cytochrome P-450 enzymes (3A4); active metabolites, peak plasma levels 2-3 hr; highly protein bound (95%-98%), urinary excretion

Drug interactions of concern to dentistry:
- Risk of interaction with other platelet aggregation inhibitors possible, not established
- Risk of drug interaction with cytochrome P-450 3A4 inhibitors: erythromycin, ketoconazole, itraconazole, diltiazem, clarithromycin, grapefruit juice
- Risk of drug interaction with cytochrome P4502C19 inhibitors: omeprazole (see Appendix I)

DENTAL CONSIDERATIONS

General:
- Determine why patient is taking the drug.
- Avoid products that affect platelet function, such as aspirin and NSAIDs.

Consultations:
- Consultation with physician may be needed if excessive bleeding occurs during dental treatment.
- Consultation should include data on bleeding time.

Teach patient/family:
- Importance of updating health and drug history if physician makes any changes in evaluation or drug regimens
- To inform dentist of unusual bleeding episodes following dental treatment
- To prevent trauma when using oral hygiene aids
- Importance of good oral hygiene to prevent soft tissue inflammation

cimetidine

(sye-met'i-deen)
Tagamet, Tagamet HB (OTC)
Apo-Cimetidine, Gen-Cimetidine, Novo-Cimetidine, PMS-Cimetidine, Peptol, Nu-Cimet

Drug class.: H_2 histamine receptor antagonist

Action: Inhibits histamine at H_2-receptor site in parietal cells, which inhibits gastric acid secretion

Uses: Short-term treatment of duodenal and benign gastric ulcers and maintenance; gastroesophageal reflux disease, upper GI bleeding, pathologic hypersecretory diseases and heartburn with acid indigestion

Dosage and routes:

Duodenal ulcer:
- *Adult:* PO preferred dose 800 mg hs for 4-8 wk, heavy smokers and conditions involving larger ulcers may require 1600 mg hs; other regimens are 300 mg qid at meals and hs; or 400 mg bid (AM and hs); treatment should continue 4-8 wk;

maintenance dose is 400 mg hs; IV bol 300 mg/20 ml 0.9% NaCl over 1-2 min q6h; IV inf 300 mg/50 ml D_5W over 15-20 min; IM 300 mg q6h, not to exceed 2400 mg

Heartburn/acid indigestion (OTC dose): PO 200 mg qd up to bid

GERD:

• *Adult:* PO 800 mg bid or 400 mg qd × 12 wk

Available forms include: Tabs (100 mg OTC) 200, 300, 400, 800 mg; liq 300 mg/5 ml; inj 150 mg/ml, 300 mg/2 ml, 300 mg/50 ml 0.9% NaCl

Side effects/adverse reactions:

▼ *ORAL:* Lichenoid reaction

CNS: Confusion, headache, ***convulsions,*** depression, dizziness, anxiety, weakness, psychosis, tremors

CV: Bradycardia, tachycardia

GI: Diarrhea, ***paralytic ileus, jaundice,*** abdominal cramps

HEMA: ***Agranulocytosis, thrombocytopenia, neutropenia, aplastic anemia,*** increase in PT

GU: Gynecomastia, galactorrhea, impotence, increase in BUN, creatinine

INTEG: ***Exfoliative dermatitis,*** urticaria, rash, alopecia, sweating, flushing

Contraindications: Hypersensitivity, concurrent use with dofetilide

Precautions: Pregnancy category B, lactation, child <12 yr, organic brain syndrome, hepatic disease, renal disease, smoking

Pharmacokinetics:

PO: Peak 1-1.5 hr, half-life 1.5 hr; metabolized by liver; excreted in urine (unchanged); crosses placenta; enters breast milk

Drug interactions of concern to dentistry:

• GI ulceration, bleeding: aspirin, NSAIDs

• Decreased absorption: sodium bicarbonate, anticholinergics

• Decreased absorption of fluconazole, ketoconazole, tetracycline (take doses 2 hr apart), ferrous salts

• Increased blood levels of metronidazole, alcohol, lidocaine, narcotic analgesics, benzodiazepines, carbamazepine

DENTAL CONSIDERATIONS

General:

• Monitor vital signs at every appointment because of cardiovascular side effects.

• Consider semisupine chair position for patient comfort because of GI effects of disease.

• Avoid prescribing aspirin- or NSAID-containing products in patients with active upper GI disease; there is a risk of irritation and ulceration.

• Sodium bicarbonate products can be used 1 hr before or 1 hr after cimetidine dose.

Teach patient/family:

• Importance of good oral hygiene to prevent soft tissue inflammation

• Caution to prevent injury when using oral hygiene aids

---

cinoxacin

(sin-ox'a-sin)

Cinobac

Drug class.: Urinary tract antibacterial

Action: Interferes with DNA replication

Uses: UTIs caused by *E. coli, Klebsiella, Enterobacter, P. mirabi-*

lis, P. vulgaris, P. morganii, Serratia, Citrobacter

Dosage and routes:

• *Adult:* PO 1 g/day in 2-4 divided doses × 1-2 wk

Available forms include: Caps 250, 500 mg

Side effects/adverse reactions:

CNS: Dizziness, headache, agitation, insomnia, confusion

GI: Nausea, vomiting, anorexia, abdominal cramps, diarrhea

EENT: Sensitivity to light, visual disturbances, blurred vision, tinnitus

INTEG: Pruritus, rash, urticaria, photosensitivity, edema

Contraindications: Hypersensitivity to this drug or other quinolones, anuria, CNS damage

Precautions: Renal disease, hepatic disease, pregnancy category B, lactation, safety and efficacy in children <18 yr not established

Pharmacokinetics:

PO: Duration 6-8 hr, half-life 1.5 hr; excreted in urine (unchanged/inactive metabolites)

DENTAL CONSIDERATIONS

General:

• Be aware that the patient has a UTI.

• Avoid dental light in patient's eyes; offer dark glasses for patient comfort.

• Advise patient if dental drugs prescribed have a potential for photosensitivity.

Consultations:

• May need to consult with physician when it is necessary to prescribe antiinfectives for a dental infection.

ciprofloxacin

(sip-roe-flox'a-sin)

Cipro, Cipro IV, Cipro XR

Drug class.: Fluoroquinolone antiinfective

Action: A broad-spectrum bactericidal agent that inhibits the enzymes topoisomerase II (DNA gyrase) and topoisomerase IV, which are required for bacterial DNA replication, transcription, repair, and recombination

Uses: Adult UTIs (including complicated) caused by *E. coli, E. cloacae, P. mirabilis, K. pneumoniae, C. freundi, S. epidermidis,* and others; lower respiratory tract infections caused by *H. parainfluenzae, H. influenzae, K. pneumoniae, E. coli, E. cloacae;* chronic bacterial prostatitis; skin and skin structure infections, bone/joint infections caused by *E. cloacae, S. marcescens, P. aeruginosa,* infectious diarrhea, typhoid fever, STDs, and acute uncomplicated cystitis in females; postexposure inhalational anthrax

Dosage and routes:

Uncomplicated UTIs:

• *Adult:* PO 250 mg q12h; IV 200 mg q12h for 7-14 days; 3-day regimen: PO 100 mg bid q3d

Complicated/severe UTIs/nosocomial pneumonia:

• *Adult:* PO 500 mg q12h for 7-14 days; IV 400 mg q12h

Lower respiratory tract infections (mild to moderate):

• *Adult:* PO 500 mg q12h, IV 400 mg q12h

Bone and joint infections:

• *Adult:* PO 500-750 mg q12h for 4-6 wk (mild to moderate); 750 mg q12h for 4-6 wk (severe or complicated)

Postexposure inhalational anthrax:

• *Adult:* PO 500 mg bid up to 60 days

Available forms include: Tabs 100, 250, 500, 750 mg; ext rel tab 500 mg; IV 200 mg/100 ml D_5W, 400 mg/200 ml D_5W; 200, 400 mg vial; powder for oral susp 5 g/100 ml, 10 g/100 ml

Side effects/adverse reactions:

▼ *ORAL:* Candidiasis, unpleasant taste

CNS: Headache, dizziness, fatigue, insomnia, depression, restlessness, tremors, confusion, hallucinations

GI: Nausea, vomiting, diarrhea, abdominal pain, constipation, increased ALT/AST, flatulence, insomnia, heartburn, dysphagia, pseudomembranous colitis

INTEG: Rash, pruritus, urticaria, photosensitivity, flushing, fever, chills

GU: Vaginitis, crystalluria (rare)

EENT: Blurred vision, diplopia, tinnitus, phototoxicity

MS: Tendinitis, tendon rupture, arthralgia

META: Elevation of liver enzymes ALT, AST

MISC: ***Anaphylaxis,*** superinfections

Contraindications: Hypersensitivity to quinolines

Precautions: Pregnancy category C, lactation, children, renal disease, tendon ruptures of shoulder, hand, and Achilles tendons, epilepsy, severe cerebral arteriosclerosis; monitor blood glucose levels, extended release tablets can be taken with meals, defects in glucose-6-phosphate dehydrogenase activity, myasthenia gravis

Pharmacokinetics:

PO: Peak 1 hr, half-life 3-4 hr; steady state 2 days; excreted in urine as active drug, metabolites

Drug interactions of concern to dentistry:

• Decreased absorption: divalent, trivalent antacids, iron and zinc salts, calcium fortified juices

• Increased serum levels: probenecid

• Increased risk of bleeding with warfarin (monitor)

• Serious adverse effects with theophylline, caffeine

DENTAL CONSIDERATIONS

General:

• Determine why the patient is taking the drug.

• Avoid dental light in patient's eyes; offer dark glasses for patient comfort.

• Minimize exposure to sunlight and wear sunscreen if sun exposure is planned.

• Ruptures of the shoulder, hand, and Achilles tendon that required surgical repair or resulted in prolonged disability have been reported with this drug.

Consultations:

• Consult with patient's physician if an acute dental infection occurs and another antiinfective is required.

Teach patient/family:

• To discontinue treatment and inform dentist immediately if patient experiences pain or inflammation of a tendon, and to rest and refrain from exercise

ciprofloxacin HCl

(sip-roe-flox'a-sin)
Ciloxan

Drug class.: Topical fluoroquinolone antiinfective

Action: A broad-spectrum bactericidal agent that inhibits the enzyme DNA gyrase needed for bacterial DNA replication
Uses: Infections caused by susceptible strains of microorganisms in conjunctivitis or corneal ulcers
Dosage and routes:
Bacterial conjunctivitis:
• *Adult:* TOP solution 1-2 drops q2h while awake × 2 days; then 1-2 gtt q4h while awake for 5 days; ointment: apply ½-inch ribbon of ointment tid × 2 days; then ½-inch ribbon bid for 5 days
Corneal ulcers:
• *Adult:* TOP solution 2 drops in affected eye q15min × 6 hr, then 2 drops q30min for rest of the day; on day 2, 2 drops hourly; on days 3 through 14, 2 drops q4h
Available forms include: Sol 3.5 mg/ml in 2.5, 5 ml; oint 3.5 mg
Side effects/adverse reactions:
▼ *ORAL:* Bad taste
GI: Nausea
EENT: Burning, discomfort, eyelid crusting, scale, white crystalline deposits, itching, foreign body sensation, blurred vision, eye pain
INTEG: Dermatitis
MISC: Allergic reactions
Contraindications: Hypersensitivity to fluoroquinolones or any ingredient in these preparations
Precautions: Prolonged use and risk of resistant microorganisms, do not contaminate sterile product, pregnancy category B, safety and efficacy has not been established for ointment use in children <2yr and <1 yr for solution
Pharmacokinetics:
TOP: Minimal systemic absorption with oral solution; no other data available
Drug interactions of concern to dentistry:
• Specific studies have not been conducted with topical ciprofloxacin. See systemic drug for interactions.

DENTAL CONSIDERATIONS
General:
• Protect patient's eyes from accidental spatter during dental treatment.
• Avoid dental light in patient's eyes; offer dark glasses for patient comfort.

citalopram hydrobromide

(ce'tal-o-pram)
Celexa

Drug class.: Antidepressant

Action: Selectively inhibits the reuptake of serotonin
Uses: Major depression
Dosage and routes:
• *Adult:* PO initial 20 mg once daily; can increase dose in 20 mg increments at intervals of at least 1 wk; doses >40 mg once daily generally not recommended
Elderly or hepatic impairment:
• *Elderly:* PO 20 mg qd/daily limit
Available forms include: Tabs 10, 20, 40 mg; oral sol 10 mg/5 ml
Side effects/adverse reactions:
▼ *ORAL: Dry mouth,* unspecified dysphagia, teeth grinding, gingivitis
CNS: Dizziness, insomnia, somno-

lence, agitation, fatigue, anxiety, decreased libido
CV: Tachycardia, postural hypotension, hypotension
GI: Nausea, vomiting, dyspepsia, abdominal pain
RESP: URI, cough
HEMA: Purpura, anemia
GU: Ejaculation disorder, impotence
EENT: Rhinitis, sinusitis
INTEG: Rash, pruritus
MS: Asthenia, tremor, arthralgia, myalgia
MISC: Sweating, fever, alcohol intolerance

Contraindications: Hypersensitivity, concurrent use of MAOI

Precautions: Activation of mania, hypomania, seizure disorders, hepatic impairment, pregnancy category C, lactation, safe use in children unknown, reduce doses in elderly, risk of serotonin syndrome with other drugs that increase serotonin (5-HT) activity

Pharmacokinetics:
PO: Peak blood levels approximately 4 hr, bioavailability 80%, hepatic metabolism, involves CYP3A4, CYP2C19 isoenzymes, active metabolites, enterohepatic circulation, fecal and renal excretion

Drug interactions of concern to dentistry:

- Possibly increased CNS depression: all CNS depressants, alcohol
- Decrease in plasma levels: carbamazepine
- Increase in plasma levels: macrolide antibiotics, ketoconazole, itraconazole, omeprazole (see Appendix I)
- First-time users of SSRIs also taking NSAIDs may have a higher risk of GI side effects; until more data are available, it may be advisable to avoid use of NSAIDs in these patients (*Br J Clin Pharmacol* 55:591-595, 2003)

DENTAL CONSIDERATIONS

General:

- Evaluate for TMJ therapy if bruxism causes symptoms of pain.
- Assess salivary flow as a factor in caries, periodontal disease, and candidiasis.
- Monitor vital signs at every appointment because of cardiovascular and respiratory side effects.
- After supine positioning, have patient sit upright for 2 min or more to avoid orthostatic hypotension.
- Consider semisupine chair position for patient comfort because of GI side effects of drug.
- Short appointments and a stress reduction protocol may be required for anxious patients.

Consultations:

- Medical consultation may be required to assess disease control and patient's ability to tolerate stress.
- Physician should be informed if significant xerostomic side effects occur (e.g., increased caries, sore tongue, problems eating or swallowing, difficulty wearing prosthesis) so that a medication change can be considered.

Teach patient/family:

- Importance of good oral hygiene to prevent soft tissue inflammation
- Use of electric toothbrush if patient has difficulty holding conventional devices

When chronic dry mouth occurs, advise patient:

- To avoid mouth rinses with high

alcohol content because of drying effects
• To use daily home fluoride products for anticaries effect
• To use sugarless gum, frequent sips of water, or saliva substitutes

clarithromycin

(kla-rith'roe-mye-sin)

Biaxin, Biaxin Filmtab, Biaxin XL

Drug class.: Macrolide antibiotic

Action: Binds to 50S ribosomal subunits of susceptible bacteria and suppresses protein synthesis

Uses: Mild-to-moderate infections of the upper/lower respiratory tract; community-acquired pneumonia caused by *H. influenzae;* uncomplicated skin and skin structure infections caused by *S. pneumoniae, M. pneumoniae, C. diphtheriae, B. pertussis, L. monocytogenes, H. influenzae, S. pyogenes, S. aureus;* otitis media; maxillary sinusitis, bronchitis (XL dose form); middle ear infection; disseminated *Mycobacterium avium* complex (MAC); in combination with other drugs for *H. pylori* duodenal ulcer

Dosage and routes:
• *Adult:* PO 250-500 mg bid × 7-14 days; ext rel tab 1000 mg once daily × 7 days (bronchitis) or 14 days (sinusitis), to be taken with food

Bacterial endocarditis prophylaxis:
• *Adult:* PO for patients allergic to amoxicillin, 500 mg 1 hr before dental procedure
• *Child:* PO for patients allergic to amoxicillin, 15 mg/kg of body weight not to exceed the adult dose 1 hr before dental procedure

Eradicating H. pylori (double therapy):
• *Adult:* PO (days 1-14) 500 mg clarithromycin tid plus omeprazole 20 mg bid qAM ; days 15-28 omeprazole 20 mg qAM

Eradicating H. pylori (triple therapy):
• *Adult:* PO 500 mg clarithromycin plus 30 mg lansoprazole plus 1 g amoxicillin q12h × 10-14 days, or 500 mg clarithromycin plus omeprazole 20 mg plus 1 g amoxicillin × 10 days

Available forms include: Tabs 250, 500 mg; ext rel 500 mg; susp 125 mg/5 ml and 250 mg/ml in 50, 100 ml

Side effects/adverse reactions:
▼ *ORAL: Abnormal taste,* candidiasis, stomatitis
GI: Nausea, abdominal pain, diarrhea, ***hepatotoxicity,*** heartburn, anorexia, vomiting
GU: Vaginitis, moniliasis
INTEG: Rash, urticaria, pruritus
MISC: Headache

Contraindications: Hypersensitivity, indinavir

Precautions: Pregnancy category C, lactation, hepatic and renal disease

Pharmacokinetics:
PO: Peak 2 hr, duration 12 hr, half-life 4-6 hr; metabolized by the liver; excreted in bile, feces

Drug interactions of concern to dentistry:
• Decreased effect: anticholinergic drugs
• Increased effects of cyclosporine, warfarin, cilostazol, tacrolimus, pimozide, methylprednisolone, fluconazole, buspirone

• Decreased action of clindamycin, penicillins, lincomycin, rifabutin, rifampin, zidovudine
• Increased serum levels of carbamazepine, theophylline, digoxin
• Contraindicated with indinavir
• Suspected risk of increased CNS depression with alprazolam, diazepam, midazolam, triazolam
• Oral contraceptives: advise patient of a potential risk for decreased contraceptive action, to maintain compliance with oral contraceptive use while using antibiotics, and to consider the use of additional nonhormonal contraception
• Suspected increase in plasma levels of repaglinide
• Risk of severe myopathy or rhabdomyolysis: atorvastatin, fluvastatin, lovastatin, pravastatin

DENTAL CONSIDERATIONS

General:

• Determine why the patient is taking the drug.
• May prove to be an alternative drug of choice for mild infections caused by a susceptible organism in patients who are allergic to penicillin.

Teach patient/family:

• Importance of good oral hygiene to prevent soft tissue inflammation

When used for dental infection, advise patient:

• To report sore throat, oral burning sensation, fever, fatigue, any of which could indicate superinfection
• To take at prescribed intervals and complete dosage regimen
• To immediately notify the dentist if signs or symptoms of infection increase

clemastine fumarate

(klem'as-teen)

Dayhist-1, Tavist Allergy

✤ Tavist

Drug class.: Antihistamine, H_1-receptor antagonist

Action: Acts on blood vessels, GI, respiratory system by competing with histamine for H_1-receptor site; decreases allergic response by blocking histamine

Uses: Allergy symptoms, rhinitis, angioedema, urticaria, common cold

Dosage and routes:

• *Adult and child >12 yr:* PO 1.34-2.68 mg bid-tid, not to exceed 8.04 mg/day

Available forms include: Tabs 1.34, 2.68 mg; syr 0.67 mg/5 ml

Side effects/adverse reactions:

▼ *ORAL:* Dry mouth

CNS: Dizziness, drowsiness, poor coordination, fatigue, anxiety, euphoria, confusion, paresthesia, neuritis

CV: Hypotension, palpitation, tachycardia

GI: Constipation, nausea, vomiting, anorexia, diarrhea

RESP: Increased thick secretions, wheezing, chest tightness

HEMA: ***Thrombocytopenia,*** agranulocytosis, hemolytic anemia

GU: Retention, dysuria, frequency

EENT: Blurred vision, dilated pupils, tinnitus, nasal stuffiness, dry nose/throat

INTEG: Rash, urticaria, photosensitivity

Contraindications: Hypersensitivity to H_1-receptor antagonists, acute asthma attack, lower respiratory tract disease

Precautions: Increased intraocular pressure, renal disease, cardiac disease, hypertension, bronchial asthma, seizure disorder, stenosed peptic ulcers, hyperthyroidism, prostatic hypertrophy, bladder neck obstruction, pregnancy category B, elderly

Pharmacokinetics:

PO: Peak 5-7 hr, duration 10-12 hr or more; metabolized in liver; excreted by kidneys

Drug interactions of concern to dentistry:

• Increased CNS depression: all CNS depressants, alcohol

• Increased anticholinergic effect of anticholinergics, phenothiazines, tricyclic antidepressants

DENTAL CONSIDERATIONS

General:

• Assess salivary flow as a factor in caries, periodontal disease, and candidiasis.

• Determine why the patient is taking the drug.

Teach patient/family:

• Importance of good oral hygiene to prevent soft tissue inflammation

• Caution to prevent injury when using oral hygiene aids

When chronic dry mouth occurs, advise patient:

• To avoid mouth rinses with high alcohol content because of drying effects

• To use daily home fluoride products for anticaries effect

• To use sugarless gum, frequent sips of water, or saliva substitutes

clindamycin HCl/ clindamycin palmitate HCl/clindamycin phosphate

(klin-da-mye'sin)

Cleocin, Cleocin Pediatric

♣ Dalacin C Flavored Granules, Dalacin C, Dalacin C Phosphate

Drug class.: Lincomycin derivative antiinfective

Action: Binds to 50S subunit of bacterial ribosomes, suppresses protein synthesis

Uses: Indications for use include serious infections caused by susceptible anaerobic bacteria and the treatment of serious infections caused by susceptible strains of pneumococci and streptococci; includes infections of the respiratory tract, serious skin and soft tissue infections, intraabdominal abscess, and infections of the female GU tract

Dosage and routes:

• *Adult:* PO 150-450 mg q6h; IM/IV 300 mg q6-12h, not to exceed 4800 mg/day; dose and duration determined by seriousness of the infection

• *Child >1 mo:* PO 8-25 mg/kg/day in divided doses q6-8h; IM/IV 15-40 mg/kg/day in divided doses q6-8h in 3-4 equal doses; dose and duration determined by seriousness of the infection

PID:

• *Adult:* IV 600 mg qid plus gentamicin

Bacterial endocarditis prophylaxis:

• *Adult:* PO in patients allergic to amoxicillin, 600 mg 1 hr before dental procedure; IV for patients unable to take oral medications, 600 mg 1 hr before dental procedure

• *Child:* PO in patients allergic to amoxicillin, 20 mg/kg of body weight, not to exceed the adult dose, 1 hr before dental procedure; IV for patients unable to take oral medications, 20 mg/kg of body weight, not to exceed the adult dose, 1 hr before dental procedure

Prosthetic joint prophylaxis (when indicated):

• *Adult:* PO 600 mg 1 hr before dental procedure; IV for patients unable to take oral medications, 600 mg 1 hr before dental procedure

Available forms include: Inj 150 mg/ml, 2, 4, 6, 60 and 100 ml; caps 75, 150, 300 mg; oral sol 75 mg/ml

Side effects/adverse reactions:

▼ *ORAL:* Candidiasis

GI: Nausea, vomiting, abdominal pain, diarrhea, ***pseudomembranous colitis,*** anorexia, weight loss

HEMA: ***Leukopenia, eosinophilia, agranulocytosis, thrombocytopenia***

GU: Vaginitis, increased AST/ALT, bilirubin, alk phosphatase, jaundice, urinary frequency

EENT: Rash, urticaria, pruritus, erythema, pain, abscess at injection site

Contraindications: Hypersensitivity to this drug or lincomycin, ulcerative colitis/enteritis, infants <1 mo

Precautions: Renal disease, liver disease, GI disease, elderly, pregnancy category B, lactation, tartrazine sensitivity

Pharmacokinetics:

PO: Peak 45 min, duration 6 hr, plasma protein binding 92%-94%, hepatic metabolism

IM: Peak 3 hr, duration 8-12 hr, half-life 2.5 hr; metabolized in liver; excreted in urine, bile, feces as active/inactive metabolites; crosses placenta; excreted in breast milk

Drug interactions of concern to dentistry:

• Decreased action: erythromycin, absorbent antidiarrheals

• Increased effects of nondepolarizing muscle relaxants, hydrocarbon inhalation anesthetics

• Avoid antiperistaltic drugs if diarrhea occurs

• Possible reduced blood levels of cyclosporine

• Oral contraceptives: advise patient of a potential risk for decreased contraceptive action, to maintain compliance with oral contraceptive use while using antibiotics, and to consider the use of additional nonhormonal contraception

DENTAL CONSIDERATIONS

General:

• Determine why the patient is taking the drug.

Consultations:

• Medical consultation may be required to assess disease control.

Teach patient/family:

• Importance of good oral hygiene to prevent soft tissue inflammation

• Caution to prevent injury when using oral hygiene aids

When used for dental infection, advise patient:

• To report sore throat, oral burning sensation, fever, fatigue, any of which could indicate superinfection

• To take at prescribed intervals and complete dosage regimen

• To immediately notify the dentist if signs or symptoms of infection increase

clobetasol propionate (topical foam)

(kloe-bay'ta-sol)

Olux

Drug class.: Topical corticosteroid, very high potency

Action: Glucocorticoids have multiple actions that include anti-inflammatory and immunosuppressant effects. They inhibit phospholipase A_2, interfering with or reducing the synthesis of prostaglandins and leukotrienes. They also bind to cytoplasmic GRs and enter the cell nucleus to bind with DNA. This results in the synthesis of various enzymes such as collagenase, elastase, and cytokines that play important roles in inflammation and immunosuppression. They also suppress the production of lymphocytes, monocytes, and eosinophils.

Uses: Treatment of inflammatory and pruritic manifestations of moderate to severe corticosteroid-responsive dermatitis of the scalp; other uses include psoriasis

Dosage and routes:

• *Adult:* TOP apply small amount of foam to affected scalp area bid (AM and PM)

Available forms include: Foam 0.05% in 100 g container

Side effects/adverse reactions:

INTEG: Burning, stinging, irritation, pruritus, erythema, folliculitis, contact allergy, dry skin, telangiactasia

ENDO: Possible hypothalamic-pituitary-adrenal cortex suppression

MISC: Finger numbness

Contraindications: Hypersensitivity

Precautions: Occlusive dressings, lactation, adrenal cortical suppression, avoid use in infection, not for use in rosacea or perioral dermatitis, pregnancy category C, lactation, children more susceptible to systemic absorption

Pharmacokinetics:

TOP: Absorbed through skin, especially if abraded

Drug interactions of concern to dentistry:

• None reported.

DENTAL CONSIDERATIONS

General:

• Determine why patient is taking the drug.

• Avoid use of systemic corticosteroids unless a consultation is made.

clobetasol propionate

(klo-bay'ta-sol)

Embeline-E, Temovate, Temovate Emollient Cream, Temovate Gel, Temovate Scalp Application

Dermovate, Dermovate Scalp Lotion

Drug class.: Topical corticosteroid, group I very high potency

Action: Glucocorticoids have multiple actions that include anti-inflammatory and immunosuppressant effects. They inhibit phospholipase A_2, interfering with or reducing the synthesis of prostaglandins and leukotrienes. They also bind to cytoplasmic GRs and enter the cell nucleus to bind with DNA. This results in the synthesis of various enzymes such as collagenase, elastase, and cytokines that play important roles in inflammation and immunosuppression. They also suppress the production of lymphocytes, monocytes, and eosinophils.

Uses: Psoriasis, eczema, contact dermatitis, pruritus, symptomatic relief of ulcerative inflammatory lesions; usually reserved for severe dermatoses that have not responded to less potent formulations

Dosage and routes:

• *Adult and child >12 yrs:* TOP apply to affected area bid, tid

Available forms include: Oint 0.05%; cream 0.05% in 15, 30, 45 g; gel 0.05% in 15, 30, 60 g; scalp application 0.05% in 25, 50 ml

Side effects/adverse reactions:

INTEG: Burning, dryness, itching, irritation, acne, folliculitis, hypertrichosis, perioral dermatitis, hypopigmentation, atrophy, striae, miliaria, allergic contact dermatitis, secondary infection

Contraindications: Hypersensitivity to corticosteroids, fungal infections, viral infections

Precautions: Pregnancy category C, lactation, bacterial infections

DENTAL CONSIDERATIONS

General:

• Place on frequent recall to evaluate healing response.

• Topical adrenocorticosteroids are not indicated for treating plaque-related gingivitis, which should be treated by removal of local irritants and improved oral hygiene.

Teach patient/family:

• Importance of good oral hygiene to prevent soft tissue inflammation

• That use on oral herpetic ulcerations is contraindicated

• To apply at bedtime or after meals for maximum effect

• To apply with cotton-tipped applicator by pressing, not rubbing, paste on lesion

• When used for oral lesions, advise patient to return for oral evaluation if response of oral tissues has not occurred in 7-14 days

clocortolone pivalate

(klo-kort′o-lone)

Cloderm

Drug class.: Topical corticosteroid, group III medium potency

Action: Glucocorticoids have multiple actions that include anti-inflammatory and immunosuppressant effects. They inhibit phospholipase A_2, interfering with or reducing the synthesis of prostaglandins and leukotrienes. They also bind to cytoplasmic GRs and enter the cell nucleus to bind with DNA. This results in the synthesis of various enzymes such as collagenase, elastase, and cytokines that play important roles in inflammation and immunosuppression. They also suppress the production of lymphocytes, monocytes, and eosinophils.

Uses: Psoriasis, eczema, contact dermatitis, pruritus

Dosage and routes:

• *Adult and child:* Apply to affected area tid or qid

Available forms include: Cream 0.1% in 15, 45 gm

Side effects/adverse reactions:

▼ *ORAL:* Perioral dermatitis

INTEG: Burning, dryness, itching, irritation, acne, folliculitis, hypertrichosis, hypopigmentation, atrophy, striae, miliaria, allergic contact dermatitis, secondary infection

Contraindications: Hypersensi-

tivity to corticosteroids, fungal infections

Precautions: Pregnancy category C, lactation, viral infections, bacterial infections

DENTAL CONSIDERATIONS

General:

• Determine why the patient is taking the drug.

• Place on frequent recall to evaluate healing response if used on a chronic basis.

• Apply lubricant to dry lips for patient comfort before dental procedures.

---

clofazimine

(kloe-fa'zi-meen)

Lamprene

Drug class.: Leprostatic

Action: Inhibits mycobacterial growth, binds to mycobacterial DNA

Uses: Lepromatous leprosy, dapsone-resistant leprosy, lepromatous leprosy complicated by erythema nodosum leprosum

Dosage and routes:

Erythema nodosum leprosum:

• *Adult:* PO 100-200 mg qd × 3 mo, then taper dosage to 100 mg when disease is controlled, do not exceed 300 mg/day

Dapsone-resistant leprosy:

• *Adult:* PO 100 mg/day in combination with at least one other antileprosy drug × 3 yr, then 100 mg qd clofazimine (only)

Available forms include: Caps 50 mg

Side effects/adverse reactions:

▼ *ORAL: Stomatitis (rarely)*

CNS: Dizziness, headache, fatigue, drowsiness

GI: Diarrhea, nausea, vomiting, abdominal pain, intolerance, ***GI bleeding, obstruction, hepatitis,*** anorexia, constipation, jaundice

EENT: Pigmentation of cornea, conjunctiva, drying, burning, itching, irritation

INTEG: Pink or brown discoloration, dryness, pruritus, rash, photosensitivity, acne, monilial cheilosis

MISC: Discolored urine, feces, sputum, sweat

Precautions: Pregnancy category C, lactation, children, abdominal pain, diarrhea, depression

Pharmacokinetics:

PO: Half-life 70 days; deposited in fatty tissue, reticuloendothelial system; small amount excreted in feces, sputum, sweat

Drug interactions of concern to dentistry:

• None reported

DENTAL CONSIDERATIONS

General:

• Develop awareness of the patient's disease.

Teach patient/family:

• Importance of good oral hygiene to prevent soft tissue inflammation

• To avoid mouth rinses with high alcohol content because of drying effects

---

clofibrate

(kloe-fye'brate)

Abitrate, Atromid-S

♣ Claripex, Novofibrate

Drug class.: Antihyperlipidemic

Action: Inhibits biosynthesis of VLDL and LDL, which are responsible for triglyceride development; mobilizes triglycerides from tissue; increases excretion of neutral sterols

Uses: Hyperlipidemia (types III, IV, V)

Dosage and routes:

• *Adult:* PO 1.5-2 g/day in 2-4 divided doses

Available forms include: Caps 500 mg, 1 g

Side effects/adverse reactions:

▼ *ORAL: Stomatitis*

CNS: Fatigue, weakness, drowsiness, dizziness

CV: ***Pulmonary emboli,*** angina, dysrhythmias, thrombophlebitis

GI: Nausea, vomiting, dyspepsia, increased liver enzymes, flatulence

HEMA: ***Leukopenia, eosinophilia,*** anemia, bleeding

GU: ***Hematuria,*** decreased libido, impotence, dysuria, proteinuria, oliguria

INTEG: Rash, urticaria, pruritus, dry hair and skin, alopecia

MS: Myalgias, arthralgias

MISC: Polyphagia, weight gain

Contraindications: Severe hepatic disease, severe renal disease, primary biliary cirrhosis, pregnancy, lactation, children

Precautions: Peptic ulcer, pregnancy category C

Pharmacokinetics:

PO: Peak 2-6 hr, half-life 6-25 hr; plasma protein binding >96%; metabolized in liver; excreted in urine

DENTAL CONSIDERATIONS

General:

• Consider semisupine chair position for patient comfort if GI side effects occur.

• Patients on chronic drug therapy may rarely have symptoms of blood dyscrasias, which can include infection, bleeding, and poor healing.

• No dental drug interactions have been reported.

Consultations:

• In a patient with symptoms of blood dyscrasias, request a medical consultation for blood studies and postpone treatment until normal values are reestablished.

Teach patient/family:

• Importance of good oral hygiene to prevent soft tissue inflammation

---

clomiphene citrate

(kloe′mi-feen)

Clomid, Milophene, Serophene

Drug class.: Nonsteroidal ovulatory stimulant, antiestrogen

Action: Binds to hypothalamic estrogen receptors, resulting in increase of LH and FSH release from the pituitary, which increases maturation of ovarian follicle, ovulation, and development of corpus luteum

Uses: Female infertility

Dosage and routes:

• ***Initial adult:*** PO 50 mg qd × 5 days; may be repeated until conception occurs or 3-4 cycles of therapy have been completed

• *Second trial adult:* PO 100 mg/day × 5 days, can repeat third time

Available forms include: Tabs 50 mg

Side effects/adverse reactions:

CNS: Headache, depression, restlessness, anxiety, nervousness, fatigue, insomnia, dizziness, flushing

CV: Vasomotor flushing, phlebitis, deep vein thrombosis

GI: Nausea, vomiting, constipation, abdominal pain, bloating

GU: Polyuria, frequency, birth defects, spontaneous abortions, multiple ovulation, breast pain, oliguria, abnormal uterine bleeding

EENT: Blurred vision, diplopia, photophobia

INTEG: Rash, dermatitis, urticaria, alopecia
Contraindications: Hypersensitivity, pregnancy category X, hepatic disease, undiagnosed bleeding, uncontrolled thyroid or adrenal dysfunction, intracranial lesion, ovarian cyst, abnormal uterine bleeding
Precautions: Hypertension, depression, convulsions, diabetes mellitus
Pharmacokinetics:
PO: Metabolized in liver, excreted in feces
DENTAL CONSIDERATIONS
General:
- Consider semisupine chair position for patient comfort because of GI effects of drug.
- Avoid dental light in patient's eyes; offer dark glasses for patient comfort.
- Be aware that patient may be in early stage of pregnancy.
- No dental drug interactions reported

clomipramine HCl

(kloe-mi'pra-meen)
Anafranil
Drug class.: Tricyclic antidepressant

Action: Inhibits both norepinephrine and serotonin (5-HT) uptake in the brain, although the precise antidepressant mechanism remains unclear
Uses: Obsessive-compulsive disorder; unapproved: depression, panic disorder, narcolepsy, and neurogenic pain
Dosage and routes:
Obsessive-compulsive disorder:
- *Adult:* PO 25 mg hs; increase gradually over 4 wk to a dose of 75-300 mg/day in divided doses
- *Child 10-18 yr:* PO 25 mg/day gradually increased; not to exceed 200 mg/day

Available forms include: Caps 25, 50, 75 mg; tabs 10, 25, 50 mg (Canada only)
Side effects/adverse reactions:
▼ *ORAL: Dry mouth, unpleasant taste,* bleeding
CNS: Dizziness, tremors, mania, ***seizures,*** aggressiveness
CV: ***Cardiac arrest,*** orthostatic hypotension, tachycardia, prolonged QT interval
GI: Constipation
HEMA: ***Agranulocytosis, neutropenia, pancytopenia***
GU: Delayed ejaculation, anorgasmy, retention
INTEG: Diaphoresis
ENDO: Galactorrhea, hyperprolactinemia
META: Increased hyponatremia, hyperthermia, AST, ALT
MISC: Weight gain
Contraindications: Hypersensitivity, generally contraindicated with concurrent use or within 14 days of discontinuing MAOI, acute recovery phase of MI
Precautions: Seizures, suicidal patients, elderly, MAOIs, pregnancy category C, not for use in children <10 yr, renal or hepatic dysfunction
Pharmacokinetics:
PO: Half-life: 21 hr parent compound, 36 hr metabolite; extensively bound to tissue and plasma proteins; demethylated in liver (active metabolites); excreted in urine (metabolites)
Drug interactions of concern to dentistry:
- Increased anticholinergic effects: muscarinic blockers, antihistamines, phenothiazines

• Increased effects of direct-acting sympathomimetics (epinephrine, levonordefrin)
• Potential risk of CNS depression: alcohol, barbiturates, benzodiazepines, and other CNS depressants
• Decreased antihypertensive effects: clonidine, guanadrel, guanethidine
• Use with caution, possible reduced metabolism: drugs metabolized by CYP450 2D6 isoenzymes (see Appendix I)
• Avoid concurrent use with St. John's wort (herb)

DENTAL CONSIDERATIONS

General:

• Take vital signs at every appointment because of cardiovascular side effects.
• Assess salivary flow as a factor in caries, periodontal disease, and candidiasis.
• Patients on chronic drug therapy may rarely have symptoms of blood dyscrasias, which can include infection, bleeding, and poor healing.
• After supine positioning, have patient sit upright for at least 2 min before standing to avoid orthostatic hypotension.
• Use vasoconstrictor with caution, in low doses, and with careful aspiration. Avoid use of gingival retraction cord with epinephrine.
• Place on frequent recall because of oral side effects.
• A stress reduction protocol may be required.

Consultations:

• In a patient with symptoms of blood dyscrasias, request a medical consultation for blood studies and postpone dental treatment until normal values are reestablished.
• Physician should be informed if significant xerostomic side effects occur (e.g., increased caries, sore tongue, problems eating or swallowing, difficulty wearing prosthesis) so that a medication change can be considered.
• Medical consultation may be required to assess disease control.

Teach patient/family:

• Importance of good oral hygiene to prevent soft tissue inflammation
• Caution to prevent injury when using oral hygiene aids

When chronic dry mouth occurs, advise patient:

• To avoid mouth rinses with high alcohol content because of drying effects
• To use daily home fluoride products for anticaries effect
• To use sugarless gum, frequent sips of water, or saliva substitutes

---

clonazepam

(kloe-na'zi-pam)

Klonopin

♣ Alti-Clonazepam, Apo-Clonazepam, Clonapam, Gen-Clonazepam, PMS-Clonazepam, Rivotril

Drug class.: Anticonvulsant, benzodiazepine derivative

Controlled Substance Schedule IV

Action: Inhibits spike and wave formation in absence seizures (petit mal); decreases amplitude, frequency, duration, spread of discharge in minor motor seizures; acts on benzodiazepine receptors in the CNS to enhance the activity of γ-aminobutyric acid (GABA)

Uses: Absence, atypical absence, akinetic, myoclonic seizures; unlabeled uses Parkinson's dysarthria, adjunct in schizophrenia, neuralgias

Dosage and routes:

Seizures:

- *Adult:* PO not to exceed 1.5 mg/day in 3 divided doses; may be increased 0.5-1 mg q3d until desired response; not to exceed 20 mg/day
- *Child up to 10 yr or 30 kg:* PO 0.01-0.03 mg/kg/day in divided doses q8h, not to exceed 0.05 mg/kg/day; may be increased 0.25-0.5 mg q3d until desired response, not to exceed 0.1-0.2 mg/kg/day

Available forms include: Tabs 0.5, 1, 2 mg

Side effects/adverse reactions:

▼ *ORAL:* Dry mouth or increased salivation, bleeding

CNS: Drowsiness, dizziness, confusion, behavioral changes, tremors, insomnia, headache, suicidal tendencies, slurred speech

CV: Palpitation, bradycardia

GI: Nausea, constipation, polyphagia, anorexia, xerostomia, diarrhea, gastritis

RESP: ***Respiratory depression,*** dyspnea, congestion

HEMA: ***Thrombocytopenia, leukocytosis, eosinophilia***

GU: Dysuria, enuresis, nocturia, retention

EENT: Nystagmus, diplopia, abnormal eye movements

INTEG: Rash, alopecia, hirsutism

Contraindications: Hypersensitivity to benzodiazepines, acute narrow-angle glaucoma, ritonavir, saquinavir, significant liver impairment

Precautions: Open-angle glaucoma, chronic respiratory disease, pregnancy category C, renal, hepatic disease, elderly, interferes with cognitive and motor performance, withdrawal symptoms

Pharmacokinetics:

PO: Absolute bioavailability 90%, plasma protein binding 85%, peak 1-4 hr, half-life 18-50 hr; extensively metabolized by liver (CYP 3A); excreted in urine

Drug interactions of concern to dentistry:

- Increased sedation: alcohol, all CNS depressants, indinavir, kava (herb)
- Risk of increased serum levels: drugs that inhibit CYP3A4 isoenzymes, ketoconazole, itraconazole, fluconazole, protease inhibitor, nefazodone (see Appendix I)
- Risk of decreased effect: St. John's wort (herb)

DENTAL CONSIDERATIONS

General:

- Patients on chronic drug therapy may rarely have symptoms of blood dyscrasias, which can include infection, bleeding, and poor healing.
- Assess salivary flow as a factor in caries, periodontal disease, and candidiasis.
- Psychologic and physical dependence may occur with chronic administration.
- Geriatric patients are more susceptible to drug effects; use lower dose.
- Ask about type of epilepsy, seizure frequency, and quality of seizure control.

Consultations:

- Medical consultation may be required to assess disease control.
- In a patient with symptoms of blood dyscrasias, request a medical

consultation for blood studies and postpone dental treatment until normal values are reestablished.

Teach patient/family:

- Importance of good oral hygiene to prevent soft tissue inflammation
- Caution to prevent injury when using oral hygiene aids

When chronic dry mouth occurs, advise patient:

- To avoid mouth rinses with high alcohol content because of drying effects
- To use daily home fluoride products for anticaries effect
- To use sugarless gum, frequent sips of water, or saliva substitutes

clonidine HCl/clonidine transdermal

(kloe'ni-deen)

Catapres, Catapres-TTS, Duraclon

🍁 Dixarit

Drug class.: Antihypertensive, central α-adrenergic agonist

Action: Inhibits sympathetic vasomotor center in CNS, thus reducing impulses in sympathetic nervous system; decreases blood pressure, pulse rate, and cardiac output; analgesic action associated with α_2-adrenergic receptors in the spinal cord preventing pain signal transmission to higher centers

Uses: Hypertension, severe pain in combination with opioids for cancer patients; unapproved: opioid abstinence syndrome, nicotine withdrawal, vascular headache, alcohol withdrawal, ADHD, postherpetic neuralgia

Dosage and routes:

Hypertension:

- *Adult:* PO/TRANSDERMAL 0.1 mg bid, then increase by 0.1 mg/day or 0.2 mg/day until desired response; range 0.2-0.8 mg/day in divided doses

Severe pain:

- *Adult:* INF continuous epidural infusion 30 μg/hr

Available forms include: Tabs 0.1, 0.2, 0.3 mg; transderm sys 2.5, 5, 7.5 mg delivering 0.1, 0.2, 0.3 mg/24 hr, respectively; 100 μg/ml in 10 ml vials (Duraclon)

Side effects/adverse reactions:

▼ *ORAL:* Dry mouth, taste changes, salivary pain or swelling

CNS: Drowsiness, sedation, headache, fatigue, nightmares, insomnia, mental changes, anxiety, depression, hallucinations, delirium

CV: Orthostatic hypotension, palpitation, ***CHF,*** ECG abnormalities

GI: Nausea, vomiting, malaise, constipation

GU: Impotence, nocturia, dysuria, gynecomastia

EENT: Parotid pain

INTEG: Rash, alopecia, facial pallor, pruritus, hives, edema, burning papules, excoriation (transdermal patches)

ENDO: Hyperglycemia

MS: Muscle/joint pain, leg cramps

Contraindications: Hypersensitivity to this drug or any component of the transdermal system

Precautions: MI (recent), cerebrovascular disease, chronic renal failure, Raynaud's disease, thyroid disease, depression, COPD, child <12 yr (patches), asthma, pregnancy category C, lactation, elderly

Pharmacokinetics:

PO: Peak 3-5 hr, half-life 12-16 hr; metabolized by liver (metabolites); excreted in urine (unchanged, inactive metabolites), feces; crosses blood-brain barrier; excreted in breast milk

Drug interactions of concern to dentistry:

• Increased CNS depression: alcohol, all CNS depressants

• Decreased hypotensive effects: NSAIDs, especially indomethacin, sympathomimetics, tricyclic antidepressants

DENTAL CONSIDERATIONS

General:

• Monitor vital signs at every appointment because of cardiovascular side effects.

• After supine positioning, have patient sit upright for at least 2 min before standing to avoid orthostatic hypotension.

• Limit use of sodium-containing products such as saline IV fluids for patients with a dietary salt restriction.

• Assess salivary flow as a factor in caries, periodontal disease, and candidiasis.

• Stress from dental procedures may compromise cardiovascular function; determine patient risk.

• Short appointments and a stress reduction protocol may be required for anxious patients.

• Consider drug in diagnosis of taste alterations.

Consultations:

• Medical consultation may be required to assess disease control.

Teach patient/family:

When chronic dry mouth occurs, advise patient:

• To avoid mouth rinses with high alcohol content because of drying effects

• To use daily home fluoride products for anticaries effect

• To use sugarless gum, frequent sips of water, or saliva substitutes

clopidogrel bisulfate

(kloe-pid-o'grel)

Plavix

Drug class.: Platelet aggregation inhibitor

Action: Irreversibly inhibits adenosine diphosphate (ADP)–induced platelet aggregation, binds to the ADP platelet receptors

Uses: Adjunctive treatment in recent MI, ischemic stroke, and peripheral vascular disease in patients with atherosclerosis; treatment of acute coronary syndrome (unstable angina with non–Q wave MI)

Dosage and routes:

Recent MI, ischemic stroke, or peripheral vascular disease:

• *Adult:* PO 75 mg qd with or without food

Acute coronary syndrome:

• *Adult:* PO initial loading dose 300 mg; then 75 mg qd; also use 75 mg to 325 mg aspirin qd

Available forms include: Tabs 75 mg

Side effects/adverse reactions:

CNS: Headache, dizziness, depression

CV: Fatigue, chest pain, edema, hypertension

GI: Diarrhea, abdominal pain, nausea, gastritis with bleeding, dyspepsia

RESP: URTI, bronchitis, coughing

EENT: Epistaxis, rhinitis

HEMA: Bleeding, neutropenia (rare), ***thrombotic thrombocytopenia purpura***

INTEG: Rash, urticaria, purpura, pruritus

META: Liver function abnormalities, hepatotoxicity, hypercholesterolemia

GU: UTI
MS: Arthralgia, back pain
MISC: Flulike symptoms
Contraindications: Hypersensitivity, active bleeding, bleeding disorders, anticoagulants, antiplatelet agents
Precautions: Hepatic impairment, renal impairment, hypertension, history of bleeding disorders, major surgery, pregnancy category B, safety and efficacy during lactation or use in children not established
Pharmacokinetics:
PO: Well absorbed, peak levels <1 hr, hepatic metabolism, active metabolite, plasma protein binding 94%-98%, excreted in both urine and feces, maximal effect on bleeding time 5-7 days
Drug interactions of concern to dentistry:
• Caution in use with NSAIDs
DENTAL CONSIDERATIONS
General:
• Effects on platelet aggregation return to normal in 5-7 days.
• Patients on chronic drug therapy may rarely have symptoms of blood dyscrasias, which can include infection, bleeding, and poor healing.
• Consider local hemostasis measures to prevent excessive bleeding.
• Question patient about concurrent aspirin use.
• Monitor vital signs at every appointment because of cardiovascular disease.
• Consider semisupine chair position for patient comfort if GI side effects occur.
Consultations:
• Medical consultation may be required to assess disease control and patient's ability to tolerate stress.
• Consultation should include data on bleeding time.
• In a patient with symptoms of blood dyscrasias, request a medical consultation for blood studies and postpone treatment until normal values are reestablished.
Teach patient/family:
• Importance of updating health and drug history if physician makes any changes in evaluation or drug regimens
• Caution to prevent trauma when using oral hygiene aids
• To report any unusual or prolonged bleeding episodes after dental treatment

clorazepate dipotassium

(klor-az'e-pate)
Gen-Xene, Tranxene-SD, Tranxene-SD Half Strength, Traxene T-Tab
♣ Apo-Chlorazepate, Novo-Clopate, Tranxene
Drug class.: Benzodiazepine

Controlled Substance Schedule IV
Action: Produces CNS depression by interacting with a benzodiazepine receptor to facilitate the action of the inhibitory neurotransmitter γ-aminobutyric acid (GABA)
Uses: Anxiety, acute alcohol withdrawal, adjunctive treatment of partial seizures
Dosage and routes:
Anxiety:
• *Adult:* PO 15-60 mg/day in divided doses

• *Elderly or debilitated:* PO 7.5-15 mg/day or lower if required

Alcohol withdrawal:

• *Adult:* PO 30 mg initially, then 30-60 mg in divided doses; day 2, 45-90 mg in divided doses; day 3, 22.5-45 mg in divided doses; day 4, 15-30 mg in divided doses; then reduce daily dose to 7.5-15 mg

Partial seizures:

• *Adult and child >12 yr:* PO initial dose 7.5 mg tid; can increase by 7.5 mg qwk, limit 90 mg/day

• *Child 9-12 yr:* PO initial dose 7.5 mg bid; can increase by 7.5 mg qwk, limit 60 mg/day

Available forms include: Caps 3.75, 7.5, 15 mg; tabs 3.75, 7.5, 15 mg, single-dose tab 11.25, 22.5 mg

Side effects/adverse reactions:

▼ *ORAL:* Dry mouth

CNS: Dizziness, drowsiness, confusion, headache, anxiety, tremors, stimulation, fatigue, depression, insomnia, hallucinations

CV: Orthostatic hypotension, ***ECG changes, tachycardia,*** hypotension

GI: Constipation, nausea, vomiting, anorexia, diarrhea

EENT: Blurred vision, tinnitus, mydriasis

INTEG: Rash, dermatitis, itching

Contraindications: Hypersensitivity to benzodiazepines, narrow-angle glaucoma, psychosis, pregnancy category D, child <18 yr; ritonavir, saquinavir

Precautions: Elderly, debilitated, hepatic disease, renal disease

Pharmacokinetics:

PO: Onset 15 min, peak 1-2 hr, duration 4-6 hr, half-life 30-100 hr; metabolized by liver; excreted by kidneys; crosses placenta, excreted in breast milk

Drug interactions of concern to dentistry:

• Increased effects: CNS depressants, alcohol, opioid analgesics, general anesthetics, indinavir

• Increased serum levels and prolonged effect of benzodiazepines: fluconazole, ketoconazole, itraconazole, miconazole (systemic)

• Possible increase in CNS side effects: kava (herb)

• Contraindicated with saquinavir

DENTAL CONSIDERATIONS

General:

• Monitor vital signs at every appointment because of cardiovascular side effects.

• Assess salivary flow as a factor in caries, periodontal disease, and candidiasis.

• After supine positioning, have patient sit upright for at least 2 min to avoid orthostatic hypotension.

• Psychologic and physical dependence may occur with chronic administration.

• Geriatric patients are more susceptible to drug effects; use a lower dose.

• Short appointments and a stress reduction protocol may be required for anxious patients

• Seizure: ask about type of epilepsy, seizure frequency and quality of seizure control

Consultations:

• Medical consultation may be required to assess disease control and the patient's ability to tolerate stress patient.

Teach patient/family:

When chronic dry mouth occurs, advise patient:

• To avoid mouth rinses with high alcohol content because of drying effects

• To use daily home fluoride products for anticaries effect
• To use sugarless gum, frequent sips of water, or saliva substitutes

clotrimazole

(kloe-trim'a-zole)

Vaginal products: Gyne-Lotrimin 3, Gyne-Lotrimin 7, Gye-Lotrimin 3 Combination Pack, Mycelex-7, Mycelex-7 Combination Pack

Topical products: Cruex, Desenex, Fungoid, Lotrimin, Lotrimin AF

Oral products: Mycelex Lozenges

✤ Canesten, Myclo-Gyne, Neo-Zol

Drug class.: Imidazole antifungal

Action: Interferes with fungal DNA replication; binds sterols in fungal cell membrane, which increases permeability, leaking of cell nutrients; fungicidal

Uses: Tinea pedis; tinea cruris; tinea corporis; tinea versicolor; *C. albicans* infection of the vagina, vulva, throat, mouth

Dosage and routes:

• *Adult and child:* TOP use OTC products daily for 4 wk; prescription products use bid AM and PM up to 4 wk

VAG SUPP one intravaginally at hs for 3 consecutive days

VAG CREAM one full applicator daily at hs for 3-7 consecutive days

• *Adult and child:* ORAL LOZ dissolve 1 oral troche in mouth 5 × day for 14 days

Available forms include: Cream, sol, lotion 1%; vag supp 100, 200 mg; vag cream 1%, 2%; troche 10 mg; combo products include cream 1% with 100, 200 mg suppository

Side effects/adverse reactions:

INTEG: Rash, urticaria, stinging, burning, peeling, blistering

MISC: Abdominal cramps, bloating, urinary frequency, dyspareunia

Contraindications: Hypersensitivity

Precautions: Pregnancy category B, lactation

Drug interactions of concern to dentistry:

• None reported

DENTAL CONSIDERATIONS

General:

• Determine why the patient is taking the drug.
• Examine oral mucous membranes for signs of fungal infection.

Teach patient/family:

• If used for oral infection: to soak full or partial dentures in an antifungal solution overnight until lesions are absent; prolonged infections may require fabrication of new prosthesis
• To dispose of toothbrush used during oral infection after oral lesions are absent to prevent reinoculation
• That long-term therapy may be needed to clear infection; to complete entire course of medication

clozapine

(klo'za-pin)

Clozaril

Drug class.: Antipsychotic, atypical

Action: Interferes with binding of dopamine at D_1 and D_2 receptors with low extrapyramidal symptoms; also acts as an adrenergic, cholinergic, histaminergic, and serotonergic antagonist; antipsychotic mechanism not established

Uses: Management of psychotic symptoms in schizophrenic patients for whom other antipsychotics have failed (available only through the Clozaril Patient Management System)

Dosage and routes:

• *Adult:* PO initial dose 12.5 mg qd or bid, then 25 mg qd or bid, may increase by 25-50 mg/day; normal range 300-450 mg/day after 2 wk; do not increase dose more than 2 × weekly; do not exceed 900 mg/day; use lowest dose to control symptoms

Available forms include: Tabs 25, 100 mg

Side effects/adverse reactions:

▼ *ORAL: Dry mouth, increased salivation,* glossitis

CNS: Sedation, dizziness, headache, tremors, sleep problems, akinesia, fever, ***seizures,*** sweating, akathisia, confusion, fatigue, insomnia, depression, slurred speech, anxiety

CV: Tachycardia, orthostatic hypotension, hypertension, chest pain, ECG changes

GI: Constipation, nausea, abdominal discomfort, vomiting, diarrhea, anorexia

RESP: Dyspnea, nasal congestion, throat discomfort

HEMA: ***Leukopenia, neutropenia, agranulocytosis, eosinophilia***

GU: Urinary abnormalities, incontinence, ejaculation dysfunction, frequency, urgency, retention

MS: Weakness; pain in back, neck, legs; spasm

Contraindications: Hypersensitivity, myeloproliferative disorders, severe granulocytopenia, CNS depression, coma, narrow-angle glaucoma

Precautions: Pregnancy category B; lactation; children <16 yr; hepatic, renal, cardiac disease; seizures; prostatic enlargement; elderly; increased incidence of cardiomyopathy

Pharmacokinetics:

PO: Steady state 2.5 hr, half-life 8-12 hr; 95% protein bound; completely metabolized by the liver; excreted in urine and feces (metabolites)

Drug interactions of concern to dentistry:

• Increased anticholinergic effects: anticholinergics

• Increased CNS depression: alcohol, all CNS depressant drugs

• Increased serum concentration, leukocytosis: erythromycin base

• Possible decreased effects: carbamazepine

• Increased plasma levels: ciprofloxacin

DENTAL CONSIDERATIONS

General:

• Monitor vital signs at every appointment because of cardiovascular and respiratory side effects.

• Patients on chronic drug therapy may rarely have symptoms of blood dyscrasias, which can include infection, bleeding, and poor healing.

• After supine positioning, have patient sit upright for at least 2 min before standing to avoid orthostatic hypotension.

• Assess salivary flow as a factor in caries, periodontal disease, and candidiasis.

• Determine why the patient is taking the drug.

• Place on frequent recall because of oral side effects.

Consultations:

• In a patient with symptoms of blood dyscrasias, request a medical consultation for blood studies and postpone dental treatment until normal values are reestablished.

• Medical consultation may be required to assess disease control and stress tolerance of patient.

• Physician should be informed if significant xerostomic side effects occur (e.g., increased caries, sore tongue, problems eating or swallowing, difficulty wearing prosthesis) so that a medication change can be considered.

Teach patient/family:

• Importance of good oral hygiene to prevent soft tissue inflammation

• Caution to prevent injury when using oral hygiene aids

• To use electric toothbrush if patient has difficulty holding conventional devices

When chronic dry mouth occurs, advise patient:

• To avoid mouth rinses with high alcohol content because of drying effects

• To use daily home fluoride products for anticaries effect

• To use sugarless gum, frequent sips of water, or saliva substitutes

codeine sulfate/ codeine phosphate

(koe'deen)

generic codeine

Drug class.: Narcotic analgesic

Controlled Substance Schedule II, Canada N

Action: Depresses pain impulse transmission in CNS by interacting with opioid receptors

Uses: Mild-to-moderate pain, nonproductive cough

Dosage and routes:

Pain:

• *Adult:* PO 15-60 mg q4h prn; IM/SC 15-60 mg q4h prn

• *Child >1 yr:* PO 0.5 mg/kg/day q4-6h prn

Cough:

• *Adult:* PO 10-20 mg q4-6h, not to exceed 120 mg/day

• *Child 6-12 yr:* PO 5-10 mg q4-6h (24 hr limit 60 mg)

• *Child 2-6 yr:* PO 2.5-5 mg q4-6h (24 hr limit 30 mg)

Available forms include: Inj IM/SC 15, 30, 60 mg/ml; tabs 15, 30, 60 mg

Side effects/adverse reactions:

▼ *ORAL: Dry mouth,* lichenoid reaction

CNS: Drowsiness, sedation, dizziness, agitation, dependency, lethargy, restlessness

CV: Bradycardia, palpitation, orthostatic hypotension, tachycardia

GI: Nausea, vomiting, anorexia, constipation

RESP: ***Respiratory depression, respiratory paralysis***

GU: Urinary retention

INTEG: Flushing, rash, urticaria

Contraindications: Hypersensitivity to opiates, respiratory depression, increased intracranial pressure, seizure disorders, severe respiratory disorders

Precautions: Elderly, cardiac dysrhythmias, pregnancy category C

Pharmacokinetics:

PO: Onset 15-30 min, peak 1-2 hr, duration 4-6 hr, half-life 2.5-4 hr; metabolized by liver; excreted by kidneys; crosses placenta; excreted in breast milk

Drug interactions of concern to dentistry:

- Increased sedation with other CNS depressants and alcohol
- Increased effects of anticholinergics

DENTAL CONSIDERATIONS

General:

- Monitor vital signs at every appointment because of cardiovascular and respiratory side effects.
- After supine positioning, have patient sit upright for at least 2 min to avoid orthostatic hypotension.
- Assess salivary flow as a factor in caries, periodontal disease, and candidiasis.
- Psychologic and physical dependence may occur with chronic administration.

Teach patient/family:

When chronic dry mouth occurs, advise patient:

- To avoid mouth rinses with high alcohol content because of drying effects
- To use daily home fluoride products for anticaries effect
- To use sugarless gum, frequent sips of water, or saliva substitutes

colchicine

(kol'chi-seen)

generic colchicine

Drug class.: Antigout agent

Action: Inhibits deposition of uric acid crystals in soft tissues; mechanism unclear

Uses: Gout, gouty arthritis (prevention, treatment), unlabeled uses: hepatic cirrhosis, Behcet's disease, scleroderma, Sweet's syndrome

Dosage and routes:

Prevention:

- *Adult:* PO 0.5-1.8 mg qd depending on severity

Treatment:

- *Adult:* PO 0.6-1.2 mg, then 0.6 mg q1h until pain decreases or side effects occur

Available forms include: Tabs 0.6 mg

Side effects/adverse reactions:

▼ *ORAL:* Metallic taste, lichenoid reaction

GI: Nausea, vomiting, anorexia, malaise, cramps, peptic ulcer, diarrhea

HEMA: ***Agranulocytosis, thrombocytopenia, aplastic anemia, pancytopenia***

GU: Hematuria, oliguria, renal damage

INTEG: Chills, dermatitis, pruritus, purpura, erythema

MISC: Myopathy, alopecia, reversible azoospermia, peripheral neuritis

Contraindications: Hypersensitivity; serious GI, renal, hepatic, cardiac disorders; blood dyscrasias

Precautions: Severe renal disease, blood dyscrasias, pregnancy category C, hepatic disease, elderly, lactation, children, retards B_{12} absorption

Pharmacokinetics:

PO: Peak 0.5-2 hr, half-life 20 min; deacetylates in liver; excreted in feces (metabolites/active drug)

Drug interactions of concern to dentistry:

• Increased risk of GI side effects: NSAIDs, alcohol

• Possible increased serum levels: erythromycin

DENTAL CONSIDERATIONS

General:

• Consider drug in diagnosis of taste alteration.

• Patients on chronic drug therapy may rarely have symptoms of blood dyscrasias, which can include infection, bleeding, and poor healing.

• Avoid prescribing aspirin-containing products.

Consultations:

• Medical consultation may be required to assess disease control.

• In a patient with symptoms of blood dyscrasias, request a medical consultation for blood studies and postpone dental treatment until normal values are reestablished.

Teach patient/family:

• Importance of good oral hygiene to prevent soft tissue inflammation

• Caution to prevent injury when using oral hygiene aids

• To avoid mouth rinses with high alcohol content because of drying effects

colesevelam HCl

(koh-le-sev′-e-lam)

Welchol

Drug class.: Antihyperlipidemic

Action: Combines with bile acids to form insoluble complexes that are excreted through the feces; loss of bile acids lowers cholesterol levels

Uses: Adjunctive therapy to diet and exercise, alone or in combination with an HMG-Co A reductase inhibitor (statin) in patients with primary hypercholesterolemia (type IIa) to reduce elevated LDL cholesterol

Dosage and routes:

• *Adult:* PO initial dose 3 tabs (187 mg) bid with meals and a full glass of water; or 6 tabs once/day with meals. Dose may be increased to 7 tabs depending on need.

Combination therapy with HMG-Co A reductase inhibitor:

• *Adult:* PO 3 tabs (1875 mg) bid with meals or 6 tabs once/day taken with a meal

Available forms include: Tabs 625 mg

Side effects/adverse reactions:

CNS: Headache

GI: Constipation, dyspepsia, flatulence diarrhea, abdominal pain, nausea

RESP: Increased cough

EENT: Sinusitis, rhinitis, pharyngitis

MS: Myalgia, back pain

MISC: Flulike syndrome

Contraindications: Hypersensitivity, bowel obstruction

Precautions: Preexisting GI diseases, primary biliary cirrhosis, biliary obstruction, hypertriglyceridemia, pregnancy category B, use in children not established

Pharmacokinetics: Drug is not absorbed from GI tract

Drug interactions of concern to dentistry:

• None reported, but monitor if drugs with narrow therapeutic index are prescribed for dental conditions

DENTAL CONSIDERATIONS

General:

• Consider semisupine chair position for patient comfort because of GI side effects of drug.

• Monitor vital signs at every appointment because of possibility of cardiovascular disease.

colestipol HCl

(koe-les'ti-pole)

Colestid

Drug class.: Antihyperlipidemic

Action: Absorbs, combines with bile acids to form insoluble complex that is excreted through feces; loss of bile acids lowers cholesterol levels

Uses: Adjunctive therapy to diet and exercise for the reduction of elevated serum total and LDL cholesterol in patients with primary hypercholesterolemia

Dosage and routes:

• *Adult:* PO (granules) initial dose 5 g/day or bid, then 5-30 g/day in 2-4 divided doses

• *Adult:* PO (tablets) 2-16 g/day once or in divided doses bid

Available forms include: Tabs 1 g, granules for oral suspension 5 g powder/packet

Side effects/adverse reactions:

ORAL: Glossitis

GI: Constipation, abdominal pain, nausea, fecal impaction, hemorrhoids, flatulence, vomiting, steatorrhea, peptic ulcer

HEMA: Decreased vitamins A, D, K red folate content; ***hyperchloremic acidosis;*** bleeding; decreased protime

INTEG: Rash, irritation of perianal area, skin

Contraindications: Hypersensitivity, biliary obstruction

Precautions: Pregnancy category B, lactation, children, bleeding disorders

Pharmacokinetics:

PO: Not absorbed; excreted in feces

Drug interactions of concern to dentistry:

• Decreased absorption of tetracyclines, cephalexin, phenobarbital, corticosteroids, clindamycin, penicillins; administer doses several hours apart

DENTAL CONSIDERATIONS

General:

• Consider semisupine chair position for patient comfort because of GI effects of disease.

cortisone acetate

(kor'ti-sone)

Cortone

Drug class.: Glucocorticoid, short-acting

Action: Glucocorticoids have multiple actions that include anti-inflammatory and immunosuppressant effects. They inhibit phospholipase A_2, interfering with or reducing the synthesis of prostaglandins and leukotrienes. They also bind to cytoplasmic GRs and enter the cell nucleus to bind with DNA. This results in the synthesis of various enzymes such as collagenase, elastase, and cytokines that play important roles in inflammation and immunosuppression. They also suppress the production of lymphocytes, monocytes, and eosinophils.

Uses: Inflammation, severe allergy, adrenal insufficiency, collagen disorders, respiratory, dermatologic disorders

Dosage and routes:

• *Adult:* PO 25-300 mg qd or q2d, titrated to patient response

Available forms include: Tabs 5, 10, 25 mg; inj 50 mg/ml in 10 ml

Side effects/adverse reactions:

▼ *ORAL:* Dry mouth, poor wound healing, petechiae, candidiasis

CNS: Depression, flushing, sweating, headache, mood changes

CV: Hypertension, ***circulatory collapse, thrombophlebitis, embolism, necrotizing angiitis, CHF,*** tachycardia, edema

GI: Diarrhea, nausea, abdominal distention, ***GI hemorrhage, pancreatitis,*** increased appetite

HEMA: ***Thrombocytopenia***

EENT: Fungal infections, increased intraocular pressure, blurred vision

INTEG: Acne, poor wound healing, ecchymosis, bruising, petechiae

MS: Fractures, osteoporosis, weakness

Contraindications: Psychosis, hypersensitivity, idiopathic thrombocytopenia, acute glomerulonephritis, amebiasis, fungal infections, nonasthmatic bronchial disease, child <2 yr, AIDS, TB

Precautions: Pregnancy category C, diabetes mellitus, glaucoma, osteoporosis, seizure disorders, ulcerative colitis, CHF, myasthenia gravis, renal disease, esophagitis, peptic ulcer, rifampin

Pharmacokinetics:

PO: Peak 2 hr, duration 1.5 days

IM: Peak 20-48 hr, duration 1.5 days

Drug interactions of concern to dentistry:

• Decreased action: barbiturates, rifabutin, rifampin

• Increased GI side effects: alcohol, salicylates, NSAIDs

• Increased action: ketoconazole, macrolide antibiotics

• Hepatotoxicity: acetaminophen (chronic, high doses)

DENTAL CONSIDERATIONS

General:

• Monitor vital signs at every appointment because of cardiovascular side effects.

• Patients on chronic drug therapy may rarely have symptoms of blood dyscrasias, which can include infection, bleeding, and poor healing.

• Assess salivary flow as a factor in caries, periodontal disease, and candidiasis.

• Avoid prescribing aspirin-containing products.

• Symptoms of oral infections may be masked.

• Place on frequent recall to evaluate healing response.

• Prophylactic antibiotics may be indicated to prevent infection if surgery or deep scaling is planned.

• Determine dose and duration of steroid therapy for each patient to assess risk for stress tolerance and immunosuppression.

• Patients who have been or are currently on chronic steroid therapy (>2 wk) may require supplemental steroids for dental treatment.

• Determine why the patient is taking the drug.

Consultations:

• In a patient with symptoms of blood dyscrasias, request a medical consultation for blood studies and postpone dental treatment until normal values are reestablished.

• Medical consultation may be required to assess disease control and stress tolerance of patient.

• Consultation may be required to confirm steroid dose and duration of use.

Teach patient/family:

• Importance of good oral hygiene to prevent soft tissue inflammation

• Caution to prevent injury when using oral hygiene aids

When chronic dry mouth occurs, advise patient:

• To avoid mouth rinses with high alcohol content because of drying effects

• To use daily home fluoride products for anticaries effect

• To use sugarless gum, frequent sips of water, or saliva substitutes

cromolyn sodium (disodium cromoglycate)

(kroe'moe-lin)

Gastrocrom, Intal, Nasalcrom

🍁 Novo-Cromolyn, PMS-Sodium Gen-Chromglycate, Intal Inhaler, Intal Syncroner

Drug class.: Antiasthmatic, mast cell stabilizer

Action: Stabilizes the membrane of the sensitized mast cell, preventing release of chemical mediators after an antigen-Ig E interaction

Uses: Allergic rhinitis, severe perennial bronchial asthma, exercise-induced bronchospasm (prevention), prevention of acute bronchospasm induced by environmental pollutants, mastocytosis

Dosage and routes:

Allergic rhinitis:

• *Adult and child >6 yr:* NASAL SOL 1 spray in each nostril tid-qid, not to exceed 6 doses/day

Bronchospasm prevention:

• *Adult and child >5 yr:* INH 20 mg <1 hr before exercise by nebulizer

Bronchial asthma prophylaxis:

• *Adult and child >5 yr:* INH 20 mg qid; NEBULIZ 20 mg qid by nebulization

Mastocytosis (Gastrocrom product only):

• *Adult and child ≥13 yr:* PO 200 mg qid 30 min ac and hs

• *Child 2-12 yr:* PO 100 mg qid 30 min ac and hs

Available forms include: Nasal sol 40 mg/ml; sol for inf 20 mg/2 ml; neb sol 20 mg; aerosol 800 µ/actuation; oral conc 5 ml/100 mg in ampules

Side effects/adverse reactions:

▼ *ORAL:* Dry, burning mouth, bitter taste (aerosol)

GI: Nausea, vomiting, anorexia

GU: Frequency, dysuria

INTEG: Rash, urticaria, angioedema

MS: Joint pain/swelling

Contraindications: Hypersensitivity to this drug or lactose, status asthmaticus

Precautions: Pregnancy category B, lactation, renal disease, hepatic disease, child <5 yr

Pharmacokinetics:
INH: Peak 15 min, duration 4-6 hr, half-life 80 min; excreted unchanged in feces

DENTAL CONSIDERATIONS

General:
- Assess salivary flow as a factor in caries, periodontal disease, and candidiasis.
- Consider semisupine chair position for patients with respiratory disease.
- A stress reduction protocol may be required.
- Midday appointments and a stress reduction protocol may be required for anxious patients.
- Be aware that aspirin or sulfite preservatives in vasoconstrictor-containing products can exacerbate asthma.

Consultations:
- Consider drug in diagnosis of taste alteration and burning mouth syndrome.
- Medical consultation may be required to assess disease control and stress tolerance of patient.

Teach patient/family:
- For inhalation dosage forms, rinse mouth with water after each dose to prevent dryness

When chronic dry mouth occurs, advise patient:
- To avoid mouth rinses with high alcohol content because of drying effects
- To use daily home fluoride products for anticaries effect
- To use sugarless gum, frequent sips of water, or saliva substitutes

cyanocobalamin (vitamin B_{12})/ hydroxocobalamin (vitamin $B_{12}a$)

(sye-an-oh-koe-bal'a-min)

Crystamine, Crysti- 1000, Cyanoject, Cyomin, HydroCobex, Hydro-Crysti-12, LA-12, Nascobal, Rubesol-1000

♣ Anacobin, Bedoz

Intranasal gel: Nascobal

Drug class.: Vitamin B_{12}, water-soluble vitamin

Action: Needed for adequate nerve functioning, protein and carbohydrate metabolism, normal growth, RBC development, cell reproduction

Uses: Vitamin B_{12} deficiency, pernicious anemia, vitamin B_{12} malabsorption syndrome, Schilling test, increased requirements with pregnancy thyrotoxicosis, hemolytic anemia, hemorrhage, renal and hepatic disease; intranasal gel: maintaining vitamin B_{12} levels in patients with HIV, multiple sclerosis, or Crohn's disease

Dosage and routes:
- *Adult:* PO 25 μg qd × 5-10 days, maintenance 100-200 μg IM qmo; IM/SC 30-100 μg qd × 5-10 days, maintenance 100-200 μg IM qmo
- *Child:* PO 1 μg qd × 5-10 days, maintenance 60 μg IM qmo or more; IM/SC 1-30 μg qd × 5-10 days, maintenance 60 μg IM qmo or more

Pernicious anemia/malabsorption syndrome:
- *Adult:* IM 100-1000 μg qd × 2 wk, then 100-1000 μg IM qmo

• *Child:* IM 100-500 μg over 2 wk or more given in 100-500 μg doses, then 60 μg IM/SC qmo
Schilling test:
• *Adult and child:* IM 1000 μg in one dose
Intranasal:
• *Adult and child:* TOP after appropriate vitamin B_{12} dose is determined; administer 1 hr before or 1 hr after ingestion of hot foods or liquids
Available forms include: Tabs 500, 1000 μg; inj IM 100, 1000 μg/ml; intranasal gel 500 μg/0.1 ml in 5 ml
Side effects/adverse reactions:
CNS: Flushing, optic nerve atrophy
CV: ***CHF, pulmonary edema,*** peripheral vascular thrombosis
GI: Diarrhea
INTEG: Itching, rash, pain at site
META: Hypokalemia
Contraindications: Hypersensitivity, optic nerve atrophy
Precautions: Pregnancy category A, lactation, children
Pharmacokinetics:
PO: Stored in liver, kidneys, stomach; 50%-90% excreted in urine; crosses placenta, excreted in breast milk
Drug interactions of concern to dentistry:
• Increased absorption: prednisone
DENTAL CONSIDERATIONS
General:
• Deficiency in vitamin B_{12} and other B-complex vitamins may cause oral symptomatology.

cyclizine HCl

(sye'kli-zeen)
Marezine
Drug class.: Antiemetic, antihistaminic, anticholinergic

Action: May act centrally by blocking chemoreceptor trigger zone, which in turn acts on vomiting center; also antagonizes histamine peripherally
Uses: Motion sickness
Dosage and routes:
• *Adult:* PO 50 mg 30 min before departure, then q4-6h prn, not to exceed 200 mg/day (HCl)
• *Child 6-12 yr:* PO 25 mg up to three times daily
Available forms include: Tabs 50 mg
Side effects/adverse reactions:
▼ *ORAL:* Dry mouth
CNS: Drowsiness, dizziness, convulsions in children, vertigo, fatigue, restlessness, headache, insomnia, hallucinations (auditory/visual)
GI: Nausea, anorexia
EENT: Blurred vision, tinnitus
Contraindications: Hypersensitivity to cyclizines, shock
Precautions: Children, narrow-angle glaucoma, urinary retention, lactation, prostatic hypertrophy, elderly, pregnancy category B, lactation
Pharmacokinetics:
PO: Duration 4-6 hr, other pharmacokinetics not known
Drug interactions of concern to dentistry:
• Increased CNS depression: alcohol, all CNS depressants

• May increase effect of anticholinergic drugs

DENTAL CONSIDERATIONS

General:

• Monitor vital signs at every appointment because of cardiovascular side effects.

• Assess salivary flow as a factor in caries, periodontal disease, and candidiasis.

Teach patient/family:

When chronic dry mouth occurs, advise patient:

• To avoid mouth rinses with high alcohol content because of drying effects

• To use daily home fluoride products for anticaries effect

• To use sugarless gum, frequent sips of water, or saliva substitutes

---

cyclobenzaprine HCl

(sye-kloe-ben'za-preen)

Flexeril

Drug class.: Skeletal muscle relaxant, centrally acting tricyclic

---

Action: Unknown; may be related to antidepressant effects, has actions similar to those of tricyclic antidepressants

Uses: Adjunct for relief of muscle spasm and pain in musculoskeletal conditions; unlabeled use: fibromyalgia syndrome

Dosage and routes:

• *Adult:* PO 10 mg tid × 1 wk, not to exceed 60 mg/day × 3 wk

Available forms include: Tabs 10 mg

Side effects/adverse reactions:

▼ *ORAL:* Dry mouth, unpleasant taste

CNS: Dizziness, weakness, drowsiness, headache, tremor, depression, insomnia, confusion, paresthesia

CV: Postural hypotension, tachycardia, dysrhythmias

GI: Nausea, vomiting, hiccups

GU: Urinary retention, frequency, change in libido

EENT: Diplopia, temporary loss of vision

INTEG: Rash, pruritus, fever, facial flushing, sweating

Contraindications: Acute recovery phase of MI, dysrhythmias, heart block, CHF, hypersensitivity, child <12 yr, intermittent porphyria, thyroid disease, concomitant use with or within 14 days of discontinuing MAOIs

Precautions: Renal disease, hepatic disease, addictive personality, pregnancy category B, elderly

Pharmacokinetics:

PO: Onset 1 hr, peak 3-8 hr, duration 12-24 hr, half-life 1-3 days; metabolized by liver; excreted in urine; crosses placenta; excreted in breast milk

Drug interactions of concern to dentistry:

• Increased CNS depression: alcohol, narcotics, barbiturates, sedatives, hypnotics

• Increased effects of anticholinergic drugs

• Increased effects of direct-acting sympathomimetics (epinephrine, levonordefrin)

DENTAL CONSIDERATIONS

General:

• Monitor vital signs at every appointment because of cardiovascular side effects.

• Assess salivary flow as a factor in caries, periodontal disease, and candidiasis.

• After supine positioning, have patient sit upright for at least 2 min to avoid orthostatic hypotension.

• Use vasoconstrictors with cau-

tion, in low doses, and with careful aspiration. Avoid use of gingival retraction cord with epinephrine.
• Place on frequent recall because of oral side effects.
• Consider drug in diagnosis of taste alterations.
Consultations:
• Medical consultation may be required to assess disease control.
Teach patient/family:
When chronic dry mouth occurs, advise patient:
• To avoid mouth rinses with high alcohol content because of drying effects
• To use daily home fluoride products for anticaries effect
• To use sugarless gum, frequent sips of water, or saliva substitutes

cyclophosphamide

(sye-kloe-foss'fa-mide)

Cytoxan, Cytoxan Lyophilized, Neosar

🍁 Procytox

Drug class.: Antineoplastic alkylating agent

Action: Alkylates DNA, RNA; inhibits enzymes that allow synthesis of amino acids in proteins; is also responsible for cross-linking DNA strands
Uses: Hodgkin's disease; lymphomas; leukemia; cancer of female reproductive tract, lung, prostate; multiple myeloma; neuroblastoma, retinoblastoma; Ewing's sarcoma, Burkett's lymphoma, advanced mycosis fungoides, nephrotic syndrome (children)
Dosage and routes:
• *Adult:* PO initially 1-5 mg/kg over 2-5 days, maintenance 1-5 mg/kg; IV initially 40-50 mg/kg in divided doses over 2-5 days, maintenance 10-15 mg/kg q7-10d or 3-5 mg/kg q3d
• *Child:* PO/IV 2-8 mg/kg or 60-250 mg/m^2 in divided doses for at least 6 days; maintenance 10-15 mg/kg q7-10d or 30 mg/kg q3-4wk; dose should be reduced by half when bone marrow depression occurs
Available forms include: Powder for inj IV 100 mg in vial; tabs 25, 50 mg
Side effects/adverse reactions:
▼ *ORAL:* Stomatitis, swelling of lips, tongue
CNS: Headache, dizziness
CV: ***Cardiotoxicity*** (high doses)
GI: Nausea, vomiting, diarrhea, weight loss, ***hepatotoxicity,*** colitis
RESP: ***Fibrosis***
HEMA: ***Thrombocytopenia, leukopenia, pancytopenia, myelosuppression***
GU: ***Hemorrhagic cystitis, hematuria, neoplasms,*** amenorrhea, azoospermia, impotence, sterility, ovarian fibrosis
INTEG: Alopecia, dermatitis
ENDO: Syndrome of inappropriate antidiuretic hormone (SIADH)
Contraindications: Lactation, pregnancy category D
Precautions: Radiation therapy
Pharmacokinetics:
PO: Half-life 4-6.5 hr; 50% bound to plasma proteins; metabolized by liver; excreted in urine
Drug interactions of concern to dentistry:
• Increased blood dyscrasia: NSAIDs, dapsone, phenothiazines, corticosteroids
• Increased metabolism: phenobarbital

DENTAL CONSIDERATIONS

General:

• Monitor vital signs at every appointment because of cardiovascular and respiratory side effects.

• Patients on chronic drug therapy may rarely have symptoms of blood dyscrasias, which can include infection, bleeding, and poor healing.

• Avoid prescribing aspirin-containing products.

• Prophylactic antibiotics may be indicated to prevent infection if surgery or deep scaling is planned because of leukopenic drug side effects.

• Patients receiving chemotherapy may require palliative treatment for stomatitis.

Consultations:

• In a patient with symptoms of blood dyscrasias, request a medical consultation for blood studies and postpone dental treatment until normal values are reestablished.

• Take precautions if dental surgery is anticipated and anesthesia is required.

Teach patient/family:

• Importance of good oral hygiene to prevent soft tissue inflammation

• Caution to prevent injury when using oral hygiene aids

---

cycloserine

(sye-kloe-ser'een)

Seromycin Pulvules

Drug class.: Antitubercular

Action: Inhibits cell wall synthesis, analog of D-alanine

Uses: Pulmonary TB, extrapulmonary as adjunctive

Dosage and routes:

• *Adult:* PO 250 mg q12h × 14 days, then 250 mg q8h × 2 wk if there are no signs of toxicity, then 250 mg q6h if there are no signs of toxicity, not to exceed 1 g/day

Available forms include: Caps 250 mg

Side effects/adverse reactions:

CNS: ***Convulsions,*** headache, anxiety, drowsiness, tremors, lethargy, depression, confusion, psychosis, aggression

CV: ***CHF***

HEMA: ***Megaloblastic anemia,*** vitamin B_{12} deficiency, folic acid deficiency, leukocytosis

INTEG: Dermatitis, photosensitivity

Contraindications: Hypersensitivity, seizure disorders, renal disease, alcoholism (chronic), depression, severe anxiety, lactation, anemia

Precautions: Pregnancy category C, children

Pharmacokinetics:

PO: Peak 3-8 hr; excreted unchanged in urine; crosses placenta; excreted in breast milk

Drug interactions of concern to dentistry:

• Seizures: alcohol

• Drowsiness is a common side effect; although no drug interactions with sedatives are reported, increased drowsiness might be possible

DENTAL CONSIDERATIONS

General:

• Patients on chronic drug therapy may rarely have symptoms of blood dyscrasias, which can include infection, bleeding, and poor healing.

• Examine for evidence of oral signs of disease.
• Determine why the patient is taking the drug (i.e., for preventive or therapeutic therapy).

Consultation:
• Medical consultation may be required to assess patient's ability to tolerate stress.
• In a patient with symptoms of blood dyscrasias, request a medical consultation for blood studies and postpone dental treatment until normal values are reestablished.
• *Determine that noninfectious status exists by ensuring that:*
• Anti-TB drugs have been taken for more than 3 wk
• Culture confirms antibiotic susceptibility to TB microorganism
• Patient has had three consecutive negative sputum smears
• Patient is not in the coughing stage

Teach patient/family:
• To avoid mouth rinses with high alcohol content
• Caution to prevent injury when using oral hygiene aids
• Importance of good oral hygiene to prevent soft tissue inflammation
• Importance of taking medication for full length of prescribed therapy to ensure effectiveness of treatment and prevent the emergence of resistant forms of microbe

cyclosporine

(sye'kloe-spor-een)

Neoral, Sandimmune, SangCya

Drug class.: Immunosuppressant

Action: Exact mechanism is not clear; may be related to the inhibition of synthesis and release of interleukin 2 leading to inhibition of T lymphocytes; both T-helper cells and T-suppressor cells are suppressed

Uses: To prevent rejection of tissues/allogenic organ transplants; severe recalcitrant psoriasis; rheumatoid arthritis (Neoral only); NOTE: Sandiimmune and Neoral are not bioequivalent

Dosage and routes:
• *Adult and child:* PO 15 mg/kg several hours before surgery, daily for 2 wk, reduce dosage by 2.5 mg/kg/wk to 5-10 mg/kg/day; IV 5-6 mg/kg several hours before surgery, daily, switch to PO form as soon as possible

Rheumatoid arthritis (Neoral only):
• *Adult:* PO initial dose 2.5 mg/kg/day bid, after 8 wk dose may be increased by 0.5-0.75 mg/kg/day and again at 12 wk, max dose 4 mg/kg/day

Psoriasis (Neoral only):
• *Adult:* PO initial dose 2.5 mg/kg/day in a twice-daily dose; if no progress is seen in 4 wk can increase dose in 2 wk intervals, 0.5 mg/kg/day, to a max of 4 mg/kg/day

Available forms include: Oral sol 100 mg/ml; inj IV 50 mg/ml; caps 25, 50, 100 mg; oral sol for microemulsion 100 μg/ml in 50 ml; cap for microemulsion 25, 50 mg

Side effects/adverse reactions:
▼ *ORAL: Candidiasis, gingival overgrowth*
CNS: Tremors, headache
CV: Hypertension
GI: ***Hepatotoxicity,*** nausea, vomiting, diarrhea, pancreatitis
GU: ***Albuminuria, hematuria, proteinuria, renal failure***

INTEG: Hirsutism, rash, acne
Contraindications: Hypersensitivity
Precautions: Severe renal disease, severe hepatic disease, pregnancy category C
Pharmacokinetics:
PO: Peak 4 hr, half-life (biphasic) 1.2 hr, 25 hr; highly protein bound; metabolized in liver; crosses placenta; excreted in feces, breast milk
Drug interactions of concern to dentistry:
- Hepatotoxicity/nephrotoxicity: erythromycin, azithromycin, clarithromycin
- Decreased action: barbiturates, carbamazepine
- Possibly reduced blood levels: clindamycin
- Increased infection and immunosuppression: corticosteroids
- Increased blood levels and risk of toxicity: fluconazole, ketoconazole, and itraconazole

DENTAL CONSIDERATIONS
General:
- Monitor vital signs at every appointment because of cardiovascular side effects.
- Patients on chronic drug therapy may rarely have symptoms of blood dyscrasias, which can include infection, bleeding, and poor healing.
- Place on frequent recall to evaluate gingival condition and healing response.
- Monitor time since organ/tissue transplant.

Consultations:
- Antibiotic prophylaxis is usually recommended in patients with organ transplants and immunosuppression.
- In a patient with symptoms of blood dyscrasias, request a medical consultation for blood studies and postpone dental treatment until normal values are reestablished.
- Request baseline blood pressure in renal transplant patients for patient evaluation before dental treatment.

Teach patient/family:
- Importance of good oral hygiene to prevent soft tissue inflammation
- Caution to prevent injury when using oral hygiene aids

cyclosporine ophthalmic
(sye'kloe- spor-een)
Restasis
Drug class.: Immunosuppressant

Action: Produces immunosuppression by inhibiting T lymphocytes
Uses: Increases tear production in patient with suppressed tear production caused by ocular inflammation associated with keratoconjunctivitis sicca
Dosage and routes:
- *Adult and child >16 yr:* TOP after thorough mixing instill 1 drop bid (12 hr apart), then discard vial; if needed, artificial tears product can be used 15 min later

Available forms include: Ophth sol 0.05% in single-use vial 0.4 ml
Side effects/adverse reactions:
EENT: Burning, conjunctival hyperemia, eye pain, epiphora, foreign body sensation, pruritus, blurred vision
Contraindications: Hypersensitivity, active ocular infection
Precautions: Single-use vials are intended to be used for one application only and then discarded; do not wear contact lenses, pregnancy

category C, lactation (no data on this product), safety and efficacy in children <16 yr not established

Pharmacokinetics:

TOP: No detectable drug accumulation in blood

Drug interactions of concern to dentistry:

- None reported

DENTAL CONSIDERATIONS

General:

- Determine why the patient is taking the drug.
- Protect the patient's eyes from accidental spatter during dental treatment.
- Avoid dental light in the patient's eyes; offer dark glasses for patient comfort.

---

cyproheptadine HCl

(si-proe-hep'ta-deen)

Periactin

PMS-Cyproheptadine

Drug class.: Antihistamine, H_1-receptor antagonist

Action: Acts on blood vessels, GI, respiratory system by competing with histamine for H_1 receptor site; decreases allergic response by blocking histamine

Uses: Allergy symptoms, rhinitis, pruritus, cold urticaria

Dosage and routes:

- *Adult:* PO 4 mg tid-qid, not to exceed 0.5 mg/kg/day
- *Child 7-14 yr:* PO 4 mg bid-tid, not to exceed 16 mg/day
- *Child 2-6 yr:* PO 2 mg bid-tid, not to exceed 12 mg/day

Available forms include: Tabs 4 mg; syr 2 mg/5 ml

Side effects/adverse reactions:

▼ *ORAL: Dry mouth*

CNS: Dizziness, drowsiness, poor coordination, fatigue, anxiety, euphoria, confusion, paresthesia, neuritis

CV: Hypotension, palpitation, tachycardia

GI: Constipation, nausea, vomiting, anorexia, diarrhea, weight gain

RESP: Increased thick secretions, wheezing, chest tightness

GU: Retention, dysuria, frequency, increased appetite

EENT: Blurred vision, dilated pupils, tinnitus, nasal stuffiness, dry nose/throat

INTEG: Rash, urticaria, photosensitivity

Contraindications: Hypersensitivity to H_1-receptor antagonist, acute asthma attack, lower respiratory tract disease

Precautions: Increased intraocular pressure, renal disease, cardiac disease, hypertension, bronchial asthma, seizure disorder, stenosed peptic ulcers, hyperthyroidism, prostatic hypertrophy, bladder neck obstruction, pregnancy category B, elderly

Pharmacokinetics:

PO: Duration 4-6 hr; metabolized in liver; excreted by kidneys; excreted in breast milk

Drug interactions of concern to dentistry:

- Increased CNS depression: alcohol, CNS depressants
- Increased effect of anticholinergic drugs

DENTAL CONSIDERATIONS

General:

- Assess salivary flow as a factor in caries, periodontal disease, and candidiasis.
- Determine why the patient is taking the drug.

C

Teach patient/family:
When chronic dry mouth occurs, advise patient:
• To avoid mouth rinses with high alcohol content because of drying effects
• To use daily home fluoride products for anticaries effect
• To use sugarless gum, frequent sips of water, or saliva substitutes

daclizumab

(dac-klye′zue-mab)
Zenapax

Drug class.: Immunosuppressive, Ig G1 monoclonal antibody

Action: Acts as an interleukin-2 (IL-2) receptor antagonist binding to the Tac subunit of IL-2 receptor
Uses: Prophylaxis of acute organ rejection in patients with renal transplants; used in combination with cyclosporine and glucocorticoids
Dosage and routes:
• *Adult:* IV infusion; 1 mg/kg of body weight as an initial dose no more than 24 hr before transplant surgery and an additional 4 doses given at intervals of 14 days
Available forms include: Vials 25 mg/5 ml
Side effects/adverse effects:
CNS: Tremor, headache, dizziness, insomnia
CV: Peripheral edema, aggravated hypertension
GI: Diarrhea, vomiting, constipation, abdominal pain
RESP: Cough, dyspnea, pulmonary edema
HEMA: Bleeding, lymphocele
GU: Oliguria, dysuria, urinary tract bleeding
EENT: Blurred vision
INTEG: Impaired wound healing, acne, pruritus, rash
MS: Myalgia, back pain
MISC: Fever, pain, fatigue
Contraindications: Hypersensitivity
Precautions: Risk of lymphoproliferative disease and opportunistic infections, anaphylaxis risk unknown, long-term effects unknown, pregnancy category C, lactation, children, geriatric patients
Pharmacokinetics:
IV: Required serum levels for Tac saturation 5-10 μg/ml, terminal elimination half-life 20 days with a range of 11-38 days, renal clearance
Drug interactions of concern to dentistry:
• None reported
DENTAL CONSIDERATIONS
General:
• This is a hospital-type drug, but because some dosing is continued, patients may appear in the dental office while receiving this drug.
• Transplant patients may also be taking cyclosporine and glucocorticoids; review each transplant patient's medications.
• Short appointments and a stress reduction protocol may be required for anxious patients.
Consultations:
• Antibiotic prophylaxis is usually recommended in patients with organ transplants and immunosuppression.
• Medical consultation may be required to assess disease control and patient's ability to tolerate stress.
Teach patient/family:
• Importance of good oral hygiene to prevent soft tissue inflammation
• To prevent trauma when using oral hygiene aids

• Importance of updating health and drug history if physician makes any changes in evaluation or drug regimens

dalteparin sodium

(dal-te'pa-rin)

Fragmin

Drug class.: Heparin-type anticoagulant

Action: Low-molecular-weight heparin having antithrombotic actions with higher anti–factor X_a activity compared with anti–factor II_a

Uses: Prevention of deep vein thrombosis following abdominal surgery, treatment of life-threatening conditions such as unstable angina, non–q-wave MI; prevention of ischemia complications caused by blood clot formation in patients on aspirin therapy; in combination with warfarin in deep vein thrombosis with or without pulmonary embolism

Dosage and routes:

Deep vein thrombosis prophylaxis:

• *Adult:* SC 2500 IU each day starting 1-2 hr before surgery and repeated once daily for 5-10 days postoperatively

Unstable angina; non–Q-wave angina:

• *Adult:* SC 120 IU/kg q12hr with 75-165 mg oral aspirin per day for 5-8 days

Available forms include: Prefilled syringe 2500 IU, 5000 IU in 0.2 ml; vial 10,000 IU in 9.5 ml

Side effects/adverse reactions:

HEMA: Bleeding after surgery, thrombocytopenia

INTEG: Skin necrosis

MISC: Local pain, irritation, ***anaphylaxis*** (rare)

Contraindications: Hypersensitivity, active major bleeding, thrombocytopenia, IM administration

Precautions: Hemorrhage, cannot be used interchangeably with other forms of heparin, pregnancy category B, lactation, children, requires monitoring, GI bleeding

Pharmacokinetics: *SC inj only:* Good absorption, peak levels of anti–factor X_a activity 4 hr, renal excretion

Drug interactions of concern to dentistry:

• Avoid concurrent use of aspirin (except as noted), NSAIDs, dipyridamole, and sulfinpyrazone

DENTAL CONSIDERATIONS

General:

• Product may be used in outpatient therapy. Delay elective dental treatment until patient completes anticoagulant therapy.

• Determine why patient is taking the drug.

• Consider local hemostasis measures to prevent excessive bleeding.

• Avoid prescribing aspirin-containing products.

Consultations:

• Medical consultation should include routine blood counts, including platelet counts and bleeding time.

Teach patient/family:

• Importance of good oral hygiene to prevent soft tissue inflammation

• To prevent trauma when using oral hygiene aids

• To report oral lesions, soreness, or bleeding to dentist

danaparoid

(da-nap′a-roid)

Orgaran

Drug class.: Heparinoid-type anticoagulant

Action: Low-molecular-weight heparin-like product having antithrombotic actions with higher anti–factor X_a activity compared with anti–factor II_a

Uses: Prevention of deep vein thrombosis following hip or knee replacement surgery; unapproved: thromboembolism, hemodialysis, and cardiovascular surgery

Dosage and routes:

• *Adult:* SC 750 anti–factor X_a units bid; 1-4 hr preoperatively and not sooner than 2 hr after surgery; may be used for 7-12 days

Available forms include: Inj 750 anti–factor X_a U/0.6 ml, amps and prefilled syringes

Side effects/adverse reactions:

CNS: Insomnia, headache, dizziness

CV: Peripheral edema

GI: Nausea, vomiting, constipation

HEMA: Bleeding after surgery, anemia

GU: UTI, urinary retention

INTEG: Rash, pruritus

MS: Asthenia

MISC: Fever, injection site pain, joint disorder

Contraindications: Hypersensitivity, severe bleeding disorders, type II thrombocytopenia, IM administration

Precautions: Cannot interchange with heparin, hemorrhage, thrombocytopenia, renal or hepatic impairment, pregnancy category B, lactation, children, antidotes not available, GI bleeding

Pharmacokinetics: *SC inj only:* Bioavailability 100%, maximum activity 2-5 hr; renal excretion; half-life based on plasma anti–factor X_a activity is 18-28 hr

Drug interactions of concern to dentistry:

• Avoid concurrent use of platelet aggregation antagonist such as aspirin, NSAIDs, dipyridamole

DENTAL CONSIDERATIONS

General:

• Determine why patient is taking the drug.

• Consider local hemostasis measures to prevent excessive bleeding if dental treatment must be performed.

• Antibiotic prophylaxis before dental treatment may be required for joint prosthesis. See 2003 ADA guidelines.

• Delay elective dental treatment until patient completes danaparoid therapy.

Consultations:

• Medical consultation should include routine blood counts, including platelet counts and bleeding time.

Teach patient/family:

• Importance of good oral hygiene to prevent soft tissue inflammation

• Caution to prevent trauma when using oral hygiene aids

• To report oral lesions, soreness, or bleeding to dentist

danazol

(da'na-zole)
Danocrine
✤ Cyclomen

Drug class.: Androgen, α-ethinyl testosterone derivative

Action: Decreases FSH and LH output and inhibits output of pituitary gonadotropins, leading to amenorrhea/anovulation, also decreases IgG, IgM, and IgA levels

Uses: Endometriosis, prevention of hereditary angioedema, fibrocystic breast disease

Dosage and routes:

Endometriosis:

• *Adult:* PO initial dose 400 mg bid, then decreased to 200-400 mg bid × 3-9 mo

Fibrocystic breast disease:

• *Adult:* PO 100-400 mg qd in 2 divided doses × 2-6 mo

Hereditary angioedema:

• *Adult:* PO 200 mg bid-tid until desired response, then decrease dose to 100 mg at 1-3 mo intervals

Available forms include: Caps 50, 100, 200 mg

Side effects/adverse reactions:

ORAL: Gingival bleeding (rare), stomatitis, Stevens-Johnson syndrome (rare)

CNS: Dizziness, headache, fatigue, tremors, paresthesia, flushing, sweating, anxiety, lability, insomnia

CV: Increased BP

GI: ***Cholestatic jaundice,*** nausea, vomiting, constipation, weight gain

GU: Hematuria, amenorrhea, atrophic vaginitis, decreased libido, decreased breast size, clitoral hypertrophy, testicular atrophy

EENT: Carpal tunnel syndrome, conjunctional edema, nasal congestion

INTEG: Rash, acneiform lesions, oily hair/skin, flushing, sweating, acne vulgaris, alopecia, hirsutism

ENDO: Abnormal GTT

MS: Cramps, spasms

Contraindications: Severe renal disease, severe cardiac disease, severe hepatic disease, hypersensitivity, genital bleeding (abnormal), pregnancy

Precautions: Migraine headaches, seizure disorders, pregnancy category X

Pharmacokinetics: Limited data available; oral absorption variable; metabolized in the liver

Drug interactions of concern to dentistry:

• Increased serum concentration of carbamazepine; consider avoiding concurrent administration

DENTAL CONSIDERATIONS

General:

• Patients on chronic drug therapy may rarely have symptoms of blood dyscrasias, which can include infection, bleeding, and poor healing.

Consultations:

• In a patient with symptoms of blood dyscrasias, request a medical consultation for blood studies and postpone dental treatment until normal values are reestablished.

Teach patient/family:

• Importance of good oral hygiene to prevent soft tissue inflammation

• To avoid mouth rinses with high alcohol content because of drying and irritating effects

dantrolene sodium

(dan'troe-leen)

Dantrium, Dantrium Intravenous

Drug class.: Skeletal muscle relaxant, direct acting

Action: Interferes with intracellular release of the calcium necessary to initiate contraction

Uses: Spasticity in multiple sclerosis, stroke, spinal cord injury, cerebral palsy, malignant hyperthermia

Dosage and routes:

Spasticity:

- *Adult:* PO 25 mg/day; may increase by 25-100 mg bid-qid, not to exceed 400 mg/day × 1 wk
- *Child:* PO 1 mg/kg/day given in divided doses bid-tid; may increase gradually, not to exceed 100 mg qid

Malignant hyperthermia prophylaxis:

- *Adult and child:* IV 1 mg/kg, may repeat to total dose of 10 mg/kg; PO 4-8 mg/kg/day in 4 divided doses × 3 days to prevent further hyperthermia; PO 4 to 8 mg/kg/day in 3 or 4 divided doses 1-2 days before surgery; give last dose 3-4 hr before surgery

Available forms include: Caps 25, 50, 100 mg; powder for inj IV 20 mg/vial

Side effects/adverse reactions:

▼ *ORAL:* Alteration of taste

CNS: Dizziness, weakness, fatigue, drowsiness, headache, disorientation, insomnia, paresthesia, tremors

CV: Hypotension, chest pain, palpitation, tachycardia

GI: Nausea, ***hepatotoxicity,*** constipation, vomiting, abdominal pain, diarrhea, anorexia; increased AST, alk phosphatase

HEMA: ***Eosinophilia***

GU: Urinary frequency, nocturia, impotence, crystalluria

EENT: Nasal congestion, blurred vision, mydriasis

INTEG: Rash, pruritus, photosensitivity

MS: Myalgia, backache

Contraindications: Hypersensitivity, compromised pulmonary function, active hepatic disease, impaired myocardial function, lactation

Precautions: Peptic ulcer disease, renal disease, hepatic disease, stroke, seizure disorder, diabetes mellitus, pregnancy category C, elderly; monitor liver enzymes

Pharmacokinetics:

PO: Peak 5 hr, half-life 8 hr; highly protein bound; metabolized in liver; excreted in urine (metabolites)

Drug interactions of concern to dentistry:

- None reported

DENTAL CONSIDERATIONS

General:

- Monitor vital signs at every appointment because of cardiovascular and respiratory side effects.
- Patients on chronic drug therapy may rarely have symptoms of blood dyscrasias, which can include infection, bleeding, and poor healing.
- Requires proficiency in IV administration technique when used for emergency treatment of malignant hyperthermia.

Consultations:

- In a patient with symptoms of blood dyscrasias, request a medical

consultation for blood studies and postpone dental treatment until normal values are reestablished.

Teach patient/family:

• Importance of good oral hygiene to prevent soft tissue inflammation

• To avoid mouth rinses with high alcohol content because of drying effects

---

dapsone (DDS)

(dap'sone)

Drug class.: Leprostatic, antibacterial

Action: Bactericidal and bacteriostatic against *M. leprae;* may also be immunosuppressant

Uses: Leprosy (Hansen's disease); dermatitis herpetiformis; unapproved: cicatricial pemphigoid, LE, pemphigoid, malaria, *P. carinii*

Dosage and routes:

Leprosy:

• *Adult:* PO 50-100 mg qd with rifampin 600 mg qd × 6 mo

• *Child:* PO 1-2 mg/kg/day for minimum of 3 yr; not to exceed adult dose

Dermatitis herpetiformis:

• *Adult:* PO initial dose 50 mg/day; can increase by 50 mg q1-2wk until remission; dose limit 500 mg/day; gradually reduce dose to lowest effective maintenance dose

Available forms include: Tabs 25, 100 mg

Side effects/adverse reactions:

▼ *ORAL:* Oral ulceration (erythema multiforme), lichenoid drug reaction

CNS: ***Convulsions,*** peripheral neuropathy, headache, anxiety, drowsiness, tremors, lethargy, depression, confusion, psychosis, aggression

GI: Nausea, vomiting, abdominal pain, anorexia

HEMA: ***Megaloblastic anemia***

GU: Proteinuria, nephrotic syndrome, renal papillary necrosis

EENT: Blurred vision, optic neuritis, photophobia

INTEG: ***Exfoliative dermatitis,*** photosensitivity

Contraindications: Hypersensitivity to sulfones, severe anemia

Precautions: Renal disease, hepatic disease, G6PD deficiency, pregnancy category C, lactation

Pharmacokinetics:

PO: Half-life 10-50 hr; rapid complete absorption; highly bound to plasma protein; metabolized in liver; excreted in urine

Drug interactions of concern to dentistry:

• None reported

DENTAL CONSIDERATIONS

General:

• Patients on chronic drug therapy may rarely have symptoms of blood dyscrasias, which can include infection, bleeding, and poor healing.

• Avoid dental light in patient's eyes; offer dark glasses for patient comfort.

• Advise patient if dental drugs prescribed have a potential for photosensitivity.

Consultations:

• In a patient with symptoms of blood dyscrasias, request a medical consultation for blood studies and postpone dental treatment until normal values are reestablished.

Teach patient/family:

• Importance of good oral hygiene to prevent soft tissue inflammation

• Caution to prevent injury when using oral hygiene aids

daptomycin

(dap' toe-mye-sin)

Cubicin

Drug class.: Antiinfective (polypeptide)

Action: Binds to bacterial membranes causing a rapid depolarization of membrane potential leading to inhibition of protein, DNA, and RNA synthesis resulting in bacterial cell death

Uses: Complicated skin and skin structure infections caused by susceptible strains of *S. aureus* (including methicillin-resistant *S. aureus*), *S. pyogenes, S. agalactiae, S. dysgalactiae, E. coli,* and *E. faecalis* (vancomycin-susceptible strains only)

Dosage and routes:

• *Adult:* IV infusion 4 mg/kg over 30 min; q24h × 7-14 days

Available forms include: Vials 250, 500 mg/10 ml

Side effects/adverse reactions:

▼ *ORAL:* Bell's palsy, taste disturbance

CNS: Paresthesias, headache, insomnia, dizziness, anxiety, fatigue

CV: Hypotension, hypertension, edema, chest pain

GI: ***Pseudomembranous colitis,*** constipation, nausea, diarrhea, vomiting, dyspepsia

RESP: Dyspnea

HEMA: Anemia

GU: ***Renal failure,*** UTI

EENT: Rash, pruritus, sore throat

META: ↑ CPK, abnormal liver function tests (↑ AST, ↑ ALT), hypoglycemia

MS: Myalgia, arthralgia, muscle weakness

MISC: Fever, injection site pain, fungal infections

Contraindications: Hypersensitivity

Precautions: Reduce dose in renal impairment, risk of superinfection, monitor for muscle weakness, pain and ↑ CPK levels, pregnancy category B, lactation, safety and efficacy in children <18 yr not established, elderly

Pharmacokinetics:

IV: Maximum blood levels 0.5-0.8 hr; half-life 8-9 hr, plasma protein binding 92%, site of metabolism unknown, excreted primarily in urine (78%), lesser amounts in feces

Drug interactions of concern to dentistry:

• None reported

DENTAL CONSIDERATIONS

General:

• Used in the hospital environment for serious infections.

• Determine why patient is taking the drug.

• Monitor vital signs at every appointment, including temperature, blood pressure, and respiration qualities and rate.

Consultations:

• Consult with patient's physician if an acute dental infection occurs and another antiinfective is required.

darbepoetin alfa

(dar-be-poe'e-tin)

Aranesp

Drug class.: Hematopoietic agent

Action: An erythropoiesis-stimulating protein; stimulates the division and differentiation of erythroid progenitors in bone marrow

Uses: Anemia associated with chronic renal failure; chemotherapy-induced anemia in patients with nonmyeloid malignancies

Dosage and routes:

- *Adult:* IV or SC start with low dose and slowly adjust upward depending on hemoglobin levels, give once weekly; to correct anemia the starting dose is 0.45 μg/kg; titrate dose to target of 12 g/L of hemoglobin

Available forms include: 25, 40, 60, 100, 150, 200, 300, 500 μg/ml in 1 ml single-use vials

Side effects/adverse reactions:

CNS: Headache, fatigue, dizziness

CV: Hypertension, hypotension, ***CHF, acute MI, stroke,*** TIA, peripheral edema, arrhythmias, angina pain

GI: Diarrhea, nausea, vomiting, abdominal pain, constipation

RESP: URI, dyspnea, cough, bronchitis

HEMA: ***Thrombosis***

MS: Myalgia, chest pain, asthenia, limb pain

MISC: Infection, fever, flulike syndrome

Contraindications: Uncontrolled hypertension, hypersensitivity

Precautions: Increased risk of serious cardiovascular events, seizures in CRF, albumin formula has risk of viral diseases, pregnancy category C, safety in lactation or pediatric patients not established

Pharmacokinetics: *SC:* Slow absorption, half life 27-89 hr, peak levels 34 hr

Drug interactions of concern to dentistry:

- No studies reported

DENTAL CONSIDERATIONS

General:

- Monitor vital signs at every appointment because of cardiovascular side effects.
- Consider semisupine chair position for patient comfort if GI side effects occur.
- Monitor disease control and date of last dialysis.
- Prophylactic antibiotics may be indicated to prevent infection if surgery or deep scaling is planned.

Consultations:

- Medical consultation may be required to assess disease control and patient's ability to tolerate stress.

Teach patient/family:

- Importance of good oral hygiene to prevent soft tissue inflammation/infection
- Importance of updating health and drug history if physician makes any changes in evaluation or drug regimens

---

delavirdine mesylate

(de-la-vir'deen)

Rescriptor

Drug class.: Antiviral, nonnucleoside

Action: Inhibits HIV-I reverse transcriptase enzymes; inhibits both DNA- and RNA-directed polymerase activity

Uses: HIV infection in combination with appropriate antiretroviral agents when therapy is warranted

Dosage and routes:

- *Adult:* PO 400 mg tid; may be given with or without food

Available forms include: Tabs 100, 200 mg

Side effects/adverse reactions:

▼ *ORAL:* Dry mouth (<2%), stomatitis, mouth ulcers, taste perversion

CNS: Headache, fatigue, agitation, confusion
CV: Bradycardia, palpitation, orthostatic hypotension, syncope
GI: Nausea, vomiting, abdominal pain, dyspepsia, diarrhea
RESP: Cough, congestion
HEMA: Neutropenia, leukopenia, thrombocytopenia, anemia, granulocytopenia
GU: Proteinuria
EENT: Dry eyes, conjunctivitis, diplopia
INTEG: Skin rash, pruritus
META: Altered liver function tests, elevated serum creatinine, alcohol intolerance
MS: Myalgia, cramps

Contraindications: Hypersensitivity

Precautions: Modify dose in liver disease; children <16 yr, pregnancy category C, lactation; rapid development of viral resistance if used as a single drug

Pharmacokinetics:
PO: Peak plasma levels 1.0 hr, highly protein bound (98%), hepatic metabolism (CYP3A4 isoenxyme), excreted in both urine and feces, plasma half-life 2-11 hr

Drug interactions of concern to dentistry:
- Reduced absorption: antacids, cimetidine, other H_2-receptor antagonists
- Increased plasma levels of both delavirdine and clarithromycin
- Increased plasma levels of alprazolam, triazolam, midazolam
- Avoid coadministration with carbamazepine, phenobarbital, ketoconazole, fluoxetine

DENTAL CONSIDERATIONS

General:
- Examine for oral manifestation of opportunistic infection.
- Patients on chronic drug therapy may rarely have symptoms of blood dyscrasias, which can include infection, bleeding, and poor healing.
- Assess salivary flow as a factor in caries, periodontal disease, and candidiasis.
- After supine positioning, have patient sit upright for at least 2 min before standing to avoid orthostatic hypotension.
- Do not use ingestible sodium bicarbonate products, such as the air polishing system Prophy
- Jet, within 2 hr of drug use.

Consultations:
- In a patient with symptoms of blood dyscrasias, request a medical consultation for blood studies and postpone treatment until normal values are reestablished.
- Medical consultation may be required to assess disease control and patient's ability to tolerate stress.

Teach patient/family:
- Importance of good oral hygiene to prevent soft tissue inflammation
- Caution to prevent trauma when using oral hygiene aids
- That secondary oral infection may occur; must see dentist immediately if infection occurs

When chronic dry mouth occurs, advise patient:
- To avoid mouth rinses with high alcohol content because of drying effects
- To use daily home fluoride products for anticaries effect

• To use sugarless gum, frequent sips of water, or saliva substitutes

demeclocycline HCl

(dem-e-kloe-sye'kleen)

Declomycin

Drug class.: Tetracycline

Action: Inhibits protein synthesis and phosphorylation in microorganisms by binding to 30S ribosomal subunits, reversibly binding to 50S ribosomal subunits; bacteriostatic

Uses: A wide variety of gram-positive and gram-negative bacteria, protozoa, *Rickettsia, Mycoplasma,* agents of psittacosis and ornithosis, actinomyces species

Dosage and routes:

• *Adult:* PO 150 mg q6h or 300 mg q12h

• *Child >8 yr:* PO 3-6 mg/kg/day in divided doses q6-12h

Gonorrhea:

• *Adult:* PO 600 mg, then 300 mg q12h × 4 days, total 3 g

Syndrome of inappropriate antidiuretic hormone:

• *Adult:* PO 600-1200 mg/day in divided doses

Available forms include: Tabs 150, 300 mg

Side effects/adverse reactions:

▼ *ORAL:* Candidiasis, tooth discoloration, increased thirst, discolored tongue, lichenoid reaction

CNS: Fever, headache, paresthesia

CV: Pericarditis

GI: Nausea, vomiting, diarrhea, ***hepatotoxicity, pseudomembranous colitis,*** anorexia, enterocolitis, flatulence, abdominal cramps, epigastric burning

HEMA: ***Eosinophilia, neutropenia, thrombocytopenia, leukocytosis, hemolytic anemia***

GU: Increased BUN, ***renal failure, nephrotoxicity,*** polyuria, polydipsia

EENT: Dysphagia, abdominal pain

INTEG: Rash, urticaria, photosensitivity, increased pigmentation, ***exfoliative dermatitis,*** pruritus, angioedema

Contraindications: Hypersensitivity to tetracyclines, children <8 yr, pregnancy category D, isotretinoin

Precautions: Renal disease, hepatic disease, lactation, nephrogenic diabetes insipidus

Pharmacokinetics:

PO: Peak 3-6 hr, duration 48-72 hr, half-life 10-17 hr; 36%-91% bound to serum protein; crosses placenta; excreted in urine, breast milk

Drug interactions of concern to dentistry:

• Decreased effect of penicillins, cephalosporins, oral contraceptives

• Oral contraceptives: advise patient of a potential risk for decreased contraceptive action, to maintain compliance with oral contraceptive use while using antibiotics, and to consider the use of additional nonhormonal contraception

• Contraindicated with isotretinoin (Accutane)

DENTAL CONSIDERATIONS

General:

• Examine oral cavity for side effects if on long-term drug therapy.

• Determine why the patient is taking the drug.

• Do not prescribe during pregnancy or before age 8 yr because of tooth discoloration.

• Absorption is reduced by dairy products, metals, and antacids.

Consultations:

• Medical consultation may be required to assess disease control.

Teach patient/family:

• Importance of good oral hygiene to prevent soft tissue inflammation

• Caution to prevent injury when using oral hygiene aids

When used for dental infection, advise patient:

• To report sore throat, oral burning sensation, fever, fatigue, any of which could indicate superinfection

• To take at prescribed intervals and complete dosage regimen

• To immediately notify the dentist if signs or symptoms of infection increase

---

desipramine HCl

(des-ip′ra-meen)

Norpramin

Drug class.: Antidepressant, tricyclic

Action: Inhibits both norepinephrine and serotonin (5-HT) uptake in the brain, although the precise antidepressant mechanism remains unclear

Uses: Depression; unapproved: neurogenic pain

Dosage and routes:

• *Adult:* PO 100-200 mg/day in divided doses, may increase to 300 mg/day or may give daily dose hs

• *Adolescent/geriatric:* PO 25-50 mg/day, may increase to 100 mg/day

Available forms include: Tabs 10, 25, 50, 75, 100, 150 mg

Side effects/adverse reactions:

▼ *ORAL: Dry mouth, unpleasant taste,* bleeding, stomatitis

CNS: Dizziness, drowsiness, confusion, headache, anxiety, tremors, stimulation, weakness, insomnia, nightmares, EPS (elderly), increased psychiatric symptoms, paresthesia

CV: Orthostatic hypotension, ECG changes, tachycardia, ***hypertension,*** palpitation, prolonged QT interval

GI: Diarrhea, ***paralytic ileus, hepatitis,*** increased appetite, cramps, epigastric distress, jaundice, nausea, vomiting

HEMA: ***Agranulocytosis, thrombocytopenia, eosinophilia, leukopenia***

GU: Retention, ***acute renal failure***

EENT: Blurred vision, tinnitus, mydriasis, ophthalmoplegia

INTEG: Rash, urticaria, sweating, pruritus, photosensitivity

Contraindications: Hypersensitivity to tricyclic antidepressants, recovery phase of MI, narrow-angle glaucoma, convulsive disorders, prostatic hypertrophy, child <12 yr

Precautions: Suicidal patients, severe depression, increased intraocular pressure, narrow-angle glaucoma, elderly, pregnancy category C, MAOIs

Pharmacokinetics:

PO: Steady state 2-11 days, half-life 14-62 hr; metabolized by liver; excreted by kidneys; crosses placenta

Drug interactions of concern to dentistry:

• Increased anticholinergic effects: muscarinic blockers, antihistamines, phenothiazines

• Increased effects of direct-acting sympathomimetics: epinephrine, levonordefrin
• Potential risk for increased CNS depression: alcohol, barbiturates, benzodiazepines, and other CNS depressants
• Decreased antihypertensive effects: clonidine, guanadrel, guanethidine
• At higher tricyclic doses, serum levels of fluconazole and ketoconazole may be elevated
• Avoid concurrent use with St. John's wort

DENTAL CONSIDERATIONS
General:
• Take vital signs at every appointment because of cardiovascular side effects.
• Assess salivary flow as a factor in caries, periodontal disease, and candidiasis.
• Patients on chronic drug therapy may rarely have symptoms of blood dyscrasias, which can include infection, bleeding, and poor healing.
• After supine positioning, have patient sit upright for at least 2 min to avoid orthostatic hypotension.
• Use vasoconstrictors with caution, in low doses, and with careful aspiration. Avoid use of gingival retraction cord with epinephrine.
• Place on frequent recall because of oral side effects.

Consultations:
• In a patient with symptoms of blood dyscrasias, request a medical consultation for blood studies and postpone dental treatment until normal values are reestablished.
• Medical consultation may be required to assess disease control.
• Physician should be informed if significant xerostomic side effects occur (e.g., increased caries, sore tongue, problems eating or swallowing, difficulty wearing prosthesis) so that a medication change can be considered.

Teach patient/family:
• Importance of good oral hygiene to prevent soft tissue inflammation
• Caution to prevent injury when using oral hygiene aids

When chronic dry mouth occurs, advise patient:
• To avoid mouth rinses with high alcohol content because of drying effects
• To use daily home fluoride products for anticaries effect
• To use sugarless gum, frequent sips of water, or saliva substitutes

D

desloratadine

(des-lor-at'-a-deen)

Clarinex, Clarinex RediTabs

Drug class.: Antihistamine, histamine H_1-receptor antagonist

Action: Antagonism of H_1-receptors, blocking typical allergic manifestations of histamine release
Use: Seasonal allergic rhinitis; chronic idiopathic urticaria
Dose and routes:
• *Adult and child >12 yr:* PO 5 mg once daily; RAP DISINTEGR TAB place on tongue immediately after opening foil, tablet disintegrates on tongue; adjust dose to 5 mg every other day if hepatic/renal impairment is present

Available forms include: Tab 5 mg; rap disintegr tab 5 mg
Side effects/adverse reactions:
▼ *ORAL: Dry mouth*
CNS: Somnolence, fatigue, headache, dizziness
CV: Tachycardia

GI: Nausea, dyspepsia
METAB: Elevated liver enzymes, elevated bilirubin
EENT: Pharyngitis
INTEG: Rash, pruritus, urticaria
MS: Myalgia
MISC: Rarely edema, anaphylaxis, dyspnea

Contraindications: Hypersensitivity to this drug or loratadine

Precautions: Pregnancy category B, distributed to breast milk (caution in nursing), incomplete dosing studies in the elderly, safety has not been established in children <12 yr, dosage adjustment required in hepatic impairment

Pharmacokinetics:
PO: Good oral absorption; peak levels 3 hr; metabolized to 3-hydroxydesloratadine (active metabolite), highly plasma protein bound (desloratadine, 82%-87%; –3-hydroxydesloratadine, 85%-87%); glucuronidated metabolites excreted in urine

Drug interactions of concern to dentistry:
- Limited studies with concurrent doses of erythromycin; ketoconazole and azithromycin show slight elevations of plasma levels, but no clinically relevant changes in electrocardiographic parameters
- One report indicated a potential for increased anticholinergic effects with other anticholinergic drugs and increased somnolence with CNS depressants; however, data are lacking

DENTAL CONSIDERATIONS

General:
- Assess salivary flow as a factor in caries, periodontal disease, and candidiasis.

Teach patient/family:
- Importance of good oral hygiene to prevent soft tissue inflammation

When chronic dry mouth occurs, advise patient:
- To avoid mouth rinses with high alcohol content because of drying effects
- To use sugarless gum, frequent sips of water, or saliva substitutes
- To use daily home fluoride products for anticaries effect

---

desmopressin acetate

(des-moe-press'in)

DDAVP, DDAVP Nasal Solution, Stimate Nasal Solution

♣ DDAVP Rhinal Tube, DDAVP Rhinyl Nasal Solution, DDAVP Spray, Octostim

Drug class.: Synthetic antidiuretic hormone (a synthetic analog of vasopressin)

Action: Promotes reabsorption of water by action on renal tubular epithelium; also causes an increase in factor VIII levels

Uses: Primary nocturnal enuresis, hemophilia A with factor VIII levels >5%, von Willebrand's disease, neurogenic diabetes insipidus, renal concentration capacity

Dosage and routes:

Diabetes insipidus:
- *Adult:* INTRANASAL 0.1-0.4 ml qd in divided doses; IV/SC 0.5-1 ml qd in divided doses
- *Adult:* PO initial dose 0.05 mg bid, increase to 0.1-1.2 mg in divided doses as required
- *Child 3 mo-12 yr:* INTRANASAL 0.05-0.3 ml qd in divided doses

Hemophilia/von Willebrand's disease
• *Adult and child:* IV 0.3 μg/kg in NaCl over 15-30 min; may repeat if needed
Available forms include: Nasal sol 1.5 mg/ml; nasal spray pump 0.1 mg/ml; intranasal test 0.1 mg/ml; inj IV/SC 4, 15 μg/ml; tab 0.1 and 0.2 mg
Side effects/adverse reactions:
CNS: Headache, drowsiness, lethargy, flushing
CV: Increased BP
GI: Nausea, *mild abdominal cramps,* heartburn
GU: Vulval pain
EENT: Nasal irritation, congestion, rhinitis
Contraindications: Hypersensitivity, nephrogenic diabetes insipidus
Precautions: Pregnancy category B, CAD, lactation, hypertension
Pharmacokinetics:
NASAL: Onset 1 hr, peak 1-2 hr, duration 8-20 hr, half-life 8 min, 76 min (terminal)
Drug interactions of concern to dentistry:
• Decreased antidiuretic effects: demeclocycline
• Increased antidiuretic effects: carbamazepine

DENTAL CONSIDERATIONS
General:
• Monitor vital signs at every appointment because of cardiovascular side effects.
• Avoid prescribing aspirin-containing products if treatment is for bleeding disorder.
• Consider local hemostasis measures to prevent excessive bleeding.
• Determine why the patient is taking the drug.
• Consider semisupine chair position for patient comfort because of GI effects of disease.
Consultations:
• Medical consultation may be required to assess disease control; definite consultation for patients with chronic bleeding disorders.
• Medical consultation should include partial prothrombin time or prothrombin time.
Teach patient/family:
• To advise dentist if excessive bleeding occurs or continues after dental treatment

desonide

(dess'oh-nide)
DesOwen, Tridesilon
Drug class.: Topical corticosteroid, group IV low potency

Action: Glucocorticoids have multiple actions that include anti-inflammatory and immunosuppressant effects. They inhibit phospholipase A_2, interfering with or reducing the synthesis of prostaglandins and leukotrienes. They also bind to cytoplasmic GRs and enter the cell nucleus to bind with DNA. This results in the synthesis of various enzymes such as collagenase, elastase, and cytokines that play important roles in inflammation and immunosuppression. They also suppress the production of lymphocytes, monocytes, and eosinophils.
Uses: Psoriasis, eczema, contact dermatitis, pruritus
Dosage and routes:
• *Adult and child:* TOP apply to affected area bid-tid
Available forms include: Cream 0.05%; oint 0.05%; lotion 0.05%

Side effects/adverse reactions:
▼ *ORAL:* Perioral dermatitis
INTEG: Burning, dryness, itching, irritation, acne, folliculitis, hypertrichosis, hypopigmentation, atrophy, striae, miliaria, allergic contact dermatitis, secondary infection
Contraindications: Hypersensitivity to corticosteroids, fungal infections
Precautions: Pregnancy category C, lactation, viral infections, bacterial infections

DENTAL CONSIDERATIONS
General:
• Determine why the patient is taking the drug.
• Place on frequent recall to evaluate healing response if used on chronic basis.
• Apply lubricant to dry lips for patient comfort before dental procedures.

desoximetasone

(des-ox-i-met'a-sone)
Topicort, Topicort LP

Drug class.: Topical corticosteroid, group II potency (0.25%), group III potency (0.05%)

Action: Glucocorticoids have multiple actions that include anti-inflammatory and immunosuppressant effects. They inhibit phospholipase A_2, interfering with or reducing the synthesis of prostaglandins and leukotrienes. They also bind to cytoplasmic GRs and enter the cell nucleus to bind with DNA. This results in the synthesis of various enzymes such as collagenase, elastase, and cytokines that play important roles in inflammation and immunosuppression. They also suppress the production of lymphocytes, monocytes, and eosinophils.
Uses: Psoriasis, eczema, contact dermatitis, pruritus
Dosage and routes:
• *Adult and child:* TOP apply to affected area bid
Available forms include: Cream 0.05%, 0.25%; oint 0.25%; gel 0.05% in 15 and 60 g tubes
Side effects/adverse reactions:
▼ *ORAL:* Thinning of mucosa, stinging sensation (oral application)
INTEG: Burning, dryness, itching, irritation, acne, folliculitis, hypertrichosis, perioral dermatitis, hypopigmentation, atrophy, striae, miliaria, allergic contact dermatitis, secondary infection
Contraindications: Hypersensitivity to corticosteroids, fungal infections
Precautions: Pregnancy category C, lactation, viral infections, bacterial infections

DENTAL CONSIDERATIONS
General:
• Gel formulations are used in the treatment of oral lichen planus lesions when the diagnosis has been confirmed by immunofluorescent biopsy testing.
• Place on frequent recall to evaluate healing response.
Teach patient/family:
• When used for oral lesions, to return for oral evaluation if response of oral tissues has not occurred in 7-14 days
• Importance of good oral hygiene to prevent soft tissue inflammation
• That use on oral herpetic ulcerations is contraindicated

• To apply at bedtime or after meals for maximum effect
• To apply with cotton-tipped applicator, dabbing gently, not rubbing medication on lesion

dexamethasone/ dexamethasone sodium phosphate

(dex-a-meth'a-sone)

dexamethasone: Aeroseb-Dex, Decaspray

✤ dexamethasone sodium phosphate: Decadron Phosphate

Drug class.: Synthetic topical corticosteroid

Action: Glucocorticoids have multiple actions that include anti-inflammatory and immunosuppressant effects. They inhibit phospholipase A_2, interfering with or reducing the synthesis of prostaglandins and leukotrienes. They also bind to cytoplasmic GRs and enter the cell nucleus to bind with DNA. This results in the synthesis of various enzymes such as collagenase, elastase, and cytokines that play important roles in inflammation and immunosuppression. They also suppress the production of lymphocytes, monocytes, and eosinophils.

Uses: Corticosteroid-responsive dermatoses, oral ulcerative inflammatory lesions

Dosage and routes:
• *Adult and child:* TOP apply to affected area bid-qid

Available forms include: Aerosol 0.01%, 0.04%; cream 0.1%

Side effects/adverse reactions:
▼ *ORAL:* Thinning of mucosa, stinging sensation (oral application)
INTEG: Burning, dryness, itching, irritation, acne, folliculitis, hypertrichosis, perioral dermatitis, hypopigmentation, atrophy, striae, miliaria, allergic contact dermatitis, secondary infection

Contraindications: Hypersensitivity to corticosteroids, fungal infections, viral infections

Precautions: Pregnancy category C, lactation, viral infections, bacterial infections

DENTAL CONSIDERATIONS

General:
• Place on frequent recall to evaluate healing response.

Teach patient/family:
• When used for oral lesions, to return for oral evaluation if response of oral tissues has not occurred in 7-14 days
• Importance of good oral hygiene to prevent soft tissue inflammation
• To apply approximately 0.25 inch; measure and apply with cotton-tipped applicator by gently dabbing, not rubbing, medication on lesion
• To apply at bedtime or after meals for maximum effect
• That use on oral herpetic ulcerations is contraindicated

dexamethasone/ dexamethasone acetate/ dexamethasone sodium phosphate

(dex-a-meth'a-sone)

Dexamethasone oral tab: *Decadron, Dexameth Unipak, Dexameth, Dexaone, Hexadrol, Hexadrol Therapeutic Pack*

✤ Deronil, Dexasone, Oradexan

Dexamethasone elixir: Decadron, Hexadrol

Dexamethasone oral solution: Intensol

Dexamethasone acetate (long-lasting injection, NOT FOR IV USE): Dalalaone DP, Dalalone LA, Decadron LA, Decaject-LA, Dexasone-LA, Dexone LA, Solurex-LA

Dexamethasone sodium phosphate (inj): Cortastat, Dalaone, Decadron Phosphate, Decaject, Dexone, Hexadrol Phosphate, Solurex

Drug class.: Glucocorticoid, long acting

Action: Glucocorticoids have multiple actions that include anti-inflammatory and immunosuppressant effects. They inhibit phospholipase A_2, interfering with or reducing the synthesis of prostaglandins and leukotrienes. They also bind to cytoplasmic GRs and enter the cell nucleus to bind with DNA. This results in the synthesis of various enzymes such as collagenase, elastase, and cytokines that play important roles in inflammation and immunosuppression. They also suppress the production of lymphocytes, monocytes, and eosinophils.

Uses: Inflammation, allergies, neoplasms, cerebral edema, shock, collagen disorders

Dosage and routes:

Inflammation:

- *Adult:* PO 0.25-4 mg bid-qid; IM 4-16 mg q1-3wk (acetate)

Shock:

- *Adult:* IV 1-6 mg/kg or 40 mg q2-6h (phosphate)

Cerebral edema:

- *Adult:* IV 10 mg, then 4-6 mg q6h × 2-4 days, then taper over 1 wk
- *Child:* PO 0.2 mg/kg/day in divided doses

Available forms include: Tabs 0.25, 0.5, 0.75, 1, 1.5, 2, 4, 6 mg; inj IM acetate 8, 16 mg/ml; inj IV phosphate 4, 10, 20, 24 mg/ml; elix 0.5 mg/5 ml; oral sol 0.5 mg/5 ml, 0.5 mg/0.5 ml

Side effects/adverse reactions:

▼ *ORAL: Candidiasis,* dry mouth

CNS: Depression, flushing, sweating, headache, mood changes

CV: Hypertension, ***circulatory collapse, thrombophlebitis, embolism,*** tachycardia, edema

GI: Diarrhea, nausea, abdominal distention, ***GI hemorrhage, pancreatitis,*** increased appetite

HEMA: ***Thrombocytopenia***

EENT: Fungal infections, increased intraocular pressure, blurred vision

INTEG: Acne, poor wound healing, ecchymosis, petechiae

MS: Fractures, osteoporosis, weakness

Contraindications: Psychosis, hypersensitivity, idiopathic thrombocytopenia, acute glomerulonephritis, amebiasis, fungal infections, nonasthmatic bronchial disease, child <2 yr, AIDS, TB

Precautions: Pregnancy category C, diabetes mellitus, glaucoma, osteoporosis, seizure disorders, ulcerative colitis, CHF, myasthenia gravis, renal disease, peptic ulcer, esophagitis

Pharmacokinetics:

PO: Peak 1-2 hr, duration 2.33 days
IM: Peak 8 hr, duration 6 days
Half-life 3-4.5 hr

Drug interactions of concern to dentistry:

- Decreased action: barbiturates
- Increased side effects: alcohol, salicylates, and other NSAIDs
- Increased action: ketoconazole, macrolide antibiotics

DENTAL CONSIDERATIONS

General:

- Monitor vital signs at every appointment because of cardiovascular side effects.
- Patients on chronic drug therapy may rarely have symptoms of blood dyscrasias, which can include infection, bleeding, and poor healing.
- Symptoms of oral infections may be masked.
- Patients who have been or are currently on chronic steroid therapy (>2 wk) may require supplemental steroids for dental treatment.
- Avoid prescribing aspirin-containing products.
- Place on frequent recall to evaluate healing response.
- Prophylactic antibiotics may be indicated to prevent infection if surgery or deep scaling is planned.

Consultations:

- In a patient with symptoms of blood dyscrasias, request a medical consultation for blood studies and postpone dental treatment until normal values are reestablished.
- Medical consultation may be required to assess disease control.
- Consultation may be required to confirm steroid dose and duration of use.

Teach patient/family:

- Importance of good oral hygiene to prevent soft tissue inflammation
- Caution to prevent injury when using oral hygiene aids
- To avoid mouth rinses with high alcohol content because of drug interaction

dexchlorpheniramine maleate

(dex-klor-fen-eer′a-meen)

Polaramine, Polaramine Repetabs

Drug class.: Antihistamine

Action: Acts on blood vessels, GI system, respiratory system by competing with histamine for H_1-receptor site; decreases allergic response by blocking histamine

Uses: Allergy symptoms, rhinitis, pruritus, contact dermatitis

Dosage and routes:

- *Adult and child ≥12 yr:* PO repeat action 4-6 mg q8-10h, or at hs
- *Child 6-12 yr:* PO time rel 4 mg hs

Available forms include: Time rel tab 4, 6 mg

Side effects/adverse reactions:

ORAL: Dry mouth

CNS: Dizziness, drowsiness, poor coordination, fatigue, anxiety, euphoria, confusion, paresthesia, neuritis

CV: Hypotension, palpitations, tachycardia
GI: Constipation, nausea, vomiting, anorexia, diarrhea
RESP: Increased thick secretions, wheezing, chest tightness
GU: Retention, dysuria, frequency
EENT: Blurred vision, dilated pupils, tinnitus, nasal stuffiness, dry nose/throat
INTEG: Rash, urticaria, photosensitivity

Contraindications: Hypersensitivity to H_1-receptor antagonist; acute asthma attack, lower respiratory tract disease

Precautions: Increased intraocular pressure, renal disease, cardiac disease, hypertension, bronchial asthma, seizure disorder, stenosed peptic ulcers, hyperthyroidism, prostatic hypertrophy, bladder neck obstruction, pregnancy category B, elderly

Pharmacokinetics: *PO (except extended-action dose forms):* Onset 15 min, peak 3 hr, duration ≈8 hr; metabolized in liver; excreted by kidneys (inactive metabolites); excreted in breast milk (small amounts)

Drug interactions of concern to dentistry:
- Increased CNS depression: barbiturates, narcotics, hypnotics, tricyclic antidepressants, alcohol
- Increased anticholinergic effect: anticholinergic drugs

DENTAL CONSIDERATIONS

General:
- Assess salivary flow as a factor in caries, periodontal disease, and candidiasis.
- Consider semisupine chair position for patient comfort because of respiratory effects of disease.

Teach patient/family:

When chronic dry mouth occurs, advise patient:
- To avoid mouth rinses with high alcohol content because of drying effects
- To use sugarless gum, frequent sips of water, or saliva substitutes
- To use daily home fluoride products for anticaries effect

---

dexmethylphenidate HCl

(dex-meth-il-fen'-i-date)
Focalin

Drug class.: CNS stimulant; related to the amphetamines

Controlled Substance Schedule II

Action: Blocks the reuptake of norepinephrine and dopamine in the presynaptic neuron and is presumed to increase the release of these neurotransmitters

Uses: Treatment of attention deficit hyperactivity disorder (ADHD)

Dosage and routes:

Patients new to methylphenidate:
- *Adults and children >6 yr:* PO 2.5 mg bid; dosage may be adjusted at weekly intervals in 2.5-5 mg increments up to 20 mg/day

Patients currently using methylphenidate:
- *Adults and children >6 yr:* PO starting dose is half the dose of racemic methylphenidate, not to exceed 20 mg/day

Available forms include: Tabs 2.5, 5, and 10 mg

Side effects/adverse reactions:

▼ *ORAL:* Dry mouth
CNS: Anorexia, insomnia, mood alteration

CV: Tachycardia, angina, arrhythmias, palpitation
GI: Abdominal pain, nausea
HEMA: ***Thrombocytopenia purpura,*** leukopenia
EENT: Blurred vision
INTEG: ***Exfoliative dermatitis,*** skin rash, urticaria, erythema multiforme
MS: Twitching (includes vocal tics), arthralgia
MISC: Fever, weight loss

Contraindications: Hypersensitivity to methylphenidate, glaucoma, marked anxiety, tension, agitation, tics, Gilles de la Tourette's syndrome, concurrent use or use within the past 14 days of MAOI

Precautions: Long-term effect on growth in children unknown, exacerbation of psychotic behavior, history of seizures, hypertension, heart failure, recent MI, hyperthyroidism, use in child <6 yr not established, drug dependence, pregnancy category C, lactation

Pharmacokinetics:
PO: Readily absorbed, peak plasma levels 1-1.5 hr; mean plasma half-life 2.2 hr; readily metabolized, excreted in urine (80%)

Drug interactions of concern to dentistry:
- May inhibit metabolism of phenobarbital, tricyclic antidepressants, and SSRIs
- Increased effects of anticholinergics, CNS stimulants, tricyclic antidepressants, and sympathomimetics

DENTAL CONSIDERATIONS

General:
- Monitor vital signs at every appointment because of cardiovascular side effects.
- Assess salivary flow as a factor in caries, periodontal disease, and candidiasis.
- Patients on chronic drug therapy may rarely have symptoms of blood dyscrasias, which can include infection, bleeding, and poor healing.
- Use vasoconstrictor with caution, in low doses, and with careful aspiration.
- Determine why the patient is taking the drug.

Consultations:
- In a patient with symptoms of blood dyscrasias, request a medical consultation for blood studies and postpone treatment until normal values are reestablished.
- Medical consultation may be required to assess disease control

Teach patient/family:
- Importance of good oral hygiene to prevent soft tissue inflammation/infection
- To prevent injury when using oral hygiene aids
- Importance of updating health and drug history if physician makes any changes in evaluation/drug regimens

When chronic dry mouth occurs, advise patient:
- To avoid mouth rinses with high alcohol content because of drying effects
- To use daily home fluoride products for anticaries effect
- To use sugarless gum, frequent sips of water, or saliva substitutes

dextroamphetamine sulfate

(dex-troe-am-fet'a-meen)

Dexedrine, Dexedrine Spansules, DextroStat

Drug class.: Amphetamine

Controlled Substance Schedule II, Canada C

Action: Increases release of norepinephrine, dopamine in cerebral cortex to reticular activating system

Uses: Narcolepsy, attention deficit disorder with hyperactivity

Dosage and routes:

Narcolepsy:

• *Adult:* PO 5-60 mg qd in divided doses

• *Child >12 yr:* PO 10 mg qd, increasing by 10 mg/day at weekly intervals, limit usually 40 mg/day

• *Child 6-12 yr:* PO 5 mg qd increasing by 5 mg/wk

Attention deficit disorder:

• *Child >6 yr:* PO 5 mg qd-bid increasing by 5 mg/day at weekly intervals

• *Child 3-5 yr:* PO 2.5 mg qd increasing by 2.5 mg/day at weekly intervals

Available forms include: Tabs 5, 10 mg; sus rel caps 5, 10, 15 mg

Side effects/adverse reactions:

▼ *ORAL:* Dry mouth, metallic taste

CNS: Hyperactivity, insomnia, restlessness, talkativeness, dizziness, headache, chills, stimulation, dysphoria, irritability, aggressiveness, tremor

CV: Palpitation, tachycardia, hypertension, decrease in heart rate, dysrhythmias

GI: Anorexia, diarrhea, constipation, weight loss

GU: Impotence, change in libido

INTEG: Urticaria

Contraindications: Hypersensitivity to sympathomimetic amines, hyperthyroidism, hypertension, glaucoma hypertrophy, severe arteriosclerosis, drug abuse, cardiovascular disease, anxiety, MAOIs, or within 14 days of MAOI use

Precautions: Gilles de la Tourette's syndrome, pregnancy category C, lactation, child <3 yr

Pharmacokinetics:

PO: Onset 30 min, peak 1-3 hr, duration 4-20 hr, half-life 10-30 hr; metabolized by liver; urine excretion pH dependent; crosses placenta, excreted in breast milk

Drug interactions of concern to dentistry:

• Increased risk of serious side effects: meperidine, propoxyphene, tricyclic antidepressants

DENTAL CONSIDERATIONS

General:

• Monitor vital signs at every appointment because of cardiovascular side effects.

• Assess salivary flow as a factor in caries, periodontal disease, and candidiasis.

• Psychologic and physical dependence may occur with chronic administration.

Consultations:

• Medical consultation may be required to assess disease control.

Teach patient/family:

When chronic dry mouth occurs, advise patient:

• To avoid mouth rinses with high alcohol content because of drying effects

• To use daily home fluoride products for anticaries effect

• To use sugarless gum, frequent sips of water, or saliva substitutes

dextromethorphan hydrobromide

(dex-troe-meth-or'fan)

Benylin Adult, Benylin Pediatric, Creo-Terpin, Dexalone, Delsyn, Hold DM, Robitussin Maximum Strength, Robitussin Pediatric, Silphen DM, Scot-Tussin DM, Trocal, Vicks 44 Cough

♣ Benylin DM Syrup, Balamil DM, Broncho-Grippo-DM, Calmylin HI, Delsym, Koflex, NovoHistadex, Novahistine DM, Robidex, Sedatuss, Triaminic DM

Drug class.: Antitussive, nonnarcotic

Action: Depresses cough center in medulla

Uses: Nonproductive cough

Dosage and routes:

• *Adult:* PO 10-20 mg q4h or 30 mg q6-8h, not to exceed 120 mg/day; con rel liq 60 mg bid, not to exceed 120 mg/day

• *Child 6-12 yr:* PO 5-10 mg q4h; con rel liq 30 mg bid, not to exceed 60 mg/day

• *Child 2-6 yr:* PO 2.5-5 mg q4h or 7.5 mg q6-8h, not to exceed 30 mg/day

Available forms include: Loz 5 mg; sol 5, 7.5, 10, 15 mg/5 ml

Side effects/adverse reactions:

CNS: Dizziness

GI: Nausea

Contraindications: Hypersensitivity, asthma/emphysema, productive cough, MAOI

Precautions: Nausea, vomiting, increased temperature, persistent headache, pregnancy category C, drug abuse

Pharmacokinetics:

PO: Onset 15-30 min, duration 3-6 hr

Drug interactions of concern to dentistry:

• Inhibition of metabolism: terbinafine

DENTAL CONSIDERATIONS

General:

• Consider semisupine chair position for patients with respiratory disease.

diazepam

(dye-az'e-pam)

Diastat, Diazepam Intensol, Valium

♣ Apo-Diazepam, Novo-Dipam, PMS Diazepam, Vivol

Drug class.: Benzodiazepine, anxiolytic

Controlled Substance Schedule IV

Action: Produces CNS depression, interacts with a benzodiazepine receptor to facilitate the action of the inhibitory neurotransmitter γ-aminobutyric acid (GABA)

Uses: Anxiety, acute alcohol withdrawal, adjunct in seizure disorders, skeletal muscle spasm; conscious sedation in dentistry

Dosage and routes:

Anxiety, convulsive disorders, sedation:

• *Adult:* PO 2-10 mg tid-qid; elderly or debilitated PO 2-2.5 mg once or twice daily, may increase as tolerated

• *Child >6 mo:* PO 1-2.5 mg tid-qid

Mild anxiety:

• *Adult:* IV titrate doses to desired response, give slowly (reduce narcotic dose, if used, by one half), up to 20 mg may be used; IM 5-10 mg 30 min before procedure

Tetanic muscle spasms:

- *Child >5 yr:* IM/IV 5-10 mg q3-4h prn
- *Infant >30 days:* IM/IV 1-2 mg q3-4h prn

Status epilepticus:

- *Adult:* IV BOLUS 5-20 mg, 2 mg/min; may repeat q5-10min, not to exceed 60 mg; may repeat in 30 min if seizures reappear
- *Child:* IV BOLUS 0.1-0.3 mg/kg (1 mg/min over 3 min); may repeat q15min × 2 doses

Adjunct in skeletal muscle spasm:

- *Adult:* PO 2-10 mg tid-qid

Available forms include: Tabs 2, 5, 10 mg; IM/IV inj 5 mg/ml; oral sol 5 mg/ml; gel (DIASTAT only) 5, 10, 15, 20 mg

Side effects/adverse reactions:

▼ *ORAL:* Dry mouth, ulcerations

CNS: Dizziness, drowsiness, confusion, headache, anxiety, tremors, stimulation, fatigue, depression, insomnia, hallucinations

CV: Orthostatic hypotension, ***ECG changes, tachycardia,*** hypotension

GI: Constipation, nausea, vomiting, anorexia, diarrhea

EENT: Blurred vision, tinnitus, mydriasis

INTEG: Rash, dermatitis, itching

Contraindications: Hypersensitivity to benzodiazepines, narrow-angle glaucoma, psychosis, ritonavir, indinavir, saquinavir

Precautions: Elderly, debilitated, hepatic disease, renal disease, pregnancy category D

Pharmacokinetics:

PO: Onset 30 min, duration 2-3 hr

IM: Onset 15-30 min, duration 1-1.5 hr

IV: Onset 1-5 min, duration 15 min, half-life 20-50 hr; metabolized by liver enzymes including CYP2C19 and CYP3A4; excreted by kidneys; crosses placenta, excreted in breast milk; more effective by mouth

Drug interactions of concern to dentistry:

- Increased CNS depression of diazepam: alcohol, all CNS depressants, kava (herb)
- Increased serum levels and prolonged effect of benzodiazepines: erythromycin, clarithromycin, ketoconazole, itraconazole, fluconazole, miconazole (systemic), cimetidine, rifamycins (see Appendix I)
- Contraindicated with saquinavir
- Possible increase in CNS side effects: kava (herb)

DENTAL CONSIDERATIONS

General:

- Assess salivary flow as a factor in caries, periodontal disease, and candidiasis.
- After supine positioning, have patient sit upright for at least 2 min before standing to avoid orthostatic hypotension.
- Psychologic and physical dependence may occur with chronic administration.
- Geriatric patients are more susceptible to drug effects; use lower dose.
- Have someone drive patient to and from dental appointment when used for conscious sedation.
- Provide assistance when escorting patient to and from dental chair when dizziness occurs.
- Avoid the use of this drug in a patient with a history of drug abuse or alcoholism.

Teach patient/family:

- Importance of good oral hygiene to prevent soft tissue inflammation

When chronic dry mouth occurs, advise patient:
• To avoid mouth rinses with high alcohol content because of drying effects
• To use daily home fluoride products for anticaries effect
• To use sugarless gum, frequent sips of water, or saliva substitutes

diclofenac

(dye-kloe'fen-ak)

Diclofenac potassium: Cataflam
✦ Voltaren Rapide
Diclofenac sodium delayed release: Voltaren
✦ Novo-Difenac Apo-Diclo, Nu-Diclo
Diclofenac sodium extended release: Voltaren XR
✦ Novo-Difenac SR

Drug class.: Nonsteroidal antiinflammatory

Action: Inhibits prostaglandin synthesis by interfering with cyclooxygenase needed for biosynthesis; possesses analgesic, antiinflammatory, antipyretic properties

Uses: Acute, chronic rheumatoid arthritis, osteoarthritis, ankylosing spondylitis, analgesia

Dosage and routes:

Osteoarthritis (immediate or delayed release tablets):
• *Adult:* PO 100-150 mg/day in divided doses; chronic therapy EXT REL 100 mg/day

Rheumatoid arthritis (immediate or delayed release tablets):
• *Adult:* PO 150-200 mg/day in divided doses; chronic therapy EXT REL 100 mg/day

Ankylosing spondylitis (delayed release tablets):
• *Adult:* PO 100-125 mg/day; give 25 mg qid and 25 mg hs if needed

Analgesia and dysmenorrhea (immediate release tablets):
• *Adult:* PO 50 mg tid or 100 mg first dose followed by 50 mg with a daily first day limit of 200 mg; do not exceed 150 mg/day thereafter

Available forms include: Tabs 50 mg, del rel tabs 25, 50, 75 mg; ext rel tabs 100 mg

Side effects/adverse reactions:

▼ *ORAL:* Dry mouth, stomatitis, bitter taste, lichenoid reaction
CNS: Dizziness, drowsiness, fatigue, tremors, confusion, insomnia, anxiety, depression, nervousness, paresthesia, muscle weakness, headache
CV: ***CHF, dysrhythmias,*** tachycardia, peripheral edema, palpitation, hypotension, hypertension, fluid retention
GI: ***Jaundice, cholestatic hepatitis*** constipation, flatulence, cramps, peptic ulcer, GI bleeding, nausea, anorexia, vomiting, diarrhea
RESP: *Laryngeal edema,* asthma, rhinitis, shortness of breath, dyspnea, hemoptysis, pharyngitis
HEMA: ***Blood dyscrasias,*** epistaxis, bruising
GU: ***Nephrotoxicity, hematuria,*** oliguria, azotemia, cystitis, UTI
EENT: Tinnitus, hearing loss, blurred vision
INTEG: Purpura, rash, pruritus, sweating, erythema, petechiae, photosensitivity, alopecia, eczema, ***erythema multiforme, angioedema***
META: ↑AST, ↑ALT

Contraindications: Hypersensi-

D

tivity to aspirin, iodides, other nonsteroidal antiinflammatory agents, asthma

Precautions: Pregnancy category B (first, second trimester), lactation, children, bleeding disorders, GI disorders, cardiac disorders, hypersensitivity to other antiinflammatory agents

Pharmacokinetics:

PO: Peak 2-3 hr, elimination half-life 1-2 hr; 90% bound to plasma proteins; metabolized in liver to metabolite; excreted in urine

Drug interactions of concern to dentistry:

- GI ulceration, bleeding: aspirin, alcohol, corticosteroids, potassium supplements
- Nephrotoxicity: acetaminophen (prolonged use)
- Possible risk of decreased renal function: cyclosporine

When prescribed for dental pain:

- Risk of increased effects: oral anticoagulants, oral antidiabetics, lithium, methotrexate
- Decreased antihypertensive effects of diuretics, β-adrenergic blockers, and ACE inhibitors
- First-time users of SSRIs also taking NSAIDs may have a higher risk of GI side effects; until more data are available, it may be advisable to avoid use of NSAIDs in these patients (*Br J Clin Pharmacol* 55:591-595, 2003)

DENTAL CONSIDERATIONS

General:

- Patients on chronic drug therapy may rarely have symptoms of blood dyscrasias, which can include infection, bleeding, and poor healing.
- Assess salivary flow as a factor in caries, periodontal disease, and candidiasis.
- Avoid prescribing for dental use in last trimester of pregnancy.
- Avoid prescribing aspirin-containing products.
- Consider semisupine chair position for patients with rheumatic disease.
- Advise patient if dental drugs prescribed have a potential for photosensitivity.

Consultations:

- In a patient with symptoms of blood dyscrasias, request a medical consultation for blood studies and postpone dental treatment until normal values are reestablished.
- Medical consultation may be required to assess disease control.

Teach patient/family:

- Importance of good oral hygiene to prevent soft tissue inflammation
- Caution to prevent injury when using oral hygiene aids

When chronic dry mouth occurs, advise patient:

- To avoid mouth rinses with high alcohol content because of drying effects
- To use daily home fluoride products for anticaries effect
- To use sugarless gum, frequent sips of water, or saliva substitutes

dicloxacillin sodium

(dye-klox-a-sil'in)

Dycill, Dynapen, Pathocil

Drug class.: Penicillinase-resistant penicillin

Action: Interferes with cell wall replication of susceptible organisms; the cell wall, rendered osmot-

ically unstable, swells and bursts from osmotic pressure
Uses: Infections caused by penicillinase-producing *Staphylococcus*
Dosage and routes:
• *Adult:* PO 125-250 mg q6h
• *Child up to 40 kg:* PO 12.5-25 mg/kg in divided doses q6h
Available forms include: Caps 250, 500 mg
Side effects/adverse reactions:
▼ *ORAL: Candidiasis* (superinfection)
CNS: ***Coma, convulsions,*** lethargy, hallucinations, anxiety, depression, twitching
GI: Nausea, vomiting, diarrhea, increased AST/ALT, abdominal pain, colitis
HEMA: ***Bone marrow depression, granulocytopenia,*** anemia, increased bleeding time
GU: ***Oliguria, proteinuria, hematuria, vaginitis, moniliasis, glomerulonephritis***
Contraindications: Hypersensitivity to penicillins; neonates
Precautions: Hypersensitivity to cephalosporins, pregnancy category B
Pharmacokinetics:
PO: Peak 1 hr, duration 4-6 hr; metabolized in liver; excreted in urine, bile, breast milk; crosses placenta
Drug interactions of concern to dentistry:
• Decreased antimicrobial effectiveness: tetracyclines, erythromycins
When prescribed for dental infection:
• Decreased effect of oral contraceptives
• Increased dicloxacillin concentration: probenecid

DENTAL CONSIDERATIONS
General:
• Take precautions regarding allergy to medication.
• Determine why the patient is taking the drug.
Consultations:
• Concern for drug of choice if dental infection is also present.
Teach patient/family:
• Importance of good oral hygiene to prevent soft tissue inflammation
• Caution to prevent trauma when using oral hygiene aids
When used for dental infection, advise patient:
• Taking birth control pill to use additional method of contraception for duration of cycle
• To report sore throat, oral burning sensation, fever, fatigue, any of which could indicate superinfection
• To take at prescribed intervals and complete dosage regimen
• To immediately notify the dentist if signs or symptoms of infection increase

dicyclomine HCl

(dye-sye'kloe-meen)
Antispas, Bentyl, Di-Spaz, Byclomine, Or-Tyl, Dibent, Dilomine
♣ Bentylol, Formulex, Spasmoban
Drug class.: GI anticholinergic

Action: Inhibits muscarinic actions of acetylcholine at postganglionic parasympathetic neuroeffector sites
Uses: Treatment of irritable bowel syndrome

Dosage and routes:
• *Adult:* PO 40 mg qid; limit 160 mg/day; IM 20 mg

Available forms include: Caps 10, 20 mg; tabs 20 mg; syr 10 mg/5 ml; inj IM 10 mg/ml

Side effects/adverse reactions:

▼ *ORAL: Dry mouth*

CNS: Confusion, stimulation in elderly, ***seizures, coma*** (child <3 mo), headache, insomnia, dizziness, drowsiness, anxiety, weakness, hallucination

CV: Palpitation, tachycardia

GI: Constipation, ***paralytic ileus,*** heartburn, nausea, vomiting, dysphagia

GU: Hesitancy, retention, impotence

EENT: Blurred vision, photophobia, mydriasis, cycloplegia, increased ocular tension

SYST: Urticaria, rash, pruritus, anhidrosis, fever, allergic reactions

Contraindications: Hypersensitivity to anticholinergics, narrow-angle glaucoma, GI obstruction, myasthenia gravis, paralytic ileus, GI atony, toxic megacolon

Precautions: Hyperthyroidism, CAD, dysrhythmias, CHF, ulcerative colitis, hypertension, hiatal hernia, hepatic disease, renal disease, pregnancy category B, urinary retention, prostatic hypertrophy

Pharmacokinetics:

PO: Onset 1-2 hr, duration 3-4 hr; metabolized by liver; excreted in urine

Drug interactions of concern to dentistry:
• Increased anticholinergic effect: atropine, scopolamine, other anticholinergics, and meperidine
• Decreased effect of ketoconazole

DENTAL CONSIDERATIONS

General:
• Assess salivary flow as a factor in caries, periodontal disease, and candidiasis.
• Avoid dental light in patient's eyes; offer dark glasses for patient comfort.

Consultation:
• Physician should be informed if significant xerostomic side effects occur (e.g., increased caries, sore tongue, problems eating or swallowing, difficulty wearing prosthesis) so that a medication change can be considered.

Teach patient/family:
• Importance of good oral hygiene to prevent soft tissue inflammation

When chronic dry mouth occurs, advise patient:
• To avoid mouth rinses with high alcohol content because of drying effects
• To use daily home fluoride products for anticaries effect
• To use sugarless gum, frequent sips of water, or saliva substitutes

---

didanosine (also called ddI, dideoxyinosine)

(dye-dan'o-seen)

Videx, Videx EC

Drug class.: Synthetic antiviral, nucleoside analog

Action: Converted by cellular enzymes to active form, which acts as an antimetabolite to inhibit HIV reverse transcriptase and viral replication

Uses: Advanced HIV infections in adults and children who have been unable to use zidovudine or who have not responded to treatment; used in combination with other antiretroviral drugs

Dosage and routes:

• *Adult:* PO >60 kg: 200 mg bid tabs or 250 mg bid buffered powder or TAB (EC) 400 mg qd, tabs must be chewed or crushed in water; <60 kg: 125 mg bid or 167 mg bid buffered powder or tablet (EC) 250 mg qd

Enteric-coated capsule:

• *Child:* PO 120 mg/m^2 bid

Available forms include: Tabs, buffered, chewable/dispersible 25, 50, 100, 150, 200 mg; powder for oral sol, buffered 100, 167, 250, 375 mg; powder for oral sol, pedi 2, 4 g; del rel caps 125, 200, 250, 400 mg

Side effects/adverse reactions:

▼ *ORAL:* Stomatitis, dry mouth, taste perversion, candidiasis

CNS: ***Peripheral neuropathy, seizures, CNS depression,*** confusion, anxiety, hypertonia, abnormal thinking, asthenia, insomnia, pain, dizziness, chills, fever, headache

CV: Hypertension, vasodilation, dysrhythmia, syncope, CHF, palpitation

GI: ***Pancreatitis,*** diarrhea, nausea, vomiting, abdominal pain, constipation, dyspepsia, liver abnormalities, flatulence, melena, increased ALT/AST, alk phosphatase, amylase

RESP: Cough, pneumonia, dyspnea, asthma, epistaxis, hypoventilation, sinusitis

HEMA: ***Leukopenia, granulocytopenia, thrombocytopenia, anemia***

GU: Increased bilirubin, uric acid

EENT: Ear pain, otitis, photophobia, visual impairment

INTEG: Rash, pruritus, alopecia, ecchymosis, hemorrhage, petechiae, sweating

MS: Myalgia, arthritis, myopathy, muscular atrophy

Contraindications: Hypersensitivity

Precautions: Renal disease, hepatic disease, pregnancy category B, lactation, children, sodium-restricted diets; pancreatitis (in combination with stavudine); lactic acidosis, severe hepatomegaly

Pharmacokinetics:

PO: Rapidly absorbed, bioavailability ≈42%, elimination half-life 1.62 hr; extensive metabolism is thought to occur; administration within 5 min of food decreases absorption

Drug interactions of concern to dentistry:

• Decreased absorption of the following drugs: ketoconazole, dapsone, itraconazole, tetracyclines, fluoroquinolone antibiotics

• Increased risk of pancreatitis: metronidazole, sulfonamides, sulindac, tetracyclines

• Increased risk of peripheral neuropathy: metronidazole, nitrous oxide

DENTAL CONSIDERATIONS

General:

• Monitor vital signs at every appointment because of cardiovascular side effects.

• Avoid dental light in patient's eyes; offer dark glasses for patient comfort.

• Patients on chronic drug therapy may rarely have symptoms of blood dyscrasias, which can include infection, bleeding, and poor healing.

Consultations:

• Medical consultation may be required to assess patient's ability to tolerate stress.

• In a patient with symptoms of blood dyscrasias, request a medical consultation for blood studies and postpone dental treatment until normal values are reestablished.

Teach patient/family:

• Importance of good oral hygiene to prevent soft tissue inflammation

• Caution to prevent injury when using oral hygiene aids

When chronic dry mouth occurs, advise patient:

• To avoid mouth rinses with high alcohol content because of drying effects

• To use daily home fluoride products for anticaries effect

• To use sugarless gum, frequent sips of water, or saliva substitutes

---

diethylpropion HCl

(dye-eth-il-proe'pee-on)

Tenuate, Tenuate Dospan

Drug class.: Anorexiant, amphetamine-like

Controlled Substance Schedule IV

Action: Exact mechanism of action on appetite suppression unknown, but may have an effect on satiety center of hypothalamus

Uses: Exogenous obesity

Dosage and routes:

• *Adult:* PO 25 mg/1 hr ac; con rel 75 mg qd midmorning

Available forms include: Tabs 25 mg; susp rel tabs 75 mg

Side effects/adverse reactions:

▼ *ORAL:* Dry mouth, unpleasant taste

CNS: Hyperactivity, restlessness, anxiety, insomnia, dizziness, dysphonia, depression, tremors, headache, blurred vision, incoordination, fatigue, malaise, euphoria, depression, tremor, confusion

CV: Palpitation, tachycardia, hypertension, dysrhythmias, pulmonary hypertension, ECG changes

GI: Nausea, vomiting, anorexia, diarrhea, constipation

HEMA: ***Bone marrow depression,*** leukopenia, agranulocytosis

GU: Impotence, change in libido, menstrual irregularities, dysuria, polyuria

INTEG: Urticaria

Contraindications: Hypersensitivity, hyperthyroidism, hypertension, glaucoma, angina pectoris, drug abuse, cardiovascular disease, children <12 yr, severe arteriosclerosis, agitated states

Precautions: Convulsive disorders, pregnancy category B, lactation

Pharmacokinetics:

PO: Duration 4 hr

CON REL: Duration 10-14 hr, half-life 1-3.5 hr; metabolized by liver; excreted by kidneys; crosses placenta, excreted in breast milk

Drug interactions of concern to dentistry:

• Dysrhythmia: hydrocarbon inhalation anesthetics

• Decreased effects: barbiturates, tricyclic antidepressants, phenothiazines

DENTAL CONSIDERATIONS

General:

• Monitor vital signs at every appointment because of cardiovascular and respiratory side effects.

• Examine for evidence of oral manifestations of blood dyscrasias (infection, bleeding, poor healing).

• Assess salivary flow as a factor in caries, periodontal disease, and candidiasis.
• Psychologic and physical dependence may occur with chronic administration.
• Consider semisupine chair position for patient comfort because of GI effects of disease.

Consultations:
• Medical consultation for blood studies (CBC); leukopenic or thrombocytopenic side effects may result in infection, delayed healing, and excessive bleeding. Postpone dental treatment until normal values are maintained.

Teach patient/family:
• Importance of good oral hygiene to prevent soft tissue inflammation
• Caution in use of oral hygiene aids to prevent injury

When chronic dry mouth occurs, advise patient:
• To avoid mouth rinses with high alcohol content because of drying effects
• To use daily home fluoride products for anticaries effect
• To use sugarless gum, frequent sips of water, or saliva substitutes

---

difenoxin HCl with atropine sulfate

(dye-fen-ox'in)
Motofen
Drug class.: Antidiarrheal

Controlled Substance Schedule IV

Action: Inhibits gastric motility by acting on mucosal receptors responsible for peristalsis

Uses: Acute nonspecific and acute exacerbations of chronic functional diarrhea

Dosage and routes:
• *Adult:* PO 2 tabs, then 1 tab after each loose stool; or 1 tab q3-4h as needed, not to exceed 8 tabs/24 hr

Available forms include: Tabs 1 mg difenoxin HCl with 0.025 mg atropine sulfate

Side effects/adverse reactions:
▼ *ORAL: Dry mouth*
CNS: Dizziness, drowsiness, headache, fatigue, nervousness, insomnia, confusion
GI: Nausea, vomiting, epigastric distress, constipation
EENT: Burning eyes, blurred vision

Contraindications: Hypersensitivity, pseudomembranous enterocolitis, jaundice, glaucoma, child <2 yr, severe electrolyte imbalances, diarrhea associated with organisms that penetrate intestinal mucosa, MAOI

Precautions: Hepatic disease, renal disease, ulcerative colitis, pregnancy category C, lactation, severe liver disease

Pharmacokinetics:
PO: Peak 40-60 min, duration 3-4 hr, terminal half-life 12-14 hr; metabolized in liver to inactive metabolite; excreted in urine, feces

Drug interactions of concern to dentistry:
• Increased effects of alcohol: all CNS depressants, opioid analgesics, and anticholinergics

DENTAL CONSIDERATIONS

General:
• This drug product is normally used only for a few doses for acute problems; however, some patients may have to take it for longer time periods as dictated by a contributing disease.
• Assess salivary flow as a factor in caries, periodontal disease, and candidiasis.

Teach patient/family:

When chronic dry mouth occurs, advise patient:

• To avoid mouth rinses with high alcohol content because of drying effects

• To use daily home fluoride products for anticaries effect

• To use sugarless gum, frequent sips of water, or saliva substitutes

---

diflorasone diacetate

(die-floor'a-sone)

Florone, Florone E, Maxiflor, Psorcon, Psorcon E

Drug class.: Topical corticosteroid, group II high potency

Action: Glucocorticoids have multiple actions that include antiinflammatory and immunosuppressant effects. They inhibit phospholipase A_2, interfering with or reducing the synthesis of prostaglandins and leukotrienes. They also bind to cytoplasmic GRs and enter the cell nucleus to bind with DNA. This results in the synthesis of various enzymes such as collagenase, elastase, and cytokines that play important roles in inflammation and immunosuppression. They also suppress the production of lymphocytes, monocytes, and eosinophils.

Uses: Psoriasis, eczema, contact dermatitis, pruritus

Dosage and routes:

• *Adult and child:* Apply to affected area qd-tid

Available forms include: Cream 0.05%; oint 0.05% in 15, 30, 60 g

Side effects/adverse reactions:

▼ *ORAL:* Perioral dermatitis

INTEG: Burning, dryness, itching, irritation, acne, folliculitis, hypertrichosis, hypopigmentation, atrophy, striae, miliaria, allergic contact dermatitis, secondary infection

Contraindications: Hypersensitivity to corticosteroids, fungal infections

Precautions: Pregnancy category C, lactation, viral infections, bacterial infections

DENTAL CONSIDERATIONS

General:

• Determine why the patient is taking the drug.

• Apply lubricant to dry lips for patient comfort before dental procedures.

• Place on frequent recall to evaluate healing response if used on chronic basis.

---

diflunisal

(dye-floo'ni-sal)

Dolobid

✤ Apo-Diflunisal, Novo-Diflunisal

Drug class.: Salicylate derivative, nonsteroidal antiinflammatory

Action: Inhibits prostaglandin synthesis by interfering with cyclooxygenase needed for biosynthesis; possesses analgesic, antiinflammatory, antipyretic properties

Uses: Mild-to-moderate pain, symptoms of rheumatoid arthritis and osteoarthritis

Dosage and routes:

Pain/fever:

• *Adult:* PO loading dose 1 g, then 500-1000 mg/day in 2 divided doses q12h, not to exceed 1500 mg/day

Available forms include: Tabs 250, 500 mg

Side effects/adverse reactions:
▼ *ORAL:* Dry mouth, lichenoid reaction
CNS: ***Convulsions,*** stimulation, drowsiness, dizziness, confusion, headache, flushing, hallucinations, coma
CV: ***Pulmonary edema,*** rapid pulse
GI: Nausea, vomiting, GI bleeding, diarrhea, heartburn, ***hepatitis,*** anorexia
RESP: Wheezing, hyperpnea
HEMA: ***Thrombocytopenia, agranulocytosis, leukopenia, neutropenia, hemolytic anemia,*** increased pro-time
EENT: Blurred vision, decreased acuity, corneal deposits
INTEG: Rash, urticaria, bruising
ENDO: Hypoglycemia, hyponatremia, hypokalemia

Contraindications: Hypersensitivity to salicylates, GI bleeding, bleeding disorders, children <3 yr, vitamin K deficiency

Precautions: Anemia, hepatic disease, renal disease, Hodgkin's disease, pregnancy category C, lactation

Pharmacokinetics:
PO: Onset 15-30 min, peak 2-3 hr, half-life up to 6 hr; 99% protein bound; metabolized by liver; excreted by kidneys; crosses placenta; excreted in breast milk

Drug interactions of concern to dentistry:
- Increased risk of GI ulceration and bleeding: aspirin, steroids, alcohol, indomethacin, and other NSAIDs
- Hepatotoxicity, nephrotoxicity: acetaminophen (prolonged use)
- Suspected increase in potential toxic effects: probenecid

DENTAL CONSIDERATIONS
General:
- Patients on chronic drug therapy may rarely have symptoms of blood dyscrasias, which can include infection, bleeding, and poor healing.
- Assess salivary flow as a factor in caries, periodontal disease, and candidiasis.
- Avoid prescribing for dental use in first and last trimester of pregnancy.

Consultations:
- Medical consultation may be required to assess disease control.
- In a patient with symptoms of blood dyscrasias, request a medical consultation for blood studies and postpone dental treatment until normal values are reestablished.

Teach patient/family:
- Importance of good oral hygiene to prevent soft tissue inflammation
- Caution to prevent injury when using oral hygiene aids

When chronic dry mouth occurs, advise patient:
- To avoid mouth rinses with high alcohol content because of drying effects
- To use daily home fluoride products for anticaries effect
- To use sugarless gum, frequent sips of water, or saliva substitutes

---

digoxin

(di-jox'in)
Digitek, Lanoxicaps, Lanoxin
🍁 Novo-digoxin, Lanoxin Pediatric Elixir

Drug class.: Cardiac glycoside

Action: Acts by inhibiting the sodium-potassium ATPase, which makes more calcium available for contractile proteins, resulting in increased cardiac contractility and cardiac output

Uses: CHF, atrial fibrillation, atrial flutter, paroxysmal atrial tachycardia, rapid digitalization in these disorders

Dosage and routes:

Rapid digitalization:

• *Adult:* IV give slowly over 5 min or longer; dose selected must be based on projected peak digoxin stores and can vary from 6-12 μg/kg; initial doses may range from 0.4-0.6 mg, followed by 0.1-0.3 mg q6-8h until the desired response is reached

• *Adult:* PO (capsules only) loading dose must be based on projected peak digoxin body stores; initial doses can vary from 0.4-0.6 mg, then 0.1-0.3 mg q6h until desired response is achieved; maintenance doses range from 0.35-0.5 mg/day; all doses should be titrated for each patient

• *Adult:* PO (tablets only) loading doses must be based on projected peak digoxin body stores and can vary from 0.5-0.75 mg initially; then 0.125-0.375 mg q6-8h until desired response is achieved; maintenance doses range from 0.065-0.5 mg/day; all doses should be titrated for each patient

• *Child:* PO (elixir) dosages must be individualized by age, weight, renal clearance, and intended therapeutic outcome; refer to individual package insert for complete details

Available forms include: Caps 0.05, 0.1, 0.2 mg; elix 0.05 mg/ml; tabs 0.125, 0.25, 0.50 mg; inj 0.1, 0.25 mg/ml

Side effects/adverse reactions:

▼ *ORAL:* Sensitive gag reflex

CNS: Headache, drowsiness, apathy, confusion, disorientation, fatigue, depression, hallucinations

CV: ***Dysrhythmias, hypotension,*** bradycardia, ***AV block***

GI: Nausea, vomiting, anorexia, abdominal pain, diarrhea

EENT: Blurred vision, yellowish-green halos, photophobia, diplopia

MS: Muscular weakness

Contraindications: Hypersensitivity to digitalis, ventricular fibrillation, ventricular tachycardia, carotid sinus syndrome, second- or third-degree heart block

Precautions: Renal disease, acute MI, AV block, severe respiratory disease, hypothyroidism, elderly, pregnancy category C, sinus nodal disease, lactation, hypokalemia

Pharmacokinetics:

IV: Onset 5-30 min, peak 1-5 hr, duration variable, half-life 1.5 days; excreted in urine

Drug interactions of concern to dentistry:

• Hypokalemia: corticosteroids

• Increased digoxin blood levels: erythromycin, clarithromycin, tetracyclines, itraconazole, propantheline

• Cardiac dysrhythmias: adrenergic agonists, succinylcholine

DENTAL CONSIDERATIONS

General:

• Monitor vital signs at every appointment because of cardiovascular side effects.

• After supine positioning, have patient sit upright for at least 2 min to avoid orthostatic hypotension.

• Avoid dental light in patient's eyes; offer dark glasses for patient comfort.

• An increased gag reflex may

make dental procedures such as taking radiographs or impressions difficult.

• Use vasoconstrictors with caution, in low doses, and with careful aspiration. Avoid use of gingival retraction cord with epinephrine.

Consultations:

• Stress from dental procedures may compromise cardiovascular function; determine patient risk.

• Medical consultation may be required to assess disease control and stress tolerance of patient.

dihydrocodeine bitartrate

(dye-hye-droe-koe' deen)

Combination products (see Appendix F)

Drug class.: Narcotic analgesic

Controlled Substance Schedule III (applies to combination products only)

Action: Decreases pain impulse transmission in the CNS by interacting with opioid receptors

Uses: Relief of moderate to moderately severe pain

Dosage and routes:

• *Adult:* PO dose range of combination product 1 or 2 caps q4h, usual dose is 10-30 mg tid when used alone

Available forms include: See Appendix F for combination products.

Side effects/adverse reactions: NOTE: Side effects from other ingredients in combination product must be considered in addition to those of dihydrocodeine.

▼ *ORAL:* Dry mouth

CNS: Dizziness, drowsiness, fatigue, vivid dreams, anxiety

CV: Palpitation, hypotension

GI: Nausea, vomiting, abdominal pain, indigestion, constipation

RESP: Respiratory depression

GU: Urinary retention

INTEG: Urticaria, diaphoresis

MISC: ***Anaphylaxis, angioedema,*** impairment of reaction time, dependence with withdrawal symptoms

Contraindications: Hypersensitivity to this drug, other opioids, or any ingredient in the combination products; respiratory depression, long-term use, seizure disorders

Precautions: Renal impairment (risk of more severe side effects), hepatic failure, elderly, head injury with increased intracranial pressure, opiate dependency, pregnancy category B, lactation, children <12 yr

Pharmacokinetics:

PO: peak blood levels 0.5-1.7 hr; rapid absorption, substantial first-pass metabolism and the hepatic demethylation to dihydromorphine, renal excretion

Drug interactions of concern to dentistry:

• Drug interactions caused by other ingredients in combination products must be considered

• Do not use with partial opioid antagonist

• Increased sedation with other CNS depressants and alcohol

• Increased effects of anticholinergics

• Decreased effects: rifabutin, rifampin

• Risk of priapism: sildenafil

DENTAL CONSIDERATIONS

General:

• Monitor vital signs at every appointment because of cardiovascular and respiratory side effects.

• After supine positioning, have

patient sit upright for at least 2 min before standing to avoid orthostatic hypotension.

• Assess salivary flow as a factor in caries, periodontal disease, and candidiasis.

• Psychologic and physical dependence may occur with chronic administration.

Teach patient/family:

When chronic dry mouth occurs, advise patient:

• To avoid mouth rinses with high alcohol content because of drying effects

• To use daily home fluoride products for anticaries effect

• To use sugarless gum, frequent sips of water, or saliva substitutes

dihydrotachysterol (DHT)

(dye-hye-droe-tak-iss'ter-ole)

DHT Intensol, Hytakerol

Drug class.: Vitamin D analog

Action: Increases intestinal absorption of calcium for bones, increases renal tubular absorption of phosphate

Uses: Nutritional supplement, rickets, hypoparathyroidism, pseudohypoparathyroidism, postoperative tetany

Dosage and routes:

Hypoparathyroidism/tetany:

• *Adult:* PO initial dose 0.75-2.5 mg day, given for several days; maintenance dose 0.2-1.75 mg qd as required

Available forms include: Tabs 0.125, 0.2, 0.4 mg; caps 0.125 mg; intensol sol 0.2 mg/ml

Side effects/adverse reactions:

▼ *ORAL:* Dry mouth, metallic taste

CNS: Drowsiness, headache, vertigo, fever, lethargy

GI: Nausea, diarrhea, vomiting, jaundice, anorexia, constipation, cramps

GU: ***Polyuria, hematuria,*** hypercalciuria, hyperphosphatemia

EENT: Tinnitus

MS: Myalgia, arthralgia, decreased bone development

Contraindications: Hypersensitivity, renal disease, hyperphosphatemia, hypercalcemia

Precautions: Pregnancy category C, renal calculi, lactation, cardiovascular disease

Pharmacokinetics:

PO: Onset 2 wk; metabolized by liver; excreted in feces (active/inactive)

Drug interactions of concern to dentistry:

• Decreased effect of dihydrotachysterol: prolonged use of corticosteroids, barbiturates

DENTAL CONSIDERATIONS

General:

• Consider semisupine chair position for patient comfort because of GI effects of drug.

• Assess salivary flow as a factor in caries, periodontal disease, and candidiasis.

Teach patient/family:

When chronic dry mouth occurs, advise patient:

• To avoid mouth rinses with high alcohol content because of drying effects

• Of need for daily home fluoride to prevent caries

• To use sugarless gum, frequent sips of water, or saliva substitutes

diltiazem HCl

(dil-tye'a-zem)

Cardizem, Cardizem CD, Cardizem SR, Cartia XT, Diacor XR, Dilitia XT, Tiazac

✦ Apo-Diltaz, Novo-Diltiazem, Nu-Dilitaz, Syn-Diltiazem

Drug class.: Calcium channel blocker

Action: Inhibits calcium ion influx across cell membrane during cardiac depolarization; produces relaxation of coronary vascular smooth muscle; dilates coronary arteries; slows SA/AV node conduction; dilates peripheral arteries

Uses: Chronic stable angina pectoris, vasospastic angina, coronary artery spasm, hypertension, supraventricular tachydysrhythmias

Dosage and routes:

• *Adult:* PO (tablet) 30 mg qid, increasing dose gradually to 180-360 mg/day in divided doses or 60-120 mg bid; may increase to 240-360 mg/day

• *Adult:* PO (capsules) ext rel in hypertension 180-240 mg once daily; angina initial dose 120 mg, range may vary from 180-480 mg/day

Available forms include: Tabs 30, 60, 90, 120 mg; sus rel caps 60, 90, 120 mg; ext rel caps 60, 90, 120, 180, 240, 300, 360, 420 mg; inj 5 mg/ml in 5, 10, 25 ml vials; powder for inj 25, 100 mg

Side effects/adverse reactions:

▼ *ORAL:* Dry mouth, gingival overgrowth, altered taste, ulcers

CNS: Headache, fatigue, drowsiness, dizziness, depression, weakness, insomnia, tremor, paresthesia

CV: Dysrhythmia, edema, ***CHF,*** bradycardia, hypotension, palpitation, heart block, peripheral edema, angina

GI: Nausea, vomiting, diarrhea, gastric upset, constipation, increased liver function studies

GU: ***Acute renal failure,*** nocturia, polyuria

HEMA: Postoperative hemorrhage

INTEG: Rash, pruritus, flushing, photosensitivity

Contraindications: Sick sinus syndrome, second- or third-degree heart block, hypotension <90 mm Hg systolic, acute MI, pulmonary congestion

Precautions: CHF, hypotension, hepatic injury, pregnancy category C, lactation, children, renal disease

Pharmacokinetics:

PO: Onset 30-60 min, peak 2-3 hr (immediate rel), 6-11 hr (sus rel), half-life 3.5-9 hr; metabolized by liver; excreted in urine (96% as metabolites)

Drug interactions of concern to dentistry:

• Decreased effect: indomethacin, possibly other NSAIDs, phenobarbital

• Increased effect: parenteral and inhalational general anesthetics or other drugs with hypotensive actions

• Increased effects of carbamazepine, midazolam, triazolam, buspirone

DENTAL CONSIDERATIONS

General:

• Monitor cardiac status; take vital signs at each appointment because of CV side effects. Consider a stress reduction protocol to prevent stress-induced angina during the dental appointment.

• After supine positioning, have patient sit upright for at least 2 min to avoid orthostatic hypotension.
• Place on frequent recall to monitor gingival condition.
• Limit use of sodium-containing products such as saline IV fluids for patients with a dietary salt restriction.
• Assess salivary flow as a factor in caries, periodontal disease, and candidiasis.
• Consider drug in diagnosis of taste alterations.

Consultations:

• Medical consultation may be required to assess disease control.

Teach patient/family:

• Importance of good oral hygiene to prevent soft tissue inflammation and to minimize gingival overgrowth
• Need for frequent oral prophylaxis if gingival overgrowth occurs

When chronic dry mouth occurs, advise patient:

• To avoid mouth rinses with high alcohol content because of drying effects
• To use daily home fluoride products for anticaries effect
• To use sugarless gum, frequent sips of water, or saliva substitutes

dimenhydrinate

(dye-men-hye'dri-nate)

Calm-X, Children's Dramamine, Dinate, Dimetabs, Dramamine, Dramanate, Dymenate, Hydrate, Triptone Caplets

🍁 Apo-Dimenhydrinate, Gravol, Traveltabs, PMS-Dimenhydrinate

Drug class.: H_1-receptor antagonist (equal parts diphenhydramine and chlorotheophylline)

Action: Acts on blood vessels, GI system, respiratory system by competing with histamine for H_1-receptor site; decreases allergic response by blocking histamine

Uses: Motion sickness, nausea, vomiting, vertigo

Dosage and routes:

• *Adult:* PO 50-100 mg q4h; IM/IV 50 mg as needed
• *Child 6-12 yr:* PO 25-50 mg q6-8h, limit 150 mg/day
• *Child 2-6 yr:* PO 1.25-25 mg q6-8h, limit 75 mg/day

Available forms include: Tabs 50 mg; inj 50 mg/ml; liq 12.5/4 ml, 15.62 mg/5ml; chew tab 50 mg

Side effects/adverse reactions:

▼ *ORAL: Dry mouth*

CNS: Drowsiness, ***convulsions*** (young children), restlessness, headache, dizziness, insomnia, confusion, nervousness, tingling, vertigo, hallucinations

CV: Hypertension, hypotension, palpitation

GI: Nausea, anorexia, diarrhea, vomiting, constipation

EENT: Blurred vision, diplopia, nasal congestion, photosensitivity

SYST: Rash, urticaria, fever, chills, flushing

Contraindications: Hypersensitivity to narcotics, shock

Precautions: Children, cardiac dysrhythmias, elderly, asthma, pregnancy category B, prostatic hypertrophy, bladder neck obstruction, narrow-angle glaucoma, stenosing peptic ulcer, pyloroduodenal obstruction, may mask ototoxicity of ototoxic antibiotics

Pharmacokinetics:

IM/PO: Duration 4-6 hr

Drug interactions of concern to dentistry:

- Increased photosensitization: tetracycline
- Increased effects of alcohol, other CNS depressants, anticholinergics

DENTAL CONSIDERATIONS

General:

- Assess salivary flow as a factor in caries, periodontal disease, and candidiasis.

Teach patient/family:

When chronic dry mouth occurs, advise patient:

- To avoid mouth rinses with high alcohol content because of drying effects
- To use daily home fluoride products for anticaries effect
- To use sugarless gum, frequent sips of water, or saliva substitutes

diphenhydramine HCl

(dye-fen-hye'dra-meen)

AllerMax, Banophen, Benadryl, Calm-X, Diphen AF, Diphenhist, Dormin, Genahist, Miles Nervene, Nytol Sleep-Eze, Siladryl, sominex, Tusstat, Scot-Tussin Allergy Relief

♣ Allerdryl

Drug class.: Antihistamine, H_1-receptor antagonist

Action: Acts on blood vessels, GI system, respiratory system by competing with histamine for H_1-receptor site; decreases allergic response by blocking histamine

Uses: Allergy symptoms, rhinitis, motion sickness, antiparkinsonism, nighttime sedation, infant colic, nonproductive cough; unlabeled use for dental local anesthesia

Dosage and routes:

- *Adult:* PO 25-50 mg q4-6h, not to exceed 400 mg/day; IM/IV 10-50 mg, not to exceed 400 mg/day
- *Child >12 kg:* PO/IM/IV 5 mg/kg/day in 4 divided doses, not to exceed 300 mg/day
- *Local anesthetic (unapproved use):* INTRAORAL INJ use *only* the 10 mg/ml solution and never >1.5 ml per injection per patient; risk of tissue irritation if more is used; must use sterile technique at all times; no data to support combined use with vasoconstrictor

Available forms include: Caps 25, 50 mg; tabs 25, 50 mg; elix 12.5 mg/5 ml; syr 12.5 mg/5 ml; liquid 12.5 mg/5 ml; inj IM/IV 10, 50 mg/ml

Side effects/adverse reactions:

▼ *ORAL:* Dry mouth

CNS: Dizziness, drowsiness, poor

coordination, fatigue, anxiety, euphoria, confusion, paresthesia, neuritis
GI: Nausea, anorexia, diarrhea
RESP: Increased thick secretions, wheezing, chest tightness
HEMA: ***Thrombocytopenia, agranulocytosis, hemolytic anemia***
GU: Retention, dysuria, frequency
EENT: Blurred vision, dilated pupils, tinnitus, nasal stuffiness, dry nose/throat
INTEG: Photosensitivity
Contraindications: Hypersensitivity to H_1-receptor antagonist, acute asthma attack, lower respiratory tract disease
Precautions: Increased intraocular pressure, renal disease, cardiac disease, hypertension, bronchial asthma, seizure disorder, stenosed peptic ulcers, hyperthyroidism, prostatic hypertrophy, bladder neck obstruction, pregnancy category C
Pharmacokinetics:
PO: Peak 1-3 hr, duration 4-7 hr
IM: Onset 0.5 hr, peak 1-4 hr, duration 4-7 hr
IV: Onset immediate, duration 4-7 hr, half-life 2-7 hr
Metabolized in liver; excreted by kidneys; crosses placenta; excreted in breast milk
Drug interactions of concern to dentistry:
• Increased CNS depression: all CNS depressants, alcohol
• Increased anticholinergic effect: anticholinergics
• Increased plasma levels of labetalol
DENTAL CONSIDERATIONS
General:
• Patients on chronic drug therapy may rarely have symptoms of blood dyscrasias, which can include infection, bleeding, and poor healing.
• Assess salivary flow as a factor in caries, periodontal disease, and candidiasis.
• Consider semisupine chair position for patients with respiratory disease.
Consultations:
• In a patient with symptoms of blood dyscrasias, request a medical consultation for blood studies and postpone dental treatment until normal values are reestablished.
Teach patient/family:
• Importance of good oral hygiene to prevent soft tissue inflammation
• Caution to prevent injury when using oral hygiene aids
When chronic dry mouth occurs, advise patient:
• To avoid mouth rinses with high alcohol content because of drying effects
• To use daily home fluoride products for anticaries effect
• To use sugarless gum, frequent sips of water, or saliva substitutes

diphenoxylate HCl with atropine sulfate

(dye-fen-ox'i-late)
Logen, Lomanate, Lomotil, Lonox
Drug class.: Antidiarrheal (opioid with atropine)

Controlled Substance Schedule V
Action: Inhibits gastric motility by acting on mucosal receptors responsible for peristalsis
Uses: Simple diarrhea

Dosage and routes:
• *Adult:* PO 2.5-5 mg qid, titrated to patient response
• *Child 2-12 yr:* PO 0.3-0.4 mg/kg/day in divided doses
Available forms include: Tabs 2.5 mg with atropine 0.025 mg; liquid 2.5 mg with atropine 0.025 mg/5 ml in 60 ml
Side effects/adverse reactions:
▼ *ORAL:* Dry mouth
CNS: Drowsiness, headache, sedation, depression, weakness, lethargy, flushing, hyperthermia
CV: Tachycardia
GI: Nausea, vomiting, ***paralytic ileus, toxic megacolon,*** abdominal pain, colitis
GU: Urinary retention
EENT: Blurred vision, nystagmus, mydriasis
SYST: ***Angioneurotic edema,*** rash, urticaria, pruritus
Contraindications: Hypersensitivity, severe liver disease, pseudomembranous enterocolitis, glaucoma, child <2 yr, electrolyte imbalances
Precautions: Hepatic disease, renal disease, ulcerative colitis, pregnancy category C, lactation, elderly, not recommended for children <2 yr, Down syndrome
Pharmacokinetics:
PO: Onset 45-60 min, peak 2 hr, duration 3-4 hr, half-life 2.5 hr, terminal half-life 12-14 hr; metabolized in liver to active form; excreted in urine, feces, breast milk
Drug interactions of concern to dentistry:
• Contraindication: MAOIs
• Increased effects of alcohol, all CNS depressants, opioid analgesics, anticholinergics

DENTAL CONSIDERATIONS
General:
• Assess salivary flow as a factor in caries, periodontal disease, and candidiasis.
• Psychologic and physical dependence may occur with chronic administration.
• Consider semisupine chair position for patient comfort because of GI effects of disease.
• This drug product is normally used only for a few doses for acute problems; however, some patients may have to take it for longer periods as dictated by a contributing disease.
Teach patient/family:
• To avoid mouth rinses with high alcohol content because of drying effects

dipivefrin HCl

(dye-pi've-frin)
AKPro, Propine
♣ Ophtho-Dipivefrin
Drug class.: Adrenergic agonist

Action: Converted to epinephrine, which decreases aqueous production and increases outflow
Uses: Open-angle glaucoma
Dosage and routes:
• *Adult:* Instill 1 drop q12h
Available forms include: Sol 0.1%
Side effects/adverse reactions:
CV: Hypertension, tachycardia, dysrhythmias
EENT: Burning, stinging, mydriasis, photophobia
Contraindications: Hypersensitivity, narrow-angle glaucoma
Precautions: Pregnancy category B, lactation, children, aphakia

Pharmacokinetics:
INSTILL: Onset 30 min, peak 1 hr, duration 12 hr

Drug interactions of concern to dentistry:

• Avoid use of anticholinergics such as atropine, scopolamine, and propantheline; use benzodiazepines with caution

DENTAL CONSIDERATIONS

General:

• Avoid dental light in patient's eyes; offer dark glasses for patient comfort.

---

dipyridamole

(dye-peer-id'a-mole)

Persantine

Apo-Dipyridamole, Novo-Dipiradol

Drug class.: Platelet aggregation inhibitor

Action: Specific action unclear; inhibits ability of platelets to aggregate, possibly through effects on adenosine, cAMP, or thromboxane A_2

Uses: Adjunctive therapy with warfarin in prosthetic heart valve replacement

Dosage and routes:

Adjunctive therapy:

• *Adult:* PO 50-75 mg qid in combination with warfarin

Available forms include: Tabs 25, 50, 75 mg

Side effects/adverse reactions:

ORAL: Gingival bleeding

CNS: Headache, dizziness, weakness, fainting, syncope

CV: Postural hypotension

GI: Nausea, vomiting, anorexia, diarrhea

INTEG: Rash, flushing

Contraindications: Hypersensitivity, hypotension

Precautions: Pregnancy category B, children <12 yr

Pharmacokinetics:
PO: Peak 2-2.5 hr, duration 6 hr; therapeutic response may take several months; metabolized in liver; excreted in bile; undergoes enterohepatic recirculation

Drug interactions of concern to dentistry:

• Additive antiplatelet effects: aspirin and other NSAIDs

DENTAL CONSIDERATIONS

General:

• Monitor vital signs at every appointment because of cardiovascular side effects.

• After supine positioning, have patient sit upright for at least 2 min to avoid orthostatic hypotension.

• Avoid prescribing aspirin-containing products, even though ASA/dipyridamole combination drugs are used in some patients.

• Patients with prosthetic valves require antibiotic prophylaxis

• Evaluate for clotting ability during gingival instrumentation, because inhibition of platelet aggregation may occur.

• Consider local hemostatic measures to prevent excessive bleeding during instrumentation.

Consultations:

• Medical consultation should include partial prothrombin time or prothrombin time.

• Medical consultation may be required to assess disease control.

Teach patient/family:

• Importance of good oral hygiene to prevent gingival inflammation

diirithromycin

(dye-rith'roe-mye-sin)

Dynabac

Drug class.: Macrolide antibiotic

Action: Active product (erythromycylamine) binds to 50S ribosomal subunits of susceptible bacteria to inhibit bacterial growth

Uses: Treatment of acute and secondary bacterial infection of acute bronchitis, community-acquired pneumonia, streptococcal pharyngitis, and uncomplicated skin and skin structure infections

Dosage and routes:

- *Adult and child >12 yr:* PO 500 mg/day for 7-14 days; give with food or within 1 hr of eating; do not crush or chew tablets

Available forms include: Tabs 250 mg

Side effects/adverse reactions:

▼ *ORAL:* Dry mouth, taste alteration, mouth ulcers (all <1%); although not documented, it is reasonable to assume opportunistic oral candidiasis

CNS: Headache, somnolence, dizziness, insomnia

GI: Diarrhea, abdominal pain, nausea, dyspepsia, pseudomembranous colitis

RESP: Dyspnea, cough

GU: Vaginal candidiasis

INTEG: Rash, pruritus, urticaria

MS: Asthenia

Contraindications: Hypersensitivity to macrolide antibiotics

Precautions: Not for *H. influenzae* or *S. pyogenes* infections, pregnancy category C, lactation, child <12 yr

Pharmacokinetics:

PO: Half-life 30-44 hr; after absorption, parent drug is converted to erythromycylamine; plasma protein binding low (15%-30%); excreted in bile

Drug interactions of concern to dentistry:

- Other drug interactions: data are limited; antacids and histamine H_2 antagonists tend to enhance absorption; refer to erythromycin for potential interacting drugs

DENTAL CONSIDERATIONS

General:

- Do not use in patients at risk for bacteremias caused by inadequate serum levels.
- Potential value in dental infections is unknown.
- Determine why the patient is taking the drug.
- Examine for oral manifestations of opportunistic infections.

Consultations:

- Medical consultation may be required to assess disease control.

Teach patient/family:

- To be aware of the possibility of secondary oral infection and the need to see dentist immediately if infection occurs

disopyramide phosphate

(dye-soe-peer'a-mide)

Norpace, Norpace CR

♣ Rythmodan-LA

Drug class.: Antidysrhythmic (class Ia)

Action: Prolongs action potential duration and effective refractory period; reduces disparity in refractoriness between normal and infarcted myocardium

Uses: PVCs, ventricular tachycardia

Dosage and routes:

• *Adult:* PO 100-200 mg q6h, in renal dysfunction 100 mg q6h; ext rel caps 200 mg q12h

• *Child 12-18 yr:* PO 6-15 mg/kg/day, in divided doses q6h

• *Child 4-12 yr:* PO 10-15 mg/kg/day, in divided doses q6h

• *Child 1-4 yr:* PO 10-20 mg/kg/day, in divided doses q6h

• *Child <1 yr:* PO 10-30 mg/kg/day, in divided doses q6h

Available forms include: Caps 100, 150 mg (as phosphate); ext rel caps 100, 150 mg

Side effects/adverse reactions:

▼ *ORAL: Dry mouth*

CNS: Headache, dizziness, psychosis, fatigue, depression, paresthesia, anxiety, insomnia

CV: Hypotension, bradycardia, ***CHF, cardiac arrest,*** angina, PVCs, tachycardia, increase in QRS and QT segments, edema, weight gain, AV block, syncope, chest pain

GI: Constipation, nausea, anorexia, flatulence, diarrhea, vomiting

HEMA: ***Thrombocytopenia, agranulocytosis,*** anemia (rare), decreased hemoglobin, hematocrit

GU: Retention, hesitancy, impotence, urinary frequency, urgency

EENT: Blurred vision, dry nose/throat/eyes, narrow-angle glaucoma

INTEG: Rash, pruritus, urticaria

MS: Weakness, pain in extremities

META: Hypoglycemia

Contraindications: Hypersensitivity, second- or third-degree heart block, cardiogenic shock, CHF (uncompensated), sick sinus syndrome, QT prolongation

Precautions: Pregnancy category C, lactation, diabetes mellitus, renal disease, children, hepatic disease, myasthenia gravis, narrow-angle glaucoma, cardiomyopathy, conduction abnormalities

Pharmacokinetics:

PO: Peak 30 min-3 hr, duration 6-12 hr, half-life 4-10 hr; metabolized in liver; excreted in feces, urine, breast milk; crosses placenta

Drug interactions of concern to dentistry:

• Possible increased risk of prolonged QT interval: clarithromycin, erythromycin

• Increased side effects: anticholinergics, alcohol

• Decreased effects: barbiturates, corticosteroids

DENTAL CONSIDERATIONS

General:

• Monitor vital signs at every appointment because of cardiovascular side effects.

• After supine positioning, have patient sit upright for at least 2 min before standing to avoid orthostatic hypotension.

• Patients on chronic drug therapy may rarely have symptoms of blood dyscrasias, which can include infection, bleeding, and poor healing.

• Assess salivary flow as a factor in caries, periodontal disease, and candidiasis.

Consultations:

• In a patient with symptoms of blood dyscrasias, request a medical consultation for blood studies and postpone dental treatment until normal values are reestablished.

• Medical consultation may be required to assess disease control and patient's ability to tolerate stress.

Teach patient/family:

• Importance of good oral hygiene to prevent soft tissue inflammation

When chronic dry mouth occurs, advise patient:

• To avoid mouth rinses with high alcohol content because of drying effects

• To use daily home fluoride products for anticaries effect

• To use sugarless gum, frequent sips of water, or saliva substitutes

---

disulfiram

(dye-sul'fi-ram)

generic

Drug class.: Aldehyde dehydrogenase inhibitor

Action: Blocks oxidation of alcohol at acetaldehyde stage; accumulation of acetaldehyde produces the disulfiram-alcohol reaction

Uses: Chronic alcoholism (as adjunct)

Dosage and routes:

• *Adult:* PO 500 mg qd × 1-2 wk, then 125-500 mg qd

Available forms include: Tabs 250, 500 mg

Side effects/adverse reactions:

▼ *ORAL:* Metallic taste

CNS: Headache, drowsiness, restlessness, dizziness

CV: ***Dysrhythmias,*** tachycardia, chest pain, hypotension

GI: ***Hepatotoxicity,*** nausea, vomiting

RESP: ***Respiratory depression,*** hyperventilation, dyspnea

INTEG: Rash, dermatitis, urticaria

Disulfiram-alcohol reaction: Flushing, throbbing, headache, respiratory difficulty, nausea, vomiting, sweating, thirst, chest pain, palpitation, dyspnea, hyperventilation, tachycardia, confusion, CV collapse, MI, CHF, convulsions, death

Contraindications: Hypersensitivity, alcohol intoxication, psychoses, CV disease, pregnancy category not listed

Precautions: Hypothyroidism, hepatic disease, diabetes mellitus, seizure disorders, nephritis, cerebral damage

Pharmacokinetics:

PO: Onset 1-2 hr; oxidized by liver; excreted unchanged in feces; can affect alcohol metabolism for 1-2 wk after last dose

Drug interactions of concern to dentistry:

• Increased CNS depression: long-acting benzodiazepines

• Increased disulfiram reaction: alcohol

• Risk of psychosis: metronidazole (do not use), tricyclic antidepressants

DENTAL CONSIDERATIONS

General:

• Be aware of the needs of patients who are in recovery from substance abuse.

• Avoid other addictive drugs, including opioids and benzodiazepines.

Consultations:

• Medical consultation may be required to assess disease control.

Teach patient/family:

• To avoid mouth rinses with high alcohol content because of drying effects and drug-drug interaction

docosanol

(do-cos′a-nole)

Abreva

Drug class.: Synthetic lipophilic alcohol

Action: A highly lipophilic, fatty alcohol that prevents fusion of lipid-enveloped viruses with cell membranes, thereby blocking viral replication

Uses: Treatment of recurrent herpes labialis (cold sores, fever blisters) on the face or lips; appears to shorten healing time by at least 1 day

Dosage and routes:

• *Adult and child >12 yr:* TOP apply small amount to affected area on face or lips or at the first sign of lesion for 5 × daily until healed

Available forms include: Cream 10%, 2 g tube (OTC product)

Side effects/adverse reactions:

CNS: Headache

INTEG: Site reaction, rash, pruritus, dry skin, acne

Contraindications: Hypersensitivity

Precautions: External use only (not for intraoral use), children <12 yr, avoid application to eyes, pregnancy category B

Pharmacokinetics:

TOP: Negligible absorption

Drug interactions of concern to dentistry:

• None reported

DENTAL CONSIDERATIONS

Teach patient/family:

• Apply with finger cot; wash hands before and after use.

• Do not share this medication to prevent potential cross contamination of virus.

• Replace toothbrush after resolution of lesion to prevent reinfection of virus.

dofetilide

(doe-fet′il-ide)

Tikosyn

Drug class.: Antidysrhythmic (class III)

Action: Blockade of the cardiac ion channel carrying the rapid components of the delayed rectifier potassium current (I_{kr}); increases the monophasic action potential duration; increases effective refractory period; increases QT interval on ECG; and terminates induced reentrant tachyarrhythmias

Uses: Maintenance of normal sinus rhythm in patients with atrial fibrillation/atrial flutter >1 wk duration, who have been converted to normal sinus rhythm; conversion of atrial fibrillation/atrial flutter to normal sinus rhythm

Dosage and routes:

• *Adult:* PO initial doses are started only in patients placed in an appropriate facility for 3 days for ECG monitoring; must be individualized according to creatinine clearance and QT interval. Usual dose is 0.5 mg bid. Available only to hospitals or other limited institutions and to physicians who have completed proper training program.

Available forms include: Caps 0.125, 0.25, 0.50 mg

Side effects/adverse reactions:

▼ *ORAL:* Angioedema, facial paralysis

CNS: Headache, dizziness, insomnia, anxiety, syncope

CV: Chest pain, ***ventricular tachycardia, torsade de pointes,*** AV

block, angina pectoris, hypertension, palpitation
GI: Diarrhea, flatulence, abdominal pain
RESP: RTI, dyspnea, cough
GU: UTI
INTEG: Rash, sweating
MS: Back pain, arthralgia, asthenia
MISC: Flulike syndrome
Contraindications: Hypersensitivity, congenital or acquired QT syndromes (QT interval greater than 440 ms), severe renal impairment, contraindicated with cimetidine, trimethoprim, ketoconazole, prochlorperazine, megestrol, or verapamil
Precautions: Requires dose adjustment in renal impairment, can cause life-threatening ventricular arrhythmias, caution in use with CYP450 3A4 isoenzyme inhibitors, hepatic impairment, abnormal serum potassium or magnesium levels, pregnancy category C, lactation, children <18 yr
Pharmacokinetics:
PO: Bioavailability >90%, peak plasma levels 2-3 hr, steady-state levels 2-3 days, plasma protein binding 60%-70%, excreted (80%) in urine unchanged, excretion involves both glomerular filtration and active tubular secretion, limited metabolism by CYP450 3A4 isoenzymes
Drug interactions of concern to dentistry:
- Decreased renal excretion: ketoconazole (contraindicated use)
- Not recommended with concurrent use of phenothiazines, tricyclic antidepressants, SSRIs, macrolide antiinfectives (erythromycin, clarithromycin), azole antifungals, or other drugs that inhibit CYP3A4 isoenzymes (see Appendix I)
- Contraindicated with cimetidine, trimethoprim, ketoconazole, prochlorperazine, megestrol, or verapamil

DENTAL CONSIDERATIONS
General:
- Monitor vital signs at every appointment because of cardiovascular side effects.
- Delay or avoid dental treatment if patient shows signs of cardiac symptoms or respiratory distress.
- Ensure that the patient is compliant with drug therapy.

Consultations:
- Patient's physician should be informed about any use of dental drugs.
- Medical consultation may be required to assess disease control and patient's ability to tolerate stress.

Teach patient/family:
- Importance of updating health and drug history if physician makes any changes in evaluation or drug regimens

---

dolasetron mesylate
(dol-a'se-tron)
Anzemet
Drug class.: Antinauseant and antiemetic

Action: Acts as an antagonist for serotonin ($5HT_3$) receptors in the CNS; may also reduce afferent stimulus from GI tract
Uses: Control of nausea and vomiting associated with cancer chemotherapy and prevention of postoperative nausea and vomiting
Dosage and routes:
Cancer chemotherapy:
- *Adult:* PO 100 mg given 1 hr before chemotherapy
- *Child 2-16 yr:* PO 1.8 mg/kg

given 1 hr before chemotherapy not to exceed 100 mg

Parenteral chemotherapy:

• *Adult:* IV 1.8 mg/kg as a single dose about 30 min before chemotherapy, alternatively for most patients, a fixed dose of 100 mg can be given over 30 sec

• *Child 2-16 yr:* IV 1.8 mg/kg as a single dose approximately 30 min before chemotherapy up to a maximum of 100 mg

Prevention or treatment of postoperative nausea and vomiting:

• *Adult:* PO 100 mg given 2 hr before surgery

• *Child 2-16 yr:* PO 1.2 mg/kg given 2 hr before surgery, not to exceed 100 mg

• *Adult:* IV 12.5 mg as a single dose 15 min before the end of anesthesia or as soon as nausea and vomiting are evident

• *Child 2-16 yr:* IV 0.35 mg/kg with a maximum dose of 12.5 mg (single dose) approximately 15 min before cessation of anesthesia or as soon as nausea and vomiting are present

Available forms include: Tabs 50, 100 mg; inj 20 mg/ml in 0.625 ml, 5 ml vials

Side effects/adverse reactions:

▼ *ORAL: Taste alteration*

CNS: Headache, fatigue, sedation, dizziness, light-headedness, nervousness, paresthesia

CV: Bradycardia, tachycardia, alteration of ECG, orthostatic hypotension, hypertension

GI: Increased appetite, nausea, constipation, diarrhea, dyspepsia, flatulence

EENT: Blurred vision

INTEG: Pruritus

META: Elevation of aminotransferases

MISC: Fever, chills

Contraindications: Hypersensitivity

Precautions: Previous hypersensitivity to other 5-HT_3 antagonists, cardiovascular disease, seizure disorders, ECG changes, hypokalemia, hypomagnesemia, diuretics, antiarrhythmics, pregnancy category B, lactation

Pharmacokinetics:

IV: Metabolized to active metabolite, peak plasma concentrations 1 hr, urinary excretion mostly, some fecal excretion

PO: Well absorbed, rapidly metabolized to active metabolite

Drug interactions of concern to dentistry:

• Does not influence anesthesia recovery time

DENTAL CONSIDERATIONS

General:

• Monitor patients in recovery to avoid untoward events.

• Patients taking opioids for acute or chronic pain should be given alternative analgesics for dental pain.

• Chlorhexidine mouth rinse before and during chemotherapy may reduce severity of mucositis.

• Palliative medication may be required for management of oral side effects from chemotherapy.

Teach patient/family:

• To be aware of possible oral side effects from concurrent cancer chemotherapy

• To report excessive nausea and vomiting to dentist for patients recovering from anesthesia after dental treatment

donepezil HCl

(doe-nep'e-zeel)

Aricept

Drug class.: Cholinesterase inhibitor

Action: A centrally acting reversible inhibitor of choline esterase enzyme

Uses: Mild to moderate dementia associated with Alzheimer's disease

Dosage and routes:

• *Adult:* PO initial 5 mg/day; can increase to 10 mg/day after 4-6 wk evaluation at 5 mg dose; take dose in evening just before retiring

Available forms include: Tabs 5, 10 mg

Side effects/adverse reactions:

▼ *ORAL:* Toothache (1%), dry mouth, bad taste, gingivitis, tongue edema, coated tongue

CNS: Insomnia, anorexia, headache, dizziness, depression, abnormal dreams

CV: Syncope, hot flashes, hypotension, hypertension

GI: Nausea, diarrhea, vomiting, anorexia

RESP: Dyspnea

HEMA: Thrombocytopenia, ecchymosis, anemia

GU: Frequency of urination

EENT: Sore throat, dry eyes, blurred vision, earache, tinnitus

INTEG: Pruritus, urticaria

META: Weight decrease, dehydration

MS: Muscle cramps, arthritis

MISC: Fatigue, generalized pain

Contraindications: Hypersensitivity

Precautions: Bradycardia, sick sinus syndrome, GI ulcer disease, bladder obstruction, seizures, asthma, obstructive pulmonary disease, pregnancy category C, lactation, children, hepatic impairment

Pharmacokinetics:

PO: Bioavailability 100%, peak plasma levels 3-4 hr, 96% bound to plasma proteins, hepatic metabolism (CYP3A4, CYP2D6 isoenzymes), active metabolites, urinary excretion

Drug interactions of concern to dentistry:

• Enhanced succinylcholine muscle relaxation during anesthesia

• Risk of GI side effects: NSAIDs

• Action may be inhibited by anticholinergic drugs or enhanced by cholinergic agonists

• Increased blood levels: ketoconazole, paroxetine

• Use with caution drugs that inhibit CYP3A4 or CYP2D6 isoenzymes (see Appendix I)

DENTAL CONSIDERATIONS

General:

• Determine why patient is taking the drug.

• Monitor vital signs at every appointment because of cardiovascular side effects.

• After supine positioning, have patient sit upright for at least 2 min before standing to avoid orthostatic hypotension.

• Use precaution if sedation or general anesthesia is required.

• Patients on chronic drug therapy may rarely have symptoms of blood dyscrasias, which can include infection, bleeding, and poor healing.

• Drug is used early in the disease; ensure that patient or care giver understands informed consent.

D

• Place on frequent recall because early attention to dental health is important for Alzheimer's patients.
• Assess salivary flow as factor in caries, periodontal disease, and candidiasis.
• Consider semisupine chair position for patient comfort if GI side effects occur.

Consultations:
• Consultation with physician may be needed if sedation or general anesthesia is required.
• Medical consultation may be required to assess disease control and patient's ability to tolerate stress.
• In a patient with symptoms of blood dyscrasias, request a medical consultation for blood studies and postpone treatment until normal values are reestablished.

Teach patient/family:
• Importance of good oral hygiene to prevent soft tissue inflammation
• To prevent trauma when using oral hygiene aids
• Use of electric toothbrush if patient has difficulty holding conventional devices

When chronic dry mouth occurs, advise patient:
• To avoid mouth rinses with high alcohol content because of drying effects
• To use daily home fluoride products for anticaries effect
• To use sugarless gum, frequent sips of water, or saliva substitutes

dornase alfa

(dor'nase)

Pulmozyme

Drug class.: Recombinant human deoxyribonuclease (rh DNase)

Action: Reduces sputum viscosity by hydrolyzing extracellular DNA in sputum

Uses: Cystic fibrosis; reduces incidence of pulmonary infections; improves pulmonary function

Dosage and routes:
• *Adult and child >5 yr:* INH inhale 2.5 mg once daily with recommended nebulizer

Available forms include: INH 1.0 mg/ml in 2.5 ml ampules

Side effects/adverse reactions:
CV: Chest pain, ***cardiac failure***
GI: Intestinal obstruction, abdominal pain
RESP: Apnea, bronchitis, dyspnea, coughing
EENT: Pharyngitis, laryngitis, conjunctivitis, voice alteration, sinusitis
INTEG: Rash, urticaria
MISC: Flulike symptoms, malaise, weight loss

Contraindications: Hypersensitivity, allergy to Chinese hamster ovary cell products

Precautions: Pregnancy category B, lactation, child <5 yr

Pharmacokinetics:
INH: Peak sputum levels 15 min

Drug interactions of concern to dentistry:
• None documented

DENTAL CONSIDERATIONS

General:
• Consider semisupine chair position for patients with respiratory disease.
• Monitor vital signs at every appointment because of respiratory and cardiovascular side effects.
• A stress reduction protocol may be required.

Consultations:
• A medical consultation may be required to assess disease control.

Teach patient/family:
• Importance of good oral hygiene to prevent soft tissue inflammation

dorzolamide HCl

(dor-zole'a-mide)
Trusopt
Drug class.: Carbonic anhydrase inhibitor

Action: Reduces intraocular pressure through inhibition of carbonic anhydrase enzyme
Uses: Ocular hypertension, open-angle glaucoma
Dosage and routes:
• *Adult:* Instill 1 gtt in affected eye(s) tid; if other ophthalmic drug products are also used, give the drugs at least 10 min apart
Available forms include: Sol 2% in 5, 10 ml
Side effects/adverse reactions:
ORAL: Bitter taste
CNS: Headache
GI: Nausea
EENT: Ocular burning, stinging, conjunctivitis, lid reactions, keratitis, blurred vision, photophobia
INTEG: Skin rashes
Contraindications: Hypersensitivity
Precautions: Allergy to sulfonamides, renal or hepatic impairment, pregnancy category C, lactation, children, oral carbonic anhydrase inhibitors, contact lenses
Pharmacokinetics: Systemically absorbed from the eye
Drug interactions of concern to dentistry:
• Avoid drugs that may exacerbate glaucoma (anticholinergic drugs)
• High-dose salicylates to avoid systemic toxicity

DENTAL CONSIDERATIONS
General:
• Avoid dental light in patient's eyes; offer dark glasses for patient comfort.
• Protect patient's eyes from accidental spatter during dental treatment.
• Check patient's compliance with prescribed drug regimen for glaucoma.
Consultations:
• Medical consultation may be required to assess disease control.

doxazosin mesylate

(dox-ay'zoe-sin)
Cardura
Cardura-1, Cardura-2, Cardura-3
Drug class.: Peripheral α-adrenergic blocker

Action: Selectively blocks α_1-adrenergic receptors, which results in peripheral vasodilation and lowering of blood pressure; also causes relaxation of smooth muscles of the bladder, prostate, and prostate capsule in benign prostatic hyperplasia; also lowers total cholesterol, LDL, and triglycerides
Uses: Hypertension, benign prostatic hypertrophy
Dosage and routes:
Hypertension:
• *Adult:* PO 1 mg qd, increasing up to 16 mg qd if required; usual range 4-16 mg/day
Benign prostatic hypertrophy:
• *Adult:* PO initial dose 1 mg/day, depending on symptoms dose can be increased to 2 mg/day; then to 4 mg/day up to a maximum of 8 mg/day

Available forms include: Tabs 1, 2, 4, 8 mg

Side effects/adverse reactions:

▼ *ORAL:* Dry mouth

CNS: Dizziness, headache, weakness, fatigue, asthenia, drowsiness, anxiety, depression, vertigo

CV: Palpitation, orthostatic hypotension, tachycardia, edema, dysrhythmias, chest pain

GI: Nausea, vomiting, diarrhea, constipation, abdominal pain

GU: Incontinence, polyuria

EENT: Epistaxis, tinnitus, red sclera, pharyngitis, rhinitis

INTEG: Lichen planus

Contraindications: Hypersensitivity to quinazolines

Precautions: Pregnancy category B, children, lactation, hepatic disease

Pharmacokinetics:

PO: Onset 2 hr, peak 2-6 hr, duration 24 hr, half-life 22 hr; extensively protein bound (98%); metabolized in liver; excreted via bile, feces (<63%) and in urine (9%)

Drug interactions of concern to dentistry:

- Increased hypotensive effects: all CNS depressants
- Reduced effects with indomethacin, NSAIDs, sympathomimetics
- Caution in use of drugs that may cause urinary retention: anticholinergics, opioids

DENTAL CONSIDERATIONS

General:

- Monitor vital signs at every appointment because of cardiovascular side effects.
- After supine positioning, have patient sit upright for at least 2 min before standing to avoid orthostatic hypotension.
- Assess salivary flow as a factor in caries, periodontal disease, and candidiasis.

Consultations:

- Medical consultation may be required to assess disease control and patient's ability to tolerate stress.

Teach patient/family:

When chronic dry mouth occurs, advise patient:

- To avoid mouth rinses with high alcohol content because of drying effects
- To use daily home fluoride products for anticaries effect
- To use sugarless gum, frequent sips of water, or saliva substitutes

---

doxepin HCl (topical)

(dox'e-pin)

Zonalon

Drug class.: Topical antipruritic (tricyclic antidepressant)

Action: Antipruritic mechanism unknown; has antihistaminic activity; also produces drowsiness

Uses: Pruritus associated with eczema, atopic dermatitis, lichen simplex chronicus

Dosage and routes:

- *Adult:* TOP apply to affected area qid with intervals of 3-4 days between applications for up to 8 days

Available forms include: Cream 5% in 30 g tube

Side effects/adverse reactions:

▼ *ORAL: Dry mouth, taste alteration, dry lips*

CNS: Drowsiness, headache, fatigue, dizziness, anxiety

INTEG: Burning, stinging, dryness of skin, edema, paresthesia

MISC: Fever

Contraindications: Hypersensi-

tivity, untreated glaucoma, tendency for urinary retention

Precautions: Pregnancy category B, lactation, children, for external use only, caution in driving car, concurrent use with alcohol or MAOI

Pharmacokinetics:

TOP: Variable absorption, half-life 28-52 hr; hepatic metabolism; widely distributed; renal excretion

Drug interactions of concern to dentistry:

• Potential for interactions depends on how much drug is absorbed and duration of use (>8 days)

• Increased anticholinergic effects: anticholinergics, antihistamines, phenothiazines, other tricyclic antidepressants

• Potential risk for increased CNS depression: all CNS depressants

• Increased effects of direct-acting sympathomimetics: epinephrine, levonordefrin

• Avoid concurrent use with St. John's wort

DENTAL CONSIDERATIONS

General:

• Doxepin may be absorbed and produce typical systemic side effects of tricyclic drugs.

• Monitor vital signs at every appointment because of cardiovascular side effects.

• Use vasoconstrictors with caution, in low doses, and with careful aspiration.

• Place on frequent recall because of oral side effects.

• Apply lubricant to dry lips for patient comfort before dental procedures.

• Assess salivary flow as a factor in caries, periodontal disease, and candidiasis.

Consultations:

• Medical consultation may be required to assess disease control.

Teach patient/family:

• To avoid mouth rinses with high alcohol content because of interaction with alcohol (see precautions) and drying effects

When chronic dry mouth occurs, advise patient:

• Of need for daily home fluoride for anticaries effect

• To use sugarless gum, frequent sips of water, or saliva substitutes

doxepin HCl

(dox'e-pin)

Sinequan

Novo-Doxepin, Triadapin

Drug class.: Antidepressant, tricyclic

Action: Inhibits both norepinephrine and serotonin (5-HT) reuptake in synapses in the brain, but the precise antidepressant mechanism remains unclear

Uses: Major depression, anxiety; unapproved: panic disorders

Dosage and routes:

• *Adult:* PO 50-75 mg/day in divided doses; may increase to 150 mg/day or may give daily dose hs; severe depression up to 300 mg

Available forms include: Caps 10, 25, 50, 75, 100, 150 mg; oral conc 10 mg/ml

Side effects/adverse reactions:

ORAL: Dry mouth, unpleasant taste, bleeding, stomatitis, lichenoid reaction

CNS: Dizziness, drowsiness, confusion, headache, anxiety, tremors, stimulation, weakness, insomnia, nightmares, EPS (elderly), increased psychiatric symptoms, paresthesia

CV: Orthostatic hypotension, ECG changes, tachycardia, ***hypertension,*** palpitation

GI: Diarrhea, ***paralytic ileus, hepatitis,*** increased appetite, cramps, epigastric distress, jaundice, nausea, vomiting

HEMA: ***Agranulocytosis, thrombocytopenia, eosinophilia, leukopenia***

GU: Retention, ***acute renal failure***

EENT: Blurred vision, tinnitus, mydriasis, ophthalmoplegia

INTEG: Rash, urticaria, sweating, pruritus, photosensitivity

Contraindications: Hypersensitivity to tricyclic antidepressants, urinary retention, narrow-angle glaucoma, prostatic hypertrophy

Precautions: Suicidal patients, elderly, pregnancy category C, MAOIs

Pharmacokinetics:

PO: Steady-state 2-8 days, half-life 8-24 hr; metabolized by liver; excreted by kidneys; crosses placenta; excreted in breast milk

Drug interactions of concern to dentistry:

- Increased anticholinergic effects: anticholinergic blockers, antihistamines, phenothiazines
- Increased effects of direct-acting sympathomimetics (epinephrine, levonordefrin)
- Potential risk of increased CNS depression: alcohol, barbiturates, benzodiazepines, and other CNS depressants
- Decreased antihypertensive effects: clonidine, guanadrel, guanethidine

DENTAL CONSIDERATIONS

General:

- Monitor vital signs at every appointment because of cardiovascular side effects.
- Assess salivary flow as a factor in caries, periodontal disease, and candidiasis.
- Patients on chronic drug therapy may rarely have symptoms of blood dyscrasias, which can include infection, bleeding, and poor healing.
- After supine positioning, have patient sit upright for at least 2 min before standing to avoid orthostatic hypotension.
- Use vasoconstrictors with caution, in low doses, and with careful aspiration. Avoid use of gingival retraction cord with epinephrine.
- Place on frequent recall because of oral side effects.

Consultations:

- In a patient with symptoms of blood dyscrasias, request a medical consultation for blood studies and postpone dental treatment until normal values are reestablished.
- Medical consultation may be required to assess disease control.
- Physician should be informed if significant xerostomic side effects occur (e.g., increased caries, sore tongue, problems eating or swallowing, difficulty wearing prosthesis) so that a medication change can be considered.

Teach patient/family:

- Importance of good oral hygiene to prevent soft tissue inflammation

When chronic dry mouth occurs, advise patient:

- To avoid mouth rinses with high alcohol content because of drying effects

• To use daily home fluoride products for anticaries effect
• To use sugarless gum, frequent sips of water, or saliva substitutes

doxycycline hyclate (dental-systemic)

(dox-i-sye'kleen)
Periostat

Drug class.: Tetracycline derivative for nonantibacterial use

Action: Reduces elevated collagenase activity in gingival crevicular fluid of patients with adult periodontitis; no antibacterial effect reported at this dose
Uses: Adjunct to scaling and root planing to promote attachment level gain and reduce pocket depth in adult periodontitis
Dosage and routes:
• *Adult:* PO 20 mg bid as an adjunct to scaling and root planing; may be administered for up to 9 mo; exceeding the recommended dosage may increase risk of side effects, including the development of resistant organisms
Available forms include: Caps 20 mg, tabs 20 mg
Side effects/adverse reactions: NOTE: In a clinical study of 428 patients there was little to no difference in the incidence of side effects reported between this drug and a placebo. See doxycycline hyclate monograph for typical side effects associated with oral administration. Whether these side effects would occur at doses used in this product is unknown.
Contraindications: Hypersensitivity to tetracyclines
Precautions: Children <8 yr, pregnant and nursing mothers, predisposition to oral or vaginal candidiasis, pregnancy category D; not to be used for antimicrobial effect in periodontitis
Pharmacokinetics: No data available
Drug interactions of concern to dentistry:
• No data reported for this dose form; see doxycycline hyclate monograph for drug interactions reported with tetracyclines
DENTAL CONSIDERATIONS
General:
• Examine for oral manifestation of opportunistic infection
• Should be administered at least 1 hr before or 2 hr after morning or evening meals
Teach patient/family:
• To avoid using ingestible sodium bicarbonate products, such as the air polishing system ProphyJet, within 2 hr of drug use

doxycycline hyclate/ doxycycline calcium

(dox-i-sye'kleen)
Doxycycline calcium: Vibramycin
Doxycycline hyclate: Adoxa, Doryx, Doxy100, Doxy200, Monodox, Vibramycin, Vibra-Tabs
♣ Apo-Doxy, Novo-doxylin, Alti-Doxycycline, Doxycin, Doxytec, Nu-Doxycycline, Apo-Doxy Tabs

Drug class.: Tetracycline, broad-spectrum antiinfective

Action: Inhibits protein synthesis and phosphorylation in microorganisms by binding to 30S ribosomal subunits, reversibly binding to 50S ribosomal subunits; bacteriostatic
Uses: Syphilis, *C. trachomatis,*

gonorrhea, lymphogranuloma venereum, uncommon gram-negative/gram-positive organisms, necrotizing ulcerative gingivostomatitis; cutaneous or inhalational anthrax exposure

Dosage and routes:

• *Adult:* PO 100 mg q12h on day 1, then 100 mg/day; IV 200 mg in 1-2 inf on day 1, then 100-200 mg/day

• *Child >8 yr:* PO/IV 4.4 mg/kg/day in divided doses q12h on day 1, then 2.2-4.4 mg/kg/day

Gonorrhea (uncomplicated):

• *Adult:* PO 200 mg, then 100 mg hs and 100 mg bid × 3 days or 300 mg, then 300 mg in 1 hr

• *Disseminated:* 100 mg PO bid × at least 7 days

Chlamydia trachomatis:

• *Adult:* PO 100 mg bid × 7 days

Syphilis:

• *Adult:* PO 300 mg/day in divided doses × 10 days

Anthrax exposure:

• *Adults and children ≥100 lb:* PO 100 mg bid × 60 days (tetracyclines used in this age-group for anthrax only)

• *Child <100 lb:* PO 2.2 mg/kg given bid × 60 days (tetracyclines used in this age-group for anthrax only)

Available forms include: Tabs 50, 100 mg; caps 50, 100 mg; syr 50 mg/ml; powder for inj IV 100, 200 mg; powder for oral susp 25 mg/5 ml in 60 ml; syrup 50 mg/5 ml in 60 ml

Side effects/adverse reactions:

▼ *ORAL:* Candidiasis, tooth discoloration, tongue discoloration, dry mouth

CNS: Fever

CV: Pericarditis

GI: Nausea, abdominal pain, vomiting, diarrhea, ***hepatotoxicity,*** anorexia, enterocolitis, flatulence, abdominal cramps, gastric burning, pancreatitis

HEMA: ***Depression of plasma prothrombin activity, eosinophilia, neutropenia, thrombocytopenia, hemolytic anemia***

EENT: Dysphagia

INTEG: Rash, urticaria, photosensitivity, increased pigmentation, ***exfoliative dermatitis, angioedema,*** pruritus

Contraindications: Hypersensitivity to tetracyclines, children <8 yr, pregnancy category D, isotretinoin

Precautions: Hepatic disease, lactation

Pharmacokinetics:

PO: Peak 1.5-4 hr, half-life 15-22 hr; 25%-93% protein bound; excreted in bile

Drug interactions of concern to dentistry:

• Decreased absorption: $NaHCO_3$, other antacids

• Increased rate of metabolism: barbiturates, carbamazepine, hydantoins

• Decreased effect of penicillins, cephalosporins

• May increase the effectiveness of anticoagulants, methotrexate, digoxin

• Oral contraceptives: advise patient of a potential risk for decreased contraceptive action, to maintain compliance with oral contraceptive use while using antibiotics, and to consider the use of additional nonhormonal contraception

• Contraindicated with isotretinoin (Accutane)

DENTAL CONSIDERATIONS

General:

• Determine why the patient is taking tetracycline.

• Broad-spectrum antibiotics may promote oral or vaginal *Candida* infection.

Consultations:

• Medical consultation may be required to assess disease control.

Teach patient/family:

• That tetracycline can be taken with milk, food; take with a full glass of water

• To take tetracycline doses 1 hr before or 2 hr after air polishing device (ProphyJet), if used

When used for dental infection, advise patient:

• To report sore throat, oral burning sensation, fever, fatigue, any of which could indicate superinfection

• To take at prescribed intervals and complete dosage regimen

• To immediately notify the dentist if signs or symptoms of infection increase

doxycycline hyclate gel

(dox-i-sye'kleen)

Atridox

Drug class.: Tetracycline, antiinfective

Action: Inhibits bacterial protein synthesis by disruption of transfer RNA and messenger RNA

Uses: For adjunctive treatment of chronic adult periodontitis to increase clinical attachment, reduce probing depth, and reduce bleeding on probing

Dosage and routes:

• *Adult:* TOP mix contents of syringes according to detailed instructions, completing 100 cycles; attach blunt cannula to syringe A and fill the pocket; after it becomes firm, the mixture may be packed further into the pocket with a dental instrument

Available forms include: Syringe 50 mg and delivery system syringe (450 mg), blunt cannula; refrigerate

Side effects/adverse reactions:

▼ *ORAL: Gingival discomfort, pain, loss of attachment, toothache, periodontal abscess, exudate, infection, drainage, swelling, thermal tooth sensitivity, extreme mobility, localized allergic reaction*

CNS: Headache

CV: High blood pressure

GI: Diarrhea

GU: PMS

EENT: Skin infection, photosensitivity

MS: Muscle aches, backache

MISC: Common cold

Contraindications: Hypersensitivity

Precautions: Pregnancy category D, children (tooth staining), lactation, photosensitivity, predisposition to candidiasis

Pharmacokinetics: Gingival crevicular fluid levels peak 2 hr, sustained levels up to 18 hr and decline over 7 days; low serum levels not exceeding 0.1 g/ml

Drug interactions of concern to dentistry:

• None specifically identified for this product; unknown whether typical tetracycline interactions occur

DENTAL CONSIDERATIONS

General:

• Examine for oral manifestation of opportunistic infection.

Teach patient/family:

• To be alert to the possibility of secondary oral infection and the need to see dentist immediately if signs of infection occur

• Caution against oral hygiene procedures in treated areas of mouth for 7 days to avoid dislodging product

---

dronabinol

(droe-nab'i-nol)

Marinol

Drug class.: Antiemetic, appetite stimulant

Controlled Substance Schedule III, Canada N

Action: Orally active cannabinoid (*a*D[9]-tetrahydrocannabinol) with varying effects in the CNS; exact mechanism unknown, may be due to inhibition of vomiting control mechanism in medulla oblongata

Uses: Control nausea, vomiting in selected patients receiving emetogenic cancer chemotherapy; stimulate appetite in AIDS-associated anorexia

Dosage and routes:

Chemotherapy prophylaxis for emesis:

• *Adult:* PO 5 mg/m^2 1-3 hr before chemotherapy, then q2-4h for total of 6 doses per day; dose may be increased by 2.5 mg/m^2 if response is not adequate; do not exceed 15 mg/m^2 per dose

Appetite stimulant:

• *Adult:* PO initially 2.5 mg bid, before lunch and supper, or 2.5 mg single dose in PM or hs; max dose 20 mg/day; 5 mg doses may be given if tolerated

Available forms include: Gelcaps 2.5, 5, 10 mg

Side effects/adverse reactions:

▼ *ORAL:* Dry mouth

CNS: Dizziness, drowsiness, poor concentration, ataxia, confusion, paranoid reactions, unsteadiness, restlessness, sleep disturbances, psychotomimetic effects

CV: Palpitation, tachycardia, flushing, orthostatic hypotension

GI: Nausea, vomiting, abdominal pain, diarrhea

EENT: Blurred vision, changes in vision

MS: Asthenia, myalgia

MISC: Abstinence syndrome (hot flashes, sweating, rhinorrhea, loose stools, hiccups, anorexia)

Contraindications: Hypersensitivity: marijuana, sesame oil

Precautions: Pregnancy category C, lactation, children, elderly; cardiac disorders, drug abuse, alcoholism, hypertension, manic or depressive state, schizophrenia

Pharmacokinetics:

PO: 90%-95% absorbed after single dose, only 10%-20% reaches systemic circulation because of first-pass hepatic metabolism and high lipid solubility; protein binding (97%); half-life alpha 4 hr; effects 4-24 hr; fecal elimination

Drug interactions of concern to dentistry:

• Increased CNS depression: alcohol, CNS depressants, tricyclic antidepressants

• Additive hypertension, tachycardia, possible cardiotoxicity: tricyclic antidepressants, amphetamines, other sympathomimetics

• Additive tachycardia, drowsiness: atropine, scopolamine, antihistamines, anticholinergic drugs

DENTAL CONSIDERATIONS

General:

• Monitor vital signs at every appointment because of cardiovascular side effects.

• After supine positioning, have patient sit upright for at least 2 min to avoid orthostatic hypotension.

• Patients taking opioids for acute or chronic pain should be given alternative analgesics for dental pain.

• Assess salivary flow as a factor in caries, periodontal disease, and candidiasis.

• Consider semisupine chair position for patient comfort if GI side effects occur.

Teach patient/family:

When chronic dry mouth occurs, advise patient:

• To avoid mouth rinses with high alcohol content because of drying effects

• To use daily home fluoride products for anticaries effect

• To use sugarless gum, frequent sips of water, or saliva substitutes

---

dutasteride

(doo- tas'teer-ide)

Avodart

Drug class.: Synthetic steroid

Action: Selectively inhibits steroid 5α-reductase enzymes (types 1 and 2), thereby inhibiting the conversion of testosterone to 5α-dihydrotestosterone (DHT).

Uses: Treatment of benign prostate hyperplasia (BPH) in men to improve symptoms, reduce the risk of urinary retention, and reduce the need for BPH-related surgery

Dosage and routes:

• *Adult:* PO 0.5 mg daily with or without food

Available forms include: Caps 0.5 mg

Side effects/adverse reactions:

GU: Impotence, ejaculation disorder

MISC: Decreased libido, gynecomastia

Contraindications: Hypersensitivity to this drug or other 5α-reductase inhibitors, women, and children; women who are pregnant or might be pregnant should not handle capsules, potential risk of fetal abnormality for male fetus

Precautions: Hepatic impairment, men cannot donate blood until at least 6 mo after last dose, drug also found in semen, no data on use in patients <18 yr or in renal impairment, pregnancy category X, nursing mothers (not used in women)

Pharmacokinetics:

PO: Absolute bioavailability ≈60%, peak plasma levels 2-3 hr, highly bound to plasma proteins (99%), extensively metabolized mainly by CYP3A4 isoenzymes; one metabolite (6B-hydroxydutastride), unchanged dutasteride and metabolites excreted in the feces

Drug interactions of concern to dentistry:

• No drug interaction studies have been conducted; however, caution should be observed when used in combination with potent and chronically used CYP3A4 inhibitors (see Appendix I)

• Opioids and anticholinergic drugs may enhance urinary retention; use alternative analgesics (NSAIDs)

DENTAL CONSIDERATIONS

General:

• Determine why patient is taking the drug.

Consultations:

• Medical consultation may be required to assess disease control in the patient.

Teach patient/family:

• Importance of updating health and drug history if physician makes any changes in evaluation/ drug regimens

---

dyclonine hydrochloride

(dye'kloe-neen)

Dyclone

Drug class.: Topically acting local anesthetic (ketone)

Action: Inhibits nerve impulses from sensory nerves, thus producing local anesthesia; nerve impulses are blocked as a result of decreased nerve membrane permeability to sodium influx

Uses: Topical anesthesia of mucous membranes of mouth, pharynx, larynx, trachea, esophagus, and urethra before a variety of procedures; 0.5% solution may be used to block the gag reflex to relieve the pain of oral ulcers or stomatitis secondary to antineoplastic chemotherapy or radiation

Dosage and routes:

• *Adult:* TOP individualized dose depending on disease or patient need; use lowest effective dose; max recommended dose is 30 ml of a 1% solution (300 mg); usual dosage range is 4-20 ml; reduced dosage is recommended for elderly and pediatric patients

Available forms include: Topical solution 0.5%, 1.0% in 30 ml bottles

(NOTE: Astra no longer makes this product.)

Side effects/adverse reactions:

INTEG: Allergic reactions (urticaria, edema, contact dermatitis)

MISC: ***Anaphylaxis***

More severe systemic reactions can be observed if excessive absorption leads to toxic doses

Contraindications: Hypersensitivity

Precautions: Do not inject or apply to nasal or conjunctival mucous membranes, pregnancy category C, lactation, children <12 yr

Pharmacokinetics:

TOP: Rapid onset and relatively short duration of action

DENTAL CONSIDERATIONS

General:

• Low incidence of side effects following topical application.

• Expectorate excess solution when used topically.

• Limit area of application, especially in inflamed or denuded areas.

• Dry mucous membranes in area of application before applying solution.

• Symptoms of systemic toxicity include nervousness, nausea, excitement followed by drowsiness, convulsions, and cardiac and respiratory depression.

• Symptoms may vary because they depend on the amount of drug actually absorbed.

Teach patient/family

• To prevent injury while numbness is present

• To avoid chewing gum or eating after dental treatment

dyphylline

(dye'fi-lin)

Dilor, Dilor-400, Lufyllin, Lufyllin-400

Drug class.: Xanthine derivative

Action: Relaxes smooth muscle of respiratory system by blocking phosphodiesterase, which increases intracellular AMP

Uses: Bronchial asthma, bronchospasm in chronic bronchitis, COPD, emphysema

Dosage and routes:

- *Adult:* PO 200-800 mg q6h; IM 250-500 mg q6h injected slowly; dose limit 15 mg/kg q6h
- *Child >6 yr:* PO 4-7 mg/kg/day in 4 divided doses

Available forms include: Tabs 200, 400 mg; elix 100, 160 mg/15 ml; inj IM 250 mg/ml

Side effects/adverse reactions:

▼ *ORAL:* Bitter taste

CNS: Anxiety, restlessness, insomnia, dizziness, ***convulsions,*** headache, light-headedness, muscle twitching

CV: Palpitation, sinus tachycardia, hypotension, flushing, dysrhythmias

GI: Nausea, vomiting, anorexia, dyspepsia, epigastric pain

RESP: Tachypnea

INTEG: Flushing, urticaria

MISC: ***Albuminuria,*** fever, dehydration, hyperglycemia

Contraindications: Hypersensitivity to xanthines, tachydysrhythmias

Precautions: Elderly, CHF, cor pulmonale, hepatic disease, active peptic ulcer disease, diabetes mellitus, hyperthyroidism, hypertension, children, renal disease, pregnancy category C, glaucoma

Pharmacokinetics:

PO: Peak 1 hr, half-life 2 hr; excreted in urine unchanged

Drug interactions of concern to dentistry:

- Increased action: erythromycin, ciprofloxacin, tetracyclines
- Increased risk of cardiac dysrhythmia: halothane-inhalation anesthesia, CNS stimulants
- Decreased effect: barbiturates, carbamazepine, ketoconazole
- May decrease sedative effects of benzodiazepines

DENTAL CONSIDERATIONS

General:

- Monitor vital signs at every appointment because of cardiovascular and respiratory side effects.
- Consider semisupine chair position for patients with respiratory disease.

econazole nitrate (topical)

(e-kone'a-zole)

Spectazole

✤ Ecostatin Cream

Drug class.: Local antifungal

Action: Interferes with fungal cell membrane, increasing permeability and leading to leaking of cell nutrients

Uses: Tinea pedis, tinea cruris, tinea corporis, tinea versicolor, cutaneous candidiasis

Dosage and routes:

- *Adult and child:* TOP apply to affected area once daily

Cutaneous candidiasis:

- *Adult and child:* TOP apply to affected area bid (AM and PM)

Available forms include: Cream 1% in 15, 30, 85 g

Side effects/adverse reactions:

INTEG: Rash, urticaria, stinging, burning, pruritus

Contraindications: Hypersensitivity

Precautions: Pregnancy category C, lactation

DENTAL CONSIDERATIONS

• None

efalizumab

(e-fa-li-zoo′-mab)

Raptiva

Drug class.: Monoclonal antibody

Action: A humanized IgG 1 kappa monoclonal antibody that binds to human CD 11a; inhibits the binding of leukocyte function antigen-1 (LFA-1) thereby affecting T-lymphocyte activity in inflammation; thus it acts as an immunosuppressive drug

Uses: Treatment of chronic moderate to severe plaque psoriasis in patients (>18 yr) who are candidates for systemic therapy or phototherapy

Doses and routes:

• *Adults and adolescents >18 yr:* SC 0.7 mg/kg in a single dose; then 1 mg/kg weekly; maximum single dose limit 200 mg

Available dose forms: Powder for inj: 150 mg

Side effects/adverse reactions:

CNS: Headache

CV: Peripheral edema

GI: Nausea

HEMA: ***Thrombocytopenia***

INTEG: Acne, worsening of psoriasis

METAB: Increase in alkaline phosphatase, lymphocytosis

MS: Back pain, myalgia

MISC: ***Infections,*** *fever, flu syndrome, chills,* ***malignancies,*** hypersensitivity reactions

Contraindications: Hypersensitivity

Precautions: Increased risk of infections, malignancies, worsening of psoriasis, use in elderly, pregnancy category C, safety and efficacy have not been established in lactation or children

Pharmacokinetics: *SC:* Time to peak levels 1-5 days, other data not established

Drug interactions of concern to dentistry:

• None reported

DENTAL CONSIDERATIONS

General:

• Understand the disease and the patient's need to use this drug.

• Rarely oral lesions and geographic tongue may occur in patients with psoriasis.

efavirenz

(ef-a-vir′enz)

Sustiva

Drug class.: Antiviral (nonnucleoside)

Action: Acts as a reverse transcriptase inhibitor in HIV-1

Uses: For use in HIV-1 infection, only in combination with other HIV-1 antiretroviral agents

Dosage and routes:

• *Adult:* PO 600 mg qd in combination with a protease inhibitor or nucleoside reverse transcriptase inhibitor or both; avoid high-fat meals with dosing

• *Child >3 yr weighing 10-40 kg:* PO:

Weight (kg)	Dose (daily)
10-<15	200 mg
15-<20	250 mg
20-<25	300 mg
25-<32.5	350 mg
32.5-<40	400 mg
>40	600 mg

Available forms include: Caps 50, 100, 200 mg; tab 600 mg

Side effects/adverse reactions:

▼ *ORAL:* Dry mouth, altered taste

CNS: Dizziness, somnolence, insomnia, abnormal dreams, confusion, abnormal thinking, impaired concentration, amnesia, agitation, depersonalization, hallucinations, euphoria

CV: Flushing, palpitation, tachycardia, thrombophlebitis

GI: Nausea, vomiting, diarrhea

RESP: Cough, asthma

EENT: Tinnitus, blurred vision

INTEG: Rash, eczema, urticaria

META: Elevation of AST and ALT enzymes

MS: Arthralgia, myalgia

MISC: Fever, fatigue, alcohol intolerance

Contraindications: Hypersensitivity: concurrent use with midazolam, triazolam, or ergot derivatives

Precautions: Must not be used as a single agent for HIV, avoid pregnancy with use, pregnancy category C, lactation, mental illness, substance abuse, caution with alcohol or psychotropic drugs, driving or other hazardous tasks, monitor cholesterol, hepatic impairment

Pharmacokinetics:

PO: Peak plasma levels 5 hr, avoid high-fat meals, hepatic metabolism by cytochrome P-450 enzymes (CYP3A4, CYP2B6 isoenzymes), excreted in both urine and feces; high plasma protein binding (99%)

Drug interactions of concern to dentistry:

• Contraindicated drugs: midazolam, triazolam (see Appendix I)

• Decreased plasma levels of clarithromycin, carbamazepine, St. John's wort (herb)

• Potential for increased levels with ketoconazole, itraconazole (no studies)

• Increased risk of CNS side effects with CNS depressants

DENTAL CONSIDERATIONS

General:

• Examine for oral manifestation of opportunistic infection.

• Monitor vital signs at every appointment because of cardiovascular and respiratory side effects.

• Consider semisupine chair position for patient comfort because of GI side effects of drug.

• Assess salivary flow as a factor in caries, periodontal disease, and candidiasis.

• Short appointments and a stress reduction protocol may be required for anxious patients.

Consultations:

• Medical consultation may be required to assess disease control.

Teach patient/family:

• To prevent trauma when using oral hygiene aids

• Importance of good oral hygiene to prevent soft tissue inflammation

• To be alert for the possibility of

secondary oral infection and to see dentist immediately if signs of infection occur

When chronic dry mouth occurs, advise patient:

• To avoid mouth rinses with high alcohol content because of drying effects

• To use daily home fluoride products for anticaries effect

• To use sugarless gum, frequent sips of water, or saliva substitutes

eletriptan hydrobromide

(el-e-trip'tan)

Relpax

Drug class.: Serotonin receptor agonist

Action: Serotonin agonist that binds to multiple 5-HT receptors including 5-HT_{1B}, 5-HT_{1D}, and 5-HT_{1F} and others located on intracranial blood vessels

Uses: Treatment of acute migraine with or without aura in adults

Dosage and routes:

• *Adult:* PO individualize dose; starting dose is 20 or 40 mg; second dose may be given if required no sooner than 2 hr after the initial dose; maximum single dose 40 mg; maximum daily dose 80 mg

Available forms include: Tabs 20, 40 mg

Side effects/adverse reactions:

▼ *ORAL: Dry mouth,* facial edema

CNS: Asthenia, dizziness, somnolence, headache, anorexia, paresthesia

CV: Flushing, ***risk of severe cardiac events,*** chest pain, palpitation, peripheral edema

GI: Nausea, abdominal discomfort, dyspepsia, peripheral edema, palpitation, diarrhea

HEMA: Anemia, lymphadenopathy, leukopenia (all rare)

EENT: Vertigo, pharyngitis

INTEG: Sweating

META: ↑ creatine phosphokinase

MS: Back pain, arthralgia, bone pain, myalgia

MISC: Chills

Contraindications: Hypersensitivity, various types of ischemic heart disease (angina pectoris, hypertension, MI, or CAD), cerebrovascular syndromes, peripheral vascular disease, ischemic bowel disease, uncontrolled hypertension; other 5-HT_1 agonists, ergotamine or ergot-type medications, severe hepatic impairment, hemiplegic or basilar migraine

Precautions: Do not use within 72 hr of treatment with strong CYP3A4 enzyme inhibitors, pregnancy category C, caution in lactation, safety and use in children <18 yr has not been established

Pharmacokinetics:

PO: Absolute bioavailability 50%, peak plasma levels ≈1.5 hr, plasma protein binding 85%, active metabolite is an *N*-demethylated product, metabolized mainly by CYP3A4 isoenzymes, renal excretion

Drug interactions of concern to dentistry:

• Avoid use of strong CYP3A4 drugs concurrently or within 72 hr of use of eletriptan: ketoconazole, itraconazole, erythromycin, clarithromycin, and others (see Appendix I)

DENTAL CONSIDERATIONS

General:

• This is an acute-use drug; it is

doubtful that patients will seek dental treatment during acute migraine attacks.

• Be aware of the patient's disease, its severity, and its frequency, when known.

• Monitor vital signs at every appointment because of cardiovascular side effects.

• Assess salivary flow as a factor in caries, periodontal disease, and candidiasis.

• Consider semisupine chair position for patient comfort if GI side effects occur.

Consultations:

• If treating chronic orofacial pain, consult with patient's physician.

Teach patient/family:

• That oral symptoms will disappear when drug is discontinued

emedastine difumarate (optic)

(em-e-das'teen)

Emadine

Drug class.: Ophthalmic antihistamine

Action: Selective H_1-receptor antagonist

Uses: Temporary relief of signs and symptoms of allergic conjunctivitis

Dosage and routes:

• *Adult:* Ophth 1 drop in affected eye up to qid

Available forms include: Ophth sol 0.05% in 5 ml

Side effects/adverse reactions:

▼ *ORAL:* Bad taste

CNS: Headache, abnormal dreams

EENT: Blurred vision, burning, stinging, corneal staining, dry eyes, rhinitis, sinusitis, tearing

INTEG: Dermatitis, pruritus

MS: Asthenia

Contraindications: Hypersensitivity

Precautions: Avoid wearing contact lens if eye is red, wait at least 10 min after application to insert contact lens, pregnancy category B, lactation, no data for use in children <3 yr

Pharmacokinetics:

TOP: Systemic absorption below level for assay; any absorbed drug is metabolized and excreted in urine

Drug interactions of concern to dentistry:

• None reported

DENTAL CONSIDERATIONS

General:

• Protect patient's eyes from accidental spatter during dental treatment.

emtricitabine

(em-trye-sye' ta-been)

Emtriva

Drug class.: Antiviral, nucleoside reverse transcriptase inhibitor

Action: Converted to emtricitabine 5-triphosphate by cellular enzymes and inhibits the action of HIV-1 reverse transcriptase thereby terminating DNA chain formation

Uses: Treatment of HIV-1 infection in adults; used in combination with other antiretroviral medications

Dosage and routes:

• *Adult and adolescents 18 yr and older:* PO 200 mg/day

Available forms include: Caps 200 mg

Side effects/adverse reactions:

CNS: Headache, asthenia, dizziness, sleep disorders

GI: Diarrhea, nausea, ***hepatotoxicity,*** abdominal pain, vomiting
RESP: Increased cough
HEMA: ↑ neutrophils
EENT: Rhinitis
INTEG: Rash, discoloration of palms or soles
META: ***Lactic acidosis,*** elevated AST, ALT, creatine kinase, triglycerides
MS: Arthralgia, myalgia
MISC: Change in body fat distribution

Contraindications: Hypersensitivity

Precautions: Possible risk of lactic acidosis, severe hepatomegaly with steatosis, use not established in HIV/HBV infections, renal impairment (dose reduction required), pregnancy category B, avoid nursing when taking this drug, safety and efficacy in pediatric patients have not been established

Pharmacokinetics:
PO: Absolute bioavailability 95%, peak plasma levels 1-2 hr, plasma protein binding <4%, half-life 10 hr, excreted mainly in urine (86%) and to lesser extent in feces (14%)

Drug interactions of concern to dentistry:
• None reported

DENTAL CONSIDERATIONS

General:
• Examine for oral manifestation of opportunistic infection.
• Consider semisupine chair position for patient comfort if GI side effects occur.
• Patient history should include all medications and herbal or nonherbal remedies taken by the patient.

Consultations:
• Medical consultation may be required to assess disease control and patient's ability to tolerate stress.

Teach patient/family:
• Importance of good oral hygiene to prevent soft tissue inflammation/infection
• To prevent trauma when using oral hygiene aids
• Importance of updating health and drug history, reporting changes in health status, drug regimen changes, or disease/treatment status

---

enalapril maleate

(e-nal'a-pril)
Vasotec, Vasotec IV

Drug class.: Angiotensin-converting enzyme (ACE) inhibitor

Action: Selectively suppresses renin-angiotensin-aldosterone system; inhibits ACE; prevents conversion of angiotensin I to angiotensin II, leading to dilation of arterial and venous vessels

Uses: Hypertension, heart failure adjunct, asymptomatic left ventricular dysfunction

Dosage and routes:
• *Adult:* PO 5 mg/day; may increase or decrease to desired response range 10-40 mg/day; lower initial dose with a diuretic

Hypertension:
• *Adult:* IV 1.25 mg q6h over 5 min

Patients on diuretics:
• *Adult:* IV 0.625 over 5 min; may give additional doses of 1.25 mg q6h

Renal impairment:
• *Adult:* 1.25 mg q6h with CrCl <3 mg/dl or 0.625 mg if CrCl >3 mg/dl

Available forms include: Tabs 2.5, 5, 10, 20 mg; inj 1.25 mg/ml

Side effects/adverse reactions:

▼ *ORAL:* Loss of taste, oral ulceration (Stevens-Johnson syndrome, rare), dry mouth, angioedema (lips, tongue, mucous membranes), lichenoid drug reaction

CNS: Insomnia, dizziness, paresthesia, headache, fatigue, anxiety

CV: Hypotension, chest pain, tachycardia, dysrhythmias

GI: Nausea, vomiting, colitis, cramps, diarrhea, constipation, pancreatitis, flatulence

RESP: Dyspnea, cough, rales, angioedema

HEMA: ***Agranulocytosis, neutropenia***

GU: ***Proteinuria, renal failure,*** increased frequency of polyurea or oliguria

INTEG: Rash, purpura, alopecia

META: Hyperkalemia

Contraindications: Pregnancy category D; can cause serious reactions in second and third trimester; lactation

Precautions: Renal disease, hyperkalemia

Pharmacokinetics:

PO: Peak 1 hr, half-life 11 hr; metabolized by liver to active metabolite; excreted in urine

IV: Onset 5-15 min, peak up to 4 hr

Drug interactions of concern to dentistry:

• Increased hypotension: alcohol, phenothiazines

• Decreased hypotensive effects: indomethacin and possibly other NSAIDs, sympathomimetics

• Suspected reduction in the antihypertensive and vasodilator effects by salicylates; monitor blood pressure if used concurrently

DENTAL CONSIDERATIONS

General:

• Monitor vital signs at every appointment because of cardiovascular side effects.

• After supine positioning, have patient sit upright for at least 2 min before standing to avoid orthostatic hypotension.

• Patients on chronic drug therapy may rarely have symptoms of blood dyscrasias, which can include infection, bleeding, and poor healing.

• Assess salivary flow as a factor in caries, periodontal disease, and candidiasis.

• Limit use of sodium-containing products such as saline IV fluids for those patients with a dietary salt restriction.

• Use vasoconstrictors with caution, in low doses, and with careful aspiration.

• Stress from dental procedures may compromise cardiovascular function; determine patient risk.

• Short appointments and a stress reduction protocol may be required for anxious patients.

Consultations:

• Medical consultation may be required to assess patient's ability to tolerate stress.

• In a patient with symptoms of blood dyscrasias, request a medical consultation for blood studies and postpone dental treatment until normal values are reestablished.

• Take precautions if dental surgery is anticipated and sedation or general anesthesia is required; risk of hypotensive episode.

Teach patient/family:

• Importance of good oral hygiene to prevent soft tissue inflammation

When chronic dry mouth occurs, advise patient:

• To avoid mouth rinses with high alcohol content because of drying effects

• To use daily home fluoride products for anticaries effect

• To use sugarless gum, frequent sips of water, or saliva substitutes

enfuvirtide

(en'floo-veer-tide)

Fuzeon

Drug class.: Antiviral

Action: Inhibits fusion of viral and cellular membranes interfering with viral (HIV-1) entry into cells

Uses: Used in combination with other antiretroviral agents for the treatment of HIV-1 infection in treatment-experienced patients with HIV-1 replication despite ongoing antiretroviral therapy

Dosage and routes:

• *Adult:* SC 90 mg bid in the upper arm, anterior thigh, or abdomen

• *Child:* SC 2 mg/kg (maximum dose 90 mg) bid in the upper arm, anterior thigh, or abdomen

Available forms include: Lyophilized powder 108 mg in a single-use vial in cartons of 60 vials with water for injection, syringes, and alcohol wipes

Side effects/adverse reactions:

▼ *ORAL:* Taste disturbance

CNS: Peripheral neuropathy, ***Guillain-Barré syndrome,*** asthenia, anorexia

CV: Fatigue, insomnia, depression, anxiety

GI: Diarrhea, nausea, constipation, pancreatitis

RESP: Influenza, pneumonia

HEMA: Lymphadenopathy, eosinophilia

GU: Glomerulonephritis

EENT: Sinusitis, conjunctivitis

INTEG: Local injection site reactions, erythema, induration, nodules or cysts, pruritus, ecchymosis, abscess, cellulitis, skin papilloma

META: Weight variation, hyperglycemia, elevated liver enzymes (ALT, AST, lipase, GGT), ↑ creatine phosphokinase, ↑ triglycerides

MS: Myalgia

MISC: Hypersensitivity reactions, herpes simplex, flulike symptoms

Contraindications: Hypersensitivity

Precautions: Patients should be instructed in recognizing local injection site reactions and trained in aseptic technique, pregnancy category B, HIV-infected mothers must not nurse, use in children under 6 yr has not been established

Pharmacokinetics: *SC:* Absolute bioavailability 84%, plasma protein binding 92%, elimination pathways have not been studied, effects of hepatic or renal impairment have not been studied

Drug interactions of concern to dentistry:

• None reported

DENTAL CONSIDERATIONS

General:

• Patients taking this drug will be taking other antiviral drugs that may interact with some dental drugs. Be sure to take a complete drug history.

• Patients on chronic drug therapy may rarely have symptoms of blood dyscrasias, which can include infection, bleeding, and poor healing.

• Examine for oral manifestation of opportunistic infection.

Consultations:

• Medical consultation may be required to assess disease control in the patient.

• In a patient with symptoms of blood dyscrasias, request a medical consultation for blood studies and postpone treatment until normal values are reestablished.

Teach patient/family:

• Importance of good oral hygiene to prevent soft tissue inflammation

• To prevent trauma when using oral hygiene aids

• Importance of updating health and drug history if physician makes any changes in evaluation/ drug regimens

---

enoxaparin sodium

(ee-nox-a-pa′rin)

Lovenox

Drug class.: Heparin-type anticoagulant

Action: Low-molecular-weight heparin having antithrombotic actions with higher anti–factor X_a activity compared with anti–factor II_a

Uses: Prevention and treatment of deep vein thrombosis following hip or knee replacement surgery; also used in abdominal and gynecologic surgery; with aspirin in the prevention of ischemic complications of unstable angina and non–Q-wave MI; in combination with warfarin for deep vein thrombosis, with or without pulmonary embolism

Dosage and routes:

• *Adult:* SC 30 mg bid with first dose given 12-24 hr after surgery; or SC 40 mg qd with first dose given 2 hr before surgery

Available forms include: Prefilled syringes 30, 40, 60, 80, 90, 100, 120, 150 mg

Side effects/adverse reactions:

CNS: Confusion

GI: Nausea

HEMA: Bleeding after surgery, ***thrombocytopenia,*** hemorrhage, anemia

INTEG: Edema, hematoma, erythema

MISC: Local pain, irritation, fever

Contraindications: Hypersensitivity, active major bleeding, thrombocytopenia, IM administration

Precautions: Hemorrhage, thrombocytopenia, renal impairment, elderly, pregnancy category B, lactation, children, requires monitoring, GI bleeding

Pharmacokinetics: *SC INJ ONLY:* Maximum anti–factor X_a and antithrombin effect 3-5 hr, activity lasts up to 12 hr; renal excretion

Drug interactions of concern to dentistry:

• Avoid concurrent use of aspirin, NSAIDs, dipyridamole, sulfinpyrazone

• Use with caution in patients taking olanzapine

DENTAL CONSIDERATIONS

General:

• Determine why patient is taking the drug.

• Product may be used in outpatient therapy. Delay elective dental treatment until patient completes enoxaparin therapy.

• Consider local hemostasis measures to prevent excessive bleeding if dental treatment must be performed.

• Avoid products that affect platelet function, such as aspirin and NSAIDs.
• Antibiotic prophylaxis before dental treatment may be required for joint prosthesis. See 2003 ADA guidelines.

Consultations:
• Medical consultation should include routine blood counts, including platelet counts and bleeding time.

Teach patient/family:
• Importance of good oral hygiene to prevent soft tissue inflammation
• Caution to prevent trauma when using oral hygiene aids
• To report oral lesions, soreness, or bleeding to dentist

---

entacapone

(en-tak'a-pone)

Comtan

Drug class.: Antiparkinsonian

Action: Inhibits catechol-*O*-methyltransferase (COMT), decreases peripheral conversion of levodopa to 3-*O*-methyldopa

Uses: Adjunct to levodopa/carbidopa in the treatment of Parkinson's disease, not used alone

Dosage and routes:
• *Adult:* PO 200 mg with each levodopa/carbidopa dose not to exceed 8 times daily; adjust dose downward as symptoms improve

Available forms include: Tabs 200 mg

Side effects/adverse reactions:

▼ *ORAL:* Taste alteration, dry mouth (1%)

CNS: Dyskinesia, hyperkinesia, psychiatric reactions, hallucinations, aggravation of Parkinson's symptoms, hypokinesia, dizziness, anxiety

CV: Orthostatic hypotension, syncope

GI: Nausea, diarrhea, abdominal pain

RESP: Dyspnea

HEMA: Purpura

GU: Discolored urine (brown-orange)

INTEG: Sweating

META: May decrease serum iron levels

MS: ***Rhabdomyolysis,*** back pain, fatigue

Contraindications: Hypersensitivity, nonselective MAOIs

Precautions: Enhanced orthostatic hypotension with levodopa/carbidopa, hepatic impairment, caution in driving, pregnancy category C, lactation, children

Pharmacokinetics:
PO: Rapid absorption, bioavailability 35%, highly plasma protein bound (98%), hepatic metabolism, metabolites excreted mostly (90%) in feces

Drug interactions of concern to dentistry:
• Increased heart rate, arrhythmias, hypertension: with epinephrine, norepinephrine, levonordefrin, or other sympathomimetics metabolized by COMT
• Possible decrease in urinary excretion: erythromycin

DENTAL CONSIDERATIONS

General:
• Monitor vital signs at every appointment because of cardiovascular side effects.
• Short appointments and a stress reduction protocol may be required for anxious patients.

• Consider semisupine chair position for patient comfort if GI side effects occur.
• Use vasoconstrictor with caution, in low doses, and with careful aspiration. Avoid using gingival retraction cord containing epinephrine.
• Assess for presence of extrapyramidal motor symptoms, such as tardive dyskinesia and akathisia. Extrapyramidal motor activity may complicate dental treatment.
• After supine positioning, have patient sit upright for at least 2 min to avoid orthostatic hypotension.
• Assess salivary flow as a factor in caries, periodontal disease, and candidiasis.

Consultations:
• Medical consultation may be required to assess disease control and patient's ability to tolerate stress.

Teach patient/family:
• Use of electric toothbrush if patient has difficulty holding conventional devices
• Importance of updating health and drug history if physician makes any changes in evaluation or drug regimens

When chronic dry mouth occurs, advise patient:
• To avoid mouth rinses with high alcohol content because of drying effects
• To use daily home fluoride products for anticaries effect
• To use sugarless gum, frequent sips of water, or saliva substitutes

ephedrine sulfate

(e-fed'rin)
generic

Drug class.: Adrenergic, mixed direct and indirect effects

Action: Causes increased contractility and heart rate by acting on β-receptors in the heart; also acts on α-receptors, causing vasoconstriction in blood vessels

Uses: Shock, increased perfusion, hypotension, bronchodilation, nasal decongestant

Dosage and routes:
• *Adult:* IM/SC 25-50 mg, not to exceed 150 mg/24 hr; IV 10-25 mg, not to exceed 150 mg/24 hr
• *Child:* SC/IV 3 mg/kg/day in divided doses q4-6h

Bronchodilation:
• *Adults and child >12 yr:* PO 12.5-50 mg bid-qid, not to exceed 150 mg/24 hr

Acute hypotensive events:
• *Adult:* SC, IM, or slow IV 25-50 mg; may also use slow IV push 5-25 mg
• *Child:* SC, IM 16.7 mg/m^2 q4-6h

Available forms include: Inj IM/SC/IV 50 mg/ml; caps 25 mg

Side effects/adverse reactions:
▼ *ORAL:* Dry mouth
CNS: Tremors, anxiety, ***convulsions, CNS depression,*** insomnia, headache, dizziness, confusion, hallucinations
CV: ***Dysrhythmias,*** palpitation, tachycardia, hypertension, chest pain
GI: Anorexia, nausea, vomiting
GU: Dysuria, urinary retention

Contraindications: Hypersensitivity to sympathomimetics, narrow-angle glaucoma

Precautions: Pregnancy category C, cardiac disorders, hyperthyroidism, diabetes mellitus, prostatic hypertrophy

Pharmacokinetics:

PO: Onset 15-60 min, duration 2-4 hr

IV: Onset 5 min, duration 2 hr

Metabolized in liver; excreted in urine (unchanged); crosses blood-brain barrier, placenta, excreted in breast milk

Drug interactions of concern to dentistry:

- Decreased pressor effect: haloperidol, phenothiazines, thioxanthenes
- Dysrhythmia: halogenated general anesthetics

DENTAL CONSIDERATIONS

General:

- Monitor vital signs at every appointment because of cardiovascular side effects.
- Assess salivary flow as a factor in caries, periodontal disease, and candidiasis.
- Consider semisupine chair position for patients with respiratory disease.
- Consider short appointments and a stress reduction protocol for anxious patients.

Consultations:

- Medical consultation may be required to assess disease control and patient's tolerance for stress.

Teach patient/family:

When chronic dry mouth occurs, advise patient:

- To avoid mouth rinses with high alcohol content because of drying effects
- To use daily home fluoride products for anticaries effect
- To use sugarless gum, frequent sips of water, or saliva substitutes

epinastine HCl

(ep-i-nas'teen)

Elestat

Drug class.: Ophthalmic antihistamine

Action: Selective H_1-receptor antagonist, inhibits histamine release from mast cells

Uses: Prevention of itching associated with allergic conjunctivitis

Dosage and routes:

- *Adult:* TOP 1 drop in each eye bid

Available forms include: Sol 0.05% in 5, 10 ml

Side effects/adverse reactions:

CNS: Headache

RESP: URI, cough

EENT: Burning sensation in eye, rhinitis, pharyngitis

INTEG: Pruritus, hyperemia

MISC: Folliculosis, coldlike symptoms

Contraindications: Hypersensitivity

Precautions: Do not wear contact lens if the eye is red, otherwise contact may be placed in eye 10 min after dosing; pregnancy category C, use in nursing and in children <3 yr has not been established

Pharmacokinetics:

TOP: Some absorption, low plasma levels, plasma protein binding 64%, excreted via renal tubular secretion; mostly in the urine; some fecal excretion.

Drug interactions of concern to dentistry:

- None reported

DENTAL CONSIDERATIONS

General:

- Protect patient's eyes from accidental spatter during dental treatment.

• Avoid dental light in patient's eyes; offer dark glasses for patient comfort.

epinephrine/ epinephrine bitartrate/ epinephrine HCl

(ep-i-nef'rin)

Epinephrine HCl inj: *Adrenalin Chloride, EpiPen Auto-Injector, EpiPen Jr.*

♣ *Epinephrine HCl inh:* Adrenalin, Primatine Mist

Racemic epinephrine: Asthma Nefrin, MicroNefrin, Nephron S-2

♣ Vaponefrin

Epinephrine HCl ophthalmic: Epiferin, Glaucon

Epinephrine borate ophthalmic: Epinal

Epinephrine HCl nasal sol: Adrenalin

Drug class.: Adrenergic agonist, catecholamine

Action: Acts on both α- and β-adrenergic receptors; magnitude of response depends on specific receptors activated, tissue innervated, and the dose and rate of administration; effects on the cardiovascular system include peripheral vasoconstriction, stimulation of cardiac muscle, and, in the pulmonary system, relaxation of bronchial smooth muscles. Epinephrine elevates systemic blood pressure, increases the strength and rate of cardiac contraction; action on β_2-adrenergic receptors reduces bronchial congestion by relaxing bronchial smooth muscle mediated through cyclic AMP; application to the eye results in mydriasis and reduction in intraocular pressure.

Uses: Acute asthmatic attacks, hemostasis, bronchospasm, anaphylaxis, allergic reactions, cardiac arrest, vasopressor, open-angle glaucoma, nasal congestion

Dosage and routes:

• *Adult:* Bronchial asthma, allergic reactions, angioedema, urticaria, serum sickness, anaphylaxis (give SC: 0.1-0.25 mg; if given IM do not administer in buttocks)

Cardiopulmonary resuscitation: applicable when other CPR measures have failed; IV or intracardially administer 1-10 ml of a 1:10,000 solution (use diluted solutions or dilute more concentrated solutions) and support with CPR measures

• *Child:* Bronchial asthma and allergic reactions–usual dose is 0.01 mg/kg or 0.3 mg/m^2 to a maximum of 0.5 mg

Asthma:

• *Adult and child:* INH 1-2 puffs of 1:100 or 2.25% racemic q15min

Hemostasis:

• *Adult:* TOP 1:50,000-1:1000 applied as needed to stop bleeding

Glaucoma:

• *Adult:* OPHTH: 1 drop in affected eye(s) once or twice daily

Nasal congestion:

• *Adult and child >6 yr:* TOP apply locally prn (avoid excessive use)

Available forms include: Aerosol 0.16, 0.2, 0.25 mg/spray; inj IM/IV/SC 1:1000 (1 mg/ml), inj 1:2000 (0.5 mg/ml), 1:10.000 (0.1 mg/ml); sol for nebuliz 1:100, 1.25% 2.25% (base); ophth sol 0.5%, 1%, 2%; nasal sol 1 mg/ml, 10 mg/ml

Side effects/adverse reactions:

CNS: Tremors, anxiety, ***cerebral hemorrhage,*** insomnia, headache, dizziness, confusion, hallucinations

CV: ***Dysrhythmias,*** palpitations, tachycardia, hypertension, increased T wave

GI: Anorexia, nausea, vomiting

RESP: Dyspnea

GU: Urinary retention

Contraindications: Hypersensitivity to sympathomimetics, narrow-angle glaucoma

Precautions: Pregnancy category C, cardiac disorders, hyperthyroidism, diabetes mellitus, prostatic hypertrophy

Pharmacokinetics: *SC:* Onset 3-5 min, duration 20 min *PO/ INH:* Onset 1 min

Drug interactions of concern to dentistry:

• Hypotension, tachycardia: haloperidol, loxapine, phenothiazines, thioxanthenes

• Ventricular dysrhythmia: hydrocarbon-inhalation anesthetics, CNS stimulants, tricyclic antidepressants

• With larger doses of epinephrine risk of hypertension followed by bradycardia with β-adrenergic antagonists

DENTAL CONSIDERATIONS

General:

• Monitor vital signs at every appointment because of cardiovascular side effects.

• Assess salivary flow as a factor in caries, periodontal disease, and candidiasis.

• Consider semisupine chair position for patients with respiratory disease.

• Acute asthmatic episodes may be precipitated in the dental office. Sympathomimetic inhalants should be available for emergency use; a stress reduction protocol may be required.

---

eplerenone

(e-pler'en-one)

Inspra

Drug class.: Antihypertensive, aldosterone antagonist

Action: Acts as a selective aldosterone receptor antagonist; thereby inhibiting aldosterone's effects on blood pressure and sodium reabsorption; chemically related to spironolactone

Uses: Treatment of hypertension as a single drug or in combination with other antihypertensive drugs; improved survival of CHF patients following an acute heart attack

Dosage and routes:

• *Adult:* PO starting dose 50 mg/day; for patients with an inadequate response after a trial period dose can be increased to 50 mg bid

Available forms include: Tabs 25, 50, 100 mg

Side effects/adverse reactions:

CNS: Headache, dizziness, fatigue

CV: Angina pectoris, ***myocardial infarction***

GI: Diarrhea, abdominal pain

RESP: Cough

GU: Albuminuria, abnormal vaginal bleeding

META: Increased GGT, hypercholesterolemia, hypertriglyceridemia, hyperkalemia, increased ALT, BUN, creatinine, uric acid

MISC: Influenza-like symptoms, gynecomastia

Contraindications: Hypersensitivity, serum potassium >5.5 meq/L, type 2 diabetes with microalbuminuria, serum creatinine >2.0 mg/dl in males or >1.8 mg/dl in females, creatinine clearance <50 ml/min; potassium supplements, potassium-sparing diuretics, ketoconazole, itraconazole.

Precautions: Hyperkalemia, monitor serum potassium periodically, impaired hepatic or renal function, ACE inhibitors, angiotensin II antagonists, pregnancy category B, lactation, use in children has not been established

Pharmacokinetics:

PO: Bioavailability unknown, peak plasma levels 1.5 hr, plasma protein binding 50%, metabolized by CYP450 3A4 isoenzymes, no active metabolites, excreted in urine (67%) and feces (32%)

Drug interactions of concern to dentistry:

• See contraindications; use with caution in patients taking strong inhibitors of CYP 3A4 isoenzymes (erythromycin) (see Appendix I)

• Monitor blood pressure if NSAIDs are required

DENTAL CONSIDERATIONS

General:

• Monitor vital signs at every appointment because of cardiovascular side effects.

• Short appointments and a stress reduction protocol may be required for anxious patients.

• Take precautions if dental surgery is anticipated and general anesthesia is required.

Consultations:

• Medical consultation may be required to assess disease control and patient's ability to tolerate stress.

• Consultation with physician may be needed if sedation or general anesthesia is required.

Teach patient/family:

• Importance of updating health and drug history if physician makes any changes in evaluation/drug regimens

---

epoetin alfa (erythropoietin)

(e-poe'e-tin)

Epogen, Procrit

Drug class.: Hematinic, antianemic

Action: Stimulates production of red blood cells by action on erythroid progenitor cells and peripheral hemopoietic progenitor cells

Uses: Anemia of chronic renal failure, end-stage renal disease, anemia in zidovudine-treated HIV patients, anemia in cancer patients on chemotherapy, reduction of allogenic blood transfusion in surgery patients

Dosage and routes:

Chronic renal failure:

• *Adult:* IV or SC initial dose 50-100 U/kg 3 ×/wk, maintenance dose individually adjusted

• *Pediatric:* IV or SC 50 U/kg 3 ×/wk, maintenance dose individually adjusted

Zidovudine-treated HIV infection (erythropoietin levels <500 mu/ml):

• *Adult:* IV or SC 100 U/kg 3 times weekly × 8 wk

Dialysis (CRF):

• *Adult:* IV or SC initial dose 50 U/kg 3 ×/wk, maintenance dose individually adjusted

Chemotherapy for malignancy:

• *Adult:* IV or SC initial dose 150 U/kg 3 ×/wk, adjust dose to patient response

• *Child 6 mo-18 yr:* IV or SC dose range 25-300 U/kg, 3-7 ×/wk

Surgery:

• *Adult:* SC 300 U/kg for 10 days before surgery, on the day of surgery, and 4 days after surgery

Available forms include: Vials 2000, 3000, 4000, 10,000, 20,000, 40,000 U/ml

Side effects/adverse reactions:

CNS: Headache, fatigue, asthenia, dizziness, seizure (CRF patient)

CV: Hypertension, edema, chest pain, tachycardia

GI: Nausea, diarrhea, vomiting, constipation

RESP: Shortness of breath, URI, cough

HEMA: Thrombotic events (A-V shunt)

EENT: Pharyngitis

INTEG: Injection site reaction, rash, urticaria

META: Hyperkalemia

MS: Arthralgias

MISC: Allergic reactions, immunogenicity, flulike symptoms

Contraindications: Hypersensitivity to mammalian cell-derived products, human albumin, uncontrolled hypertension

Precautions: Contains benzyl alcohol (risk of complications in premature infants), increased thrombosis risk in CHF, ischemic heart disease, coronary artery bypass, pure red cell aplasia, monitor and control BP, seizures in CRF, thrombosis during hemodialysis, porphyria, pregnancy category C, lactation, safety and efficacy in children <1 mo have not been established, monitor renal function, monitor hematocrit

Pharmacokinetics: *SC:* Peak levels 5-24 hr, bioavailability 22%-31%, IV use 20%, half-life (4-13 hr)

Drug interactions of concern to dentistry:

• None reported

DENTAL CONSIDERATIONS

General:

• Patient's disease, treatment history, and use of other drugs will affect patient evaluation and management.

• Determine why patient is taking the drug.

• Monitor vital signs at every appointment because of cardiovascular and respiratory side effects.

• Take precautions if dental surgery is anticipated and general anesthesia is required.

• Patient history should include all medications and herbal or nonherbal remedies taken by the patient.

• Consider semisupine chair position for patient comfort if GI side effects occur.

• Place on frequent recall because of oral side effects, depending on chemotherapy regimen or HIV immunologic status.

Consultations:

• Medical consultation should include hematocrit and routine blood counts, including platelet counts and bleeding time.

• Consultation with physician may be needed if sedation or general anesthesia is required.

• Medical consultation may be required to assess disease control and patient's ability to tolerate stress.

Teach patient/family:

• Importance of good oral hygiene to prevent soft tissue inflammation/infection

eprosartan mesylate

(ep-roe-sar'tan)

Teveten

Drug class.: Antihypertensive, angiotensin II receptor (AT_1) antagonist

Action: A selective antagonist for angiotensin II receptor sites (AT_1); antagonizes the vasoconstrictor- and aldosterone-secreting effects of angiotensin

Uses: Hypertension as a single drug or in combination with other antihypertensive drugs

Dosage and route:

• *Adult:* PO initial 600 mg qd, can also be given bid in total daily doses ranging from 400-800 mg

Available forms include: Tabs 400, 600 mg

Side effects/adverse reactions:

▼ *ORAL:* ***Angioedema,*** facial edema, dry mouth

CNS: Fatigue, depression, headache, dizziness, anxiety, nervousness

CV: Chest pain, peripheral edema, angina pectoris, arrhythmias, postural hypotension

GI: Abdominal pain, diarrhea, constipation, nausea, vomiting

RESP: URI, coughing, bronchitis, dyspnea, asthma

HEMA: Anemia, purpura

GU: UTI

EENT: Rhinitis, pharyngitis, sinusitis, epistaxis

INTEG: Eczema, rash

META: Hypertriglyceridemia, ↑ AST, ↑ ALT, ↑ CPK

MS: Arthralgia, myalgia, leg cramps

MISC: Viral infection, herpes simplex

Contraindications: Hypersensitivity, pregnancy (second and third trimesters)

Precautions: Renal impairment maximum daily dose is 600 mg, risk of renal impairment, pregnancy category C (first trimester) and pregnancy category D (second and third trimesters); safety and efficacy in lactation and patients <18 yr have not been established

Pharmacokinetics:

PO: Absolute bioavailability 13%, peak plasma levels 1-2 hr, plasma protein binding 98%, little metabolism, excreted mostly unchanged by biliary and renal routes

Drug interactions of concern to dentistry:

• None reported

DENTAL CONSIDERATIONS

General:

• Monitor vital signs at every appointment because of cardiovascular side effects.

• Stress from dental procedures may compromise cardiovascular function; determine patient risk.

• Limit use of sodium-containing products such as saline IV fluids for those patients with a dietary salt restriction.

• Short appointments and a stress reduction protocol may be required for anxious patients.

• Use precaution if sedation or general anesthesia is required; risk of hypotensive episode.

• Assess salivary flow as a factor in caries, periodontal disease, and candidiasis.

• After supine positioning, have

patient sit upright for at least 2 min before standing to avoid orthostatic hypotension.

Consultations:

• Medical consultation may be required to assess disease control and patient's ability to tolerate stress.

Teach patient/family:

• Importance of updating health and drug history if physician makes any changes in evaluation or drug regimens

When chronic dry mouth occurs, advise patient:

• To avoid mouth rinses with high alcohol content because of drying effects

• To use daily home fluoride products for anticaries effect

• To use sugarless gum, frequent sips of water, or saliva substitutes

ergoloid mesylate

(er'goe-loid) (mess'i-late)

Gerimal, Hydergine, Hydergine LC

Drug class.: Ergot alkaloids

Action: Actual mechanism unknown, may increase cerebral metabolism and blood flow

Uses: Senile dementia, Alzheimer's dementia, multiinfarct dementia, primary progressive dementia

Dosage and routes:

• *Adult:* PO/SL 1 mg tid; may increase to 4.5-12 mg/day

Available forms include: Tabs SL 0.5, 1 mg; tabs 0.5, 1 mg; caps 1 mg; liq 1 mg/ml

Side effects/adverse reactions:

▼ *ORAL:* Sublingual irritation (SL tablet)

CNS: Dizziness, syncope, headache, anorexia

CV: Bradycardia, orthostatic hypotension

GI: Nausea, vomiting

EENT: Blurred vision, nasal stuffiness

INTEG: Skin rash, flushing

Contraindications: Hypersensitivity to ergot preparations; psychosis

Precautions: Acute intermittent porphyria, pregnancy category C

Pharmacokinetics:

PO: Peak 1 hr, half-life 3.5 hr; metabolized in liver; excreted as metabolites in feces; crosses blood-brain barrier

DENTAL CONSIDERATIONS

General:

• Monitor vital signs at every appointment because of cardiovascular side effects.

• After supine positioning, have patient sit upright for at least 2 min before standing to avoid orthostatic hypotension.

• Consider semisupine chair position for patient comfort because of GI effects of drug.

Teach patient/family:

• Use of electric toothbrush if patient is unable to carry out oral hygiene procedures

ergotamine tartrate

(er-got'a-meen)

Ergomar

🍁 Gynergen

Drug class.: α-adrenergic blocker

Action: By a direct action, constricts vascular smooth muscle in peripheral and cranial blood vessels; relaxes uterine muscle

Uses: Vascular headache (migraine or histamine), cluster headache

Dosage and routes:

• *Adult:* SL 2 mg, then 1-2 mg qh or q0.5h, not to exceed 6 mg/day or 10 mg/wk

Available forms include: SL tabs 2 mg

Side effects/adverse reactions:

CNS: Numbness in fingers/toes, headache, weakness, visual changes

CV: Transient tachycardia, chest pain, bradycardia, edema, claudication, increase or decrease in BP

GI: Nausea, vomiting

MS: Muscle pain

Contraindications: Hypersensitivity to ergot preparations, occlusion (peripheral, vascular), CAD, hepatic disease, renal disease, peptic ulcer, hypertension, pregnancy category X

Precautions: Lactation, children, anemia

Pharmacokinetics:

PO: Peak 30 min-3 hr; metabolized in liver; excreted as metabolites in feces; crosses blood-brain barrier; excreted in breast milk

Drug interactions of concern to dentistry:

• Increased vasoconstriction: vasoconstrictor in local anesthetics

• Suspected increased risk of ergotism: erythromycin, clarithromycin, troleandomycin

• Use anticholinergic with caution in the elderly

DENTAL CONSIDERATIONS

General:

• This is an acute-use drug; patients are unlikely to seek dental treatment while using this drug.

• Monitor vital signs at every appointment because of cardiovascular side effects.

Teach patient/family:

• Use of electric toothbrush if patient has difficulty holding conventional devices

E

erythromycin (ophthalmic)

(er-ith-roe-mye'sin)

Ilotycin Ophthalmic

Drug class.: Antiinfective

Action: Inhibits bacterial protein synthesis

Uses: Infection of external eye, prophylaxis of neonatal conjunctivitis and ophthalmia neonatorum

Dosage and routes:

• *Adult and child:* Oint apply qd-qid as needed

Ophthalmia neonatorum:

• *Neonates:* Apply oint to conjunctival sacs immediately after delivery

Available forms include: Oint 0.5% in 3.5 g

Side effects/adverse reactions:

EENT: Poor corneal wound healing, temporary visual haze, irritation, overgrowth of nonsusceptible organisms, irritation

Contraindications: Hypersensitivity

Precautions: Antibiotic hypersensitivity, pregnancy category B, lactation

DENTAL CONSIDERATIONS

General:

• Avoid dental light in patient's eyes; offer dark glasses for patient comfort.

• Protect patient's eyes from accidental spatter during dental treatment.

erythromycin (topical)

(er-ith-roe-mye'sin)

Akne-mycin, Emgel, Erygel

Drug class.: Macrolide antibacterial (topical)

Action: Interferes with bacterial protein synthesis to inhibit bacterial growth

Uses: Acne vulgaris

Dosage and routes:

• *Adult and child >12 yr:* Top apply to affected area tid to qid

Available forms include: Top oint 2%; gel 2%

Side effects/adverse reactions:

INTEG: Rash, urticaria, stinging, burning, pruritus, dry/scaly/oily skin

EENT: Eye irritation, tenderness

Contraindications: Hypersensitivity

Precautions: Pregnancy category C, lactation

DENTAL CONSIDERATIONS

• None indicated

erythromycin base/ erythromycin estolate/ erythromycin ethylsuccinate/ erythromycin gluceptate/ erythromycin lactobionate/ erythromycin stearate

(er-ith-roe-mye'sin)

Erythromycin base: E-Base, E-Mycin, Eryc, Ery-Tab, Erythromycin Filmtabs, PCE Dispertab

♣ Apo-Erythro, Apo-Erythro-EC, Erybid, Erythromid, Novo-Rythro EnCap, ERYC-333

Erythromycin estolate: Ilosone

♣ Novo-Erythro

Erythromycin stearate: Erythrocin Stearate

♣ Apo-Erythro-S, Novo-rytho

Erythromycin ethylsuccinate: EES 200, EES 400, EES Granules, EryPed, EryPed Drops

♣ Apo-Erythro-ES, Novo-Rythro

Erythromycin lactobionate inj: Erythrocin

Erythromycin glucepate inj: Ilotycin

Drug class.: Macrolide antibiotic

Action: Binds to 50S ribosomal subunits of susceptible bacteria and suppresses protein synthesis

Uses: Infections caused by *N. gonorrhoeae;* mild-to-moderate respiratory tract, skin, soft tissue infections caused by *S. pneumoniae, M. pneumoniae, C. diphtheriae, B. pertussis, L. monocytogenes, S. pyogenes;* syphilis; legionnaires' disease; *C. trachomatis; H. influenzae;* endocarditis prophylaxis

Dosage and routes:
Soft tissue infections:
• *Adult:* PO 250-500 mg q6h (base, estolate, stearate) or 500 mg q12h or 333 mg q8h; PO 400-800 mg q6h (ethylsuccinate); IV inf 15-20 mg/kg/day (lactobionate)
• *Child:* PO 30-50 mg/kg/day in divided doses q6h (salts); IV 15-20 mg/kg/day in divided doses q4-6h (lactobionate)
Available forms include: Base: enteric-coated tabs 250, 333, 500 mg; film-coated tabs 250, 500 mg; caps 250, 500 mg; estolate: tabs 500 mg; caps 250 mg; susp 125, 250 mg/5 ml; stearate: film-coated tabs 250, 500 mg; ethylsuccinate: chew tabs 200 mg; susp 100 mg/2.5 ml, 200, 400 mg/5 ml; powder for inj; 500 mg and 1 g
Side effects/adverse reactions:
▼ *ORAL:* Candidiasis, lichenoid reaction
GI: Nausea, vomiting, diarrhea, ***hepatotoxicity,*** abdominal pain, heartburn, anorexia, pruritus ani, pseudomembranous colitis
GU: Vaginitis, moniliasis
EENT: Hearing loss, tinnitus
INTEG: Rash, urticaria, pruritus, thrombophlebitis (IV site), hypersensitivity
Contraindications: Hypersensitivity, erythromycin estolate in preexisting hepatic disease, cisipride, sparfloxacin, pimozide
Precautions: Pregnancy category B, hepatic disease, lactation
Pharmacokinetics:
PO: Peak 4 hr, duration 6 hr, half-life 1-3 hr; metabolized in liver; excreted in bile, feces
Drug interactions of concern to dentistry:
• Increased duration of alfentanil, cyclosporine
• Increased serum levels: indinavir, digoxin
• Decreased action of clindamycin, penicillins, lincomycin
• Increased serum levels of alfentanil, carbamazepine, theophylline (and other methylxanthines) and felodipine (possibly with other calcium blockers in the dihydropyridine class), ergot alkaloids, oral anticoagulants, buspirone, tacrolimus
• Risk of rhabdomyolysis: HMG-CoA reductase inhibitors
• Oral contraceptives: advise patient of a potential risk for decreased contraceptive action, to maintain compliance with oral contraceptive use while using antibiotics, and to consider the use of additional nonhormonal contraception
• May increase the effects of certain benzodiazepines: alprazolam, diazepam, midazolam, andtriazolam (see Appendix I)
• Risk of increased QT interval–use with caution in patients taking gatifloxacin, moxifloxacin, pimozide, disopyramide
• Possible serotonin syndrome with SSRIs
• Suspected increase in plasma levels of repaglinide

DENTAL CONSIDERATIONS
General:
• Alternative drug of choice for mild infection caused by a susceptible organism in patients who are allergic to penicillin.
• Determine why the patient is taking the drug.
• Estolate salt form is not indicated for adults because of risk of cholestatic jaundice.
Teach patient/family:
• To take oral drug with full glass

of water; take with food if GI symptoms occur (estolate, ethylsuccinate, and coated tabs only)

When used for dental infection, advise patient:

- To report sore throat, oral burning sensation, fever, fatigue, any of which could indicate superinfection
- To take at prescribed intervals and complete dosage regimen
- To immediately notify the dentist if signs or symptoms of infection increase

---

escitalopram oxalate

(es-sye-tal'oh-pram)

Lexapro

Drug class.: Antidepressant, selective serotonin reuptake inhibitor

---

Action: Inhibits CNS neuronal reuptake of serotonin, minimal effects on reuptake of norepinephrine or dopamine

Uses: Treatment of major depressive disorder; maintenance treatment of major depressive disorder

Dosage and routes:

- *Adult:* PO 10 mg daily; dose may be increased to 20 mg/day after a minimum of 1 wk; dose limit in elderly is 10 mg/day

Available forms include: Tabs 5, 10, 20 mg

Side effects/adverse reactions:

▼ *ORAL: Dry mouth*

CNS: Insomnia, dizziness, somnolence, anorexia, headache

GI: Nausea, diarrhea, abdominal pain, constipation, indigestion

RESP: Rhinitis, sinusitis

GU: Ejaculation disorder, decreased libido, impotence

META: Hyponatremia

MISC: Sweating, fatigue, flulike symptoms

Contraindications: Hypersensitivity to this drug or citalopram, concurrent use of MAOI and up to 2 wk after discontinuing use of MAOI

Precautions: Hyponatremia, activation of mania/hypomania, seizures, suicide, hepatic impairment, renal impairment, concurrent use of citalopram, pregnancy category C, lactation, use in children has not been established

Pharmacokinetics:

PO: Absolute bioavailability 80%, plasma protein binding 56%, hepatic metabolism (CYP3A4, CYP2D6, and CYP2C19 isoenzymes); renal excretion

Drug interactions of concern to dentistry:

- Increased sedation: alcohol and other CNS depressants
- Drugs that inhibit CYP3A4 or other CYP isoenzymes may or may not affect plasma levels, but should be used with observation and caution
- Modest inhibitor of CYP 2D6
- First-time users of SSRIs also taking NSAIDs may have a higher risk of GI side effects; until more data are available, it may be advisable to avoid use of NSAIDs in these patients (*Br J Clin Pharmacol* 55:591-595, 2003)

DENTAL CONSIDERATIONS

General:

- Assess salivary flow as a factor in caries, periodontal disease, and candidiasis.
- Consider semisupine chair position for patient comfort if GI side effects occur.

• Question patient about tolerance of NSAIDs or aspirin related to GI disease.
• Evaluate respiration characteristics and rate.

Consultations:
• Medical consultation may be required to assess disease control and patient's ability to tolerate stress.
• Physician should be informed if significant xerostomia occurs (e.g., increased caries, sore tongue, problems eating or swallowing, difficulty wearing prosthesis) so that a medication change can be considered.

Teach patient/family:
• Importance of good oral hygiene to prevent soft tissue inflammation/infection

When chronic dry mouth occurs, advise patient:
• To avoid mouth rinses with high alcohol content because of drying effects
• To use daily home fluoride products for anticaries effect
• To use sugarless gum, frequent sips of water, or saliva substitutes
• Importance of compliance with recommended regimens for oral care

esomeprazole magnesium

(es-oh-me'pray-sol)

Nexium

Drug class.: Antisecretory, proton pump inhibitor

Action: Suppresses gastric acid secretion by inhibiting hydrogen/potassium ATPase enzyme system in the gastric parietal cell; characterized as a gastric acid pump inhibitor because it blocks the final step of acid production

Uses: Gastroesophageal reflux disease (GERD), healing and maintenance of erosive esophagitis and *H. pylori* eradication in combination with antibiotics

Dosage and routes:

Healing of erosive esophagitis:
• *Adult:* PO 20 or 40 mg/day × 4-8 wk; some may require 16 wk

Maintenance of healing of erosive esophagitis:
• *Adult:* PO 20 mg/day × 4 wk

Symptomatic GERD:
• *Adult:* PO 20 mg/day × 4 wk

H. pylori eradication to reduce risk of duodenal ulcer recurrence:
• *Adult:* PO 40 mg/day × 10 days, with amoxicillin 1000 mg bid × 10 days and clarithromycin 500 mg bid × 10 days

Available forms include: Del rel caps 20, 40 mg (do not chew or crush)

Side effects/adverse reactions:

▼ *ORAL: Dry mouth,* ulcerative stomatitis, taste loss

CNS: Headache, anorexia, apathy, nervousness, sleep disorder

CV: Flushing, hypertension, tachycardia

GI: Nausea, diarrhea, flatulence, abdominal pain, constipation, dyspepsia

RESP: Asthma aggravated, cough, dyspnea, laryngeal swelling

HEMA: Anemia, leukocytosis, leukopenia, thrombocytopenia

GU: Dysmenorrhea, vaginitis, dysuria, polyuria

EENT: Earache, tinnitus, conjunctivitis, abnormal vision

INTEG: Acne, dermatitis, pruritus, urticaria, angioedema

ENDO: Goiter

META: Glycosuria, hyperuricemia, hyponatremia, ↑alkaline phosphatase
MS: Back pain, chest pain, arthralgia
MISC: Asthenia, flulike symptoms

Contraindications: Hypersensitivity

Precautions: Presence of gastric malignancy, atrophic gastritis, pregnancy category B, lactation, use in pediatric patients has not been studied, severe hepatic impairment, allergic reactions to related proton pump inhibitors

Pharmacokinetics:
PO: Take 1 hr before meals; peak plasma levels 1.5 hr; bioavailability ~90%, highly plasma protein bound (97%); extensive hepatic metabolism (CYP 2C19 major, CYP 3A4 lesser); 80% of metabolites excreted in urine and 2% in feces

Drug interactions of concern to dentistry:
• May interfere with absorption of drugs where gastric pH is an important factor in bioavailability (e.g., iron products, ketoconazole, trovafloxacin, ampicillin)

DENTAL CONSIDERATIONS
General:
• Assess salivary flow as a factor in caries, periodontal disease, and candidiasis.
• Question patient about tolerance of NSAIDs or aspirin related to GI disease.
• Consider semisupine chair position for patient comfort because of GI side effects of disease.
• Patients on chronic drug therapy may rarely have symptoms of blood dyscrasias, which can include infection, bleeding, and poor healing.
• Place on frequent recall because of oral side effects and oral effects of reflux disease

Consultations:
• In a patient with symptoms of blood dyscrasias, request a medical consult for blood studies and postpone treatment until normal values are reestablished.

Teach patient/family:
• To be aware of oral side effects and potential sequelae.
• To prevent trauma when using oral hygiene aids
• Importance of good oral hygiene to prevent soft tissue inflammation/infection

When chronic dry mouth occurs, advise patient:
• To avoid mouth rinses with high alcohol content because of drying effects
• To use daily home fluoride products for anticaries effect
• To use sugarless gum, frequent sips of water, or saliva substitutes

---

estazolam

(es-ta'zoe-lam)
ProSom

Drug class.: Benzodiazepine, sedative-hypnotic

Controlled Substance Schedule IV (US)

Action: Produces CNS depression by interacting with a benzodiazepine receptor to facilitate the action of the inhibitory neurotransmitter γ-aminobutyric acid (GABA)

Uses: Insomnia

Dosage and routes:
• *Adult:* PO 1-2 mg hs

Available forms include: Tabs 1, 2 mg

Side effects/adverse reactions:
▼ *ORAL:* Dry mouth, taste alteration, oral ulceration
CNS: Lethargy, drowsiness, daytime sedation, dizziness, confusion, light-headedness, headache, anxiety, irritability, weakness, tremors, depression, lack of coordination
CV: Chest pain, pulse changes, palpitation, tachycardia
GI: Nausea, vomiting, diarrhea, heartburn, abdominal pain, constipation, anorexia
HEMA: ***Leukopenia, granulocytopenia*** (rare)
INTEG: Dermatitis, allergy, sweating, flushing, pruritus
MISC: Joint pain, congestion
Contraindications: Hypersensitivity to benzodiazepines, pregnancy category X, sleep apnea, ritonavir, saquinavir
Precautions: Hepatic disease, renal disease, suicidal individuals, drug abuse, elderly, psychosis, child <18 yr, lactation, depression, pulmonary insufficiency, narrow-angle glaucoma
Pharmacokinetics:
PO: Onset 15-45 min, peak 1.5-2 hr, duration 7-8 hr; metabolized by liver; excreted by kidneys (inactive/active metabolites); crosses placenta; excreted in breast milk
Drug interactions of concern to dentistry:
• Increased CNS depression: alcohol, all CNS depressants
• Increased serum levels and prolonged effect of benzodiazepines: ketoconazole, itraconazole, fluconazole, and miconazole (systemic), indinavir
• Contraindicated with saquinavir
• Possible increase in CNS side effects: kava (herb)
• Decreased plasma levels: St. John's wort (herb)

DENTAL CONSIDERATIONS
General:
• Psychologic and physical dependence may occur with chronic administration.
• Geriatric patients are more susceptible to drug effects; use lower dose.
• Avoid the use of this drug in a patient with a history of drug abuse or alcoholism.
Teach patient/family:
• To avoid mouth rinses with high alcohol content because of drying effects

---

esterified estrogens
Menest
🍁 Neo-Estrone
Drug class.: Synthetic estrogen

Action: Required for the development, maintenance, and adequate function of the female reproductive system by increasing synthesis of DNA, RNA, and selected proteins; decreases the release of gonadotropin-releasing hormone; inhibits ovulation and helps maintain bone structure
Uses: Menopause, breast cancer, prostatic cancer, hypogonadism, ovariectomy, primary ovarian failure, osteoporosis prevention
Dosage and routes:
Menopause:
• *Adult:* PO 0.30-1.25 mg qd 3 wk on, 1 wk off
Hypogonadism/ovariectomy/ovarian failure:
• *Adult:* PO 2.5 mg qd-tid 3 wk on, 1 wk off
Prostatic cancer:
• *Adult:* PO 1.25-2.50 mg tid

E

Breast cancer:
- *Adult:* PO 10 mg tid × 3 mo or longer

Available forms include: Tabs 0.3, 0.625, 1.25, 2.5 mg

Side effects/adverse reactions:

▼ *ORAL:* Exacerbates gingivitis, bleeding

CNS: Dizziness, headache, migraines, depression

CV: ***Thromboembolism, stroke, pulmonary embolism, MI,*** hypertension, thrombophlebitis, edema

GI: Nausea, cholestatic jaundice, vomiting, diarrhea, anorexia, pancreatitis, cramps, constipation, increased appetite, increased weight

GU: Gynecomastia, testicular atrophy, impotence, amenorrhea, cervical erosion, breakthrough bleeding, dysmenorrhea, vaginal candidiasis, breast changes

EENT: Contact lens intolerance, increased myopia, astigmatism

INTEG: Rash, urticaria, acne, hirsutism, alopecia, oily skin, seborrhea, purpura, melasma

META: Folic acid deficiency, hypercalcemia, hyperglycemia

Contraindications: Breast cancer, thromboembolic disorders, reproductive cancer, vaginal bleeding (abnormal, undiagnosed), pregnancy category X

Precautions: Hypertension, asthma, blood dyscrasias, gallbladder disease, CHF, diabetes mellitus, bone disease, depression, migraine headache, convulsive disorders, hepatic disease, renal disease, family history of cancer of breast or reproductive tract

Pharmacokinetics:

PO: Degraded in liver, excreted in urine, crosses placenta, excreted in breast milk

Drug interactions of concern to dentistry:
- Increased action of corticosteroids

DENTAL CONSIDERATIONS

General:
- Place on frequent recall to evaluate gingival condition.
- Monitor vital signs at every appointment because of cardiovascular side effects.

Teach patient/family:
- Importance of good oral hygiene to prevent gingival inflammation

---

estradiol/estradiol cypionate/estradiol valerate

(es-tra-dye'ole)

Estradiol: Estrace, Gynodiol

✤ Estring

Estradiol cypionate: depGynogen, Depo-Estriadol, DepoGen

Estradiol valerate: Delestrogen

✤ Femogex

Estradiol topical emulsion: Estrasorb

Drug class.: Estrogen

Action: Required for the development, maintenance, and adequate function of the female reproductive system by increasing synthesis of DNA, RNA, and selected proteins; decreases the release of gonadotropin-releasing hormone; inhibits ovulation and helps maintain bone structure

Uses: Menopause, breast cancer, prostatic cancer, atrophic vaginitis, kraurosis vulvae, hypogonadism, ovariectomy, primary ovarian failure, prevention of osteoporosis and menopause-related vasomotor symptoms

Dosage and routes:
Menopause/hypogonadism/ovariectomy/ovarian failure:
• *Adult:* PO 1-2 mg qd 3 wk on, 1 wk off or 5 days on, 2 days off; IM 0.2-1 mg qwk
Prostatic cancer:
• *Adult:* IM 30 mg q1-2wk (valerate); PO 1-2 mg tid (oral estradiol)
Breast cancer:
• *Adult:* PO 10 mg tid × 3 mo or longer
Atrophic vaginitis:
• *Adult:* Vag cream 2-4 g qd × 1-2 wk, then 1 g 1-3× weekly
Osteoporosis prevention:
• *Adult:* PO 0.5 mg/day; 23 days on drug, 5 days off drug
Vasomotor symptoms associated with menopause:
• *Adult:* TOP apply 2 pouches daily to legs according to attached instructions
Available forms include: Estradiol–tabs 0.5, 1, 1.5, 2 mg; cypionate–inj IM 5 mg/ml; valerate–inj IM 10, 20, 40 mg/ml; top emulsion 2.5 mg/g in foil pouches
Side effects/adverse reactions:
▼ *ORAL:* Exacerbates gingivitis, bleeding
CNS: Dizziness, headache, migraines, depression
CV: ***Thromboembolism, stroke, pulmonary embolism, MI,*** hypertension, thrombophlebitis, edema
GI: Nausea, ***cholestatic jaundice,*** vomiting, diarrhea, anorexia, pancreatitis, cramps, constipation, increased appetite, increased weight
GU: Gynecomastia, testicular atrophy, impotence, amenorrhea, cervical erosion, breakthrough bleeding, dysmenorrhea, vaginal candidiasis, breast changes
EENT: Contact lens intolerance, increased myopia, astigmatism
INTEG: Rash, urticaria, acne, hirsutism, alopecia, oily skin, seborrhea, purpura, melasma
META: Folic acid deficiency, hypercalcemia, hyperglycemia
Contraindications: Breast cancer, thromboembolic disorders, reproductive cancer, vaginal bleeding (abnormal, undiagnosed), pregnancy category X
Precautions: Hypertension, asthma, blood dyscrasias, gallbladder disease, CHF, diabetes mellitus, bone disease, depression, migraine headache, convulsive disorders, hepatic disease, renal disease, family history of cancer of breast or reproductive tract
Pharmacokinetics:
PO: Well absorbed; moderate-to-high protein binding; hepatic metabolism with primary renal excretion
Drug interactions of concern to dentistry:
• Increased action of corticosteroids
DENTAL CONSIDERATIONS
General:
• Place on frequent recall to evaluate gingival condition.
• Monitor vital signs because of cardiovascular side effects.
Teach patient/family:
• Importance of good oral hygiene to prevent gingival inflammation

estradiol transdermal system

(es-tra-dye′ole)
Alora, Climara, Esclim, Estraderm, Vivelle-Dot, Vivelle
Drug class.: Estrogen

Action: Required for the development, maintenance, and adequate function of the female reproductive system by increasing synthesis of DNA, RNA, and selected proteins; decreases the release of gonadotropin-releasing hormone; inhibits ovulation and helps maintain bone structure

Uses: Menopause symptoms, postmenopausal osteoporosis prophylaxis

Dosage and routes:

Menopause:

• *Adult:* 0.025-0.05 mg once or twice weekly; apply patch to skin of buttocks or abdomen

Postmenopausal bone loss:

• *Adult:* 0.025-0.05 mg daily (one patch weekly); apply patch to skin on buttocks or abdomen

Available forms include: Transdermal system patches with release rates of 0.025, 0.0375, 0.05, 0.075, 0.1 mg/24 hr

Side effects/adverse reactions:

▼ *ORAL:* Exacerbates gingivitis, bleeding

CNS: Dizziness, headache, migraines, depression

CV: ***Thromboembolism, stroke, pulmonary embolism, MI,*** hypertension, thrombophlebitis, edema

GI: Nausea, ***cholestatic jaundice,*** vomiting, diarrhea, anorexia, pancreatitis, cramps, constipation, increased appetite, increased weight

GU: Gynecomastia, testicular atrophy, impotence, amenorrhea, cervical erosion, breakthrough bleeding, dysmenorrhea, vaginal candidiasis, breast changes

EENT: Contact lens intolerance, increased myopia, astigmatism

INTEG: Rash, urticaria, acne, hirsutism, alopecia, oily skin, seborrhea, purpura, melasma

META: Folic acid deficiency, hypercalcemia, hyperglycemia

Contraindications: Breast cancer, thromboembolic disorders, reproductive cancer, genital bleeding (abnormal, undiagnosed), pregnancy category X

Precautions: Hypertension, asthma, blood dyscrasias, gallbladder disease, CHF, diabetes mellitus, bone disease, depression, migraine headache, convulsive disorders, hepatic disease, renal disease, family history of cancer of the breast or reproductive tract

Pharmacokinetics:

TOP: Absorbed through the skin at a release rate of 0.05 or 1.0 mg/24 hr; hepatic metabolism and renal excretion; serum levels in 4 hr

Drug interactions of concern to dentistry:

• Increased action of corticosteroids

DENTAL CONSIDERATIONS

General:

• Place on frequent recall to evaluate gingival condition.

• Monitor vital signs because of cardiovascular side effects.

Teach patient/family:

• Importance of good oral hygiene to prevent gingival inflammation

---

estrogenic substances, conjugated

Premarin

✤ CES, Congest

Drug class.: Estrogen

Action: Required for the development, maintenance, and adequate function of the female reproductive system by increasing synthesis of DNA, RNA, and selected proteins;

decreases the release of gonadotropin-releasing hormone; inhibits ovulation and helps maintain bone structure

Uses: Menopause, breast cancer, prostatic cancer, abnormal uterine bleeding, hypogonadism, ovariectomy, primary ovarian failure, osteoporosis

Dosage and routes:

Menopause:

• *Adult:* PO 0.3-1.25 mg qd 3 wk on, 1 wk off

Prostatic cancer:

• *Adult:* PO 1.25-2.5 mg tid

Breast cancer:

• *Adult:* PO 10 mg tid × 3 mo or longer

Abnormal uterine bleeding:

• *Adult:* IV/IM 25 mg, repeat in 6-12 hr

Ovariectomy/primary ovarian failure/osteoporosis:

• *Adult:* PO 1.25 mg qd 3 wk on, 1 wk off

Hypogonadism:

• *Adult:* PO 0.3-0.625 mg/day; 3 wk on, 1 wk off

Available forms include: Tabs 0.3, 0.45, 0.625, 0.9, 1.25, 2.5 mg; inj 25 mg/5ml vial

Side effects/adverse reactions:

▼ *ORAL:* Exacerbates gingivitis, bleeding

CNS: Dizziness, headache, migraine, depression

CV: ***Thromboembolism, stroke, pulmonary embolism, MI,*** hypertension, thrombophlebitis, edema

GI: Nausea, ***cholestatic jaundice,*** vomiting, diarrhea, anorexia, pancreatitis, cramps, constipation, increased appetite, increased weight

GU: Gynecomastia, testicular atrophy, impotence, amenorrhea, cervical erosion, breakthrough bleeding, dysmenorrhea, vaginal candidiasis, breast changes

EENT: Contact lens intolerance, increased myopia, astigmatism

INTEG: Rash, urticaria, acne, hirsutism, alopecia, oily skin, seborrhea, purpura, melasma

META: Folic acid deficiency, hypercalcemia, hyperglycemia

Contraindications: Breast cancer, thromboembolic disorders, reproductive cancer, vaginal bleeding (abnormal, undiagnosed), pregnancy category X, lactation

Precautions: Hypertension, asthma, blood dyscrasias, gallbladder disease, CHF, diabetes mellitus, bone disease, depression, migraine headache, convulsive disorders, hepatic disease, renal disease, family history of cancer of breast or reproductive tract

Pharmacokinetics:

PO: Well absorbed; moderate-to-high protein binding; hepatic metabolism with primary renal excretion

Drug interactions of concern to dentistry:

• Increased action of corticosteroids

DENTAL CONSIDERATIONS

General:

• Place on frequent recall to evaluate gingival condition.

• Monitor vital signs because of cardiovascular side effects.

Teach patient/family:

• Importance of good oral hygiene to prevent gingival inflammation

estrogens A, conjugated synthetic

(es'troe-jenz)

Cenestin

Drug class.: Estrogens (nine synthetic estrogens expressed as alphabetical A for this combination)

Action: Reacts with estrogenic receptors; responsible for development and maintenance of female reproductive system and secondary sex characteristics, acts to reduce elevated levels of LH and FSH in postmenopausal women

Uses: Control of vasomotor symptoms, such as hot flashes and sweating in menopausal women

Dosage and routes:

• *Adult:* PO initial dose 0.625 mg; doses can be titrated to 1.25 mg; reassess use q3-6mo; discontinue as soon as possible

Available forms include: Tabs 0.3, 0.625, 0.9, 1.25 mg

Side effects/adverse reactions:

CNS: Headache

CV: Depression, insomnia, dizziness, nervousness, paresthesia

GI: Abdominal pain, flatulence, nausea, diarrhea

GU: Metrorrhagia, vagal bleeding changes

MS: Back pain, myalgia

MISC: Breast pain

Contraindications: Undiagnosed genital bleeding, breast cancer, estrogen-dependent neoplasm, active thrombophlebitis or thromboembolic disorders; pregnancy

Precautions: Endometrial cancer risk, venous thromboembolism, gallbladder disease, elevated BP, hyperlipoproteinemia, impaired liver function, lactation, pediatric patients, hypercalcemia

Pharmacokinetics:

PO: Well absorbed, maximum plasma levels in 4-16 hr; metabolized in liver, enterohepatic circulation

Drug interactions of concern to dentistry:

• None reported

DENTAL CONSIDERATIONS

General:

• Consider semisupine chair position for patient comfort if GI side effects occur.

Teach patient/family:

• Importance of good oral hygiene to prevent soft tissue inflammation

estropipate

(es'troe-pih-pate)

Ogen, Ortho-Est

Drug class.: Estrogen (piperazine estrone sulfate)

Action: Required for the development, maintenance, and adequate function of the female reproductive system by increasing synthesis of DNA, RNA, and selected proteins; decreases the release of gonadotropin-releasing hormone; inhibits ovulation and helps maintain bone structure

Uses: Vasomotor symptoms of menopause, atrophic vaginitis, primary female hypogonadism, primary ovarian failure, estrogen imbalance, ovariectomy

Dosage and routes:

Menopause:

• *Adult:* PO 0.75-6 mg daily; discontinue or reduce dose at 3-6 mo intervals

Hypogonadism:

• *Adult:* PO 1.5-9 mg/day × 3 wk; rest 8-10 days

Osteoporosis prevention:

• *Adult:* PO 0.75 mg/day × 25 days

Available forms include: Tabs 0.75, 1.5, 3, 6 mg

Side effects/adverse reactions:

▼ *ORAL:* Exacerbates gingivitis, bleeding

CNS: Dizziness, headache, migraine, depression

CV: ***Thromboembolism, stroke, pulmonary embolism, MI,*** hypertension, thrombophlebitis, edema

GI: Nausea, ***cholestatic jaundice,*** vomiting, diarrhea, anorexia, pancreatitis, cramps, constipation, increased appetite, increased weight

GU: Gynecomastia, testicular atrophy, impotence, amenorrhea, cervical erosion, breakthrough bleeding, dysmenorrhea, vaginal candidiasis, breast changes

EENT: Contact lens intolerance, increased myopia, astigmatism

INTEG: Rash, urticaria, acne, hirsutism, alopecia, oily skin, seborrhea, purpura, melasma

META: Folic acid deficiency, hypercalcemia, hyperglycemia

Contraindications: Breast cancer, thromboembolic disorders, reproductive cancer, vaginal bleeding (abnormal, undiagnosed), pregnancy category X, lactation

Precautions: Hypertension, asthma, blood dyscrasias, gallbladder disease, CHF, diabetes mellitus, bone disease, depression, migraine headache, convulsive disorders, hepatic disease, renal disease, family history of cancer of breast or reproductive tract

Pharmacokinetics:

PO: Well absorbed; moderate-to-high protein binding; hepatic metabolism with primary renal excretion

Drug interactions of concern to dentistry:

• Increased action of corticosteroids

DENTAL CONSIDERATIONS

General:

• Place on frequent recall to evaluate gingival condition.

• Monitor vital signs because of cardiovascular side effects.

Teach patient/family:

• Importance of good oral hygiene to prevent gingival inflammation

---

etanercept

(e-tan'er-cept)

Enbrel

Drug class.: Antiinflammatory and immunomodulator; biologic response modifier

---

Action: This drug consists of the extracellular ligand-binding protein of tumor necrosis factor (TNF) receptor linked to the Fc portion of human IgG1 that specifically binds to TNF and blocks its interaction with cell surface TNF receptors.

Uses: Reduction in signs and symptoms of moderately to severely active rheumatoid arthritis in patients with an inadequate response to one or more disease-modifying antirheumatic drugs; polyarticular-course juvenile rheumatoid arthritis; psoriatic arthritis; also approved for initial therapy

Dosage and routes:

• *Adult:* SC 25 mg twice weekly; 72-96 hr apart; can be given with other drugs used in rheumatoid arthritis treatment

• *Child 4-17 yr:* SC limited use in

children at doses of 0.4 mg/kg (limit 25 mg) given twice weekly
Available forms include: 25 mg single-use vial kit
Side effects/adverse reactions:
CNS: Headache, dizziness, asthenia
CV: ***MI, myocardial ischemia, cerebral ischemia*** (all rare but life-threatening reactions)
GI: Abdominal pain, vomiting in children
RESP: Sinusitis, URI, cough, pharyngitis, rhinitis
INTEG: Injection site reactions, rash
MISC: Infections, positive ANA readings, ***pancytopenia,*** allergic reactions
Contraindications: Hypersensitivity, use of live vaccines
Precautions: Risk of new malignancies and infrequent severe cardiovascular events, discontinue if serious infection occurs, immunosuppression risk, caution with preexisting demyelinating disorders, pregnancy category B, lactation, viral infections, children <4 yr
Pharmacokinetics:
SC: Half-life 115 hr, maximum plasma levels 72 hr, no information on metabolism or excretion
Drug interactions of concern to dentistry:
• No studies have been conducted.
DENTAL CONSIDERATIONS
General:
• Monitor vital signs at every appointment because of potential cardiovascular side effects
• Consider semisupine chair position for patient comfort because of GI side effects of drug
• If acute oral infection occurs, inform physician.
• Note elevated ANA levels if diagnosing Sjögren's syndrome.
Consultations:
• Consult if needed.
Teach patient/family:
• Importance of good oral hygiene to prevent soft tissue inflammation
• Use of electric toothbrush if patient has difficulty holding conventional devices

---

ethacrynate sodium/ ethacrynic acid

(eth-a-kri'nate)
Edecrin, Edecrin Sodium
Drug class.: Loop diuretic

Action: Acts on loop of Henle by increasing excretion of chloride, sodium
Uses: Pulmonary edema, edema in CHF, liver disease, nephrotic syndrome, ascites, hypertension
Dosage and routes:
• *Adult:* PO 50-200 mg/day; may give up to 200 mg bid
• *Child:* PO 25 mg, increased by 25 mg/day until desired effect occurs
Pulmonary edema:
• *Adult:* IV 50 mg given over several minutes or 0.5-1.0 mg/kg
Available forms include: Tabs 25, 50 mg; powder for inj 50 mg
Side effects/adverse reactions:
▼ *ORAL:* Dry mouth, increased thirst
CNS: Headache, fatigue, weakness, vertigo
CV: ***Circulatory collapse,*** chest pain, hypotension, ECG changes
GI: ***GI bleeding, severe diarrhea, acute pancreatitis,*** nausea, vomiting, anorexia, cramps, upset stomach, abdominal pain, jaundice
HEMA: ***Thrombocytopenia, agran-***

ulocytosis, leukopenia, neutropenia
GU: Polyuria, renal failure, glycosuria
EENT: ***Loss of hearing,*** ear pain, tinnitus, blurred vision
INTEG: Rash, pruritus, ***Stevens-Johnson syndrome,*** sweating, purpura, photosensitivity
ENDO: Hyperglycemia
MS: Cramps, arthritis, stiffness
ELECT: Hypokalemia, hypochloremic alkalosis, hypomagnesemia, hyperuricemia, hypocalcemia, hyponatremia
Contraindications: Hypersensitivity to sulfonamides, anuria, hypovolemia, lactation, electrolyte depletion, infants
Precautions: Dehydration, ascites, severe renal disease, pregnancy category D, hypoproteinemia
Pharmacokinetics:
PO: Onset 0.5 hr, peak 2 hr, duration 6-8 hr
IV: Onset 5 min, peak 15-30 min, duration 2 hr
Half-life 30-70 min, excreted by kidneys, crosses placenta
Drug interactions of concern to dentistry:
• Masked ototoxicity: phenothiazines
• Decreased antihypertensive effect: NSAIDs, especially indomethacin
DENTAL CONSIDERATIONS
General:
• Monitor vital signs at every appointment because of cardiovascular side effects.
• Patients on chronic drug therapy may rarely have symptoms of blood dyscrasias, which can include infection, bleeding, and poor healing.
• Assess salivary flow as a factor in caries, periodontal disease, and candidiasis.
• After supine positioning, have patient sit upright for at least 2 min before standing to avoid orthostatic hypotension.
• Patients on high-potency diuretics should be monitored for serum K^+ levels.
Consultations:
• In a patient with symptoms of blood dyscrasias, request a medical consultation for blood studies and postpone dental treatment until normal values are reestablished.
• Medical consultation may be required to assess disease control.
Teach patient/family:
• Importance of good oral hygiene to prevent gingival inflammation
When chronic dry mouth occurs, advise patient:
• To avoid mouth rinses with high alcohol content because of drying effects
• To use daily home fluoride products for anticaries effect
• To use sugarless gum, frequent sips of water, or saliva substitutes

ethambutol HCl

(e-tham'byoo-tole)
Myambutol
Etibi
Drug class.: Antitubercular

Action: Inhibits RNA synthesis, decreases tubercle bacilli replication
Uses: Pulmonary TB, as an adjunct
Dosage and routes:
• *Adult and child >13 yr:* PO 15 mg/kg/day as a single dose

Re-treatment:

• *Adult and child >13 yr:* PO 25 mg/kg/day as single dose × 2 mo with at least one other drug, then decrease to 15 mg/kg/day as single dose

Available forms include: Tabs 100, 400 mg

Side effects/adverse reactions:

▼ *ORAL:* Lichenoid reaction

CNS: Headache, confusion, fever, malaise, dizziness, disorientation, hallucinations, peripheral neuritis

GI: Abdominal distress, anorexia, nausea, vomiting

EENT: Blurred vision, optic neuritis, photophobia, decreased visual acuity

INTEG: Dermatitis, pruritus

META: Elevated uric acid, acute gout, liver function impairment

MISC: ***Thrombocytopenia,*** joint pain

Contraindications: Hypersensitivity, optic neuritis, child <13 yr

Precautions: Pregnancy category D, renal disease, diabetic retinopathy, cataracts, ocular defects, hepatic disorders, hematopoietic disorders

Pharmacokinetics:

PO: Peak 2-4 hr, half-life 3 hr; metabolized in liver; excreted in urine (unchanged drug/inactive metabolites); excreted unchanged in feces

Drug interactions of concern to dentistry:

• None reported

DENTAL CONSIDERATIONS

General:

• Examine for evidence of oral signs of disease.

• Avoid dental light in patient's eyes; offer dark glasses for patient comfort.

• Determine why the patient is taking the drug.

Consultations:

• Medical consultation is required to assess patient's current status; avoid elective dental procedures in active infections.

Determine that noninfectious status exists by ensuring the following:

• Anti-TB drugs have been taken for longer than 3 wk.

• Culture confirms antibiotic susceptibility to TB microorganisms.

• Patient has had three consecutive negative sputum smears.

• Patient is not in the coughing stage.

Teach patient/family:

• Importance of taking medication for full length of prescribed therapy to ensure effectiveness of treatment and to prevent the emergence of resistant forms of microbes

---

ethionamide

(e-thye-on-am'ide)

Trecator-SC

Drug class.: Antitubercular

Action: Bacteriostatic against *M. tuberculosis;* may inhibit protein synthesis

Uses: Pulmonary, extrapulmonary tuberculosis when other antitubercular drugs have failed

Dosage and routes:

• *Adult:* PO 15-20 mg/kg/day (limit 1 g/day)

• *Child:* PO 10-20 mg/kg/day in 2-3 doses, not to exceed 1 g

Available forms include: Tabs 250 mg

Side effects/adverse reactions:

▼ *ORAL:* Metallic taste, stomatitis, salivation

CNS: Anorexia, ***convulsions,*** headache, drowsiness, tremors, depression, psychosis, dizziness, peripheral neuritis
CV: Severe postural hypotension
GI: Anorexia, nausea, vomiting, diarrhea, hepatitis, jaundice, hypoglycemia
HEMA: ***Thrombocytopenia,*** purpura
EENT: Blurred vision, optic neuritis
INTEG: Dermatitis, alopecia, acne
MS: Asthenia
MISC: Gynecomastia, impotence, menorrhagia, difficulty managing diabetes mellitus, hypothyroidism

Contraindications: Hypersensitivity, severe hepatic disease

Precautions: Pregnancy category C, lactation, renal disease, diabetic retinopathy, cataracts, ocular defects, child <12 yr; pyridoxine concurrent use is recommended, resistance may develop

Pharmacokinetics:
PO: Peak 3 hr, duration 9 hr, half-life 3 hr; metabolized in liver; excreted in urine (unchanged drug/ inactive); crosses placenta

Drug interactions of concern to dentistry:
- None reported

DENTAL CONSIDERATIONS

General:
- Monitor vital signs at every appointment because of cardiovascular side effects.
- After supine positioning, have patient sit upright for at least 2 min before standing to avoid orthostatic hypotension.
- Consider semisupine chair position for patient comfort because of GI effects of disease.
- Evaluate for clotting ability during gingival instrumentation.
- Examine for evidence of oral manifestations of blood dyscrasias (infection, bleeding, poor healing).
- Palliative treatment may be required for oral side effects.
- Examine for evidence of oral signs of disease.

Consultations:
- Medical consultation for blood studies (CBC); leukopenic or thrombocytopenic side effects may result in infection, delayed healing, and excessive bleeding. Postpone elective dental treatment until normal values are maintained. Instruct patient to take with meals to decrease GI symptoms.
- Medical consultation may be required to assess disease control and determine infectious nature of disease.

Teach patient/family:
- Importance of good oral hygiene to prevent soft tissue inflammation
- Caution in use of oral hygiene aids to prevent injury

---

ethosuximide

(eth-oh-sux'i-mide)
Zarontin
Drug class.: Anticonvulsant

Action: Suppresses spike and wave formation in absence seizures (petit mal); decreases amplitude, frequency, duration, spread of discharge in minor motor seizures

Uses: Absence seizures (petit mal); unapproved: complex partial seizures

Dosage and routes:
- *Adult and child >6 yr:* PO 250 mg bid initially; may increase by 250 mg q4-7d, not to exceed 1.5 g/day
- *Child 3-6 yr:* PO 250 mg/day or 125 mg bid; may increase by 250

mg q4-7d, not to exceed 1.5 g/day
Available forms include: Caps 250 mg; syr 250 mg/5 ml
Side effects/adverse reactions:
▼ *ORAL:* Gingival bleeding, ulcerations (Stevens-Johnson syndrome); swelling of tongue and gingival enlargement (rare)
CNS: Drowsiness, dizziness, fatigue, euphoria, lethargy, anxiety, aggressiveness, irritability, depression, insomnia, headache
GI: Nausea, vomiting, heartburn, anorexia, diarrhea, abdominal pain, cramps, constipation, hiccups, weight loss
HEMA: ***Agranulocytosis, aplastic anemia, thrombocytopenia, leukocytosis, eosinophilia, pancytopenia***
GU: ***Hematuria, renal damage,*** vaginal bleeding
EENT: Myopia
INTEG: ***Stevens-Johnson syndrome,*** urticaria, pruritic erythema, hirsutism
Contraindications: Hypersensitivity to succinimide derivatives, blood dyscrasias
Precautions: Lactation, pregnancy category not established, hepatic disease, renal disease
Pharmacokinetics:
PO: Peak 1-7 hr, steady state 4-7 days, half-life 24-60 hr; metabolized by liver; excreted in urine, bile, feces
Drug interactions of concern to dentistry:
• Enhanced CNS depression: CNS depressants, alcohol
DENTAL CONSIDERATIONS
General:
• Patients on chronic drug therapy may rarely have symptoms of blood dyscrasias, which can include infection, bleeding, and poor healing.
• Talk with patient to ascertain seizure frequency and how well seizures are controlled. A stress reduction protocol may be required.
Consultations:
• In a patient with symptoms of blood dyscrasias, request a medical consultation for blood studies and postpone dental treatment until normal values are reestablished.
• Medical consultation may be required to assess disease control and patient's ability to tolerate stress.
Teach patient/family:
• Importance of good oral hygiene to prevent gingival inflammation
• To avoid mouth rinses with high alcohol content because of drying effects

---

ethotoin
(eth'oh-toyin)
Peganone
Drug class.: Hydantoin derivative anticonvulsant

Action: Inhibits spread of seizure activity in motor cortex
Uses: Generalized tonic-clonic or complex-partial seizures
Dosage and routes:
• *Adult:* PO 250 mg qid initially; may increase over several days to 3 g/day in divided doses
• *Child:* PO 250 mg bid; may increase to 250 mg qid, not to exceed 3 g/day
Available forms include: Tabs 250, 500 mg
Side effects/adverse reactions:
▼ *ORAL:* Gingival overgrowth (rare), gingival bleeding

CNS: *Fatigue, insomnia, numbness, fever, headache, dizziness*
CV: Chest pain
GI: *Nausea, vomiting, diarrhea*
HEMA: ***Agranulocytosis, thrombocytopenia, leukopenia, pancytopenia, megaloblastic anemia,*** lymphadenopathy
EENT: *Nystagmus, diplopia*
INTEG: Rash

Contraindications: Hypersensitivity to hydantoins, blood dyscrasias, hematologic disease, hepatic disease

Precautions: Pregnancy category C, lactation, geriatric patients

Pharmacokinetics:
PO: Half-life 3-9 hr, rapid oral absorption; metabolized by liver; excreted in urine

Drug interactions of concern to dentistry:

- Decreased effects: barbiturates
- Increased effects: ketoconazole, fluconazole, itraconazole, metronidazole
- Hepatotoxicity: acetaminophen or aspirin (chronic, high doses only)
- Decreased effects of corticosteroids, doxycycline, carbamazepine, itraconazole

DENTAL CONSIDERATIONS

General:

- Patients on chronic drug therapy may rarely have symptoms of blood dyscrasias, which can include infection, bleeding, and poor healing.
- Place on frequent recall to evaluate gingival condition and self-care.
- Short appointments and a stress reduction protocol may be required for anxious patients.
- Determine type of epilepsy, seizure frequency, and quality of seizure control.
- Consider semisupine chair position for patient comfort if GI side effects occur.

Consultations:

- In a patient with symptoms of blood dyscrasias, request a medical consultation for blood studies and postpone dental treatment until normal values are reestablished.
- Medical consultation may be required to assess disease control and patient's ability to tolerate stress.

Teach patient/family:

- Importance of good oral hygiene to prevent soft tissue inflammation and minimize gingival overgrowth
- Caution patient to prevent trauma when using oral hygiene aids

---

etidronate disodium

(e-ti-droe'nate)
Didronel, Didronel IV
Drug class.: Antihypercalcemic

Action: Exact mechanism unclear; chemisorbs to calcium phosphate surfaces of hydroxyapatite and interferes with aggregation, growth, and mineralization of hydroxyapatite crystals; slows resorption and new bone development (accretion)

Uses: Paget's disease, heterotopic ossification, hypercalcemia of malignancy

Dosage and routes:

Paget's disease:

- *Adult:* PO 5-10 mg/kg/day as a single dose with water, not to exceed 20 mg/kg/day, max 6 mo

Heterotropic ossification (spinal cord injury):

- *Adult:* PO 20 mg/kg qd × 2 wk, then 10 mg/kg/day for 10 wk, total 12 wk

Heterotropic ossification (total hip replacement):
• *Adult:* PO 20 mg/kg/d, up to 4 mo
Hypercalcemia of pregnancy:
• *Adult:* IV infusion only 7.5 mg/day over 2 hr for at least 3 days; 7 days of therapy may be used if required
Available forms include: Tabs 200, 400 mg; inj 50 mg/ml in 6 ml
Side effects/adverse reactions:
▼ *ORAL:* Altered taste (parenteral administration), glossitis
GI: Nausea, diarrhea, esophagitis, exacerbation of peptic ulcer
CNS: Amnesia, confusion, depression, headache
HEMA: ***Agranulocytosis (rare),*** leukopenia
INTEG: Alopecia, rash, pruritus, urticaria
RESP: Aggravation of asthma
MS: Bone pain, hypocalcemia, decreased mineralization of nonaffected bones, arthropathies, leg pain
MISC: Hypersensitivity reactions
Contraindications: Pathologic fractures, children, colitis, severe renal disease with creatinine >5 mg/dl, cardiac failure, osteomalacia
Precautions: Pregnancy category C, renal disease, lactation, adequate intake of vitamin D and calcium, safety and efficacy in children have not been established
Pharmacokinetics: Therapeutic response: 1-3 mo; not metabolized; excreted in urine
Drug interactions of concern to dentistry:
• Possible increased risk of gastric ulceration: NSAIDs

DENTAL CONSIDERATIONS
General:
• Be aware of the oral manifestations of Paget's disease (macrognathia, alveolar pain).
Consultations:
• Medical consultation may be required to assess disease control.

etodolac

(e-toe-doe'lack)
Lodine, Lodine XL
Drug class.: Nonsteroidal antiinflammatory

Action: Inhibits prostaglandin synthesis by interfering with cyclooxygenase needed for biosynthesis; possesses analgesic, antiinflammatory, antipyretic properties
Uses: Mild-to-moderate pain, osteoarthritis, rheumatoid arthritis
Dosage and routes:
Osteoarthritis:
• *Adult:* PO initial dose 300 mg bid or 400-500 mg bid, then adjust dose to 600-1200 mg/day in divided doses; do not exceed 1200 mg/day; patients <60 kg, not to exceed 20 mg/kg; ext rel 400-1200 mg qd
Analgesia:
• *Adult:* PO 200-400 q6-8h prn for acute pain; do not exceed 1200 mg/day; patients <60 kg, not to exceed 20 mg/kg (immediate release doseform only)
Available forms include: Caps 200, 300 mg; ext rel tabs 400, 500, 600 mg; tabs 400, 500 mg
Side effects/adverse reactions:
▼ *ORAL:* Stomatitis, lichenoid reaction, dry mouth, bitter taste
CNS: Dizziness, headache, drowsiness, fatigue, tremors, confusion, insomnia, anxiety, depression, light-headedness, vertigo

CV: Tachycardia, peripheral edema, fluid retention, palpitation, dysrhythmias, CHF

GI: Nausea, anorexia, ***cholestatic hepatitis, GI bleeding,*** vomiting, diarrhea, jaundice, constipation, flatulence, cramps, peptic ulcer, dyspepsia

RESP: Bronchospasm

HEMA: ***Blood dyscrasias***

GU: ***Nephrotoxicity: dysuria, hematuria, oliguria, azotemia,*** cystitis, UTI

EENT: Tinnitus, hearing loss, blurred vision

INTEG: Erythema, urticaria, purpura, rash, pruritus, sweating, angioedema

Contraindications: Hypersensitivity; patients in whom aspirin, iodides, or other nonsteroidal anti-inflammatories have produced asthma, rhinitis, urticaria, nasal polyps, angioedema, bronchospasm

Precautions: Pregnancy category C, lactation, children, bleeding disorders, GI disorders, cardiac disorders, elderly, renal, hepatic disorders

Pharmacokinetics:

PO: Onset 30 min, peak 1-2 hr, half-life 7 hr; serum protein binding >90%; metabolized by liver (metabolites excreted in urine)

Drug interactions of concern to dentistry:

- GI ulceration, bleeding: aspirin, alcohol, corticosteroids, biphosphonates
- Decreased action: salicylates
- Nephrotoxicity: acetaminophen (prolonged use)
- Possible risk of decreased renal function: cyclosporine
- First-time users of SSRIs also taking NSAIDs may have a higher risk of GI side effects; until more data are available, it may be advisable to avoid use of NSAIDs in these patients (*Br J Clin Pharmacol* 55:591-595, 2003)

When prescribed for dental pain:

- Risk of increased effects: oral anticoagulants, oral antidiabetics, lithium, methotrexate
- Decreased effects of diuretics
- Increased risk of methotrexate toxicity

DENTAL CONSIDERATIONS

General:

- Patients on chronic drug therapy may rarely have symptoms of blood dyscrasias, which can include infection, bleeding, and poor healing.
- Assess salivary flow as a factor in caries, periodontal disease, and candidiasis.
- Avoid prescribing for dental use in last trimester of pregnancy.
- Avoid prescribing aspirin-containing products.
- Consider semisupine chair position for patients with arthritic disease.

Consultations:

- In a patient with symptoms of blood dyscrasias, request a medical consultation for blood studies and postpone dental treatment until normal values are reestablished.
- Medical consultation may be required to assess disease control.

Teach patient/family:

- To avoid mouth rinses with high alcohol content because of drying effects

ezetimibe

(ez-et'i-mibe)

Zetia

Drug class.: Cholesterol-lowering agent

Action: Selectively inhibits the intestinal absorption of cholesterol and chemically related phytosterols

Uses: Adjunctive therapy to diet for reduction of cholesterol in patients with primary hypercholesterolemia

Dosage and routes:

• *Adult:* PO 10 mg daily with or without food; can also be taken with an HMG-CoA reductase inhibitor

Available forms include: Tabs 10 mg

Side effects/adverse reactions:

CNS: Fatigue

GI: Abdominal pain, diarrhea

RESP: Coughing, pharyngitis, sinusitis

META: Increase in serum transaminases (when combined with HMG-CoA reductase inhibitor)

MS: Arthralgia, back pain

MISC: Viral infection

Contraindications: Hypersensitivity; concurrent use with an HMG-Co A reductase inhibitor in patients with active liver disease or in patients with unexplained, persistent increase in serum transaminases, hepatic impairment

Precautions: When used with an HMG-CoA reductase inhibitor must follow all precautions for use (including pregnancy risk, risk of increased serum transaminase or myopathy); pregnancy category C, pregnancy, lactation and children <10 yr not established

Pharmacokinetics:

PO: absorbed with or without food; peak plasma levels 4-12 hr, primarily metabolized in small intestine and liver; extensive glucuronide conjugation, highly plasma protein bound (>90%); excreted in feces (78%) and urine (11%)

Drug interactions of concern to dentistry:

• None reported

DENTAL CONSIDERATIONS

General:

• Consider semisupine chair position for patient comfort if GI, respiratory, or musculoskeletal side effects occur.

• Monitor vital signs at every appointment because of possible cardiovascular disease.

Teach patient/family:

• Importance of updating health and drug history if physician makes any changes in evaluation/drug regimens

famciclovir

(fam-sye'kloe-veer)

Famvir

Drug class.: Antiviral

Action: Converted to active metabolite, penciclovir triphosphate, which inhibits DNA viral synthesis and replication; shows antiviral activity against herpes simplex virus (HSV-1, HSV-2), varicella zoster virus (VZV), and Epstein-Barr virus

Uses: Acute herpes zoster (shingles) infection; recurrent genital herpes; recurrent herpes simplex virus infections in HIV-infected patients

Dosage and routes:

Shingles:

• *Adult:* PO 500 mg tid × 7 days, start soon after symptoms appear; reduce doses in renal impairment

Recurrent genital herpes:

• *Adult:* PO 125 mg bid × 5 days; initiate therapy at first sign or symptom

Available forms include: Tabs 125, 250, 500 mg

Side effects/adverse reactions:

CNS: Headache, fatigue, dizziness, paresthesia

GI: Nausea, diarrhea, vomiting

EENT: Sinusitis, pharyngitis

INTEG: Pruritus

MS: Arthralgia, back pain

MISC: Fever

Contraindications: Hypersensitivity

Precautions: Pregnancy category B, children <18 yr, lactation, elderly, hepatic and renal function impairment

Pharmacokinetics:

PO: Peak plasma levels less than 1 hr; after PO absorption, converted to penciclovir; low plasma protein binding (20%-25%); renal excretion

Drug interactions of concern to dentistry:

• None reported in otherwise uncompromised patients

DENTAL CONSIDERATIONS

General:

• Determine why the patient is taking the drug.

• Consider semisupine chair position for patient comfort because of GI effects of drug.

• Be aware of general discomfort associated with shingles; acute symptoms may preclude patient's routine dental visit or mandate short appointments.

Consultations:

• Medical consultation may be required to assess patient's ability to tolerate stress.

• Medical consultation may be required to assess disease control.

famotidine

(fa-moe'te-deen)

Pepcid, Pepcid IV, Pepcid RPD

♣ Acid Control, Apo-Famotidine, Gen-Famotidine, Nu-Famotidine

OTC: Mylanta-AR, Pepcid AC

♣ Acid Control, Act, DysepHB, Gen-Famotidine, Maalox H2 Acid Controller, Ucidine HB

Drug class.: Histamine H_2-receptor antagonist

Action: Inhibits histamine at H_2-receptor site in parietal cells, which inhibits gastric acid secretion

Uses: Short-term treatment of active duodenal ulcer, maintenance therapy for duodenal ulcer, Zollinger-Ellison syndrome, multiple endocrine adenomas, benign gastric ulcers, gastroesophageal reflux disease; OTC: heartburn, acid indigestion

Dosage and routes:

Duodenal ulcer:

• *Adult:* PO 40 mg qd hs × 4-8 wk, then 20 mg qd hs if needed (maintenance); IV 20 mg q12h if unable to take PO

Benign gastric ulcer:

• *Adult:* PO 40 mg/day hs

Hypersecretory conditions:

• *Adult:* PO 20 mg q6h, may give 160 mg q6h if needed; if unable to take PO; IV 20 mg q12h given over 15-30 min

GERD:

• *Adult:* PO 20 mg bid up to 6

wk, if ulcerations/erosions present 20-40 mg bid up to 12 wk

Heartburn, acid indigestion (OTC):

• *Adult and child >12 yr:* PO prophylaxis 10 mg 15 min ac; treatment 10 mg once or twice daily (limit 20 mg/day)

Available forms include: Tabs 10 mg (OTC) and 20, 40 mg; powder for oral susp 40 mg/5 ml; oral disintegrating tab 20, 40 mg, inj IV 10 mg/ml; tabs chewable 10 mg (OTC); gelcaps 10 mg (OTC)

Side effects/adverse reactions:

▼ *ORAL: Dry mouth,* taste changes

CNS: Headache, dizziness, paresthesia, seizure, depression, anxiety, somnolence, insomnia, fever

GI: Constipation, nausea, vomiting, anorexia, cramps, abnormal liver enzymes

RESP: ***Bronchospasm***

HEMA: ***Thrombocytopenia***

EENT: Tinnitus, orbital edema

INTEG: Rash

MS: Myalgia, arthralgia

Contraindications: Hypersensitivity

Precautions: Pregnancy category B, lactation, children, severe renal disease, severe hepatic function, elderly, RPD tablets contain aspartame (caution: phenylketonuria)

Pharmacokinetics:

PO: Peak 1-3 hr, half-life 2.5-3.5 hr; plasma protein binding 15%-20%; metabolized in liver (active metabolites); excreted by kidneys

Drug interactions of concern to dentistry:

• Decreased absorption of ketoconazole or itraconazole (take doses 2 hr apart)

DENTAL CONSIDERATIONS

General:

• Avoid prescribing aspirin-containing products in patients with active GI disease.

• Consider semisupine chair position for patient comfort because of GI effects of disease.

• Assess salivary flow as a factor in caries, periodontal disease, and candidiasis.

Teach patient/family:

• Importance of good oral hygiene to prevent gingival inflammation

When chronic dry mouth occurs, advise patient:

• To avoid mouth rinses with high alcohol content because of drying effects

• To use daily home fluoride products for anticaries effect

• To use sugarless gum, frequent sips of water, or saliva substitutes

---

felbamate

(fel'ba-mate)

Felbatol

Drug class.: Anticonvulsant (carbamate derivative)

Action: Anticonvulsant action is unclear

Uses: Used alone or as adjunct therapy in partial seizures; also for partial seizures associated with Lennox-Gastaut syndrome in children; because of severe side effects use only for severe seizures when other therapy is inadequate

Dosage and routes:

• *Adult and child >14 yr:* PO (used alone) 1200 mg/day in 3 or 4 divided doses; increase dose by 600 mg increments q2wk; 3600 mg/day usual dose

• *Child 2-14 yr:* PO with Lennox-Gastaut syndrome (adjunctive) 15 mg/kg/day in 3-4 divided doses; reduce dose of other anticonvulsant drugs by 20%; increase dose by 15 mg/kg/day up to 45 mg/kg/day while further reducing the dose of other anticonvulsant drugs

Adjunctive therapy: PO reduce doses of other anticonvulsants by one third; then 1200 mg/day in 3 or 4 divided doses with 1200 mg increments to 3600 mg; doses of other anticonvulsants must be further reduced

Available forms include: Tabs 400, 600 mg; susp 600 mg/5 ml in 240, 960 ml sizes

Side effects/adverse reactions:

▼ *ORAL: Facial edema,* buccal mucous membrane swelling (rare), dry mouth

CNS: Insomnia, headache, somnolence, dizziness, ataxia, fatigue, anorexia, abnormal gait

CV: Palpitation, tachycardia

GI: Vomiting, diarrhea, nausea, constipation, dyspepsia

RESP: Dyspnea, upper respiratory infection, rhinitis

HEMA: ***Aplastic anemia,*** agranulocytosis, granulocytopenia, lymphadenopathy, leukopenia, thrombocytopenia

GU: UTI, incontinence (children)

EENT: Blurred vision

INTEG: Acne, rash, pruritus, photosensitivity reaction

MS: Tremor, abnormal gait

Contraindications: Hypersensitivity, hepatic impairment

Precautions: Pregnancy category C, lactation, warning of increased risk of aplastic anemia, hepatic failure, safety and efficacy in children with other types of seizures has not been established

Pharmacokinetics:

PO: Peak plasma levels 1-3 hr; 20%-25% protein bound; up to 40% excreted in urine unchanged

Drug interactions of concern to dentistry:

• Decreased effects of carbamazepine

• Increased photosensitization: drugs causing photosensitivity (e.g., tetracyclines)

DENTAL CONSIDERATIONS

General:

• Examine for evidence of oral manifestations of blood dyscrasia (infection, bleeding, poor healing).

• Short appointments and a stress reduction protocol may be required for anxious patients.

• Determine type of epilepsy, seizure frequency, and quality of seizure control. A stress reduction protocol may be required.

• Assess salivary flow as a factor in caries, periodontal disease, and candidiasis.

• Monitor vital signs at every appointment because of cardiovascular side effects.

• Advise patient if dental drugs prescribed have a potential for photosensitivity.

Consultations:

• Medical consultation may be required to assess disease control.

• Medical consultation may be required to assess patient's ability to tolerate stress.

Teach patient/family:

• Importance of good oral hygiene to prevent soft tissue inflammation

• Caution to prevent injury when using oral hygiene aids

• Use of electric toothbrush if patient has difficulty holding conventional devices

When chronic dry mouth occurs, advise patient:

• To avoid mouth rinses with high alcohol content because of drying effects

F

• To use daily home fluoride products for anticaries effect
• To use sugarless gum, frequent sips of water, or saliva substitutes

felodipine

(fel-loe'di-peen)
Plendil
♣ Renedil

Drug class.: Calcium channel blocker

Action: Inhibits calcium ion influx across cell membrane during cardiac depolarization; produces relaxation of coronary vascular smooth muscle, dilates coronary arteries, decreases SA/AV node conduction, dilates peripheral arteries

Uses: Essential hypertension, alone or with other antihypertensives, chronic angina pectoris

Dosage and routes:
• *Adult:* PO 5 mg qd initially, usual range 5-10 mg qd; do not exceed 20 mg qd; do not adjust dosage at intervals of <2 wk

Available forms include: Ext rel tabs 2.5, 5, 10 mg

Side effects/adverse reactions:
▼ *ORAL:* Gingival enlargement, dry mouth
CNS: Headache, fatigue, drowsiness, dizziness, anxiety, depression, nervousness, insomnia, lightheadedness, paresthesia, tinnitus, psychosis, somnolence
CV: ***MI, pulmonary edema,*** dysrhythmia, edema, CHF, hypotension, palpitation, tachycardia, syncope, AV block, angina
GI: Nausea, vomiting, diarrhea, gastric upset, constipation, increased liver function studies
HEMA: Anemia
GU: Nocturia, polyuria
INTEG: Rash, pruritus
MISC: Flushing, sexual difficulties, cough, nasal congestion, shortness of breath, wheezing, epistaxis, respiratory infection, chest pain

Contraindications: Hypersensitivity, sick sinus syndrome, second- or third-degree heart block

Precautions: CHF, hypotension <90 mm Hg systolic, hepatic injury, pregnancy category C, lactation, children, renal disease, elderly

Pharmacokinetics:
PO: Absolute bioavailability 20%, peak plasma levels 2.5-5 hr, elimination half-life 11-16 hr; highly protein bound; >99% metabolized in liver (CYP3A4 isoenzymes); excreted in urine (70%)

Drug interactions of concern to dentistry:
• Decreased effect: indomethacin, possibly other NSAIDs, phenobarbital, carbamazepine
• Increased effect: parenteral and inhalational general anesthetics or other drugs with hypotensive actions
• Increased effects of nondepolarizing muscle relaxants, diazepam, midazolam
• Increased plasma levels: itraconazole, erythromycin, carbamazepine (see Appendix I)

DENTAL CONSIDERATIONS

General:
• Monitor cardiac status; take vital signs at each appointment because of CV side effects. Consider a stress reduction protocol to prevent stress-induced angina during the dental appointment.
• After supine positioning, have patient sit upright for at least 2 min before standing to avoid orthostatic hypotension at dismissal.

• Place on frequent recall to monitor gingival condition.
• Limit use of sodium-containing products such as saline IV fluids for patients with a dietary salt restriction.
• Assess salivary flow as a factor in caries, periodontal disease, and candidiasis.
• Use vasoconstrictors with caution, in low doses, and with careful aspiration. Avoid use of gingival retraction cord with epinephrine.
• Use precaution if sedation or general anesthesia is required; risk of hypotensive episode.

Consultations:
• Medical consultation may be required to assess disease control.
• Consultation with physician may be needed if sedation or general anesthesia is required.

Teach patient/family:
• Importance of good oral hygiene to prevent gingival inflammation and minimize hyperplasia
• Need for frequent oral prophylaxis if hyperplasia occurs

When chronic dry mouth occurs, advise patient:
• To avoid mouth rinses with high alcohol content because of drying effects
• To use daily home fluoride products for anticaries effect
• To use sugarless gum, frequent sips of water, or saliva substitutes

---

fenofibrate (micronized)

(fen-o-fye'brate)
Tricor

Drug class.: Antihyperlipidemic

Action: Inhibits biosynthesis of triglyceride synthesis, reducing VLDL, and stimulates the catabolism of triglyceride-rich lipoprotein (ULDL); reduces serum uric acid levels

Uses: Hyperlipidemia, types IV and V, as an adjunct to diet therapy

Dosage and routes:
• *Adult:* PO initial dose 54-160 mg daily in conjunction with triglyceride-lowering diet
• *Elderly:* Limit initial dose to 54 mg daily

Available forms include: Tabs 54, 160 mg

Side effects/adverse reactions:
CNS: Headache, dizziness, paresthesia, insomnia, increased appetite
CV: Arrhythmia
GI: Dyspepsia, flatulence, nausea, vomiting, abdominal pain, constipation, diarrhea, pancreatitis
RESP: Flulike syndrome, cough
HEMA: ***Thrombocytopenia, agranulocytosis*** (very rare)
GU: Decreased libido, polyuria, vaginitis
EENT: Rhinitis, sinusitis, earache, blurred vision, photosensitivity
INTEG: Pruritus, rash
META: Elevated BUN and creatinine
MS: Asthenia, myositis, rhabdomyolysis (rare)
MISC: Fatigue, localized pain, hypersensitivity

Contraindications: Hypersensitivity, hepatic or severe renal dysfunction, primary biliary cirrhosis, preexisting gallbladder disease

Precautions: Monitor liver function; may lead to cholelithiasis; can be associated with myositis, myopathy, or rhabdomyolysis; pregnancy category C, avoid if lactating; safe use in children unknown;

F

discontinue use if no response in 2 mo; increased anticoagulant effect with oral anticoagulants

Pharmacokinetics:

PO: Well absorbed, increased absorption with food, peak plasma levels 6-8 hr, highly plasma protein bound (99%); hepatic metabolism, active metabolite; excreted largely in urine (60%)

Drug interactions of concern to dentistry:

• None reported

DENTAL CONSIDERATIONS

General:

• Monitor vital signs at every appointment because of cardiovascular and respiratory side effects.

• Consider semisupine chair position for patient comfort because of GI side effects of drug.

• Patients on chronic drug therapy may rarely have symptoms of blood dyscrasias, which can include infection, bleeding, and poor healing.

• Avoid dental light in patient's eyes; offer dark glasses for patient comfort.

Consultations:

• In a patient with symptoms of blood dyscrasias, request a medical consultation for blood studies and postpone treatment until normal values are reestablished.

Teach patient/family:

• Use of electric toothbrush if patient has difficulty holding conventional devices

• To prevent trauma when using oral hygiene aids

fenoprofen calcium

(fen-oh-proe'fen)

Nalfon

Drug class.: Nonsteroidal antiinflammatory, propionic acid derivative

Action: Inhibits prostaglandin synthesis by interfering with cyclooxygenase needed for biosynthesis; possesses analgesic, antiinflammatory, antipyretic properties

Uses: Mild-to-moderate pain, osteoarthritis, rheumatoid arthritis, acute gout, arthritis, ankylosing spondylitis, nonrheumatic inflammation, dysmenorrhea

Dosage and routes:

Pain (mild to moderate):

• *Adult:* PO 200 mg q4-6h as needed

Arthritis:

• *Adult:* PO 300-600 mg tid/qid, not to exceed 3.2 g/day

Available forms include: Caps 200, 300 mg; tabs 600 mg

Side effects/adverse reactions:

ORAL: Dry mouth, bleeding, stomatitis, lichenoid reaction

CNS: Dizziness, headache, drowsiness, fatigue, tremors, confusion, insomnia, anxiety, depression

CV: Tachycardia, peripheral edema, palpitation, dysrhythmias

GI: ***Cholestatic hepatitis,*** nausea, anorexia, vomiting, diarrhea, jaundice, constipation, flatulence, cramps, peptic ulcer

HEMA: ***Blood dyscrasias,*** increased bleeding time

GU: ***Nephrotoxicity: dysuria, hematuria, oliguria, azotemia***

EENT: Tinnitus, hearing loss, blurred vision

INTEG: Purpura, rash, pruritus, sweating

Contraindications: Hypersensitivity, asthma, severe renal disease, severe hepatic disease

Precautions: Pregnancy category not established (use not recommended); lactation, children, bleeding disorders, GI disorders, cardiac disorders, hypersensitivity to other antiinflammatory agents

Pharmacokinetics:

PO: Peak 2 hr, half-life 3-3.5 hr; 99% plasma protein binding; metabolized in liver; excreted in urine (metabolites), breast milk

Drug interactions of concern to dentistry:

- GI bleeding, ulceration: salicylates, alcohol, corticosteroids, other NSAIDs, biphosphonates
- May decrease effects of fenoprofen: phenobarbital
- Nephrotoxicity: acetaminophen (prolonged use)
- Possible risk of decreased renal function: cyclosporine
- Probable increased bleeding risk: warfarin
- Suspected increased risk for methotrexate toxicity
- First-time users of SSRIs also taking NSAIDs may have a higher risk of GI side effects; until more data are available, it may be advisable to avoid use of NSAIDs in these patients (*Br J Clin Pharmacol* 55:591-595, 2003)

DENTAL CONSIDERATIONS

General:

- Assess salivary flow as a factor in caries, periodontal disease, and candidiasis.
- Avoid prescribing for dental use in pregnancy.
- Possibility of cross-allergenicity when patient is allergic to aspirin.

Consultations:

- Medical consultation may be required to assess disease control.

Teach patient/family:

- Importance of good oral hygiene to prevent gingival inflammation
- Caution to prevent injury when using oral hygiene aids

When chronic dry mouth occurs, advise patient:

- To avoid mouth rinses with high alcohol content because of drying effects
- To use daily home fluoride products for anticaries effect
- To use sugarless gum, frequent sips of water, or saliva substitutes

---

fentanyl transdermal system

(fen'ta-nil)

Duragesic 25, 50, 75, 100 Transdermal Patches, Fentanyl Oralet

Oral transmucosal fentanyl citrate: Actiq (lozenges)

Drug class.: Narcotic analgesics

Controlled Substance Schedule II, Canada N

Action: Interacts with opioid receptors in the CNS to alter pain perception

Uses: Management of chronic pain when opioids are necessary; transmucosal form: only for management of breakthrough cancer pain in patients with malignancies who are using or tolerant to opioids; not appropriate for acute postoperative pain

Dosage and routes:

Chronic pain:

- *Adult only:* One patch every 72 hr; dose depends on need for pain control; titrate as required

F

Transmucosal form:

• *Adult only (patch and lozenge on a stick only [Actiq]):* Dose must be titrated starting with lowest dose size (must be kept secure from children)

Conscious sedation or anesthesia (Oralet only) in hospital setting:

• *Adult:* Doses must match patient, usually no more than 5 μg/kg (400 μg); doses for children must be adjusted for weight; see package insert directions for use

Available forms include: Number on patch (25, 50, 75, and 100) refers to μg/hr fentanyl-release rate; lozenges to be dissolved in mouth 100, 200, 300, 400 μg; lozenges on a stick 200, 400, 600, 800, 1200, 1600 μg

Side effects/adverse reactions:

▼ *ORAL:* Dry mouth

CNS: Dizziness, delirium, euphoria

CV: ***Bradycardia, arrest,*** hypotension or hypertension

GI: Nausea, vomiting

RESP: ***Respiratory depression, arrest, laryngospasm***

EENT: Blurred vision, miosis

MS: Muscle rigidity

Contraindications: Hypersensitivity to opiates, myasthenia gravis

Precautions: Elderly, respiratory depression, increased intracranial pressure, seizure disorders, severe respiratory disorders, cardiac dysrhythmias, pregnancy category C, children

Pharmacokinetics:

TD: Dosage adjusted according to opioid tolerance if patient has been taking opioids (2.5 mg of transdermal fentanyl is equivalent to approximately 90 mg of oral morphine in 24 hr); peak serum levels take up to 24 hr after applied; liver metabolism; renal excretion of metabolites

Drug interactions of concern to dentistry:

• Effects may be increased with other CNS depressants: alcohol, narcotics, sedative/hypnotics, skeletal muscle relaxants, chlorpromazine

• Additive hypotension: nitrous oxide, benzodiazepines, phenothiazines

• Increased anticholinergic effect: anticholinergics

• Contraindication: MAOIs

DENTAL CONSIDERATIONS

General:

• Monitor vital signs at every appointment because of cardiovascular and respiratory side effects.

• After supine positioning, have patient sit upright for at least 2 min before standing to avoid orthostatic hypotension.

• Assess salivary flow as a factor in caries, periodontal disease, and candidiasis.

• Psychologic and physical dependence may occur with chronic administration.

• Determine why the patient is taking the drug.

• Consider alternative drugs to opioids and NSAIDs for management of dental pain.

Consultations:

• Medical consultation may be required to assess disease control.

Teach patient/family:

• Importance of good oral hygiene to prevent gingival inflammation

• To avoid mouth rinses with high alcohol content because of drying effects

ferrous fumarate/ ferrous gluconate/ ferrous sulfate

(fer'us fyoo'ma-rate; gloo'koe-nate)

Ferrous sulfate: Fer-in-Sol, Feosol, Ed-In-sol, Fer-gen-sol, Fer-Iron, Feratab, Slow-Fe

Ferrous gluconate: Fergon

Ferrous fumarate: Femiron, Ircon, Hemocyte, Nephro-Fer, Feostat, Vitron-C

✤ Neo-Fer, Novofumar, Palafer

Drug class.: Hematinic, iron preparation

Action: Replaces iron stores needed for red blood cell development, energy and O_2 transport, utilization

Uses: Iron deficiency anemia, prophylaxis for iron deficiency in pregnancy

Dosage and routes:

Fumarate:

- *Adult:* PO 200 mg tid-qid
- *Child 2-12 yr:* PO 3 mg/kg/day (elemental iron) tid-qid
- *Child 6 mo-2 yr:* PO up to 6 mg/kg/day (elemental iron) tid-qid
- *Infants:* PO 10-25 mg/day (elemental iron) tid-qid

Gluconate:

- *Adult:* PO 200-600 mg tid
- *Child 6-12 yr:* 300-900 mg qd
- *Child <6 yr:* 100-300 mg qd

Sulfate:

- *Adult:* PO 0.750-1.5 g/day in divided doses tid
- *Child 6-12 yr:* 600 mg/day in divided doses

Pregnancy:

- *Adult:* PO 300-600 mg/day in divided doses

Available forms include:

- *Fumarate:* Tabs 63, 200, 324, 325, 350 mg; chew tabs 100 mg; oral susp 100 mg/5 ml, drops 45 mg/0.6 ml
- *Gluconate:* Tabs 240, 325 mg
- *Sulfate:* Tabs 324, 325 mg; syr 90 mg/5 ml; elixir 220 mg/5 ml; drops 75 mg/0.6 ml

Side effects/adverse reactions:

▼ *ORAL:* Extrinsic stain on teeth (liquid form)

GI: Nausea, constipation, epigastric pain, black and red tarry stools, vomiting, diarrhea

Contraindications: Hypersensitivity, ulcerative colitis/regional enteritis, hemosiderosis/hemochromatosis, peptic ulcer disease, hemolytic anemia, cirrhosis

Precautions: Long-term anemia, pregnancy category A

Pharmacokinetics:

PO: Excreted in feces, urine, skin, breast milk; enters bloodstream; bound to transferrin; crosses placenta

Drug interactions of concern to dentistry:

- Decreased absorption of tetracycline, zinc, ciprofloxacin

DENTAL CONSIDERATIONS

Teach patient/family:

- If patient is using hydrogen peroxide as a dentifrice to remove extrinsic stain, caution against frequent use to avoid peroxide-related soft tissue injury
- That liquid iron preparation taken through straw followed by rinsing mouth can reduce staining

fexofenadine HCl

(fex-oh-fen'a-deen)

Allegra

Drug class.: Antihistamine, nonsedating

Action: Antagonist for histamine (H_1) receptors; active metabolite of terfenadine

Uses: Seasonal allergic rhinitis, chronic idiopathic urticaria

Dosage and routes:

• *Adult and child >12 yr:* PO 60 mg bid or 180 mg qd

• *Child 6-11 yr:* PO 30 mg bid

• *Adult >65 yr:* PO 60 mg qd

Renal dysfunction:

• *Adult and child >12 yr:* PO 60 mg/day

• *Child 6-11 yr:* PO 30 mg/day

Chronic idiopathic urticaria:

• *Adult and child >12 yr:* PO 60 mg bid

• *Child 6-11 yr:* PO 30 mg bid

Available forms include: Caps 60 mg; tabs 30, 60, 180 mg

Side effects/adverse reactions:

CNS: Drowsiness, headache

GI: Nausea, dyspepsia

GU: Dysmenorrhea

EENT: Throat irritation

MISC: Fatigue

Contraindications: Hypersensitivity; troglitazone

Precautions: Reduce dose in elderly, renally impaired, pregnancy category C, lactation, child <12 yr

Pharmacokinetics:

PO: Well absorbed, peak plasma levels 2.6 hr; 60%-70% plasma protein bound; excreted mainly in feces; only 5% of dose is metabolized

Drug interactions of concern to dentistry:

• Elevated plasma levels with erythromycin, ketoconazole

• Decreased absorption: grapefruit juice

• Suspected decreased antihistaminic effects: rifampin

DENTAL CONSIDERATIONS

General:

• Consider semisupine chair position for patient comfort because of GI effects of drug.

finasteride

(fi-nas'ter-ide)

Propecia (hair growth product), Proscar

Drug class.: Synthetic steroid

Action: Competitive inhibitor of type II 5-α-reductase, an enzyme that converts testosterone to 5-α-dihydrotestosterone; this enzyme is found in the liver, skin, and scalp

Uses:

Proscar: Symptomatic benign prostatic hyperplasia, reduce risk for acute urinary retention and surgery

Propecia: Treatment of male pattern baldness (androgenic alopecia) in men 18-41 yr

Dosage and routes:

Prostatic hypertrophy (Proscar):

• *Adult:* PO 5 mg day, reassess in 6-12 mo

Male pattern baldness (Propecia):

• *Adult:* PO 1 mg daily; several months of therapy may be required, minimum 3 mo

Available forms include: Tabs 1 mg (Propecia), 5 mg (Proscar)

Side effects/adverse reactions:
GU: Impotence, decreased libido, decreased ejaculate volume
INTEG: Skin rash
MISC: Gynecomastia, allergic reactions

Contraindications: Hypersensitivity, pregnancy, lactation, children, prostate cancer, obstructive urinary disease; women should avoid handling broken tablets

Precautions: Pregnancy category X, lactation, lower PSA levels do not suggest absence of prostate cancer; women should avoid drug/semen contact, hepatic impairment

Pharmacokinetics:
PO: Bioavailability 63%-80%, peak levels 1-2 hr, half-life 6 hr; highly protein bound; liver metabolism; metabolites excreted in feces, urine

Drug interactions of concern to dentistry:
- Opioids and anticholinergic drugs may enhance urinary retention; use alternative analgesics (NSAIDs)

DENTAL CONSIDERATIONS
Consultations:
- Determine why patient is taking the drug; for prostatic hyperplasia or male pattern baldness.
- Medical consultation may be required to assess disease control.

flavoxate HCl

(fla-vox'ate)
Urispas
Drug class.: Antispasmodic

Action: Relaxes smooth muscles in urinary tract

Uses: Relief of nocturia, incontinence, suprapubic pain, dysuria, frequency associated with urologic conditions (symptomatic only)

Dosage and routes:
- *Adult and child >12 yr:* PO 100-200 mg tid-qid

Available forms include: Tabs 100 mg

Side effects/adverse reactions:
▼ *ORAL: Dry mouth*
CNS: Anxiety, restlessness, dizziness, convulsions, headache, drowsiness, confusion, decreased concentration
CV: Palpitation, sinus tachycardia, hypotension
GI: Nausea, vomiting, anorexia, abdominal pain, constipation
HEMA: ***Leukopenia, eosinophilia***
GU: Dysuria
EENT: Blurred vision, increased intraocular tension, dry throat
INTEG: Urticaria, dermatitis

Contraindications: Hypersensitivity, GI obstruction, GI hemorrhage, GU obstruction

Precautions: Pregnancy category B, lactation, suspected glaucoma, children <12 yr

Pharmacokinetics: Excreted in urine

Drug interactions of concern to dentistry:
- Increased anticholinergic effect: anticholinergic drugs
- Drug may cause drowsiness or blurred vision: advise patients when other CNS depressants are used

DENTAL CONSIDERATIONS
General:
- Assess salivary flow as a factor in caries, periodontal disease, and candidiasis.

Teach patient/family:
• Importance of good oral hygiene to prevent gingival inflammation
• To avoid mouth rinses with high alcohol content because of drying effects

flecainide acetate

(fle-kay'nide)
Tambocor

Drug class.: Antidysrhythmic (Class IC)

Action: Decreases conduction in all parts of the heart, with greatest effect on His-Purkinje system, which stabilizes cardiac membrane

Uses: Prevention of life-threatening ventricular dysrhythmias, sustained supraventricular tachycardia; prevention of paroxysmal atrial flutter, fibrillation, or paroxysmal atrial tachycardia

Dosage and routes:
• *Adult:* PO 100 mg q12h, may increase q4d by 50 mg q12h to desired response, not to exceed 300 mg/day

Available forms include: Tabs 50, 100, 150 mg

Side effects/adverse reactions:
▼ *ORAL:* Changes in taste, dry mouth
CNS: Headache, dizziness, involuntary movement, confusion, psychosis, restlessness, irritability, paresthesia, ataxia, flushing, somnolence, depression, anxiety, malaise
CV: Hypotension, bradycardia, ***heart block, cardiovascular collapse, cardiac arrest,*** dysrhythmias, CHF, fatal ventricular tachycardia, angina, PVC
GI: Nausea, vomiting, anorexia, constipation, abdominal pain, flatulence
RESP: ***Respiratory depression,*** dyspnea
HEMA: ***Leukopenia, thrombocytopenia***
GU: Impotence, decreased libido, polyuria, urinary retention
EENT: Blurred vision, hearing loss, tinnitus
INTEG: Rash, urticaria, edema, swelling

Contraindications: Hypersensitivity, severe heart block, cardiogenic shock, nonsustained ventricular dysrhythmias, frequent PVCs, non–life-threatening dysrhythmias

Precautions: Pregnancy category C, lactation, children, renal disease, liver disease, CHF, respiratory depression, myasthenia gravis

Pharmacokinetics:
PO: Peak 3 hr, half-life 12-27 hr; metabolized by liver; excreted unchanged by kidneys (10%); excreted in breast milk

Drug interactions of concern to dentistry:
• No specific interactions are reported with dental drugs; however, any drug that could affect the cardiac action of flecainide (e.g., other local anesthetics, vasoconstrictors, and anticholinergics) should be used in the lowest effective dose.

DENTAL CONSIDERATIONS

General:
• Monitor vital signs at every appointment because of cardiovascular and respiratory side effects.
• Assess salivary flow as a factor in caries, periodontal disease, and candidiasis.

• Stress from dental procedures may compromise cardiovascular function; determine patient risk.
• Use vasoconstrictors with caution, in low doses, and with careful aspiration. Avoid use of gingival retraction cord with epinephrine.

Consultations:
• Medical consultation may be required to assess disease control and patient's ability to tolerate stress.

Teach patient/family:
• Importance of good oral hygiene to prevent gingival inflammation
• To avoid mouth rinses with high alcohol content because of drying effects

---

fluconazole

(floo-koe'na-zole)
Diflucan
Drug class.: Antifungal

Action: A triazole antifungal that inhibits CYP450 enzymes and sterol C-14 alpha demethylation in fungi; this leads to ergosterol depletion and direct damage to the cell membrane

Uses: Oropharyngeal candidiasis, chronic mucocutaneous candidiasis, vaginal candidiasis, cryptococcal meningitis, esophageal candidiasis and prophylaxis in patients receiving bone marrow transplants with chemotherapy or radiation

Dosage and routes:
Esophageal candidiasis:
• *Adult:* PO 200 mg first day, then 100 mg daily
• *Child:* PO 6 mg/kg on day 1, then 3 mg/kg qd up to 3 wk minimum, then for 2 wk following resolution

Oropharyngeal candidiasis:
• *Adult:* PO 200 mg first day, then 100 mg daily
• *Child:* PO 6 mg/kg on day 1, then 3 mg/kg qd up to 2 wk

Cryptococcal meningitis:
• *Adult:* PO/IV 400 mg initially, then 200 mg/day; adjust dose downward for renal impairment
• *Child:* PO/IV 12 mg/kg on day 1, then 6 mg/kg qd

Prevention in bone marrow transplants:
• *Adult:* PO/IV 400 mg/day

Vaginal candidiasis:
• *Adult:* PO 150 mg as a single dose

Available forms include: Tabs 50, 100, 150, 200 mg; IV inj 200, 400 mg; powder oral susp 10 mg/ml, 40 mg/ml; inj 2 ml/ml in 100 and 200 ml

Side effects/adverse reactions:
CNS: ***Headache,*** seizures
GI: Nausea, vomiting, diarrhea, cramping, flatus, increased AST/ALT
HEMA: ***Agranulocytosis, hepatic failure,*** leukopenia, thrombocytopenia, hepatitis
INTEG: ***Toxic epidermal necrolysis*** (Stevens-Johnson syndrome, rare), *skin rash,* exfoliative skin disorders
META: Rare abnormal liver function, elevated cholesterol, triglycerides
MS: ***Anaphylaxis***

Contraindications: Hypersensitivity

Precautions: Renal disease, pregnancy category C

Pharmacokinetics:
PO/IV: Bioavailability more than 90%, peak plasma levels 1-2 hr, with loading doses see quicker steady-state levels; low plasma protein binding (12%); minimal metabolism; 80% excreted unchanged in urine

Drug interactions of concern to dentistry:

• Caution: a potent inhibitor of cytochrome P450 3A4 isoenzymes (see Appendix I)

• Increased plasma levels of oral hypoglycemics: theophylline, cyclosporine, tacrolimus, corticosteroids

• Inhibits metabolism of certain benzodiazepines: alprazolam, chlordiazepoxide, clonazepam, clorazepate, diazepam, estazolam, flurazepam, halazepam, midazolam, triazolam, quazepam, zolpidem (see Appendix I)

• Increased anticoagulant effect: may inhibit metabolism of warfarin

• Suspected risk of increased neurologic side effects: haloperidol, tricyclic antidepressants

• May increase levels and side effects of HMG-CoA reductase inhibitors

• Suspected increase in antihypertensive effects of losartan; if used concurrently monitor blood pressure

• Decreased renal clearance: hydrochlorothiazide

• Suspected decrease in oral contraceptive effectiveness: may want to suggest additional contraception

DENTAL CONSIDERATIONS

General:

• Culture may be required to confirm fungal organism.

• Patients on chronic drug therapy may rarely have symptoms of blood dyscrasias, which can include infection, bleeding, and poor healing.

Consultations:

• In a patient with symptoms of blood dyscrasias, request a medical consultation for blood studies and postpone treatment until normal values are reestablished.

Teach patient/family:

• That long-term therapy may be needed to clear infection

• To prevent reinoculation of *Candida* infection by disposing of toothbrush or other contaminated oral hygiene devices used during period of infection

---

flucytosine

(floo-sye'toe-seen)

Ancobon

Ancotil

Drug class.: Antifungal

Action: Converted to fluorouracil after entering fungi, thus inhibiting DNA and RNA synthesis

Uses: *Candida* infections (septicemia, endocarditis, pulmonary and urinary tract infections), *Cryptococcus* (meningitis, pulmonary and urinary tract infections)

Dosage and routes:

• *Adult and child >50 kg:* PO 50-150 mg/kg/day q6h

Available forms include: Caps 250, 500 mg

Side effects/adverse reactions:

ORAL: Bleeding (if bone marrow depression occurs), stomatitis

CNS: Headache, confusion, dizziness, sedation

GI: Nausea, vomiting, anorexia, ***bowel perforation*** (rare), diarrhea, cramps, enterocolitis, increased AST/ALT, alk phosphatase

RESP: ***Respiratory arrest,*** chest pain, dyspnea

HEMA: ***Thrombocytopenia, agranulocytosis, anemia, leukopenia, pancytopenia***

GU: Increased BUN, creatinine

INTEG: Rash, photosensitivity, urticaria

Contraindications: Hypersensitivity

Precautions: Renal disease, bone marrow depression, blood dyscrasias, radiation therapy or chemotherapy, pregnancy category C

Pharmacokinetics:

PO: Peak 2.5-6 hr, half-life 3-6 hr; excreted in urine (unchanged); well distributed to CSF, aqueous humor, joints

Drug interactions of concern to dentistry:

- None

DENTAL CONSIDERATIONS

General:

- Patients on chronic drug therapy may rarely have symptoms of blood dyscrasias, which can include infection, bleeding, and poor healing.
- Examine for evidence of oral *Candida* infection.

Consultations:

- Medical consultation may be required to assess disease control.
- In a patient with symptoms of blood dyscrasias, request a medical consultation for blood studies and postpone dental treatment until normal values are reestablished.

Teach patient/family:

- Importance of good oral hygiene to prevent gingival inflammation

---

fludrocortisone acetate

(floo-droe-kor'ti-sone)

Florinef Acetate

Drug class.: Glucocorticoid and mineralocorticoid

Action: Glucocorticoids have multiple actions that include antiinflammatory and immunosuppressant effects. They inhibit phospholipase A_2, interfering with or reducing the synthesis of prostaglandins and leukotrienes. They also bind to cytoplasmic GRs and enter the cell nucleus to bind with DNA. This results in the synthesis of various enzymes such as collagenase, elastase, and cytokines that play important roles in inflammation and immunosuppression. They also suppress the production of lymphocytes, monocytes, and eosinophils.

Uses: Adrenal insufficiency (Addison's disease), salt-losing adrenogenital syndrome

Dosage and routes:

- *Adult:* PO 0.1-0.2 mg/day
- *Pediatric:* PO 0.05-0.10 mg/day

Available forms include: Tabs 0.1 mg

Side effects/adverse reactions:

CNS: ***Flushing, sweating,*** headache

CV: Hypertension, ***circulatory collapse, thrombophlebitis, embolism,*** tachycardia, edema, enlargement of heart

MS: Fractures, osteoporosis, weakness

Contraindications: Hypersensitivity, acute glomerulonephritis, amebiasis

Precautions: Pregnancy category C, lactation, osteoporosis, CHF, safety and use in children has not been established

Pharmacokinetics:

PO: Half-life 3.5 hr, duration 1-2 days; highly protein bound; metabolized by liver; excreted in urine

Drug interactions of concern to dentistry:

- Decreased action: barbiturates

• Increased side effects: sodium-containing food or sodium-containing polishing devices
• Decreased effects of salicylates

DENTAL CONSIDERATIONS

General:

• Patients with Addison's disease are more susceptible to stress and may require supplemental systemic glucocorticoids before dental treatment.
• Patients who have been or are currently on chronic steroid therapy (>2 wk) may require supplemental steroids for dental treatment.
• Monitor vital signs at every appointment because of nature of disease.
• Short appointments and a stress reduction protocol may be required for anxious patients.
• Patients with Addison's disease must be evaluated closely for presence of oral infection.
• Do not use ingestible sodium bicarbonate products, such as the air polishing system Prophy
• Jet, or IV saline fluids for patients on a salt-restriction regimen.
• Use precautions if dental surgery is anticipated and conscious sedation or general anesthesia is required.
• Monitor patient for any signs of inadequate management of disease such as potassium depletion, muscle weakness, paresthesia, fatigue, nausea, depression, polyuria, and edema.

Consultations:

• Medical consultation is required to assess disease control and stress tolerance of the patient.
• Consultation may be required to confirm steroid dose and duration of use.

Teach patient/family:

• That identification as a steroid user should be carried
• To report to the dental office any signs that might indicate an oral infection

---

flumazenil

(floo-may'ze-nil)

Romazicon

Drug class.: Benzodiazepine receptor antagonist

Action: Antagonizes the actions of benzodiazepines on the CNS; competitively inhibits the activity at the benzodiazepine recognition site on the GABA–benzodiazepine receptor complex

Uses: Reversal of the sedative effects of benzodiazepines

Dosage and routes:

Reversal of conscious sedation or in general anesthesia:

• *Adult:* IV 0.2 mg (2 ml) given over 15-30 sec; wait 45-60 sec for desired response, then give 0.2 mg (2 ml) if consciousness does not occur; may be repeated at 60 sec intervals as needed, up to 4 additional times (max total dose 1 mg); dose is to be individualized

Management of suspected benzodiazepine overdose:

• *Adult:* IV 0.2 mg (2 ml) given over 15-30 sec; wait 45-60 sec for desired response, then give 0.2 mg (2 ml) over 30 sec if consciousness does not occur; further doses of 0.5 mg (5 ml) can be given over 30 sec at intervals of 1 min up to cumulative dose of 3 mg in 1 hr

Available forms include: Inj 0.1 mg/ml in 5 ml and 10 ml vials

Side effects/adverse reactions:
CNS: ***Convulsions,*** dizziness, agitation, emotional lability, confusion, somnolence
CV: Hypertension, palpitation, cutaneous vasodilation, dysrhythmias, bradycardia, tachycardia, chest pain
GI: Nausea, vomiting, hiccups
EENT: Abnormal vision, blurred vision, tinnitus
SYST: Headache, injection site pain, increased sweating, fatigue, rigors

Contraindications: Hypersensitivity to this drug or benzodiazepines, serious cyclic antidepressant overdose, patients given benzodiazepine for control of life-threatening condition

Precautions: Pregnancy category C, lactation, elderly, renal disease, seizure disorders, head injury, labor and delivery, hepatic disease, hypoventilation, panic disorder, drug and alcohol dependency, ambulatory patients; no risk-benefits have been established for children

Pharmacokinetics:
IV: Terminal half-life 41-79 min; metabolized in liver

Drug interactions of concern to dentistry:
• May not be effective: mixed drug overdosage

DENTAL CONSIDERATIONS

General:
• Monitor vital signs at every appointment because of cardiovascular side effects.
• Monitor for resedation; duration of antagonism is short compared with benzodiazepines.

Teach patient/family:
• To be alert for possible resedation when discharged from office

flunisolide

(floo-niss'oh-lide)

Oral inh aerosol: Aerobid, Aerobid-M
Bronalide
Nasal sol: Nasalide, Nasarel
Rhinalar

Drug class.: Synthetic glucocorticoid

Action: Glucocorticoids have multiple actions that include antiinflammatory and immunosuppressant effects. They inhibit phospholipase A_2, interfering with or reducing the synthesis of prostaglandins and leukotrienes. They also bind to cytoplasmic GRs and enter the cell nucleus to bind with DNA. This results in the synthesis of various enzymes such as collagenase, elastase, and cytokines that play important roles in inflammation and immunosuppression. They also suppress the production of lymphocytes, monocytes, and eosinophils.

Uses: Oral inhalation for prophylaxis or maintenance treatment of chronic asthma; nasal solution for seasonal or perennial rhinitis

Dosage and routes:
• *Adult:* INSTILL 2 sprays in each nostril bid, then increase to tid if needed; not to exceed 8 sprays in each nostril per day; INH 2 inhalations bid (AM and PM), limit to 4 inh/day
• *Child 6-15 yr:* INSTILL 1 spray in each nostril tid or 2 sprays bid; not to exceed 4 sprays in each nostril per day
• *Child 6-14 yr:* INH 2 inhalations bid

F

Available forms include: Aerosol 250 μg/spray; nasal sol 0.025% in 25 ml

Side effects/adverse reactions:

▼ *ORAL:* Dry mouth, candidiasis, loss of taste sensation

CNS: Headache, dizziness

EENT: Nasal irritation, dryness, rebound congestion, epistaxis, sneezing

INTEG: Urticaria

SYST: ***CHF, convulsions,*** increased sodium, hypertension

Contraindications: Hypersensitivity, child <12 yr, fungal, bacterial infection of nose

Precautions: Lactation, pregnancy category C; warning: switching patients from systemic steroids to inhalation must be done carefully to avoid severe adrenal insufficiency

Pharmacokinetics:

AERO: Effective response time 1-4 wk; metabolized in liver; excreted in urine and feces

DENTAL CONSIDERATIONS

General:

- Examine oral cavity for evidence of drug side effects.
- Assess salivary flow as a factor in caries, periodontal disease, and candidiasis.
- Evaluate respiration characteristics and rate.
- Consider semisupine chair position for patients with respiratory disease.
- Determine dose and duration of steroid therapy for each patient to assess risk for stress tolerance and immunosuppression.
- Acute asthmatic episodes may be precipitated in the dental office. Sympathomimetic inhalants should be available for emergency use. A stress reduction protocol may be required.
- Consider the drug in the diagnosis of taste alterations.

Consultations:

- Medical consultation may be required to assess disease control.

Teach patient/family:

- Importance of good oral hygiene to prevent soft tissue inflammation
- Caution to prevent injury when using oral hygiene aids
- Importance of gargling, rinsing mouth with water, and expectorating after each aerosol dose

When chronic dry mouth occurs, advise patient:

- To use daily home fluoride products for anticaries effect
- To avoid mouth rinses with high alcohol content because of drying effects
- To use sugarless gum, frequent sips of water, or saliva substitutes

---

fluocinonide

(floo-oh-sin'oh-nide)

Cream: Fluonex, Lidex, Lidex-E

♣ Lidemol, Lyderm

Ointment: Lidex

Solution: Lidex

Gel: Lidex

♣ Topsyn

Drug class.: Topical corticosteroid, synthetic fluorinated agent, group II potency

Action: Glucocorticoids have multiple actions that include antiinflammatory and immunosuppressant effects. They inhibit phospholipase A_2, interfering with or reducing the synthesis of prostaglandins and leukotrienes. They also bind to cytoplasmic GRs and enter the cell nucleus to bind with

DNA. This results in the synthesis of various enzymes such as collagenase, elastase, and cytokines that play important roles in inflammation and immunosuppression. They also suppress the production of lymphocytes, monocytes, and eosinophils.

Uses: Psoriasis, eczema, contact dermatitis, pruritus, oral lichen planus lesions

Dosage and routes:

• *Adult and child:* Apply to affected area tid-qid

Available forms include: Oint 0.5%; cream 0.05%; sol 0.05% in 20, 60 ml; gel 0.05% in 15, 30, 60, and 120 g tubes

Side effects/adverse reactions:

▼ *ORAL:* Thinning of mucosa, stinging sensation (oral application)

INTEG: Burning, dryness, itching, irritation, acne, folliculitis, hypertrichosis, perioral dermatitis, hypopigmentation, atrophy, striae, miliaria, allergic contact dermatitis, secondary infection

Contraindications: Hypersensitivity tocorticosteroids, fungal infections

Precautions: Pregnancy category C, lactation, viral infections, bacterial infections

DENTAL CONSIDERATIONS

General:

• Place on frequent recall to evaluate healing response.

Teach patient/family:

• When used for oral lesions, to return for oral evaluation if response of oral tissues has not occurred in 7-14 days

• That use on oral herpetic ulcerations is contraindicated

• Importance of good oral hygiene to prevent soft tissue inflammation

• To apply at bedtime or after meals for maximum effect

• To apply with cotton-tipped applicator by pressing, not rubbing, paste on lesion

fluorouracil (topical)

(flure-oh-yoor'a-sil)

Efudex, Fluoroplex

Drug class.: Topical antineoplastic

Action: Inhibits synthesis of DNA and RNA in susceptible cells

Uses: Keratosis (multiple/actinic), basal cell carcinoma; unapproved: condyloma acuminatum

Dosage and routes:

• *Adult and child:* TOP apply to affected area bid

Available forms include: Sol 1%, 2%, 5%; cream 1%, 5%

Side effects/adverse reactions:

▼ *ORAL:* Stomatitis, medicinal taste, lichenoid reaction

CNS: Insomnia, irritability

EENT: Lacrimation, soreness

INTEG: Pain, burning, pruritus, contact dermatitis, scaling, swelling, soreness, hyperpigmentation

Contraindications: Hypersensitivity, pregnancy

Precautions: Pregnancy category X, occlusive dressings, lactation, children, excessive exposure to sunlight

Pharmacokinetics:

TOP: No significant absorption, onset 2-3 days; treatment may last up to 12 wk; healing may be delayed for 1-2 mo

Drug interactions of concern to dentistry:

• None reported, but limit drugs that may also produce photosensitivity reaction

DENTAL CONSIDERATIONS

General:

• Be aware of patient's disease and avoid treated areas to prevent further irritation.

fluoxetine

(floo-ox'e-teen)

Prozac, Prozac Weekly, Sarafem

Drug class.: Antidepressant

Action: Selectively inhibits the uptake of serotonin (5-HT) in the brain

Uses: Major depressive disorder, bulimia, obsessive-compulsive disorder, premenstrual tension, geriatric depression in patients >65 yr, panic disorder with or without agoraphobia; premenstrual dysphoric disorder (Sarafem)

Dosage and routes:

Depression:

• *Adult:* PO 20 mg qd in AM; after several weeks if no clinical improvement is noted, dose may be increased to 20 mg bid, not to exceed 80 mg/day; Prozac Weekly 90 mg del rel capsule only for stabilized patients requiring maintenance therapy

Obsessive-compulsive disorder:

• *Adult:* PO initial 20 mg qd in AM; if no improvement after several weeks dose may be increased to 20 mg bid, not to exceed 80 mg/day

• *Children 8-17 yr:* PO initial 10 mg/day in AM; after 2 wk dose may be increased to 20 mg/day, other dose increases may be used depending on patient response; range 20-60 mg/day

Bulimia:

• *Adult:* PO 60 mg qd in AM; can start with lower dose and gradually increase to 60 mg/day

Panic disorder:

• *Adult:* PO initial dose 10 mg/day; after 1 wk dose may be increased to 20 mg/day; total dose should not exceed 60 mg/day

Premenstrual dysphoric disorder (Sarafem):

• *Adult:* PO 20 mg/day each day of menstruation or intermittent doses starting 14 days before onset of menses through first full day of menses; repeat each cycle

Available forms include: Tabs 10, 20 mg; caps 10, 20, 40 mg; del rel caps 90 mg; oral sol 20 mg/5ml in 120 ml

Side effects/adverse reactions:

▼ *ORAL: Dry mouth, taste changes*

CNS: Headache, nervousness, insomnia, drowsiness, anxiety, tremor, dizziness, fatigue, sedation, poor concentration, abnormal dreams, agitation, convulsions, apathy, euphoria, hallucinations, delusions, psychosis

CV: Hot flashes, palpitation, MI, angina pectoris, hemorrhage, tachycardia, first-degree AV block, bradycardia, thrombophlebitis

GI: Nausea, diarrhea, anorexia, dyspepsia, constipation, cramps, vomiting, flatulence, decreased appetite

RESP: Infection, pharyngitis, nasal congestion, sinus headache, sinusitis, cough, dyspnea, bronchitis, asthma, hyperventilation, pneumonia

GU: Dysmenorrhea, decreased libido, abnormal ejaculation, urinary frequency, UTI, amenorrhea, cystitis, impotence

EENT: Visual changes, ear/eye pain, photophobia, tinnitus

INTEG: Sweating, rash, pruritus, urticaria, acne, alopecia

MS: Pain, arthritis, twitching
SYST: Asthenia, viral infection, fever, allergy, chills
Contraindications: Hypersensitivity, MAOIs, thioridazine
Precautions: Pregnancy category B, lactation, children, elderly; treatment-emergent adverse effects, hepatic impairment, interference with cognitive or motor performance
Pharmacokinetics:
PO: Peak 6-8 hr, half-life 2-7 days, plasma protein binding 94.5%; metabolized in liver by CYP2D6 isoenzymes; excreted in urine
Drug interactions of concern to dentistry:
• Increased CNS depression: alcohol, all CNS depressants, tricyclic antidepressants, benzodiazepines, St. John's wort (herb)
• Increased side effects: highly protein-bound drugs (aspirin)
• Caution: can inhibit cytochrome P4502D6 isoenzymes (see Appendix I)
• Increased serum levels of carbamazepine
• Possible "serotonin syndrome" with macrolide antibiotics
• First-time users of SSRIs also taking NSAIDs may have a higher risk of GI side effects; until more data are available, it may be advisable to avoid use of NSAIDs in these patients (*Br J Clin Pharmacol* 55:591-595, 2003)
DENTAL CONSIDERATIONS
General:
• Monitor vital signs at every appointment because of cardiovascular side effects.
• Assess salivary flow as a factor in caries, periodontal disease, and candidiasis.
Consultations:
• Medical consultation may be required to assess disease control and patient's ability to tolerate stress.
• Physician should be informed if significant xerostomic side effects occur (e.g., increased caries, sore tongue, problems eating or swallowing, difficulty wearing prosthesis) so that a medication change can be considered.
Teach patient/family:
• To use electric toothbrush if patient has difficulty holding conventional devices
When chronic dry mouth occurs, advise patient:
• To avoid mouth rinses with high alcohol content because of drying effects
• To use daily home fluoride products for anticaries effect
• To use sugarless gum, frequent sips of water, or saliva substitutes

fluoxymesterone

(floo-ox-i-mes'te-rone)
Halotestin
Drug class.: Androgenic anabolic steroid

Controlled Substance Schedule III
Action: Increases weight by building body tissue; increases potassium, phosphorus, chloride, nitrogen levels; increases bone development
Uses: Impotence from testicular deficiency, hypogonadism, palliative treatment of female breast cancer
Dosage and routes:
Hypogonadism/impotence:
• *Adult:* PO 2-20 mg qd

Breast cancer:
• *Adult:* PO 10-40 mg qd in divided doses until therapeutic effect occurs; dosage should then be reduced
Available forms include: Tabs 2, 5, 10 mg
Side effects/adverse reactions:
▼ *ORAL:* Reddish spots on mucosa (high dose)
CNS: Dizziness, headache, fatigue, tremors, paresthesia, flushing, sweating, anxiety, lability, insomnia
CV: Increased BP
GI: ***Cholestatic jaundice,*** nausea, vomiting, constipation, weight gain
GU: ***Hematuria,*** amenorrhea, vaginitis, decreased libido, decreased breast size, clitoral hypertrophy, testicular atrophy
EENT: Carpal tunnel syndrome, conjunctional edema, nasal congestion
INTEG: Rash, acneiform lesions, oily hair/skin, flushing, sweating, acne vulgaris, alopecia, hirsutism
ENDO: Abnormal GTT
MS: Cramps, spasms
Contraindications: Severe renal disease, severe cardiac disease, severe hepatic disease, hypersensitivity, pregnancy category X, lactation, genital bleeding (abnormal)
Precautions: Diabetes mellitus, CV disease, MI
Pharmacokinetics:
PO: Metabolized in liver; excreted in urine; crosses placenta; excreted in breast milk
Drug interactions of concern to dentistry:
• Edema: corticosteroids
DENTAL CONSIDERATIONS
General:
• Monitor vital signs at every appointment because of cardiovascular side effects.
• Patients receiving chemotherapy may require palliative treatment for stomatitis.
Teach patient/family:
• Importance of good oral hygiene to prevent soft tissue inflammation
• To prevent trauma when using oral hygiene aids

fluphenazine decanoate/ fluphenazine HCl

(floo-fen'a-zeen)
Prolixin Decanoate
🍁 Apo-Fluphenazine, Modecate, Modecate Concentrate, Moditen HCl, PMS Fluphenazine
Drug class.: Phenothiazine antipsychotic

Action: Blocks neurotransmission at dopaminergic synapses in the cerebral cortex, hypothalamus, and limbic system; exhibits strong peripheral α-adrenergic, anticholinergic blocking action; mechanism for antipsychotic effects is unclear
Uses: Psychotic disorders, schizophrenia; unapproved: adjunct to tricyclic antidepressants in neurogenic pain
Dosage and routes:
Decanoate:
• *Adult and child >12 yr:* SC 12.5-25 mg q1-3wk
HCl:
• *Adult:* PO 2.5-10 mg in divided doses q6-8h, not to exceed 20 mg qd; IM initially 1.25 mg, then 2.5-10 mg in divided doses q6-8h
Available forms include: HCl: tabs 1, 2.5, 5, 10 mg; inj 2.5 mg/ml; decanoate: inj SC/IM 25 mg/ml

Side effects/adverse reactions:
▼ *ORAL: Dry mouth,* lichenoid reaction
CNS: Extrapyramidal symptoms: pseudoparkinsonism, akathisia, dystonia, tardive dyskinesia, drowsiness, headache, ***neuroleptic malignant syndrome,*** seizures
CV: Orthostatic hypotension, ***cardiac arrest, tachycardia,*** hypertension, ECG changes
GI: ***Paralytic ileus, hepatitis,*** nausea, vomiting, anorexia, constipation, diarrhea, jaundice, weight gain
RESP: ***Respiratory depression,*** laryngospasm, dyspnea
HEMA: ***Leukopenia, leukocytosis, agranulocytosis,*** anemia
GU: Urinary retention, urinary frequency, enuresis, impotence, amenorrhea, gynecomastia
EENT: Blurred vision, glaucoma, dry eyes
INTEG: Rash, photosensitivity, dermatitis

Contraindications: Hypersensitivity, circulatory collapse, liver damage, cerebral arteriosclerosis, coronary disease, severe hypertension/hypotension, blood dyscrasias, coma, child <12 yr, brain damage, bone marrow depression, alcohol and barbiturate withdrawal states

Precautions: Pregnancy category not established, lactation, seizure disorders, hypertension, hepatic disease, cardiac disease

Pharmacokinetics:
PO/IM: HCl–onset 1 hr, peak 2-4 hr, duration 6-8 hr
SC: decanoate–onset 1-3 days, peak 1-2 days, duration >4 wk, half-life (single dose) 6.8-9.6 days, half-life (multiple dose) 14.3 days; metabolized by liver; excreted in urine (metabolites); crosses placenta; excreted in breast milk

Drug interactions of concern to dentistry:
- Increased sedation: other CNS depressants, alcohol, barbiturate anesthetics, opioid analgesics
- Hypotension, tachycardia: epinephrine
- Increased extrapyramidal effects: phenothiazines and related drugs (haloperidol, droperidol), metoclopramide
- Additive photosensitization: tetracyclines
- Increased anticholinergic effects: anticholinergics

DENTAL CONSIDERATIONS

General:
- Monitor vital signs at every appointment because of cardiovascular side effects.
- Patients on chronic drug therapy may rarely have symptoms of blood dyscrasias, which can include infection, bleeding, and poor healing.
- After supine positioning, have patient sit upright for at least 2 min before standing to avoid orthostatic hypotension.
- Assess salivary flow as a factor in caries, periodontal disease, and candidiasis.
- Avoid dental light in patient's eyes; offer dark glasses for patient comfort.
- Assess for presence of extrapyramidal motor symptoms, such as tardive dyskinesia and akathisia. Extrapyramidal motor activity may complicate dental treatment.
- Geriatric patients are more susceptible to drug effects; use a lower dose.

• Use vasoconstrictors with caution, in low doses, and with careful aspiration.

Consultations:

• In a patient with symptoms of blood dyscrasias, request a medical consultation for blood studies and postpone dental treatment until normal values are reestablished.

• Take precautions if dental surgery is anticipated and anesthesia is required.

• If signs of tardive dyskinesia or akathisia are present, refer to physician.

• Physician should be informed if significant xerostomic side effects occur (e.g., increased caries, sore tongue, problems eating or swallowing, difficulty wearing prosthesis) so that a medication change can be considered.

Teach patient/family:

• Importance of good oral hygiene to prevent soft tissue inflammation

• Caution to prevent injury when using oral hygiene aids

• To use electric toothbrush if patient has difficulty holding conventional devices

When chronic dry mouth occurs, advise patient:

• To avoid mouth rinses with high alcohol content because of drying effects

• To use daily home fluoride products for anticaries effect

• To use sugarless gum, frequent sips of water, or saliva substitutes

flurandrenolide

(flure-an-dren'oh-lide)

Cordran, Cordran SP

✤ Drenison, Drenisone-1/4

Drug class.: Topical corticosteroid, group III medium potency

Action: Glucocorticoids have multiple actions that include antiinflammatory and immunosuppressant effects. They inhibit phospholipase A_2, interfering with or reducing the synthesis of prostaglandins and leukotrienes. They also bind to cytoplasmic GRs and enter the cell nucleus to bind with DNA. This results in the synthesis of various enzymes, such as collagenase, elastase, and cytokines, that play important roles in inflammation and immunosuppression. They also suppress the production of lymphocytes, monocytes, and eosinophils.

Uses: Corticosteroid-responsive dermatoses, pruritus

Dosage and routes:

• *Adult and child:* TOP apply to affected area tid-qid; apply tape q12-24h

Available forms include: Oint 0.025%, 0.05%; cream 0.025%, 0.05%; lotion 0.05%; tape 4 µg/cm^2

Side effects/adverse reactions:

▼ *ORAL:* Perioral dermatitis

INTEG: Burning, dryness, itching, irritation, acne, folliculitis, hypertrichosis, hypopigmentation, atrophy, striae, miliaria, allergic contact dermatitis, secondary infection

Contraindications: Hypersensitivity to corticosteroids, fungal infections, viral infections

Precautions: Pregnancy category C, lactation, viral infections, bacterial infections

DENTAL CONSIDERATIONS

General:

• Determine why the patient is taking the drug.

• Apply lubricant to dry lips for patient comfort before dental procedures.

• Place on frequent recall to evaluate healing response when used on chronic basis.

---

flurazepam HCl

(flur-az'e-pam)

Dalmane

♣ Apo-Flurazepam, Novo-flupam, Somnol

Drug class.: Benzodiazepine, sedative-hypnotic

Controlled Substance Schedule IV

Action: Produces CNS depression by interacting with a benzodiazepine receptor to facilitate the action of the inhibitory neurotransmitter γ-aminobutyric acid (GABA)

Uses: Insomnia

Dosage and routes:

• *Adult:* PO 15-30 mg hs, may repeat dose once if needed

• *Geriatric:* PO 15 mg hs, may increase if needed

Available forms include: Caps 15, 30 mg

Side effects/adverse reactions:

▼ *ORAL:* Dry mouth (infrequent)

CNS: Lethargy, drowsiness, daytime sedation, dizziness, confusion, light-headedness, headache, anxiety, irritability

CV: Chest pain, pulse changes

GI: Nausea, vomiting, diarrhea, heartburn, abdominal pain, constipation

HEMA: ***Leukopenia, granulocytopenia*** (rare)

Contraindications: Hypersensitivity to benzodiazepines, pregnancy category X, lactation, intermittent porphyria, uncontrolled pain, ritonavir, saquinavir

Precautions: Anemia, hepatic disease, renal disease, suicidal individuals, drug abuse, elderly, psychosis, child <15 yr

Pharmacokinetics:

PO: Onset 15-45 min, duration 7-8 hr, half-life 47-100 hr, additional 100 hr for active metabolites; metabolized by liver; excreted by kidneys (inactive/active metabolites); crosses placenta; excreted in breast milk

Drug interactions of concern to dentistry:

• Increased sedation: alcohol, CNS depressants

• Increased serum levels and prolonged effect of benzodiazepines: ketoconazole, itraconazole, fluconazole, and miconazole (systemic), indinavir

• Contraindicated with saquinavir

• Possible increase in CNS side effects: kava (herb)

DENTAL CONSIDERATIONS

General:

• Assess salivary flow as a factor in caries, periodontal disease, and candidiasis.

• Psychologic and physical dependence may occur with chronic administration.

• Geriatric patients are more susceptible to drug effects; use lower dose.

Consultations:
• Medical consultation may be required to assess disease control.
Teach patient/family:
• To avoid mouth rinses with high alcohol content because of drying effects

---

flurbiprofen

(flure-bi'proe-fen)
Ansaid
♣ Apo-Flurbiprofen, Froben, Froben SR, Novo-Flurbiprofen, Nu-Flurbiprofen

Drug class.: Nonsteroidal antiinflammatory

Action: Inhibits prostaglandin synthesis by interfering with cyclooxygenase needed for biosynthesis; possesses analgesic, antiinflammatory, antipyretic properties
Uses: Acute, long-term treatment of rheumatoid arthritis, osteoarthritis; unapproved: mild-to-moderate pain
Dosage and routes:
• *Adult:* PO 200-300 mg daily in divided doses bid, tid, or qid
Available forms include: Tabs 50, 100 mg
Side effects/adverse reactions:
▼ *ORAL:* Dry mouth, stomatitis, lichenoid reaction
CNS: Dizziness, drowsiness, fatigue, tremors, confusion, anxiety, myalgia, insomnia, depression, convulsions, malaise, nervousness, paresthesias
CV: Tachycardia, peripheral edema, palpitation, chest pain
GI: ***Jaundice, cholestatic hepatitis,*** nausea, anorexia, vomiting, diarrhea, constipation, flatulence, cramps, peptic ulcer, dyspepsia, indigestion
RESP: ***Bronchospasm,*** dyspnea, hemoptysis, rhinitis, shortness of breath
HEMA: ***Blood dyscrasias, bone marrow depression***
GU: ***Nephrotoxicity: dysuria, hematuria, oliguria, azotemia, cystitis, UTI, nocturia, renal insufficiency***
EENT: Tinnitus, hearing loss, blurred vision
INTEG: Purpura, rash, pruritus, erythema, urticaria, petechiae, ecchymosis, photosensitivity, exfoliative dermatitis, alopecia, eczema
Contraindications: Hypersensitivity; hypersensitivity to other antiinflammatory agents
Precautions: Pregnancy category B, first or second trimester, lactation, children, bleeding disorders, GI disorders, cardiac disorders, severe renal disease, severe hepatic disease
Pharmacokinetics:
PO: Peak 1.5 hr, half-life 6 hr; metabolized in liver; excreted in urine (metabolites), breast milk
Drug interactions of concern to dentistry:
• GI ulceration, bleeding: aspirin, alcohol, corticosteroids
• Decreased action: salicylates
• Nephrotoxicity: acetaminophen (prolonged use)
When prescribed for dental pain:
• Risk of increased effects: oral anticoagulants, oral antidiabetics, lithium, methotrexate
• Decreased effects of diuretics
• First-time users of SSRIs also taking NSAIDs may have a higher risk of GI side effects; until more data are available, it may be advisable to avoid use of NSAIDs in these patients (*Br J Clin Pharmacol* 55:591-595, 2003)

DENTAL CONSIDERATIONS

General:

• Patients on chronic drug therapy may rarely have symptoms of blood dyscrasias, which can include infection, bleeding, and poor healing.

• Assess salivary flow as a factor in caries, periodontal disease, and candidiasis.

• Avoid prescribing for dental use in last trimester of pregnancy.

• Avoid prescribing aspirin-containing products.

• Consider semisupine chair position for patients with arthritic disease.

Consultations:

• Medical consultation may be required to assess disease control.

• In a patient with symptoms of blood dyscrasias, request a medical consultation for blood studies and postpone dental treatment until normal values are reestablished.

Teach patient/family:

• Importance of good oral hygiene to prevent soft tissue inflammation

• Caution to prevent injury when using oral hygiene aids

When chronic dry mouth occurs, advise patient:

• To avoid mouth rinses with high alcohol content because of drying effects

• To use daily home fluoride products for anticaries effect

• To use sugarless gum, frequent sips of water, or saliva substitutes

flurbiprofen sodium

(flure-bi'proe-fen)

Ocufen

Drug class.: Nonsteroidal antiinflammatory ophthalmic

Action: Inhibits enzyme system necessary for biosynthesis of prostaglandins; inhibits miosis

Uses: Inhibition of intraoperative miosis, corneal edema

Dosage and routes:

• *Adult:* 1 drop q0.5h 2 hr before surgery (4 drop total)

Available forms include: Sol 0.03%

Side effects/adverse reactions:

EENT: Burning, stinging in the eye, eye irritation/bleeding/redness

Contraindications: Hypersensitivity, epithelial herpes simplex keratitis

Precautions: Pregnancy category C, lactation, child, aspirin or NSAID hypersensitivity, allergy, bleeding disorder

DENTAL CONSIDERATIONS

General:

• Avoid dental light in patient's eyes; offer dark glasses for patient comfort.

flutamide

(floo'ta-mide)

Eulexin

🍁 Euflex

Drug class.: Antineoplastic

Action: Interferes with testosterone at the cellular level; inhibits androgen uptake by inhibiting nuclear binding or by interfering with androgen in target tissues

Uses: Metastatic prostatic carcinoma, stage D2; early-stage prostate cancer, stages B2 and C, in combination with LHRH agonistic analogs (leuprolide) and radiation

Dosage and routes:

- *Adult:* PO 250 mg q8h, for a daily dose of 750 mg

Available forms include: Caps 125 mg

Side effects/adverse reactions:

CNS: Hot flashes, drowsiness, confusion, depression, anxiety

GI: Diarrhea, nausea, vomiting, ***hepatitis, liver failure,*** increased liver function studies, anorexia

GU: Decreased libido, impotence, gynecomastia

INTEG: Irritation at site, rash, photosensitivity

MISC: Edema, hematopoietic symptoms, neuromuscular and pulmonary symptoms, hypertension

Contraindications: Hypersensitivity, severe hepatic impairment, pregnancy category D

Precautions: Liver toxicity, monitoring requirements for hepatic injury, women

Pharmacokinetics: Rapidly and completely absorbed, half-life 6 hr, geriatric half-life 8 hr; 94% bound to plasma proteins; excreted in urine and feces as metabolites

DENTAL CONSIDERATIONS

General:

- Talk with patient about any pain medication being taken.
- Avoid drugs (anticholinergics) that could exacerbate urinary retention (if present).

fluticasone propionate

(floo-tik'a-sone)

Nasal spray: Flonase, *oral inhalation:* Flovent, Flovent Rotadisk, Flovent Diskus

Drug class.: Synthetic corticosteroid, medium potency

Action: Glucocorticoids have multiple actions that include anti-inflammatory and immunosuppressant effects. They inhibit phospholipase A_2, interfering with or reducing the synthesis of prostaglandins and leukotrienes. They also bind to cytoplasmic GRs and enter the cell nucleus to bind with DNA. This results in the synthesis of various enzymes such as collagenase, elastase, and cytokines that play important roles in inflammation control and immunosuppression. They also suppress the production of lymphocytes, monocytes, and eosinophils.

Uses:

Nasal spray: For management of nasal symptoms of seasonal and perennial allergic and nonallergic rhinitis in adults and pediatric patient 4 yr and older

Oral inhalation: For maintenance treatment of asthma as prophylactic therapy; also indicated for patients requiring oral glucocorticoid therapy

Dosage and routes:

Nasal spray:

- *Adult:* Initial dose, 2 sprays in each nostril once daily; initial dose can also be given in 2 equal doses (8 AM and 8 PM); reduce to 1 spray per nostril for maintenance

Oral inhalation:

- *Adults and adolescents with previous asthma therapy (Rotadisk or*

Diskus): INH 100 to 250 μg bid; max dose 500 μg bid
• *Child 4-11 yr:* INH 50 μg bid; max dose 100 μg bid
• *Adults and child >12 yr (Flovent inhaler):* INH 88-220 μg bid; max dose 440 μg bid

Available forms include: Nasal spray 50 μg per actuation (16 g); Flovent inh 44, 110, 220 μg per actuation in 7.9, 13 g; Rotadisk inh powder 50, 100, 250 μg per actuation (15 disk per pkg); Diskus inh powder 50, 100, 250 μg per actuation (device with 28 or 60 blisters)

Side effects/adverse reactions:
▼ *ORAL:* Oral candidiasis (INH product)
CNS: Headache
GI: Nausea, vomiting
RESP: URI, cough, bronchitis
HEMA: Epistaxis (nasal use)
EENT: Pharyngitis, throat irritation, rhinitis
INTEG: Rash
MS: Muscle pain (nonspecific)
MISC: Angioedema (rare)

Contraindications: Hypersensitivity, oral INH as a primary drug for status asthmaticus or other acute asthmatic episodes

Precautions: Suppression of hypothalamic-pituitary-adrenal axis, warning of manifestation of HPA suppression when switching drug from oral to inhaled steroids, suppression of growth in children <4 yr; use is restricted for some dose forms to children >12 yr; pregnancy category C, lactation

Pharmacokinetics:
INH/spray: Bioavailability of nasal spray <2%, oral inhalation <1%; high plasma protein binding (91%), metabolized by CYP3A4 enzymes, metabolites excreted in urine and feces

Drug interactions of concern to dentistry:
• No specific interactions reported, but use inhibitors of CYP3A4 with caution (see Appendix I)

DENTAL CONSIDERATIONS
General:
• Examine oral cavity for evidence of opportunistic candidiasis in patients using the inhaler.
• Allergic rhinitis may be a factor in mouth breathing and drying of oral tissues.
• Be aware that aspirin or sulfite preservatives in vasoconstrictor-containing products can exacerbate asthma.
• Acute asthmatic episodes may be precipitated in the dental office. Rapid-acting sympathomimetic inhalants should be available for emergency use. A stress reduction protocol may be required.
• Consider semisupine chair position for patients with respiratory disease.

Consultations:
• Consultation may be required to confirm steroid dose and duration of use.

Teach patient/family:
• Importance of updating health and drug history if physician makes any changes in drug regimens
• Importance of gargling, rinsing mouth with water, and expectorating after each aerosol use

fluticasone propionate

(floo-tik'a-sone)
Cutivate

Drug class.: Synthetic glucocorticoid, medium potency

Action: Glucocorticoids have multiple actions that include antiinflammatory and immunosuppressant effects. They inhibit phospholipase A_2, interfering with or reducing the synthesis of prostaglandins and leukotrienes. They also bind to cytoplasmic GRs and enter the cell nucleus to bind with DNA. This results in the synthesis of various enzymes such as collagenase, elastase, and cytokines that play important roles in inflammation control and immunosuppression. They also suppress the production of lymphocytes, monocytes, and eosinophils.

Uses: Relief of inflammatory and pruritic manifestations of glucocorticoid-responsive dermatoses

Dosage and routes:

Cream only:

• *Adult and pediatric patients >3 mo:* TOP apply a thin film of cream to affected area of skin bid; do not use occlusive dressing or on diapered area of infants

Ointment:

• *Adults:* TOP apply a thin film of ointment to affected areas of the skin bid; not for use in children

Available forms include: Cream 0.05%; oint 0.005% in 15, 30, 60 g tubes

Side effects/adverse reactions:

INTEG: Pruritus, dryness, burning, infection, eczema, atopic dermatitis, folliculitis, perioral dermatitis

MISC: Finger numbness

Contraindications: Hypersensitivity

Precautions: Suppression of the hypothalamic-pituitary-adrenal axis, concurrent skin infections, skin atrophy, pregnancy category C, caution when nursing; ointment not approved for use in pediatric patients; cream can be used in children 3 mo or older, but limit use to no longer than 4 wk

Pharmacokinetics:

TOP: Measureable absorption from skin sites (occlusive dressing enhances systemic absorption); any absorbed drug is metabolized by CYP3A4 enzymes, excretion routes include renal and fecal

DENTAL CONSIDERATIONS

Teach patient/family:

• That use of topical preparations on fungal or herpetic lesions is contraindicated

fluvastatin sodium

(floo'va-sta-tin)

Lescol, Lescol XL

Drug class.: Cholesterol-lowering agent, antihyperlipidemic

Action: Inhibits HMG-Co A reductase enzyme, which reduces cholesterol synthesis; reduced synthesis of VLDL; plasma triglyceride levels may also be decreased

Uses: As an adjunct in homozygous familial hypercholesterolemia, mixed hyperlipidemia, elevated serum triglyceride levels and type IV hyperproteinemia, also reduces total cholesterol LDL-C, apo B and triglyceride levels; patient should first be placed on cholesterol-lowering diet; to reduce risk in coronary artery revascularization procedures; prevention of secondary coronary events

Dosage and routes:

• *Adult:* PO initial 20-40 mg/day hs; dosage range 20-80 mg/day; ext rel tabs 80 mg as starting dose; with larger goal for LDL reduction 80 mg/day hs can be used

Risk reduction in coronary artery revascularization procedures:
• *Adult:* PO 40 mg bid or 80 mg/day
Available forms include: Caps 20, 40 mg; ext rel tabs 80 mg
Side effects/adverse reactions:
▼ *ORAL:* Taste alteration (rare)
CNS: Fatigue, headache, dizziness, insomnia
GI: ***Nausea, diarrhea, dyspepsia, abdominal pain, constipation, flatulence,*** elevated transaminase levels
RESP: Upper respiratory infection, bronchitis, coughing
GU: Decreased libido
EENT: Rhinitis, sinusitis, pharyngitis
INTEG: Rash, pruritus
MS: Muscle pain, back pain, arthropathy, ***rhabdomyolysis,*** myopathy
MISC: Photosensitivity, ***anaphylaxis***
Contraindications: Hypersensitivity, active liver disease, pregnancy, lactation, child <18 yr
Precautions: Pregnancy category X; liver dysfunction; alcoholism; severe acute infection; metabolic, endocrine, or electrolyte disorders; uncontrolled seizures; alterations in liver function tests may be observed with use
Pharmacokinetics:
PO: Absolute bioavailability 24%, peak plasma levels <1 hr, first-pass metabolism; highly protein bound (8%), hepatic metabolism (CYP2C9 and to a lesser extent CYP2C8, CYP3A4 isoenzymes); excreted in feces
Drug interactions of concern to dentistry:
• Increased plasma levels: alcohol, fluconazole, itraconazole, ketoconazole, erythromycin (see Appendix I)
DENTAL CONSIDERATIONS
General:
• Consider semisupine chair position for patient comfort because of GI, musculoskeletal, and respiratory side effects.

F

fluvoxamine maleate

(floo-vox'a-meen)
Luvox
Drug class.: Selective serotonin reuptake inhibitor, antidepressant

Action: Selectively inhibits the reuptake of serotonin in CNS neurons
Uses: Obsessive-compulsive disorder and panic disorder
Dosage and routes:
• *Adult:* PO initial dose 50 mg hs, increase by 50 mg increments slowly q4-7d as required in 2 divided doses; limit 300 mg/day
• *Child 8-17 yr:* PO 25 mg hs; can increase dose in 25 mg increments q 4-7 days in two divided doses, limit 200 mg/day
Available forms include: Tabs 25, 50, 100 mg
Side effects/adverse reactions:
▼ *ORAL: Dry mouth,* dysphagia, increased salivation (rare)
CNS: Somnolence, asthenia, nervousness, dizziness, headache, agitation, anxiety, suicidal ideation, anorexia
CV: Postural hypotension, palpitation, hypertension, syncope, tachycardia
GI: Nausea, dyspepsia, diarrhea
GU: Sexual dysfunction
RESP: Dyspnea
MS: Dystonic symptoms

Contraindications: Hypersensitivity, MAOIs, alcohol
Precautions: Pregnancy category C, lactation, renal and hepatic impairment, epilepsy, elderly
Pharmacokinetics:
PO: Rapid absorption, peak plasma levels 5 hr; plasma protein binding 77%; hepatic metabolism; urinary excretion
Drug interactions of concern to dentistry:
• Increased plasma levels of tricyclic antidepressants, carbamazepine, benzodiazepine; reduce doses of alprazolam, diazepam, midazolam, and triazolam by one half
• Risk of serotonin syndrome: SSRIs
• First-time users of SSRIs also taking NSAIDs may have a higher risk of GI side effects; until more data are available, it may be advisable to avoid use of NSAIDs in these patients (*Br J Clin Pharmacol* 55:591-595, 2003)
DENTAL CONSIDERATIONS
General:
• After supine positioning, have patient sit upright for at least 2 min to avoid orthostatic hypotension.
• Assess salivary flow as a factor in caries, periodontal disease, and candidiasis.
• Consider semisupine chair position for patient comfort because of GI effects of drug.
Consultations:
• Medical consultation may be required to assess patient's ability to tolerate stress.
• Physician should be informed if significant xerostomic side effects occur (e.g., increased caries, sore tongue, problems eating or swallowing, difficulty wearing prosthesis) so that a medication change can be considered.
Teach patient/family:
When chronic dry mouth occurs, advise patient:
• To avoid mouth rinses with high alcohol content because of drying effects
• To use daily home fluoride products for anticaries effect
• To use sugarless gum, frequent sips of water, or saliva substitutes

---

folic acid (vitamin B_9)

(foe'lic)
Folvite
✦ Apo-Folic, Novo-Folacid
Drug class.: Water-soluble B vitamin

Action: Needed for erythropoiesis; increases RBC, WBC, and platelet formation in megaloblastic anemias
Uses: Megaloblastic or macrocytic anemia caused by folic acid deficiency; liver disease; alcoholism; hemolysis; intestinal obstruction; pregnancy
Dosage and routes:
Recommended dietary allowance:
• *Adult male:* PO 0.15-0.2 mg/day
• *Adult female:* PO 0.15-0.18 mg/day
Chemical supplement:
• *Adult:* PO/IM/SC 0.1 mg qd
• *Child:* PO 0.05 mg qd
Megaloblastic/macrocytic anemia:
• *Adult and child 4 yr and older:* PO/SC/IM 0.4 mg/day
• *Child <4 yr:* PO/SC/IM 0.3 mg or less qd
• *Infant:* PO/SC/IM 0.1 mg qd
• *Pregnancy/lactation:* PO/SC/IM 0.8 mg qd

Prevention of megaloblastic/macrocytic anemia:
• *Pregnancy:* PO/SC/IM 1 mg qd
Available forms include: Tabs 0.4, 0.8, 1 mg; inj SC/IM 5 mg/ml
Side effects/adverse reactions:
RESP: ***Bronchospasm*** (rare allergic reaction)
Contraindications: Hypersensitivity, anemias other than megaloblastic/macrocytic anemia, vitamin B_{12} deficiency anemia
Precautions: Pregnancy category A
Pharmacokinetics:
PO: Peak 0.5-1 hr; bound to plasma proteins; excreted in breast milk; methylated in liver; excreted in urine (small amounts)
Drug interactions of concern to dentistry:
• Increased metabolism of phenobarbital
DENTAL CONSIDERATIONS
General:
• Deficiency in folic acid; glossitis may be a symptom of folic acid deficiency.

---

fondaparinux sodium
(fon-da'-par-in-no)
Arixtra
Drug class.: Synthetic anticoagulant

Action: Selectively binds to antithrombin III (ATIII) to inhibit activated factor Xα resulting in inhibition of thrombus formation and development
Uses: Prophylaxis of deep vein thrombosis in patients undergoing hip fracture surgery, hip replacement surgery, or knee replacement surgery
Dosage and routes:
• *Adult:* SC after establishment of hemostasis, 2.5 mg once daily 6-8 hr after surgery; duration of use 6-9 days
Available forms include: Single-dose syringe 2.5 mg/0.5 ml
Side effects/adverse reactions:
CNS: Insomnia, dizziness, confusion, headache
CV: Edema, hypotension
GI: Nausea, constipation, vomiting, diarrhea, dyspepsia
HEMA: ***Hemorrhage,*** injection site bleeding, anemia, hematoma, postoperative bleeding, major bleeding events
GU: UTI
INTEG: Rash, pruritus, bullous eruption
META: Increase in AST, ALT, hypokalemia
MISC: Fever, pain
Contraindications: Hypersensitivity, renal impairment, body weight <50 kg, major bleeding problems, endocarditis, thrombocytopenia
Precautions: Neuroaxial (spinal/epidural) anesthesia, avoid IM use, anticoagulant effects persist for 2-4 days after administration, elderly patients, pregnancy category B, no data available for nursing mothers, use in children has not been established
Pharmacokinetics:
SC: Absolute bioavailability 100%, peak levels ≈2 hr; excreted unchanged in urine (77% over 72 hr)
Drug interactions of concern to dentistry:
• Avoid concurrent use of aspirin and NSAIDs

DENTAL CONSIDERATIONS

General:

• Determine why patient is taking the drug.

• Monitor vital signs at every appointment because of cardiovascular side effects.

• Consider local hemostasis measures to prevent excessive bleeding.

• Antibiotic prophylaxis before dental treatment may be required for joint prosthesis. See 2003 ADA guidelines.

• Delay elective dental treatment until patient completes anticoagulant therapy.

Consultations:

• Medical consultation should include routine blood counts, including platelet counts and bleeding time.

Teach patient/family:

• Importance of good oral hygiene to prevent soft tissue inflammation/infection

• To prevent injury when using oral hygiene aids

• To report oral lesions, soreness, or bleeding to dentist

---

formoterol fumarate inhalation powder

(for-moh'te-rol)

Foradil Aerolizer

🍁 Oxeze

Drug class.: Selective β_2-adrenergic bronchodilator

Action: A long-acting, selective β_2-adrenergic agonist that acts locally in the lung as a bronchodilator, resulting in bronchial smooth muscle relaxation and inhibition of release of inflammatory mediators

Uses: Long-term treatment of asthma and prevention of bronchospasm in adults and children >5 yr; prevention of exercise-induced bronchospasm in adults and children >12 yr; maintenance treatment of COPD

Dosage and routes:

Maintenance treatment of asthma/bronchospasm:

• *Adult and child >5 yr:* INH: inhale the contents of one capsule (12 μg) q12h using the Aerolizer Inhaler System; , do not exceed this dose; not for oral use

Prevention of exercise-induced bronchospasm (EIB):

• *Adult and child >12 yr:* INH: inhale the contents of one capsule (12 mg) 15 min before exercise, administered on prn basis

COPD maintenance treatment:

• *Adult:* INH inhale the contents of one capsule (12 μg) q12h using the Aerolizer Inhaler System

Available forms include: Caps 12 μg for use only by inhalation in the Aerolizer Inhaler System

Side effects/adverse reactions:

▼ *ORAL:* Dry mouth, irritation of mouth and throat, taste alteration

CNS: Tremor, dizziness, insomnia, nervousness, headache

CV: Angina, hypertension, tachycardia, arrhythmias, palpitation

GI: Nausea, dyspepsia, abdominal pain, vomiting

RESP: Bronchitis, URI, dyspnea, exacerbation of asthma, coughing

EENT: Tonsillitis

INTEG: Rash, urticaria

META: Hypokalemia, hyperglycemia, metabolic acidosis

MISC: Viral infection, ***immediate hypersensitivity reaction (anaphylaxis), angioedema***

Contraindications: Hypersensitivity

Precautions: Not for acute asthma symptoms, not for use in life-threatening situations; paradoxic bronchospasm may occur with use; not a substitute for corticosteroids; cardiovascular disease (coronary insufficiency, cardiac arrhythmias, hypertension), hyperthyroidism, seizures, hypokalemia, pregnancy category C, lactation

Pharmacokinetics:

INH: Rapid absorption, peak plasma levels 5 min; plasma protein binding 61%-64%; extensive hepatic metabolism (CYP2D6, CYP2C19, CYP2C9, CYP2A6 isoenzymes), excreted mostly in urine (62%) and in feces (34%), onset 1-3 min, peak effects 2 hr with duration 8-12 hr

Drug interactions of concern to dentistry:

• Avoid MAOIs, tricyclic antidepressants, and drugs that prolong the QT interval (phenothiazines, procainamide) (see Appendix I)

• Adrenergic agents/sympathomimetics may potentiate effects

• Beta-adrenergic blockers may antagonize sympathomimetic effects

DENTAL CONSIDERATIONS

General:

• Monitor vital signs at every appointment because of cardiovascular side effects.

• Assess salivary flow as a factor in caries, periodontal disease, and candidiasis.

• Consider semisupine chair position for patient comfort because of respiratory side effects of disease.

• Short midday appointments and a stress reduction protocol may be required for anxious patients.

• Have patient bring personal short-acting bronchodilator to appointment for use in emergency.

• Acute asthmatic episodes may be precipitated in the dental office. Rapid-acting sympathomimetic inhalants should be available for emergency use.

• Avoid prescribing aspirin-containing products.

Consultations:

• Medical consultation may be required to assess disease control and patient's ability to tolerate stress.

Teach patient/family:

• Importance of gargling, rinsing mouth with water, and expectorating after each aerosol dose

When chronic dry mouth occurs, advise patient:

• To avoid mouth rinses with high alcohol content because of drying effects

• To use daily home fluoride products for anticaries effect

• To use sugarless gum, frequent sips of water, or saliva substitutes

---

foscarnet sodium (phosphonoformic acid)

(foss-car'net)

Foscavir

Drug class.: Antiviral

Action: Antiviral activity is produced by selective inhibition at the pyrophosphate binding site of viral DNA polymerase, preventing replication of herpes simplex virus (HSV)

Uses: Treatment of cytomegalovirus (CMV) retinitis in AIDS, acyclovir-resistant herpes simplex I mucocutaneous diseases, and acyclovir-resistant HSV in immunocompromised patients; unapproved: life-threatening CMV disease

Dosage and routes:

CMV retinitis:

• *Adult:* IV inf 90 mg/kg given over at least 1.5-2 hr q12h × 2-3 wk initially, then 90-120 mg/kg/day over 2 hr; or 60 mg/kg given over 1 hr q8h × 2-3 wk

HSV:

• *Adult:* IV inf 40 mg/kg bid/tid × 2-3 wk

Available forms include: Inj 24 mg/ml in 250, 500 ml bottles

Side effects/adverse reactions:

▼ *ORAL:* Glossitis, stomatitis, facial edema, dry mouth, ulcerative stomatitis, taste perversion

CNS: ***Seizures, coma, paralysis, tetany,*** fever, dizziness, headache, fatigue, neuropathy, tremor, ataxia, dementia, stupor, EEG abnormalities, vertigo, abnormal gait, hypertonia, extrapyramidal disorders, hemiparesis, hyperreflexia, paraplegia, hyporeflexia, neuralgia, neuritis, cerebral edema, paresthesia, depression, confusion, anxiety, insomnia, somnolence, amnesia, hallucinations, agitation

CV: ***Cardiac arrest,*** hypertension, palpitations, ECG abnormalities, first-degree AV block, nonspecific ST-T segment changes, hypotension, cerebrovascular disorder, cardiomyopathy, bradycardia, dysrhythmias

GI: ***Pseudomembranous colitis, paralytic ileus, esophageal ulceration, hepatitis,*** nausea, vomiting, anorexia, abdominal pain, constipation, dysphagia, rectal hemorrhage, melena, flatulence, pancreatitis, enteritis, enterocolitis, proctitis, increased amylases, gastroenteritis, duodenal ulcer, abnormal A-G ratio, increased AST/ALT, cholecystitis, dyspepsia, tenesmus, hepatosplenomegaly, jaundice

RESP: ***Pulmonary infiltration, pneumothorax, hemoptysis, bronchospasm, respiratory depression, pleural effusion, pulmonary hemorrhage,*** rhinitis, coughing, dyspnea, pneumonia, sinusitis, pharyngitis, bronchitis, stridor

HEMA: ***Granulocytopenia, leukopenia, thrombocytopenia, thrombosis, pulmonary embolism, coagulation disorders, decreased prothrombin, hypochromic anemia, pancytopenia, hemolysis, leukocytosis,*** lymphadenopathy, epistaxis, lymphopenia, anemia, platelet abnormalities

GU: ***Acute renal failure, glomerulonephritis, toxic nephropathy, nephrosis, renal tubular disorders, pyelonephritis, uremia, hematuria, albuminuria,*** dysuria, polyuria, decreased CCr, increased serum creatinine

EENT: Visual field defects, vocal cord paralysis, speech disorders, eye pain, conjunctivitis, tinnitus, otitis

INTEG: Rash, sweating, pruritus, skin ulceration, seborrhea, skin discoloration, alopecia, acne, dermatitis, pain/inflammation at injection site, facial edema, dry skin, urticaria

MS: Arthralgia, myalgia

SYST: ***Sepsis, death, ascites,*** hypokalemia, hypocalcemia, hypomagnesemia, increased alk phosphatase, LDH, BUN, acidosis, hypophosphatemia, hyperphosphatemia, dehydration, glycosuria, increased creatine phosphokinase, hypervolemia, infection, hyponatremia, hypochloremia, hypercalcemia

Contraindications: Hypersensitivity

Precautions: Pregnancy category C, lactation, children, elderly, renal disease, seizure disorders, electrolyte/mineral imbalances, severe anemia; monitor for renal impairment

Pharmacokinetics:

IV: Half-life 2-8 hr in normal renal function; 14%-17% plasma protein bound

Drug interactions of concern to dentistry:

• Avoid nephrotoxic drugs (amphotericin B)

• Possible increased risk of seizures: fluoroquinolones

DENTAL CONSIDERATIONS

General:

• Examine for oral manifestations of opportunistic infections.

• Examine for evidence of oral manifestations of blood dyscrasias (infection, bleeding, poor healing).

• Consider local hemostasis measures to prevent excessive bleeding.

• Assess salivary flow as a factor in caries, periodontal disease, and candidiasis.

• Monitor vital signs at every appointment because of cardiovascular and respiratory side effects.

• Place on frequent recall to evaluate healing response.

Consultations:

• Medical consultation for blood studies (CBC); leukopenic or thrombocytopenic side effects may result in infection, delayed healing, and excessive bleeding. Postpone elective dental treatment until normal values are maintained.

• Medical consultation may be required to assess disease control.

Teach patient/family:

• Caution in use of oral hygiene aids to prevent injury

• That secondary oral infection may occur; must see dentist immediately if infection occurs

• Importance of good oral hygiene to prevent soft tissue inflammation

• Use of electric toothbrush if patient has difficulty holding conventional devices because of extrapyramidal side effects

When chronic dry mouth occurs, advise patient:

• To avoid mouth rinses with high alcohol content because of drying effects

• To use daily home fluoride products for anticaries effect

• To use sugarless gum, frequent sips of water, or saliva substitutes

---

fosfomycin tromethamine

(fos-foe-mye'sin)

Monurol

Drug class.: Antiinfective (phosphonic acid derivative)

Action: Broad-spectrum and bactericidal against a wide range of gram-positive aerobic microorganisms associated with GU infections; inactivates the enzyme diphosphate acetylglucosamine to interfere with cell wall synthesis

Uses: Uncomplicated UTIs in women caused by susceptible strains of *E. coli* and *Enterococcus faecalis*

Dosage and routes:

Women >18 yr: PO one sachet with or without food; mix contents of one sachet with water and drink mixture

Available forms include: Sachet 3 g

Side effects/adverse reactions:

▼ *ORAL:* Dry mouth (<1%)

CNS: Headache, dizziness, migraine, somnolence
GI: Diarrhea, nausea, dyspepsia
RESP: Asthma (rare)
HEMA: ***Angioedema (rare), aplastic anemia***
GU: Vaginitis
EENT: Rhinitis, pharyngitis
INTEG: Rash
ENDO: Menstrual disorder
MS: Asthenia, myalgia
MISC: Fever
Contraindications: Hypersensitivity
Precautions: Renal impairment, one dose per single episode of cystitis, pregnancy category B, lactation, children <12 yr
Pharmacokinetics:
PO: Peak plasma levels >2 hr; not plasma protein bound; widely distributed to GU tissues; excreted unchanged in urine and feces
Drug interactions of concern to dentistry:
• Lowered serum concentrations: metoclopramide
DENTAL CONSIDERATIONS
General:
• Determine why patient is taking the drug.
• Consider semisupine chair position for patient comfort if GI side effects occur.
Teach patient/family:
When chronic dry mouth occurs, advise patient:
• To avoid mouth rinses with high alcohol content because of drying effects
• To use daily home fluoride products for anticaries effect
• To use sugarless gum, frequent sips of water, or saliva substitutes

fosinopril

(foe-sin'oh-pril)
Monopril
Drug class.: Angiotension-converting enzyme (ACE) inhibitor

Action: Selectively suppresses renin-angiotensin-aldosterone system; inhibits ACE; prevents conversion of angiotensin I to angiotensin II; results in dilation of arterial, venous vessels
Uses: Hypertension, alone or in combination with thiazide diuretics, management of heart failure
Dosage and routes:
• *Adult:* PO 10 mg qd initially, then 20-40 mg/day divided bid or qd
Available forms include: Tabs 10, 20, 40 mg
Side effects/adverse reactions:
▼ *ORAL:* Taste disturbances, angioedema (lips, tongue), dry mouth
CNS: Insomnia, paresthesia, headache, dizziness, fatigue, memory disturbance, tremor, mood change
CV: Hypotension, chest pain, palpitation, angina, orthostatic hypotension
GI: Nausea, constipation, vomiting, diarrhea
RESP: **Bronchospasm,** cough, sinusitis, dyspnea
HEMA: ***Eosinophilia, leukopenia, neutropenia,*** decreased Hct/Hgb
GU: ***Proteinuria,*** increased BUN/creatinine, decreased libido
INTEG: **Angioedema,** rash, flushing, sweating, photosensitivity, pruritus
MS: Arthralgia, myalgia
META: Hyperkalemia
Contraindications: Hypersensitivity to ACE inhibitors, pregnancy category D, lactation, children

Precautions: Impaired liver function, hypovolemia, blood dyscrasias, CHF, COPD, asthma, elderly

Pharmacokinetics:

PO: Onset 1 hr, peak 3 hr, half-life 12 hr; serum protein binding 97%; metabolized by liver; metabolites excreted in urine, feces

Drug interactions of concern to dentistry:

• Increased hypotension: alcohol, phenothiazines

• Decreased hypotensive effects: indomethacin and possibly other NSAIDs, sympathomimetics

• Suspected reduction in the antihypertensive and vasodilator effects by salicylates; monitor blood pressure if used concurrently

DENTAL CONSIDERATIONS

General:

• Monitor vital signs at every appointment because of cardiovascular and respiratory side effects.

• After supine positioning, have patient sit upright for at least 2 min before standing to avoid orthostatic hypotension.

• Patients on chronic drug therapy may rarely have symptoms of blood dyscrasias, which can include infection, bleeding, and poor healing.

• Assess salivary flow as a factor in caries, periodontal disease, and candidiasis.

• Limit use of sodium-containing products such as saline IV fluids for patients with a dietary salt restriction.

• Stress from dental procedures may compromise cardiovascular function; determine patient risk.

• Short appointments and a stress reduction protocol may be required for anxious patients.

Consultations:

• Medical consultation may be required to assess disease control and patient's ability to tolerate stress.

• In a patient with symptoms of blood dyscrasias, request a medical consultation for blood studies and postpone dental treatment until normal values are reestablished.

• Take precautions if dental surgery is anticipated and sedation or general anesthesia is required (risk of hypotensive episode).

Teach patient/family:

• Importance of good oral hygiene to prevent soft tissue inflammation

• Caution to prevent injury when using oral hygiene aids

When chronic dry mouth occurs, advise patient:

• To avoid mouth rinses with high alcohol content because of drying effects

• To use daily home fluoride products for anticaries effect

• To use sugarless gum, frequent sips of water, or saliva substitutes

---

fosphenytoin sodium

(fos'fen-i-toyn)

Cerebyx

Drug class.: Hydantoin-anticonvulsant

Action: Prodrug converted to phenytoin after injection; phenytoin inhibits spread of seizure activity in motor cortex

Uses: Control of generalized convulsive status epilepticus; prevention and treatment of seizures during neurosurgery; short-term substitute for oral phenytoin

Dosage and routes:

• *Adult:* IV loading dose, 15-20 mg phenytoin sodium equivalents (PE/kg) at 100-150 mg PE/min; effect is not immediate, may require use of IV benzodiazepine

• *Adult:* IV maintenance dose, IM 4-6 mg/PE/kg per day

Substitution for oral phenytoin:

• *Adult:* IV, IM at the same total daily dose for phenytoin

Available forms include: Inj 10 ml (750 mg of fosphenytoin sodium equivalent to 500 mg phenytoin); 2 ml (150 mg of fosphenytoin equivalent to 100 mg of phenytoin)

Side effects/adverse reactions:

▼ *ORAL:* Dry mouth, taste perversion, gingival overgrowth

CNS: Nystagmus, dizziness, paresthesia, headache, somnolence, ataxia, tremor, extrapyramidal syndrome

CV: Hypotension, bradycardia, vasodilation, tachycardia

GI: Nausea, vomiting, constipation

HEMA: ***Thrombocytopenia, anemia, leukopenia,*** petechia

EENT: Tinnitus, diplopia

INTEG: Pruritus, rash

MS: Asthenia, back pain

META: Hypokalemia

Contraindications: Hypersensitivity to hydantoin drugs; sinus bradycardia, S-A block, second- and third-degree AV block; Adams-Stokes syndrome, abrupt discontinuation

Precautions:

IV: Do not exceed injection rate of 150 mg PE/min, risk of seizures with abrupt withdrawal; hypotension, severe myocardial insufficiency, phosphate restriction; thyroid, renal, or hepatic disease; elderly, pregnancy category D, lactation, pediatric use

Pharmacokinetics:

IV: Highly protein bound (95%-99%); converted to phenytoin; metabolized in liver; renal excretion

IM: Completely bioavailable, peak levels 30 min

Drug interactions of concern to dentistry:

• Increased phenytoin levels: benzodiazepines (chlordiazepoxide, diazepam), halothane, salicylates

• Increased CNS depression: benzodiazepines, H_1-blocker antihistamines, opiate agonists

• Decreased phenytoin levels: carbamazepine, ciprofloxacin

• Decreased effectiveness of corticosteroids

• Suspected risk of hepatic toxicity: chronic use of acetaminophen and phosphenytoin

DENTAL CONSIDERATIONS

General:

• This drug is intended for short-term use in an emergency department or hospital setting. Patient will probably return to oral phenytoin or other anticonvulsant after hospital care.

• Use precaution if sedation or general anesthesia is required; risk of hypotensive episode.

Consultations:

• Determine type of epilepsy, seizure frequency, and quality of seizure control. A stress reduction protocol may be required.

• Medical consultation may be required to assess disease control and patient's ability to tolerate stress.

Teach patient/family:

• Importance of updating health and drug history if physician makes any changes in evaluation or drug regimens

frovatriptan succinate

(froe-va-trip'tan)

Frova

Drug class.: Serotonin receptor agonist

Action: A selective serotonin agonist for 5-HT_{1D} and 5-HT_{1B} serotonin receptors on intracranial blood vessels

Uses: Acute treatment of migraine with or without aura

Dosage and routes:

• *Adult:* PO 2.5 mg; if headache recurs after initial dose, a second tablet may be taken with an interval between doses of at least 2 hr; maximum daily dose 3 tabs

Available forms include: Tab 2.5 mg

Side effects/adverse reactions:

▼ *ORAL: Dry mouth,* taste alteration

CNS: Dizziness, fatigue, insomnia, anxiety

CV: Flushing, chest pain, ***risk of serious CV events (MI, ventricular tachycardia),*** palpitation

GI: Dyspepsia, vomiting, nausea, diarrhea, abdominal pain

EENT: Sinusitis, rhinitis, vision abnormalities, tinnitus

INTEG: Sweating

MS: Musculoskeletal pain

MISC: Peripheral paresthesia, hot or cold sensation

Contraindications: Hypersensitivity, ischemic heart disease (angina, MI), Prinzmetal's variant angina, cerebrovascular syndrome, uncontrolled hypertension within 24 hr of use of ergotamine or other 5HT_1 agonists, hemiplegic or basilar migraine, prophylactic therapy of migraine, Wolff-Parkinson-White syndrome, accessory conduction arrhythmias, MAOIs, peripheral vascular disease

Precautions: Renal impairment, hypertension, coronary artery disease, hypercholesterolemia, smoking, diabetes mellitus, men >40 yr, asthma, allergies, pregnancy category C, lactation, children, serotonin syndrome, risk of myocardial ischemia

Pharmacokinetics:

PO: Peak blood levels 2-4 hr; bioavailability 24%-30%; hepatic metabolism; urinary excretion

Drug interactions of concern to dentistry:

• Potential serotonin crisis: SSRIs, ergot-containing drugs (avoid use within 24 hr of taking this drug)

• Decreased plasma levels: cimetidine

DENTAL CONSIDERATIONS

General:

• This is an acute-use drug; it is doubtful that patients will seek dental treatment during acute migraine attacks.

• Be aware of patient's disease, its severity, and its frequency, when known.

• Advise patient if dental drugs prescribed have a potential for photosensitivity.

Consultations:

• If treating chronic orofacial pain, consult with physician of record.

• Medical consultation may be required to assess disease control and patient's ability to tolerate stress.

Teach patient/family:

• That dryness of the mouth may occur when taking this drug; avoid mouth rinses with high alcohol content because of additional drying effects

• Importance of updating health

and drug history if physician makes any changes in evaluation or drug regimens

furosemide

(fur-oh'se-mide)

Lasix

✤ Apo-Furosemide, Furoside, Lasix Special, Novosemide, Uritol

Drug class.: Loop diuretic

Action: Acts on loop of Henle to decrease the reabsorption of chloride and sodium with resultant diuresis

Uses: Pulmonary edema, edema in CHF, liver disease, nephrotic syndrome, ascites, hypertension

Dosage and routes:

Edema:

• *Adult:* PO 20-80 mg/day in AM, may give another dose in 6 hr, up to 600 mg/day; IM/IV 20-40 mg, increased by 20 mg q2h until desired response

Hypertension:

• *Adult:* PO 40 mg bid

• *Child:* PO/IM/IV 2 mg/kg, may increase by 1-2 mg/kg q6-8h up to 6 mg/kg

Pulmonary edema:

• *Adult:* IV 40 mg given over several minutes, repeated in 1 hr; increase to 80 mg if needed

Available forms include: Tabs 20, 40, 80 mg; oral sol 10 mg/ml, 40 mg/5 ml; inj IM/IV 10 mg/ml

Side effects/adverse reactions:

▼ *ORAL:* Dry mouth, increased thirst, lichenoid drug reaction

CNS: Headache, fatigue, weakness, vertigo, paresthesia

CV: ***Circulatory collapse,*** orthostatic hypotension, chest pain, ECG changes

GI: Nausea, diarrhea, vomiting, anorexia, cramps, gastric irritations, pancreatitis

HEMA: ***Thrombocytopenia, agranulocytosis, leukopenia, neutropenia, anemia***

GU: Polyuria, **renal failure,** glycosuria

EENT: Loss of hearing, ear pain, tinnitus, blurred vision

INTEG: ***Rash, pruritus, Stevens-Johnson syndrome,*** purpura, sweating, photosensitivity, urticaria

ENDO: ***Hyperglycemia***

MS: Cramps, arthritis, stiffness

ELECT: Hypokalemia, hypochloremic alkalosis, hypomagnesemia, hyperuricemia, hypocalcemia, hyponatremia

Contraindications: Hypersensitivity to sulfonamides, anuria, hypovolemia, infants, lactation, electrolyte depletion

Precautions: Diabetes mellitus, dehydration, ascites, severe renal disease, pregnancy category C

Pharmacokinetics:

PO: Onset 1 hr, peak 1-2 hr, duration 6-8 hr

IV: Onset 5 min, peak 0.5 hr, duration 2 hr

Excreted in urine, feces, breast milk; crosses placenta

Drug interactions of concern to dentistry:

• Increased electrolyte imbalance: corticosteroids

• Masked ototoxicity: phenothiazines

• Decreased antihypertensive effect: NSAIDs, especially indomethacin

DENTAL CONSIDERATIONS

General:

• Monitor vital signs at every appointment because of cardiovascular side effects.

• Patients on chronic drug therapy may rarely have symptoms of blood dyscrasias, which can include infection, bleeding, and poor healing.

• Assess salivary flow as a factor in caries, periodontal disease, and candidiasis.

• After supine positioning, have patient sit upright for at least 2 min before standing to avoid orthostatic hypotension.

• Patients on high-potency diuretics should be monitored for serum K^+ levels.

Consultations:

• In a patient with symptoms of blood dyscrasias, request a medical consultation for blood studies and postpone dental treatment until normal values are reestablished.

• Medical consultation may be required to assess disease control.

Teach patient/family:

• Importance of good oral hygiene to prevent soft tissue inflammation

• Caution to prevent injury when using oral hygiene aids

When chronic dry mouth occurs, advise patient:

• To use daily home fluoride products for anticaries effect

• To avoid mouth rinses with high alcohol content because of drying effects

• To use sugarless gum, frequent sips of water, or saliva substitutes

gabapentin

(ga'ba-pen-tin)

Neurontin

Drug class.: Anticonvulsant, analgesic

Action: Neither the anticonvulsant nor the analgesic mechanism of action has been described, although these effects are observed in laboratory models

Uses: Adjunctive therapy in patients 12 yr or older with partial seizures with or without secondary generalization and as adjunctive therapy for partial seizures in children 3-12 yr; postherpetic neuralgia in adults; unlabeled use: bipolar disorder, migraine prophylaxis, tremors of multiple sclerosis

Dosage and routes:

Epilepsy:

• *Adult and child >12 yr:* PO titration to 900-1800 mg/day in 3 equal doses; start 300 mg on day 1, 300 mg bid on day 2, 300 mg tid on day 3, can be increased to 1800 mg/day with titration of doses

• *Child 3-12 yr:* PO initial dose 10-15 mg/kg/day in 3 equal doses; titrated dose upward over 3-day period

Postherpetic neuralgia:

• *Adult:* PO initiate dose with 300 mg on day 1, 300 mg bid on day 2, and 300 mg tid on day 3; doses can be titrated up to 1800 mg/day

Available forms include: Caps 100, 300, 400 mg; tabs 600 mg; oral sol 250 mg/5 ml

Side effects/adverse reactions:

▼ *ORAL:* Dry mouth, glossitis, gingivitis, stomatitis (infrequent)

CNS: Somnolence, dizziness, ataxia, fatigue, nystagmus

CV: Hypertension, palpitation, tachycardia
GI: Dyspepsia, constipation
RESP: Pharyngitis, coughing
HEMA: Leukopenia, purpura
GU: Impotence
EENT: Rhinitis, blurred vision
INTEG: Pruritus
MS: Myalgia
MISC: Edema

Contraindications: Hypersensitivity

Precautions: Pregnancy category C, lactation, renal function impairment, children <12 yr, elderly

Pharmacokinetics: Bioavailability decreases as dose increases; low protein binding, 3%; primarily renal excretion

Drug interactions of concern to dentistry:

• None reported at this time, but, because CNS side effects are common, the use of anxiolytic sedative drugs may potentially increase the CNS side effects.

DENTAL CONSIDERATIONS

General:

• Early-morning appointments and a stress reduction protocol may be required for anxious patients.

• Place on frequent recall because of oral side effects.

• Monitor vital signs at every appointment because of cardiovascular side effects.

• Assess salivary flow as a factor in caries, periodontal disease, and candidiasis.

• Determine type of epilepsy and quality of seizure control.

Consultations:

• Medical consultation may be required to assess disease control.

• Medical consultation may be required to assess patient's ability to tolerate stress.

Teach patient/family:

• Importance of good oral hygiene to prevent soft tissue inflammation

• Caution in use of oral hygiene aids to prevent injury

When chronic dry mouth occurs, advise patient:

• To avoid mouth rinses with high alcohol content because of drying effects

• To use daily home fluoride products for anticaries effect

• To use sugarless gum, frequent sips of water, or saliva substitutes

---

galantamine HBr

(ga-lan'ta-meen)

Reminyl

Drug class.: Cholinesterase inhibitor

Action: Exact mechanism unclear, but it is thought to be a competitive, long-acting, and reversible inhibitor of acetylcholinesterase enzyme; inhibits acetylcholinesterase activity at peripheral and central cholinergic synapses and in PNS; potentiates nicotinic receptor response to acetylcholine

Uses: Mild to moderate dementia of Alzheimer's disease

Dosage and routes:

• *Adult:* PO starting dose is 4 mg bid; increase dose to 8 mg bid after a 4 wk minimum treatment period; increases to 12 mg bid should be attempted only after a minimum of 4 wk; increase dose only if the lower dose is tolerated; dose range 16-24 mg/day in two equal doses preferably with AM and PM meals;

with moderate renal or hepatic impairment dose should not exceed 16 mg/day (severe impairment do not use)

Available forms include: Tabs 4, 8, 12 mg; oral sol 4 mg/ml in 100 ml

Side effects/adverse reactions:

CNS: Anorexia, dizziness, headache, tremor, depression, insomnia, somnolence, agitation, confusion, fatigue

CV: Syncope, bradycardia, peripheral edema, chest pain

GI: Nausea, vomiting, diarrhea, abdominal pain, dyspepsia, constipation, flatulence

RESP: URI, bronchitis

HEMA: Anemia

GU: UTI, hematuria, incontinence

EENT: Rhinitis

ENDO: Weight loss, sweating

Contraindications: Hypersensitivity, severe hepatic or renal impairment

Precautions: Potentiation of succinylcholine-like neuromuscular blocking drugs, obstructive GI disease, Parkinson's disease, epilepsy, cardiac conduction disorders, AV block, bradycardia, history of GI ulcer, hypersecretory disorders (gastric), bladder outflow obstruction, COPD, asthma, moderate hepatic impairment, moderate renal impairment, pregnancy category B, lactation, pediatric use

Pharmacokinetics:

PO: Absolute bioavailability ~90%, peak plasma levels 1 hr, plasma protein binding 18%; hepatic metabolism (CYP450 2D6 and CYP450 3A4 isoenzymes); unchanged drug and glucuronate metabolites, excreted in urine

Drug interactions of concern to dentistry:

- Increased plasma levels: ketoconazole
- Increased bioavailability: cimetidine, paroxetine
- Enhanced succinylcholine muscle relaxation during anesthesia
- Action may be inhibited by anticholinergic drugs or enhanced by cholinergic agonists

DENTAL CONSIDERATIONS

General:

- Monitor vital signs at every appointment because of cardiovascular side effects.
- After supine positioning, have patient sit upright for 2 min or longer to avoid orthostatic hypotension.
- Drug is used early in the disease; ensure that patient or care giver understands informed consent.
- Place on frequent recall because early attention to dental health is important for Alzheimer's patients.
- Consider semisupine chair position for patient comfort if GI side effects occur.

Consultations:

- Consultation with physician may be needed if sedation or general anesthesia is required.
- Medical consultation may be required to assess disease control and patient's ability to tolerate stress.

Teach patient/family:

- Importance of good oral hygiene to prevent soft tissue inflammation
- To assist patient or care giver with oral home-care regimen as cognitive ability declines
- Use of electric toothbrush if patient has difficulty holding conventional devices
- Importance of updating health

and drug history if physician makes any changes in evaluation or drug regimens

ganciclovir (DHPG)

(gan-sye'kloe-veer)

Cytovene, Cytovene IV, Vitrasert implant

Drug class.: Antiviral, nucleoside analog

Action: Inhibits replication of most herpes viruses in vitro; phosphorylated by CMV protein kinase to triphosphate forms; inhibits viral DNA polymerase and is incorporated into viral DNA, resulting in termination of elongation of viral DNA

Uses: Prevention and treatment of CMV retinitis in patients with AIDS or organ transplants; life-threatening CMV disease

Dosage and routes:

Induction treatment:

• *Adult:* IV 5 mg/kg given over 1 hr, q12h × 2-3 wk

Maintenance treatment:

• *Adult:* IV inf 5 mg/kg given over 1 hr, qd × 7 days/wk; or 6 mg/kg qd × 5 days/wk; dosage must be reduced in renal impairment

• *Adult:* PO 1000 mg tid with food or 500 mg q3h (for 6 doses) during waking hours and with food

Available forms include: Caps 250, 500 mg; vials 500 mg; intraocular implant 4.5 mg

Side effects/adverse reactions:

CNS: Fever, ***coma,*** chills, confusion, abnormal thoughts, dizziness, bizarre dreams, headache, psychosis, tremors, somnolence, paresthesia

CV: Dysrhythmia, hypertension/hypotension

GI: Abnormal LFTs, ***hemorrhage,*** nausea, vomiting, anorexia, diarrhea, abdominal pain

RESP: Dyspnea

HEMA: ***Granulocytopenia, thrombocytopenia, irreversible neutropenia, anemia, eosinophilia***

GU: ***Hematuria,*** increased creatinine/BUN

EENT: Retinal detachment in CMV retinitis

INTEG: Rash, alopecia, pruritus, urticaria, pain at site, phlebitis

Contraindications: Hypersensitivity to acyclovir or ganciclovir

Precautions: Preexisting cytopenia, renal function impairment, pregnancy category C, lactation, children <6 mo, elderly, platelet count <25,000/mm^3

Pharmacokinetics: *PO/IV:* Half-life 3-4.5 hr; excreted by the kidneys (unchanged drug); crosses blood-brain barrier

Drug interactions of concern to dentistry:

• Increased risk of blood dyscrasias: dapsone, carbamazepine, phenothiazines

• Increased risk of seizures: imipenem/cilastatin (Primaxin)

• Low platelet counts may prevent the use of aspirin, NSAIDs

DENTAL CONSIDERATIONS

General:

• Examine for oral manifestations of opportunistic infection.

• Examine for evidence of oral manifestations of blood dyscrasias (infection, bleeding, poor healing).

• Place on frequent recall to evaluate healing response.

• Consider local hemostasis measures to prevent excessive bleeding.

• Monitor vital signs at every appointment because of cardiovascular and respiratory side effects.

Consultations:

• Medical consultation for blood studies (CBC); leukopenic or thrombocytopenic side effects may result in infection, delayed healing, and excessive bleeding. Postpone elective dental treatment until normal values are maintained.

• Medical consultation may be required to assess disease control.

Teach patient/family:

• Caution in use of oral hygiene aids to prevent injury

• That secondary oral infection may occur; must see dentist immediately if infection occurs

• Importance of good oral hygiene to prevent soft tissue inflammation

---

gatifloxacin

(gat-i-flox'a-sin)

Tequin

Drug class.: Fluoroquinolone anti-infective

Action: A broad-spectrum bactericidal agent that inhibits the enzymes topoisomerase II (DNA gyrase) and topoisomerase IV required for bacterial DNA replication, transcription repair, and recombination

Uses: Acute bacterial exacerbation of chronic bronchitis caused by *S. pneumoniae, H. influenzae, H. parainfluenzae, M. catarrhalis,* or *S. aureus;* acute sinusitis *(S. pneumoniae, H. influenzae);* community-acquired pneumonia (*S. pneumoniae, H. influenzae, H. parainfluenzae, M. catarrhalis, M. pneumoniae, C. pneumoniae, L. pneumoniae,* or *S. aureus;* complicated or uncomplicated UTI *(E. coli, K. pneumoniae, P. mirabilis);* pyelonephritis *(E. coli),* acute uncomplicated rectal infections in women or uncomplicated urethral or cervical gonorrhea *(N. gonorrhoeae);* uncomplicated skin and skin structure infections

Dosage and routes:

Uncomplicated uretheral gonorrhea in men or rectal gonorrhea in women:

• *Adult and child >18 yr:* PO or IV inf 200-400 mg qd as a single dose; for PO doses take at least 4 hr before or 8 hr after antacids (Mg^{2+}, Al^{3+}), sucralfate, metal cations (Fe^{2+}, Zn^{2+}), or didanosine

Other infections:

• *Adult and child >18 yr:* PO or IV inf 200-400 mg qd for 3-14 days depending on type of infection; for PO doses take at least 4 hr before or 8 hr after antacids (Mg^{2+}, Al^{3+}), sucralfate, metal cations (Fe^{2+}, Zn^{2+}), or didanosine

Available forms include: Tabs 200, 400 mg; single-use vials 400 mg; premix parenteral sol 200, 400 mg

Side effects/adverse reactions:

▼ *ORAL:* Candidiasis, glossitis, stomatitis, mouth ulcers, taste perversion

CNS: **Headache, dizziness,** insomnia, tremor, nervousness

CV: ***Prolonged QT interval,*** palpitation, peripheral edema, vasodilation

GI: Nausea, diarrhea, abdominal pain, antibiotic associated pseudomembranous colitis

RESP: Dyspnea, bronchospasm

HEMA: Neutropenia

GU: Vaginitis, dysuria, hematuria

EENT: Vertigo, pharyngitis, abnormal vision, tinnitus

INTEG: Rash, sweating, photosensitivity

META: Increased ALT, AST, alk phosphatase levels
MS: Back pain, chest pain, risk of tendon rupture
MISC: *Injection site reactions,* chills fever, allergic reaction
Contraindications: Hypersensitivity to fluoroquinolones
Precautions: Reduce dose with creatinine clearance <40 ml/min; probenecid increases half life; children <18 yr, pregnancy category C, lactation, seizure history, avoid use with class IA and III antiarrhythmics; many prolong QT interval; cross resistance with other fluoroquinolones, monitor blood glucose in diabetes
Pharmacokinetics:
PO: Well absorbed, bioavailability 96%, peak plasma levels 1-2 hr, kinetics of IV dose after 1 hr inf are similar to oral doses; steady-state levels in 3 days PO or third dose IV; plasma protein binding 20%, widely distributed, limited metabolism; excreted unchanged mainly in urine

Drug interactions of concern to dentistry:
- Caution: use with erythromycin and tricyclic antidepressants (no data, risk of ↑ QT interval)
- Decreased absorption: divalent and trivalent cations, iron and zinc salts
- Increased risk of CNS stimulation and seizures: NSAIDs
- Increased risk of life-threatening arrhythmias: procainamide

DENTAL CONSIDERATIONS
General:
- Determine why patient is taking the drug.
- Monitor vital signs at every appointment because of cardiovascular side effects.
- Examine for oral manifestation of opportunistic infection.
- Advise patient if dental drugs prescribed have a potential for photosensitivity.
- Ruptures of the shoulder, hand, and Achilles tendons that required surgical repair or resulted in prolonged disability have been reported with the use of fluoroquinolones. Question patient about history of side effects associated with fluoroquinolone use.

Consultations:
- Physician consultation is advised in the presence of an acute dental infection requiring another antibiotic.

Teach patient/family:
- *If used for dental infection:*
- To minimize exposure to sunlight and wear sunscreen if sun exposure is planned
- To discontinue treatment and inform dentist immediately if patient experiences pain or inflammation of a tendon, and to rest and refrain from exercise

---

gatifloxacin ophthalmic

(gat-i-flox'a-sin)
Zymar
Drug class.: Fluoroquinolone anti-infective

Action: A broad-spectrum bactericidal agent that inhibits the enzymes topoisomerase II (DNA gyrase) and topoisomerase IV required for bacterial DNA replication, transcription repair, and recombination
Uses: Bacterial conjunctivitis

caused by susceptible organisms including *C. propinquum, S. aureus, S. epidermidis, S. mitis, S. pneumoniae,* and *H. influenzae*

Dosage and routes:

• *Adult:* TOP on days 1 and 2, place 1 drop in affected eye(s) q2h while awake; on days 3-7, place 1 drop in affected eye(s) qid while awake

Available forms include: Sol 0.3% in 2.5, 5 ml

Side effects/adverse reactions:

▼ *ORAL:* Taste disturbance

CNS: Headache

EENT: Conjunctival irritation, increased lacrimation, keratitis and papillary conjunctivitis, chemosis, dry eyes, eye pain

MISC: Hypersensitivity reactions

Contraindications: Hypersensitivity to this drug or other fluoroquinolones

Precautions: Avoid prolonged use, do not wear contact lens when infection is present, do not contaminate applicator tip, pregnancy category C, lactation, child <1 yr

Pharmacokinetics:

TOP: Serum levels below quantification

Drug interactions of concern to dentistry:

• None reported

DENTAL CONSIDERATIONS

General:

• Protect patient's eyes from accidental spatter during dental treatment.

• Avoid dental light in patient's eyes; offer dark glasses for patient comfort.

gemfibrozil

(jem-fi'broe-zil)

Lopid

♣ Apo-Gemfibrozil, Gen-Fibro, Novo-Gemfibrozil, Nu-Gemfibrozil

Drug class.: Antihyperlipidemic

Action: Reduces plasma triglyceride and very-low-density lipoprotein (VLDL) levels, possibly through inhibition of peripheral lipolysis and decreased hepatic extraction of free fatty acids; HDL levels increase

Uses: Types IIb, IV, V hyperlipidemia

Dosage and routes:

• *Adult:* PO 1200 mg in divided doses bid 30 min before AM and PM meals

Available forms include: Tabs 600 mg

Side effects/adverse reactions:

CNS: Dizziness, blurred vision

GI: Nausea, vomiting, dyspepsia, diarrhea, abdominal pain

HEMA: ***Leukopenia, anemia, eosinophilia***

INTEG: Rash, urticaria, pruritus

Contraindications: Severe hepatic disease, preexisting gallbladder disease, severe renal disease, primary biliary cirrhosis, hypersensitivity

Precautions: Monitor hematologic and hepatic function, pregnancy category B, lactation

Pharmacokinetics:

PO: Peak 1-2 hr, half-life 1.5 hr; plasma protein binding >90%; excreted in urine; metabolized in liver

Drug interactions of concern to dentistry:

- None reported

DENTAL CONSIDERATIONS

General:

- Patients on chronic drug therapy may rarely have symptoms of blood dyscrasias, which can include infection, bleeding, and poor healing.

Consultations:

- In a patient with symptoms of blood dyscrasias, request a medical consultation for blood studies and postpone dental treatment until normal values are reestablished.

---

gemifloxacin mesylate

(je-mi-flox'-a-sin)

Factive

Drug class.: Fluoroquinolone anti-infective

Action: A broad-spectrum bactericidal agent that inhibits the enzymes topoisomerase II (DNA gyrase) required for bacterial DNA replication, transcription repair, and recombination

Uses: Acute bacterial exacerbation of chronic bronchitis caused by susceptible strains of *S. pneumoniae, H. influenzae, H. parainfluenzae,*or *M. catarrhalis;* community-acquired pneumonia caused by susceptible strains of *S. pneumoniae* (except drug-resistant strains), *H. influenzae, M. catarrhalis, M. pneumoniae, C. pneumoniae,* or *K. pneumoniae*

Dosage and routes:

- *Adult:* PO 320 mg/day for 5-7 days as dictated by infection

Available forms include: Tabs 320 mg

Side effects/adverse reactions:

▼ *ORAL: Altered taste,* ***angioedema,*** dry mouth

CNS: Headache, CNS reactions

CV: ECG changes

GI: Nausea, diarrhea, vomiting, ***antibiotic-associated colitis,*** anorexia, abdominal pain

GU: Candida infection

EENT: Pharyngitis

INTEG: Rash, urticaria, photosensitivity, risk of severe dermatologic reactions

META: Bilirubinemia; ↑ ALT, AST, GGT

MS: Arthralgia, back pain, myalgia

MISC: ***Anaphylaxis***

Contraindications: Hypersensitivity to this drug or any fluoroquinolone, patients with prolonged QT interval or uncorrected electrolyte disorders, or patients taking quinidine, procainamide, amiodarone, or sotalol

Precautions: Safety and efficacy in children <18 yr, pregnancy and nursing not established; may prolong QT interval, risk of tendinitis and tendon rupture, epilepsy, pregnancy category C, cerebral arteriosclerosis, renal dysfunction

Pharmacokinetics:

PO: Rapid absorption, oral availability 75%-95%, plasma protein binding 60%-70%, peak plasma levels 0.5-2 hr, limited hepatic metabolism, excretion mainly in feces (61%) and lesser amount in urine (36%)

Drug interactions of concern to dentistry:

- Decreased absorption: divalent or trivalent antacids, iron or zinc salts
- Use with caution or avoid drugs that affect QT interval: erythromycin, antipsychotics, tricyclic antidepressants

---

DENTAL CONSIDERATIONS

General:

• Determine why patient is taking the drug.

• Avoid dental light in patient's eyes; offer dark glasses for patient comfort.

• Examine for oral manifestation of opportunistic infection.

• Advise patient if dental drugs prescribed have a potential for photosensitivity.

• As with other fluoroquinolones there is a risk of tendinitis and tendon rupture.

• Consider semisupine chair position for patient comfort if GI side effects occur.

Consultations:

• Consult with patient's physician if an acute dental infection occurs and another antiinfective is required.

Teach patient/family:

When chronic dry mouth occurs, advise patient:

• To avoid mouth rinses with high alcohol content because of drying effects

• To use daily home fluoride products for anticaries effect

• To use sugarless gum, frequent sips of water, or saliva substitutes

---

gentamicin sulfate (ophthalmic)

(jen-ta-mye'sin)

Garamycin Ophthalmic, Genoptic, Genoptic SOP, Gentacidin, Gentak

Drug class.: Aminoglycoside antiinfective ophthalmic

Action: Inhibits bacterial protein synthesis

Uses: Infection of external eye

Dosage and routes:

• *Adult and child:* Instill 1 drop q4h; top apply oint to conjunctival sac bid (can use 1 drop qh for severe infections)

Available forms include: Oint, sol 3%

Side effects/adverse reactions:

EENT: Poor corneal wound healing, temporary visual haze, overgrowth of nonsusceptible organisms

Contraindications: Hypersensitivity

Precautions: Antibiotic hypersensitivity, pregnancy category C

DENTAL CONSIDERATIONS

General:

• Avoid dental light in patient's eyes; offer dark glasses for patient comfort.

• Protect patient's eyes from accidental spatter during dental treatment.

---

glimepiride

(glye'me-pye-ride)

Amaryl

Drug class.: Oral antidiabetic (second generation)

Action: Causes functioning β-cells in pancreas to release insulin, leading to drop in blood glucose levels; may also play a role in increased sensitivity of peripheral tissues to insulin

Uses: Stable adult-onset diabetes mellitus (type II); may also be used with insulin or metformin where diet and exercise are not effective in controlling hyperglycemia

Dosage and routes:

• *Adult:* PO usual initial dose 1-2 mg once daily with breakfast or first meal of the day; maintenance

G

dose range 1-4 mg daily; max daily dose 8 mg; adjust dose increments at no more than 2 mg every 1-2 wk

Insulin supplementation:

• *Adult:* PO 8 mg daily with first main meal; start low-dose insulin and adjust dose according to patient response

Available forms include: Tabs 1, 2, 4 mg

Side effects/adverse reactions:

CNS: Dizziness, headache

GI: Nausea, abdominal pain, cholestatic jaundice, vomiting, diarrhea

HEMA: ***Leukopenia, agranulocytosis, thrombocytopenia, hemolytic anemia, pancytopenia***

EENT: Blurred vision, changes in accommodation

INTEG: Pruritus, erythema, urticaria, rash, photosensitivity

META: Hyponatremia, hypoglycemia

MISC: Asthenia

Contraindications: Hypersensitivity, diabetic ketoacidosis

Precautions: Malnourished; adrenal, pituitary, or hepatic insufficiency; hypoglycemia recognition in elderly or in those taking β-blockers; increased risk of cardiovascular mortality has been reported in patients using oral hypoglycemics; alcohol use; pregnancy category C, lactation; children

Pharmacokinetics:

PO: Good oral absorption, peak plasma levels 2-3 hr; plasma protein binding 99.5%; extensive hepatic metabolism; excreted in urine (60%) and feces (40%)

Drug interactions of concern to dentistry:

• Risk of potentiation of hypoglycemic effects: NSAIDs, salicylates, sulfonamides, β-adrenergic blockers, ketoconazole

DENTAL CONSIDERATIONS

General:

• Short appointments and a stress reduction protocol may be required for anxious patients.

• Question patient about self-monitoring of drug's antidiabetic effect, including blood glucose values or finger-stick records.

• Ensure that patient is following prescribed diet and regularly takes medication.

• Patients on chronic drug therapy may rarely have symptoms of blood dyscrasias, which can include infection, bleeding, and poor healing.

• Diabetics may be more susceptible to infection and have delayed wound healing.

• Place on frequent recall to evaluate healing response.

• Advise patient if dental drugs prescribed have a potential for photosensitivity.

Consultations:

• Medical consultation may be required to assess disease control.

• In a patient with symptoms of blood dyscrasias, request a medical consultation for blood studies and postpone treatment until normal values are reestablished.

• Medical consultation may include data from patient's blood glucose monitoring, including glycosylated hemoglobin or HbA_{1c} testing.

Teach patient/family:

• Importance of good oral hygiene to prevent soft tissue inflammation

• Caution to prevent trauma when using oral hygiene aids

• Importance of updating health

and drug history if physician makes any changes in evaluation or drug regimens

glipizide

(glip'i-zide)

Glucotrol, Glucotrol XL

Drug class.: Oral antidiabetic (second generation)

Action: Causes functioning β-cells in pancreas to release insulin, leading to drop in blood glucose levels; may improve insulin binding to insulin receptors or increase the number of insulin receptors; not effective if patient lacks functioning β-cells

Uses: Stable adult-onset diabetes mellitus (type II)

Dosage and routes:

• *Adult:* PO 5 mg/day initially, then increased to desired response; max 15 mg once-a-day dose, 40 mg/day in divided doses

• *Elderly:* PO 2.5 mg initially, then increased to desired response; max 40 mg/day in divided doses or 15 mg once-a-day dose

Available forms include: Tabs 5, 10 mg; ext rel 5, 10 mg

Side effects/adverse reactions:

CNS: Headache, weakness, dizziness, drowsiness, tinnitus, fatigue, vertigo

GI: ***Hepatotoxicity, cholestatic jaundice,*** nausea, vomiting, diarrhea, heartburn

HEMA: ***Leukopenia, thrombocytopenia, agranulocytosis, aplastic anemia,*** pancytopenia, hemolytic anemia, increased AST/ALT, alk phosphatase

INTEG: Rash, allergic reactions, pruritus, urticaria, eczema, photosensitivity, erythema

ENDO: ***Hypoglycemia***

Contraindications: Hypersensitivity to sulfonylureas, juvenile or brittle diabetes

Precautions: Pregnancy category C, elderly, cardiac disease, severe renal disease, severe hepatic disease, thyroid disease

Pharmacokinetics:

PO: Completely absorbed by GI route, onset 1-1.5 hr, duration 10-24 hr, half-life 2-4 hr; 90%-95% is plasma protein bound; metabolized in liver; excreted in urine

Drug interactions of concern to dentistry:

• Increased hypoglycemic effects: salicylates, ketoconazole

• Decreased action of glipizide: corticosteroids

• Disulfiram-like reaction: alcohol

DENTAL CONSIDERATIONS

General:

• Monitor vital signs at every appointment because of cardiovascular side effects.

• Patients on chronic drug therapy may rarely have symptoms of blood dyscrasias, which can include infection, bleeding, and poor healing.

• Short appointments and a stress reduction protocol may be required for anxious patients.

• Place on frequent recall to evaluate healing response.

• Diabetics may be more susceptible to infection and have delayed wound healing.

• Question patient about self-monitoring of drug's antidiabetic effect, including blood glucose values or finger-stick records.

• Ensure that patient is following prescribed diet and regularly takes medication.

G

• Avoid prescribing aspirin-containing products.

Consultations:

• In a patient with symptoms of blood dyscrasias, request a medical consultation for blood studies and postpone dental treatment until normal values are reestablished.

• Medical consultation may be required to assess disease control.

• Medical consultation may include data from patient's blood glucose monitoring, including glycosylated hemoglobin or HbA_{1c} testing.

Teach patient/family:

• Importance of good oral hygiene to prevent soft tissue inflammation

• Caution to prevent injury when using oral hygiene aids

• To avoid mouth rinses with high alcohol content because of drying effects

---

glucagon

(gloo'ka-gon)

Glucagon Emergency Kit

Drug class.: Antihypoglycemic, hormone

Action: A (rDNA) polypeptide hormone, identical to human pancreatic glucagon, that increases blood glucose and relaxes the smooth muscle of the GI tract

Uses: Severe hypoglycemia; as a diagnostic aid to facilitate in the radiologic examination of the GI tract by relaxing smooth muscle

Dosage and routes:

Severe hypoglycemia:

• *Adult and child >20 kg (44 lb):* IV, SC, or IM 1 mg

• *Child <20 kg (44 lb):* IV, SC, or IM 0.5 mg; use only freshly reconstituted, water-clear solution; discard any unused quantity; do not exceed concentration of 1 mg/ml

Available forms include: Emergency and diagnostic kits: each contains 1 mg powder with 1 ml diluent

Side effects/adverse reactions:

CV: Transient increase in blood pressure, pulse rate

GI: Nausea, vomiting

MISC: Generalized allergic reactions

Contraindications: Hypersensitivity; patients with known pheochromocytoma

Precautions: For type I diabetes give supplemental carbohydrates as soon as possible; insulinoma, starvation, glycogen depletion, adrenal insufficiency, chronic hypoglycemia, pregnancy category B, lactation

Pharmacokinetics:

PARENTERAL: Peak levels in 20 min (SC) or 13 min (IM); extensively metabolized in liver, kidney, and plasma

Drug interactions of concern to dentistry:

• Patients taking β-adrenergic blockers: may be expected to have a transient but greater increase in blood pressure and pulse

DENTAL CONSIDERATIONS

General:

• Glucagon may be used as an emergency drug for severe hypoglycemia. Patients should be closely monitored and referred immediately for evaluation.

• IV glucose may be required for patients nonresponsive to glucagon.

• Unconscious patients should awaken within 15 min or less.

glyburide

(glye'byoor-ide)

DiaBeta, Glynase PresTab, Micronase

♣ Albert Glyburide, Apo-Glyburide, Euglucon, Gen-Glybe, Novo-Glyburide, Nu-Glyburide

Drug class.: Oral antidiabetic (second generation)

Action: Causes functioning β-cells in pancreas to release insulin, leading to drop in blood glucose levels; may improve insulin binding to insulin receptors and increase number of insulin receptors; not effective if patient lacks functioning β-cells

Uses: Stable adult-onset diabetes mellitus (type II)

Dosage and routes:

• *Adult:* PO 2.5-5 mg/day initially, then increased to desired response; limit 20 mg/day

• *Elderly:* PO 1.25 mg initially, then increased to desired response; max 20 mg/day; maintenance 20 mg qd

Available forms include: Tabs 1.25, 1.5, 2.5, 3, 4.5, 5, 6 mg

Side effects/adverse reactions:

CNS: ***Headache, weakness,*** paresthesia, tinnitus, fatigue, vertigo

GI: ***Hepatotoxicity, cholestatic jaundice,*** nausea, fullness, heartburn, vomiting, diarrhea

HEMA: ***Leukopenia, thrombocytopenia, agranulocytosis, aplastic anemia,*** increased AST/ALT, alk phosphatase

INTEG: Rash, allergic reactions, pruritus, urticaria, eczema, photosensitivity, erythema

ENDO: ***Hypoglycemia***

MS: Joint pains

Contraindications: Hypersensitivity to sulfonylureas, juvenile or brittle diabetes

Precautions: Pregnancy category B, elderly, cardiac disease, severe renal disease, severe hepatic disease, thyroid disease, severe hypoglycemia reactions

Pharmacokinetics:

PO: Completely absorbed by GI route, onset 2-4 hr, peak 2-8 hr, duration 24 hr, half-life 10 hr; 90%-95% is plasma protein bound; metabolized in liver; excreted in urine, feces (metabolites); crosses placenta

Drug interactions of concern to dentistry:

• Increased hypoglycemic effects: NSAIDs, salicylates, ketoconazole

• Decreased action of glyburide: corticosteroids

• Disulfiram-like reaction: alcohol

DENTAL CONSIDERATIONS

General:

• Monitor vital signs at every appointment because of cardiovascular side effects.

• Patients on chronic drug therapy may rarely have symptoms of blood dyscrasias, which can include infection, bleeding, and poor healing.

• Place on frequent recall to evaluate healing response.

• Ensure that patient is following prescribed diet and regularly takes medication.

• Short appointments and stress reduction protocol may be required for anxious patients.

• Patients with diabetes may be more susceptible to infection and have delayed wound healing.

• Question patient about self-monitoring of drug's antidiabetic effect, including blood glucose values or finger-stick records.

- Avoid prescribing aspirin-containing products.

Consultations:

- In a patient with symptoms of blood dyscrasias, request a medical consultation for blood studies and postpone dental treatment until normal values are reestablished.
- Medical consultation may be required to assess disease control.
- Medical consultation may include data from patient's blood glucose monitoring, including glycosylated hemoglobin or HbA_{1c} testing.

Teach patient/family:

- Importance of good oral hygiene to prevent soft tissue inflammation
- Caution to prevent injury when using oral hygiene aids
- To avoid mouth rinses with high alcohol content because of drying effects

---

glycopyrrolate

(glye-koe-pye'roe-late)
Robinul, Robinul Forte

Drug class.: Anticholinergic

Action: Inhibits acetylcholine at receptor sites in autonomic nervous system, which controls secretions, free acids in stomach

Uses: Decreased secretions before surgery, reversal of neuromuscular blockade, peptic ulcer disease, irritable bowel syndrome

Dosage and routes:

Preoperatively:

- *Adult:* IM 0.002 mg/lb 0.5-1 hr before surgery
- *Child 2-12 yr:* IM 0.002-0.004 mg/lb
- *Child <2 yr:* IM 0.004 mg/lb

Reversal of neuromuscular blockage:

- *Adult:* IV 0.2 mg for each 1 mg of neostigmine or 5 mg IV of pyridostigmine simultaneously

GI disorders:

- *Adult:* PO 1-3 mg bid-tid; IM/IV 0.1-0.2 mg tid-qid, titrated to patient response

Available forms include: Tabs 1, 2 mg; inj 0.2 mg/ml

Side effects/adverse reactions:

▼ *ORAL: Dry mouth*

CNS: Confusion, anxiety, restlessness, irritability, delusions, hallucinations, headache, sedation, depression, incoherence, dizziness, lethargy, flushing, weakness

CV: Palpitation, tachycardia, postural hypotension, paradoxic bradycardia

GI: Constipation, nausea, vomiting, abdominal distress, paralytic ileus

GU: Hesitancy, retention, impotence

EENT: Blurred vision, photophobia, dilated pupils, difficulty swallowing, increased intraocular pressure, mydriasis, cycloplegia

INTEG: Urticaria, allergic reactions

MISC: Suppression of lactation, nasal congestion, decreased sweating

Contraindications: Hypersensitivity, narrow-angle glaucoma, myasthenia gravis, GI/GU obstruction, child <3 yr, tachycardia, myocardial ischemia, hepatic disease, ulcerative colitis, toxic megacolon

Precautions: Pregnancy category C, elderly, lactation, prostatic hypertrophy, renal disease, CHF, pulmonary disease, hyperthyroidism

Pharmacokinetics:
PO: Peak 1 hr, duration 6 hr
IM: Peak 30-45 min, duration 7 hr
IV: Peak 10-15 min, duration 4 hr, excreted in urine, bile, feces (unchanged)

Drug interactions of concern to dentistry:
• Increased anticholinergic effect: antihistamines, phenothiazines, meperidine, haloperidol, scopolamine, atropine
• Do not mix with diazepam, pentobarbital, in syringe or solution
• Constipation, urinary retention: opioid analgesics
• Reduced absorption of ketoconazole

DENTAL CONSIDERATIONS
General:
• Avoid dental light in patient's eyes; offer dark glasses for patient comfort.
• Assess salivary flow as a factor in caries, periodontal disease, and candidiasis.

Consultation: Physician should be informed if significant xerostomic side effects occur (e.g., increased caries, sore tongue, problems eating or swallowing, difficulty wearing prosthesis) so that a medication change can be considered.

Teach patient/family:
When chronic dry mouth occurs, advise patient:
• To avoid mouth rinses with high alcohol content because of drying effects
• To use daily home fluoride products for anticaries effect
• To use sugarless gum, frequent sips of water, or saliva substitutes

guaifenesin

(gwye-fen'e-sin)
Anti-Tuss, Duratuss-G, Fenesin, Guaifenex LA, Guaituss, Humibid LA, Hytuss, Hytuss 2X, Liquibid, Mucinex, MucoFen, Organidin NR, Robitussin, Scot-Tussin, Siltussin, Touro-Ex
Balminil, Benylin-E, Resyl

Drug class.: Expectorant, glyceryl guaiacolate

Action: Acts as an expectorant by stimulating a mucosal reflex to increase the production of less-viscous lung mucus

Uses: Dry, nonproductive cough

Dosage and routes:
• *Adult:* PO 200-400 mg q4-6h, not to exceed 1-2 g/day
• *Child 6-12 yr:* PO 100-200 mg q4h; max dose 1200 mg day

Available forms include: Tabs 100, 200, 1200 mg; caps 200 mg; syr 100 mg/5 ml; ext rel caps 300, 600 mg; ext rel tabs 600 mg; liquid 100, 200 mg/5 ml

Side effects/adverse reactions:
CNS: Drowsiness
GI: Nausea, anorexia, vomiting

Contraindications: Hypersensitivity, persistent cough

Precautions: Pregnancy category C

DENTAL CONSIDERATIONS
General:
• Consider semisupine chair position for patients with respiratory disease.
• Elective dental treatment may be precluded by significant coughing episodes.

G

guanabenz acetate

(gwahn'a-benz)

Wytensin

Drug class.: Centrally acting antihypertensive

Action: Stimulates central α_2-adrenergic receptors, resulting in decreased sympathetic outflow from brain

Uses: Hypertension

Dosage and routes:

• *Adult:* PO 4 mg bid, increasing in increments of 4-8 mg/day q1-2wk, not to exceed 32 mg bid

Available forms include: Tabs 4, 8 mg

Side effects/adverse reactions:

▼ *ORAL: Dry mouth*

CNS: Drowsiness, dizziness, sedation, headache, depression, weakness

CV: ***Severe rebound hypertension,*** chest pain, dysrhythmias, palpitation

GI: Nausea, diarrhea, constipation

GU: Impotence

EENT: Nasal congestion, blurred vision

Contraindications: Hypersensitivity to guanabenz

Precautions: Pregnancy category C, lactation, children <12 yr, severe coronary insufficiency, recent MI, cerebrovascular disease, severe hepatic or renal failure

Pharmacokinetics:

PO: Peak 2-4 hr, half-life 6 hr; excreted in urine

Drug interactions of concern to dentistry:

• Increased CNS depression: alcohol, all CNS depressants

• Decreased hypotensive effects: NSAIDs, especially indomethacin, sympathomimetics

DENTAL CONSIDERATIONS

General:

• Monitor vital signs at every appointment because of cardiovascular side effects.

• Limit use of sodium-containing products such as saline IV fluids for patients with a dietary salt restriction.

• Assess salivary flow as a factor in caries, periodontal disease, and candidiasis.

• Stress from dental procedures may compromise cardiovascular function; determine patient risk.

• Short appointments and a stress reduction protocol may be required for anxious patients.

Consultations:

• Medical consultation may be required to assess disease control and patient's ability to tolerate stress.

Teach patient/family:

When chronic dry mouth occurs, advise patient:

• To avoid mouth rinses with high alcohol content because of drying effects

• To use daily home fluoride products for anticaries effect

• To use sugarless gum, frequent sips of water, or saliva substitutes

guanadrel sulfate

(gwahn'a-drel)

Hylorel

Drug class.: Antihypertensive

Action: Inhibits sympathetic vasoconstriction by inhibiting release of norepinephrine; depletes norepinephrine stores in adrenergic nerve endings

Uses: Hypertension

Dosage and routes:

• *Adult:* PO 5 mg bid, adjusted to desired response, may need 20-75 mg/day in divided doses

Available forms include: Tabs 10, 25 mg

Side effects/adverse reactions:

▼ *ORAL:* Dry mouth

CNS: Drowsiness, fatigue, weakness, feeling of faintness, insomnia, dizziness, mental changes, memory loss, hallucinations, *depression,* anxiety, *confusion, paresthesias, headache*

CV: Orthostatic hypotension, bradycardia, ***CHF,*** palpitation, chest pain, tachycardia, dysrhythmias

GI: Nausea, cramps, diarrhea, constipation, anorexia, indigestion

RESP: ***Bronchospasm,*** dyspnea, cough, rales, shortness of breath

GU: Ejaculation failure, impotence, dysuria, nocturia, frequency

EENT: Nasal stuffiness, tinnitus, visual changes, sore throat, double vision, dry/burning eyes

INTEG: Rash, purpura, alopecia

MS: Leg cramps, aching, pain, inflammation

Contraindications: Hypersensitivity, pregnancy category B, pheochromocytoma, lactation, CHF, child <18 yr

Precautions: Elderly, bronchial asthma, peptic ulcer, electrolyte imbalances, vascular disease

Pharmacokinetics:

PO: Onset 0.5-2 hr, peak 1.5-2 hr, duration 4-14 hr, half-life 10-12 hr; excreted in urine (50% unchanged)

Drug interactions of concern to dentistry:

• Increased orthostatic hypotension: alcohol, opioid analgesics, barbiturates, phenothiazines, haloperidol

• Decreased hypotensive effect: ephedrine, sympathomimetics, NSAIDs, indomethacin, tricyclic antidepressants

DENTAL CONSIDERATIONS

General:

• Monitor vital signs at every appointment because of cardiovascular side effects.

• After supine positioning, have patient sit upright for at least 2 min before standing to avoid orthostatic hypotension.

• Limit use of sodium-containing products such as saline IV fluids for patients with a dietary salt restriction.

• Stress from dental procedures may compromise cardiovascular function; determine patient risk.

• Short appointments and a stress reduction protocol may be required for anxious patients.

• Assess salivary flow as a factor in caries, periodontal disease, and candidiasis.

Consultations:

• Medical consultation may be required to assess disease control and patient's ability to tolerate stress.

Teach patient/family:

When chronic dry mouth occurs, advise patient:

• To avoid mouth rinses with high alcohol content because of drying effects

• To use daily home fluoride products for anticaries effect

• To use sugarless gum, frequent sips of water, or saliva substitutes

guanethidine sulfate

(gwahn-eth'i-deen)
Ismelin
♣ Apo-Guanethidine
Drug class.: Antihypertensive

Action: Inhibits norepinephrine release, depleting norepinephrine stores in adrenergic nerve endings
Uses: Moderate-to-severe hypertension
Dosage and routes:
• *Adult:* PO 10 mg qd, increase by 10 mg qwk at monthly intervals; may require 25-50 mg qd
• *Adult (hospitalized):* 25-50 mg; may increase by 25-50 mg/day or qod
• *Child:* PO 200 μg/kg/day; increase q7-10d; not to exceed 3000 μg/kg/24 hr
Available forms include: Tabs 10, 25 mg
Side effects/adverse reactions:
▼ *ORAL:* Dry mouth, salivary gland pain or swelling
CNS: Depression
CV: Orthostatic hypotension, dizziness, weakness, lassitude, bradycardia, CHF, fatigue, angina, heart block, chest paresthesia
GI: Nausea, vomiting, *diarrhea,* constipation, weight gain, anorexia
RESP: Dyspnea
HEMA: ***Thrombocytopenia, leukopenia***
GU: Ejaculation failure, impotence, nocturia, edema, retention, increased BUN
EENT: Nasal congestion, ptosis, blurred vision
INTEG: Dermatitis, loss of scalp hair
Contraindications: Hypersensitivity, pheochromocytoma, recent MI, CHF, cardiac failure, sinus bradycardia
Precautions: Pregnancy category C, lactation, children; peptic ulcer, asthma, frequent orthostatic hypotension, fever, renal impairment
Pharmacokinetics:
PO: Therapeutic level 1-3 wk, half-life 5 days; metabolized by liver; excreted in urine (metabolites), breast milk
Drug interactions of concern to dentistry:
• Increased orthostatic hypotension: alcohol, opioid analgesics, barbiturates, phenothiazines, haloperidol
• Decreased hypotensive effect: ephedrine, NSAIDs, indomethacin, sympathomimetics, tricyclic antidepressants

DENTAL CONSIDERATIONS
General:
• Monitor vital signs at every appointment because of cardiovascular and respiratory side effects.
• Patients on chronic drug therapy may rarely have symptoms of blood dyscrasias, which can include infection, bleeding, and poor healing.
• Assess salivary flow as a factor in caries, periodontal disease, and candidiasis.
• After supine positioning, have patient sit upright for at least 2 min before standing to avoid orthostatic hypotension.
• Limit use of sodium-containing products such as saline IV fluids for patients with a dietary salt restriction.
• Stress from dental procedures may compromise cardiovascular function; determine patient risk.

• Short appointments and a stress reduction protocol may be required for anxious patients.
• Use vasoconstrictors with caution, in low doses, and with careful aspiration. Avoid using gingival retraction cord with epinephrine.
• Consider semisupine chair position for patients with respiratory distress.

Consultations:
• Medical consultation may be required to assess disease control and patient's ability to tolerate stress.
• In a patient with symptoms of blood dyscrasias, request a medical consultation for blood studies and postpone dental treatment until normal values are reestablished.

Teach patient/family:
• Importance of good oral hygiene to prevent soft tissue inflammation
• Caution to prevent injury when using oral hygiene aids

When chronic dry mouth occurs, advise patient:
• To avoid mouth rinses with high alcohol content because of drying effects
• To use daily home fluoride products for anticaries effect
• To use sugarless gum, frequent sips of water, or saliva substitutes

---

halcinonide

(hal-sin'oh-nide)
Halog, Halog-E

Drug class.: Corticosteroid, synthetic topical

Action: Glucocorticoids have multiple actions that include anti-inflammatory and immunosuppressant effects. They inhibit phospholipase A_2, interfering with or reducing the synthesis of prostaglandins and leukotrienes. They also bind to cytoplasmic GRs and enter the cell nucleus to bind with DNA. This results in the synthesis of various enzymes such as collagenase, elastase, and cytokines that play important roles in inflammation and immunosuppression. They also suppress the production of lymphocytes, monocytes, and eosinophils.

Uses: Inflammation of corticosteroid-responsive dermatoses

Dosage and routes:
• *Adult:* TOP apply to affected area bid-tid

Available forms include: Cream 0.025%, 0.1%; oint 0.1%; sol 0.1%

Side effects/adverse reactions:
▼ *ORAL:* Thinning of mucosa, stinging sensation (local application)
INTEG: Acne, atrophy, epidermal thinning, purpura, striae

Contraindications: Hypersensitivity, viral infections, fungal infections

Precautions: Pregnancy category C

DENTAL CONSIDERATIONS

General:
• Place on frequent recall to evaluate healing response when used on chronic basis.

Teach patient/family:
• Importance of good oral hygiene to prevent soft tissue inflammation
• When used for oral lesions, to return for oral evaluation if response of oral tissues has not occurred in 7-14 days
• To apply at bedtime or after meals for maximum effect
• To apply with cotton-tipped applicator by pressing, not rubbing, paste on lesion

• That use on oral herpetic ulcerations is contraindicated

halobetasol propionate

(hal-oh-bay'ta-sol)

Ultravate

Drug class.: Topical corticosteroid, group VI potency

Action: Glucocorticoids have multiple actions that include anti-inflammatory and immunosuppressant effects. They inhibit phospholipase A_2, interfering with or reducing the synthesis of prostaglandins and leukotrienes. They also bind to cytoplasmic GRs and enter the cell nucleus to bind with DNA. This results in the synthesis of various enzymes such as collagenase, elastase, and cytokines that play important roles in inflammation and immunosuppression. They also suppress the production of lymphocytes, monocytes, and eosinophils.

Uses: Psoriasis, eczema, contact dermatitis, pruritus

Dosage and routes:

• *Adult and child:* Apply to affected area tid-qid

Available forms include: Cream 0.05%; oint 0.05%

Side effects/adverse reactions:

INTEG: Burning, dryness, itching, irritation, acne, folliculitis, hypertrichosis, perioral dermatitis, hypopigmentation, atrophy, striae, miliaria, allergic contact dermatitis, secondary infection

Contraindications: Hypersensitivity to corticosteroids, fungal infections

Precautions: Pregnancy category C, lactation, viral infections, bacterial infections

DENTAL CONSIDERATIONS

Teach patient/family:

• That use on oral herpetic ulcerations is contraindicated

haloperidol/haloperidol decanoate

(ha-loe-per'i-dole)

Haldol, Haldol Deconate

✤ Apo-Haloperidol, Novoperidol, Peridol

Drug class.: Antipsychotic/butyrophenone

Action: Blocks neurotransmission at dopaminergic synapses in the cerebral cortex, hypothalamus, and limbic system; exhibits strong peripheral α-adrenergic and anticholinergic blocking action; mechanism for antipsychotic effects is unclear

Uses: Psychotic disorders, control of tics and vocal utterances in Tourette's syndrome, short-term treatment of hyperactive children showing excessive motor activity; unapproved: autism and chemotherapy-induced nausea and vomiting

Dosage and routes:

Psychosis:

• *Adult:* PO 0.5-2 mg bid or tid initially, depending on severity of condition, dose is increased to desired dose, max 100 mg/day; IM 2-5 mg q1-8h

• *Child 3-12 yr:* PO/IM 0.05-0.075 mg/kg/day

• *Decanoate:* Initial dose IM is 10-15 × daily PO dose q4wk; do not administer IV; not to exceed 100 mg

Tics/vocal utterances:

- *Adult:* PO 0.5-1.5 mg bid or tid, increased until desired response occurs
- *Child 3-12 yr:* PO 0.05-0.075 mg/kg/day

Available forms include: Tabs 0.5, 1, 2, 5, 10, 20 mg; conc 2 mg/ml; inj IM 5 mg/ml, 50, 100 mg in 1 ml amps; 5 ml vials

Side effects/adverse reactions:

▼ *ORAL: Dry mouth, tardive dyskinesia (tongue, lip movements),* sore throat, mouth

CNS: Extrapyramidal symptoms: pseudoparkinsonism, akathisia, dystonia, tardive dyskinesia, drowsiness, headache, ***seizures, neuroleptic malignant syndrome,*** confusion

CV: Orthostatic hypotension, ***cardiac arrest, tachycardia,*** hypertension, ECG changes

GI: Nausea, vomiting, anorexia, constipation, ***ileus, hepatitis,*** diarrhea, jaundice, weight gain

RESP: ***Laryngospasm, respiratory depression,*** dyspnea

GU: Urinary retention, urinary frequency, enuresis, impotence, amenorrhea, gynecomastia

EENT: Blurred vision, glaucoma, dry eyes

INTEG: Rash, photosensitivity, dermatitis

Contraindications: Hypersensitivity, blood dyscrasias, coma, child <3 yr, brain damage, bone marrow depression, alcohol and barbiturate withdrawal states, Parkinson's disease, angina, epilepsy, urinary retention, narrow-angle glaucoma

Precautions: Pregnancy category C, lactation, seizure disorders, hypertension, hepatic disease, cardiac disease

Pharmacokinetics:

PO: Onset erratic, peak 2-6 hr, half-life 24 hr

IM: Onset 15-30 min, peak 15-20 min, half-life 21 hr; decanoate–peak 4-11 days, half-life 3 wk

Metabolized by liver; excreted in urine, bile; crosses placenta; excreted in breast milk

Drug interactions of concern to dentistry:

- Increased sedation: other CNS depressants, alcohol, barbiturate anesthetics, opioid analgesics
- Hypotension, tachycardia: epinephrine
- Increased extrapyramidal effects: phenothiazines and related drugs (haloperidol, droperidol), metoclopramide
- Additive photosensitization: tetracyclines
- Increased anticholinergic effects: anticholinergics
- Suspected increase in neurologic side effects: fluconazole, itraconazole, ketoconazole

DENTAL CONSIDERATIONS

General:

- Monitor vital signs at every appointment because of cardiovascular side effects.
- After supine positioning, have patient sit upright for at least 2 min before standing to avoid orthostatic hypotension.
- Assess salivary flow as a factor in caries, periodontal disease, and candidiasis.
- Avoid dental light in patient's eyes; offer dark glasses for patient comfort.
- Assess for presence of extrapy-

ramidal motor symptoms, such as tardive dyskinesia and akathisia. Extrapyramidal motor activity may complicate dental treatment.

- Geriatric patients are more susceptible to drug effects; use lower dose.
- Use vasoconstrictors with caution, in low doses, and with careful aspiration. Avoid use of gingival retraction cord with epinephrine.

Consultations:

- Take precautions if dental surgery is anticipated and anesthesia is required.
- If signs of tardive dyskinesia or akathisia are present, refer to physician.
- Physician should be informed if significant xerostomic side effects occur (e.g., increased caries, sore tongue, problems eating or swallowing, difficulty wearing prosthesis) so that a medication change can be considered.

Teach patient/family:

- Importance of good oral hygiene to prevent soft tissue inflammation
- Caution to prevent injury when using oral hygiene aids
- To use electric toothbrush if patient has difficulty holding conventional devices

When chronic dry mouth occurs, advise patient:

- To avoid mouth rinses with high alcohol content because of drying effects
- To use daily home fluoride products for anticaries effect
- To use sugarless gum, frequent sips of water, or saliva substitutes

heparin calcium/ heparin sodium

(hep'a-rin)

Heparin sodium: *generic, Hep Lock, Hep-Lock Flush, Hep-Lock U/P*

🍁 *Heparin calcium:* Calcilean, Calciparine

Drug class.: Anticoagulant

Action: Acts in combination with antithrombin III (heparin cofactor) to inhibit thrombosis; inactivates factor Xa and inhibits conversion of prothrombin to thrombin; affects both intrinsic and extrinsic clotting pathways

Uses: Anticoagulant in thrombosis, embolism (both prevention and treatment), coagulopathies, deep vein thrombosis, prevention of clotting when extracorporeal circulation is required (cardiac surgery), dialysis, maintenance of patency of indwelling IV lines

Dosage and routes:

General doses listed; all doses must be individualized to patient and circumstance:

- *Adult:* SC 10,000-20,000 U (USP) initially, then 8000-10,000 U q8h or 15,000 U q12h; IV 10,000 U initially, then 5000-10,000 U q4-6h; IV inf 20,000-40,000 U in 1 L of normal saline over 24 hr
- *Child:* IV 50 U/kg initially, then 100 U/kg by IV drip q4h or 20,000 U/m^2 over 24 hr by continuous infusion

Available forms include: Amps 1000, 5000, 10,000 U/ml; vials 1000, 2000, 2500, 5000, 10,000, 20,000, 40,000 U/ml; unit dose 1000, 2500, 5000, 7500, 10,000,

20,000 U/dose; heparin lock flush 10, 100 U/ml; heparin calcium 5000 U/dose

Side effects/adverse reactions:
▼ *ORAL:* Bleeding, stomatitis
CNS: Fever, chills
GI: Diarrhea, ***hepatitis,*** nausea, vomiting, anorexia, abdominal cramps
GU: ***Hematuria***
HEMA: ***Hemorrhage, thrombocytopenia***
INTEG: Rash, hives, itching, allergies

Contraindications: Hypersensitivity, hemophilia, leukemia with bleeding, peptic ulcer disease, thrombocytopenic purpura, hepatic disease (severe), renal disease (severe), blood dyscrasias, pregnancy, severe hypertension, subacute bacterial endocarditis, acute nephritis

Precautions: Hematoma (IM); elderly; pregnancy category C; lactation; hyperkalemia; monitor APTT, PTT, WBC, ACT; endocarditis; trauma; alcoholism; prolongs intrinsic clotting pathway approximately 4-6 hr after each dose

Pharmacokinetics:
IV: Peak 5 min, duration 2-6 hr
SC: Onset 20-60 min, duration 8-12 hr, half-life 1.5 hr (variable depending on dose); 95% bound to plasma proteins; excreted in urine

Drug interactions of concern to dentistry:
- Increased risk of bleeding: salicylates, NSAIDs, parenteral penicillins, glucocorticoids, certain cephalosporins (cefamandole, cefoperazone, cefotetan)

DENTAL CONSIDERATIONS

General:
- Heparin is used only in hospitalized patients or during dialysis. A medical consultation is necessary if oral and maxillofacial surgery or trauma treatment is required. May need to defer treatment.
- Avoid products that affect platelet function, such as aspirin and NSAIDs.
- Consider local hemostasis measures to prevent excessive bleeding.
- Take precautions if dental surgery or intubation for general anesthesia is anticipated.

Consultations:
- Medical consultation may be required to assess disease control and patient's ability to tolerate stress.
- Medical consultation should include ACT, partial prothrombin, and prothrombin times.

Teach patient/family:
- Caution to prevent trauma when using oral hygiene aids
- Importance of good oral hygiene to prevent soft tissue inflammation
- To report oral lesions, soreness, or bleeding

homatropine HBr (optic)

(hoe-ma'troe-peen)
Isopto Homatropine
✤ Minims Homatropine
Drug class.: Mydriatic (topical)

Action: Blocks response of iris sphincter muscle and muscle of accommodation of ciliary body to cholinergic stimulation, resulting in dilation and paralysis of accommodation

Uses: Cycloplegic refraction, uveitis, mydriatic lens opacities

Dosage and routes:
- *Adult and child:* Instill 1 drop, repeat in 5-10 min for refraction or

1 drop bid or tid for uveitis; use 2% for children

Available forms include: Sol 2%, 5%

Side effects/adverse reactions:

CNS: Confusion, somnolence, flushing, fever

CV: Tachycardia

EENT: Blurred vision, photophobia, increased intraocular pressure, irritation, edema

Contraindications: Hypersensitivity, children <6 yr, narrow-angle glaucoma, increased intraocular pressure, infants

Precautions: Children, elderly, hypertension, hyperthyroidism, diabetes, pregnancy category C

Pharmacokinetics:

INSTILL: Peak 0.5-1 hr, duration 1-3 days

Drug interactions of concern to dentistry:

- Avoid concurrent use with pilocarpine
- Increased anticholinergic effects with other anticholinergic drugs (when significant absorption from the eye occurs)

DENTAL CONSIDERATIONS

General:

- Avoid dental light in patient's eyes; offer dark glasses for patient comfort.
- Protect patient's eyes from accidental spatter during dental treatment.

hydralazine HCl

(hye-dral'a-zeen)

Apresoline

Apo-Hydral, Novo-Hylazin

Drug class.: Antihypertensive, direct-acting peripheral vasodilator

Action: Dilates arteriolar smooth muscle by direct relaxation; reduction in blood pressure with reflex increases cardiac function

Uses: Essential hypertension; parenteral: severe essential hypertension

Dosage and routes:

- *Adult:* PO 10 mg qid 2-4 days, then 25 mg for rest of first wk, then 50 mg qid individualized to desired response, not to exceed 300 mg; IV/IM bol 20-40 mg q4-6h, administer PO asap; IM 20-40 mg q4-6h
- *Child:* PO 0.75 mg/kg/day in 4 divided doses; max 7.5 mg/kg/24 hr; IV 0.1-0.2 mg/kg q4-6h; IM 0.1-0.2 mg/kg q4-6h

Available forms include: Inj IV/IM 20 mg/ml; tabs 10, 25, 50, 100 mg

Side effects/adverse reactions:

CNS: Headache, tremors, dizziness, anxiety, peripheral neuritis, depression

CV: Palpitation, reflex tachycardia, angina, ***shock,*** edema, rebound hypertension

GI: Nausea, vomiting, anorexia, diarrhea, constipation

HEMA: ***Leukopenia, agranulocytosis,*** anemia

GU: Impotence, urinary retention, sodium, water retention

INTEG: Rash, pruritus

MISC: Lupus-like symptoms, nasal congestion, muscle cramps

Contraindications: Hypersensitivity to hydralazines, CAD, mitral valvular rheumatic heart disease, rheumatic heart disease

Precautions: Pregnancy category C, CVA, advanced renal disease

Pharmacokinetics:

PO: Onset 20-45 min, peak 1-2 hr, duration 2-4 hr

IV: Onset 5-20 min, peak 10-80 min, duration 2-6 hr, half-life 2-8 hr

Metabolized by liver; <10% present in urine

Drug interactions of concern to dentistry:

• Reduced effects: NSAIDs, indomethacin, sympathomimetics

DENTAL CONSIDERATIONS

General:

• Monitor vital signs at every appointment because of cardiovascular side effects.

• Patients on chronic drug therapy may rarely have symptoms of blood dyscrasias, which can include infection, bleeding, and poor healing.

• Limit use of sodium-containing products such as saline IV fluids for patients with a dietary salt restriction.

• After supine positioning, have patient sit upright for at least 2 min to avoid orthostatic hypotension.

Consultations:

• In a patient with symptoms of blood dyscrasias, request a medical consultation for blood studies and postpone dental treatment until normal values are reestablished.

• Medical consultation may be required to assess disease control and patient's ability to tolerate stress.

Teach patient/family:

• Importance of good oral hygiene to prevent soft tissue inflammation

• Caution to prevent injury when using oral hygiene aids

---

hydrochlorothiazide (HTCZ)

(hye-droe-klor-oh-thye'a-zide)

Esidrix, Ezide, HydroDIURIL, Hydro-Par, Microzide, Oretic

♣ Apo-Hydro, Diuchlor H, Neo-Codema, Novo-Hydrazide, Urozide

Drug class.: Thiazide diuretic

Action: Acts on distal tubule by increasing excretion of water, sodium, chloride, potassium

Uses: Edema, hypertension, diuresis, CHF

Dosage and routes:

• *Adult:* PO 12.5-50 mg/day

• *Child >6 mo:* PO 2.2 mg/kg/day in divided doses

• *Child <6 mo:* PO up to 3.3 mg/kg/day in divided doses

Available forms include: Tabs 12.5, 25, 50, 100 mg; caps 12.5 mg; sol 50 mg/5 ml, 100 mg/ml

Side effects/adverse reactions:

▼ *ORAL: Dry mouth, increased thirst,* lichenoid reaction

CNS: Dizziness, fatigue, weakness, drowsiness, paresthesia, anxiety, depression, headache

CV: Irregular pulse, orthostatic hypotension, palpitation, volume depletion

GI: Nausea, vomiting, anorexia, hepatitis, constipation, diarrhea, cramps, pancreatitis, GI irritation

HEMA: ***Aplastic anemia, hemolytic anemia, leukopenia, agranulocytosis, thrombocytopenia, neutropenia***

GU: Frequency, uremia, glucosuria, polyuria

EENT: Blurred vision
INTEG: Rash, urticaria, purpura, photosensitivity, fever
META: Hyperglycemia, hyperuricemia, increased creatinine, BUN
ELECT: Hypokalemia, hypercalcemia, hyponatremia, hypochloremia, hypomagnesemia
Contraindications: Hypersensitivity to thiazides or sulfonamides, anuria, renal decompensation, hypomagnesemia
Precautions: Hypokalemia, renal disease, pregnancy category B, hepatic disease, gout, COPD, lupus erythematosus, diabetes mellitus
Pharmacokinetics:
PO: Onset 2 hr, peak 4 hr, duration 6-12 hr; excreted unchanged by kidneys; crosses placenta; enters breast milk
Drug interactions of concern to dentistry:
- Decreased hypotensive response: NSAIDs, especially indomethacin

DENTAL CONSIDERATIONS
General:
- Monitor vital signs at every appointment because of cardiovascular side effects.
- Patients on chronic drug therapy may rarely have symptoms of blood dyscrasias, which can include infection, bleeding, and poor healing.
- After supine positioning, have patient sit upright for at least 2 min before standing to avoid orthostatic hypotension.
- Assess salivary flow as a factor in caries, periodontal disease, and candidiasis.
- Limit use of sodium-containing products such as saline IV fluids for patients with a dietary salt restriction.
- Stress from dental procedures may compromise cardiovascular function; determine patient risk.
- Short appointments and a stress reduction protocol may be required for anxious patients.
- Patients taking diuretics should be monitored for serum K^+ levels.

Consultations:
- In a patient with symptoms of blood dyscrasias, request a medical consultation for blood studies and postpone dental treatment until normal values are reestablished.
- Medical consultation may be required to assess disease control and patient's ability to tolerate stress.
- Physician should be informed if significant xerostomic side effects occur (e.g., increased caries, sore tongue, problems eating or swallowing, difficulty wearing prosthesis) so that a medication change can be considered.

Teach patient/family:
- Importance of good oral hygiene to prevent soft tissue inflammation
- Caution to prevent injury when using oral hygiene aids

When chronic dry mouth occurs, advise patient:
- To avoid mouth rinses with high alcohol content because of drying effects
- To use daily home fluoride products for anticaries effect
- To use sugarless gum, frequent sips of water, or saliva substitutes

hydrocodone bitartrate

(hye-droe-koe'done)
Hycodan
Robidone

Drug class.: Narcotic analgesic

Controlled Substance Schedule III, Canada N1

Action: Interacts with opioid receptors in the CNS to alter pain perception; acts directly on cough center in medulla to suppress cough

Uses: Hyperactive and nonproductive cough; mild-to-moderate pain; normally used in combination with aspirin or acetaminophen for post-treatment pain control

Dosage and routes:

• *Adult:* PO 5 mg q4h prn or 10 mg q12h (long-acting)

• *Child:* PO 0.15 mg/kg q6h

Available forms include: Caps 5 mg; susp 5 mg/ml; tabs 5, 10 mg (long-acting); some dose forms not available in United States

NOTE: Hycodan tablets (USA) are combined with 1.5 mg of homatropine methylbromide.

Side effects/adverse reactions:

ORAL: Dry mouth

CNS: ***Convulsions,*** drowsiness, dizziness, light-headedness, confusion, headache, sedation, euphoria, dysphoria, weakness, hallucinations, disorientation

CV: ***Circulatory depression,*** palpitation, tachycardia, bradycardia, change in BP, syncope

GI: Nausea, vomiting, anorexia, constipation, cramps

RESP: ***Respiratory depression***

GU: Increased urinary output, dysuria, urinary retention

EENT: Tinnitus, blurred vision, miosis, diplopia

INTEG: Rash, urticaria, flushing, pruritus

Contraindications: Hypersensitivity, addiction (narcotic)

Precautions: Addictive personality, pregnancy category C, lactation, increased intracranial pressure, MI (acute), severe heart disease, respiratory depression, hepatic disease, renal disease, child <18 yr

Pharmacokinetics: Onset 10-20 min, duration 3-6 hr, half-life 3-4 hr; metabolized in liver; excreted in urine; crosses placenta

Drug interactions of concern to dentistry:

• Increased CNS depression: alcohol, other opioids, phenothiazines, sedative/hypnotics, skeletal muscle relaxants, general anesthetics

• Contraindication: MAOIs

• Increased effects of anticholinergics

DENTAL CONSIDERATIONS

General:

• Monitor vital signs at every appointment because of cardiovascular and respiratory side effects.

• After supine positioning, have patient sit upright for at least 2 min to avoid orthostatic hypotension.

• Psychologic and physical dependence may occur with chronic administration.

• Determine why the patient is taking the drug.

Teach patient/family:

• To avoid mouth rinses with high alcohol content because of drying effects

H

hydrocortisone/ hydrocortisone acetate/hydrocortisone buteprate/ hydrocortisone butyrate/ hydrocortisone valerate

(hye-droe-kor'ti-sone)

Hydrocortisone: Ala-Cort, Articort, Bactine Hydrocortisone, Cortaid, Cort-Dome, Cortizone-5, Cortizone-10, Delcort, Dermacort, Dermolate, Dermtex HC, Hi-Cor 1.0, Hycort, Hydro-Tex, Hytone, Nutracort, Penecort, Procort, Scalpicin, St-Coat, Synacort, Tegrin-HC

♣ Cortef, Emo-Cort, Lemoderm Cortate, Prevex-HC, Unicort

Hydrocortisone acetate: Anusol HC, Cortaid with aloe, Corticaine, Cortef Feminine, Gynecort, Lanacort-5

♣ Novohydrocort

Hydrocortisone buteprate: Pandel

Hydrocortisone butyrate: Locoid Cream, Locoid Ointment

Hydrocortisone valerate: Wescort Cream, Westcort Ointment

Drug class.: Topical corticosteroid

Action: Interacts with steroid cytoplasmic receptors to induce antiinflammatory effects; possesses antipruritic, antiinflammatory actions

Uses: Psoriasis, eczema, contact dermatitis, pruritus

Dosage and routes:

• *Adult and child >2 yr:* Apply to affected area qd-qid

Available forms include: Hydrocortisone: oint 0.5%, 1%, 2.5%; cream 0.5%, 1%, 2.5%; lotion 0.25%, 0.5%, 1%, 2%, 2.5%; gel 1%; sol 1%; aerosol/pump spray 1.0%; acetate: oint 0.5%, 1%; cream 0.5%; valerate: oint 0.2%; cream 0.2%; buteprate: cream 0.1%, 1% in 15 and 45 g; butyrate: oint 0.1%, cream 0.1%; sol 0.1%

Side effects/adverse reactions:

▼ *ORAL:* Thinning of mucosa, stinging sensation (oral application site)

INTEG: Burning, dryness, itching, irritation, acne, folliculitis, hypertrichosis, perioral dermatitis, hypopigmentation, atrophy, striae, miliaria, allergic contact dermatitis, secondary infection

Contraindications: Hypersensitivity to corticosteroids, fungal infections, herpetic infections

Precautions: Pregnancy category C, lactation, viral infections, bacterial infections

DENTAL CONSIDERATIONS

General:

• Place on frequent recall to evaluate healing response if used on a chronic basis.

Teach patient/family:

• Importance of good oral hygiene to prevent soft tissue inflammation

• To apply at bedtime or after meals for maximum effect

• That use on oral herpetic ulcerations is contraindicated

• To apply with cotton-tipped applicator by pressing, not rubbing, paste on lesion

• That when used for oral lesions, to return for oral evaluation if response of oral tissues has not occurred in 7-14 days

hydrocortisone/ hydrocortisone acetate/hydrocortisone cypionate/ hydrocortisone sodium phosphate/ hydrocortisone sodium succinate

(hye-dro-kor'ti-sone)

Hydrocortisone (tab): Cortef, Hydrocortone

Hydrocortisone cypionate (oral susp): Cortef

Hydrocortisone sodium phosphate (IV/IM/SC): Hydrocortone Phosphate

Hydrocortisone sodium succinate (IV/IM): A-Hydrocort, Solu-Cortef

Hydrocortisone acetate (intraarticular, soft tissue only): Hydrocortone Acetate

Hydrocortisone acetate (rectal): Cortiform

Hydrocortisone (rectal): Cortenema

Drug class.: Corticosteroid

Action: Glucocorticoids have multiple actions that include anti-inflammatory and immunosuppressant effects. They inhibit phospholipase A_2, interfering with or reducing the synthesis of prostaglandins and leukotrienes. They also bind to cytoplasmic GRs and enter the cell nucleus to bind with DNA. This results in the synthesis of various enzymes such as collagenase, elastase, and cytokines that play important roles in inflammation and immunosuppression. They also suppress the production of lymphocytes, monocytes, and eosinophils.

Uses: Severe inflammation, shock, adrenal insufficiency, ulcerative colitis, collagen disorders

Dosage and routes:

Adrenal insufficiency/inflammation:

• *Adult:* PO 5-30 mg bid-qid; IM/IV 100-250 mg (succinate), then 50-100 mg IM as needed; IM/IV 15-240 mg q12h (phosphate)

Shock:

• *Adult:* 500 mg-2 g q2-6h (succinate)

• *Child:* IM/IV 0.16-1 mg/kg bid-tid (succinate)

Colitis:

• *Adult:* Enema 100 mg nightly for 21 days

Available forms include: Retention enema 100 mg/60 ml; tabs 5, 10, 20 mg; inj 50 mg/ml; succinate inj 100, 250, 500, 1000 mg/vial; phosphate inj 50 mg/ml; acetate inj 25, 50 mg/ml; oral susp 10 mg/5 ml in 120 ml

Side effects/adverse reactions:

▼ *ORAL:* Dry mouth, poor wound healing, petechiae, candidiasis

CNS: Depression, flushing, sweating, headache, mood changes

CV: Hypertension, ***circulatory collapse, thrombophlebitis, embolism,*** tachycardia, edema

GI: Diarrhea, nausea, ***pancreatitis, GI hemorrhage,*** increased appetite, abdominal distention

HEMA: ***Thrombocytopenia***

EENT: Fungal infections, increased intraocular pressure, blurred vision

INTEG: Acne, poor wound healing, ecchymosis, petechiae

MS: Fractures, osteoporosis, weakness

Contraindications: Psychosis, hypersensitivity, idiopathic thrombocytopenia, acute glomerulonephritis, amebiasis, fungal infections, nonasthmatic bronchial disease, child <2 yr, AIDS, TB

Precautions: Pregnancy category C, diabetes mellitus, glaucoma, osteoporosis, seizure disorders, ulcerative colitis, CHF, myasthenia gravis, renal disease, esophagitis, peptic ulcer, rifampin

Pharmacokinetics:

PO: Onset 1-2 hr, peak 1 hr, duration 1-1.5 days

IM/IV: Onset 20 min, peak 4-8 hr, duration 1-1.5 days

REC: Onset 3-5 days

Metabolized by liver, excreted in urine (17-OHCH, 17-KS), crosses placenta

Drug interactions of concern to dentistry:

- Decreased action: barbiturates, rifabutin, rifampin
- Increased GI side effects: alcohol, salicylates, NSAIDs
- Increased action: ketoconazole, macrolide antibiotics

DENTAL CONSIDERATIONS

General:

- Monitor vital signs at every appointment because of cardiovascular side effects.
- Patients on chronic drug therapy may rarely have symptoms of blood dyscrasias, which can include infection, bleeding, and poor healing.
- Assess salivary flow as a factor in caries, periodontal disease, and candidiasis.
- Place on frequent recall to evaluate healing response.
- Prophylactic antibiotics may be indicated to prevent infection if surgery or deep scaling is planned.
- Avoid prescribing aspirin-containing products.
- Symptoms of oral infections may be masked.
- Determine dose and duration of steroid therapy for each patient to assess the risk for stress tolerance and immunosuppression.
- Patients who have been or are currently on chronic steroid therapy >2 wk may require supplemental steroids for dental treatment.
- Determine why the patient is taking the drug.

Consultations:

- In a patient with symptoms of blood dyscrasias, request a medical consultation for blood studies and postpone dental treatment until normal values are reestablished.
- Medical consultation may be required to assess disease control and patient's ability to tolerate stress.
- Consultation may be required to confirm steroid dose and duration of use.

Teach patient/family:

- Importance of good oral hygiene to prevent soft tissue inflammation
- Caution to prevent injury when using oral hygiene aids

When chronic dry mouth occurs, advise patient:

- To avoid mouth rinses with high alcohol content because of drying effects
- To use sugarless gum, frequent sips of water, or saliva substitutes
- To use daily home fluoride products for anticaries effect

hydromorphone HCl

(hye-droe-mor'fone)

Dilaudid, Dilaudid-5, Dilaudid HP

♣ PMS-Hydromorphone

Drug class.: Synthetic narcotic analgesic

Controlled Substance Schedule II, Canada N

Action: Inhibits ascending pain pathways in CNS, increases pain threshold, alters pain perception

Uses: Moderate-to-severe pain

Dosage and routes:

• *Adult:* PO 1-10 mg q3-6h depending on pain severity and dose form; IM/SC/IV 2-4 mg q4-6h; rec 3 mg hs prn

Available forms include: Inj IM/IV 1, 2, 3, 4, 10 mg/ml; tabs 1, 2, 3, 4, 8 mg; rec supp 3 mg; liquid 5 mg/5 ml

Side effects/adverse reactions:

▼ *ORAL:* Dry mouth

CNS: Drowsiness, dizziness, confusion, headache, sedation, euphoria

CV: Palpitation, bradycardia, change in BP

GI: Nausea, vomiting, anorexia, constipation, cramps

RESP: ***Respiratory depression***

GU: Increased urinary output, dysuria, urinary retention

EENT: Tinnitus, blurred vision, miosis, diplopia

INTEG: Rash, urticaria, bruising, flushing, diaphoresis, pruritus

Contraindications: Hypersensitivity, addiction (narcotic), MAOIs

Precautions: Addictive personality, pregnancy category C, lactation, increased intracranial pressure, MI (acute), severe heart disease, respiratory depression, hepatic disease, renal disease, child <18 yr

Pharmacokinetics:

PO: Onset 15-30 min, peak 0.5-1.5 hr, duration 4-5 hr; metabolized by liver; excreted by kidneys; crosses placenta; excreted in breast milk

Drug interactions of concern to dentistry:

• Effects may be increased with other CNS depressants: alcohol, narcotics, sedative/hypnotics, skeletal muscle relaxants

• Increased effects of anticholinergic drugs

DENTAL CONSIDERATIONS

General:

• Monitor vital signs at every appointment because of cardiovascular and respiratory side effects.

• After supine positioning, have patient sit upright for at least 2 min to avoid orthostatic hypotension.

• Assess salivary flow as a factor in caries, periodontal disease, and candidiasis.

• Psychologic and physical dependence may occur with chronic administration.

• Determine why the patient is taking the drug.

• Avoid in patients with chronic obstructive pulmonary disease.

Teach patient/family:

• To avoid mouth rinses with high alcohol content because of drying effects

H

hydroxychloroquine sulfate

(hye-drox-ee-klor'oh-kwin)

Plaquenil Sulfate

Drug class.: Antimalarial

Action: Inhibits parasite replications and transcription of DNA to RNA by forming complexes with DNA of parasite

Uses: Malaria caused by *P. vivax, P. malariae, P. ovale, P. falciparum* (some strains); lupus erythematosus; rheumatoid arthritis

Dosage and routes:

Malaria (suppressive therapy):

• *Adult:* PO 400 mg once q7d

• *Child:* PO 6.4 mg/kg once q7d

Malaria (therapeutic therapy):

• *Adult:* PO 800 mg single dose, or give an initial dose of 800 mg followed by 400 mg in 6-8 hr, then 400 mg qd for next 2 days

• *Child:* PO 10 mg/kg as an initial dose, followed by 5 mg/kg 6 hr later, then 5 mg/kg on the next 2 days; do not exceed the adult dose

Lupus erythematosus:

• *Adult:* PO up to 6.5 mg/kg of lean body weight/day

Rheumatoid arthritis:

• *Adult:* PO 400-600 mg qd, then 200-300 mg qd after good response

Available forms include: Tabs 200 mg

Side effects/adverse reactions:

▼ *ORAL:* Discoloration of mucosa, lichenoid lesions

CNS: ***Convulsions,*** headache, stimulation, fatigue, irritability, bad dreams, dizziness, confusion, psychosis, decreased reflexes

CV: ***Asystole with syncope,*** hypotension, heart block

GI: Nausea, vomiting, anorexia, diarrhea, cramps

HEMA: ***Thrombocytopenia, agranulocytosis, hemolytic anemia, leukopenia***

EENT: Blurred vision, corneal changes, retinal changes, difficulty focusing, tinnitus, vertigo, deafness, photophobia, corneal edema

INTEG: ***Exfoliative dermatitis,*** alopecia, pruritus, pigmentation changes, skin eruptions, lichen planus–like eruptions, eczema

Contraindications: Hypersensitivity, retinal field changes, porphyria, children (long-term use)

Precautions: Blood dyscrasias, severe GI disease, neurologic disease, alcoholism, hepatic disease, G6PD deficiency, psoriasis, eczema, pregnancy category C

Pharmacokinetics:

PO: Peak 1-2 hr, half-life 3-5 days; metabolized in liver; excreted in urine, feces, breast milk; crosses placenta

Drug interactions of concern to dentistry:

• None reported

DENTAL CONSIDERATIONS

General:

• Patients on chronic drug therapy may rarely have symptoms of blood dyscrasias, which can include infection, bleeding, and poor healing.

• Avoid dental light in patient's eyes; offer dark glasses for patient comfort.

• Determine why the patient is taking the drug.

Consultations:

• In a patient with symptoms of blood dyscrasias, request a medical consultation for blood studies and postpone dental treatment until normal values are reestablished.

Teach patient/family:

• Importance of good oral hygiene to prevent soft tissue inflammation

• To avoid mouth rinses with high alcohol content because of drying effects

---

hydroxyurea

(hye-drox-ee-your-ee'a)

Hydrea

Drug class.: Antineoplastic

Action: Acts by inhibiting DNA synthesis without interfering with the synthesis of RNA or protein

Uses: Melanoma, chronic myelocytic leukemia, recurrent or metastatic ovarian cancer, in combination with irradiation therapy for carcinomas of the head and neck (except the lip); sickle cell anemia; unapproved use in thrombocythemia

Dosage and routes:

Sickle cell anemia:

• *Child:* PO 15 mg/kg/day single dose, titrated at 12 wk up to 35 mg/kg/day; monitor CBC q2wk

Solid tumors:

• *Adult:* PO 80 mg/kg as a single dose q3d or 20-30 mg/kg as a single dose daily for continuous therapy

With radiation:

• *Adult:* PO 80 mg/kg as a single dose q3d

Available forms include: Caps 500 mg

Side effects/adverse reactions:

▼ *ORAL:* Stomatitis, mucositis (with irradiation), lichenoid reaction

CNS: ***Convulsions,*** anorexia, headache, confusion, hallucinations, dizziness

CV: Angina, ischemia

GI: Nausea, vomiting, anorexia, diarrhea, constipation

HEMA: ***Leukopenia, anemia, thrombocytopenia***

GU: Increased BUN, uric acid, creatinine, temporary renal function impairment

INTEG: *Rash,* urticaria, pruritus, dry skin, facial erythema

Contraindications: Hypersensitivity, leukopenia (<2500/mm^3), thrombocytopenia (<100,000/mm^3), anemia (severe), marked bone marrow depression

Precautions: Pregnancy category D, monitor blood counts and hemoglobin, renal impairment, elderly

Pharmacokinetics:

PO: Readily absorbed with PO use, peak level in 2 hr; 80% excreted in urine

Drug interactions of concern to dentistry:

• None reported

DENTAL CONSIDERATIONS

General:

• Patients receiving chemotherapy may be taking chronic opioids for pain. Consider NSAIDs for dental pain management.

• Patients receiving chemotherapy may require palliative therapy for stomatitis.

• Patients on chronic drug therapy may rarely have symptoms of blood dyscrasias, which can include infection, bleeding, and poor healing.

Consultations:

• Medical consultation may be required to assess disease control.

• In a patient with symptoms of blood dyscrasias, request a medical consultation for blood studies and postpone dental treatment until normal values are reestablished.

Teach patient/family:

• That secondary oral infection may occur; must see dentist immediately if infection occurs

When chronic dry mouth occurs, advise patient:

• To avoid mouth rinses with high alcohol content because of drying effects

• To use sugarless gum, frequent sips of water, or saliva substitutes

• To use daily home fluoride products for anticaries effect

---

hydroxyzine HCl/ hydroxyzine pamoate

(hye-drox'i-zeen)

Atarax, Vistaril, Vistaril IM, Vistazine 50

✦ Apo-Hydroxyzine, Multipax, Novo-Hydroxyzin

Drug class.: Antianxiety, antihistamine

Action: Depresses subcortical levels of CNS, antagonist for histamine H_1-receptors

Uses: Anxiety, preoperatively/postoperatively to prevent nausea and vomiting, to potentiate narcotic analgesics, sedation, pruritus

Dosage and routes:

Pruritus:

• *Adult:* PO 25 mg tid-qid

Anxiety:

• *Adult:* PO 50-100 mg qid

• *Child 6 yr or older:* 50-100 mg/day in divided doses

• *Child <6 yr:* Up to 50 mg/day in divided doses

Preoperatively/postoperatively:

• *Adult:* IM 25-100 mg q4-6h

• *Child:* IM 1.1 mg/kg q4-6h

Available forms include: Tabs 10, 25, 50, 100 mg; caps 25, 50, 100 mg; syr 10 mg/5 ml; oral susp 25 mg/5 ml; inj IM 25 mg/ml, 50 mg/5 ml

Side effects/adverse reactions:

▼ *ORAL:* Dry mouth

CNS: Dizziness, drowsiness, confusion, headache, tremors, fatigue, depression, convulsions

Contraindications: Hypersensitivity, pregnancy category not established, avoid in pregnancy

Precautions: Elderly, debilitated, hepatic disease, renal disease

Pharmacokinetics:

PO: Onset 15-30 min, duration 4-6 hr, half-life 3 hr

Drug interactions of concern to dentistry:

• Increased CNS depressant effect: alcohol, all CNS depressants

• Increased anticholinergic effects: other antihistamines, anticholinergics, opioid analgesics

DENTAL CONSIDERATIONS

General:

• Potentiates other CNS depressant drugs. When used in combination, the dose of other CNS depressants should be reduced by one half.

• Assess salivary flow as a factor in caries, periodontal disease, and candidiasis.

• Geriatric patients are more susceptible to drug effects; use lower dose.

• Have someone drive patient to and from dental appointment if the drug is prescribed for dental therapy.

Teach patient/family:

When chronic dry mouth occurs, advise patient:

• To avoid mouth rinses with high alcohol content because of drying effects

• To use sugarless gum, frequent sips of water, or saliva substitutes
• To use daily home fluoride products for anticaries effect

hyoscyamine sulfate

(hye-oh-sye'a-meen)

Anaspaz, A-Spas S/L, Cystospaz, Cystospaz-M, Donnamar, ED-Spaz, Gastrosed, Levbid, Levsin, Levsin S/L, Levsinex, Neoquess

Drug class.: Anticholinergic

Action: Inhibits muscarinic actions of acetylcholine at postganglionic parasympathetic neuroeffector sites

Uses: Treatment of peptic ulcer disease in combination with other drugs, other GI disorders, other spastic disorders such as parkinsonism, preoperatively to reduce secretions, GU disorders (cystitis, renal colic), partial heart block

Dosage and routes:

• *Adult:* PO/SL 0.125-0.25 mg tid-qid ac, hs; time rel 0.375 q12h; IM/SC/IV 0.25-0.5 mg q6h

• *Child 2-10 yr:* One-half adult dose

• *Child <2 yr:* One-fourth adult dose

Available forms include: Tabs 0.125, 0.15 mg; time rel caps 0.375 mg; ext rel tabs 0.375; sol 0.125 mg/ml; elix 0.125 mg/5 ml; inj IM/IV/SC 0.5 mg/ml

Side effects/adverse reactions:

▼ *ORAL: Dry mouth*

CNS: Confusion, stimulation in elderly, headache, insomnia, dizziness, drowsiness, anxiety, weakness, hallucination

CV: Palpitation, tachycardia

GI: Constipation, paralytic ileus, heartburn, nausea, vomiting, dysphagia

GU: Hesitancy, retention, impotence

EENT: Blurred vision, photophobia, mydriasis, cycloplegia, increased ocular tension

INTEG: Urticaria, rash, pruritus, anhidrosis, fever, allergic reactions

Contraindications: Hypersensitivity to anticholinergics, narrow-angle glaucoma, GI obstruction, myasthenia gravis, paralytic ileus, GI atony, toxic megacolon, prostatic hypertrophy

Precautions: Hyperthyroidism, CAD, dysrhythmias, CHF, ulcerative colitis, hypertension, hiatal hernia, hepatic disease, renal disease, pregnancy category C, urinary retention

Pharmacokinetics:

PO: Duration 4-6 hr; metabolized by liver, excreted in urine, half-life 3.5 hr

Drug interactions of concern to dentistry:

• Increased anticholinergic effect: other anticholinergics, opioid analgesics

• Decreased effect of phenothiazines

DENTAL CONSIDERATIONS

General:

• After supine positioning, have patient sit upright for at least 2 min to avoid orthostatic hypotension.

• Assess salivary flow as a factor in caries, periodontal disease, and candidiasis.

• Avoid dental light in patient's eyes; offer dark glasses for patient comfort.

Consultation: Physician should be informed if significant xerostomic side effects occur (e.g., in-

H

creased caries, sore tongue, problems eating or swallowing, difficulty wearing prosthesis) so that a medication change can be considered.

Teach patient/family:

• Importance of good oral hygiene to prevent soft tissue inflammation

When chronic dry mouth occurs, advise patient:

• To avoid mouth rinses with high alcohol content because of drying effects

• To use sugarless gum, frequent sips of water, or artificial saliva substitutes

• To use daily home fluoride products for anticaries effect

---

ibuprofen

(eye-byoo-proe'fen)

Ibifon, IBU, Ibuprohm, Motrin, Rufen

♣ Amersol

OTC: Advil, Advil Migraine, Advil Liqui-Gels, Children's Advil, Children's Motrin, Genpril, Haltran, Junior Strength Advil, Menadol, Midol Maximum, Motrin IB, Motrin Junior Strength, Motrin Migraine Pain, Nuprin

♣ Actiprofen, Apo-Ibuprofen, Novo-Profen, Nu-Ibuprofen

Susp: Children's Advil, Infant's Motrin, Pediatric Advil, PediaCare Fever

♣ Children's Apo-Ibuprofen

Drug class.: Nonsteroidal antiinflammatory

Action: Inhibits prostaglandin synthesis by interfering with cyclooxygenase needed for biosynthesis; possesses analgesic, antiinflammatory, antipyretic properties

Uses: Rheumatoid arthritis, osteoarthritis, primary dysmenorrhea, gout, mild to moderate pain, fever

Dosage and routes:

Arthritis:

• *Adult:* PO 200-800 mg qid, not to exceed 3.2 g/day

• *Child 2-11 yr:* PO oral suspension (OTC) for fever and minor aches and pain, toothache; 7.5 mg/kg up to qid; max daily dose 30 mg/kg

Mild to moderate pain:

• *Adult:* PO 400 mg q4-6h

Dysmenorrhea:

• *Adult:* PO 400 mg q4h

Antipyretic use only:

• *Child 6 mo-12 yr:* 5 mg/kg for temperature <102.5° F; 10 mg/kg for higher temperature q4-6h, max dose 40 mg/kg

Available forms include: Tabs 100, 200 (OTC), 300, 400, 600, 800 mg; OTC chew tabs 50, 100 mg; OTC susp 100 mg/2.5, 5 ml in 7.5, 60, 120, and 480 ml volumes; caps 200 mg; oral drops 40 mg/ml in 15 ml

Side effects/adverse reactions:

▼ *ORAL:* Dry mouth, bleeding, stomatitis, lichenoid reaction

CNS: Dizziness, drowsiness, fatigue, tremors, confusion, insomnia, anxiety, depression

CV: Tachycardia, peripheral edema, palpitation, dysrhythmias

GI: ***Cholestatic hepatitis,*** nausea, anorexia, vomiting, diarrhea, jaundice, constipation, flatulence, cramps, peptic ulcer

HEMA: ***Blood dyscrasias***

GU: ***Nephrotoxicity: dysuria, hematuria, oliguria, azotemia***

EENT: Tinnitus, hearing loss, blurred vision

INTEG: Purpura, rash, pruritus, sweating

Contraindications: Hypersensitivity, asthma, severe renal disease, severe hepatic disease, alcohol

Precautions: Pregnancy category not established (use not recommended), lactation, children, bleeding disorders, GI disorders, cardiac disorders, hypersensitivity to other antiinflammatory agents

Pharmacokinetics:

PO: Peak 1-2 hr, half-life 2-4 hr; 90%-99% plasma-protein binding; metabolized in liver (inactive metabolites); excreted in urine (inactive metabolites)

Drug interactions of concern to dentistry:

- GI ulceration, bleeding: aspirin, alcohol (3 or more drinks/day), corticosteroids
- Decreased action: salicylates
- Nephrotoxicity: acetaminophen (prolonged use)
- Possible risk of decreased renal function: cyclosporine
- First-time users of SSRIs also taking NSAIDs may have a higher risk of GI side effects; until more data are available, it may be advisable to avoid use of NSAIDs in these patients (*Br J Clin Pharmacol* 55:591-595, 2003)

When prescribed for dental pain:

- Risk of increased effects: oral anticoagulants, oral antidiabetics, lithium, methotrexate
- Decreased antihypertensive effects of diuretics, β-adrenergic blockers, and ACE inhibitors

DENTAL CONSIDERATIONS

General:

- Patients on chronic drug therapy may rarely have symptoms of blood dyscrasias, which can include infection, bleeding, and poor healing.
- Assess salivary flow as a factor in caries, periodontal disease, and candidiasis.
- Avoid prescribing aspirin-containing products.
- Consider semisupine chair position for patients with arthritic disease.

Consultations:

- In a patient with symptoms of blood dyscrasias, request a medical consultation for blood studies and postpone dental treatment until normal values are reestablished.
- Medical consultation may be required to assess disease control.

Teach patient/family:

- To follow labeled directions for OTC products
- Importance of good oral hygiene to prevent soft tissue inflammation
- Caution to prevent injury when using oral hygiene aids

When chronic dry mouth occurs, advise patient:

- To avoid mouth rinses with high alcohol content because of drying effects
- To use sugarless gum, frequent sips of water, or saliva substitutes
- To use daily home fluoride products for anticaries effect

---

imatinib mesylate

(im-at'i-nib)

Gleevec

Drug class.: Antineoplastic

Action: Inhibits protein-tyrosine kinase, notably Bcr-Abl tyrosine kinase (the abnormal tyrosine kinase) in chronic myeloid leukemia; inhibits proliferation and induces apoptosis (programmed cell death) in Bcr-Abl–positive cell lines

Uses: Chronic myeloid leukemia

(CML) in blast crisis, accelerated phase or chronic phase after failure of interferon-alpha therapy; gastrointestinal stromal tumors

Dosage and routes:

• *Adult:* PO 400 mg/day for patients in chronic phase; 600 mg/day for patients in blast crisis or accelerated phases; dose is administered once daily with a meal and large glass of water

Available forms include: Caps 100 mg; tabs 100, 400 mg

Side effects/adverse reactions:

CNS: Headache, fatigue, anorexia, weakness

CV: Neutropenia, thrombocytopenia, anemia, potentially serious edema

GI: Nausea, vomiting, diarrhea, dyspepsia, abdominal pain

RESP: ***Pleural effusion,*** pulmonary edema, cough, dyspnea, pneumonia

HEMA: Hemorrhage (CNS, GI), epistaxis

EENT: Nasopharyngitis

INTEG: Rash, pruritus, petechiae

ENDO: Hypokalemia, elevation of transaminase, bilirubin, AST, ALT, creatinine, alk phosphatase

META: Weight gain

MS: Muscle cramps, pain, arthralgia

MISC: Edema (lower limbs, periorbital tissues), ascites, fever

Contraindications: Hypersensitivity, pregnancy not advised while taking this drug

Precautions: Fluid retention, edema risk; neutropenia, thrombocytopenia, GI irritation, liver function abnormalities; pregnancy category D, safety in lactation or pediatric patients has not been studied

Pharmacokinetics:

PO: Mean absolute bioavailability 95%; plasma protein binding 95%; metabolized by cytochrome P450 3A4 enzymes; active metabolite, excreted mainly in feces 68%, urine 13%

Drug interactions of concern to dentistry:

• Increased plasma levels with CYP 3A4 isoenzyme inhibitors: ketoconazole; possibly macrolide antibiotics, itraconazole, benzodiazepines (see Appendix I)

• Use acetaminophen with caution or avoid if hepatotoxicity is present

• Possible decrease in plasma concentrations: dexamethasone, carbamazepine, St. John's wort (herb)

DENTAL CONSIDERATIONS

General:

• Prophylactic or therapeutic antibiotics may be indicated to prevent or treat infection if surgery or periodontal debridement is required.

• Patients taking opioids for acute or chronic pain should be given alternative analgesics for dental pain.

• Short appointments and a stress reduction protocol may be required for anxious patients.

• Consider local hemostasis measures to control excessive bleeding.

• Patients on chronic drug therapy may rarely have symptoms of blood dyscrasias, which can include infection, bleeding, and poor healing.

• Consider semisupine chair position for patient comfort if GI side effects occur.

Consultations:

• In a patient with symptoms of blood dyscrasias, request a medical consultation for blood studies and postpone treatment until normal values are reestablished.

• Consultation with physician may be needed if sedation or general anesthesia is required.

• Medical consultation should include routine blood counts, including platelet counts and bleeding time.

Teach patient/family:

• Importance of good oral hygiene to prevent soft tissue inflammation/infection

• To inform dentist of unusual bleeding episodes following dental treatment

imipramine HCl/imipramine pamoate

(im-ip'ra-meen)

Imipramine HCl: Tofranil

♣ Apo-Imipramine, Impril, Novopramine

Imipramine pamoate: Tofranil-PM Capsules

Drug class.: Antidepressant (tricyclic)

Action: Inhibits both norepinephrine and serotonin (5-HT) uptake in the brain, although the precise antidepressant mechanism remains unclear

Uses: Depression, enuresis in children; unapproved: neurogenic pain, panic disorder, migraine headache

Dosage and routes:

• *Adult:* PO/IM 75-100 mg/day in divided doses; may increase by 25-50 mg to 200 mg, not to exceed 200 mg/day; may give daily dose hs

• *Adolescent and geriatric:* PO 30-40 mg/day; do not exceed 100 mg/day

Enuresis:

• *Child >6 yr:* PO initial dose 25 mg/day 1 hr before bedtime; dose may be increased to 50 mg if response is unsatisfactory; children >12 yr may use up to 75 mg/day

Available forms include: Tabs 10, 25, 50 mg; caps 75, 100, 125, 150 mg

Side effects/adverse reactions:

▼ *ORAL: Dry mouth, unpleasant taste,* stomatitis

CNS: Dizziness, drowsiness, confusion, headache, anxiety, tremors, stimulation, weakness, insomnia, nightmares, EPS (elderly), increased psychiatric symptoms, paresthesia

CV: Orthostatic hypotension, ECG changes, tachycardia, ***hypertension,*** palpitation

GI: Diarrhea, ***paralytic ileus, hepatitis,*** nausea, vomiting, increased appetite, cramps, epigastric distress, jaundice

HEMA: ***Agranulocytosis, thrombocytopenia, eosinophilia, leukopenia***

GU: Retention, ***acute renal failure***

EENT: Blurred vision, tinnitus, mydriasis

INTEG: Rash, urticaria, sweating, pruritus, photosensitivity

Contraindications: Hypersensitivity to tricyclic antidepressants, recovery phase of MI, convulsive disorders, prostatic hypertrophy

Precautions: Suicidal patients, severe depression, increased intraocular pressure, narrow-angle glaucoma, urinary retention, cardiac disease, hepatic disease, hyperthyroidism, electroshock therapy, elective surgery, elderly, pregnancy category C, MAOIs

I

Pharmacokinetics:
PO: Steady state 2-5 days, half-life 6-20 hr; metabolized by liver; excreted by kidneys, feces; crosses placenta; excreted in breast milk

Drug interactions of concern to dentistry:
- Increased anticholinergic effects: muscarinic blockers, antihistamines, phenothiazines
- Increased effects of direct-acting sympathomimetics (epinephrine, levonordefrin)
- Potential risk of increased CNS depression: alcohol, barbiturates, benzodiazepines, and other CNS depressants
- Decreased antihypertensive effects: clonidine, guanadrel, guanethidine
- Avoid concurrent use with St. John's wort (herb)
- Suspected increased tricyclic antidepressant effects: fluconazole, ketoconazole
- Increased serum levels of carbamazepine
- Caution in using drugs metabolized by CYP2D6: increased effects (see Appendix I)

DENTAL CONSIDERATIONS

General:
- Monitor vital signs at every appointment because of cardiovascular side effects.
- Assess salivary flow as a factor in caries, periodontal disease, and candidiasis.
- Patients on chronic drug therapy may rarely have symptoms of blood dyscrasias, which can include infection, bleeding, and poor healing.
- After supine positioning, have patient sit upright for at least 2 min to avoid orthostatic hypotension.
- Use vasoconstrictors with caution, in low doses, and with careful aspiration. Avoid use of gingival retraction cord with epinephrine.
- Place on frequent recall because of oral side effects.

Consultations:
- In a patient with symptoms of blood dyscrasias, request a medical consultation for blood studies and postpone dental treatment until normal values are reestablished.
- Medical consultation may be required to assess disease control.
- Physician should be informed if significant xerostomic side effects occur (e.g., increased caries, sore tongue, problems eating or swallowing, difficulty wearing prosthesis) so that a medication change can be considered.

Teach patient/family:
- Importance of good oral hygiene to prevent soft tissue inflammation
- Caution to prevent injury when using oral hygiene aids

When chronic dry mouth occurs, advise patient:
- To avoid mouth rinses with high alcohol content because of drying effects
- To use sugarless gum, frequent sips of water, or saliva substitutes
- To use daily home fluoride products for anticaries effect

---

imiquimod

(i-mi-kwi'mod)

Aldara

Drug class.: Immune response modifier

Action: Mechanism is unknown; imiquimod induces cytokines including interferon-α in animal studies

Uses: External genital and perianal

warts, condylomata acuminata; unapproved: refractory common and plantar warts

Dosage and routes:

• *Adult and children 12 yr and older:* TOP apply cream 3 days per week at bedtime, leave on the skin for 6-10 hr; remove cream with mild soap and water after treatment; max duration of treatment 16 wk; cream is applied in a thin layer to the wart and rubbed in until no longer visible

Available forms include: Cream 5% in packets containing 250 mg of cream, 12 packets/box

Side effects/adverse reactions:

CNS: Headache, fatigue, fever

GI: Diarrhea

INTEG: Erythema, erosion, flaking, edema, induration, ulceration, scabbing, vesicles

MS: Myalgia

MISC: Fungal infection, flulike symptoms

Contraindications: None listed

Precautions: Has not been evaluated in papilloma viral diseases, cream may weaken condoms and diaphragms, external use only, pregnancy category B, lactation, children <18 yr

Pharmacokinetics:

TOP: Minimal cutaneous absorption

Drug interactions of concern to dentistry:

• None reported

DENTAL CONSIDERATIONS

General:

• Oral manifestations of the disease may occur in the oral mucosa.

• Patient may have history of other STDs.

Consultations:

• Medical consultation may be required to assess disease control.

Teach patient/family:

• To report oral lesions to the dentist

• Importance of updating health and drug history if physician makes any changes in evaluation or drug regimens

indapamide

(in-dap'a-mide)

Lozol

Apo-indapamide, Gen-indapamide, Lozide, Novo-indapamide, Nu-indapamide

Drug class.: Diuretic, thiazide-like

Action: Acts on distal tubule by increasing excretion of water, sodium, chloride, potassium

Uses: Edema, hypertension

Dosage and routes:

• *Adult:* PO 2.5 mg qd in AM, may be increased to 5 mg qd if needed

Available forms include: Tabs 1.25, 2.5 mg

Side effects/adverse reactions:

ORAL: Dry mouth

CNS: Headache, dizziness, fatigue, weakness, paresthesia, depression

CV: Orthostatic hypotension, volume depletion, palpitation

GI: Nausea, diarrhea, vomiting, anorexia, cramps, constipation, pancreatitis, abdominal pain, jaundice, hepatitis

HEMA: ***Thrombocytopenia, agranulocytosis, leukopenia, neutropenia, anemia***

GU: Polyuria, dysuria, frequency

EENT: Loss of hearing, tinnitus, blurred vision, nasal congestion, increased intraocular pressure

INTEG: Rash, pruritus, photosensitivity, alopecia, urticaria

MS: Cramps

ELECT: Hypochloremic alkalosis,

hypomagnesemia, hyperuricemia, hypercalcemia, hyponatremia, hypokalemia, hyperglycemia

Contraindications: Hypersensitivity, anuria

Precautions: Hypokalemia, dehydration, ascites, hepatic disease, severe renal disease, pregnancy category B

Pharmacokinetics:

PO: Onset 1-2 hr, peak 2 hr, duration up to 36 hr, half-life 14-18 hr; excreted in urine, feces

Drug interactions of concern to dentistry:

• Decreased hypotensive response: NSAIDs, especially indomethacin

DENTAL CONSIDERATIONS

General:

• Monitor vital signs at every appointment because of cardiovascular side effects.

• Patients on chronic drug therapy may rarely have symptoms of blood dyscrasias, which can include infection, bleeding, and poor healing.

• After supine positioning, have patient sit upright for at least 2 min before standing to avoid orthostatic hypotension.

• Assess salivary flow as a factor in caries, periodontal disease, and candidiasis.

• Limit use of sodium-containing products such as saline IV fluids for patients with a dietary salt restriction.

• Stress from dental procedures may compromise cardiovascular function; determine patient risk.

• Short appointments and a stress reduction protocol may be required for anxious patients.

• Patients on diuretic therapy should be monitored for serum K^+ levels.

Consultations:

• In a patient with symptoms of blood dyscrasias, request a medical consultation for blood studies and postpone dental treatment until normal values are reestablished.

• Medical consultation may be required to assess disease control and patient's ability to tolerate stress.

Teach patient/family:

• Importance of good oral hygiene to prevent soft tissue inflammation

• Caution to prevent injury when using oral hygiene aids

When chronic dry mouth occurs, advise patient:

• To avoid mouth rinses with high alcohol content because of drying effects

• To use sugarless gum, frequent sips of water, or saliva substitutes

• To use daily home fluoride products for anticaries effect

---

indinavir sulfate

(in-din'a-veer)

Crixivan

Drug class.: Antiviral

Action: Inhibits HIV protease enzyme, preventing cleavage of viral polyproteins and formation of immature noninfectious viral particles

Uses: HIV infection; prophylaxis after needle stick with AZT and lamivudine within 2 hr of needle stick

Dosage and routes:

• *Adult:* PO 800 mg q8h without food, 1 hr before or 2 hr after meal, force fluids; reduce dose to 600 mg q8h with concurrent use of ketoconazole; dose reduction is also required when given with delavirdine; increase dose when given with efavirenz

Available forms include: Caps 100, 200, 333 mg, 400 mg

Side effects/adverse reactions:

▼ *ORAL: Dry mouth, taste alteration,* aphthous stomatitis, gingivitis

CNS: Headache, insomnia, dizziness, somnolence

CV: Palpitation

GI: Abdominal pain, nausea, diarrhea, vomiting, acid regurgitation

RESP: Upper respiratory infection, cough

HEMA: ***Hyperbilirubinemia,*** anemia, lymphadenopathy

GU: Nephrolithiasis, flank pain, hematuria

EENT: Pharyngitis, blurred vision

INTEG: Rash, dry skin, dermatitis

MS: Asthenia, fatigue, back pain

Contraindications: Hypersensitivity; concurrent use with triazolam, midazolam, alprazolam, chlordiazepoxide, clonazepam, chlorazepate, diazepam, estazolam, flurazepam, halazepam, quazepam

Precautions: Nephrolithiasis (requires adequate hydration), hyperbilirubinemia, serum transaminase elevation, hepatic impairment, dose reduction of rifabutin required, pregnancy category C, lactation, children

Pharmacokinetics:

PO: Rapid absorption, food reduces absorption, 60% plasma protein bound, peak plasma levels 1 hr, hepatic metabolism, urinary and GI excretion

Drug interactions of concern to dentistry:

• Contraindicated with triazolam, midazolam (see Appendix I)

• Reduce dose when given with ketoconazole

DENTAL CONSIDERATIONS

General:

• Consider semisupine chair position when GI side effects occur.

• Assess salivary flow as a factor in caries, periodontal disease, and candidiasis.

• Monitor vital signs at every appointment because of cardiovascular side effects.

• Examine for oral manifestation of opportunistic infection.

• Patients with gastroesophageal reflux may have oral symptoms, including burning mouth, secondary candidiasis, and signs of tooth erosion.

Consultations:

• Medical consultation may be required to assess disease control.

Teach patient/family:

• Importance of good oral hygiene to prevent soft tissue inflammation

• To report oral lesions, soreness, or bleeding to dentist

• Importance of updating health history/drug record if physician makes any changes in evaluation or drug regimens

When chronic dry mouth occurs, advise patient:

• To avoid mouth rinses with high alcohol content because of drying effects

• To use daily home fluoride products for anticaries effect

• To use sugarless gum, frequent sips of water, or saliva substitutes

indomethacin

(in-doe-meth'a-sin)

Indocin, Indocin SR

♣ Apo-Indomethacin, Indocid, Indocid SR, Novo-Methacin, Nu-Indo

Drug class.: Nonsteroidal antiinflammatory

Action: Inhibits prostaglandin synthesis by interfering with cyclooxygenase needed for biosynthesis; possesses analgesic, antiinflammatory, and antipyretic properties

Uses: Rheumatoid arthritis, osteoarthritis, ankylosing rheumatoid spondylitis, acute gouty arthritis; unapproved: closure of patent ductus arteriosus in premature infants

Dosage and routes:

Arthritis:

• *Adult:* PO/REC 25 mg bid-tid, may increase by 25 mg/day q1wk, not to exceed 200 mg/day; sus rel 75 mg qd, may increase to 75 mg bid

Acute gouty arthritis:

• *Adult:* PO/REC 50 mg tid; use only for acute attack, then reduce dose

Available forms include: Caps 25, 50 mg; ext rel caps 75 mg; susp 25 mg/5 ml; rec supp 50 mg

Side effects/adverse reactions:

▼ *ORAL:* Dry mouth, bleeding, stomatitis, lichenoid reaction

CNS: Dizziness, drowsiness, fatigue, tremors, confusion, insomnia, anxiety, depression

CV: Tachycardia, peripheral edema, palpitation, dysrhythmias

GI: ***Cholestatic hepatitis,*** nausea, anorexia, vomiting, diarrhea, jaundice, constipation, flatulence, cramps, peptic ulcer

HEMA: ***Blood dyscrasias***

GU: ***Nephrotoxicity: dysuria, hematuria, oliguria, azotemia***

EENT: Tinnitus, hearing loss, blurred vision

INTEG: Purpura, rash, pruritus, sweating

Contraindications: Hypersensitivity, asthma, severe renal disease, severe hepatic disease

Precautions: Pregnancy category not listed (use not recommended), lactation, children, bleeding disorders, GI disorders, cardiac disorders, hypersensitivity to other antiinflammatory agents, depression

Pharmacokinetics:

PO: Onset 1-2 hr, peak 3 hr, duration 4-6 hr; 99% plasma-protein binding; metabolized in liver, kidneys; excreted in urine, bile, feces, breast milk; crosses placenta

Drug interactions of concern to dentistry:

• Increased GI bleeding, ulceration: corticosteroids, alcohol, aspirin, other NSAIDs

• Renal toxicity: acetaminophen (high doses, prolonged use)

• Possible risk of decreased renal function: cyclosporine

• *When prescribed for dental pain:*

• Risk of increased effects: oral anticoagulants, oral antidiabetics, lithium, methotrexate

• Decreased antihypertensive effects of diuretics, β-adrenergic blockers, and ACE inhibitors

• Increased toxicity of zidovudine

• First-time users of SSRIs also taking NSAIDs may have a higher risk of GI side effects; until more data are available, it may be advisable to avoid use of NSAIDs in these patients (*Br J Clin Pharmacol* 55:591-595, 2003)

DENTAL CONSIDERATIONS

General:

• Avoid prescribing aspirin-containing products.

• Patients on chronic drug therapy may rarely have symptoms of blood dyscrasias, which can include infection, bleeding, and poor healing.

• Assess salivary flow as a factor in caries, periodontal disease, and candidiasis.

• Consider semisupine chair position for patients with arthritic disease.

Consultations:

• In a patient with symptoms of blood dyscrasias, request a medical consultation for blood studies and postpone dental treatment until normal values are reestablished.

• Medical consultation may be required to assess disease control.

Teach patient/family:

• Importance of good oral hygiene to prevent soft tissue inflammation

• Caution to prevent injury when using oral hygiene aids

When chronic dry mouth occurs, advise patient:

• To avoid mouth rinses with high alcohol content because of drying effects

• To use sugarless gum, frequent sips of water, or saliva substitutes

• To use daily home fluoride products for anticaries effect

infliximab

(in-flix'i-mab)

Remicade

Drug class.: Antiinflammatory

Action: A monoclonal antibody to tumor necrosis factor alpha (TNFα) that is believed to prevent TNFα receptor binding resulting in reduced infiltration of inflammatory cells and reduced cytokine levels

Uses: Reduces signs and symptoms, progression of structural damage in rheumatoid arthritis in combination with methotrexate; improvement of physical function in moderate to severe rheumatoid arthritis in combination with methotrexate; reduction in signs and symptoms in patients with Crohn's disease with inadequate response to conventional therapy, long-term control of remission-level Crohn's disease; reduces and maintains fistulas in Crohn's disease

Dosage and routes:

Rheumatoid arthritis:

• *Adult:* IV 3 mg/kg infusion followed by additional doses at 2 and 6 wk, then q8wk; used with methotrexate; doses up to 10 mg/kg have been used

Crohn's disease with fistualizing disease:

• *Adult:* IV 5 mg/kg infusion at 0, 2, and 6 wk; maintenance dose q8wk thereafter

Available forms include: Vial 100 mg in 20 ml

Side effects/adverse reactions:

▼ *ORAL: Facial lip edema*

CNS: Headache, dizziness, fatigue

CV: Syncope (rare), hypotension or hypertension, chest pain, arrhythmia

GI: Nausea, diarrhea, abdominal pain, vomiting, dyspepsia

RESP: UTI, sinusitis, bronchitis, ***latent TB,*** coughing, pneumonia

HEMA: Development of antinuclear antibodies (ANAs), ***lymphoma***

I

GU: UTI
EENT: Sore throat, pharyngitis, rhinitis
INTEG: Rash, pruritus, LE
META: Transient elevation of AST, ALT
MS: Myalgia, arthralgia
MISC: Infusion reaction, fever

Contraindications: Hypersensitivity to murine proteins, active infection

Precautions: Risk of serious infections, risk of autoimmunity, chronic use increases risk of lymphoma, do not give live vaccines to patients taking this drug, patients should be tested for TB before starting therapy, pregnancy category B, no data on lactation or pediatric use

Pharmacokinetics:
IV: Peak levels at end of infusion; detectable levels up to 12 wk, no data on metabolism or excretion

Drug interactions of concern to dentistry:
- No drug interaction studies conducted

DENTAL CONSIDERATIONS

General:
- Determine why patient is taking the drug.
- Question patient about other drugs being taken.
- Examine for oral manifestation of opportunistic infection.
- Report oral infections to patient's physician, treat infections aggressively.

Consultations:
- Medical consultation may be required to assess disease control and patient's ability to tolerate stress.

Teach patient/family:
- Importance of good oral hygiene to prevent soft tissue inflammation/infection
- To immediately report any signs/symptoms of oral infection

---

insulin

(in'su-lin)

rapid-acting insulin

Insulin injection USP (pork): Regular Iletin II

Insulin human injection USP: Humulin-R, Novolin R, Novolin R Pen Fill, Novolin R Prefilled, Velosulin BR

✤ Novolin ge Toronto, Novolin ge Toronto Penfill

Insulin analog solution: insulin lispro (Humalog) and insulin aspart (Novolog)

intermediate-acting insulin

Isophane insulin suspension (pork): NPH Iletin II

Isophane insulin suspension, human: Humulin N, Novolin N, Novolin N Pen Fill, Novolin N Prefilled

✤ Novolin ge NPH

Insulin zinc suspension (pork): Lente Iletin II

Insulin zinc suspension, human: Humulin L

✤ Novolin ge Lente

long-acting insulin

Insulin zinc suspension, human extended: Humulin U Ultralente

✤ Novolin ge Ultralente

Insulin analog solution: insulin glargine solution: Lantus

combination insulin products

Isophane insulin suspension and insulin, human: Humulin 50/50, Humulin 70/30, Novolin 70/30, Novolin 70/30 Pen Fill, Novolin 70/30 Prefilled

✤ Humulin 10/90; Novolin ge

10/90 Penfill, Humulin 20/80, Novolin ge 20/80 Penfill, Humulin 30/70, Novolin ge 30/70, Humulin 40/60, Novolin ge 40/60 Penfill, Humulin 50/50, Novolin ge 50/50 Penfill
Insulin analog with protamine: Humalog Mix 75/25

insulin injection concentrated, human

Insulin (human): Humulin R Regular U-500

Drug class.: Hormone, antidiabetic

Action: Decreases blood glucose; stimulates glucose uptake in skeletal muscle, fat, and other tissues, decreases hepatic glucose production, inhibits lipolysis and proteolysis

Uses: Severe ketoacidosis, type 1 (IDDM) and type 2 (NIDDM; when diet, weight control, exercise, or oral hypoglycemics are not sufficient); hyperkalemia, hyperalimentation

Dosage and routes:
- *Adult:* SC/IV/IM dosage individualized by blood, urine glucose qd-tid; dose range for adults or child 0.5-1.0 U/kg/day; type of insulin selected varies with patient need

Available forms include: 100 U/ml in multiple-dose vials (10 ml) or prefilled pens and cartridges for NovoPen units; concentrate 500U/ml in 20 ml

Side effects/adverse reactions: These reactions may reflect either the disease or inappropriate insulin doses.

▼ *ORAL:* Dry mouth (rarely a problem)
CNS: Headache, lethargy, tremors, weakness, fatigue, delirium, sweating
CV: Tachycardia, palpitation
GI: Hunger, nausea
EENT: Blurred vision
INTEG: Flushing, rash, urticaria, warmth, lipodystrophy, lipohypertrophy
META: Hypoglycemia
SYST: ***Anaphylaxis,*** local allergic reactions

Contraindications: Hypersensitivity to protamine or animal source insulin (or both); hypoglycemia

Precautions: Change in type of insulin requires monitoring, dose adjustment for human insulin in renal failure, pregnancy category B, glargine and aspart pregnancy category C, dose intervals in elderly, insulin resistance, lipodystrophy, lipohypertrophy, changes in thyroid function

Pharmacokinetics: Depends on type of insulin used; regular insulin, insulin lispro, insulin aspart, and prompt insulin zinc suspension have rapid onset and short duration; NPH insulin and zinc insulin suspensions are intermediate acting, and protamine zinc insulin and extended zinc insulin are long acting

Drug interactions of concern to dentistry:
- Increased hypoglycemia: salicylates and NSAIDs (large doses and chronic use), alcohol
- Hyperglycemia: corticosteroids, epinephrine

DENTAL CONSIDERATIONS

General:
- Monitor vital signs at every appointment because of cardiovascular effects of hypoglycemia.

• Place on frequent recall to evaluate healing response.
• Diabetics may be more susceptible to infection and have delayed wound healing.
• Assess salivary flow as a factor in caries, periodontal disease, and candidiasis.
• Prophylactic antibiotics may be indicated in uncontrolled diabetics to prevent infection if surgery or deep scaling is planned.
• Ensure that patient is following prescribed diet and regularly takes medication.
• Question patient about self-monitoring of drug's antidiabetic effect, including blood glucose values or finger-stick records.
• Keep a readily available source of sugar or fruit juice in case of insulin overdose.

Consultations:
• Medical consultation may be required to assess disease control and patient's tolerance for stress.
• Medical consultation may include data from patient's blood glucose monitoring, including glycosylated hemoglobin or HbA_{1c} testing.

Teach patient/family:
• Importance of good oral hygiene to prevent soft tissue inflammation
• Caution to prevent injury when using oral hygiene aids
• To avoid mouth rinses with high alcohol content because of drying effects

---

interferon alfa-2a

(in-ter-feer'on)
Roferon A

Drug class.: Biologic response modifier

Action: Made by recombinant DNA technology; has broad antiviral and antitumor activity including inhibition of viral replication, antitumor action by suppression of cell proliferation and immunomodulating actions

Uses: Hairy cell leukemia in patients >18 yr, AIDS-related Kaposi's sarcoma, chronic hepatitis C, chronic myelogenous leukemia

Dosage and routes:

Hairy cell leukemia:
• *Adult:* SC/IM 3 million IU × 16-24 wk, then 3 million IU 3 × weekly maintenance

Chronic hepatitis C:
• *Adult:* SC/IM 3 million IU 3 × weekly for 12 mo; alternative doses or reduced doses may be required for some patients

AIDS-related Kaposi's sarcoma:
• *Adult:* SC/IM 36 million IU daily × 10-12 wk; maintenance 36 million IU 3 × weekly; alternative doses may be required for some patients

Chronic myelogenous leukemia:
• *Adult:* SC/IM initial dose 9 million IU daily; alternative doses may be required for some; limited data on use in children

Available forms include: Interferon alfa-2a inj 3, 6, 9, 36 million IU/vial; prefilled syringes 6, 9 million IU/syringe, multiple-dose vials 9, 18 million IU/vial

Side effects/adverse reactions:
▼ *ORAL: Taste changes,* dry mouth, stomatitis
CNS: Dizziness, confusion, numbness, paresthesia, headache, depression, irritability, insomnia
CV: Edema, hypertension, chest pain, flushing
GI: Weight loss, nausea, vomiting, diarrhea

RESP: Dryness of oropharynx
HEMA: ***Leukopenia, bone marrow toxicity***
GU: Impotence
EENT: Conjunctivitis, rhinitis, sinusitis
INTEG: Rash, dry skin, itching, alopecia
META: Elevation of liver enzymes, hyperglycemia, may reduce CYP450 enzymes
MISC: Flulike syndrome
Contraindications: Hypersensitivity
Precautions: Severe hypotension, dysrhythmia, tachycardia, pregnancy category C, lactation, children <18 yr, severe renal or hepatic disease, convulsion disorder, thrombophlebitis, coagulation disorders, hemophilia, GI bleeding; closely monitor patients; severe, life-threatening neuropsychiatric, autoimmune, ischemic, or infectious disorders may cause or aggravate these conditions
Pharmacokinetics:
SC/IM: Half-life (interferon alfa-2a) 3.7-8.5 hr, peak 3-4 hr; peak 6-8 hr; rapid proteolytic degradation in kidney
Drug interactions of concern to dentistry:
• Risk of hepatotoxicity in severe liver disease: acetaminophen
DENTAL CONSIDERATIONS
General:
• Determine why the patient is taking the drug.
• Monitor vital signs at every appointment because of cardiovascular side effects.
• Patients on chronic drug therapy may rarely have symptoms of blood dyscrasias, which can include infection, bleeding, and poor healing.
• Palliative medication may be required for oral side effects.
• Assess salivary flow as a factor in caries, periodontal disease, and candidiasis.
• Consider semisupine chair position for patient comfort if GI side effects occur.
• Avoid elective dental procedures if severe neutropenia (<500 cells/mm^3) or thrombocytopenia (<50,000 cell/mm^3) is present.
• In severe neutropenic patients antibiotic prophylaxis is indicated.
• Patient history should include all medications and herbal or nonherbal remedies taken by the patient.
• Severe side effects may require deferring elective dental procedures until drug therapy is completed.
• Evaluate efficacy of oral hygiene home care; preventive appointments may be necessary.
Consultations:
• Medical consultation may be required to assess disease control.
• In a patient with symptoms of blood dyscrasias, request a medical consultation for blood studies and postpone treatment until normal values are reestablished.
• Liver function tests may be required to determine chronic liver disease.
Teach patient/family:
• Importance of good oral hygiene to prevent soft tissue inflammation
• To report oral lesions, soreness, or bleeding to dentist
• Importance of updating medical/drug records if physician makes any changes in evaluation or drug regimens

When chronic dry mouth occurs, advise patient:
• To avoid mouth rinses with high alcohol content because of drying effects
• To use sugarless gum, frequent sips of water, or saliva substitutes
• To use daily home fluoride products for anticaries effect

---

interferon alfa-2b

(in-ter-feer'on)
Intron A

Drug class.: Biologic response modifier

Action: Made by recombinant DNA technology; has broad antiviral and antitumor activity including inhibition of viral replication, antitumor action by suppression of cell proliferation and immunomodulating actions

Uses: Hairy cell leukemia in persons >18 yr, malignant melanoma, chronic hepatitis B, follicular lymphoma, AIDS-related Kaposi's sarcoma, chronic hepatitis C, condylomata acuminata

Dosage and routes:

Hairy cell leukemia:
• *Adult and patients 18 yr or older:* SC/IM 2 million IU/m^2 3 × weekly × 6 mo; some patients may require a dose reduction because of side effects

Malignant melanoma:
• *Adult:* IV infusion 20 million IU/m^2 on consecutive days × 4 wk; maintenance dose SC 10 million IU/m^2 3 × weekly × 48 wk

Follicular lymphoma:
• *Adult:* SC 5 million IU 3 × weekly, up to 18 mo with an anthracycline-containing chemotherapy regimen

AIDs-related Kaposi's sarcoma:
• *Adult:* SC/IM 30 million IU/m^2; patients may require a small dose because of side effects; continue treatment until there is no further evidence of tumor; discontinue if severe opportunistic infection or adverse effects occur

Condyloma acuminatum:
• *Adult:* Intralesionally 1 million IU/lesion 3 × weekly on alternating days; up to 5 lesions can be treated at one time; give PM dose of acetaminophen to reduce side effects

Chronic hepatitis C:
• *Adult:* SC/IM 3 million IU 3 × weekly; if patients have normal ALT after 16 wk of treatment continue doses up to 24 mo; some patients may require dose adjustment because of side effects

Chronic hepatitis B:
• *Adult:* SC/IM 5 million IU daily or 10 million IU 3 × weekly for total weekly dose of 30-35 million IU × 16 wk
• *Children:* SC first week 3 million IU/m^2 3 × weekly, then 6 million IU/m^2 3 × weekly; max dose 10 million IU/m^2/wk; duration of treatment 16-24 wk

Available forms include: Powder for inj 3, 5, 10, 18, 25, 50 million IU/vial; sol for inj 3, 5, 10, 18, 25 million IU in vials; inj 3, 5, 10 million IU/multidose pens
(NOTE: Consult manufacturer's literature on the correct dose form to use for each route of administration and application.)

Side effects/adverse reactions:
▼ *ORAL: Taste changes, dry mouth,* facial edema
CNS: Fever, headache, anorexia, fatigue, depression, confusion, paresthesia
CV: Peripheral edema, hyperten-

sion, various arrhythmias, angina, palpitation, postural hypotension
GI: Nausea, vomiting, diarrhea
RESP: Dyspnea, coughing
HEMA: ***Leukopenia, granulocytopenia, thrombocytopenia,*** anemia
GU: Urinary frequency, UTI, dysmenorrhea
EENT: Sinusitis, pharyngitis, nasal congestion, blurred vision, dry eyes
INTEG: Rash, pruritus, alopecia, dermatitis, dry skin
ENDO: Hyperglycemia, ↑ triglycerides, aggravation of diabetes mellitus, thyroid abnormalities
META: Abnormal hepatic function tests, jaundice
MS: Generalized pain
MISC: Flulike syndrome, injection site pain, allergic reactions, candidiasis, herpes simplex

Contraindications: Hypersensitivity

Precautions: Preexisting psoriasis and sarcoidosis, do not use in patients with platelet counts <50,000/mm^3, preexisting CV disease, suicidal tendency, depression, preexisting psychiatric diseases, depressed bone marrow, pregnancy category C, safety and efficacy in lactation or child <18 yr have not been established

Pharmacokinetics:
SC/IM: Peak serum levels 3-12 hr; IV peak levels 30 min; metabolism, excretion data not reported

Drug interactions of concern to dentistry:

• Risk of hepatotoxicity in severe liver disease: acetaminophen

DENTAL CONSIDERATIONS

General:

• Determine why the patient is taking the drug.

• Monitor vital signs at every appointment because of cardiovascular side effects.

• After supine positioning, have patient sit upright for at least 2 min to avoid orthostatic hypotension.

• Palliative medication may be required for oral side effects.

• Assess salivary flow as a factor in caries, periodontal disease, and candidiasis.

• Patients on chronic drug therapy may rarely have symptoms of blood dyscrasias, which can include infection, bleeding, and poor healing.

• Consider semisupine chair position for patient comfort if GI side effects occur.

• Avoid elective dental procedures if severe neutropenia (<500 cells/mm^3) or thrombocytopenia (<50,000 cell/mm^3) is present.

• In severe neutropenic patients antibiotic prophylaxis is indicated.

• Patient history should include all medications and herbal or nonherbal remedies taken by the patient.

• Severe side effects may require deferring elective dental procedures until drug therapy is completed.

• Evaluate efficacy of oral hygiene home care; preventive appointments may be necessary.

Consultations:

• Medical consultation may be required to assess disease control.

• In a patient with symptoms of blood dyscrasias, request a medical consultation for blood studies and postpone treatment until normal values are reestablished

• Liver function tests may be required to determine chronic liver disease.

Teach patient/family:

• Importance of good oral hygiene to prevent soft tissue inflammation

• To report oral lesions, soreness, or bleeding to dentist

• Importance of updating medical/drug records if physician makes any changes in evaluation or drug regimens

When chronic dry mouth occurs, advise patient:

• To avoid mouth rinses with high alcohol content because of drying effects

• To use sugarless gum, frequent sips of water, or saliva substitutes

• To use daily home fluoride products for anticaries effect

interferon alfa-n3

(in-ter-feer'on)

Alferon N

Drug class.: Biologic response modifier

Action: A leukocyte-derived interferon made by recombinant DNA technology; has broad antiviral and antitumor activity including inhibition of viral replication, antitumor action by suppression of cell proliferation and immunomodulating actions

Uses: Intralesional treatment of refractory or recurring external condylomata acuminata in patients 18 yr or older

Dosage and routes:

• *Adult 18 yr or older:* Intralesional 0.05 ml (250,000 IU) per wart twice weekly × 8 wk; max dose per treatment session is 0.5 ml (2.5 million IU); doses may need to be adjusted for some patients because of side effects

Available forms include: Inj sol 1 ml (5 million IU) vial

Side effects/adverse reactions:

▼ *ORAL:* Taste changes, salivation, herpes labialis

CNS: Dizziness, headache, fever, chills, fatigue, malaise, insomnia, depression

CV: Hot flashes

GI: Vomiting, nausea, dyspepsia, diarrhea

EENT: Sinusitis, pharyngitis, visual disturbances, epistaxis

INTEG: Neck rash, pruritus, photosensitivity

MS: Myalgia, back pain

MISC: Flulike syndrome, swollen lymph nodes, risk of generalized hypersensitivity reactions

Contraindications: Hypersensitivity to human interferons, mouse immune globulin (IgG), egg protein, and neomycin

Precautions: CV disease, unstable angina, uncontrolled CHF, severe pulmonary disease, diabetes mellitus with ketoacidosis, coagulation disorders, severe myelosuppression, seizure disorders, risk of transmitting blood-borne infectious disease, pregnancy category C, lactation, use in children <18 yr has not been established

Pharmacokinetics: Plasma levels below detectable limits

Drug interactions of concern to dentistry:

• None reported

DENTAL CONSIDERATIONS

General:

• Determine why the patient is taking the drug.

• Following injection advise patient to take acetaminophen (if there are no contraindications for its use) in PM to ease flulike symptoms.

• Advise patient if dental drugs prescribed have a potential for photosensitivity.
• Consider semisupine chair position for patient comfort if GI side effects occur.

Consultations:
• Medical consultation may be required to assess disease control.

Teach patient/family:
• Importance of updating medical/drug records if physician makes any changes in evaluation or drug regimens

interferon gamma-1b

(in-ter-fer'on)
Actimmune

Drug class.: Biologic response modifier

Action: Genetically engineered gamma interferon; naturally produced by T-lymphocytes and natural killer (NK) cells as a response to various stimuli; activates macrophages, enhances antibody-dependent cellular cytotoxicity, expression of class II major histocompatibility antigens, NK cell activity, lymphocyte expression, and Fc receptor expression on monocytes

Uses: Reduces the severity and frequency of infections associated with chronic granulomatous disease; delays disease progression in patients with severe, malignant osteoporosis

Dosage and routes:
• *Adult:* SC 50 μg/m^2 (1.0 million IU/m^2) for patients with a surface area >0.5 m^2; 1.5 μg/kg/dose for patients with a surface area <0.5/m^2; give on Monday, Wednesday, Friday for dosing 3 × weekly

Available forms include: Inj 100 μg (2 million U) single-dose vial

Side effects/adverse reactions:
CNS: Headache, fatigue, fever, chills, depression, confusion, seizures
CV: Hypotension, syncope, tachycardia, heart block
GI: Nausea, anorexia, diarrhea, vomiting, abdominal pain, weight loss, GI bleeding
RESP: Bronchospasm, tachypnea
HEMA: ***Leukopenia, thrombocytopenia,*** deep vein thrombosis
INTEG: Rash, pain at injection site, erythema
MS: Myalgia, arthralgia
META: Hyponatremia, hyperglycemia, increase in CYP450 activity
MISC: Allergic reactions

Contraindications: Hypersensitivity to interferon gamma, *E. coli*–derived products

Precautions: Pregnancy category C, cardiac disease, seizure disorders, CNS disorders, myelosuppression, lactation, children <1 yr; monitor hematologic values q3mo

Pharmacokinetics:
SC: Slow absorption, peak 7 hr, elimination half-life 5.9 hr; dose absorbed 89%

Drug interactions of concern to dentistry:
• None reported

DENTAL CONSIDERATIONS

General:
• Determine why the patient is taking the drug.
• Patients on chronic drug therapy may rarely have symptoms of blood dyscrasias, which can include infection, bleeding, and poor healing.
• Ask patient about side effects associated with drug use (abnormal hematologic values).

• Consider semisupine chair position for patient comfort if GI side effects occur.
• Place on frequent recall to evaluate healing response.
• Severe side effects may require deferring elective dental procedures until drug therapy is completed.
• In severe neutropenic patients antibiotic prophylaxis is indicated.
• Avoid elective dental procedures if severe neutropenia (<500 cells/mm^3) or thrombocytopenia (<50,000 cell/mm^3) is present.

Consultations:
• In a patient with symptoms of blood dyscrasias, request a medical consultation for blood studies and postpone dental treatment until normal values are reestablished.
• Medical consultation may be required to assess disease control and patient's ability to tolerate stress.

Teach patient/family:
• Importance of good oral hygiene to prevent soft tissue inflammation
• Caution to prevent trauma when using oral hygiene aids
• Importance of updating medical history/drug records if physician makes any changes in evaluation or drug regimens

ipratropium bromide

(i-pra-troe′pee-um)
Atrovent
✤ Apo-Ipravent, Kendral-Ipratropium
Drug class.: Anticholinergic bronchodilator

Action: A synthetic cholinergic antagonist with local action in the lungs resulting in bronchial dilation; when applied to nasal mucous membranes it reduces watery secretions from glands in the nasal mucosa

Uses: Bronchodilation during bronchospasm in those with COPD, bronchitis, emphysema, asthma; not for rapid bronchodilation, maintenance treatment only; rhinorrhea, rhinorrhea associated with allergic and nonallergic perennial rhinitis in children age 6-11 yr, rhinorrhea associated with common cold

Dosage and routes:
Bronchial dilation (aerosol or INH sol):
• *Adult and child >5 yr:* INH 2 inh 4 × daily, not to exceed 12 inh/24 hr; SOLN 500 μg nebulized at 6-8 hr intervals

Rhinorrhea (nasal spray):
• *Adult:* TOP 2 sprays (0.03%) in each nostril bid or tid
• *Child:* TOP 2 sprays (0.06%) in each nostril bid or tid

Available forms include: Nasal spray 0.03% (21 μg/spray), 0.06% (42 μg/spray); aerosol 18 μg/actuation; Canada 20 μg/actuation, 200 inh/container; sol for INH 0.02% (500 μg/vial)

Side effects/adverse reactions:
▼ *ORAL: Dry mouth,* stomatitis, metallic taste
CNS: Anxiety, dizziness, headache
CV: Palpitation
GI: Nausea, vomiting, cramps
RESP: Cough, worsening of symptoms
EENT: Blurred vision, nasal dryness, nasal bleeding
INTEG: Rash

Contraindications: Hypersensi-

tivity to this drug or atropine, soy lecithin, soybean or peanut inhalation

Precautions: Pregnancy category B, lactation, children <12 yr, narrow-angle glaucoma, prostatic hypertrophy, bladder neck obstruction

Pharmacokinetics: Onset 5-15 min, duration 3-4 hr, half-life 2 hr; does not cross blood-brain barrier

Drug interactions of concern to dentistry:

- Increased effects of anticholinergic drugs

DENTAL CONSIDERATIONS

General:

- Monitor vital signs at every appointment because of cardiovascular and respiratory side effects.
- Assess salivary flow as a factor in caries, periodontal disease, and candidiasis.
- Acute asthmatic episodes may be precipitated in the dental office. Sympathomimetic inhalants should be available for emergency use.
- Consider semisupine chair position for patients with respiratory disease.
- Place on frequent recall because of oral side effects.

Consultations:

- Medical consultation may be required to assess disease control and patient's ability to tolerate stress.

Teach patient/family:

- For inhalation dosage forms, rinse mouth with water after each dose to prevent dryness

When chronic dry mouth occurs, advise patient:

- To avoid mouth rinses with high alcohol content because of drying effects
- To use sugarless gum, frequent sips of water, or saliva substitutes
- To use daily home fluoride products for anticaries effect

irbesartan

(ir-be-sar'tan)

Avapro

Drug class.: Angiotensin II receptor antagonist, antihypertensive

Action: Acts as a competitive antagonist for angiotensin II (AT_1) receptors, inhibiting both vasoconstrictor- and aldosterone-secreting effects

Uses: Hypertension alone or in combination with other antihypertensive drugs; nephropathy in type 2 diabetes

Dosage and routes:

Hypertension:

- *Adolescents 13-16 yr and adults:* PO initial 150 mg qd; some patients may require 300 mg/day; initial dose for volume- or salt-depleted patients is 75 mg/day
- *Child 6-12 yr:* PO 75 mg qd; some patients may require 150 mg/day

Nephropathy in type 2 diabetes:

- *Adult:* PO 300 mg/day

Available forms include: Tabs 75, 150, 300 mg

Side effects/adverse reactions:

CNS: Fatigue, headache, dizziness, anxiety

CV: Orthostatic hypotension, increased heart rate

GI: Diarrhea, dyspepsia, heartburn, nausea, vomiting

RESP: URI, pharyngitis

EENT: Rhinitis

INTEG: Rash, urticaria, pruritus

MS: Musculoskeletal trauma, muscle ache

Contraindications: Hypersensi-

tivity, pregnancy category D (second, third trimester)

Precautions: Hypersensitivity to other angiotensin II receptor antagonists, pregnancy category C (first trimester), volume- or salt-depleted patients, renal impairment, lactation, children

Pharmacokinetics:

PO: Bioavailability 60%-80%, rapid absorption, peak serum levels 1.5-2 hr, 90% protein bound, hepatic metabolism, both biliary and renal excretion

Drug interactions of concern to dentistry:

• None reported

DENTAL CONSIDERATIONS

General:

• Monitor vital signs at every appointment because of cardiovascular side effects.

• Limit use of sodium-containing products such as saline IV fluids for those patients with a dietary salt restriction.

• Stress from dental procedures may compromise cardiovascular function; determine patient risk.

• Short appointments and a stress reduction protocol may be required for anxious patients.

• Use precaution if sedation or general anesthesia is required; risk of hypotensive episode.

• After supine positioning, have patient sit upright for at least 2 min before standing to avoid orthostatic hypotension.

• Consider semisupine chair position for patient comfort if GI side effects occur.

Consultations:

• Consultation with physician may be needed if sedation or general anesthesia is required.

• Medical consultation may be required to assess disease control and patient's ability to tolerate stress; there is risk for a hypotensive episode.

Teach patient/family:

• Importance of updating health and drug history if physician makes any changes in evaluation or drug regimens

isocarboxazid

(eye-soe-kar-box'a-zid)

Marplan

Drug class.: Antidepressant–monoamine oxidase inhibitor

Action: Increases concentrations of endogenous norepinephrine, serotonin, and dopamine in CNS storage sites by nonselective inhibition of MAO enzymes; the precise antidepressant mechanism is unknown

Uses: Depression

Dosage and routes:

• *Adult:* PO 10 mg/bid, if tolerated can increase dose 10 mg every 2-4 days to 40 mg by end of first wk; max daily dose 60 mg in divided doses

Available forms include: Tabs 10 mg

Side effects/adverse reactions:

▼ *ORAL: Dry mouth*

CNS: Dizziness, sedation, hypomania, headache, mania, insomnia, anxiety, tremors, stimulation, weakness, agitation, convulsions, increased neuromuscular activity

CV: Orthostatic hypotension, syncope, palpitation, tachycardia

GI: Constipation, nausea, diarrhea, abdominal pain

HEMA: ***Agranulocytosis, thrombo-***

cytopenia, spider telangiectases, anemia (rare)
GU: Sexual dysfunction, urinary retention
EENT: Blurred vision, ocular toxicity
INTEG: Rash
ENDO: ***SIADH-like syndrome,*** hyperprolactinemia
META: Hepatic function abnormalities
MISC: Weight gain
Contraindications: Hypersensitivity to MAOIs, elderly, hypertension, CHF, severe hepatic disease, pheochromocytoma, severe renal disease, severe cardiac disease, foods with high tryptophan or tyramine content, excessive caffeine, sympathomimetics, meperidine, buspirone, bupropion
Precautions: Suicidal patients, concurrent use with other antidepressants (patients must stop taking MAOI 14 days before initiating therapy with other antidepressants), general anesthesia, severe depression, schizophrenia, diabetes mellitus, pregnancy category C, lactation, children <16 yr
Pharmacokinetics:
PO: Good absorption; maximum MAO inhibition 5-10 days, duration up to 2 wk; metabolized by liver; excreted by kidneys
Drug interactions of concern to dentistry:
• Increased pressor effects: indirect-acting sympathomimetics (ephedrine)
• Hyperpyretic crisis, convulsions, hypertensive episode: meperidine, possibly other opioids, carbamazepine
• Increased anticholinergic effects: anticholinergics, antihistamines
• Increased effects of alcohol, barbiturates, benzodiazepines, CNS depressants, SSRIs, tricyclic antidepressants, cyclobenzaprine, bupropion, buspirone, dextromethorphan, antihypertensives

DENTAL CONSIDERATIONS
General:
• Monitor vital signs at every appointment because of cardiovascular side effects.
• After supine positioning, have patient sit upright for at least 2 min to avoid orthostatic hypotension.
• Patients on chronic drug therapy may rarely have symptoms of blood dyscrasias, which can include infection, bleeding, and poor healing.
• Consider semisupine chair position for patient comfort if GI side effects occur.
• Assess salivary flow as a factor in caries, periodontal disease, and candidiasis.
• Hypertensive episodes are possible even though there are no specific contraindications to vasoconstrictor use in local anesthetics.
• Short appointments and a stress reduction protocol may be required for anxious patients.
Consultations:
• Medical consultation may be required to assess disease control and patient's ability to tolerate stress.
• In a patient with symptoms of blood dyscrasias, request a medical consultation for blood studies and postpone treatment until normal values are reestablished.
Teach patient/family:
When chronic dry mouth occurs, advise patient:
• To avoid mouth rinses with high alcohol content because of drying effects

• To use daily home fluoride products for anticaries effect
• To use sugarless gum, frequent sips of water, or saliva substitutes

isoetharine HCl

(eye-soe-eth'a-reen)
Isoetharine
Drug class.: Adrenergic β_2-agonist

Action: Causes bronchodilation by β_2 stimulation, resulting in increased levels of cAMP and causing relaxation of bronchial smooth muscle with little effect on heart rate

Uses: Bronchospasm, asthma

Dosage and routes:

• *Adult:* IPPB 0.5 ml diluted 1:3 with NS; nebulizer 3-7 inh (undiluted)

Available forms include: Sol for inh 1%

Side effects/adverse reactions:

▼ *ORAL:* Dry mouth

CNS: Tremors, anxiety, insomnia, headache, dizziness, stimulation

CV: ***Cardiac arrest,*** palpitation, tachycardia, hypertension, dysrhythmias

GI: Nausea

META: Hyperglycemia

Contraindications: Hypersensitivity to sympathomimetics, narrow-angle glaucoma

Precautions: Pregnancy category C, cardiac disorders, hyperthyroidism, diabetes mellitus, prostatic hypertrophy

Pharmacokinetics:

INH: Onset immediate, peak 5-15 min, duration 1-4 hr; metabolized in liver, GI tract, lungs; excreted in urine

Drug interactions of concern to dentistry:

• Increased effects of both drugs: other sympathomimetics
• Increased dysrhythmia: halogenated hydrocarbon anesthetics

DENTAL CONSIDERATIONS

General:

• Assess salivary flow as a factor in caries, periodontal disease, and candidiasis.
• Consider semisupine chair position for patients with respiratory disease.
• Acute asthmatic episodes may be precipitated in the dental office. Sympathomimetic inhalants should be available for emergency use.

Consultations:

• Medical consultation may be required to assess disease control and patient's ability to tolerate stress.

Teach patient/family:

• For inhalation dosage forms, rinse mouth with water after each dose to prevent dryness

When chronic dry mouth occurs, advise patient:

• To avoid mouth rinses with high alcohol content because of drying effects
• To use sugarless gum, frequent sips of water, or saliva substitutes
• To use daily home fluoride products for anticaries effect

isoniazid (INH)

(eye-soe-nye'a-zid)
Nydrazid
✤ Isotamine, PMS-Isoniazid
Drug class.: Antitubercular

Action: Bactericidal, inhibition of mycolic acid synthesis leading to disruption of the bacterial cell wall

Uses: Treatment/prevention of TB

Dosage and routes:

Treatment:

• *Adult:* PO/IM 5 mg/kg qd as single dose for 9 mo–2 yr, not to exceed 300 mg/day

• *Child and infant:* PO/IM 10-15 mg/kg qd as single dose for 18-24 mo, not to exceed 300 mg/day

Prevention:

• *Adult:* PO 300 mg qd as single dose for 12 mo; IM 5 mg/kg (300 mg) qd

• *Child and infant:* PO/IM 10 mg/kg qd as single dose for 12 mo, not to exceed 300 mg/day

(NOTE: Pyridoxine [vitamin B_6] is used concurrently in patients who are alcoholic or diabetic.)

Available forms include: Tabs 100, 300 mg; inj 100 mg/ml; powder, syr 50 mg/5 ml

Side effects/adverse reactions:

▼ *ORAL:* Lichenoid reaction

CNS: Peripheral neuropathy, ***toxic encephalopathy, convulsions,*** memory impairment, psychosis

GI: ***Jaundice, fatal hepatitis,*** nausea, vomiting, epigastric distress

HEMA: ***Agranulocytosis, hemolytic anemia, aplastic anemia, thrombocytopenia, eosinophilia, methemoglobinemia***

EENT: Blurred vision, optic neuritis

INTEG: Hypersensitivity: fever, skin eruptions, lymphadenopathy, vasculitis

MISC: Dyspnea, vitamin B_6 deficiency, pellagra, hyperglycemia, metabolic acidosis, gynecomastia, rheumatic syndrome, SLE-like syndrome

Contraindications: Hypersensitivity, optic neuritis

Precautions: Pregnancy category C; renal disease; diabetic retinopathy cataracts; ocular defects; hepatic disease; fatal hepatitis, especially in black women and Hispanic women; child <13 yr, monitor liver function

Pharmacokinetics:

PO: Peak 1-2 hr, duration 6-8 hr

IM: Peak 45-60 min

Metabolized in liver, excreted in urine (metabolites), crosses placenta, excreted in breast milk

Drug interactions of concern to dentistry:

• Increased hepatotoxicity: alcohol, acetaminophen, carbamazepine

• Decreased effectiveness: glucocorticoids, especially prednisolone

• Increased plasma concentration: benzodiazepines, alfentanil

• Decreased effect of ketoconazole, miconazole

DENTAL CONSIDERATIONS

General:

• Patients on chronic drug therapy may rarely have symptoms of blood dyscrasias, which can include infection, bleeding, and poor healing.

• Medical consultation may be required to assess disease control.

• Examine for evidence of oral signs of disease.

Consultations:

• In a patient with symptoms of blood dyscrasias, request a medical consultation for blood studies and postpone dental treatment until normal values are reestablished.

Teach patient/family:

• Caution to prevent injury when using oral hygiene aids

isoproterenol HCl

(eye-soe-proe-ter'e-nole)

Drug class.: Adrenergic β_1- and β_2-agonist

Action: Has β_1 and β_2 actions; relaxes bronchial smooth muscle and dilates the trachea and main bronchi by increasing levels of cAMP, which relaxes smooth muscles; causes increased contractility and heart rate by acting on β-receptors in heart

Uses: Bronchospasm during anesthesia

Dosage and routes:

Bronchospasm:

• *Adult:* IV 1 ml (1:5000) diluted to 10 ml with normal saline or D_5W: initial dose 0.5-1.0 ml of diluted solution, the 1:50,000 may be used undiluted

Available forms include: Inj IV/IM 1:5000 (0.2 mg/ml), 1:50,000 (0.2 mg/ml)

Side effects/adverse reactions:

▼ *ORAL:* Dry mouth, altered taste

CNS: Tremors, anxiety, insomnia, headache, dizziness, stimulation

CV: ***Cardiac arrest,*** palpitation, tachycardia, hypertension

GI: Nausea, vomiting

RESP: Bronchial irritation, edema, dryness of oropharynx

META: Hyperglycemia

Contraindications: Hypersensitivity to sympathomimetics, narrow-angle glaucoma

Precautions: Pregnancy category C, cardiac disorders, hyperthyroidism, diabetes mellitus, prostatic hypertrophy

Pharmacokinetics: *INH/SL:* Onset 1-2 hr *SC:* Onset 2 hr *REC:* Onset 2-4 hr

Metabolized in liver, lungs, GI tract

Drug interactions of concern to dentistry:

• Hypotension, tachycardia: haloperidol, loxapine, phenothiazines, thioxanthenes

• Increased dysrhythmia: halogenated-hydrocarbon anesthetics

DENTAL CONSIDERATIONS

General:

• This drug is used only in conjunction with general anesthesia procedures.

isosorbide dinitrate

(eye'soe-sor-bide)

Dilatrate-SR, Isordil, Isordil Tembids, Isordil Titradose, Sorbitrate

♣ Apo-ISDN, Coronex, Cedocard SR, Coradur

Drug class.: Nitrate antianginal

Action: Decreases preload/afterload, which decreases left ventricular end-diastolic pressure, systemic vascular resistance, reduces myocardial oxygen demand

Uses: Chronic stable angina pectoris

Dosage and routes:

• *Adult:* PO 5-40 mg qid; SL 2.5-10 mg, may repeat q2-3h; chew tabs 5-10 mg prn or q2-3h as prophylaxis; sus rel 40-80 mg q8-12h

Available forms include: Sus rel caps 40 mg; tabs 5, 10, 20, 30, 40 mg; chew tabs 5, 10 mg; sus rel tabs 40 mg; SL tabs 2.5, 5, 10 mg

Side effects/adverse reactions:

▼ *ORAL:* Dry mouth, burning sensation to mucosa (SL tabs)

CNS: Vascular headache, flushing, dizziness, weakness, faintness

CV: Postural hypotension, ***collapse,*** tachycardia, syncope
GI: Nausea, vomiting
INTEG: Pallor, sweating, rash
MISC: ***Methemoglobinemia,*** twitching, hemolytic anemia
Contraindications: Hypersensitivity to this drug or nitrites, severe anemia, increased intracranial pressure, cerebral hemorrhage, acute MI
Precautions: Postural hypotension, pregnancy category C, lactation, children
Pharmacokinetics: *SUS ACTION:* Duration 6-8 hr
PO: Onset 15-30 min, duration 4-6 hr
SL: Onset 2-5 min, duration 1-4 hr
SL: Onset 3 min, duration 0.5-3 hr
Metabolized by liver, excreted in urine as metabolites (80%-100%)
Drug interactions of concern to dentistry:
• Increased effects: alcohol and other drugs that can lower blood pressure
• Severe hypotension: sildenafil, vardenafil, tadalafil
DENTAL CONSIDERATIONS
General:
• Monitor vital signs at every appointment because of cardiovascular side effects.
• After supine positioning, have patient sit upright for at least 2 min before standing to avoid orthostatic hypotension.
• Assess salivary flow as a factor in caries, periodontal disease, and candidiasis.
• Stress from dental procedures may compromise cardiovascular function; determine patient risk.
• Use vasoconstrictors with caution, in low doses, and with careful aspiration. Avoid use of gingival retraction cord with epinephrine.
• Short appointments and a stress reduction protocol may be required for anxious patients.
• Nitroglycerin should be available in case of acute anginal episode.
Consultations:
• Medical consultation may be required to assess disease control and patient's ability to tolerate stress.
Teach patient/family:
• Importance of good oral hygiene to prevent soft tissue inflammation
When chronic dry mouth occurs, advise patient:
• To avoid mouth rinses with high alcohol content because of drying effects
• To use sugarless gum, frequent sips of water, or saliva substitutes
• To use daily home fluoride products for anticaries effect

isosorbide mononitrate

(eye'soe-sor-bide)
Imdur, ISMO, Monoket
Drug class.: Antianginal, organic nitrate

Action: Decreases preload/afterload, which decreases left ventricular end-diastolic pressure, systemic vascular resistance; arterial and venous dilation; decreases myocardial oxygen demand
Uses: Prevention of angina pectoris caused by coronary artery disease
Dosage and routes:
• *Adult:* PO 20 mg bid, 7 hr apart; extended rel tab 30 mg or 60 mg/day

Available forms include: Tabs 10, 20 mg; ext rel 30, 60, 120 mg

Side effects/adverse reactions:

▼ *ORAL:* Dry mouth

CNS: Vascular headache, flushing, dizziness, weakness, faintness

CV: ***Collapse,*** postural hypotension, tachycardia, syncope

GI: Nausea, vomiting

INTEG: Pallor, sweating, rash

MISC: ***Hemolytic anemia, methemoglobinemia,*** twitching

Contraindications: Hypersensitivity to nitrites, severe anemia, increased intracranial pressure, cerebral hemorrhage, acute MI, closed-angle glaucoma

Precautions: Postural hypotension, pregnancy category C, lactation, children, glaucoma

Pharmacokinetics:

PO: Metabolized by the liver, excreted in urine as metabolites (80%-100%)

Drug interactions of concern to dentistry:

• Increased effects: alcohol and other vasodilator-type drugs

• Severe hypotension: sildenafil, vardenafil, tadalafil

DENTAL CONSIDERATIONS

General:

• Monitor vital signs at every appointment because of cardiovascular side effects.

• After supine positioning, have patient sit upright for at least 2 min before standing to avoid orthostatic hypotension.

• Stress from dental procedures may compromise cardiovascular function; determine patient risk.

• Assess salivary flow as a factor in caries, periodontal disease, and candidiasis.

• Short appointments and a stress reduction protocol may be required for anxious patients.

• Consider semisupine chair position for patients with respiratory distress.

• Use vasoconstrictors with caution, in low doses, and with careful aspiration. Avoid use of gingival retraction cord with epinephrine.

• Nitroglycerin should be available in case of an acute anginal episode.

Consultations:

• Medical consultation may be required to assess disease control and patient's ability to tolerate stress.

Teach patient/family:

When chronic dry mouth occurs, advise patient:

• To avoid mouth rinses with high alcohol content because of drying effects

• To use sugarless gum, frequent sips of water, or saliva substitutes

• To use daily home fluoride products for anticaries effect

---

isotretinoin

(eye-soe-tret'i-noyn)

Accutane

♣ Accutane-Roche

Drug class.: Retinoic acid isomer, vitamin A derivative

Action: Decreases sebum secretion; improves cystic acne

Uses: Severe recalcitrant cystic acne; unapproved: severe rosacea

Dosage and routes:

• *Adult:* PO 0.5-1 mg/kg/day in 2 divided doses × 15-20 wk

Available forms include: Caps 10, 20, 40 mg

Side effects/adverse reactions:

▼ *ORAL: Dry lips/mouth, angular cheilosis*

CNS: ***Pseudotumor cerebri,*** lethargy, fatigue, headache, depression
CV: Chest pain
GI: Nausea, vomiting, anorexia, increased liver enzymes, ***pancreatitis,*** regional ileus, abdominal pain, weight loss, hepatotoxicity
HEMA: ***Thrombocytopenia,*** decreased H & H, WBC, reticulocyte count
GU: ***Hematuria, proteinuria,*** hypouricemia
EENT: Eye irritation, conjunctivitis, epistaxis, dry nose, contact lens intolerance, optic neuritis, visual impairment, corneal opacities, hearing impairment
INTEG: Dry skin, pruritus, joint/muscle pain, hair loss, photosensitivity, urticaria, bruising, hirsutism, petechiae, hypopigmentation/hyperpigmentation, nail brittleness, onycholysis
MS: Hyperostosis, arthralgia, bone/joint/muscle pain, osteoporosis
META: Hypertriglyceridemia

Contraindications: Hypersensitivity, inflamed skin, tetracyclines; must not be used by women who are pregnant, women of childbearing age who use this drug must use two methods of contraception

Precautions: Lactation, diabetes, photosensitivity, hepatic disease, depressive illness, pregnancy category X, children <12 yr; potential musculoskeletal side effects (osteoporosis, osteopenia, bone fracture and delayed healing of bone fractures) have been spontaneously reported in Accutane users

Pharmacokinetics:
PO: Peak 2.9-3.2 hr, half-life 10-20 hr; metabolized in liver; excreted in urine, feces

Drug interactions of concern to dentistry:
- Additive photosensitization: tetracycline
- Pseudotumor cerebri, intracranial hypertension: minocycline, doxycycline, or tetracycline
- Increased tissue drying: alcohol
- Contraindicated with all tetracyclines (demeclocycline, doxycycline, minocycline, tetracycline)
- Avoid additional vitamin A supplements

DENTAL CONSIDERATIONS

General:
- Patients on chronic drug therapy may rarely have symptoms of blood dyscrasias, which can include infection, bleeding, and poor healing.
- Assess salivary flow as a factor in caries, periodontal disease, and candidiasis.
- An exaggerated healing response characterized by exuberant granulation tissue has been reported.
- Apply lubricant to dry lips for patient comfort before dental procedures.

Consultations:
- In a patient with symptoms of blood dyscrasias, request a medical consultation for blood studies and postpone dental treatment until normal values are reestablished.

Teach patient/family:
- Importance of good oral hygiene to prevent soft tissue inflammation

When chronic dry mouth occurs, advise patient:
- To avoid mouth rinses with high alcohol content because of drying effects
- To use sugarless gum, frequent sips of water, or saliva substitutes
- To use daily home fluoride products for anticaries effect

isoxsuprine HCl

(eye-sox'syoo-preen)

Vasodilan, Voxsuprine

Drug class.: Peripheral vasodilator

Action: α-adrenoreceptor antagonist with β-adrenoreceptor–stimulating properties; may also act directly on vascular smooth muscle; causes cardiac stimulation, uterine relaxation

Uses: Symptoms of cerebrovascular insufficiency; peripheral vascular disease, including arteriosclerosis obliterans, thromboangiitis obliterans, Raynaud's disease

Dosage and routes:

• *Adult:* PO 10-20 mg tid or qid

Available forms include: Tabs 10, 20 mg

Side effects/adverse reactions:

CNS: Dizziness, weakness, tremors, anxiety

CV: Hypotension, ***tachycardia,*** palpitation, chest pain

GI: Nausea, vomiting, abdominal pain, distention

INTEG: Severe rash, flushing

Contraindications: Hypersensitivity, postpartum, arterial bleeding

Precautions: Pregnancy category C, tachycardia

Pharmacokinetics:

PO: Peak 1 hr, duration 3 hr, half-life 1.25 hr; excreted in urine; crosses placenta

Drug interactions of concern to dentistry:

• Increased effects: alcohol and drugs that also lower blood pressure

DENTAL CONSIDERATIONS

General:

• Monitor vital signs at every appointment because of cardiovascular and respiratory side effects.

• After supine positioning, have patient sit upright for at least 2 min before standing to avoid orthostatic hypotension.

• Short appointments and a stress reduction protocol may be required for anxious patients.

• Drugs used for conscious sedation that lower blood pressure may potentiate the hypotensive effects.

• Use vasoconstrictors with caution, in low doses, and with careful aspiration. Avoid use of gingival retraction cord with epinephrine.

Consultations:

• Medical consultation may be required to assess disease control and patient's ability to tolerate stress.

isradipine

(iz-ra'di-peen)

DynaCirc, DynaCirc CR

Drug class.: Calcium channel blocker

Action: Inhibits calcium ion influx across cell membrane during cardiac depolarization; produces relaxation of coronary vascular smooth muscle, peripheral vascular smooth muscle; dilates coronary vascular arteries; increases myocardial oxygen delivery in patients with vasospastic angina

Uses: Essential hypertension, alone or with a thiazide diuretic; unapproved: angina, Raynaud's disease

Dosage and routes:

Hypertension:

• *Adult:* PO 2.5 mg bid, increase at 3-4 wk intervals up to 10 mg bid; con rel tab 5 mg/day

Angina:

• *Adult:* PO 2.5-7.5 mg tid, maximum 20 mg/day

Available forms include: Caps 2.5, 5 mg; con rel tab 5, 10 mg

Side effects/adverse reactions:

▼ *ORAL:* Dry mouth (gingival overgrowth has not been documented with this drug)

CNS: Headache, fatigue, dizziness, fainting, sleep disturbances

CV: Peripheral edema, tachycardia, hypotension, chest pain

GI: Nausea, vomiting, diarrhea, gastric upset, constipation, hepatitis

HEMA: ***Thrombocytopenia, leukopenia, anemia***

GU: ***Acute renal failure,*** nocturia, polyuria

INTEG: Rash, pruritus, urticaria, photosensitivity, hair loss

MISC: Flushing

Contraindications: Sick sinus syndrome, second- or third-degree heart block, hypotension <90 mm Hg systolic, hypersensitivity

Precautions: CHF, hypotension, hepatic disease, pregnancy category C, lactation, children, renal disease, elderly

Pharmacokinetics:

PO: Peak plasma levels at 2-3 hr; metabolized in liver; metabolites excreted in urine, feces; excreted in breast milk

Drug interactions of concern to dentistry:

• Decreased effect: indomethacin, possibly other NSAIDs, phenobarbital

• Increased effect: parenteral and inhalational general anesthetics or other drugs with hypotensive actions, itraconazole

• Increased effects of carbamazepine

DENTAL CONSIDERATIONS

General:

• Monitor cardiac status; take vital signs at each appointment because of CV side effects. Consider a stress reduction protocol to prevent stress-induced angina during the dental appointment.

• After supine positioning, have patient sit upright for at least 2 min before standing to avoid orthostatic hypotension.

• Place on frequent recall to monitor gingival condition.

• Limit use of sodium-containing products such as saline IV fluids for patients with a dietary salt restriction.

• Assess salivary flow as a factor in caries, periodontal disease, and candidiasis.

• Use vasoconstrictors with caution, in low doses, and with careful aspiration. Avoid use of gingival retraction cord with epinephrine.

• Patients on chronic drug therapy may rarely have symptoms of blood dyscrasias, which can include infection, bleeding, and poor healing.

Consultations:

• In a patient with symptoms of blood dyscrasias, request a medical consultation for blood studies and postpone dental treatment until normal values are reestablished.

• Medical consultation may be required to assess disease control and stress tolerance of patient.

Teach patient/family:

• Importance of good oral hygiene to prevent soft tissue inflammation and minimize gingival overgrowth

• Need for frequent oral prophylaxis if overgrowth occurs

When chronic dry mouth occurs, advise patient:

- To avoid mouth rinses with high alcohol content because of drying effects
- To use sugarless gum, frequent sips of water, or saliva substitutes
- To use daily home fluoride products for anticaries effect

---

itraconazole

(i-tra-koe'na-zole)

Sporanox

Drug class.: Antifungal, systemic (triazole)

Action: Inhibits cytochrome P-450 enzymes and blocks synthesis of essential membrane sterols in fungal organism

Uses: Aspergillosis, blastomycosis, histoplasmosis (pulmonary and extrapulmonary); fungal infections of nails (onychomycosis); *Candida* infections of esophagus or mouth (oral sol only)

Dosage and routes:

Blastomycosis and histoplasmosis:

- *Adult:* PO 200 mg qd after a full meal, 200 mg bid for immunocompromised; max 400 mg day

Aspergillosis:

- *Adult:* PO 200-400 mg qd

Fungal nail infection (tinea unguium):

- *Adult:* PO 200 mg daily for 12 wk

Oral candidiasis:

- *Adult:* PO swish and swallow 200 mg/daily for 1-2 wk

Pharyngeal candidiasis:

- *Adult:* Swish and swallow 100 mg daily for a minimum of 3 wk

Available forms include: Caps 100 mg; oral sol 10 mg/ml in 150 ml volume; inj 10 mg/ml (IV infusion)

Side effects/adverse reactions:

CNS: Fatigue, headache, dizziness, anorexia, malaise

CV: Hypertension, edema, vertigo

GI: ***Hepatitis,*** nausea, vomiting, diarrhea, abdominal pain, hepatic dysfunction

GU: Impotence, albuminuria

INTEG: Rash, pruritus, ***Stevens-Johnson syndrome***

META: Hypokalemia, elevated liver enzymes

MISC: Fever, myalgia, ***anaphylaxis***

Contraindications: Hypersensitivity, triazolam, pimozide, quinidine, oral midazolam; avoid use in patients with CHF or who have a history of CHF

Precautions: Pregnancy category C, lactation, liver toxicity, oral anticoagulants (monitor patient), strong inhibitor of CYP 3A4 isoenzymes—note drug interactions

Pharmacokinetics:

PO: Peak plasma level 4 hr; highly protein bound (98.5%); take with food; metabolized by liver; 3%-18% excreted in feces, 40% in urine as metabolites

Drug interactions of concern to dentistry:

- Increased risk of rhabdomyolysis: lovastatin and simvastatin
- Increased risk of hypoglycemia: oral antidiabetics
- Increased metabolism: phenobarbital, carbamazepine
- May increase plasma levels of cyclosporine
- Contraindicated with triazolam, midazolam (see Appendix I)
- Inhibits metabolism of certain benzodiazepines: alprazolam, chlordiazepoxide, clonazepam,

chlorazepate, diazepam, estazolam, flurazepam, halazepam, midazolam, quazepam, triazolam, buspirone, zyloprim, felodipine
• Decreased effects: didanosine
• Increased plasma levels: saquinavir, nisoldipine, haloperidol, carbamazepine, erythromycin, clarithromycin
• Avoid itraconazole use with HMG-Co
• A reductase inhibitors or lower their dose
• May inhibit the metabolism of warfarin
• Suspected increase in plasma levels: cola beverages
• Decrease in plasma levels: grapefruit juice
• Decreased effects: didanosine (take 2 hr before didanosine tabs)
• May increase levels and side effects of HMG-Co
• A reductase inhibitors
• Increased plasma levels of alfentanil, buspirone, carbamazepine, corticosteroids, zolpidem
• Suspected decrease in oral contractive effectiveness; suggest alternative method of contraception

DENTAL CONSIDERATIONS

General:

• Monitor vital signs at every appointment because of cardiovascular side effects.
• Determine why the patient is taking the drug.
• Consider semisupine chair position for patient comfort because of GI effects of drug.

Consultations:

• Medical consultation may be required to assess patient's ability to tolerate stress.

ketoconazole

(kee-toe-koe'na-zole)

Nizoral, Nizoral Cream, Nizoral Shampoo

Drug class.: Imidazole antifungal

Action: Interferes with CYP450 enzymes preventing formation of ergosterol, resulting in damage to fungal cell membrane

Uses: Systemic candidiasis, chronic mucocutaneous candidiasis, cutaneous candidiasis, candiduria, coccidioidomycosis, histoplasmosis, chromomycosis, paracoccidioidomycosis, severe recalcitrant cutaneous dermatophyte infections; unapproved use: tinea pedis, tinea corporis, tinea cruris, and prostate cancer

Dosage and routes:

• *Adult and child >40 kg:* PO 200 mg qd; may increase to 400 mg qd if needed; high doses up to 1200 mg/day used in CNS fungal infections
• *Child >2 yr:* 3.3 to 6.6 mg/kg/day in a single dose

Cutaneous candidiasis:

• *Adult:* TOP apply cream once daily to affected area × 2-6 wk

Dandruff:

• *Adult:* Shampoo twice weekly at 3-day intervals for 4 wk

Available forms include: Tabs 200 mg, cream 2% in 15, 30, and 60 g tubes, shampoo 2% in 120 ml

Side effects/adverse reactions:

Side effects and interactions for PO form only:

▼ *ORAL:* Lichenoid reactions

CNS: Headache, dizziness, lethargy, anxiety, insomnia, dreams, paresthesia

GI: Nausea, vomiting, anorexia, ***severe hepatotoxicity,*** diarrhea, cramps, abdominal pain, constipation, flatulence, GI bleeding
GU: Gynecomastia, impotence
INTEG: Pruritus, fever, chills, photophobia, rash, dermatitis, purpura, urticaria
SYST: ***Anaphylaxis***

Contraindications: Hypersensitivity, pregnancy category C, lactation, fungal meningitis, loratadine, triazolam, dofetilide

Precautions: Renal disease, hepatic disease, drug-induced achlorhydria, potent inhibitor of CYP3A4 isoenzymes

Pharmacokinetics:
PO: Peak 1-2 hr, half-life 2 hr, terminal 8 hr; highly protein bound; metabolized in liver; excreted in bile, feces; requires acid pH for absorption; distributed poorly to CSF

Drug interactions of concern to dentistry:

- Hepatotoxicity: alcohol, high-dose long-term use, acetaminophen, carbamazepine, sulfonamides
- Decreased absorption: antacids (take 2 hr after ketoconazole), proton pump inhibitors
- Leukocyte disorders: tacrolimus
- Contraindicated with triazolam, lovastatin, dofetilide (see Appendix I)
- Inhibits the metabolism of certain benzodiazepines: alprazolam, chlordiazepoxide, clonazepam, clorazepate, diazepam, estazolam, flurazepam, halazepam, midazolam, quazepam, triazolam, zolpidem
- May inhibit metabolism of warfarin
- Decreased effects: didanosine (take 2 hr before didanosine tabs)
- May increase plasma levels and side effects of HMG-CoA reductase inhibitors, cyclosporine
- Increased serum levels of indinavir, saquinavir, ritonavir, nisoldipine, haloperidol, carbamazepine, tricyclic antidepressants, buspirone, zolpidem, corticosteroids
- Suspected decrease in oral contraceptive effectiveness: may need to suggest additional contraception

DENTAL CONSIDERATIONS

General:

- To prevent reinoculation of *Candida* infection, dispose of toothbrush or other contaminated oral hygiene devices used during period of infection.
- Determine if medication controls disease.
- Place on frequent recall to evaluate healing response.
- Assess salivary flow as a factor in caries, periodontal disease, and candidiasis.

Teach patient/family:

- To avoid mouth rinses with high alcohol content because of drying effects

ketoprofen

(kee-toe-proe'fen)

Orudis, Orudis KT (OTC), Oruvail
Apo-Keto, Apo-Keto-E, Novo-Keto-EC, Orudis-E, Rhodis, Rhodis-EC

Drug class.: Nonsteroidal antiinflammatory

Action: Inhibits prostaglandin synthesis by interfering with cyclooxygenase needed for biosynthesis; possesses analgesic, antiinflammatory, antipyretic properties

Uses: Osteoarthritis, rheumatoid arthritis, dysmenorrhea; OTC: minor aches and pains; unapproved: gouty arthritis, vascular headache

Dosage and routes:

• *Adult:* PO 75 mg tid or 50 mg qid, not to exceed 300 mg/day, or ext rel 200 mg/day; PO (OTC) 1 or 2 tabs q4-6h, limit 6 tabs/day or 75 mg

Available forms include: Tabs (OTC) 12.5 mg; caps 25, 50, 75 mg; ext rel caps 100, 150, 200 mg; supp 100 mg (Canada only)

Side effects/adverse reactions:

▼ *ORAL:* Stomatitis, bleeding, bitter taste, increased thirst, dry mouth, lichenoid reaction

CNS: Dizziness, drowsiness, fatigue, tremors, confusion, insomnia, anxiety, depression

CV: Tachycardia, peripheral edema, palpitation, dysrhythmias

GI: ***Cholestatic hepatitis,*** nausea, anorexia, vomiting, diarrhea, jaundice, constipation, flatulence, cramps, peptic ulcer

HEMA: ***Blood dyscrasias***

GU: ***Nephrotoxicity: dysuria, hematuria, oliguria, azotemia***

EENT: Tinnitus, hearing loss, blurred vision

INTEG: Purpura, rash, pruritus, sweating

Contraindications: Hypersensitivity, asthma, severe renal disease, severe hepatic disease, aspirin

Precautions: Pregnancy category B, lactation, children, bleeding disorders, GI disorders, cardiac disorders, hypersensitivity to other antiinflammatory agents, elderly, children <16 yr

Pharmacokinetics:

PO: Peak 2 hr, half-life 3-3.5 hr; 99% plasma-protein binding; metabolized in liver; excreted in urine (metabolites), breast milk

Drug interactions of concern to dentistry:

• GI ulceration, bleeding: aspirin, other NSAIDs, alcohol, corticosteroids

• Nephrotoxicity: acetaminophen (prolonged use)

• Possible risk of decreased renal function: cyclosporine

• Increased photosensitizing effect: tetracycline

• First-time users of SSRIs also taking NSAIDs may have a higher risk of GI side effects; until more data are available, it may be advisable to avoid use of NSAIDs in these patients (*Br J Clin Pharmacol* 55:591-595, 2003)

When prescribed for dental pain:

• Risk of increased effects: oral anticoagulants, oral antidiabetics, lithium, methotrexate

• Decreased effects of diuretics

DENTAL CONSIDERATIONS

General:

• Patients on chronic drug therapy may rarely have symptoms of blood dyscrasias, which can include infection, bleeding, and poor healing.

• Assess salivary flow as a factor in caries, periodontal disease, and candidiasis.

• Avoid prescribing for dental use in first and last trimester of pregnancy.

• Avoid prescribing aspirin-containing products or giving to patient taking aspirin.

• Consider semisupine chair position for patients with arthritic disease.

Consultations:
• In a patient with symptoms of blood dyscrasias, request a medical consultation for blood studies and postpone dental treatment until normal values are reestablished.
• Medical consultation may be required to assess disease control.
Teach patient/family:
• Importance of good oral hygiene to prevent soft tissue inflammation
• Caution to prevent injury when using oral hygiene aids
When chronic dry mouth occurs, advise patient:
• To avoid mouth rinses with high alcohol content because of drying effects
• To use sugarless gum, frequent sips of water, or saliva substitutes
• To use daily home fluoride products for anticaries effect

---

ketorolac tromethamine

(kee'toe-role-ak)
Toradol

Drug class.: Nonsteroidal antiinflammatory

Action: Inhibits prostaglandin synthesis by interfering with cyclooxygenase needed for biosynthesis; possesses analgesic, antiinflammatory, antipyretic properties
Uses: Short-term use of acute mild-to-moderate pain
Dosage and routes:
• *Adult <65 yr:* IM 60 mg (single dose); IV 30 mg (single dose; IV/IM 30 mg q6h, limit 120 mg/day (multiple-dose treatment)
• *Oral transition from parenteral doses:* PO 20 mg as the first oral dose after parenteral dose, then 10 mg q4-6h (limit 40 mg/day); combination parenteral and oral therapy must not exceed 5 days
• *Adult >65 yr or weight <110 lb or renal impairment:* IM 30 mg (single dose); IV 15 mg (single dose); IV/IM 15 mg q6h, limit 60 mg/day (multiple-dose treatment); PO 10 mg as first oral dose after parenteral doses, then 10 mg q4-6h (daily limit 40 mg)
Available forms include: Inj 15, 30 mg (prefilled syringes); tabs 10 mg
Side effects/adverse reactions:
▼ *ORAL:* Dry mouth, lichenoid reaction
CNS: Dizziness, drowsiness, fatigue, tremors, confusion, insomnia, anxiety, depression
CV: Tachycardia, peripheral edema, palpitation, dysrhythmias
GI: ***Cholestatic hepatitis,*** nausea, anorexia, vomiting, diarrhea, jaundice, constipation, flatulence, cramps, peptic ulcer
HEMA: ***Blood dyscrasias***
GU: ***Nephrotoxicity: dysuria, hematuria, oliguria, azotemia***
EENT: Tinnitus, hearing loss, blurred vision
INTEG: Purpura, rash, pruritus, sweating
Contraindications: Hypersensitivity, asthma, severe renal disease, severe hepatic disease, probenecid, patients with high risk of bleeding, prophylactic presurgery analgesia, labor and delivery, lactation, patients using ASA or NSAIDs
Precautions: Pregnancy category B, children, GI disorders, cardiac disorders, hypersensitivity to other antiinflammatory agents

Pharmacokinetics:
IM: Peak 50 min, half-life 6 hr

Drug interactions of concern to dentistry:

- GI ulceration, bleeding: aspirin, alcohol, corticosteroids
- Contraindicated with probenecid
- Possible risk of decreased renal function: cyclosporine
- First-time users of SSRIs also taking NSAIDs may have a higher risk of GI side effects; until more data are available, it may be advisable to avoid use of NSAIDs in these patients (*Br J Clin Pharmacol* 55:591-595, 2003)

When prescribed for dental pain:

- Risk of increased effects: oral anticoagulants, oral antidiabetics, lithium, methotrexate
- Decreased antihypertensive effects of diuretics, β-blockers, ACE inhibitors

DENTAL CONSIDERATIONS
General:

- Assess salivary flow as a factor in caries, periodontal disease, and candidiasis.
- Avoid prescribing for dental use in pregnancy.
- Avoid prescribing aspirin or other NSAIDs.
- Avoid long-term use for chronic pain syndromes; combined use of IV/IM and oral doses must not exceed 5 days.

Consultations:

- Medical consultation may be required to assess disease control.

Teach patient/family:

- To avoid mouth rinses with high alcohol content because of drying effects

ketotifen fumarate

(kee-toe-tye′-fen)
Zaditor
✤ Novo-Ketotifen, Zaditen
Drug class.: Antihistamine

Action: Noncompetitive antagonist for histamine (H_1) receptors, stabilizes mast cells

Uses: Temporary prevention of itching of the eyes caused by allergic conjunctivitis

Dosage and routes:

- *Adult:* Ophth 1 drop in affected eye(s) q8-12h

Available forms include: Ophth sol 5, 7.5 ml bottle with dropper (0.025%)

Side effects/adverse reactions:
CNS: Headache
EENT: Conjunctival infection, rhinitis, burning, stinging, eye pain, dry eyes, photophobia
INTEG: Rash

Contraindications: Hypersensitivity

Precautions: Prevent contamination of ophthalmic solution by careful use, do not wear contact lens if eyes are red, delay inserting contacts up to 10 min after drops are placed in eyes; pregnancy category C, lactation, children <3 yr

Pharmacokinetics: Limited information

Drug interactions of concern to dentistry:

- None reported

DENTAL CONSIDERATIONS
General:

- Protect patient's eyes from accidental spatter during dental treatment.
- Avoid dental light in patient's

eyes; offer dark glasses for patient comfort.

labetalol

(la-bet'a-lole)

Normodyne, Trandate

🍁 Trandate

Drug class.: Nonselective adrenergic β-blocker and selective α_1-blocker; antihypertensive

Action: Produces decreases in BP without reflex tachycardia or significant reduction in heart rate through mixture of α-blocking and β-blocking effects; elevated plasma renins are reduced

Uses: Mild-to-severe hypertension

Dosage and routes:

Hypertension:

• *Adult:* PO 100 mg bid; may be given with a diuretic, may increase to 200 mg bid after 2 days, may continue to increase q1-3d; usual maintenance dose 200-400 mg bid

Hypertensive crisis:

• *Adult:* IV inf 200 mg in 160 ml D_5W, run at 2 ml/min, stop infusion after desired response obtained, repeat q6-8h as needed; IV bol 20 mg over 2 min, may repeat 40-80 mg q10min, not to exceed 300 mg

Available forms include: Tabs 100, 200, 300 mg; inj 5 mg/ml in 20, 40 ml amps

Side effects/adverse reactions:

▼ *ORAL:* Dry mouth, taste changes, lichenoid reaction

CNS: Dizziness, mental changes, drowsiness, fatigue, headache, catatonia, depression, anxiety, nightmares, paresthesias, lethargy

CV: Orthostatic hypotension, bradycardia, ***CHF, ventricular dysrhythmias,*** chest pain, AV block

GI: Nausea, vomiting, diarrhea

RESP: ***Bronchospasm,*** dyspnea, wheezing

HEMA: ***Agranulocytosis, thrombocytopenia***

GU: Impotence, dysuria, ejaculatory failure

EENT: Tinnitus, visual changes, sore throat, double vision, dry/burning eyes

INTEG: Rash, alopecia, urticaria, pruritus, fever

Contraindications: Hypersensitivity to β-blockers, cardiogenic shock, second- or third-degree heart block, sinus bradycardia, CHF, bronchial asthma

Precautions: Major surgery, pregnancy category C, lactation, diabetes mellitus, renal disease, thyroid disease, COPD, well-compensated heart failure, CAD, nonallergic bronchospasm

Pharmacokinetics:

PO: Onset 1-2 hr, peak 2-4 hr, duration 8-12 hr

IV: Peak 5 min; half-life 6-8 hr; metabolized by liver (metabolites inactive); excreted in urine, bile, breast milk; crosses placenta

Drug interactions of concern to dentistry:

• Decreased metabolism: lidocaine

• Decreased effect: sympathomimetics

• Decreased hypotensive effects: indomethacin and other NSAIDs

• Increased hypotension, myocardial depression: hydrocarbon-inhalation anesthetics

• Increased plasma levels: diphenhydramine

DENTAL CONSIDERATIONS

General:

• Monitor vital signs at every appointment because of cardiovascular side effects.

• Patients on chronic drug therapy may rarely have symptoms of blood dyscrasias, which can include infection, bleeding, and poor healing.

• Assess salivary flow as a factor in caries, periodontal disease, and candidiasis.

• After supine positioning, have patient sit upright for at least 2 min before standing to avoid orthostatic hypotension.

• Limit use of sodium-containing products, such as saline IV fluids, for patients with a dietary salt restriction.

• Stress from dental procedures may compromise cardiovascular function; determine patient risk.

• Short appointments and a stress reduction protocol may be required for anxious patients.

Consultations:

• Medical consultation may be required to assess disease control and patient's ability to tolerate stress.

• In a patient with symptoms of blood dyscrasias, request a medical consultation for blood studies and postpone dental treatment until normal values are reestablished.

Teach patient/family:

When chronic dry mouth occurs, advise patient:

• To avoid mouth rinses with high alcohol content because of drying effects

• To use sugarless gum, frequent sips of water, or saliva substitutes

• To use daily home fluoride products for anticaries effect

lamivudine (3TC)

(la-mi'vyoo-deen)

Epivir, Epivir-HBV

♣ Heptovir

Drug class.: Antiviral, nucleoside analog

Action: Inhibition of HIV reverse transcriptase (by active phosphorylated metabolite); also inhibits RNA- and DNA-dependent DNA polymerase; monophosphate metabolite is incorporated into HBV DNA and results in DNA chain termination

Uses: Used in combination with zidovudine for the treatment of HIV infection and to reduce disease progression and death in AIDS; HBV dose form: chronic hepatitis B associated with evidence of hepatitis B viral replication and liver inflammation

Dosage and routes:

HIV infection (Epivir only):

• *Adult and child >16 yr:* PO 150 mg bid (in combination with other antiretroviral agents); for adults with low body weight (<50 kg), the recommended dose is 2 mg/kg bid in combination with zidovudine

• *Child 3 mo-16 yr:* PO 4 mg/kg (limit 150 mg) bid, in combination with other retroviral agents

Chronic hepatitis B:

• *Adult:* 100 mg qd (use Epivir-HBV dose forms only)

• *Child 2-17 yr:* PO 3 mg/kg once daily (limit 100 mg)

Available forms include: Epivir: Tabs 150, 300 mg; 10 mg/ml in 240 ml volume

Epivir-HBV: Tabs 100 mg; oral sol 5 mg/ml in 240 ml volume

L

Side effects/adverse reactions:
CNS: Malaise, fatigue, headache, anorexia, neuropathy, dizziness, insomnia, depression
GI: Nausea, diarrhea, vomiting, abdominal pain, ***pancreatitis, lactic acidosis, severe hepatomegaly***
RESP: Cough, nasal complaints
HEMA: ***Neutropenia,*** anemia
INTEG: Rash
MS: Pain, myalgia
MISC: Fever, chills, peripheral neuropathy, paresthesia
Contraindications: Hypersensitivity, history of pancreatitis as child
Precautions: Reduce dose in renal disease, pregnancy category C, lactation
Pharmacokinetics:
PO: Rapid absorption, wide tissue distribution, low plasma protein binding (36%), eliminated mostly unchanged in urine
Drug interactions of concern to dentistry:
• None reported
DENTAL CONSIDERATIONS
General:
• Patients on chronic drug therapy may rarely have symptoms of blood dyscrasias, which can include infection, bleeding, and poor healing.
• Examine for oral manifestation of opportunistic infections.
Consultations:
• In a patient with symptoms of blood dyscrasias, request a medical consultation for blood studies and postpone dental treatment until normal values are reestablished.
• Medical consultation may be required to assess disease control and patient's ability to tolerate stress.
Teach patient/family:
• Importance of good oral hygiene to prevent soft tissue inflammation
• Caution to prevent trauma when using oral hygiene aids
• That secondary oral infection may occur; must see dentist immediately if infection occurs

lamotrigine

(la-moe'tri-jeen)
Lamictal, Lamictal Chewable Dispersible
Drug class.: Antiepileptic

Action: Unknown, but may be due to blockage of voltage-dependent sodium channels with inhibition of excitatory amino acids
Uses: Adjunctive treatment of refractive partial seizures in adults and adjunctive treatment for Lennox-Gastaut syndrome in pediatric and adult patients; long-term maintenance of bipolar 1 disorder
Dosage and routes:
With enzyme-inducing drugs without valproic acid (enzyme-inducing drugs include phenytoin, phenobarbital, primidone, and carbamazepine):
• *Adult and child >12 yr:* PO initial dose 50 mg/day × 2 wk, then 50 mg bid for weeks 3 and 4
• *Child 2-12 yr:* PO initial dose 0.6 mg/kg/day in 1 or 2 divided doses × 1-2 wk; then 0.3 mg/kg/day in 2 divided doses for weeks 3 and 4
With non–enzyme-inducing drugs and valproic acid:
• *Adult and child >12 yr:* PO initial dose 25 mg qod × 2 wk, then 25 mg/day for weeks 3 and 4
• *Child 2-12 yr:* PO initial dose

0.15 mg/kg/day in 1 or 2 divided doses × 1-2 wk; then 0.3 mg/kg/day in 1 or 2 divided doses for weeks 3 and 4

Bipolar disorder (patient not taking carbamazepine or valproic acid):

• *Adult:* PO initial dose 25 mg/day × 2 wk, then 50 mg/day for weeks 3 and 4; 100 mg/day week 5; 200 mg/day week 6 and thereafter

Bipolar disorder (patient taking valproic acid):

• *Adult:* PO initial dose 25 mg qod × 2 wk, then 25 mg/day for weeks 3 and 4; 50 mg/day week 5; 100 mg/day week 6 and thereafter

Bipolar disorder (patient taking carbamazepine or other enzyme inhibitors):

• *Adult:* PO initial dose 50 mg/day × 2 wk, then 50 mg bid for weeks 3 and 4; 100 mg bid week 5; 150 mg bid week 6 and 200 mg bid thereafter

Available forms include: Tabs 25, 150, 100, 200 mg; chew tabs 2, 5, 25 mg

Side effects/adverse reactions:

▼ *ORAL:* Dry mouth, facial edema (rarely), halitosis, gingival overgrowth, stomatitis

CNS: Dizziness, headache, somnolence, fever, ataxia, insomnia, tremor, depression, anxiety, vertigo

CV: Hot flashes, palpitation, dysrhythmia

GI: Vomiting, nausea, abdominal pain, diarrhea

RESP: Respiratory complaints, cough

HEMA: Anemia, ***leukopenia, leukocytosis***

GU: Dysmenorrhea, vaginitis

EENT: Pharyngitis, rhinitis, blurred vision, diplopia, ear pain

INTEG: Skin rash, ***Stevens-Johnson syndrome, toxic epidermal necrolysis, angioedema,*** pruritus, photosensitivity

MS: Hyperkinesia, neck pain, myasthenia symptoms, arthralgia

Contraindications: Hypersensitivity

Precautions: Pregnancy category C, lactation, elderly, children <16 yr, dose adjustment with other anticonvulsants, seizure risk with drug withdrawal, renal or hepatic impairment; can cause Stevens-Johnson syndrome, toxic epidermal necrolysis

Pharmacokinetics:

PO: Rapid absorption, peak plasma levels 1.3-4.2 hr; 55% plasma protein bound; liver metabolism; renal excretion

Drug interactions of concern to dentistry:

• Increased excretion: chronic, high-dose acetaminophen (900 mg tid), but significance is unclear; carbamazepine

• Increased blood levels of carbamazepine

DENTAL CONSIDERATIONS

General:

• Early morning appointments and a stress reduction protocol may be required for anxious patients.

• Determine type of epilepsy, seizure frequency, and quality of seizure control. A stress reduction protocol may be required.

• Evaluate respiration characteristics and rate.

• Assess salivary flow as factor in caries, periodontal disease, and candidiasis.

• Patients on chronic drug therapy may rarely have symptoms of blood dyscrasias, which can include infection, bleeding, and poor healing.

• Place on frequent recall because of oral side effects.

Consultations:

• Medical consultation may be required to assess disease control and the patient's ability to tolerate stress.

• In a patient with symptoms of blood dyscrasias, request a medical consultation for blood studies and postpone dental treatment until normal values are reestablished.

Teach patient/family:

• Importance of good oral hygiene to prevent soft tissue inflammation

• Use of electric toothbrush if patient has difficulty holding conventional devices

When chronic dry mouth occurs, advise patient:

• To avoid mouth rinses with high alcohol content because of drying effects

• To use daily home fluoride products for anticaries effect

• To use sugarless gum, frequent sips of water, or saliva substitutes

---

lansoprazole

(lan-soe'pra-zole)

Prevacid

Drug class.: Antisecretory, proton pump inhibitor

Action: Suppresses gastric acid production by binding to the hydrogen/potassium ATPase enzyme system to inhibit the final step in gastric acid production

Uses: Short-term treatment for healing and symptomatic relief of active duodenal ulcer and benign gastric ulcer, erosive esophagitis, and GERD; maintenance of healing of duodenal ulcers; long-term treatment of pathologic hypersecretory syndromes; NSAID-associated gastric ulcers in patients who continue NSAID use; short-term treatment of symptomatic GERD

Dosage and routes:

Duodenal ulcers:

• *Adult:* PO 15 mg/day ac × 4 wk; maintenance 15 mg/day

Erosive esophagitis:

• *Adult:* PO 30 mg/day ac (up to 8 wk)

Hypersecretory syndromes:

• *Adult:* PO 60 mg/day (up to 120 mg in divided doses)

H. pylori related:

• *Adult:* PO lansoprazole 30 mg along with clarithromycin 500 mg and amoxicillin 1 g bid × 14 days; or in clarithromycin resistance, lansoprazole 30 mg and amoxicillin 1 g tid × 14 days

Gastric ulcer associated with NSAIDs:

• *Adult:* PO 30 mg qd (up to 8 wk) for healing; or 15 mg/day for risk reduction (up to 12 wk)

GERD:

• *Adult:* PO 15 mg qd (up to 8 wk)

• *Child 1-11 yr:* PO 30 kg weight or less, 15 mg qd (up to 12 wk); over 30 kg weight, 30 mg/day (up to 12 wk)

Available forms include: Caps 15, 30 mg; granules for oral susp 15, 30 mg in unit doses

Side effects/adverse reactions:

▼ *ORAL:* Candidiasis, stomatitis, halitosis (all <1%), dry mouth, taste alteration

CNS: Headache, dizziness

GI: Abdominal pain, diarrhea, nausea, vomiting

RESP: Cough, asthma, bronchitis, dyspnea

HEMA: Anemia

GU: Abnormal menses, glycosuria, gynecomastia, breast tenderness
EENT: Tinnitus, amblyopia, eye pain
MS: Myalgia, musculoskeletal pain
Contraindications: Hypersensitivity
Precautions: Pregnancy category B, lactation, children <18 yr, elderly (limit doses to 30 mg/day), severe hepatic disease
Pharmacokinetics:
PO: Peak plasma levels 1.7 hr, half-life 1.5 hr; 97% plasma protein bound; extensive liver metabolism; metabolites mainly excreted in feces, less in urine
Drug interactions of concern to dentistry:
• Drug interactions not established but potentially can interfere with absorption of amoxicillin, ketoconazole

DENTAL CONSIDERATIONS
General:
• Consider semisupine chair position for patient comfort because of GI effects of disease.
• Question the patient about tolerance of NSAIDs or aspirin related to GI problem.
• Patients with gastroesophageal reflux may have oral symptoms, including burning mouth, secondary candidiasis, and oral signs of dental erosion.
• Assess salivary flow as factor in caries, periodontal disease, and candidiasis.
Teach patient/family:
When chronic dry mouth occurs, advise patient:
• To avoid mouth rinses with high alcohol content because of drying effects
• To use daily home fluoride products for anticaries effect
• To use sugarless gum, frequent sips of water, or saliva substitutes

latanoprost

(la-ta'noe-prost)
Xalatan

Drug class.: Prostaglandin F_{2a} analogue

Action: A prostanoid F_{2a} analog believed to reduce intraocular pressure by increasing uveoscleral outflow of aqueous humor
Uses: Open-angle glaucoma and ocular hypertension in patients intolerant to other intraocular pressure–lowering drugs
Dosage and routes:
• *Adult:* Instill 1 drop in affected eye(s) qd in PM
Available forms include: Ophthalmic sol 0.005% (50 µg/ml) in 2.5 ml
Side effects/adverse reactions:
RESP: Upper respiratory infection, cold, flu
EENT: Blurred vision, burning, stinging, itching, foreign body sensation, increased iris pigmentation, dry eye, pain, edema, retinal artery embolus, retinal detachment (rare)
INTEG: Rash
MS: Muscle pain, chest pain, angina pain
Contraindications: Hypersensitivity to latanoprost or other ingredients in the sterile ophthalmic solution
Precautions: Gradual change in eye color, avoid contamination of sterile solution, renal or hepatic impairment, remove contact lens before using, administer at least 5 min apart if other ophthalmic drug is also used, pregnancy category C, nursing, pediatrics

Pharmacokinetics: *OPHTH:* Absorbed through cornea, peak conc 2 hr, hydrolyzed by esterases in cornea to active acid, metabolized in liver, half-life 17 min, renal excretion; onset 3-4 hr, maximum effect 8-12 hr

Drug interactions of concern to dentistry:

- None reported at this time; avoid use of anticholinergic drugs, atropine-like drugs, propantheline, and diazepam (benzodiazepines) in patient with glaucoma

DENTAL CONSIDERATIONS

General:

- Check compliance of patient with prescribed drug regimen for glaucoma.
- Avoid dental light in patient's eyes; offer dark glasses for patient comfort.
- Protect patient's eyes from accidental spatter during dental treatment.

Consultations:

- Medical consultation may be required to assess disease control.

---

leflunomide

(le-flu'no-mide)

Arava

Drug class.: Antiarthritic, immunosuppressive

Action: Acts as an immunomodulating agent by blocking dihydroorotate dehydrogenase enzymes, which results in inhibition of pyrimidine synthesis. This results in antiproliferative effects on cells dependent on this pathway.

Uses: To reduce signs and symptoms and to retard structural damage in active rheumatoid arthritis as demonstrated by x-ray erosion and joint space narrowing

Dosage and routes:

- *Adult:* PO loading dose 100 mg × 3 days, maintenance dose 20 mg daily, higher doses not recommended

Available forms include: Tabs 10, 20, 100 mg

Side effects/adverse reactions:

▼ *ORAL:* Mouth ulceration, candidiasis, dry mouth, taste disturbances

CNS: Headache, asthenia, dizziness, paresthesia

CV: Hypertension, palpitation

GI: Diarrhea, abdominal pain, nausea, dyspepsia, colitis

RESP: Cough, URI, bronchitis

HEMA: Anemia

GU: UTI

EENT: Rhinitis, sinusitis

INTEG: Rash, pruritus

META: Elevation of liver enzymes ALT, AST

MS: Synovitis, tenosynovitis, joint discomfort

MISC: Alopecia, allergic reactions

Contraindications: Hypersensitivity, pregnancy, woman of childbearing age not using reliable contraception, significant hepatic impairment, hepatitis B or C, lactation; severe immunodeficiency, bone marrow dysplasia or severe, uncontrolled infections

Precautions: Chronic renal or hepatic insufficiency, rifampin, pregnancy category X, child <18 yr

Pharmacokinetics:

PO: Loading dose required, converted to active metabolite, peak levels of metabolite 6-12 hr, half-life of metabolite (2 wk), highly protein bound (99%), metabolites removed by renal (43%) and fecal excretion (48%)

Drug interactions of concern to dentistry:

• None reported

DENTAL CONSIDERATIONS

General:

• Monitor vital signs at every appointment because of cardiovascular side effects.

• Consider semisupine chair position for patient comfort if GI side effects occur.

• Examine for oral manifestation of opportunistic infection.

• If acute oral infection occurs, inform physician.

• Assess salivary flow as a factor in caries, periodontal disease, and candidiasis.

Consultations:

• Consult if needed.

Teach patient/family:

• Importance of good oral hygiene to prevent soft tissue inflammation

• Use of electric toothbrush if patient has difficulty holding conventional devices

When chronic dry mouth occurs, advise patient:

• To avoid mouth rinses with high alcohol content because of drying effects

• To use daily home fluoride products for anticaries effect

• To use sugarless gum, frequent sips of water, or saliva substitutes

---

letrozole

(let'roe-zole)

Femara

Drug class.: Antineoplastic

Action: Acts as a nonsteroidal competitive inhibitor of aromatase enzyme and thereby interferes with the conversion of androgens to estrogens

Uses: Locally advanced or metastatic breast cancer in postmenopausal women either hormone receptor positive or hormone receptor unknown; advanced breast cancer in postmenopausal women with disease progression following antiestrogen therapy

Dosage and routes:

• *Adult:* PO 2.5 mg qd

Available forms include: Tabs 2.5 mg

Side effects/adverse reactions:

CNS: ***Hemorrhagic stroke, hemiparesis,*** headache, insomnia, TIA

CV: Hot flushes, ***MI, coronary heart disease,*** leg edema, hypertension, angina

GI: Nausea, constipation, diarrhea, vomiting, abdominal pain

RESP: Dyspnea, coughing

HEMA: ***Peripheral thromboembolic events***

INTEG: Rash, pruritus

ENDO: Hypercholesterolemia

META: Weight loss, elevated SGOT, SGPT, and bilirubin

MS: Fatigue, weakness

MISC: Bone pain, back pain, arthralgia, chest pain, hair loss, breast pain

Contraindications: Hypersensitivity

Precautions: Pregnancy category D, lactation, children (no studies), for postmenopausal women only, thrombocytopenia and decreased lymphocyte counts, liver impairment

Pharmacokinetics:

PO: Rapid, complete absorption; steady state plasma levels 2-6 wk; depression of serum estrogen levels in 24 hr; maximum suppression 2-3 days; weakly bound to plasma protein; metabolized by CYP450 3A4 and CYP450 2A6; excreted mainly in urine

Drug interactions of concern to dentistry:

• None reported

DENTAL CONSIDERATIONS

General:

• Patients taking opioids for acute or chronic pain should be given alternative analgesics for dental pain.

• Patients on chronic drug therapy may rarely have symptoms of blood dyscrasias, which can include infection, bleeding, and poor healing.

• Palliative medication may be required for management of oral side effects.

• Examine for oral manifestation of opportunistic infection.

• Consider semisupine chair position for patient comfort if GI side effects occur.

• Monitor vital signs at every appointment because of cardiovascular and respiratory side effects.

Consultations:

• In a patient with symptoms of blood dyscrasias, request a medical consultation for blood studies and postpone treatment until normal values are reestablished.

Teach patient/family:

• Importance of good oral hygiene to prevent soft tissue inflammation

• To be aware of the possibility of secondary oral infection and the need to see dentist immediately if signs of infection occur

leucovorin calcium (citrovorum factor/ folinic acid)

(loo-koe-vor'in)

Wellcovorin

Drug class.: Folic acid antagonist antidote, antineoplastic adjunct

Action: Chemically reduced derivative of folic acid; converted to tetrahydrofolate; counteracts folic acid antagonists

Uses: Megaloblastic or macrocytic anemia caused by folic acid deficiency, overdose of folic acid antagonist, methotrexate toxicity, toxicity caused by pyrimethamine or trimethoprim; used with fluorouracil in colorectal cancer

Dosage and routes:

Megaloblastic anemia caused by enzyme deficiency:

• *Adult and child:* PO 1 mg for life

Megaloblastic anemia caused by deficiency of folate:

• *Adult and child:* IM 1 mg or less qd, continued until adequate response

Methotrexate toxicity:

• *Adult and child:* PO/IM/IV 10 mg/m^2 q6h until methotrexate levels fall

Trimethoprim or pyrimethamine toxicity:

• *Adult and child:* PO/IM prevention 400 μg to 5 mg qd; PO treatment 5-15 mg/day

Available forms include: Tabs 5, 15, 25 mg; inj IM 3 mg/ml; powder for inj 50, 100, 350 mg/vial

Side effects/adverse reactions:

RESP: Wheezing

INTEG: Rash, pruritus, erythema

Contraindications: Hypersensi-

tivity, anemias other than megaloblastic not associated with B_{12} deficiency

Precautions: Pregnancy category C

Drug interactions of concern to dentistry:

• None reported

DENTAL CONSIDERATIONS

General:

• Signs of folate deficiency may appear in oral tissues.

• Determine why the patient is taking the drug.

• Patients with severe anemia or cancer or those receiving cancer chemotherapy may have oral complaints. Palliative therapy may be required.

Consultations:

• Medical consultation may be required to assess disease control.

Teach patient/family:

• Importance of good oral hygiene to prevent soft tissue inflammation

• Caution to prevent trauma when using oral hygiene aids

• To report oral lesions, soreness, or bleeding to dentist

• That secondary oral infection may occur; must see dentist immediately if infection occurs

• Importance of updating medical/drug records if physician makes any changes in evaluation or drug regimens

levalbuterol HCl

(lev'al-byoo-ter-ole)

Xopenex

Drug class.: Bronchodilator

Action: Selective β_2-adrenergic agonist; causes relaxation of smooth muscles of all airways

Uses: Treatment or prevention of bronchospasm in adults and children >6 yr with reversible obstructive airway disease

Dosage and routes:

• *Adult and child 12 yr or older:* INH 0.63 mg tid by nebulizer

• *Child 6-11 yr:* INH 0.31 mg tid by nebulizer; not to exceed 0.63 mg tid

Severe asthma not responding to 0.63 mg:

• *Adult and child 12 yr or older:* INH 1.25 mg tid by nebulizer

Available forms include: Inh sol 0.31, 0.63, 1.25 mg in 3 ml vials

Side effects/adverse reactions:

▼ *ORAL:* Dry mouth

CNS: Migraine, dizziness, nervousness, tremor, anxiety, insomnia, paresthesia

CV: Tachycardia, ECG changes

GI: Dyspepsia, diarrhea, nausea, gastroenteritis

RESP: Flulike syndrome, cough

EENT: Rhinitis, sinusitis, turbinate edema, dry throat

META: Increased plasma glucose, decreased serum K^+, eye itch

MS: Back pain, leg cramps

MISC: Pain

Contraindications: Hypersensitivity to this drug or racemic albuterol

Precautions: Paradoxic bronchospasm, cardiovascular disorders, seizures, diabetes, hyperthyroidism, coronary insufficiency, cardiac arrhythmias, hypertension, not to exceed recommended dose, β-adrenergic blockers, MAOIs, tricyclic antidepressants, pregnancy category C, lactation, children <12 yr

Pharmacokinetics:

INH: Relief of bronchoconstriction 20 min, half-life 3-4 hr, low plasma levels

L

Drug interactions of concern to dentistry:

• Significant reduction of effects: β-adrenergic blockers

• Potentiation of CV effects: MAOIs, tricyclic antidepressants, methylxanthines

• No specific dental drug interactions reported

DENTAL CONSIDERATIONS

General:

• Monitor vital signs at every appointment because of cardiovascular side effects.

• Assess salivary flow as a factor in caries, periodontal disease, and candidiasis.

• Consider semisupine chair position for patients with respiratory disease.

• Short, midday appointments and a stress reduction protocol may be required for anxious patients.

• Be aware that aspirin or sulfite preservatives in vasoconstrictor-containing products can exacerbate asthma.

• Acute asthmatic episodes may be precipitated in the dental office. Rapid-acting sympathomimetic inhalants should be available for emergency use. A stress reduction protocol may be required.

Consultations:

• Medical consultation may be required to assess disease control and patient's ability to tolerate stress.

Teach patient/family:

• For inhalation dosage forms, rinse mouth with water after each dose to prevent dryness

When chronic dry mouth occurs, advise patient:

• To avoid mouth rinses with high alcohol content because of drying effects

• To use daily home fluoride products for anticaries effect

• To use sugarless gum, frequent sips of water, or saliva substitutes

---

levamisole HCl

(lee-vam'i-sol)

Ergamisol

Drug class.: Immunomodulator

Action: May increase the action of macrophages, monocytes, and T cells, which will restore immune function; complete action is unknown

Uses: Treatment of Dukes' stage C colon cancer, given with fluorouracil after surgical resection

Dosage and routes:

• *Adult:* PO 50 mg q8h × 3 days, begin treatment at least 1 wk but no more than 4 wk after resection, given with fluorouracil 450 mg/m^2/day; IV given daily × 5 days beginning 21-34 days after resection, maintenance is 50 mg q8h × 3 days q2wk × 1 yr, given with fluorouracil 45 mg/m^2/day by IV push qwk starting 28 days after the initial 5-day course × 1 yr

Available forms include: Tabs 50 mg (base)

Side effects/adverse reactions:

▼ *ORAL:* Stomatitis, altered taste, lichenoid drug reaction

CNS: Dizziness, headache, paresthesia, somnolence, depression, anxiety, fatigue, fever, mental changes, ataxia, insomnia

CV: Chest pain, edema

GI: Nausea, vomiting, anorexia, diarrhea, constipation, flatulence, dyspepsia, abdominal pain

HEMA: ***Granulocytopenia, leukopenia, thrombocytopenia, agranulocytosis***

EENT: Altered sense of smell, blurred vision, conjunctivitis
INTEG: Rash, pruritus, alopecia, dermatitis, urticaria
META: Hyperbilirubinemia
MISC: Rigors, infection, arthralgia, myalgia
Contraindications: Hypersensitivity
Precautions: Pregnancy category C, lactation, children, blood dyscrasias
Pharmacokinetics:
PO: Peak 1.5-2 hr, elimination half-life 3-4 hr; metabolized by liver
Drug interactions of concern to dentistry:
• Disulfiram-like reaction: alcohol

DENTAL CONSIDERATIONS
General:
• Patients on chronic drug therapy may rarely have symptoms of blood dyscrasias, which can include infection, bleeding, and poor healing.
• Palliative treatment may be required for oral side effects.
• Place on frequent recall to evaluate healing response.
• Consider semisupine chair position when GI side effects occur.
Consultations:
• In a patient with symptoms of blood dyscrasias, request a medical consultation for blood studies and postpone dental treatment until normal values are reestablished.
• Medical consultation may be required to assess disease control.
Teach patient/family:
• To call physician if sore throat, swollen lymph nodes, malaise, or fever occur because other infections may exist
• To avoid mouth rinses with high alcohol content because of drying effects
• Importance of good oral hygiene to prevent soft tissue inflammation
• Caution to prevent injury when using oral hygiene aids
• To report oral lesions, soreness, or bleeding to dentist

---

levetiracetam
(lev-tir-a'se-tam)
Keppra
Drug class.: Antiepileptic

Action: Mechanism of action is unknown; suggestions include disruption of epileptiform burst firing and seizure propagation
Uses: Adjunctive therapy in adults with partial-onset seizures
Dosage and routes:
• *Adult:* PO initial dose 1000 mg/day given as 500 mg bid; additional doses may be given every 2 wk (1000 mg/day increments); max daily dose 3000 mg; doses must be adjusted with renal impairment; has been used in combination with other antiepileptic drugs
Available forms include: Tabs 250, 500, 750 mg; oral sol 100 mg/ml
Side effects/adverse reactions:
NOTE: Based on limited information.
▼ *ORAL:* Gingivitis (unspecified as to cause)
CNS: Drowsiness, somnolence, headache, dizziness, fatigue, amnesia, anxiety, ataxia, depression, emotional lability, hostility, vertigo
GI: Nausea, anorexia, abdominal pain, dyspepsia, diarrhea
RESP: Cough
HEMA: Decrease in mean RBC count, decrease in mean hemoglo-

bin and mean hematocrit, leukopenia
GU: Increase in serum creatinine, UTI
EENT: Pharyngitis, rhinitis, sinusitis, diplopia
INTEG: Rash
MS: Arthralgia
MISC: Asthenia, coordination difficulties, infection

Contraindications: Hypersensitivity

Precautions: Renal impairment, hemodialysis, pregnancy category C, lactation, may increase phenytoin blood levels, risk of seizures on withdrawal, children <16 yr

Pharmacokinetics:
PO: Bioavailability 100%, onset 1 hr, peak plasma levels 20 min-2 hr, half-life 6-8 hr, <10% plasma protein bound, limited hepatic metabolism, renal excretion (66%)

Drug interactions of concern to dentistry:
- None reported

DENTAL CONSIDERATIONS
General:
- Short appointments and a stress reduction protocol may be required for anxious patients.
- Ask patient about type of epilepsy, seizure frequency, and quality of seizure control.

Consultation: Medical consultation may be required to assess disease control and the patient's ability to tolerate stress. In patients with symptoms of blood dyscrasias, request a medical consultation for blood studies and postpone treatment until normal values are reestablished.

Teach patient/family:
- Importance of updating health and drug history if physician makes changes in evaluation or drug regimens

levobunolol HCl

(lee-voe-byoo'noe-lole)
AKBeta, Betagan Liquifilm
Drug class.: β-adrenergic blocker

Action: Reduces production of aqueous humor by unknown mechanisms

Uses: Chronic open-angle glaucoma, ocular hypertension

Dosage and routes:
- *Adult:* Instill 1 gtt in affected eye(s) qd or bid

Available forms include: Sol 0.25%, 0.5%

Side effects/adverse reactions:
CNS: Ataxia, dizziness, lethargy

Drug interactions of concern to dentistry:
- Patient with glaucoma: avoid use of anticholinergic drugs, atropine-like drugs, propantheline, and diazepam (benzodiazepines)

DENTAL CONSIDERATIONS
General:
- Check compliance of patient with prescribed drug regimen for glaucoma.
- Avoid dental light in patient's eyes; offer dark glasses for patient comfort.

Consultations:
- Consultation with physician may be needed if sedation or anesthesia is required.

levocabastine HCl

(lee'voe-kab-as-teen)

Livostin

Drug class.: Antihistamine, H_1-receptor antagonist

Action: Selective antagonist for histamine at H_1-receptors; little or no systemic absorption; intended for topical effect

Uses: Temporary relief of seasonal allergic conjunctivitis

Dosage and routes:

Ophthalmic:

• *Adult and child >12 yr:* Instill 1 gtt in affected eye qid; may continue for up to 2 wk

Available forms include: Ophth susp 0.05% in 2.5, 5, 10 ml dropper bottles

Side effects/adverse reactions:

▼ *ORAL:* Dry mouth

CNS: Headache, fatigue, somnolence

GI: Nausea

RESP: Dyspnea, cough

EENT: Local stinging/burning, red eyes, eyelid edema, lacrimation

INTEG: Rash, erythema

Contraindications: Hypersensitivity; avoid while contact lenses are being used

Precautions: Pregnancy category C, lactation, children <12 yr

Pharmacokinetics: *OPHTH:* Systemic absorption low; mean plasma concentration 1-2 ng/ml

Drug interactions of concern to dentistry:

• No documented interactions with dental drugs

DENTAL CONSIDERATIONS

General:

• Question patient about history of allergy to avoid using other potential allergens.

• Avoid dental light in patient's eyes; offer dark glasses for patient comfort.

• Evaluate respiration characteristics and rate.

• Using for less than 2 wk should not present a problem with dry mouth.

Teach patient/family:

When chronic dry mouth occurs, advise patient:

• To avoid mouth rinses with high alcohol content because of drying effects

• To use daily home fluoride products for anticaries effect

• To use sugarless gum, frequent sips of water, or saliva substitutes

L

levodopa

(lee-voe-doe'pa)

Dopar, Larodopa

Drug class.: Antiparkinson agent

Action: Small amounts of levodopa reach the brain where it is decarboxylated to dopamine, the dopamine then interacts with dopaminergic receptors in the striatum

Uses: Parkinsonism of various etiologies

Dosage and routes:

• *Adult:* PO 0.5-1 g qd either bid or qid with food; dose is titrated to tolerated side effects; may be increased by 0.75 g q3-7d, not to exceed 8 g/day; most often used in combination with carbidopa

Available forms include: Caps 100, 250, 500 mg; tabs 100, 250, 500 mg

Side effects/adverse reactions:
▼ *ORAL: Dry mouth,* bitter taste
CNS: Involuntary choreiform movements, hand tremors, fatigue, headache, anxiety, twitching, numbness, weakness, confusion, agitation, insomnia, nightmares, psychosis, hallucinations, hypomania, severe depression, dizziness
CV: Orthostatic hypotension, tachycardia, hypertension, palpitation
GI: Nausea, vomiting, anorexia, abdominal distress, flatulence, dysphagia, diarrhea, constipation
HEMA: ***Hemolytic anemia, leukopenia, agranulocytosis***
EENT: Blurred vision, diplopia, dilated pupils
INTEG: Rash, sweating, alopecia
MISC: Urinary retention, incontinence, weight change, dark urine

Contraindications: Hypersensitivity, narrow-angle glaucoma, undiagnosed skin lesions, MAOIs

Precautions: Renal disease, cardiac disease, hepatic disease, respiratory disease, MI with dysrhythmia, convulsions, peptic ulcer, pregnancy category C, asthma, endocrine disease, affective disorders, psychosis, lactation, children <12 yr

Pharmacokinetics:
PO: Peak 1-3 hr, metabolites excreted in urine

Drug interactions of concern to dentistry:
- Decreased absorption: anticholinergics
- Decreased therapeutic effect: benzodiazepines, pyridoxine (vitamin B_6), tricyclic antidepressants

DENTAL CONSIDERATIONS

General:
- Patients on chronic drug therapy may rarely have symptoms of blood dyscrasias, which can include infection, bleeding, and poor healing.
- Assess salivary flow as a factor in caries, periodontal disease, and candidiasis.
- After supine positioning, have patient sit upright for at least 2 min before standing to avoid orthostatic hypotension.
- Avoid dental light in patient's eyes; offer dark glasses for patient comfort.

Consultations:
- In a patient with symptoms of blood dyscrasias, request a medical consultation for blood studies and postpone dental treatment until normal values are reestablished.
- Take precautions if dental surgery is anticipated and anesthesia is required.
- Medical consultation may be required to assess disease control.

Teach patient/family:
- To use electric toothbrush if patient has difficulty holding conventional devices

When chronic dry mouth occurs, advise patient:
- To avoid mouth rinses with high alcohol content because of drying effects
- To use sugarless gum, frequent sips of water, or saliva substitutes
- To use daily home fluoride products for anticaries effect

levodopa-carbidopa

(lee-voe-doe'pa) (kar-bi-doe'pa)

Sinemet 10/100, Sinemet 25/100, Sinemet 25/250, Sinemet CR

✤ Apo-Levocarb, Nu-Levocarb

Drug class.: Antiparkinson agent

Action: Decarboxylation of levodopa in the periphery is inhibited by carbidopa; more levodopa is made available for transport to the brain and conversion to dopamine in the brain

Uses: Treatment of idiopathic, symptomatic, or postencephalitic parkinsonism

Dosage and routes:

- *Adult:* PO 1 tab of 10 mg carbidopa/100 mg levodopa tid or qid in divided doses, not to exceed 8 tabs/day; SUS REL tabs: 1 tab bid (not less than 6 hr apart) doses may require adjustment depending on patient response

Available forms include: Tabs 10/100, 25/100, 25/250; sus rel tabs 25/100 and 50/200 (carbidopa/levodopa in mg)

Side effects/adverse reactions:

▼ *ORAL: Dry mouth,* bitter taste

CNS: Involuntary choreiform movements, hand tremors, fatigue, headache, anxiety, twitching, numbness, weakness, confusion, agitation, insomnia, nightmares, psychosis, hallucinations, hypomania, severe depression, dizziness

CV: Orthostatic hypotension, tachycardia, hypertension, palpitation

GI: Nausea, vomiting, anorexia, abdominal distress, flatulence, dysphagia, diarrhea, constipation

HEMA: ***Hemolytic anemia, leukopenia, agranulocytosis***

EENT: Blurred vision, diplopia, dilated pupils

INTEG: Rash, sweating, alopecia

MISC: Urinary retention, incontinence, weight change, dark urine

Contraindications: Hypersensitivity, narrow-angle glaucoma, undiagnosed skin lesions

Precautions: Renal disease, cardiac disease, hepatic disease, respiratory disease, MI with dysrhythmias, convulsions, peptic ulcer, pregnancy category C

Pharmacokinetics:

PO: Peak 1-3 hr, excreted in urine (metabolites)

Drug interactions of concern to dentistry:

- Decreased absorption: anticholinergics
- Decreased therapeutic effect: benzodiazepines, pyridoxine (vitamin B_6)

DENTAL CONSIDERATIONS

General:

- Patients on chronic drug therapy may rarely have symptoms of blood dyscrasias, which can include infection, bleeding, and poor healing.
- Assess salivary flow as a factor in caries, periodontal disease, and candidiasis.
- After supine positioning, have patient sit upright for at least 2 min before standing to avoid orthostatic hypotension.
- Avoid dental light in patient's eyes; offer dark glasses for patient comfort.

Consultations:

- In a patient with symptoms of blood dyscrasias, request a medical

L

consultation for blood studies and postpone dental treatment until normal values are reestablished.

- Take precautions if dental surgery is anticipated and anesthesia is required.
- Medical consultation may be required to assess disease control.

Teach patient/family:

- To use electric toothbrush if patient has difficulty holding conventional devices

When chronic dry mouth occurs, advise patient:

- To avoid mouth rinses with high alcohol content because of drying effects
- To use sugarless gum, frequent sips of water, or saliva substitutes
- To use daily home fluoride products for anticaries effect

levofloxacin

(lee-voe-flox'a-sin)

Levaquin

Drug class.: Fluoroquinolone anti-infective

Action: A broad-spectrum bactericidal agent that inhibits the enzymes topoisomerase II (DNA gyrase) and topoisomerase IV required for bacterial DNA replication, transcription repair, and recombination

Uses: Acute infections caused by susceptible bacterial strains causing acute maxillary sinusitis, acute bacterial exacerbation of chronic bronchitis, community-acquired pneumonia, nosocomial pneumonia, complicated and uncomplicated skin and skin structure infections, uncomplicated UTI, and acute pyelonephritis; nosocomial pneumonia; chronic bacterial prostatitis

Dosage and routes:

- *Adult:* PO 500-750 mg q24h for 3-14 days depending on the type of infection
- *Adult:* IV 500 mg by slow infusion over 60 min q24h depending on type of infection

Reduce dose in renal impairment

Chronic bacterial prostatitis:

- *Adult:* PO 500 mg q24h

Available forms include: Tabs 250, 500, 750 mg; vials 500, 750 mg (25 mg/ml); Premix IV bags 250, 500, 750 mg in D_5W (5 mg/ml)

Side effects/adverse reactions:

▼ *ORAL:* Taste alteration, dry mouth (<0.5%)

CNS: Headache, dizziness, insomnia, anorexia, anxiety, tremor

CV: Edema

GI: Abdominal pain, dyspepsia, diarrhea, nausea, flatulence, vomiting

HEMA: Hemolytic anemia

GU: Vaginitis

EENT: Rhinitis, pharyngitis

INTEG: Pruritus, rash, photosensitivity, ***anaphylaxis,*** increased sweating, urticaria, erythema multiforme, Stevens-Johnson syndrome

ENDO: Alteration of blood glucose levels

MS: Tendon rupture

MISC: Chest and back pain

Contraindications: Hypersensitivity to quinolone antiinfectives

Precautions: Children <18 yr; seizure disorders, renal insufficiency, excessive exposure to sunlight, alterations in blood glucose (diabetes), pregnancy category C, lactation, drink fluids liberally; tendon rupture of shoulder, hand, and Achilles tendon, monitor blood glucose

Pharmacokinetics:

PO: Bioavailability 99%, peak plasma levels 1-2 hr; 24%-38% protein bound, limited metabolism, primarily excreted in urine as unchanged drug

IV: After 60 min infusion see peak plasma concentration 6.2 µg/ml; steady state in 48 hr with 500 mg/day

Drug interactions of concern to dentistry:

• Interference with absorption: solutions with multivalent cations (e.g., Mg^{2+})

• Increased seizure risk: NSAIDs

• May increase effects of warfarin (monitor bleeding)

DENTAL CONSIDERATIONS

General:

• Determine why patient is taking the drug.

• If dental drugs prescribed, advise patient of potential for photosensitivity.

Consultations:

• Consult with patient's physician if an acute dental infection occurs and another antiinfective is required.

Teach patient/family:

• To minimize exposure to sunlight and wear sunscreen if sun exposure is planned

• To discontinue treatment and inform dentist immediately if patient experiences pain or inflammation of a tendon, and to rest and refrain from exercise

levofloxacin ophthalmic

(lee-voe-flox'a-sin)

Quixin

Drug class.: Fluoroquinolone anti-infective

Action: A broad-spectrum bactericidal agent that inhibits the enzymes topoisomerase II (DNA gyrase) and topoisomerase IV required for bacterial DNA replication, transcription repair, and recombination

Uses: Bacterial conjunctivitis caused by susceptible trains of *S. aureus, S. epidermidis, S. pneumoniae,* strep groups C/F and G, viridans-group streptococci, limited *Corynebacterium* species, *H. influenzae, S. marcescens, A. levoffii*

Dosage and routes:

• *Adult:* TOP on days 1 and 2 apply 1-2 drops in affected eye(s) q2h while awake (8 ×/day); on days 3-7 apply 1 or 2 drops in affected eye(s) q4h while awake (4 ×/day)

Available forms include: Sol 0.5% in 2.5, 5 ml

Side effects/adverse reactions:

CNS: Headache

EENT: Pharyngitis

INTEG: Decreased vision, foreign body sensation, localized burning and irritation, ocular pain, photophobia

MISC: Fever, allergic reactions

Contraindications: Hypersensitivity to this drug or other fluoroquinolones

Precautions: Avoid prolonged use, do not wear contact lens when infection is present, avoid contamination of applicator tip, pregnancy

L

category C, lactation, safety and efficacy in child <1yr not established

Pharmacokinetics:

TOP: Some systemic absorption

Drug interactions of concern to dentistry:

• None reported

DENTAL CONSIDERATIONS

General:

• Protect patient's eyes from accidental spatter during dental treatment.

• Avoid dental light in patient's eyes; offer dark glasses for patient comfort.

---

levothyroxine sodium (T_4, L-thyroxine sodium)

(lee-voe-thye-rox'een)

Levothroid, Levoxyl, Synthroid, Thyro-Tabs, Unithroid

✦ Eltroxin, PMS-Levothyroxine sodium

Drug class.: Thyroid hormone

Action: Increases metabolic rate, with increase in cardiac output, O_2 consumption, body temperature, blood volume, growth/development at cellular level; suppression of pituitary TSH

Uses: Hypothyroidism, myxedema coma, thyroid hormone replacement, cretinism, chronic thyroiditis, euthyroid goiters, management of thyroid cancer

Dosage and routes:

• *Adult:* PO 0.05 mg qd, increased by 0.025-0.05 mg q2-4wk until desired response; maintenance 0.075-0.125 mg qd

• *Child (dose adjusted by age/wt):* PO range 0.002-0.006 mg qd; do not exceed adult dose

Myxedema coma:

• *Adult:* IV 0.2-0.5 mg; may increase by 0.1-0.3 mg after 24 hr; place on oral medication asap

Available forms include: Inj IV 200, 500 µg/vial; tabs 0.025, 0.05, 0.075, 0.088, 0.1, 0.112, 0.125, 0.137, 0.15, 0.175, 0.2, 0.3 mg

Side effects/adverse reactions:

CNS: Anxiety, insomnia, tremors, ***thyroid storm,*** headache

CV: Tachycardia, palpitation, angina, dysrhythmias, ***cardiac arrest,*** hypertension

GI: Nausea, diarrhea, increased or decreased appetite, cramps

MISC: Menstrual irregularities, weight loss, sweating, heat intolerance, fever

Contraindications: Adrenal insufficiency, MI, thyrotoxicosis

Precautions: Elderly, angina pectoris, hypertension, ischemia, cardiac disease, pregnancy category A, lactation

Pharmacokinetics: *IV/PO:* Peak 12-48 hr, half-life 6-7 days; distributed throughout body tissues

Drug interactions of concern to dentistry:

• Increased effects of sympathomimetics when thyroid doses are not carefully monitored or in patients with coronary artery disease

DENTAL CONSIDERATIONS

General:

• Uncontrolled hypothyroid patients may be more responsive to CNS depressants.

• Increased nervousness, excitability, sweating, or tachycardia may indicate a patient with uncontrolled hyperthyroidism or a dose of medication that is too high. Uncontrolled patients should be referred for medical treatment.

• Monitor vital signs at every appointment because of cardiovascular side effects.

Consultations:

• Medical consultation may be required to assess disease control.

lidocaine HCl (cardiac)

(lye'doe-kane)

Lidopen Auto-Injector, Xylocaine for Cardiac Arrythmias

Drug class.: Antidysrhythmic (class IB)

Action: Increases electrical stimulation threshold of ventricle and His-Purkinje system, which stabilizes cardiac membrane and decreases automaticity and excitability of ventricles

Uses: Ventricular tachycardia, ventricular dysrhythmias during cardiac surgery, MI, digitalis toxicity, cardiac catheterization; for acute management only

Dosage and routes:

• *Adult:* IV bol 50-100 mg over 2-3 min, repeat q3-5 min, not to exceed 200-300 mg in 1 hr, begin IV inf; IV inf 20-50 μg/kg/min; IM 200-300 mg in deltoid muscle (use 10% sol only for IM and when ECG equipment is not available)

• *Elderly, CHF-reduced liver function:* IV bol give one-half adult dose

• *Child:* IV bol 1 mg/kg, then IV INF 30 μg/kg/min

Available forms include: IV inf 0.2%, 0.4%, 0.8%; IV Ad 4%, 10%, 20%; IV Dir 1%, 2%, 4%; IM 300 mg/ml, 10%

Side effects/adverse reactions:

CNS: Headache, dizziness, nervousness, ***convulsions,*** involuntary movement, confusion, tremor, drowsiness, euphoria

CV: Bradycardia, ***hypotension, heart block, cardiovascular collapse, arrest***

GI: Nausea, vomiting, anorexia

RESP: ***Respiratory depression,*** dyspnea

EENT: Blurred vision, tinnitus

INTEG: Rash, urticaria, edema, swelling

MISC: Febrile response, phlebitis at injection site

Contraindications: Hypersensitivity to amides, severe heart block, supraventricular dysrhythmias, Adams-Stokes syndrome, Wolff-Parkinson-White syndrome

Precautions: Pregnancy category B, lactation, children, renal disease, liver disease, CHF, respiratory depression, malignant hyperthermia (questionable), elderly; need to monitor ECG

Pharmacokinetics:

IV: Onset immediate, duration 20 min

IM: Onset 5-15 min, duration 1-1.5 hr; half-life 1-2 hr; moderate-to-high protein binding; metabolized in liver; excreted in urine; crosses placenta

Drug interactions of concern to dentistry:

• Increased effects: cimetidine, β-blockers, other dysrhythmics

• Increased neuromuscular blockade of neuromuscular blockers, succinylcholine

DENTAL CONSIDERATIONS

General:

• Because this is an emergency drug used in ICUs, emergency

L

departments, and hospitals, patients using it would not be having elective dental treatment.
• Use of lidocaine to control dysrhythmias requires immediate medical consultation or removal of patient to emergency care facility.
• Monitor ECG when used; observe for lidocaine toxicity.
• Monitor patient's vital signs and support as required.

lidocaine HCl (local)

(lye'doe-kane)

Octocaine, Xylocaine, Xylocaine-MPF

With vasoconstrictor: Octocaine with Epinephrine, Xylocaine with Epinephrine

Drug class.: Amide local anesthetic

Action: Inhibits ion fluxes across membranes, particularly sodium transport across cell membrane; decreases rise of depolarization phase of action potential; blocks nerve action potential

Uses: Local dental anesthesia; peripheral nerve block; caudal anesthesia; epidural, spinal, surgical anesthesia

Dosage and routes:

Dental injection: infiltration or conduction block:

• *Lidocaine 2% without vasoconstrictor:* Max dose 7.0 mg/kg or 300 mg per dental appointment* for healthy adult patients; doses must be adjusted downward for medically compromised, debilitated, child, or elderly and for each individual patient. **Always use the lowest effective dose, a slow injection rate, and a careful aspiration technique.**

Example calculations illustrating amount of drug administered per dental cartridge(s)

# of cartridges (1.8 ml)	mg of lidocaine (2%)
1	36
2	72
4	144

*Maximum dose is cited from *USP-DI*, ed 23, 2003, US Pharmacopeial Convention, Inc., and from the manufacturer's package insert. Doses may differ in other published resources.

Lidocaine 2% with 1:50,000 epinephrine: Epinephrine 3 μg/kg, with a limit of 0.2 mg/patient.

Manufacturer's package insert indicates that the maximum dose of lidocaine with vasoconstrictors is 500 mg. Adjust doses for each individual patient as previously indicated. In considering the dose of local anesthesia with vasoconstrictor, the dose of epinephrine must also be considered. The recommended dose of epinephrine in a local anesthetic solution is 3 μg/kg, not to exceed a total dose of 0.2 mg per appointment for a healthy adult. For adult patients with clinically significant CV disease, the dose limit of epinephrine is 0.04 mg per appointment. The dose limits of epinephrine will affect the amount of local anesthetic allowable in a given appointment.

Example calculations illustrating amount of drug administered per dental cartridge(s)

# of cartridges (1.8 ml)	mg of lidocaine (2%)	mg (µg) of vasoconstrictor (1:50,000)
1	36	0.036 (36)
2	72	0.072 (72)
3	108	0.108 (108)
4	144	0.144 (144)
5	180	0.180 (180)
5.5	198	0.198 (198)

Lidocaine 2% with 1:100,000 epinephrine: The same doses and adjustments to doses apply as previously indicated.

Example calculations illustrating amount of drug administered per dental cartridge(s)

# of cartridges (1.8 ml)	mg of lidocaine (2%)	mg (µg) of vasoconstrictor (1:100,000)
1	36	0.018 (18)
2	72	0.036 (36)
3	108	0.054 (54)
6	216	0.108 (108)
8	288	0.144 (144)
10	360	0.180 (180)

Children's dose recommendation for lidocaine (*USP-DI,* ed 23, 2003, and *The ADA Guide to Dental Therapeutics,* ed 2, 2000): 4-5 mg/kg up to max 100-150 mg per appointment

Available forms include: Inj 0.5%, 1%, 1.5%, 2%, 4%, 5%; inj with epinephrine 0.5%, 1%, 1.5%, 2%; epinephrine concentrations range from 1:50,000 to 1:200,000; usual dental use is 2% conc with 1:100,000 epinephrine; other % sols are used in medical applications

Side effects/adverse reactions:
▼ *ORAL: Numbness, tingling,* trismus
CNS: ***Convulsions, loss of consciousness,*** drowsiness, disorientation, tremors, shivering, anxiety, restlessness
CV: ***Myocardial depression, cardiac arrest, dysrhythmias,*** bradycardia, hypotension, hypertension, fetal bradycardia
GI: Nausea, vomiting
RESP: ***Status asthmaticus, respiratory arrest, anaphylaxis***
EENT: Blurred vision, tinnitus, pupil constriction
INTEG: Rash, urticaria, allergic reactions, edema, burning, skin discoloration at injection site, tissue necrosis

Contraindications: Hypersensitivity, cross-sensitivity among amides (rare), severe liver disease

Precautions: Elderly, severe drug allergies, pregnancy category B, large doses of local anesthetics in patients with myasthenia gravis

Pharmacokinetics: Onset 2-10 min, duration 20 min-4 hr; metabolized by liver, metabolites may contribute to toxicity in one dose; excreted in urine (metabolites)

L

Drug interactions of concern to dentistry:

• CNS depressants: increased risk of CNS depression with all CNS depressants, especially in children and when larger doses are used

• Avoid placing dental cartridges in disinfectant solutions with heavy metals or surface-active agents; may see release of metal ions into local anesthetic solutions with tissue irritation following injection

• Avoid excessive exposure of dental cartridges to light or heat, which hastens deterioration of vasoconstrictor; observe for color change in local anesthetic solution

• Risk of cardiovascular side effects: rapid intravascular administration of local anesthetic containing vasoconstrictor, either alone or in patients taking tricyclic antidepressants, MAOIs, digitalis drugs, cocaine, phenothiazines, β-blockers, and in presence of halogenated hydrocarbon general anesthetics; use smallest effective vasoconstrictor dose and careful aspiration technique

• Avoid use of vasoconstrictors in patients with uncontrolled hyperthyroidism, diabetes, angina, or hypertension; refer these patients for medical treatment before elective dental procedures

DENTAL CONSIDERATIONS

General:

• Monitor vital signs at every appointment because of cardiovascular and respiratory side effects.

• Drug is often used with vasoconstrictor for increased duration of action.

• Lubricate dry lips before injection or dental treatment as required.

Teach patient/family:

• To use care to prevent injury while numbness exists and to refrain from gum chewing and eating following dental anesthesia

• To report any signs of infection, muscle pain, or fever to dentist when feeling returns

• To report any unusual soft tissue reactions

---

lidocaine HCl (topical)

(lye'doe-kane)

Xylocaine Liquid, Xylocaine Ointment, Xylocaine Spray, Xylocaine Viscous, Xylocaine Solution, Xylocaine Jelly, Anestacon JellY

OTC: Zilactin-L, Ela-Max, Derma-Flex

Drug class.: Topically acting local anesthetic, amide

Action: Inhibits nerve impulses from sensory nerves, which produces anesthesia

Uses: Topical anesthesia of inflamed or irritated mucous membranes; to reduce gag reflex in dental radiologic examination or in dental impressions

Dosage and routes:

• *Adult and older child:* Rinse with 5-15 ml sol q4h, or rinse just before meals to reduce pain of aphthous ulcers; expectorate after rinsing (viscous doseform)

• *Adult and adolescent:* TOP 2 metered sprays (20 mg) to gingival/oral mucosa per quadrant (spray dose form)

• *Adult and adolescent:* TOP apply a small amount to dry mucous membranes (ointment dose form)

Available forms include: Visc sol 2% in 100, 450 ml bottles; spray 10% in 30 ml, jelly 2% in 30 ml;

oint 5% in 2.5% (OTC), 35, 3.75 g; sol 4% in 50 ml; OTC cream 4%; OTC gel 0.5%, 2.5%

Side effects/adverse reactions:
INTEG: Rash, irritation, sensitization

Contraindications: Hypersensitivity, application to large areas

Precautions: Sepsis, pregnancy category B, denuded skin

DENTAL CONSIDERATIONS

General:

• Do not overuse; use just before eating to reduce pain of aphthous ulcers.

• If affected area is infected, do not apply.

Teach patient/family:

• To report rash, irritation, redness, or swelling to dentist

---

lidocaine transoral delivery system

(lye'doe-kane)

DentiPatch

Drug class.: Amide local anesthetic

Action: Inhibits nerve impulses from sensory nerves, which produces anesthesia

Uses: Mild topical anesthesia of mucous membranes of the mouth before superficial dental procedures

Dosage and routes:

• *Adult:* TOP apply one patch to area of application after drying with gauze; leave in place until local anesthesia is produced, but *no longer than 15 min*

Available forms include: Patches 0.5 cm^2, 2 cm^2 (containing 46.1 mg); carton of 50, 100 patches

Side effects/adverse reactions:
▼ *ORAL: Taste alteration, stomatitis, erythema, mucosa irritation*
CNS: Headache, excitatory or depressor actions, dizziness, nervousness, confusion, tinnitus, twitching, tremors (associated with excessive systemic absorption)
CV: Bradycardia, hypotension, ***cardiovascular collapse*** (with excessive systemic absorption)
GI: Nausea
MISC: Allergic reactions to this agent or to other ingredients in the formulation (rare)

Contraindications: Hypersensitivity to amide-type local anesthetics

Precautions: Local anesthetic toxicity, no pediatric (child <12 yr) or geriatric studies have been made, liver dysfunction, onset longer for maxilla, pregnancy category B, lactation, contains phenylalanine (caution phenylketonurics)

Pharmacokinetics:
TOP: Onset 2.5 min, duration of approximately 30 min after removal; blood levels <0.1 ng/ml limited absorption; hepatic metabolism, urinary excretion

Drug interactions of concern to dentistry:

• None reported with dental drugs

DENTAL CONSIDERATIONS

General:

• Use no more than one patch per area, remove after 15 min to avoid toxicity.

Teach patient/family:

• To prevent injury while numbness is present and to refrain from gum chewing and eating after dental treatment

• To report unresolved oral lesions to dentist

lincomycin HCl

(lin-koe-mye'sin)

Lincocin, Lincorex

Drug class.: Antibacterial

Action: Binds to 50S subunit of bacterial ribosomes; suppresses protein synthesis

Uses: Infections caused by group A β-hemolytic streptococci, pneumococci, staphylococci (respiratory tract, skin, soft tissue, urinary tract infections; osteomyelitis; septicemia), and anaerobes

Dosage and routes:

• *Adult:* PO 500 mg q6-8h, taken 1-2 hr before or after eating, not to exceed 8 g/day; IM 600 mg/day or q12h; IV 600 mg-1 g q8-12h, dilute in 100 ml IV sol, infuse over 1 hr, not to exceed 8 g/day

• *Child >1 mo:* PO 30-60 mg/kg/day in divided doses q6-8h; IM 10 mg/kg/day q12h; IV 10-20 mg/kg/day in divided doses q8-12h, dilute to 100 ml IV sol, infuse over 1 hr

Available forms include: Caps 500 mg; inj IM/IV 300 mg/ml in 2 ml, 10 ml vials

Side effects/adverse reactions:

▼ *ORAL:* Candidiasis

GI: Nausea, vomiting, abdominal pain, diarrhea, ***pseudomembranous colitis***

HEMA: ***Leukopenia, eosinophilia, agranulocytosis, thrombocytopenia***

GU: Vaginitis, increased AST/ALT, bilirubin, alk phosphatase, jaundice, urinary frequency

INTEG: Rash, urticaria, pruritus, erythema, pain, abscess at injection site

Contraindications: Hypersensitivity, ulcerative colitis/enteritis, infants <1 mo

Precautions: Renal disease, liver disease, GI disease, elderly, pregnancy category not listed, lactation

Pharmacokinetics:

PO: Peak 2-4 hr, duration 6 hr

IM: Peak 30 min, duration 8-12 hr

Half-life 4-6 hr; metabolized in liver; excreted in urine, bile, feces as active/inactive metabolites; crosses placenta; excreted in breast milk

Drug interactions of concern to dentistry:

• Decreased action of erythromycin

• Oral contraceptives: advise patient of a potential risk for decreased contraceptive action, to maintain compliance with oral contraceptive use while using antibiotics, and to consider the use of additional nonhormonal contraception

DENTAL CONSIDERATIONS

General:

• Determine why the patient is taking the drug.

Consultations:

• Medical consultation may be required to assess disease control.

Teach patient/family:

• Importance of good oral hygiene to prevent soft tissue inflammation

• Caution to prevent injury when using oral hygiene aids

• To notify dentist if diarrhea occurs

When used for dental infection, advise patient:

• To report sore throat, oral burning sensation, fever, fatigue, any of which could indicate superinfection

• To take at prescribed intervals and complete dosage regimen

• To immediately notify the dentist if signs or symptoms of infection increase

linezolid

(li-ne'zoh-lid)

Zyvox

Drug class.: Antibiotic, oxazolidinone derivative

Action: Binds to the 50S subunit of bacterial ribosomal RNA, preventing the functions of the initiation complex essential to bacterial translation; has both bacteriostatic and bactericidal activity depending on the bacterial species; nonantibiotic action includes inhibition of monoamine oxidase enzymes

Uses: For vancomycin-resistant *E. faeceum* infections; nosocomial pneumonia caused by *S. aureus* (methicillin resistant and susceptible) and *S. pneumoniae* (penicillin susceptible); complicated skin and skin structure infections caused by *S. aureus* (methicillin resistant and susceptible), *S. pyogenes,* or *S. agalactiae;* uncomplicated skin and skin structure infections caused by *S. aureus* (methicillin susceptible); community-acquired pneumonia caused by *S. pneumoniae* (penicillin susceptible) or *S. aureus* (methicillin susceptible); and diabetic foot infections without osteomyelitis caused by gram-positive bacteria

Dosage and routes:

• *Adult and child >11 yr:* PO/IV depending on type of infection 600 mg q12h for 10-28 days; for uncomplicated infection 400 mg orally q12h for 10-14 days

•*Birth-11 yr:* PO/IV 10 mg/kg up to 10-14 days

Available forms include: Tabs 400, 600 mg; oral susp 100 mg/5 ml in 150 ml vol; IV plastic infusion bags 200 (100 ml), 400 (200 ml), 600 mg (300 ml)

Side effects/adverse reactions:

▼ *ORAL:* Candidiasis, tongue discoloration

CNS: Headache, dizziness

CV: Hypotension

GI: Diarrhea, nausea, ***antibiotic-associated pseudomembranous colitis,*** dyspepsia, GI pain

HEMA: ***Thrombocytopenia, pancytopenia,*** anemia, leukopenia

GU: Vaginal candidiasis

INTEG: Rash, pruritus

META: Altered liver function tests, decrease in lab HgB levels

Contraindications: Hypersensitivity

Precautions: May promote overgrowth of nonsusceptible bacterial strains, monitor platelet counts in patients at risk for bleeding, pregnancy category C, lactation, pediatric doses not established, use >28 days, selectively inhibits monoamine oxidase enzymes, potentiation of serotonergic drugs, hepatic disease, hemodialysis patients; risk of myelosuppression, monitor CBC counts, avoid tyramine-containing foods

Pharmacokinetics:

PO: Rapid absorption, peak plasma levels 1-2 hr, absolute bioavailability ~100%, well distributed, plasma protein binding 31%, hepatic metabolism, renal excretion

Drug interactions of concern to dentistry:

• Potential to increase pressor effects of indirect-action sympathomimetic drugs and vasopressors,

such as dopaminergic drugs, phenylephrine, phenylpropanolamine, and pseudoephedrine
• Interactions with vasoconstrictors in local anesthetics has not been studied

DENTAL CONSIDERATIONS

General:

• Determine why patient is taking the drug.
• Use vasoconstrictor with caution, in low doses, and with careful aspiration. Avoid using gingival retraction cord containing epinephrine.
• Patients on chronic drug therapy may rarely have symptoms of blood dyscrasias, which can include infection, bleeding, and poor healing.
• Examine for oral manifestation of opportunistic infection.
• Consider semisupine chair position for patient comfort if GI side effects occur.

Consultations:

• In a patient with symptoms of blood dyscrasias, request a medical consultation for blood studies and postpone treatment until normal values are reestablished.
• Medical consultation may be required to assess disease control and patient's ability to tolerate stress.
• Physician consultation is advised in the presence of an acute dental infection requiring another antibiotic.

Teach patient/family:

• That secondary oral infection may occur; need to see dentist immediately if infection occurs
• To report sore throat, oral burning sensation, fever, fatigue, any of which could indicate presence of a superinfection

liothyronine sodium (T_3)

(lye-oh-thye'roe-neen)

Cytomel, Triostat

Drug class.: Thyroid hormone

Action: Increases metabolic rate with increase in cardiac output, O_2 consumption, body temperature, blood volume, growth/development at cellular level; pituitary TSH suppression

Uses: Hypothyroidism, myxedema coma, thyroid hormone replacement, cretinism, nontoxic goiter, T_3 suppression test; thyroiditis, euthyroid goiter

Dosage and routes:

• *Adult:* PO 25 μg qd, increased by 12.5-25 μg q1-2wk until desired response; maintenance 25-75 μg qd

Available forms include: Tabs 5, 25, 50 μg; inj 10 μg/ml in 1 ml vial

Side effects/adverse reactions:

CNS: Insomnia, tremors, ***thyroid storm (overdose),*** headache

CV: ***Tachycardia, palpitation, angina, dysrhythmias, cardiac arrest,*** hypertension

GI: Nausea, diarrhea, increased or decreased appetite, cramps

MISC: Menstrual irregularities, weight loss, sweating, heat intolerance, fever

Contraindications: Adrenal insufficiency, MI, thyrotoxicosis

Precautions: Elderly, angina pectoris, hypertension, ischemia, cardiac disease, pregnancy category A, lactation

Pharmacokinetics:

PO: Peak 12-48 hr, half-life 0.6-1.4 days

Drug interactions of concern to dentistry:

- Hypertension, tachycardia: ketamine
- Increased effects of sympathomimetics when thyroid doses are not carefully monitored or in patients with coronary artery disease

DENTAL CONSIDERATIONS

General:

- Patients with uncontrolled hypothyroidism may be more responsive to CNS depressants.
- Increased nervousness, excitability, sweating, or tachycardia may indicate a patient with uncontrolled hyperthyroidism or a dose of medication that is too high. Uncontrolled patients should be referred for medical treatment.

Consultations:

- Medical consultation may be required to assess disease control.

---

liotrix

(lye'oh-trix)

Thyrolar

Drug class.: Thyroid hormone

Action: Increases metabolic rate, cardiac output, O_2 consumption, body temperature, blood volume, growth/development at cellular level, pituitary TSH suppressant

Uses: Hypothyroidism, thyroid hormone replacement, thyroiditis, euthyroid goiter

Dosage and routes:

- *Adult and child:* PO 15-30 mg qd, increased by 15-30 mg q1-2wk until desired response, may increase by 15-30 mg q2wk in child
- *Geriatric:* PO 15-30 mg, double dose q6-8wk until desired response

Available forms include: Tabs 15, 30, 60, 120, 180 mg as thyroid equivalent

Side effects/adverse reactions:

CNS: Insomnia, tremors, headache, ***thyroid storm***

CV: Tachycardia, palpitation, angina, dysrhythmias, hypertension, cardiac arrest

GI: Nausea, diarrhea, increased or decreased appetite, cramps

MISC: Menstrual irregularities, weight loss, sweating, heat intolerance, fever

Contraindications: Adrenal insufficiency, MI, thyrotoxicosis

Precautions: Elderly, angina pectoris, hypertension, ischemia, cardiac disease, pregnancy category A, lactation

Pharmacokinetics:

PO: Peak 12-48 hr, half-life 6-7 days

Drug interactions of concern to dentistry:

- Hypertension, tachycardia: ketamine
- Increased effects of sympathomimetics when thyroid doses are not carefully monitored or in patients with coronary artery disease

DENTAL CONSIDERATIONS

General:

- Patients with uncontrolled hypothyroidism may be more responsive to CNS depressants.
- Increased nervousness, excitability, sweating, or tachycardia may indicate a patient with uncontrolled hyperthyroidism or a dose of medication that is too high. Uncontrolled patients should be referred for medical treatment.

Consultations:

- Medical consultation may be required to assess disease control.

Teach patient/family:
• Importance of good oral hygiene to prevent soft tissue inflammation
• To avoid mouth rinses with high alcohol content because of drying effects

lisinopril

(lyse-in'oh-pril)

Prinivil, Zestril

Drug class.: Angiotensin-converting enzyme (ACE) inhibitor

Action: Selectively suppresses renin-angiotensin-aldosterone system; inhibits ACE, which prevents conversion of angiotensin I to angiotensin II

Uses: Mild-to-moderate hypertension, post-MI if hemodynamically stable, heart failure

Dosage and routes:
• *Adult:* PO 10-40 mg qd; may increase to 80 mg qd if required; PO post-MI initial dose 5 mg, then 5 mg after 24 hr, 10 mg after 48 hr, and 10 mg/day for 6 wk

Heart failure: PO 5 mg/day with a diuretic, dose range 5-20 mg

Available forms include: Tabs 2.5, 5, 10, 20, 40 mg

Side effects/adverse reactions:

▼ *ORAL:* Dry mouth, angioedema

CNS: Vertigo, depression, stroke, insomnia, paresthesia, headache, fatigue, asthenia

CV: Hypotension, chest pain, palpitation, angina, dysrhythmia, syncope

GI: Nausea, vomiting, anorexia, constipation, flatulence, GI irritation

RESP: Cough, dyspnea

HEMA: ***Eosinophilia, leukopenia,*** decreased Hct/Hgb

GU: ***Proteinuria, renal insufficiency,*** sexual dysfunction, impotence

EENT: Blurred vision, nasal congestion

INTEG: Rash, pruritus

Contraindications: Hypersensitivity, pregnancy (second and third trimesters)

Precautions: Pregnancy category C (first trimester), pregnancy category D (second and third trimesters), lactation, renal disease, hyperkalemia

Pharmacokinetics: Peak 6-8 hr; excreted unchanged in urine

Drug interactions of concern to dentistry:
• Increased hypotension: alcohol, phenothiazines
• Decreased hypotensive effects: indomethacin and possibly other NSAIDs, sympathomimetics
• Suspected reduction in the antihypertensive and vasodilator effects by salicylates; monitor blood pressure if used concurrently

DENTAL CONSIDERATIONS

General:
• Monitor vital signs at every appointment because of cardiovascular and respiratory side effects.
• After supine positioning, have patient sit upright for at least 2 min before standing to avoid orthostatic hypotension.
• Patients on chronic drug therapy may rarely have symptoms of blood dyscrasias, which can include infection, bleeding, and poor healing.
• Assess salivary flow as a factor in caries, periodontal disease, and candidiasis.
• Limit use of sodium-containing

products, such as saline IV fluids, for patients with a dietary salt restriction.

• Use vasoconstrictors with caution, in low doses, and with careful aspiration.

• Short appointments and a stress reduction protocol may be required for anxious patients.

Consultations:

• Medical consultation may be required to assess disease control and patient's ability to tolerate stress.

• In a patient with symptoms of blood dyscrasias, request a medical consultation for blood studies and postpone dental treatment until normal values are reestablished.

• Take precautions if dental surgery is anticipated and sedation or general anesthesia is required; there is a risk of a hypotensive episode.

Teach patient/family:

• Importance of good oral hygiene to prevent soft tissue inflammation

• Caution to prevent injury when using oral hygiene aids

When chronic dry mouth occurs, advise patient:

• To avoid mouth rinses with high alcohol content because of drying effects

• To use sugarless gum, frequent sips of water, or saliva substitutes

• To use daily home fluoride products for anticaries effect

lithium carbonate/ lithium citrate

(lith'ee-um)

Lithium carbonate: ***Eskalith, Eskalith CR, Lithonate, Lithobid***

✤ Carbolith, Duralith, Lithizine, PMS-Lithium Carbonate

Drug class.: Antimanic, inorganic salt

Action: May alter sodium and potassium ion transport across cell membrane in nerve, muscle cells; may affect norepinephrine and serotonin in the CNS, as well as other monoamine neurotransmitters

Uses: Manic-depressive illness (manic phase), prevention of bipolar manic depressive psychosis; unapproved: depression, vascular headache, improved neutrophil count in cancer chemotherapy and in AIDS patients taking zidovudine

Dosage and routes:

• *Adult:* PO 300-600 mg tid, maintenance 300 mg tid or qid; slow rel tabs 300 mg bid, dose should be individualized to maintain blood levels at 0.5-1.5 mEq/L; slow rel 900 mg bid

Available forms include: Caps 150, 300, 600 mg; tabs 300 mg; slow rel tabs 300; con rel tabs 450 mg; syr 8 mEq/5 ml

Side effects/adverse reactions:

▼ *ORAL: Increased thirst, dry mouth*

CNS: Headache, drowsiness, dizziness, tremors, twitching, ataxia, seizures, slurred speech, restlessness, confusion, stupor, memory loss, clonic movements

CV: Hypotension, ***circulatory col-***

lapse, edema, ECG changes, dysrhythmias
GI: Anorexia, nausea, vomiting, diarrhea, incontinence, abdominal pain
HEMA: ***Leukocytosis***
GU: ***Polyuria, glycosuria, proteinuria, albuminuria,*** urinary incontinence, polydipsia, edema
EENT: Tinnitus, blurred vision
INTEG: Drying of hair, alopecia, rash, pruritus, hyperkeratosis, follicular mycosis fungoides
ENDO: Hyponatremia
MS: Muscle weakness
Contraindications: Hepatic disease, renal disease, brain trauma, OBS, pregnancy category D, lactation, children <12 yr, schizophrenia, severe cardiac disease, severe renal disease, severe dehydration
Precautions: Elderly, thyroid disease, seizure disorders, diabetes mellitus, systemic infection, urinary retention
Pharmacokinetics:
PO: Onset rapid, peak 0.5-4 hr, half-life 18-36 hr, depending on age; well absorbed by oral method; 80% of filtered lithium is reabsorbed by the renal tubules; excreted in urine; crosses placenta, blood-brain barrier; excreted in breast milk

Drug interactions of concern to dentistry:
- Increased toxicity: aspirin, indomethacin, other NSAIDs, haloperidol, metronidazole, carbamazepine
- Increased effects of neuromuscular blocking agents

DENTAL CONSIDERATIONS
General:
- Assess salivary flow as a factor in caries, periodontal disease, and candidiasis.
- After supine positioning, have patient sit upright for at least 2 min before standing to avoid orthostatic hypotension.

Consultations:
- Medical consultation may be required to assess disease control.

Teach patient/family:
- Importance of good oral hygiene to prevent soft tissue inflammation
- Caution to prevent injury when using oral hygiene aids

When chronic dry mouth occurs, advise patient:
- To avoid mouth rinses with high alcohol content because of drying effects
- To use sugarless gum, frequent sips of water, or saliva substitutes
- To use daily home fluoride products for anticaries effect

Iodoxamide tromethamine

(loe-dox'a-mide)
Alomide Ophthalmic
Drug class.: Mast cell stabilizer

Action: Prevents release of mediators of inflammation from mast cells involved with type 1 immediate hypersensitivity reactions
Uses: Vernal keratoconjunctivitis, vernal conjunctivitis, keratitis
Dosage and routes:
Opthalmic:
- *Adult and child >2 yr:* 1-2 gtt in each affected eye qid up to 3 mo

Available forms include: Sol 0.1% in 10 ml
Side effects/adverse reactions:
CNS: Headache, dizziness, somnolence
GI: Nausea
RESP: Sneezing
EENT: Burning/stinging eyes, itch-

ing, blurred vision, lacrimation, dry nose
INTEG: Rash
Contraindications: Hypersensitivity
Precautions: Pregnancy category B, child <2 yr, lactation, avoid contact lens use
Pharmacokinetics: Elimination half-life 8.5 hr, excreted in urine
Drug interactions of concern to dentistry:
• None reported
DENTAL CONSIDERATIONS
General:
• Question patient about history of allergy to avoid using other potential allergens.
• Avoid dental light in patient's eyes; offer dark glasses for patient comfort.

lomefloxacin HCl

(loe-me-flox'a-sin)
Maxaquin
Drug class.: Fluoroquinolone anti-infective

Action: A broad-spectrum bactericidal agent that inhibits the enzymes topoisomerase II (DNA gyrase) and topoisomerase IV required for bacterial DNA replication, transcription repair, and recombination
Uses: Treatment of lower respiratory tract infections (pneumonia, bronchitis); genitourinary infections (prostatitis, UTIs); preoperatively to reduce UTIs in transurethral and transrectal surgical procedures caused by susceptible gram-negative organisms
Dosage and routes:
• *Adult:* PO 400 mg/day × 7-14 days depending on type of infection
Renal impairment:
• *Adult:* PO 200 mg/dose
Prophylaxis of UTI:
• *Adult:* PO 400 mg 2-6 hr before surgery
Available forms include: Tabs 400
Side effects/adverse reactions:
ORAL: Dry mouth, candidiasis, stomatitis, glossitis
CNS: Dizziness, headache, somnolence, depression, insomnia, nervousness, confusion, agitation
GI: Diarrhea, nausea, vomiting, anorexia, flatulence, heartburn, increased AST/ALT, constipation, abdominal pain, pseudomembranous colitis
EENT: Visual disturbances, phototoxicity
INTEG: Rash, pruritus, urticaria
MS: Tendinitis, tendon rupture
Contraindications: Hypersensitivity to quinolones
Precautions: Pregnancy category C, lactation, children, elderly, renal disease, seizure disorders, excessive sunlight; tendon rupture in shoulder, hand, and Achilles tendons
Pharmacokinetics:
PO: Peak 1-2 hr, half-life 6-8 hr; excreted in urine as active drug, metabolites
Drug interactions of concern to dentistry:
• Decreased effects: antacids
• Increased levels of cyclosporine, caffeine
DENTAL CONSIDERATIONS
General:
• Because of drug interactions, do not use ingestible sodium bicarbonate products such as the air polishing system Prophy
• Jet unless 2 hr have passed since lomefloxacin was taken.

L

• Use caution in prescribing caffeine-containing analgesics.
• Determine why the patient is taking the drug.
• Avoid dental light in patient's eyes; offer dark glasses for patient comfort.
• Ruptures of the shoulder, hand, and Achilles tendons that required surgical repair or resulted in prolonged disability have been reported with this drug.

Consultations:
• Consult with patient's physician if an acute dental infection occurs and another antiinfective is required.

Teach patient/family:
• Caution to prevent injury when using oral hygiene aids
• To avoid mouth rinses with high alcohol content because of drying effects
• To minimize exposure to sunlight and wear sunscreen if sun exposure is planned
• To discontinue treatment and inform dentist immediately if patient experiences pain or inflammation of a tendon, and to rest and refrain from exercise

lomustine (CCNU)

(loe-mus'teen)
CeeNu

Drug class.: Antineoplastic alkylating agent

Action: Interferes with RNA and DNA strands, which leads to cell death

Uses: Hodgkin's disease; lymphomas; melanomas; multiple myeloma; brain, lung, bladder, kidney, colon cancer

Dosage and routes:
• *Adult:* PO 130 mg/m^2 as a single dose q6wk; titrate dose to WBC level; do not give repeat dose unless WBC count is >4000/mm^3, platelet count >100,000/mm^3

Available forms include: Caps 10, 40, 100 mg; dosepak

Side effects/adverse reactions:
ORAL: Stomatitis
GI: Nausea, vomiting, anorexia, ***hepatotoxicity***
RESP: ***Fibrosis, pulmonary infiltrate***
HEMA: ***Thrombocytopenia, leukopenia, myelosuppression, anemia***
GU: ***Azotemia, renal failure***
INTEG: Burning at injection site

Contraindications: Hypersensitivity, leukopenia, thrombocytopenia

Precautions: Radiation therapy, geriatric patient, pregnancy category D, lactation

Pharmacokinetics:
PO: Well absorbed, half-life 16-48 hr; 50% protein bound; metabolized in liver; excreted in urine; crosses blood-brain barrier; excreted in breast milk

Drug interactions of concern to dentistry:
• This drug depresses bone marrow function, which may increase risk of bleeding; avoid drugs that can increase bleeding, such as aspirin, NSAIDs

DENTAL CONSIDERATIONS
General:
• Patients on chronic drug therapy may rarely have symptoms of blood dyscrasias, which can in-

clude infection, bleeding, and poor healing.

• Consider semisupine chair position for patient comfort if GI side effects occur.

• Palliative medication may be required for oral side effects.

• Consider local hemostasis measures to prevent excessive bleeding.

• Prophylactic antibiotics may be indicated to prevent infection if surgery or deep scaling is planned.

• Patients taking opioids for acute or chronic pain should be given alternative analgesics for dental pain.

• Avoid prescribing aspirin-containing products.

Consultations:

• In a patient with symptoms of blood dyscrasias, request a medical consultation for blood studies and postpone dental treatment until normal values are reestablished.

• Patients on cancer chemotherapy should have an adequate WBC count before completing dental procedures that may produce a wound. Consult to determine blood count before appointment.

Teach patient/family:

• Importance of good oral hygiene to prevent soft tissue inflammation

• Caution to prevent trauma when using oral hygiene aids

• That secondary oral infection may occur; must see dentist immediately if infection occurs

• To report oral lesions, soreness, or bleeding to dentist

• To avoid mouth rinses with high alcohol content because of drying and irritating effects

• Importance of updating medical/drug records if physician makes any changes in evaluation or drug regimens

loperamide HCl

(loe-per'a-mide)

Diar-Aid, Imodium, Imodium A-D, Kaopectate II, Maalox Antidiarrheal, Neo-Diaral, Pepto Diarrhea Control

♣ APO-Loperamide, Nu-Loperamide, PMS-Loperamide Hydrochloride, Rho-Loperamide, Diarr-Eze

Drug class.: Antidiarrheal (opioid)

Action: Direct action on intestinal muscles to decrease GI peristalsis

Uses: Diarrhea (cause undetermined), chronic diarrhea, ileostomy discharge

Dosage and routes:

• *Adult:* PO 4 mg, then 2 mg after each loose stool, not to exceed 16 mg/day

• *Child 9-11 yr:* PO 2 mg after first loose stool, then 1 mg after each loose stool but limit to 6 mg/day and for not more than 2 days

• *Child 6-8 yr:* PO 1 mg after first loose stool, then 1 mg after each loose stool but limit to 4 mg/day and for not more than 2 days

Available forms include: Tabs 2 mg; caps 2 mg; liq 1 mg/5 ml, 1 mg/ml

Side effects/adverse reactions:

▼ *ORAL: Dry mouth*

CNS: Dizziness, drowsiness, fatigue, fever

GI: Nausea, vomiting, constipation, ***toxic megacolon,*** abdominal pain, anorexia

RESP: ***Respiratory depression***

INTEG: Rash

Contraindications: Hypersensitivity, severe ulcerative colitis, pseudomembranous colitis

Precautions: Pregnancy category B, lactation, children <2 yr, liver disease, dehydration, bacterial disease

Pharmacokinetics:

PO: Onset 0.5-1 hr, duration 4-5 hr; metabolized in liver; excreted in feces as unchanged drug; small amount in urine

Drug interactions of concern to dentistry:

- Increased action: opioid analgesics

DENTAL CONSIDERATIONS

General:

- Assess salivary flow as a factor in caries, periodontal disease, and candidiasis.
- Evaluate respiration characteristics and rate.
- Consider semisupine chair position for patient comfort because of GI effects of drug.
- This drug product is normally used only for a few doses for acute problems; however, some patients may have to take it for longer time periods as dictated by contributing disease.

Teach patient/family:

When chronic dry mouth occurs, advise patient:

- To avoid mouth rinses with high alcohol content because of drying effects
- To use sugarless gum, frequent sips of water, or saliva substitutes
- To use daily home fluoride products for anticaries effect

loracarbef

(loe-ra-kar'bef)

Lorabid

Drug class.: Antibiotic, second-generation cephalosporin

Action: Inhibits bacterial cell wall synthesis, which renders cell wall osmotically unstable

Uses: Gram-negative organisms: *H. influenzae, E. coli, P. mirabilis, Klebsiella;* gram-positive organisms: *S. pneumoniae, S. pyogenes, S. aureus;* upper/lower respiratory tract infection, acute maxillary sinusitis, pharyngitis, tonsillitis; urinary tract and skin infections; otitis media; some in vitro activity against anaerobes

Dosage and routes:

UTI:

- *Adult:* PO 200-400 mg q12h × 7-14 days depending on the infection; take 1 hr before or 2 hr after meals

Acute otitis media:

- *Child:* PO 15-30 mg/kg qd × 7 days; take 1 hr before or 2 hr after meals

Available forms include: Caps 200, 400 mg; susp 100, 200 mg/5 ml

Side effects/adverse reactions:

▼ *ORAL:* Candidiasis, glossitis

CNS: Dizziness, headache, fatigue, paresthesia, fever, chills, confusion

GI: Diarrhea, nausea, vomiting, anorexia, dysgeusia, bleeding, increased AST/ALT, bilirubin, LDH, alk phosphatase, abdominal pain, loose stools, flatulence, heartburn, stomach cramps, colitis, jaundice

RESP: Dyspnea

HEMA: ***Leukopenia, thrombocytopenia, agranulocytosis, neutrope-***

nia, lymphocytosis, eosinophilia, pancytopenia, hemolytic anemia, leukocytosis, granulocytopenia, anemia

GU: ***Nephrotoxicity, renal failure,*** pyuria, dysuria, reversible interstitial nephritis, vaginitis, pruritus, candidiasis, increased BUN

INTEG: Anaphylaxis, rash, urticaria, dermatitis

Contraindications: Hypersensitivity to cephalosporins or related antibiotics

Precautions: Pregnancy category B, lactation, children, renal disease

Pharmacokinetics:

PO: Peak 1 hr, half-life 1 hr; excreted in urine as unchanged drug

Drug interactions of concern to dentistry:

- Decreased effects: tetracyclines, erythromycins, lincomycins
- *When used for dental infection:*
- May reduce effect of oral contraceptives

DENTAL CONSIDERATIONS

General:

- Take precautions regarding allergy to medication.
- Determine why the patient is taking the drug.
- Examine for evidence of oral manifestations of blood dyscrasias (infection, bleeding, poor healing).

Consultations:

- Medical consultation may be required to assess disease control.
- Medical consultation for blood studies (CBC); leukopenic or thrombocytopenic side effects may result in infection, delayed healing, and excessive bleeding. Postpone elective dental treatment until normal values are maintained.

Teach patient/family:

- Importance of good oral hygiene to prevent soft tissue inflammation

loratadine

(lor-at'a-deen)

OTC: Claritin, Claritin RediTabs, Claritin Syrup, Claritin Non-Drowsy Allergy, Tavist ND, Alavert, Claritin Hives Relief

Drug class.: Antihistamine, H_1 histamine antagonist

Action: Acts on blood vessels, GI system, respiratory system by competing with histamine for H_1-receptor site; decreases allergic response by blocking histamine

Uses: Seasonal allergic rhinitis, idiopathic chronic urticaria

Dosage and routes:

- *Adult and child >6 yr:* PO 10 mg qd
- *Child 2-5 yr:* PO syr 5 mg qd

NOTE: Reduce dose to every other day in renal impairment.

Available forms include: Tabs 10 mg; rapid disintegration tabs 10 mg; syr 1 mg/1 ml

Side effects/adverse reactions:

▼ *ORAL:* Dry mouth

CNS: Dizziness, drowsiness, poor coordination, fatigue, anxiety, euphoria, confusion, paresthesia, neuritis, low incidence of sedation

GI: Nausea, anorexia, diarrhea

RESP: Increased thick secretions, wheezing, chest tightness

GU: Retention, dysuria

EENT: Blurred vision, dilated pupils, tinnitus, nasal stuffiness, dry nose/throat

Contraindications: Hypersensitivity, ketoconazole

Precautions: Pregnancy category B, increased intraocular pressure,

L

bronchial asthma, patients at risk for syncope or drowsiness, reduce dose in renal impairment to every other day

Pharmacokinetics:

PO: Peak 1.5 hr; metabolized in liver to active metabolites; excreted in urine

Drug interactions of concern to dentistry:

- Increased CNS depression: all CNS depressants, alcohol
- Increased anticholinergic effect: anticholinergics, antihistamines, antiparkinsonian drugs
- Increased plasma concentration: ketoconazole

DENTAL CONSIDERATIONS

General:

- Assess salivary flow as a factor in caries, periodontal disease, and candidiasis.
- Consider semisupine chair position for patients with respiratory disease.
- Conscious sedation drugs may produce synergistic, sedative action.

Teach patient/family:

- Importance of good oral hygiene to prevent soft tissue inflammation

When chronic dry mouth occurs, advise patient:

- To avoid mouth rinses with high alcohol content because of drying effects
- To use sugarless gum, frequent sips of water, or saliva substitutes
- To use daily home fluoride products for anticaries effect

lorazepam

(lor-a'ze-pam)

Ativan, Lorazepam Intensol

♣ Apo-Lorazepam, Novo-Lorazem, Nu-Loraz

Drug class.: Benzodiazepine, antianxiety

Controlled Substance Schedule IV

Action: Depresses subcortical levels of CNS, including limbic system and reticular formation

Uses: Anxiety, preoperatively in sedation, acute alcohol withdrawal symptoms, muscle spasm; unapproved: insomnia; acute alcohol withdrawal, psychogenic catatonia

Dosage and routes:

Anxiety:

- *Adult:* PO 2-6 mg/day in divided doses, not to exceed 10 mg/day; reduce dose to 1-2 mg/day for elderly or debilitated

Insomnia:

- *Adult:* PO 2-4 mg hs; only minimally effective after 2 wk continuous therapy

Preoperatively:

- *Adult:* IM/IV 2-4 mg; PO 2-4 mg (max dose 4 mg); IV initial dose not to exceed 2 mg

Available forms include: Tabs 0.5, 1, 2 mg; IM/IV inj 2, 4 mg/ml, conc oral sol 2 mg/ml; Canada only: sublingual tabs 0.5, 1, 2 mg

Side effects/adverse reactions:

▼ *ORAL:* Dry mouth

CNS: Dizziness, drowsiness, confusion, headache, anxiety, tremors, stimulation, fatigue, depression, insomnia, hallucinations, weakness, unsteadiness, anterograde amnesia

CV: Orthostatic hypotension, ***ECG changes, tachycardia,*** hypotension

GI: Constipation, nausea, vomiting, anorexia, diarrhea
EENT: Blurred vision, tinnitus, mydriasis
INTEG: Rash, dermatitis, itching
Contraindications: Hypersensitivity to benzodiazepines, narrow-angle glaucoma, psychosis, pregnancy category D, child <12 yr, history of drug abuse, COPD
Precautions: Elderly, debilitated, hepatic disease, renal disease, myasthenia gravis
Pharmacokinetics:
PO: Peak 1-3 hr, duration 3-6 hr, half-life 14 hr; metabolized by liver; excreted by kidneys; crosses placenta, excreted in breast milk
Drug interactions of concern to dentistry:
- Increased effects: alcohol, all CNS depressants, probenecid
- Increased sedation, hallucination: scopolamine
- Possible increase in CNS side effects of kava (herb)

DENTAL CONSIDERATIONS
General:
- After supine positioning, have patient sit upright for at least 2 min before standing to avoid orthostatic hypotension.
- Elderly persons are more prone to orthostatic hypotension and have increased sensitivity to anticholinergic and sedative effects; use lower dose.
- When administered with opioid analgesic, reduce dose of opioid by one third.
- Psychologic and physical dependence may occur with chronic administration.
- Have someone drive patient to and from dental office when used for conscious sedation.

Consultations:
- Medical consultation may be required to assess disease control.

Teach patient/family:
- Importance of good oral hygiene to prevent soft tissue inflammation
- To avoid mouth rinses with high alcohol content because of drying effects

---

losartan potassium
(loe-sar'tan)
Cozaar
Drug class.: Angiotensin II receptor antagonist

Action: Blocks the vasoconstrictor and aldosterone-releasing effects of angiotensin II
Uses: Hypertension, as a single drug or in combination with other antihypertensives; for reduction of stroke risk in patients with hypertension and left ventricular hypertrophy; neuropathy in type 2 diabetes mellitus
Dosage and routes:
- *Adult:* PO initial 50 mg/day; can be given once or twice daily in total daily doses ranging from 25-100 mg

Available forms include: Tabs 25, 50, 100 mg
Side effects/adverse reactions:
▼ *ORAL:* Dry mouth (<1%), taste alteration (rare)
CNS: Dizziness, insomnia
CV: Low incidence, including palpitation, hypotension; dysrhythmias
GI: Diarrhea, dyspepsia, nausea
RESP: Cough, infection, dyspnea
GU: Urinary frequency
EENT: Nasal congestion, sinusitis, blurred vision, tinnitus
INTEG: Dry skin, rash, urticaria

MS: Pain, cramps
MISC: Fatigue
Contraindications: Hypersensitivity, second or third trimester of pregnancy
Precautions: Pregnancy category C (first trimester) and pregnancy category D (second or third trimester), lactation, children, sodium- and volume-depleted patients, renal impairment
Pharmacokinetics:
PO: Good oral absorption, peak levels 1 hr, metabolites 3-4 hr; highly bound to plasma proteins; liver metabolism; partially converted to active metabolites (first-pass metabolism); excreted in urine, feces
Drug interactions of concern to dentistry:
• Potential for increased hypotensive effects with other hypotensive drugs and sedatives
• Suspected increase in antihypertensive effects: fluconazole, ketoconazole; if used concurrently monitor blood pressure
DENTAL CONSIDERATIONS
General:
• Monitor vital signs at every appointment because of cardiovascular effects.
• Limit use of sodium-containing products, such as saline IV fluids, for those patients with a dietary salt restriction.
• Stress from dental procedures may compromise cardiovascular function; determine patient risk.
• Assess salivary flow as a factor in caries, periodontal disease, and candidiasis.
• Short appointments and a stress reduction protocol may be required for anxious patients.
• Consider semisupine chair position for patient comfort because of respiratory side effects of drug.
• Use precaution if sedation or general anesthesia is required; risk of hypotensive episode.
Consultations:
• Medical consultation may be required to assess disease control and patient's ability to tolerate stress.
Teach patient/family:
• Importance of updating health and drug history if physician makes any changes in evaluation or drug regimens
When chronic dry mouth occurs, advise patient:
• To avoid mouth rinses with high alcohol content because of drying effects
• Of need for daily home fluoride use to prevent caries
• To use sugarless gum, frequent sips of water, or saliva substitutes

loteprednol etabonate (optic)

(loe-te-pred'nol)
Alrex, Lotemax
Drug class.: Topical glucocorticoid

Action: Glucocorticoids have multiple actions that include antiinflammatory and immunosuppressant effects. They inhibit phospholipase A_2, interfering with or reducing the synthesis of prostaglandins and leukotrienes. They also bind to cytoplasmic GRs and enter the cell nucleus to bind with DNA. This results in the synthesis of various enzymes such as collagenase, elastase, and cytokines that play important roles in inflammation and immunosuppression. They also suppress the production of lymphocytes, monocytes, and eosinophils.

Uses: For steroid-responsive inflammation of the conjunctiva, cornea, and anterior segments of the globe associated with allergic conjunctivitis, acne rosacea, iritis, superficial punctate keratitis, and so on when topical steroid use is acceptable to reduce inflammation and edema, postoperative inflammation after ocular surgery (Lotemax 0.5%); temporary relief of symptoms of seasonal allergic conjunctivitis (Alrex 0.2%)

Dosage and routes:

• *Adult:* TOP instill 1 or 2 drops into the conjunctival sac of the affected eye qid; during initial treatment (first week) up to 1 drop qh can be used if necessary; reevaluate if no response in 2 days; also used 24 hr after ocular surgery 1-2 drops qid for up to 2 wk

Available forms include: Sterile ophthalmic suspension 0.2% and 0.5% in 2.5, 5, 10, 15 ml plastic bottles

Side effects/adverse reactions:

CNS: Headache

RESP: Pharyngitis

EENT: Abnormal vision, blurring, burning, discharge, dry eyes, itching, photophobia, rhinitis

Contraindications: Hypersensitivity; viral diseases of cornea and conjunctiva, including herpes keratitis, vaccinia, and varicella; mycobacteria and fungal eye infections

Precautions: Prolonged use may result in glaucoma, increased risk of secondary ocular infections, delayed healing after cataract surgery; avoid contamination of sterile container; pregnancy category C, lactation, use in children not established

Pharmacokinetics:

INSTILL: Absorbed amounts are believed to be rapidly metabolized, metabolites excreted in urine; systemic effects unknown or not evident

Drug interactions of concern to dentistry:

• None reported

DENTAL CONSIDERATIONS

General:

• Avoid dental light in patient's eyes; offer dark glasses for patient comfort.

• Determine why patient is taking the drug.

---

lovastatin

(loe'va-sta-tin)

Mevacor, Altocor

Drug class.: Cholesterol-lowering agent

Action: Inhibits HMG-Co A reductase enzyme, which reduces cholesterol synthesis; reduced synthesis of VLDL; plasma triglyceride levels may also be decreased

Uses: As an adjunct in homozygous familial hypercholesterolemia, mixed hyperlipidemia, elevated serum triglyceride levels, and type IV hyperproteinemia, also reduces total cholesterol LDL-C, apoB, and triglyceride levels; patient should first be placed on cholesterol-lowering diet; primary prevention of CHD and to slow CHD progression

Dosage and routes:

• *Adult:* PO 20 mg qd with evening meal; may increase to 20-80 mg/

day in single or divided doses, not to exceed 80 mg/day; dosage adjustments should be made qmo
Heterozygous familial hypercholesterolemia:
• *Child age 10-17 yr:* PO 10-40 mg/day; limit 40 mg/day
Available forms include: Tabs 10, 20, 40 mg; ext rel tab 10, 20, 40, 60 mg
Side effects/adverse reactions:
CNS: Dizziness, headache
GI: Nausea, constipation, diarrhea, dyspepsia, flatus, abdominal pain, heartburn, ***liver dysfunction***
EENT: Blurred vision, dysgeusia, lens opacities
INTEG: Rash, pruritus
MS: Muscle cramps, myalgia, ***myositis, rhabdomyolysis***
Contraindications: Pregnancy category X, lactation, active liver disease, drugs that inhibit the enzyme CYP3A4
Precautions: Past liver disease, alcoholics, severe acute infections, trauma, hypotension, uncontrolled seizure disorders, severe metabolic disorders, electrolyte imbalances
Pharmacokinetics:
PO: Peak 2-4 hr; highly protein bound; metabolized in liver by CYP3A4 isoenzymes (metabolites); excreted in urine, feces, breast milk; crosses placenta
Drug interactions of concern to dentistry:
• Increased myalgia, rhabdomyolysis: erythromycin, cyclosporine (see Appendix I)
• Contraindicated with itraconazole, ketoconazole, erythromycin (see Appendix I)
DENTAL CONSIDERATIONS
General:
• Consider semisupine chair position for patient comfort because of GI side effects.
Teach patient/family:
• To avoid mouth rinses with high alcohol content because of drying effects

---

loxapine succinate

(lox'a-peen)
Loxitane
Loxapac
Drug class.: Antipsychotic

Action: Depresses cerebral cortex, hypothalamus, limbic system, all of which control activity and aggression; blocks neurotransmission produced by dopamine at synapse; exhibits strong α-adrenergic, cholinergic-blocking action; mechanism for antipsychotic effects is unclear
Uses: Psychotic disorders
Dosage and routes:
• *Adult:* PO 10 mg bid-qid initially, may be rapidly increased depending on severity of condition, maintenance 60-100 mg/day
Available forms include: Caps 5, 10, 25, 50 mg
Side effects/adverse reactions:
ORAL: Dry mouth
CNS: Extrapyramidal symptoms: pseudoparkinsonism, akathisia, dystonia, tardive dyskinesia, drowsiness, headache, ***seizures,*** confusion
CV: Orthostatic hypotension, ***cardiac arrest,*** ECG changes, tachycardia
GI: Nausea, vomiting, anorexia, constipation, diarrhea, jaundice, weight gain
RESP: ***Laryngospasm, respiratory depression,*** dyspnea

HEMA: ***Anemia, leukopenia, leukocytosis, agranulocytosis***
GU: Urinary retention, urinary frequency, enuresis, impotence, amenorrhea, gynecomastia
EENT: Blurred vision, glaucoma
INTEG: Rash, photosensitivity, dermatitis

Contraindications: Hypersensitivity, blood dyscrasias, coma, child, brain damage, bone marrow depression, alcohol and barbiturate withdrawal states

Precautions: Pregnancy category C, lactation, seizure disorders, hepatic disease, cardiac disease, prostatic hypertrophy, cardiac conditions, child <16 yr

Pharmacokinetics:
PO: Onset 20-30 min, peak 2-4 hr, duration 12 hr
IM: Onset 15-30 min, peak 15-20 min, duration 12 hr
Initial half-life 5 hr, terminal half-life 19 hr; metabolized by liver; excreted in urine; crosses placenta; excreted in breast milk

Drug interactions of concern to dentistry:

- Increased effects of both drugs: anticholinergics
- Increased CNS depression: alcohol, all CNS depressants
- Decreased effects of sympathomimetics, carbamazepine

DENTAL CONSIDERATIONS

General:

- Patients on chronic drug therapy may rarely have symptoms of blood dyscrasias, which can include infection, bleeding, and poor healing.
- Assess salivary flow as a factor in caries, periodontal disease, and candidiasis.
- Assess for presence of extrapyramidal motor symptoms, such as tardive dyskinesia and akathisia. Extrapyramidal motor activity may complicate dental treatment.
- After supine positioning, have patient sit upright for at least 2 min to avoid orthostatic hypotension.

Consultations:

- In a patient with symptoms of blood dyscrasias, request a medical consultation for blood studies and postpone dental treatment until normal values are reestablished.
- If signs of tardive dyskinesia or akathisia are present, refer to physician.
- Physician should be informed if significant xerostomic side effects occur (e.g., increased caries, sore tongue, problems eating or swallowing, difficulty wearing prosthesis) so that a medication change can be considered.

Teach patient/family:

- Importance of good oral hygiene to prevent soft tissue inflammation
- Caution to prevent injury when using oral hygiene aids
- To use electric toothbrush if patient has difficulty holding conventional devices

When chronic dry mouth occurs, advise patient:

- To avoid mouth rinses with high alcohol content because of drying effects
- To use sugarless gum, frequent sips of water, or saliva substitutes
- To use daily home fluoride products for anticaries effect

L

magaldrate (aluminum magnesium complex)

(mag'al-drate)

Iosopan, Riopan

Drug class.: Antacid/aluminum/magnesium hydroxide

Action: Neutralizes gastric acidity

Uses: Antacid for hyperacidity

Dosage and routes:

• *Adult:* Susp 5-10 ml (400-800 mg) with water between meals, hs, not to exceed 100 ml/day

Available forms include: Susp 540 mg/5 ml

Side effects/adverse reactions:

▼ *ORAL:* Chalky taste

GI: Constipation, diarrhea, nausea, vomiting, thirst, stomach cramps

META: Hypermagnesemia, hypophosphatemia, hypercalcemia

Contraindications: Hypersensitivity to this drug or aluminum products, intestinal obstruction

Precautions: Elderly, fluid restriction, decreased GI motility, GI obstruction, dehydration, renal disease, sodium-restricted diets, pregnancy category C, colitis, gastric outlet obstruction syndrome, colostomy

Pharmacokinetics:

PO: Onset 10-15 min, duration >3 hr

Drug interactions of concern to dentistry:

• Decreased absorption of anticholinergics, corticosteroids, sodium fluoride, tetracycline, ketoconazole, chlordiazepoxide, ciprofloxacin, metronidazole

DENTAL CONSIDERATIONS

General:

• If prescribing oral form of a drug for which risk of decreased absorption is reported, advise taking doses at least 2 hr after or before antacid use.

• Avoid drugs that could exacerbate upper GI distress (aspirin and NSAIDs).

• Consider semisupine chair position for patient comfort because of GI effects of disease.

maprotiline HCl

(ma-proe'ti-leen)

generic

Drug class.: Tetracyclic antidepressant

Action: Antidepressant action unknown; however, it blocks reuptake of norepinephrine into nerve endings, increasing action of norepinephrine at nerve endings

Uses: Depression, depression with anxiety, manic depression; unapproved: neurogenic pain, tension headache

Dosage and routes:

• *Adult:* PO 25-75 mg/day in moderate depression; may increase to 150 mg/day in 25 mg increments, not to exceed 225 mg/day

• *Elderly:* PO 25-75 mg/day

Available forms include: Tabs 25, 50, 75 mg

Side effects/adverse reactions:

▼ *ORAL: Dry mouth*

CNS: Dizziness, vertigo, nervousness, drowsiness, ***seizures,*** confusion, headache, anxiety, tremors, stimulation, weakness, insomnia, nightmares, EPS (elderly), increased psychiatric symptoms, sedation, manic hallucinations

CV: Orthostatic hypotension, ECG changes, tachycardia, ***hypertension (rare),*** palpitation

GI: Diarrhea, nausea, vomiting,

hepatitis, paralytic ileus, increased appetite, cramps, epigastric distress, jaundice

HEMA: ***Agranulocytosis, thrombocytopenia, eosinophilia, leukopenia***

GU: Retention, ***acute renal failure***

EENT: Blurred vision, tinnitus, mydriasis

INTEG: Rash, urticaria, sweating, pruritus, vasculitis, photosensitivity

Contraindications: Hypersensitivity to tricyclic antidepressants, recovery phase of MI, convulsive disorders, prostatic hypertrophy

Precautions: Suicidal patients, severe depression, increased intraocular pressure, narrow-angle glaucoma, urinary retention, cardiac disease, hepatic or renal disease, hypothyroidism, hyperthyroidism, electroshock therapy, elective surgery, elderly, pregnancy category B, lactation, prostate hypertrophy, schizophrenia, MAOIs

Pharmacokinetics:

PO: Onset 15-30 min, peak 12 hr, duration up to 3 wk, half-life 27-58 hr, steady state 6-10 days; protein binding 80%, metabolized by liver; excreted by kidneys, feces; crosses placenta

Drug interactions of concern to dentistry:

- Increased effects of direct-acting sympathomimetics (epinephrine)
- Potential risk of increased CNS depression: alcohol, and all CNS depressants
- Decreased antihypertensive effect: clonidine, guanadrel, guanethidine

DENTAL CONSIDERATIONS

General:

- Monitor vital signs at every appointment because of cardiovascular side effects.
- Patients on chronic drug therapy may rarely have symptoms of blood dyscrasias, which can include infection, bleeding, and poor healing.
- Assess salivary flow as a factor in caries, periodontal disease, and candidiasis.
- After supine positioning, have patient sit upright for at least 2 min before standing to avoid orthostatic hypotension.
- The use of epinephrine in gingival retraction cord is contraindicated. Use vasoconstrictors with caution, in low doses, and with careful aspiration.

Consultations:

- In a patient with symptoms of blood dyscrasias, request a medical consultation for blood studies and postpone dental treatment until normal values are reestablished.
- Take precautions if dental surgery is anticipated and anesthesia is required.
- Medical consultation may be required to assess disease control.
- Physician should be informed if significant xerostomic side effects occur (e.g., increased caries, sore tongue, problems eating or swallowing, difficulty wearing prosthesis) so that a medication change can be considered.

Teach patient/family:

- Importance of good oral hygiene to prevent soft tissue inflammation
- Caution to prevent injury when using oral hygiene aids

When chronic dry mouth occurs, advise patient:

- To avoid mouth rinses with high alcohol content because of drying effects

M

• To use sugarless gum, frequent sips of water, or saliva substitutes
• To use daily home fluoride products for anticaries effect

mecamylamine HCl

(mek-a-mil'a-meen)
Inversine

Drug class.: Antihypertensive, ganglionic blocker

Action: Occupies ganglionic receptor site, prevents acetylcholine from attaching to postsynaptic nerve ending in autonomic ganglia
Uses: Moderate-to-severe hypertension, malignant hypertension; unlabeled use: hyperreflexia, smoking cessation
Dosage and routes:
• *Adult:* PO 2.5 mg bid; may increase in increments of 2.5 mg × 2 days until desired response; maintenance 25 mg/day in 3 divided doses
Available forms include: Tabs 2.5 mg
Side effects/adverse reactions:
▼ *ORAL: Dry mouth,* glossitis, bitter taste
CNS: Drowsiness, sedation, dizziness, ***convulsions,*** headache, tremors, weakness, syncope, paresthesia, dizziness
CV: Postural hypotension, ***CHF,*** irregular heart rate
GI: Paralytic ileus, anorexia, nausea, vomiting, constipation
GU: Impotence, urinary retention, decreased libido
EENT: Blurred vision, nasal congestion, dilated pupils
Contraindications: Hypersensitivity, MI, coronary insufficiency, renal disease, glaucoma, organic pyloric stenosis, uremia, uncooperative patients, mild/labile hypertension
Precautions: CVA, prostatic hypertrophy, bladder neck obstruction, urethral stricture, renal dysfunction (elevated BUN), cerebral dysfunction, pregnancy category C, vigorous exercise, stress-related activity
Pharmacokinetics:
PO: Onset 0.5-2 hr, duration 6-12 hr; excreted unchanged in urine, feces, breast milk; crosses placenta
Drug interactions of concern to dentistry:
• Increased vasopressor response: sympathomimetics
• Decreased hypotensive effect: sympathomimetics, NSAIDs, especially indomethacin
• Increased hypotensive response: sedative drugs that may also lower blood pressure

DENTAL CONSIDERATIONS

General:
• Monitor vital signs at every appointment because of cardiovascular side effects.
• After supine positioning, have patient sit upright for at least 2 min before standing to avoid orthostatic hypotension.
• Assess salivary flow as a factor in caries, periodontal disease, and candidiasis.
• Consider semisupine chair position for patient comfort because of GI effects of disease.
• Early-morning appointments and a stress reduction protocol may be required for anxious patients.
• Stress from dental procedures may compromise cardiovascular function; determine patient risk.

• Use vasoconstrictors with caution, in low doses, and with careful aspiration.
• Avoid use of gingival retraction cord with epinephrine.
• Limit use of sodium-containing products (e.g., air polishing system and IV fluids) for patients with a dietary salt restriction.
• Take precautions if dental surgery is anticipated and anesthesia is required.

Consultations:
• Medical consultation may be required to assess disease control.

Teach patient/family:
• Importance of good oral hygiene to prevent soft tissue inflammation

When chronic dry mouth occurs, advise patient:
• To avoid mouth rinses with high alcohol content because of drying effects
• To use daily home fluoride products for anticaries effect
• To use sugarless gum, frequent sips of water, or saliva substitutes

---

meclizine HCl

(mek'li-zeen)

Antivert, Antivert 25, Antivert 50, Bonine, Dramamine less Drowsy, Meni-D, Vergon

♣ Bonamine

Drug class.: Antihistamine

Action: Specific mechanism unknown; has both anticholinergic and antihistamine (H_1) actions; CNS actions are believed to be related to its anticholinergic effects

Uses: Vertigo, motion sickness

Dosage and routes:
• *Adult:* PO 25-100 mg qd in divided doses or 25-50 mg 1 hr before traveling

Available forms include: Tabs 12.5, 25, 50 mg; chew tabs 25 mg; caps 25, 30 mg

Side effects/adverse reactions:
▼ *ORAL:* Dry mouth
CNS: Drowsiness, dizziness, sedation, fatigue, restlessness, headache, insomnia, extrapyramidal symptoms
GI: Nausea, anorexia, vomiting
GU: Difficult urination
INTEG: Rash, urticaria
EENT: Blurred vision

Contraindications: Hypersensitivity to cyclizines

Precautions: Children, narrow-angle glaucoma, urinary retention, lactation, prostatic hypertrophy, elderly, pregnancy category B, asthma

Pharmacokinetics:
PO: Onset 1 hr, duration 8-24 hr, half-life 6 hr

Drug interactions of concern to dentistry:
• Increased effect of alcohol, other CNS depressants, anticholinergics

DENTAL CONSIDERATIONS

General:
• Assess salivary flow as a factor in caries, periodontal disease, and candidiasis.

Teach patient/family:

When chronic dry mouth occurs, advise patient:
• To avoid mouth rinses with high alcohol content because of drying effects
• To use daily home fluoride products for anticaries effect
• To use sugarless gum, frequent sips of water, or saliva substitutes

M

meclofenamate sodium

(me-kloe-fen-am'ate)

generic

Drug class.: Nonsteroidal antiinflammatory

Action: Inhibits prostaglandin synthesis by interfering with cyclooxygenase needed for biosynthesis; possesses analgesic, antiinflammatory, antipyretic properties

Uses: Mild-to-moderate pain, osteoarthritis, rheumatoid arthritis, dysmenorrhea; unapproved: vascular headache, menorrhagia

Dosage and routes:

Analgesia:

• *Adult:* PO 50-100 mg q4-6h; not to exceed 400 mg/day

Rheumatoid and osteoarthritis:

• *Adult:* PO 200-400 mg/day, divided into 3 or 4 equal doses

Primary dysmenorrhea:

• *Adult:* PO 100 mg tid up to 6 days

Available forms include: Caps 50, 100 mg

Side effects/adverse reactions:

▼ *ORAL:* Stomatitis, bitter taste, dry mouth, lichenoid reaction

CNS: Dizziness, drowsiness, fatigue, tremors, confusion, insomnia, anxiety, depression

CV: Tachycardia, peripheral edema, palpitation, dysrhythmias

GI: ***Cholestatic hepatitis,*** diarrhea, nausea, anorexia, vomiting, jaundice, constipation, flatulence, cramps, peptic ulcer

HEMA: ***Blood dyscrasias***

GU: ***Nephrotoxicity: dysuria, hematuria, oliguria, azotemia***

EENT: Tinnitus, hearing loss, blurred vision

INTEG: Purpura, rash, pruritus, sweating

Contraindications: Hypersensitivity, asthma induced by aspirin, severe renal disease, severe hepatic disease, allergy to other NSAIDs

Precautions: Pregnancy category not listed, lactation, children <14 yr, bleeding disorders, upper GI disorders, cardiac disorders, hypersensitivity to other antiinflammatory agents

Pharmacokinetics:

PO: Peak serum levels 30 min, half-life 3-3.5 hr; metabolized in liver; excreted in urine (metabolites), less in feces and breast milk

Drug interactions of concern to dentistry:

• GI ulceration, bleeding: aspirin, alcohol, corticosteroids, biphosphonates

• Nephrotoxicity: acetaminophen (prolonged use)

• Possible risk of decreased renal function: cyclosporine

• First-time users of SSRIs also taking NSAIDs may have a higher risk of GI side effects; until more data are available, it may be advisable to avoid use of NSAIDs in these patients (*Br J Clin Pharmacol* 55:591-595, 2003)

• *When prescribed for dental pain:*

• Risk of increased effects: oral anticoagulants, oral antidiabetics, lithium, methotrexate

• Decreased effects of diuretics, β-adrenergic blockers

DENTAL CONSIDERATIONS

General:

• Patients on chronic drug therapy may rarely have symptoms of blood dyscrasias, which can include infection, bleeding, and poor healing.

• Assess salivary flow as a factor in caries, periodontal disease, and candidiasis.
• Avoid prescribing for dental use in last trimester of pregnancy.
• Avoid prescribing aspirin-containing products.
• Consider semisupine chair position for patients with rheumatic disease.

Consultations:
• In a patient with symptoms of blood dyscrasias, request a medical consultation for blood studies and postpone dental treatment until normal values are reestablished.
• Medical consultation may be required to assess disease control.

Teach patient/family:
• Importance of good oral hygiene to prevent soft tissue inflammation
• Caution to prevent injury when using oral hygiene aids

When chronic dry mouth occurs, advise patient:
• To avoid mouth rinses with high alcohol content because of drying effects
• To use sugarless gum, frequent sips of water, or saliva substitutes
• To use daily home fluoride products for anticaries effect

medroxyprogesterone acetate

(me-drox'ee-proe-jes'te-rone)
Amen, Curretab, Cycrin, Depo-Provera, Provera
♣ Alti-PMA, Gen-Medroxy, Novo-Medrone, Provera Pak
Drug class.: Progestogen

Action: Inhibits secretion of pituitary gonadotropins, preventing follicular maturation and ovulation; stimulates growth of mammary tissue; antineoplastic action against endometrial cancer

Uses: Uterine bleeding (abnormal), secondary amenorrhea, endometrial cancer, metastatic renal cancer, contraceptive; with estrogens to reduce incidence of endometrial hyperplasia, cancer

Dosage and routes:

Secondary amenorrhea:
• *Adult:* PO 5-10 mg qd × 5-10 days

Endometrial/renal cancer:
• *Adult:* IM 400-1000 mg/wk

Uterine bleeding:
• *Adult:* PO 5-10 mg qd × 5-10 days starting on day 16 of menstrual cycle

Contraception:
• *Adult female:* IM 150 mg q3mo

Available forms include: Tabs 2.5, 5, 10 mg; inj 150, 400 mg/ml

Side effects/adverse reactions:
▼ *ORAL:* Gingival bleeding, gingival overgrowth
CNS: Dizziness, headache, migraines, depression, fatigue
CV: ***Thromboembolism, stroke, pulmonary embolism, MI,*** hypotension, thrombophlebitis, edema
GI: Nausea, ***cholestatic jaundice,*** vomiting, anorexia, cramps, increased weight
GU: Gynecomastia, testicular atrophy, impotence, ***spontaneous abortion,*** endometriosis, amenorrhea, cervical erosion, breakthrough bleeding, dysmenorrhea, vaginal candidiasis, breast changes
EENT: Diplopia
INTEG: Rash, urticaria, acne, hirsutism, alopecia, oily skin, seborrhea, purpura, melasma, photosensitivity
META: Hyperglycemia

Contraindications: Breast cancer, hypersensitivity, thromboembolic

disorders, reproductive cancer, genital bleeding (abnormal, undiagnosed), pregnancy category X
Precautions: Lactation, hypertension, asthma, blood dyscrasias, gallbladder disease, CHF, diabetes mellitus, bone disease, depression, migraine headache, convulsive disorders, hepatic disease, renal disease, family history of cancer of breast or reproductive tract
Pharmacokinetics:
PO: Peak levels 2-7 hr, duration 24 hr, depot injection active up to 3 mo; metabolized in liver; excreted in urine, feces
DENTAL CONSIDERATIONS
General:
• Place on frequent recall to evaluate inflammatory and healing response.
Teach patient/family:
• Importance of good oral hygiene to prevent soft tissue inflammation

mefenamic acid

(me-fe-nam′ik)
Ponstel
✽ Ponstan
Drug class.: Nonsteroidal antiinflammatory

Action: Inhibits prostaglandin synthesis by interfering with cyclooxygenase needed for biosynthesis; possesses analgesic, antiinflammatory, antipyretic properties
Uses: Mild-to-moderate pain, dysmenorrhea, inflammatory disease
Dosage and routes:
Acute pain:
• *Adult and child >14 yr:* PO 500 mg, then 250 mg q6h; use not to exceed 1 wk
Primary dysmenorrhea:
• *Adult female:* PO 500 mg; then 250 mg q6h with onset of menstruation
Available forms include: Caps 250 mg
Side effects/adverse reactions:
▼ *ORAL:* Lichenoid reaction
CNS: Dizziness, drowsiness, fatigue, tremors, confusion, insomnia, anxiety, depression
CV: Tachycardia, peripheral edema, palpitation, dysrhythmias
GI: ***Cholestatic hepatitis,*** nausea, anorexia, vomiting, diarrhea, jaundice, constipation, flatulence, cramps, peptic ulcer
HEMA: ***Blood dyscrasias***
GU: ***Nephrotoxicity: dysuria, hematuria, oliguria, azotemia***
EENT: Tinnitus, hearing loss, blurred vision
INTEG: Purpura, rash, pruritus, sweating
Contraindications: Hypersensitivity, asthma, severe renal disease, severe hepatic disease
Precautions: Pregnancy category C, lactation, children, bleeding disorders, GI disorders, cardiac disorders, hypersensitivity to other antiinflammatory agents
Pharmacokinetics:
PO: Peak 2 hr, half-life 33.5 hr; extensive protein binding; metabolized in liver; excreted in urine (metabolites), breast milk
Drug interactions of concern to dentistry:
• GI bleeding, ulceration: aspirin, alcohol, corticosteroids
• Nephrotoxicity: acetaminophen (prolonged use and high doses)
• Possible risk of decreased renal function: cyclosporine
• First-time users of SSRIs also taking NSAIDs may have a higher

risk of GI side effects; until more data are available, it may be advisable to avoid use of NSAIDs in these patients (*Br J Clin Pharmacol* 55:591-595, 2003)

When prescribed for dental pain:

• Risk of increased effects of oral anticoagulants, oral antidiabetics, lithium, methotrexate

• Decreased effects of diuretics

DENTAL CONSIDERATIONS

General:

• Avoid prescribing for dental use in last trimester of pregnancy.

• Avoid prescribing aspirin-containing products.

Consultations:

• Medical consultation may be required to assess disease control.

---

megestrol acetate

(me-jes'trole)

Megace

♣ Apo-Megestrol

Drug class.: Progestin

Action: Affects endometrium by antiluteinizing effect, which results in antiproliferative changes in the endometrium, reduces serum levels of estrogens, causes weight gain by unknown mechanism, multiple cellular effects in tumors

Uses: Breast, endometrial cancer, renal cell cancer; AIDS wasting syndrome

Dosage and routes:

• *Adult:* PO 40-320 mg/day in divided doses

AIDS wasting syndrome:

• *Adult:* PO initial dose 800 mg/day

Available forms include: Tabs 20, 40 mg; oral susp 40 mg/5 ml

Side effects/adverse reactions:

▼ *ORAL:* Gingival bleeding, gingival overgrowth

CNS: Mood swings

CV: ***Thrombophlebitis***

GI: Nausea, vomiting, anorexia, diarrhea, abdominal cramps

GU: ***Hypercalcemia,*** gynecomastia, fluid retention

INTEG: Alopecia, rash, pruritus, purpura

Contraindications: Hypersensitivity, pregnancy category X

Pharmacokinetics:

PO: Duration 1-3 days, half-life 60 min; metabolized in liver; excreted in feces, breast milk

DENTAL CONSIDERATIONS

General:

• Place on frequent recall to evaluate inflammatory and healing response.

• Patients receiving chemotherapy may require palliative treatment for stomatitis.

Teach patient/family:

• Importance of good oral hygiene to prevent soft tissue inflammation

---

meloxicam

(mel-ox'i-cam)

Mobic

♣ Mobicox

Drug class.: Nonsteroidal antiinflammatory

Action: May be related to a nonselective inhibition of cyclooxygenase isoenzymes preventing the synthesis of prostaglandins

Uses: Relief of signs and symptoms of osteoarthritis

Dosage and routes:

• *Adult:* PO 7.5 mg daily, max daily dose 15 mg

M

Available forms include: Tabs 7.5 mg

Side effects/adverse reactions:

▼ *ORAL:* Facial edema, dry mouth, ulcerative stomatitis, taste perversion

CNS: Headache, dizziness, anxiety, insomnia, fatigue, malaise, vertigo

CV: Peripheral edema, hot flashes, syncope, variation in blood pressure, arrhythmia

GI: Abdominal pain, diarrhea, dyspepsia, nausea, flatulence, ulcer, esophagitis, GERD

RESP: URI, cough, asthma, bronchospasm

HEMA: ***Agranulocytosis, thrombocytopenia, leukopenia,*** anemia

GU: ***Renal failure,*** hematuria, interstitial nephritis, pharyngitis

EENT: Abnormal vision, tinnitus

INTEG: ***Stevens-Johnson syndrome, toxic epidermal necrolysis,*** rash, pruritus, erythema multiforme

META: ***Liver failure;*** elevations of AST, ALT, GGT, BUN; hepatitis; dehydration

MS: Arthralgia, back pain

MISC: ***Anaphylaxis,*** flulike symptoms, falling, allergic reactions

Contraindications: Hypersensitivity; patients who have experienced asthma, urticaria, or allergic-type reactions after taking aspirin or other NSAIDs; advanced renal disease

Precautions: Preexisting asthma, anaphylactic reactions to NSAIDs, serious GI side effects may occur, GI ulcer or GI bleeding; avoid in late pregnancy, liver dysfunction, dehydration, long-term use, edema, heart failure, hypertension, ACE inhibitors, pregnancy category C, lactation, elderly

Pharmacokinetics:

PO: Bioavailability 89%, max plasma levels in 4-5 hr, $T_{1/2}$ = 15-20 hr, plasma protein binding 99.4%, almost completely metabolized, CYP450 3A4 is a minor pathway for metabolism, equal excretion of metabolites in feces and urine

Drug interactions of concern to dentistry:

- Increased risk of GI side effects: long-duration NSAIDs, aspirin (except low-dose form), oral glucocorticoids, alcoholism, smoking, older age, and generally poor health
- Increased blood levels: lithium
- Reduced natriuretic effect: furosemide and other loop diuretics
- First-time users of SSRIs also taking NSAIDs may have a higher risk of GI side effects; until more data are available, it may be advisable to avoid use of NSAIDs in these patients (*Br J Clin Pharmacol* 55:591-595, 2003)

DENTAL CONSIDERATIONS

General:

- Assess salivary flow as a factor in caries, periodontal disease, and candidiasis.
- Patients on chronic drug therapy may rarely have symptoms of blood dyscrasias, which can include infection, bleeding, and poor healing.
- Consider semisupine chair position for patient comfort if GI side effects occur.

Consultations:

- In a patient with symptoms of blood dyscrasias, request a medical consultation for blood studies and postpone treatment until normal values are reestablished.

Teach patient/family:

- Use of electric toothbrush if patient has difficulty holding conventional devices
- Importance of updating health and drug history if physician makes any changes in evaluation or drug regimens
- Importance of good oral hygiene to prevent soft tissue inflammation
- To prevent trauma when using oral hygiene aids

When chronic dry mouth occurs, advise patient:

- To avoid mouth rinses with high alcohol content because of drying effects
- To use daily home fluoride products for anticaries effect
- To use sugarless gum, frequent sips of water, or saliva substitutes

melphalan

(mel'fa-lan)

Alkeran

Drug class.: Antineoplastic

Action: An alkylating agent; cytotoxic effects are due to cross-linking DNA or RNA strands and inhibition of protein synthesis, which leads to cell death

Uses: Palliative treatment of multiple myeloma and nonresectable epithelial carcinoma of the ovary

Dosage and routes:

Multiple myeloma:

- *Adult:* PO 6 mg daily for 2-3 wk while evaluating WBC counts; 2 mg maintenance doses may be used depending on blood cell count; IV 16 mg/m^2 as a single infusion at 2 wk intervals × 4 doses

Epithelial ovarian cancer:

- *Adult:* PO 0.2 mg/kg daily for 5 days as a single course; repeat q4-5wk depending on blood cell count

Available forms include: Tabs 2 mg; powder for inj 50 mg

Side effects/adverse reactions:

▼ *ORAL:* Stomatitis, oral ulceration

GI: Nausea, vomiting

RESP: ***Fibrosis, dysplasia***

HEMA: ***Thrombocytopenia, neutropenia, myelosuppression,*** anemia

GU: Amenorrhea, hyperuricemia

INTEG: Rash, urticaria

Contraindications: Cancer with prior resistance to drug, lactation, hypersensitivity

Precautions: Pregnancy category D, severe bone marrow depression risk, renal impairment

Pharmacokinetics: Half-life 1.5 hr; first-pass hepatic metabolism; plasma levels vary; metabolites excreted in urine

Drug interactions of concern to dentistry:

- Increased toxicity: antineoplastics, radiation

DENTAL CONSIDERATIONS

General:

- Patients receiving chemotherapy may be taking chronic opioids for pain. Consider NSAIDs for dental pain management.
- Patients receiving chemotherapy may require palliative therapy for stomatitis.
- Patients on chronic drug therapy may rarely have symptoms of blood dyscrasias, which can include infection, bleeding, and poor healing.

Consultations:

- Medical consultation may be required to assess disease control.
- In a patient with symptoms of blood dyscrasias, request a medical

consultation for blood studies and postpone dental treatment until normal values are reestablished.

Teach patient/family:

• About the possibility of secondary oral infection; must see dentist immediately if infection occurs

When chronic dry mouth occurs, advise patient:

• To avoid mouth rinses with high alcohol content because of drying effects

• To use sugarless gum, frequent sips of water, or saliva substitutes

• To use daily home fluoride products for anticaries effect

---

memantine HCl

(me-man'teen)

Namenda

Drug class.: NMDA receptor antagonist

Action: Acts as an NMDA (*N*-methyl-*D*-aspartate) receptor antagonist, binding preferentially to NMDA receptor–operated cation channels

Uses: Treatment of moderate to severe dementia of Alzheimer's disease

Dosage and routes:

• *Adult:* PO initial 5 mg/day, slowly increase dose by 5 mg/day in twice-daily dosing over 3-4 wk to max dose of 10 mg bid

Available forms include: Tab 5, 10 mg

Side effects/adverse reactions:

CNS: Fatigue, dizziness, headache, confusion, hallucination, somnolence, syncope

CV: Hypertension

GI: Constipation, vomiting, diarrhea, nausea

RESP: Coughing, dyspnea, bronchitis, URI

GU: Incontinence, UTI

INTEG: Rash, acne

MS: Back pain, arthralgia

MISC: Pain, falling, flulike symptoms

Contraindications: Hypersensitivity

Precautions: Moderate to severe renal impairment, alkaline urine pH, pregnancy category B, safety and efficacy in nursing mothers and pediatric patients have not been established

Pharmacokinetics:

PO: Well absorbed, peak blood levels in 3-7 hr; plasma protein binding 45%, minimal metabolism, excreted mostly unchanged by active tubular secretion in the urine

Drug interactions of concern to dentistry:

• None reported

DENTAL CONSIDERATIONS

• Monitor vital signs at every appointment because of cardiovascular side effects.

General:

• Patients with Alzheimer's disease may be taking other drugs; get a complete drug history.

• Drug may be used late in disease process; ensure caregiver or responsible person understands informed consent.

• Place on frequent recall to evaluate oral health.

Consultations:

• Consultation with physician may be needed if sedation or general anesthesia is required.

Teach patient/family:

• Use of electric toothbrush if patient has difficulty holding conventional devices

• Importance of good oral hygiene to prevent soft tissue inflammation/infection
• To prevent trauma when using oral hygiene aids
• Importance of updating health and drug history and reporting changes in health status, drug regimen, or disease/treatment status

mepenzolate bromide

(me-pen′zoe-late)
Cantil

Drug class.: Gastrointestinal anticholinergic

Action: Inhibits muscarinic actions of acetylcholine at postganglionic parasympathetic neuroeffector sites

Uses: Treatment of peptic ulcer disease, irritable bowel syndrome in combination with other drugs; other GI disorders

Dosage and routes:
• *Adult:* PO 25-50 mg qid with meals, hs; titrate to patient response

Available forms include: Tabs 25 mg

Side effects/adverse reactions:
▼ *ORAL: Dry mouth,* absence of taste
CNS: Confusion, stimulation in elderly, headache, insomnia, dizziness, drowsiness, anxiety, weakness, hallucination
CV: Palpitation, tachycardia
GI: Constipation, ***paralytic ileus,*** heartburn, nausea, vomiting, dysphagia
GU: Hesitancy, retention, impotence
EENT: Blurred vision, photophobia, mydriasis, cycloplegia, increased ocular tension
INTEG: Urticaria, rash, pruritus, anhidrosis, fever, allergic reactions

Contraindications: Hypersensitivity to anticholinergics, narrow-angle glaucoma, GI obstruction, myasthenia gravis, paralytic ileus, GI atony, toxic megacolon

Precautions: Hyperthyroidism, coronary artery disease, dysrhythmias, CHF, ulcerative colitis, hypertension, hiatal hernia, hepatic disease, renal disease, pregnancy category C, elderly, urinary retention, prostatic hypertrophy

Pharmacokinetics:
PO: Onset 1 hr, duration 3-4 hr; metabolized by liver; excreted in urine

Drug interactions of concern to dentistry:
• Increased anticholinergic effect: other anticholinergic drugs
• Constipation, urinary retention: opioid analgesics
• Decreased absorption of ketoconazole; take doses 2 hr apart

DENTAL CONSIDERATIONS

General:
• Monitor vital signs at every appointment because of cardiovascular side effects.
• Assess salivary flow as a factor in caries, periodontal disease, and candidiasis.
• Avoid dental light in patient's eyes; offer dark glasses for patient comfort.
• Consider semisupine chair position for patient comfort because of GI effects of disease.

Consultations:
• Physician should be informed if significant xerostomic side effects occur (e.g., increased caries, sore tongue, problems eating or swal-

bold italic = life-threatening conditions

lowing, difficulty wearing prosthesis) so that a medication change can be considered.

Teach patient/family:

When chronic dry mouth occurs, advise patient:

- To avoid mouth rinses with high alcohol content because of drying effects
- To use sugarless gum, frequent sips of water, or saliva substitutes
- To use daily home fluoride products for anticaries effect

meperidine HCl

(me-per'i-deen)

Demerol

✱ *International generic name:* pethidine

Drug class.: Synthetic narcotic analgesic

Controlled Substance Schedule II, Canada N

Action: Interacts with opioid receptors in the CNS to alter pain perception

Uses: Moderate-to-severe pain, preoperatively in sedation techniques

Dosage and routes:

Pain:

- *Adult:* PO/SC/IM 50-150 mg q3-4h prn; dose should be decreased if given IV
- *Child:* PO/SC/IM 1-1.75 mg/kg q4-6h prn, not to exceed adult dose

Preoperatively:

- *Adult:* IM/SC 50-100 mg 30-90 min before surgery; dose should be reduced if given IV
- *Child:* IM/SC 1-2.2 mg/kg 30-90 min before surgery

Available forms include: Inj SC/IM/IV 25, 50, 75, 100 mg/ml; tabs 50, 100 mg; syr 50 mg/5 ml

Side effects/adverse reactions:

▼ *ORAL:* Dry mouth

CNS: Drowsiness, dizziness, confusion, headache, sedation, euphoria, ***increased intracranial pressure***

CV: Palpitation, bradycardia, change in BP, tachycardia (IV)

GI: Nausea, vomiting, anorexia, constipation, cramps

RESP: ***Respiratory depression***

GU: Increased urinary output, dysuria, urinary retention

EENT: Tinnitus, blurred vision, miosis, diplopia, depressed corneal reflex

INTEG: Rash, urticaria, bruising, flushing, diaphoresis, pruritus

Contraindications: Hypersensitivity, addiction (narcotic), MAOIs, ritonavir, sibutramine

Precautions: Addictive personality, pregnancy category B, lactation, increased intracranial pressure, MI (acute), severe heart disease, respiratory depression, hepatic disease, renal disease, child <18 yr

Pharmacokinetics:

PO: Onset 15 min, peak 1 hr, duration 4-5 hr

SC/IM: Onset 10 min, peak 1 hr, duration 2-4 hr

IV: Onset 5 min, duration 2 hr

Half-life 3-4 hr; metabolized by liver (to active/inactive metabolites); excreted by kidneys; crosses placenta; excreted in breast milk; a toxic metabolite can result from regular use

Drug interactions of concern to dentistry:

- Increased effects with all CNS

depressants, neuromuscular blocking agents
• Contraindication: MAOIs, sibutramine
• Increased effects of anticholinergics
• Suspected increase in normeperidine levels: ritonavir
• Increased risk of hypotension: antihypertensive drugs

DENTAL CONSIDERATIONS

General:
• After supine positioning, have patient sit upright for at least 2 min to avoid orthostatic hypotension.
• Psychologic and physical dependence may occur with chronic administration.

Teach patient/family:
• To avoid mouth rinses with high alcohol content because of drying effects

mephobarbital

(me-foe-bar'bi-tal)

Mebaral

✤ Gemonil

Drug class.: Barbiturate anticonvulsant

Controlled Substance Schedule IV, Canada C

Action: A nonspecific depressant of the CNS; may enhance GABA activity in the brain

Uses: Generalized tonic-clonic (grand mal) or absence (petit mal) seizures, sedation

Dosage and routes:

Epilepsy:
• *Adult:* PO 400-600 mg/day or in divided doses
• *Child <5yr:* PO 16-32 tid or qid
• *Child >5yr:* PO 32-64 mg tid or qid

Sedation:
• *Adult:* PO 32-100 mg tid or qid
• *Childs:* PO 16-32 mg tid or qid

Available forms include: Tabs 32, 50, 100 mg

Side effects/adverse reactions:

CNS: Dizziness, headache, hangover, paradoxic stimulation, drowsiness, increased pain

CV: Hypotension, bradycardia

GI: Nausea, vomiting, epigastric pain

RESP: Wheezing, hyperpnea

HEMA: ***Thrombocytopenia, agranulocytosis, megaloblastic anemia***

EENT: Tinnitus, hearing loss

INTEG: Rash, urticaria, purpura, erythema multiforme, facial edema

ENDO: Hypoglycemia, hyponatremia, hypokalemia

Contraindications: Hypersensitivity to barbiturates, pregnancy category D

Precautions: Hepatic disease, renal disease, lactation, alcoholism, drug abuse, hyperthyroidism

Pharmacokinetics:

PO: Onset 20-60 min, duration 68 hr

REC: Onset slow, duration 4-6 hr, half-life 34 hr; metabolized by liver; excreted by kidneys

Drug interactions of concern to dentistry:
• Increased effects: alcohol, all CNS depressants
• Decreased effects of corticosteroids, doxycycline, carbamazepine

DENTAL CONSIDERATIONS

General:
• Determine type of epilepsy, seizure frequency, and quality of sei-

zure control. A stress reduction protocol may be required.

- Monitor vital signs at every appointment because of cardiovascular and respiratory side effects.
- Patients on chronic drug therapy may rarely have symptoms of blood dyscrasias, which can include infection, bleeding, and poor healing.
- Barbiturates induce liver microsomal enzymes, which alters the metabolism of other drugs.
- Avoid drugs that may lower seizure threshold (phenothiazines).
- Be sure patient is regularly taking medication.

Consultations:

- In a patient with symptoms of blood dyscrasias, request a medical consultation for blood studies and postpone dental treatment until normal values are reestablished.
- Medical consultation may be required to assess disease control and patient's ability to tolerate stress.

Teach patient/family:

- Importance of good oral hygiene to prevent soft tissue inflammation
- Caution to prevent injury when using oral hygiene aids
- To avoid mouth rinses with high alcohol content because of drying effects

---

mepivacaine HCl (local)

(me-piv'a-kane)

Carbocaine, Polocaine, Polocaine MPF

With vasoconstrictor: Carbocaine with Neo-Cobefrin, Polocaine/Levonordefrin

Drug class.: Amide local anesthetic

Action: Inhibits ion fluxes across membranes, particularly sodium transport across cell membrane; decreases rise of depolarization phase of action potential; blocks nerve action potential

Uses: Local dental anesthesia, nerve block, caudal anesthesia, epidural, pain relief, paracervical block, transvaginal block or infiltration

Dosage and routes:

Dental injection, infiltration, or conduction block:

- *Mepivacaine 3% without vasoconstrictor:* Max dose 6.6 mg/kg, or limit of 400 mg per dental appointment* for healthy patients; doses must be adjusted downward for medically compromised, debilitated, or elderly and for each individual patient. Always use lowest effective dose, a slow injection rate, and a careful aspiration technique.

Example calculations illustrating amount of drug administered per dental cartridge(s):

# of cartridges (1.8 ml)	mg of mepivacaine (3%)
1	54
2	108
4	216

*Maximum dose cited from *USP-DI,* ed 23, 2003, US Pharmacopeial Convention, Inc.; drug package inserts indicate max dose of 400 mg. Doses may differ from other published reference resources.

Mepivacaine 2% with levonordefrin 1:20,000: Continued availability of levonordefrin is in question. The same considerations for dose adjustment apply as previously indicated.

Example calculations illustrating amount of drug administered per dental cartridge(s):

# of cartridges (1.8 ml)	mg of mepivacaine (2%)	mg (μg) of vasoconstrictor (1:20,000)
1	36	0.090 (90)
2	72	0.180 (180)
3	108	0.270 (270)
5	180	0.450 (450)
8	288	0.720 (720)
10	360	0.900 (900)

Available forms include: Inj 1%, 1.5%, 2%, 3%; inj 2% with levonordefrin 1:20,000 (may not be available)

Side effects/adverse reactions:

▼ *ORAL:* Numbness, tingling, trismus

CNS: ***Convulsions, loss of consciousness,*** drowsiness, disorientation, tremors, shivering, anxiety, restlessness

CV: ***Myocardial depression, cardiac arrest, dysrhythmias,*** bradycardia, hypotension, hypertension, fetal bradycardia

GI: Nausea, vomiting

RESP: ***Status asthmaticus, respiratory arrest, anaphylaxis***

EENT: Blurred vision, tinnitus, pupil constriction

INTEG: Rash, urticaria, allergic reactions, edema, burning, skin discoloration at injection site, tissue necrosis

Contraindications: Hypersensitivity, cross-sensitivity among amide local anesthetics (rare), elderly, severe liver disease

Precautions: Elderly, severe drug allergies, pregnancy category C

Pharmacokinetics:

INJ: Onset 2-10 min, duration 20 min to 4 hr; metabolized by liver; excreted in urine (metabolites)

Drug interactions of concern to dentistry:

- CNS depressants: may see increased risk of CNS depression with all CNS depressants, especially in children and when larger doses are used
- Avoid placing dental cartridges in disinfectant solutions with heavy metals or surface-active agents; may see release of metal ions into local anesthetic solutions with tissue irritation following injection
- Avoid excessive exposure of dental cartridges to light or heat, which hastens deterioration of vasoconstrictor; observe for color change in local anesthetic solution
- Risk of cardiovascular side effects: rapid intravascular administration of local anesthetic containing vasoconstrictor, either alone or in patients taking tricyclic antidepressants, MAOIs, digitalis drugs, cocaine, phenothiazines, β-blockers, and in the presence of halogenated-hydrocarbon general anesthetics; use lowest effective vasoconstrictor dose and careful aspiration techniques
- Avoid use of vasoconstrictors in patients with uncontrolled hyperthyroidism, diabetes, angina, or hypertension; refer these patients for medical treatment before elective dental procedures

DENTAL CONSIDERATIONS

General:

- Drug is often used with a vasoconstrictor for increased duration of action.

• Monitor vital signs at every appointment because of cardiovascular and respiratory side effects.
• Lubricate dry lips before injection.

Teach patient/family:
• To use care to prevent injury while numbness exists and to refrain from chewing gum and eating following dental anesthesia
• To report any signs of infection, muscle pain, or fever to dentist when feeling returns
• To report any unusual soft tissue reactions

---

meprobamate

(me-proe-ba'mate)

Equanil, Miltown

✦ Apo-Meprobamate

Drug class.: Sedative-hypnotic, anxiolytic

Controlled Substance Schedule IV

Action: Nonspecific CNS depressant; acts in thalamus, limbic system, and spinal cord

Uses: Anxiety disorders

Dosage and routes:
• *Adult:* PO 1.2-1.6 g in 2-3 divided doses, not to exceed 2.4 g/day
• *Child 6-12 yr:* PO 100-200 mg bid-tid

Available forms include: Tabs 200, 400 mg

Side effects/adverse reactions:

▼ *ORAL:* Stomatitis, dry mouth

CNS: Dizziness, drowsiness, ***convulsions,*** headache

CV: ***Hyperthermia,*** hypotension, tachycardia, palpitation

GI: Nausea, vomiting, anorexia, diarrhea

HEMA: ***Thrombocytopenia, leukopenia, eosinophilia***

EENT: Blurred vision, tinnitus, mydriasis, slurred speech

INTEG: Urticaria, pruritus, maculopapular rash

Contraindications: Hypersensitivity, renal failure, porphyria, pregnancy category D, history of drug abuse or dependence

Precautions: Suicidal patients, severe depression, renal disease, hepatic disease, elderly

Pharmacokinetics:

PO: Onset 1 hr, half-life 6-16 hr; metabolized by liver; excreted by kidneys, in feces; crosses placenta, excreted in breast milk

Drug interactions of concern to dentistry
• Increased effects: CNS depressants, alcohol

DENTAL CONSIDERATIONS

General:
• Monitor vital signs at every appointment because of cardiovascular side effects.
• Patients on chronic drug therapy may rarely have symptoms of blood dyscrasias, which can include infection, bleeding, and poor healing.
• Assess salivary flow as a factor in caries, periodontal disease, and candidiasis.
• Avoid dental light in patient's eyes; offer dark glasses for patient comfort.
• Determine why the patient is taking the drug.
• Psychologic and physical dependence may occur with chronic administration.

Consultations:
• In a patient with symptoms of blood dyscrasias, request a medical

consultation for blood studies and postpone dental treatment until normal values are reestablished.
• Medical consultation may be required to assess disease control.
Teach patient/family:
• Importance of good oral hygiene to prevent soft tissue inflammation
• Caution to prevent injury when using oral hygiene aids
When chronic dry mouth occurs, advise patient:
• To avoid mouth rinses with high alcohol content because of drying effects
• To use sugarless gum, frequent sips of water, or saliva substitutes
• To use daily home fluoride products for anticaries effect

---

mercaptopurine (6-MP)

(mer-kap-toe-pyoor'een)
Purinethol

Drug class.: Antineoplastic-antimetabolite

Action: Inhibits purine metabolism at multiple sites, which inhibits DNA and RNA synthesis
Uses: Acute lymphatic leukemia, acute myelogenous leukemia
Dosage and routes:
• *Adult and child:* PO 2.5 mg/kg/day, not to exceed 5 mg/kg/day; maintenance 1.5-2.5 mg/kg/day
Available forms include: Tabs 50 mg
Side effects/adverse reactions:
▼ *ORAL:* Gingivitis, stomatitis
CNS: Fever, headache, weakness
GI: Nausea, vomiting, anorexia, diarrhea, ***hepatotoxicity (with high doses),*** jaundice, gastritis
HEMA: ***Thrombocytopenia, leukopenia, myelosuppression, anemia***
GU: ***Renal failure, oliguria, hematuria,*** crystalluria, hyperuricemia
INTEG: Rash, dry skin, urticaria
Contraindications: Patients with prior drug resistance, leukopenia (<2500/mm^3), thrombocytopenia (<100,000/mm^3), anemia, pregnancy category D
Precautions: Renal disease
Pharmacokinetics:
PO: Incompletely absorbed when taken orally; metabolized in liver; excreted in urine
Drug interactions of concern to dentistry:
• Increased risk of hepatotoxicity: hepatotoxic drugs

DENTAL CONSIDERATIONS
General:
• Patients on chronic drug therapy may rarely have symptoms of blood dyscrasias, which can include infection, bleeding, and poor healing.
• Avoid prescribing aspirin-containing products.
• Prophylactic antibiotics may be indicated to prevent infection if surgery or deep scaling is planned.
• Patients receiving chemotherapy may require palliative treatment for stomatitis.
Consultations:
• In a patient with symptoms of blood dyscrasias, request a medical consultation for blood studies and postpone dental treatment until normal values are reestablished.
Teach patient/family:
• Importance of good oral hygiene to prevent soft tissue inflammation
• Caution to prevent injury when using oral hygiene aids
• To avoid mouth rinses with high alcohol content

M

mesalamine

(me-sal'a-meen)

Asacol, Pentasa, Rowasa

🍁 Salofalk

Drug class.: Antiinflammatory

Action: Unknown, suggested to act topically in bowel to inhibit prostaglandin synthesis

Uses: Inflammatory bowel disease, ulcerative colitis, maintenance for remission of ulcerative colitis

Dosage and routes:

• *Adult:* PO TABS 800 mg tid for up to 6 wk; rec 500 mg bid for 3-6 wk; retention enema 4 g hs for 3-6 wk; CAPS 1 g qid up to 8 wk

Available forms include: Del rel tabs 400 mg; con rel caps 250 mg; supp 500 mg; rec susp 4 g/60 ml

Side effects/adverse reactions:

▼ *ORAL:* Lichenoid reactions

CNS: Headache, fever, dizziness, insomnia, asthenia, weakness, fatigue

GI: Cramps, gas, nausea, diarrhea, rectal pain, constipation

EENT: Sore throat

INTEG: Rash, itching, alopecia

SYST: *Flu, malaise,* back pain, peripheral edema, leg and joint pain, UTI

Contraindications: Hypersensitivity

Precautions: Pregnancy category B, renal disease, lactation, children, sulfite sensitivity

Pharmacokinetics:

REC: Half-life 1 hr, metabolite half-life 5-10 hr; primarily excreted in feces but some in urine as metabolites

DENTAL CONSIDERATIONS

General:

• Consider semisupine chair position for patient comfort because of GI effects of disease.

Consultations

• To reduce any potential risk of antibiotic-associated pseudomembranous colitis, a consultation is recommended before selecting an antibiotic for a dental infection.

mesoridazine besylate

(mez-oh-rid'a-zeen)

Serentil, Serentil Concentrate

Drug class.: Phenothiazine antipsychotic

Action: Blocks neurotransmission at dopaminergic synapses in the cerebral cortex, hypothalamus, and limbic system; exhibits strong peripheral α-adrenergic, cholinergic blocking action; mechanism for antipsychotic effects is unclear

Uses: Psychotic disorders, schizophrenia when inadequate response with other antipsychotic drugs

Dosage and routes:

Schizophrenia:

• *Adult:* PO 50 mg tid, optimum dose 100-400 mg/day; IM 25 mg, may repeat 0.5-1 hr; dosage range 25-200 mg/day

Behavior problems:

• *Adult:* PO 25 mg tid; optimum dose 75-300 mg/day

Alcoholism:

• *Adult:* PO 25 mg bid; optimum dose 50-200 mg/day

Schizoaffective disorders:

• *Adult:* PO 10 mg tid; optimum dose 30-150 mg/day

Available forms include: Tabs 10, 25, 50, 100 mg; conc 25 mg/ml; inj IM 25 mg/ml

Side effects/adverse reactions:

▼ *ORAL:* *Dry mouth,* lichenoid reaction

CNS: Extrapyramidal symptoms: pseudoparkinsonism, akathisia, dystonia, tardive dyskinesia, drowsiness, headache
CV: Orthostatic hypotension, ***cardiac arrest, torsades de pointes arrhythmias,*** hypertension, ECG changes, tachycardia
GI: Nausea, vomiting, anorexia, constipation, diarrhea, jaundice, weight gain
RESP: ***Laryngospasm, respiratory depression,*** dyspnea
HEMA: ***Anemia, leukopenia, leukocytosis, agranulocytosis***
GU: Urinary retention, urinary frequency, enuresis, impotence, amenorrhea, gynecomastia
EENT: Blurred vision, glaucoma
INTEG: Rash, photosensitivity, dermatitis

Contraindications: Hypersensitivity, circulatory collapse, liver damage, cerebral arteriosclerosis, coronary disease, severe hypertension/hypotension, blood dyscrasias, coma, brain damage, bone marrow depression, narrow-angle glaucoma, drugs known to prolong the QTc interval

Precautions: Pregnancy category C, lactation, seizure disorders, hypertension, hepatic disease, cardiac disease, prostatic hypertrophy, intestinal obstruction, respiratory conditions, dose-related prolongation of QTc interval

Pharmacokinetics:
PO: Onset erratic, peak 2 hr, duration 4-6 hr
IM: Onset 15-30 min, peak 30 min, duration 6-8 hr
Metabolized by liver, excreted in urine, crosses placenta, excreted in breast milk

Drug interactions of concern to dentistry:
- Increased sedation: other CNS depressants, alcohol, barbiturate anesthetics, opioid analgesics
- Hypotension, tachycardia: epinephrine
- Increased extrapyramidal effects: phenothiazines and related drugs (haloperidol, droperidol), metoclopramide
- Additive photosensitization: tetracyclines
- Increased anticholinergic effects: anticholinergics

DENTAL CONSIDERATIONS
General:
- Monitor vital signs at every appointment because of cardiovascular side effects.
- Patients on chronic drug therapy may rarely have symptoms of blood dyscrasias, which can include infection, bleeding, and poor healing.
- After supine positioning, have patient sit upright for at least 2 min before standing to avoid orthostatic hypotension.
- Assess salivary flow as a factor in caries, periodontal disease, and candidiasis.
- Avoid dental light in patient's eyes; offer dark glasses for patient comfort.
- Assess for presence of extrapyramidal motor symptoms, such as tardive dyskinesia and akathisia. Extrapyramidal motor activity may complicate dental treatment.
- Geriatric patients are more susceptible to drug effects; use lower dose.
- Use vasoconstrictors with caution, in low doses, and with careful aspiration. Avoid use of gingival retraction cord with epinephrine.

M

Consultations:

• In a patient with symptoms of blood dyscrasias, request a medical consultation for blood studies and postpone dental treatment until normal values are reestablished.

• Take precautions if dental surgery is anticipated and anesthesia is required.

• Refer to physician if signs of tardive dyskinesia or akathisia are present.

• Physician should be informed if significant xerostomic side effects occur (e.g., increased caries, sore tongue, problems eating or swallowing, difficulty wearing prosthesis) so that a medication change can be considered.

Teach patient/family:

• Importance of good oral hygiene to prevent soft tissue inflammation

• Caution to prevent injury when using oral hygiene aids

• To use electric toothbrush if patient has difficulty holding conventional devices

When chronic dry mouth occurs, advise patient:

• To avoid mouth rinses with high alcohol content because of drying effects

• To use sugarless gum, frequent sips of water, or saliva substitutes

• To use daily home fluoride products for anticaries effect

---

metaproterenol sulfate

(met-a-proe-ter'e-nol)
Alupent

Drug class.: Selective β_2-agonist

Action: Relaxes bronchial smooth muscle by direct action on β_2-adrenergic receptors

Uses: Bronchial asthma, bronchospasm

Dosage and routes:

• *Adult and child >12 yr:* Inh 2-3 puffs; may repeat q3-4h, not to exceed 12 puffs/day

• *Child <12 yr:* INH 1-3 puffs q3-4h, not to exceed 12 puffs/day

Available forms include: Aerosol 0.65 mg/dose; sol nebuliz 0.4, 0.6%, 5%

Side effects/adverse reactions:

▼ *ORAL:* Dry mouth, taste changes

CNS: Tremors, anxiety, insomnia, headache, dizziness, stimulation

CV: ***Cardiac arrest,*** palpitation, tachycardia, hypertension

GI: Nausea

RESP: Cough, throat dryness/irritation, nasal congestion

Contraindications: Hypersensitivity to sympathomimetics, narrow-angle glaucoma

Precautions: Pregnancy category C, cardiac disorders, hyperthyroidism, diabetes mellitus, prostatic hypertrophy

Pharmacokinetics:

PO: Onset 15-30 min, peak 1 hr, duration 4 hr, excreted in urine as metabolites

Drug interactions of concern to dentistry:

• Increased effects of both drugs: other sympathomimetics, CNS stimulants

• Increased dysrhythmias: halogenated hydrocarbon anesthetics

DENTAL CONSIDERATIONS

General:

• Assess salivary flow as a factor in caries, periodontal disease, and candidiasis.

- Consider semisupine chair position for patients with respiratory disease.
- Short appointments and a stress reduction protocol may be required for anxious patients.
- Be aware that aspirin or sulfite preservatives in vasoconstrictor-containing products can exacerbate asthma.
- Acute asthmatic episodes may be precipitated in the dental office. Sympathomimetic inhalants should be available for emergency use.

Consultations:

- Medical consultation may be required to assess disease control and patient's ability to tolerate stress.

Teach patient/family:

- For inhalation dosage forms: rinse mouth with water after each dose to prevent dryness

When chronic dry mouth occurs, advise patient:

- To avoid mouth rinses with high alcohol content because of drying effects
- To use sugarless gum, frequent sips of water, or saliva substitutes
- To use daily home fluoride products for anticaries effect

---

metaxalone

(me-tax'a-lone)

Skelaxin

Drug class.: Muscle relaxant

Action: Mechanism of action unknown; may cause generalized CNS depression

Uses: Adjunct to rest, physical therapy, and other measures for relief of discomfort associated with acute, painful musculoskeletal conditions

Dosage and routes:

- *Adult and child >12 yr:* PO 800 mg tid to qid

Available forms include: Tabs 400, 800

Side effects/adverse reactions:

CNS: Drowsiness, dizziness, headache, nervousness, irritability

GI: Nausea, vomiting, upset stomach, jaundice

HEMA: Leukopenia, ***hemolytic anemia***

INTEG: Rash, pruritus

Contraindications: Hypersensitivity, patient with tendency to drug-induced hemolytic or other anemias, pregnancy, renal or hepatic impairment

Precautions: Preexisting hepatic impairment, lactation, children <12 yr, alcohol use

Pharmacokinetics:

PO: Onset ~1 hr, peak effect ~2 hr, duration ~4-6 hr; metabolites excreted in urine

Drug interactions of concern to dentistry:

- No data reported; however, this drug does cause a nonspecific CNS depression: monitor patients if other CNS depressants are used

DENTAL CONSIDERATIONS

General:

- Determine why patient is taking the drug.
- Patients on chronic drug therapy may rarely have symptoms of blood dyscrasias, which can include infection, bleeding, and poor healing.
- Consider semisupine chair position for patient comfort if GI side effects occur.

Consultations:

- In a patient with symptoms of blood dyscrasias, request a medical

consultation for blood studies and postpone treatment until normal values are reestablished.

Teach patient/family:

• Importance of updating health and drug history if physician makes any changes in evaluation or drug regimens

metformin HCl

(met-for'min)

Glucophage, Glucophage XR

♣ Novo-Metformin, Apo-Metformin, Gen-Metformin, Glycon, Nu-Metformin

Drug class.: Oral hypoglycemic, biguanide derivative

Action: Exact mechanism unknown, requires insulin secretion to function properly; associated with a decrease in hepatic glucose production and a decrease in intestinal glucose absorption; improves insulin sensitivity through an increase in peripheral glucose uptake and utilization

Uses: Type 2 diabetes mellitus

Dosage and routes:

• *Adult:* Must be individualized; PO initial 500 mg bid with morning and evening meals, increase dose by 500 mg at weekly intervals, daily limit 2500 mg; or 850 mg once daily with morning meal, increase dose in increments of 850 mg every other week, administered in divided doses, max 2550 mg/day; EXT REL initial dose 500 mg/day with dinner, increase by 500 mg/day each week as needed up to 2000 mg/day

Maintenance dose:

• *Adult:* PO 500 or 850 mg bid or tid taken with meals; EXT REL 500-2000 mg once daily

Available forms include: Tabs 500, 850, 1000 mg; ext rel tabs 500 mg

Side effects/adverse reactions:

▼ *ORAL:* Unpleasant taste, metallic taste

GI: Diarrhea, nausea, vomiting, abdominal bloating, flatulence

HEMA: ***Megaloblastic anemia,*** lower vitamin B_{12} levels

ENDO: Hypoglycemia

MISC: ***Lactic acidosis*** (incidence rare)

Contraindications: Hypersensitivity, renal or hepatic disease, patients receiving radiologic examination with parenteral iodinated contrast media, diabetic ketoacidosis, acute or chronic metabolic acidosis, conditions requiring close blood glucose control; CHF, especially those at risk for hypoperfusion and hypoxemia

Precautions: Elderly, pregnancy category B, lactation, children, interferes with vitamin B_{12} absorption; avoid alcohol use

Pharmacokinetics:

PO: Slow absorption, peak concentrations 2-2.5 hr; little or no protein binding; not metabolized; excreted mainly in urine

Drug interactions of concern to dentistry:

• None reported

DENTAL CONSIDERATIONS

General:

• Short appointments and a stress reduction protocol may be required for anxious patients.

• Consider semisupine chair position for patient comfort if GI side effects occur.

• Question patient about self-monitoring of drug's antidiabetic effect, including blood glucose values or finger-stick records.

• Ensure that patient is following prescribed diet and regularly takes medication.
• Patients with diabetes may be more susceptible to infection and have delayed wound healing.
• Place on frequent recall to evaluate healing response.

Consultations:

• Medical consultation may be required to assess disease control and patient's ability to tolerate stress.
• Notify physician immediately if symptoms of lactic acidosis are observed (myalgia, respiratory distress, weakness, diarrhea, malaise, muscle cramps, somnolence).
• Medical consultation may include data from patient's blood glucose monitoring, including glycosylated hemoglobin or HbA_{1c} testing.
• Oral and maxillofacial surgical procedures associated with significantly restricted food intake require a medical consultation and temporary cessation of metformin use.

Teach patient/family:

• Importance of good oral hygiene to prevent soft tissue inflammation
• That alteration of taste may be due to drug side effects

methadone HCl

(meth'a-done)

Dolophine, Methadose

Drug class.: Synthetic narcotic analgesic

Controlled Substance Schedule II, Canada N

Action: Interacts with opioid receptors in the CNS to alter pain perception

Uses: Severe pain, opioid withdrawal program

Dosage and routes:

Pain:

• *Adult:* PO/SC/IM 2.5-10 mg q4-12h prn

Narcotic withdrawal:

• *Adult:* PO 15-40 mg/day individualized initially, then 20-120 mg/day titrated to patient response

Available forms include: Inj SC/IM 10 mg/ml; tabs 5, 10 mg; oral sol 5, 10 mg/5 ml; dispersible tabs 40 mg

Side effects/adverse reactions:

▼ *ORAL:* Dry mouth

CNS: Drowsiness, dizziness, confusion, headache, sedation, euphoria

CV: Palpitation, bradycardia, change in BP

GI: Nausea, vomiting, anorexia, constipation, cramps, biliary tract spasm

RESP: ***Respiratory depression***

GU: Increased urinary output, dysuria, urinary retention

EENT: Tinnitus, blurred vision, miosis, diplopia

INTEG: Rash, urticaria, bruising, flushing, diaphoresis, pruritus

Contraindications: Hypersensitivity, addiction (narcotic), MAOIs

Precautions: Addictive personality, pregnancy category B, lactation, increased intracranial pressure, MI (acute), severe heart disease, respiratory depression, hepatic disease, renal disease, child <18 yr

Pharmacokinetics:

PO: Onset 30-60 min, duration 6-8 hr, cumulative 22-48 hr

SC/IM: Onset 10-20 min, peak 1 hr, duration 6-8 hr, cumulative 22-48 hr

Half-life 1-1.5 days; 90% bound to plasma proteins; metabolized by

M

liver; excreted by kidneys; crosses placenta; excreted in breast milk

Drug interactions of concern to dentistry:

- Increased CNS depression: alcohol, narcotics, sedative-hypnotics, skeletal muscle relaxants, benzodiazepines, and other CNS depressants
- Increased effects of anticholinergics

DENTAL CONSIDERATIONS

General:

- Assess salivary flow as a factor in caries, periodontal disease, and candidiasis.
- Psychologic and physical dependence may occur with chronic administration.
- Determine why the patient is taking the drug.
- Be aware of the needs of patients who are in recovery from substance abuse.
- In an opioid-dependent patient, NSAIDs are the drugs of choice for posttreatment pain control.

Consultations:

- Patients in the methadone maintenance program should not receive additional opioids or other controlled substances without a consultation.

Teach patient/family:

When chronic dry mouth occurs, advise patient:

- To avoid mouth rinses with high alcohol content because of drying effects
- To use sugarless gum, frequent sips of water, or saliva substitutes
- To use daily home fluoride products for anticaries effect

methamphetamine HCl

(meth-am-fet'a-meen)

Desoxyn, Desoxyn Gradumet

Drug class.: Amphetamine

Controlled Substance Schedule II

Action: A sympathomimetic amine that increases release of norepinephrine and dopamine in the CNS; see increase in mental alertness, motor activity, appetite suppression; in ADHD see improvement in attention behavior and reduced motor restlessness; also peripheral effects on α- and β-adrenergic receptors

Uses: Exogenous obesity, minimal brain dysfunction, attention deficit disorder with hyperactivity

Dosage and routes:

Attention deficit disorder:

- *Child >6 yr:* PO 2.5-5 mg qd or bid increasing by 5 mg/wk up to 25 mg/day

Obesity:

- *Adult:* PO 2.5-5 mg, 30 min ac

Available forms include: Tabs 5 mg

Side effects/adverse reactions:

▼ *ORAL:* Dry mouth, unpleasant taste

CNS: Hyperactivity, insomnia, restlessness, talkativeness, dizziness, headache, chills, stimulation, dysphoria, irritability, aggressiveness, tremor

CV: Palpitation, tachycardia, hypertension, decreased heart rate, dysrhythmia

GI: Anorexia, diarrhea, constipation, weight loss, cramps

GU: Impotence, change in libido

INTEG: Urticaria

Contraindications: Hypersensi-

tivity to sympathomimetic amines, hyperthyroidism, hypertension, glaucoma hypertrophy, severe arteriosclerosis, drug abuse, cardiovascular disease, anxiety, concurrent use with MAOIs or within 14 days of discontinuing MAOIs

Precautions: Gilles de la Tourette's syndrome, pregnancy category C, lactation, child <6 yr

Pharmacokinetics:

PO: Duration 3-6 hr; metabolized by liver; excreted by kidneys; crosses blood-brain barrier

Drug interactions of concern to dentistry:

- Increased effect of methamphetamine: CNS stimulants, sympathomimetics
- Decreased effects of both drugs: haloperidol, sedative-hypnotics
- Ventricular dysrhythmia: inhalation anesthetics

DENTAL CONSIDERATIONS

General:

- Assess salivary flow as a factor in caries, periodontal disease, and candidiasis.

Consultations:

- Physician should be informed if significant xerostomic side effects occur (e.g., increased caries, sore tongue, problems eating or swallowing, difficulty wearing prosthesis) so that a medication change can be considered.

Teach patient/family:

When chronic dry mouth occurs, advise patient:

- To avoid mouth rinses with high alcohol content because of drying effects
- To use sugarless gum, frequent sips of water, or saliva substitutes
- To use daily home fluoride products for anticaries effect

methazolamide

(meth-a-zoe'la-mide)

Neptazane, GluacTabs

Drug class.: Carbonic anhydrase inhibitor

Action: Decreases production of aqueous humor in eye, which lowers intraocular pressure

Uses: Open-angle glaucoma or preoperatively in narrow-angle glaucoma; can be used with miotic, osmotic agents

Dosage and routes:

- *Adult:* PO initial dose 100-200 mg, then 100 mg q12h; maintenance dose PO 50-100 mg qd/tid

Available forms include: Tabs 25, 50 mg

Side effects/adverse reactions:

▼ *ORAL:* Taste alteration (tingling, burning, numbness has occurred with similar drugs)

CNS: Drowsiness, paresthesia, ***convulsions,*** stimulation, fatigue, anxiety, depression, headache, dizziness, confusion, sedation, nervousness

GI: Nausea, vomiting, anorexia, constipation, diarrhea, melena, weight loss, hepatic insufficiency

HEMA: ***Aplastic anemia, hemolytic anemia, leukopenia, agranulocytosis, thrombocytopenia, purpura, pancytopenia***

GU: Frequency, hypokalemia, ***glucosuria, hematuria,*** dysuria, polyuria, uremia

EENT: Myopia, tinnitus

INTEG: Rash, ***Stevens-Johnson syndrome,*** pruritus, urticaria, fever, photosensitivity

ENDO: Hyperglycemia

Contraindications: Hypersensitivity to sulfonamides or thiazide diuretics, severe renal disease, severe hepatic disease, electrolyte imbalances (hyponatremia, hypokalemia), hyperchloremic acidosis, Addison's disease, COPD

Precautions: Hypercalciuria, pregnancy category C, lactation, children

Pharmacokinetics:

PO: Slow absorption, onset 2-4 hr, peak 6-8 hr, duration 10-18 hr, half-life 14 hr; excreted in urine; crosses placenta

Drug interactions of concern to dentistry:

- Exacerbation of glaucoma: anticholinergics
- Toxicity: salicylates in large doses

DENTAL CONSIDERATIONS

General:

- Patients on chronic drug therapy may rarely have symptoms of blood dyscrasias, which can include infection, bleeding, and poor healing.
- Avoid prescribing aspirin-containing products.
- Consider semisupine chair position for patient comfort if GI side effects occur.
- Avoid dental light in patient's eyes; offer dark glasses for patient comfort.
- Protect patient's eyes from accidental spatter during dental treatment.

Consultations:

- In a patient with symptoms of blood dyscrasias, request a medical consultation for blood studies and postpone dental treatment until normal values are reestablished.

Teach patient/family:

- Importance of good oral hygiene to prevent soft tissue inflammation
- Caution to prevent trauma when using oral hygiene aids

methenamine hippurate/ methenamine mandelamine

(meth-en'a-meen) (hip'yoo-rate)

Methenamine hippurate: Hiprex, Urex

♣ Hip-Rex

Methenamine mandelate (generic)

Drug class.: Urinary antiinfective

Action: In acid urine, it is hydrolyzed to ammonia and formaldehyde, which are bactericidal

Uses: Prophylaxis and treatment of uncomplicated UTIs

Dosage and routes:

- *Adult and child >12 yr:* PO 1 g q12h, max 4 g/24 hr
- *Child 6-12 yr:* PO 500 mg-1 g q12h

Available forms include: Tabs 1 g; oral susp 500 mg/5 ml; enteric-coated tabs 500 mg, 1 g

Side effects/adverse reactions:

▼ *ORAL:* Stomatitis

CNS: Headache

GI: Nausea, vomiting, anorexia, abdominal pain, increased AST/ALT

GU: ***Albuminuria, hematuria,*** dysuria, bladder irritation, crystalluria

EENT: Tinnitus

INTEG: Pruritus, rash, urticaria

Contraindications: Hypersensitivity, severe dehydration, renal insufficiency

Precautions: Renal disease, pregnancy category C, lactation

Pharmacokinetics:
PO: Excreted in urine, half-life 4 hr
Drug interactions of concern to dentistry:
• None
DENTAL CONSIDERATIONS
General:
• Determine why the patient is taking the drug.
• Antibiotics for dental infections are not contraindicated, but a physician notification may be advisable.
• Palliative treatment may be required for oral side effects.
• Consider semisupine chair position for patient comfort because of GI effects of drug.

methimazole

(meth-im'a-zole)
Tapazole
Drug class.: Thyroid hormone antagonist

Action: Inhibits synthesis of thyroid hormones by decreasing iodine use in the manufacture of thyroglobulin and iodothyronine; does not affect already formed hormones
Uses: Hyperthyroidism
Dosage and routes:
• *Adult:* PO 15-60 mg/day in divided doses depending on severity of condition; continue until euthyroid; maintenance 5-15 mg qd or in divided doses
• *Child:* PO 0.4 mg/kg/day in divided doses q12h; continue until euthyroid; maintenance dose 0.2 mg/kg/day in one dose or divided doses q12h
Available forms include: Tabs 5, 10 mg
Side effects/adverse reactions:
▼ *ORAL:* Taste alteration
CNS: Drowsiness, headache, vertigo, fever, paresthesias, neuritis
GI: Nausea, diarrhea, vomiting, ***jaundice, hepatitis***
HEMA: ***Agranulocytosis, leukopenia, thrombocytopenia, hypothrombinemia, lymphadenopathy, aplastic anemia,*** bleeding, vasculitis
GU: ***Nephritis***
INTEG: Rash, urticaria, pruritus, alopecia, hyperpigmentation, lupus-like syndrome
ENDO: Enlarged thyroid
MS: Myalgia, arthralgia, nocturnal muscle cramps
Contraindications: Hypersensitivity, pregnancy category D (third trimester), lactation
Precautions: Infection, bone marrow depression, hepatic disease, pregnancy (first or second trimester)
Pharmacokinetics:
PO: Onset 30-40 min, duration 2-4 hr, half-life 1-2 hr; excreted in urine, bile, breast milk; crosses placenta
Drug interactions of concern to dentistry:
• Increased CV side effects in uncontrolled patients: anticholinergics and sympathomimetics
• Patients with uncontrolled hyperthyroidism are at risk when vasoconstrictors are used
• Patients with uncontrolled hypothyroidism may be more responsive to CNS depressants
DENTAL CONSIDERATIONS
General:
• Monitor vital signs at every appointment because of cardiovascular effects of disease.

M

• Patients on chronic drug therapy may rarely have symptoms of blood dyscrasias; examine for evidence of oral manifestations of blood dyscrasias (infection, bleeding, poor healing).
• Evaluate for clotting ability during periodontal instrumentation.
• Evaluate for control of hyperthyroidism. Patients with uncontrolled condition should not be treated in the dental office until thyroid values are normalized.
• Patients with uncontrolled condition should be referred for medical evaluation and treatment.

Consultations:
• Medical consultation may be required to assess disease control.
• Medical consultation for blood studies (CBC); leukopenic or thrombocytopenic side effects may result in infection, delayed healing, and excessive bleeding. Postpone elective dental treatment until normal values are maintained.

Teach patient/family:
• Importance of good oral hygiene to prevent soft tissue inflammation
• Caution in use of oral hygiene aids to prevent injury

---

methocarbamol

(meth-oh-kar'ba-mole)
Robaxin, Robaxin 750

Drug class.: Skeletal muscle relaxant

Action: Depresses multisynaptic pathways in the spinal cord

Uses: Adjunct for relief in painful musculoskeletal conditions

Dosage and routes:
• *Adult:* PO 1.5 g/day × 2-3 days, then 1 g qid or 750 mg q4h; IM 500 mg in each gluteal region, may repeat q8h; IV bol 1-3 g/day at 3 ml/min; IV inf 1 g/250 ml D_5W or NS, not to exceed 3 g/day

Available forms include: Tabs 500, 750 mg; inj IM/IV 100 mg/ml

Side effects/adverse reactions:
▼ *ORAL:* Metallic taste
CNS: Dizziness, weakness, drowsiness, ***seizures,*** headache, tremor, depression, insomnia
CV: Postural hypotension, bradycardia
GI: Nausea, vomiting, hiccups, anorexia
HEMA: Hemolysis, increased hemoglobin (IV only)
GU: Brown, black, or green urine
EENT: Diplopia, temporary loss of vision, blurred vision, nystagmus
INTEG: Rash, pruritus, fever, facial flushing, urticaria

Contraindications: Hypersensitivity, child <12 yr, intermittent porphyria

Precautions: Renal disease, hepatic disease, addictive personalities, pregnancy category C, myasthenia gravis, epilepsy

Pharmacokinetics:
PO: Onset 0.5 hr, peak 1-2 hr, half-life 1-2 hr; metabolized in liver; excreted in urine (unchanged); crosses placenta

Drug interactions of concern to dentistry:
• Increased CNS depression: alcohol, narcotics, sedative-hypnotics

DENTAL CONSIDERATIONS

General:
• Determine why the patient is taking the drug.
• Consider semisupine chair position if back is involved.

Teach patient/family:
• Importance of good oral hygiene to prevent soft tissue inflammation
• Caution to prevent injury when using oral hygiene aids
• To avoid mouth rinses with high alcohol content because of drying effects

methotrexate/ methotrexate sodium (amethopterin, MTX)

(meth-oh-trex'ate)

Rheumatrex Dose Pak, Trexall

Drug class.: Folic acid antagonist, antineoplastic

Action: Inhibits an enzyme that reduces folic acid, which is needed for nucleic acid synthesis in all cells

Uses: Acute lymphocytic leukemia, non-Hodgkins lymphoma; in combination with other drugs for breast, lung, head, neck cancer; lymphosarcoma; psoriasis; gestational choriocarcinoma; hydatidiform mole; rheumatoid arthritis

Dosage and routes:

Leukemia:
• *Adult and child:* PO 3.3 mg/m^2/day, maintenance 30 mg/m^2/day 2× weekly; IV 2.5 mg/kg q2wk; given in combination with prednisone

Choriocarcinoma:
• *Adult and child:* IM/PO 15-30 mg × 5 days, may repeat 3-5 × with rest periods of 1 wk or more; constantly reevaluate response

Severe, recalcitrant, or disabling psoriasis:
• *Adult:* PO/IV/IM 10 mg to 25 mg/weekly single dose or PO 2.5 mg q12h × 3 doses; limit 30 mg/wk

Rheumatoid arthritis:
• *Adult:* PO initial 7.5 mg/wk as a single dose or 2.5 mg q12h × 3 doses

Available forms include: Tabs 2.5, 5, 7.5, 10, 15 mg; powder for inj IV 20mg, 1 g

Side effects/adverse reactions:

▼ *ORAL: Ulcerative stomatitis, gingivitis,* bleeding

CNS: ***Convulsions,*** dizziness, headache, confusion, hemiparesis, malaise, fatigue, chills, fever

GI: Nausea, vomiting, anorexia, diarrhea, ***hepatotoxicity, GI hemorrhage,*** abdominal pain, cramps, ulcer, gastritis, hematemesis

HEMA: ***Leukopenia, thrombocytopenia, myelosuppression, aplastic anemia***

GU: ***Renal failure, hematuria, azotemia, uric acid nephropathy,*** urinary retention, menstrual irregularities, defective spermatogenesis

INTEG: Rash, alopecia, dry skin, urticaria, photosensitivity, folliculitis, vasculitis, petechiae, ecchymosis, acne, alopecia, painful plaque lesions in psoriasis, potentially life-threatening skin reactions

MISC: Rare reports of bone and soft tissue necrosis after radiation therapy; potentially fatal opportunistic infections, tumor lysis syndrome

Contraindications: Hypersensitivity, leukopenia (<2500/mm^3), thrombocytopenia (<100,000/mm^3), anemia, psoriasis or rheumatoid arthritis when patient is immunodeficient or has severe blood dyscrasias, severe renal/hepatic disease, pregnancy category D

Precautions: Renal disease, lactation, drugs with potential for hepatotoxicity, monitor for hepatic toxicity, methotrexate-induced lung disease

Pharmacokinetics:

PO: Readily absorbed when taken orally, peak 1-4 hr

IV/IM: Peak 0.5-2 hr

50% plasma protein bound; not metabolized; excreted in urine (unchanged); crosses placenta, blood-brain barrier

Drug interactions of concern to dentistry:

• Increased toxicity: aspirin, alcohol, NSAIDs

• Possible fatal interactions: NSAIDs, high-dose IV methotrexate

• Suspected increase in methotrexate toxicity: amoxicillin, tetracycline, doxycycline

DENTAL CONSIDERATIONS

General:

• Patients on chronic drug therapy may rarely have symptoms of blood dyscrasias, which can include infection, bleeding, and poor healing.

• Avoid prescribing aspirin- or NSAID-containing products.

• Place on frequent recall because of increased risk for infection and to evaluate healing response.

• Determine why the patient is taking the drug.

• Palliative treatment may be needed if stomatitis or oral desquamative lesions occur.

Consultations:

• In a patient with symptoms of blood dyscrasias, request a medical consultation for blood studies and postpone dental treatment until normal values are reestablished.

• Medical consultation may be required to assess disease control.

Teach patient/family:

• Importance of good oral hygiene to prevent soft tissue inflammation

• Caution to prevent injury when using oral hygiene aids

• About palliative therapy for sore mouth

• To avoid mouth rinses with high alcohol content because of drying effects

methsuximide

(meth-sux'i-mide)

Celontin

Drug class.: Anticonvulsant

Action: Inhibits spike wave formation in absence seizures (petit mal); decreases amplitude, frequency, duration, spread of discharge in minor motor seizures

Uses: Refractory absence seizures (petit mal)

Dosage and routes:

• *Adult and child:* PO 300 mg/day; may increase by 300 mg/wk, not to exceed 1.2 g/day in divided doses

Available forms include: Half-strength caps 150 mg; caps 300 mg

Side effects/adverse reactions:

ORAL: Gingival overgrowth, glossitis, ulcers (Stevens-Johnson syndrome)

CNS: Drowsiness, dizziness, fatigue, euphoria, lethargy, irritability, depression, insomnia, anxiety, aggressiveness, ataxia, headache, confusion

GI: Nausea, vomiting, heartburn, anorexia, diarrhea, abdominal pain, cramps, constipation

HEMA: ***Agranulocytosis, aplastic anemia, thrombocytopenia, leukocytosis, eosinophilia, pancytopenia***

GU: ***Hematuria, renal damage,*** vaginal bleeding
EENT: Myopia, blurred vision, photophobia
INTEG: ***Stevens-Johnson syndrome,*** urticaria, pruritic erythema, hirsutism
Contraindications: Hypersensitivity to succinimide derivatives
Precautions: Hepatic disease, renal disease, pregnancy category C, lactation
Pharmacokinetics:
PO: Onset 15-30 min, peak 1-2 hr, duration 4-6 hr
REC: Onset slow, duration 4-6 hr
Half-life 2.6-4 hr; metabolized by liver; excreted by kidneys
Drug interactions of concern to dentistry:
• Enhanced CNS depression: alcohol, CNS depressants
• Decreased effects: phenothiazines, thioxanthenes, barbiturates
• Changes in seizure pattern, frequency: haloperidol

DENTAL CONSIDERATIONS
General:
• Patients on chronic drug therapy may rarely have symptoms of blood dyscrasias, which can include infection, bleeding, and poor healing.
• Avoid dental light in patient's eyes; offer dark glasses for patient comfort.
• Determine type of epilepsy, seizure frequency, and quality of seizure control. A stress reduction protocol may be required.
• Place on frequent recall to monitor gingival condition.
Consultations:
• In a patient with symptoms of blood dyscrasias, request a medical consultation for blood studies and postpone dental treatment until normal values are reestablished.
• Take precautions if dental surgery is anticipated and anesthesia is required.
• Medical consultation may be required to assess disease control.
Teach patient/family:
• Importance of good oral hygiene to prevent soft tissue inflammation
• Caution to prevent injury when using oral hygiene aids
• To avoid mouth rinses with high alcohol content if oral side effects occur

---

methyldopa/ methyldopate

(meth-il-doe'pa)
generic only (U.S.)
♣ Apo-Methyldopa, Dopamet, Novomedopa, Nu-Medopa
Drug class.: Centrally acting antihypertensive

Action: Stimulates central inhibitory α-adrenergic receptors or acts as false transmitter (α-methylnorepinephrine) resulting in reduction of arterial pressure through action on CNS α-adrenergic receptors
Uses: Hypertension
Dosage and routes:
• *Adult:* PO 250 mg bid or tid, then adjusted q2d as needed, 0.5-3 g qd in 2-4 divided doses (maintenance), not to exceed 3 g/day; IV 250-500 mg in 100 ml D_5W q6h, run over 30-60 min, not to exceed 1 g q6h
• *Child:* PO 10 mg/kg/day in 2-4 divided doses, not to exceed 65 mg/kg or 3 g/day, whichever is

less; IV 20-40 mg/kg/day in 4 divided doses, not to exceed 65 mg/kg

Available forms include: Tabs 125, 250, 500 mg; inj IV 50 mg/ml

Side effects/adverse reactions:

▼ *ORAL: Dry mouth,* bleeding, lichenoid lesions

CNS: Drowsiness, weakness, dizziness, sedation, headache, depression, psychosis

CV: Bradycardia, myocarditis, orthostatic hypotension, angina, edema, weight gain

GI: Nausea, vomiting, diarrhea, constipation, hepatic dysfunction

HEMA: ***Leukopenia, thrombocytopenia,*** anemia, positive Coombs' test

GU: Impotence, failure to ejaculate

EENT: Nasal congestion, eczema

INTEG: Lupus-like syndrome

Contraindications: Active hepatic disease, hypersensitivity, blood dyscrasias, concurrently with or within 14 days of discontinuing MAOI drugs

Precautions: Pregnancy category C, liver disease, eclampsia, severe cardiac disease

Pharmacokinetics:

PO: Peak 4-6 hr, duration 12-24 hr

IV: Peak 2 hr, duration 10-16 hr

Metabolized by liver, excreted in urine

Drug interactions of concern to dentistry:

- Decreased effects: indomethacin and other NSAIDs
- Increased pressor response: epinephrine and other sympathomimetics
- Increased sedation: haloperidol, alcohol, CNS depressants
- Increased hypotensive action of general anesthetics

DENTAL CONSIDERATIONS

General:

- Monitor vital signs at every appointment because of cardiovascular side effects.
- Patients on chronic drug therapy may rarely have symptoms of blood dyscrasias, which can include infection, bleeding, and poor healing.
- Assess salivary flow as a factor in caries, periodontal disease, and candidiasis.
- Limit use of sodium-containing products such as saline IV fluids for patients with a dietary salt restriction.
- After supine positioning, have patient sit upright for at least 2 min before standing to avoid orthostatic hypotension.
- Stress from dental procedures may compromise cardiovascular function; determine patient risk.

Consultations:

- In a patient with symptoms of blood dyscrasias, request a medical consultation for blood studies and postpone dental treatment until normal values are reestablished.
- Medical consultation may be required to assess disease control and stress tolerance.

Teach patient/family:

- Importance of good oral hygiene to prevent soft tissue inflammation
- Caution to prevent injury when using oral hygiene aids

When chronic dry mouth occurs, advise patient:

- To avoid mouth rinses with high alcohol content because of drying effects
- To use sugarless gum, frequent sips of water, or saliva substitutes
- To use daily home fluoride products for anticaries effect

methylphenidate HCl

(meth-il-fen'i-date)

Concerta, Metadate CD, Metadate ER, Methylin, Methylin ER, Ritalin, Ritalin LA, Ritalin SR

♣ PMS-Methylphenidate, Riphenidate

Drug class.: CNS stimulant, related to amphetamines

Controlled Substance Schedule II, Canada C

Action: Blocks the reuptake and increases release of norepinephrine, dopamine in CNS; exact mode of action unknown in ADHD

Uses: Attention deficit disorder with hyperactivity, narcolepsy

Dosage and routes:

Attention deficit disorder:

- *Adult:* PO 20-30 mg/day in divided doses bid or tid, 45 min before meals
- *Child >6 yr:* 5 mg before breakfast and lunch, increasing by 5-10 mg/wk, not to exceed 60 mg/day; long acting form 18-36 mg qd in AM

Narcolepsy:

- *Adult:* PO 10 mg bid-tid, 30-45 min before meals; may increase up to 40-50 mg/day

Available forms include: Tabs 5, 10, 20 mg; ext rel tabs 10, 18, 20, 27, 36, 54 mg; chew tabs 2.5, 5, 10 mg; ext rel caps 10, 20, 30, 40 mg; sus rel tab 20 mg

Side effects/adverse reactions:

▼ *ORAL:* Dry mouth

CNS: Hyperactivity, insomnia, restlessness, talkativeness, dizziness, headache, akathisia, dyskinesia, Gilles de la Tourette's syndrome

CV: Palpitation, tachycardia, BP changes, angina, dysrhythmias

GI: Nausea, anorexia, diarrhea, constipation, weight loss, abdominal pain

HEMA: ***Thrombocytopenia***

GU: ***Uremia***

INTEG: ***Exfoliative dermatitis,*** urticaria, rash, erythema multiforme

ENDO: Growth retardation

Contraindications: Hypersensitivity, anxiety, history of Gilles de la Tourette's syndrome, history of seizures, concurrent use with or within 14 days of discontinuing MAOI drugs

Precautions: Hypertension, depression, pregnancy category C, seizures, lactation, drug abuse

Pharmacokinetics:

PO: Onset 0.5-1 hr, duration 4-6 hr; metabolized by liver; excreted by kidneys

Drug interactions of concern to dentistry:

- Increased effects of CNS stimulants, tricyclic antidepressants, SSRIs, sympathomimetics

DENTAL CONSIDERATIONS

General:

- Monitor vital signs often because of cardiovascular side effects.
- Patients on chronic drug therapy may rarely have symptoms of blood dyscrasias, which can include infection, bleeding, and poor healing.
- Assess salivary flow as a factor in caries, periodontal disease, and candidiasis.
- Use vasoconstrictors with caution, in low doses, and with careful aspiration.
- Determine why the patient is taking the drug.

Consultations:

- In a patient with symptoms of blood dyscrasias, request a medical

consultation for blood studies and postpone dental treatment until normal values are reestablished.

• Medical consultation may be required to assess disease control.

Teach patient/family:

• Importance of good oral hygiene to prevent soft tissue inflammation

• Caution to prevent injury when using oral hygiene aids

When chronic dry mouth occurs, advise patient:

• To avoid mouth rinses with high alcohol content because of drying effects

• To use sugarless gum, frequent sips of water, or saliva substitutes

• To use daily home fluoride products for anticaries effect

methylprednisolone/ methylprednisolone acetate/ methylprednisolone sodium succinate

(meth-il-pred-nis′oh-lone)

Methylprednisolone: Medrol, Medrol Dosepak

Methylprednisolone acetate: depMedalone 40, depMedalone 80, Depoject, Depo-Medrol, Depopred 40, Depopred 80, Duralone 40, Duralone 80, Medralone 40, Medralone 80, M-Prednisol 40, M-Prednisol 80

Methylprednisolone sodium succinate: A-Methapred, Solu-Medrol

Drug class.: Glucocorticoid, immediate acting

Action: Glucocorticoids have multiple actions that include anti-inflammatory and immunosuppressant effects. They inhibit phospholipase A_2 interfering with or reducing the synthesis of prostaglandins and leukotrienes. They also bind to cytoplasmic GRs and enter the cell nucleus to bind with DNA. This results in the synthesis of various enzymes such as collagenase, elastase, and cytokines that play important roles in inflammation and immunosuppression. They also suppress the production of lymphocytes, monocytes, and eosinophils.

Uses: Severe inflammation, shock, adrenal insufficiency, collagen disorders

Dosage and routes:

Intraarticular, intralesional, or soft tissue injection:

• *Adult and adolescent:* INJ 4-80 mg (acetate salt) at 1-5 wk intervals

Adrenal insufficiency/inflammation:

• *Adult:* PO 2-48 mg/day in 4 divided doses; IM 40-80 mg (acetate); IM/IV 10-250 mg (succinate); alternate-day therapy (inflammation): twice the usual dose given in AM qod

• *Child:* PO 0.18 mg/kg in 3 equal doses, IM 0.12 mg/kg/day in three equal doses (acetate) or 0.18 mg/kg/day in 3 equal doses every third day (succinate)

Shock:

• *Adult:* IV 100-250 mg q2-6h (succinate)

Acute spinal cord injury:

• *Adult and adolescent:* IV 30 mg/kg (succinate) over 15 min; after 45 min continuous infusion 0.54 mg/kg × 23 hr

Short-term inflammatory reactions:

• *Adult:* PO dose pack; follow package directions for use

Available forms include: Tabs 2, 4, 6, 8, 16, 24, 32 mg; inj (acetate) 20, 40, 80 mg/ml; inj (succinate) 40, 125, 500, 1000, 2000 mg/vial

CAUTION: *Do not administer acetate preparations IV.*

Side effects/adverse reactions:

▼ *ORAL:* ***Candidiasis,*** dry mouth, poor wound healing, petechiae

CNS: Depression, flushing, sweating, headache, mood changes

CV: Hypertension, ***circulatory collapse, thrombophlebitis, embolism,*** tachycardia

GI: Diarrhea, nausea, abdominal distention, ***GI hemorrhage, increased appetite, pancreatitis***

HEMA: ***Thrombocytopenia***

EENT: Fungal infections, increased intraocular pressure, blurred vision

INTEG: Acne, poor wound healing, ecchymosis, petechiae

MS: Fractures, osteoporosis, weakness

Contraindications: Psychosis, hypersensitivity, idiopathic thrombocytopenia, acute glomerulonephritis, amebiasis, fungal infections, nonasthmatic bronchial disease, child <2 yr, AIDS, TB

Precautions: Pregnancy category C, diabetes mellitus, glaucoma, osteoporosis, seizure disorders, ulcerative colitis, CHF, myasthenia gravis, renal disease, esophagitis, peptic ulcer, rifampin

Pharmacokinetics:

PO: Peak 1-2 hr, duration 1.5 days

IM: Peak 4-8 days, duration 1-4 wk

INTRAARTICULAR: Peak 1 wk

Half-life >3.5 hr

Drug interactions of concern to dentistry:

• Decreased action: barbiturates, rifampin, rifabutin

• Increased GI side effects: alcohol, salicylates, NSAIDs

• Increased action: ketoconazole, macrolide antibiotics

• Hepatotoxicity: acetaminophen (chronic, high doses)

DENTAL CONSIDERATIONS

General:

• Patients on chronic drug therapy may rarely have symptoms of blood dyscrasias, which can include infection, bleeding, and poor healing.

• Assess salivary flow as a factor in caries, periodontal disease, and candidiasis.

• Symptoms of oral infections may be masked.

• Place on frequent recall to evaluate healing response.

• Prophylactic antibiotics may be indicated to prevent infection if surgery or deep scaling is planned.

• Avoid prescribing aspirin-containing products.

• Determine dose and duration of steroid therapy for each patient to assess risk for stress tolerance and immunosuppression.

• Patients who have been or are currently on chronic steroid therapy (>2 wk) may require supplemental steroids for dental treatment.

Consultations:

• In a patient with symptoms of blood dyscrasias, request a medical consultation for blood studies and postpone dental treatment until normal values are reestablished.

• Medical consultation may be required to assess disease control.

• Consultation may be required to confirm steroid dose and duration of use.

Teach patient/family:

• Importance of good oral hygiene to prevent soft tissue inflammation

• Caution to prevent injury when

M

using oral hygiene aids because of reduced healing response

When chronic dry mouth occurs, advise patient:

• To avoid mouth rinses with high alcohol content because of drying effects

• To use sugarless gum, frequent sips of water, or saliva substitutes

• To use daily home fluoride products for anticaries effect

metoclopramide HCl

(met-oh-kloe-pra'mide)

Clopra, Maxolon, Octamide, Octamide PFS, Reglan, Reclomide

🍁 Apo-Metoclop, Maxeran, PMS-Metoclopramide

Drug class.: Central dopamine receptor antagonist

Action: Enhances response to cholinergic tissue in upper GI tract, which causes contraction of gastric muscle, relaxes pyloric and duodenal segments, increases peristalsis without stimulating secretions; antiemetic action presumably by dopamine antagonism in the CNS and serotonin in the peripheral nervous system; probably acts on the medullary chemoreceptor trigger zone

Uses: Prevention of nausea, vomiting induced by chemotherapy, radiation, delayed gastric emptying, gastroesophageal reflux, diabetic gastroparesis

Dosage and routes:

Nausea/vomiting:

• *Adult:* IV 2 mg/kg 30 min before administration of chemotherapy, then q2h × 2 doses, and then q3h × 3 doses

Postoperative nausea/vomiting:

• *Adult:* IM 10-20 mg

Diabetic gastroparesis:

• *Adult:* PO 10 mg 30 min before meals, hs × 2-8 wk

Gastroesophageal reflux:

• *Adult:* PO 10-15 mg qid 30 min ac

Available forms include: Tabs 5, 10 mg; syr 5 mg/5 ml; inj IV 5 mg/ml

Side effects/adverse reactions:

▼ *ORAL:* Dry mouth

CNS: Sedation, fatigue, restlessness, headache, sleeplessness, dystonia, dizziness, drowsiness, tardive dyskinesia, extrapyramidal symptoms, depression

CV: Hypotension, supraventricular tachycardia, hypertension (IV)

GI: Constipation, nausea, anorexia, vomiting

HEMA: ***Agranulocytosis, neutropenia, leukopenia***

GU: Decreased libido, prolactin secretion, amenorrhea, galactorrhea

INTEG: Urticaria, rash

Contraindications: Hypersensitivity to this drug or procaine or procainamide, seizure disorder, pheochromocytoma, breast cancer, GI obstruction

Precautions: Pregnancy category B, lactation, GI hemorrhage, CHF, asthma, hypertension, renal failure; extrapyramidal diseases, depression, concurrently with or within 14 days of discontinuing MAOIs

Pharmacokinetics:

IV: Onset 1-3 min, duration 1-2 hr

PO: Onset 0.5-1 hr, duration 1-2 hr

IM: Onset 10-15 min, duration 1-2 hr

Half-life 4 hr, metabolized by liver, excreted in urine

Drug interactions of concern to dentistry:

• Decreased GI action: anticholinergics, opioids

• Increased sedation: alcohol, other CNS depressants

• Increased effects of succinylcholine

DENTAL CONSIDERATIONS

General:

• Assess salivary flow as a factor in caries, periodontal disease, and candidiasis.

• Assess for presence of extrapyramidal motor symptoms, such as tardive dyskinesia and akathisia. Extrapyramidal motor activity may complicate dental treatment.

• Determine why the patient is taking the drug.

• Consider semisupine chair position for patient comfort because of GI effects of disease.

Teach patient/family:

When chronic dry mouth occurs, advise patient:

• To avoid mouth rinses with high alcohol content because of drying effects

• To use sugarless gum, frequent sips of water, or saliva substitutes

• To use daily home fluoride products for anticaries effect

metolazone

(me-tole'a-zone)

Mykrox, Zaroxolyn

Drug class.: Diuretic with thiazide-like effects

Action: Acts on distal tubule by increasing excretion of water, sodium, chloride, and potassium

Uses: Edema, hypertension, CHF

Dosage and routes:

Edema:

• *Adult:* PO 5-20 mg/day

Hypertension:

• *Adult:* PO 2.5-5 mg/day

Available forms include: Tabs 0.5, 2.5, 5, 10 mg

Side effects/adverse reactions:

▼ *ORAL: Dry mouth, increased thirst*

CNS: Dizziness, fatigue, weakness, drowsiness, paresthesia, anxiety, depression, headache

CV: Irregular pulse, orthostatic hypotension, palpitation, volume depletion

GI: Nausea, vomiting, anorexia, ***hepatitis,*** constipation, diarrhea, cramps, pancreatitis, GI irritation

HEMA: ***Aplastic anemia, hemolytic anemia, leukopenia, agranulocytosis, thrombocytopenia,*** neutropenia

GU: Frequency, ***uremia, glucosuria,*** polyuria

EENT: Blurred vision

INTEG: Rash, urticaria, purpura, photosensitivity, fever

META: Hyperglycemia, hyperuricemia, increased creatinine, BUN

ELECT: Hypokalemia, hypomagnesia, hypercalcemia, hyponatremia, hypochloremia

Contraindications: Hypersensitivity to thiazides or sulfonamides, anuria, pregnancy category D

Precautions: Hypokalemia, renal disease, hepatic disease, gout, COPD, lupus erythematosus, diabetes mellitus

Pharmacokinetics:

PO: Onset 1 hr, peak 2 hr, duration 12-24 hr, half-life 8 hr; excreted unchanged by kidneys; crosses placenta; enters breast milk

M

Drug interactions of concern to dentistry:
- Increased photosensitization: tetracycline
- Decreased hypotensive response: indomethacin and other NSAIDs

DENTAL CONSIDERATIONS

General:
- Patients on chronic drug therapy may rarely have symptoms of blood dyscrasias, which can include infection, bleeding, and poor healing.
- Assess salivary flow as a factor in caries, periodontal disease, and candidiasis.
- After supine positioning, have patient sit upright for at least 2 min before standing to avoid orthostatic hypotension.
- Short appointments and a stress reduction protocol may be required for anxious patients.
- Limit use of sodium-containing products, such as saline IV fluids, for those patients with a dietary salt restriction.
- Stress from dental procedures may compromise cardiovascular function; determine patient risk.

Consultations:
- In a patient with symptoms of blood dyscrasias, request a medical consultation for blood studies and postpone dental treatment until normal values are reestablished.
- Medical consultation may be required to assess disease control and patient's ability to tolerate stress.

Teach patient/family:
- Importance of good oral hygiene to prevent soft tissue inflammation
- Caution to prevent injury when using oral hygiene aids

When chronic dry mouth occurs, advise patient:
- To avoid mouth rinses with high alcohol content because of drying effects
- To use sugarless gum, frequent sips of water, or saliva substitutes
- To use daily home fluoride products for anticaries effect

---

metoprolol tartrate

(met-oh'proe-lol)

Lopressor, Toprol XL

✤ Apo-Metoprolol, Lopresor SR, Novometoprol

Drug class.: Antihypertensive, selective β_1-blocker

Action: This is a selective β_1-adrenergic antagonist. At higher doses selectivity may be lost with antagonism of β_2-receptors as well. The antihypertensive mechanism of action is unclear but may include a reduction in cardiac output and inhibition of renin release by the renal juxtaglomerular apparatus. Peripheral resistance decreases with long-term use. The antianginal action (when indicated for this use) may be related to a decrease in myocardial oxygen demand and negative chronotropic and inotropic effects. The antiarrhythmic action (when indicated for this use) has been related to a reduction in spontaneous pacemaker firing and slowing of AV nodal conduction.

Uses: Mild-to-moderate hypertension, acute MI to reduce risk of cardiovascular mortality, angina pectoris, CHF

Dosage and routes:

Hypertension:

• *Adult:* PO 50 mg bid or 100 mg qd; may give up to 200-450 mg in divided doses

Myocardial infarction:

• *Adult:* Early treatment, IV bol 5 mg q2min × 3, then 50 mg PO 15 min after last dose and q6h × 48 hr; late treatment, PO maintenance 100 mg bid × 3 mo

Angina pectoris:

• *Adult:* PO initial dose 100 mg/day in two equal doses, titrate dose upward as needed at weekly intervals; dose range 100-400 mg/day

CHF:

• *Adult:* PO before use, stabilize patient's doses of diuretics, ACE inhibitor, and digoxin; initial dose 12.5-25 mg/day × 2 wk, double the dose q2wk up to 200 mg

Available forms include: Tabs 50, 100 mg; ext rel 25, 50, 100, 200 mg; inj IV 1 mg/ml

Side effects/adverse reactions:

▼ *ORAL:* Dry mouth

CNS: Insomnia, dizziness, ***depression,*** mental changes, hallucinations, anxiety, headaches, nightmares, confusion, fatigue

CV: Bradycardia, CHF (palpitation), ***cardiac arrest, AV block,*** dysrhythmias, hypotension

GI: Nausea, vomiting, ***diarrhea,*** hiccups, constipation, flatulence, colitis, cramps

RESP: ***Bronchospasm,*** dyspnea, wheezing

HEMA: ***Agranulocytosis, eosinophilia, thrombocytopenic purpura***

GU: Impotence

EENT: Sore throat, dry/burning eyes

INTEG: Rash, purpura, alopecia, dry skin, urticaria, pruritus

Contraindications: Hypersensitivity to β-blockers, cardiogenic shock, second- or third-degree heart block, sinus bradycardia, CHF, bronchial asthma

Precautions: Major surgery, pregnancy category C, lactation, diabetes mellitus, renal disease, thyroid disease, COPD, heart failure, CAD, nonallergic bronchospasm, hepatic disease

Pharmacokinetics:

PO: Peak 2-4 hr, duration 13-19 hr, half-life 3-4 hr; metabolized in liver (metabolites); excreted in urine; crosses placenta; excreted in breast milk

Drug interactions of concern to dentistry:

• Increased hypotension, bradycardia: fentanyl derivatives, inhalation anesthetics

• Decreased antihypertensive effects: indomethacin and possibly other NSAIDs, sympathomimetics

• May slow metabolism of lidocaine

• Decreased β-blocking effects (or decreased β-adrenergic effects) of epinephrine, levonordefrin, isoproterenol, and other sympathomimetics

• Increased plasma concentrations: diphenhydramine

• Decreased effects: didanosine (take 2 hr before didanosine tabs)

DENTAL CONSIDERATIONS

General:

• Monitor vital signs at every appointment because of cardiovascular and respiratory side effects.

• After supine positioning, have patient sit upright for at least 2 min before standing to avoid orthostatic hypotension.

• Patients on chronic drug therapy

M

may rarely have symptoms of blood dyscrasias, which can include infection, bleeding, and poor healing.
• Assess salivary flow as a factor in caries, periodontal disease, and candidiasis.
• Stress from dental procedures may compromise cardiovascular function; determine patient risk.
• Short appointments and a stress reduction protocol may be required for anxious patients.
• Use vasoconstrictors with caution, in low doses, and with careful aspiration. Avoid use of gingival retraction cord with epinephrine.
• Determine why patient is taking the drug.

Consultations:
• In a patient with symptoms of blood dyscrasias, request a medical consultation for blood studies and postpone dental treatment until normal values are reestablished.
• Medical consultation may be required to assess disease control and patient's ability to tolerate stress.
• Take precautions if general anesthesia is required for dental surgery.

Teach patient/family:
• Importance of good oral hygiene to prevent soft tissue inflammation
• Caution to prevent injury when using oral hygiene aids

When chronic dry mouth occurs, advise patient:
• To avoid mouth rinses with high alcohol content because of drying effects
• To use sugarless gum, frequent sips of water, or saliva substitutes
• To use daily home fluoride products for anticaries effect

metronidazole/ metronidazole HCl

(me-troe-ni'da-zole)
Flagyl, Flagyl IV RTU, Flagyl 375, Flagyl ER, Helidac, Metric 21, Metro Gel, MetroCream, Noritate, Protostat
🍁 Apo-Metronidazole, Novonidazole, Trikacide

Drug class.: Trichomonacide, amebicide, antiinfective

Action: Direct-acting amebicide/trichomonacide binds, degrades DNA in organism leading to cell death

Uses: Intestinal amebiasis, amebic abscess, trichomoniasis, refractory trichomoniasis, bacterial anaerobic infections, giardiasis; unapproved: refractory adult periodontitis

Dosage and routes:

Bacterial vaginosis:
• *Adult:* TOP 1 applicator intravag qd or bid × 5 days

Trichomoniasis:
• *Adult:* PO 250 mg tid × 7 days, or 750 mg (ext rel)/day × 7 days or 2 g in single dose; do not repeat treatment for 2-3 wk

Refractory trichomoniasis:
• *Adult:* PO 250 mg bid × 10 days

Amebic abscess:
• *Adult:* PO 500-750 mg tid × 5-10 days
• *Child:* PO 35-50 mg/kg/day in 3 divided doses × 10 days

Intestinal amebiasis:
• *Adult:* PO 750 mg tid × 5-10 days
• *Child:* PO 35-50 mg/kg/day in 3 divided doses (not to exceed 750 mg dose) × 10 days; then give oral iodoquinol

Anaerobic bacterial infections:
• *Adult:* IV inf 15 mg/kg over 1 hr, then 7.5 mg/kg (500 mg for 70 kg adult) IV or PO q6h, not to exceed 4 g/day
Periodontitis:
• *Adult:* PO 250 mg tid for 7-10 days
Giardiasis:
• *Adult:* PO 250 mg tid × 5 days
• *Child:* PO 5 mg/kg tid × 5 days
H. pylori infection:
• *Adult:* PO 250 mg 4× daily in combination with 262 mg of bismuth subsalicylate and 500 mg of tetracycline (Helidac), with meals and hs × 14 days, combine with H_2 histamine antagonist
Available forms include: Tabs 250, 500 mg; caps 375 mg; ext rel tabs 750 mg; HCl inj IV 500 mg
Side effects/adverse reactions:
▼ *ORAL:* Dry mouth, furry tongue, bitter taste, metallic taste, glossitis, stomatitis
CNS: Headache, dizziness, ***convulsions,*** confusion, depression, fatigue, drowsiness, insomnia, paresthesia, peripheral neuropathy, incoordination, depression
CV: Flat T waves
GI: Nausea, vomiting, ***pseudomembranous colitis,*** diarrhea, epigastric distress, anorexia, constipation, abdominal cramps
HEMA: Leukopenia, bone marrow aplasia
GU: ***Albuminuria, nephrotoxicity,*** dysuria, cystitis, decreased libido, polyuria, incontinence, dyspareunia
EENT: Blurred vision, sore throat, retinal edema
INTEG: Rash, pruritus, urticaria, flushing
Contraindications: Hypersensitivity to this drug, renal disease, hepatic disease, contracted visual or color fields, blood dyscrasias, pregnancy (first trimester), lactation, CNS disorders
Precautions: *Candida* infections, pregnancy category B (second and third trimesters); avoid unnecessary use because shown to be carcinogenic in rodents
Pharmacokinetics:
IV/PO: Peak 1-2 hr, half-life 6.2-11.5 hr; crosses placenta; excreted in feces
Drug interactions of concern to dentistry:
• Antabuse-like reaction: alcohol, alcohol-containing products
• Decreased action: phenobarbital
• Possible increase in blood levels of tacrolimus
• Enhanced effects of warfarin, carbamazepine

DENTAL CONSIDERATIONS
General:
• Patients on chronic drug therapy may rarely have symptoms of blood dyscrasias, which can include infection, bleeding, and poor healing.
• Assess salivary flow as a factor in caries, periodontal disease, and candidiasis.
• Determine why the patient is taking the drug.
Consultations:
• In a patient with symptoms of blood dyscrasias, request a medical consultation for blood studies and postpone dental treatment until normal values are reestablished.
• Medical consultation may be required to assess disease control.
Teach patient/family:
• To avoid alcoholic beverages
• That taste alterations may occur

M

• Importance of good oral hygiene to prevent soft tissue inflammation
• Caution to prevent injury when using oral hygiene aids

When chronic dry mouth occurs, advise patient:

• To avoid mouth rinses with high alcohol content because of drying effects
• To use sugarless gum, frequent sips of water, or saliva substitutes
• To use daily home fluoride products for anticaries effect

mexiletine HCl

(mex'i-le-teen)

Mexitil

Drug class.: Antidysrhythmic (class IB, lidocaine analog)

Action: Blocks fast sodium channel in His-Purkinje system, decreasing the effective refractory period and shortening the duration of the action potential

Uses: Documented life-threatening ventricular dysrhythmias

Dosage and routes:

• *Adult:* PO 200-400 mg q8h

Available forms include: Caps 150, 200, 250 mg

Side effects/adverse reactions:

▼ *ORAL:* Dry mouth, altered taste, stomatitis

CNS: ***Convulsions,*** headache, dizziness, confusion, tremors, psychosis, nervousness, paresthesia, weakness, fatigue, coordination difficulties, change in sleep habits

CV: ***Heart block, cardiovascular collapse, arrest, left ventricular failure, cardiogenic shock,*** hypotension, bradycardia, angina, PVCs, sinus node slowing, syncope

GI: ***Hepatitis,*** nausea, vomiting, anorexia, diarrhea, abdominal pain, peptic ulcer, GI bleeding

RESP: ***Fibrosis, embolism,*** dyspnea, pneumonia

HEMA: ***Thrombocytopenia, leukopenia, agranulocytosis, hypoplastic anemia,*** SLE syndrome

GU: Urinary hesitancy, decreased libido

EENT: Blurred vision, hearing loss, tinnitus

INTEG: Rash, alopecia, dry skin

MISC: Edema, arthralgia, fever

Contraindications: Hypersensitivity to amides, cardiogenic shock, blood dyscrasias, severe heart block

Precautions: Pregnancy category C, lactation, children, renal disease, liver disease, CHF, respiratory depression, myasthenia gravis

Pharmacokinetics:

PO: Peak 2-3 hr, half-life 12 hr; metabolized by liver; excreted unchanged by kidneys (10%); excreted in breast milk

Drug interactions of concern to dentistry:

• No specific interactions are reported with dental drugs; however, any drug that could affect the cardiac action of mexiletine should be used in the least effective dose, such as other local anesthetics, vasoconstrictors, and anticholinergics

DENTAL CONSIDERATIONS

General:

• Monitor vital signs at every appointment because of cardiovascular side effects.
• Patients on chronic drug therapy may rarely have symptoms of

blood dyscrasias, which can include infection, bleeding, and poor healing.

• Assess salivary flow as a factor in caries, periodontal disease, and candidiasis.

• Stress from dental procedures may compromise cardiovascular function; determine patient risk.

Consultations:

• In a patient with symptoms of blood dyscrasias, request a medical consultation for blood studies and postpone dental treatment until normal values are reestablished.

• Medical consultation should be made to assess disease control.

• Medical consultation may be required to assess patient's ability to tolerate stress.

Teach patient/family:

• Importance of good oral hygiene to prevent soft tissue inflammation

• Caution to prevent injury when using oral hygiene aids

When chronic dry mouth occurs, advise patient:

• To avoid mouth rinses with high alcohol content because of drying effects

• To use sugarless gum, frequent sips of water, or saliva substitutes

• To use daily home fluoride products for anticaries effect

miconazole nitrate (topical)

(mi-kon'a-zole)

Femizol-M, Micatin, Miconazole-7, Monistat Cream, Monistat-Derm, Monistat-7, Monistat 3, M-Zole 3

♣ Novo-Miconazole

Drug class.: Antifungal

Action: Interferes with fungal cell membrane, increasing permeability and leading to leaking of nutrients

Uses: Tinea pedis, tinea cruris, tinea corporis, tinea versicolor, vaginal or vulval *Candida albicans*

Dosage and routes:

• *Adult and child:* TOP apply to affected area bid × 2-4 wk

• *Adult:* Intravag give 1 applicator or supp × 7 days hs; 3-day treatment–intravag insert 200 mg supp qd with topical cream bid

Available forms include: Cream, lotion, powder, spray 2%; vag cream 2%; vag supp 100, 200 mg

Side effects/adverse reactions:

GU: Vulvovaginal burning, itching, pelvic cramps

INTEG: Rash, urticaria, stinging, burning, contact dermatitis

Contraindications: Hypersensitivity

Precautions: Child <2 yr, pregnancy category B, lactation

DENTAL CONSIDERATIONS

General:

• Examine oral mucous membranes for signs of fungal infection.

• Broad-spectrum antibiotics may evoke vaginal yeast infections.

Teach patient/family:

• To prevent reinoculation of *Candida* infection by disposing of toothbrush or other contaminated oral hygiene devices used during period of infection

midazolam HCl

(mid'ay-zoe-lam)

Versed

Drug class.: Benzodiazepine, sedative, anesthesia adjunct

Controlled Substance Schedule IV

Action: Depresses subcortical levels in CNS; may act on limbic system, reticular formation; may potentiate γ-aminobutyric acid (GABA) by binding to specific benzodiazepine receptors

Uses: Conscious sedation, general anesthesia induction, sedation for diagnostic endoscopic procedures, intubation, preoperative sedation, amnesia

Dosage and routes:

WARNING: **Midazolam should be administered by persons trained in the administration of general anesthesia/IV conscious sedation. Patients must be continuously monitored, and facilities for the maintenance of a patent airway, ventilatory support, oxygen supplementation, and circulatory resuscitation must be immediately available. ALL DOSES MUST BE INDIVIDUALIZED**

Preoperative sedation and amnesia, ASA I and ASA II <60 yr:

• *Adult:* IM 0.07-0.08 mg/kg (usually 5 mg for average adult) 0.5-1 hr before general anesthesia

• *Child:* IM 0.08-0.2 mg/kg 0.5-1 hr before general anesthesia

Preoperative sedation and amnesia, ASA III or ASA IV or >60 yr:

• *Adult:* IM 0.02-0.05 mg/kg 30-60 min before surgery

Induction of general anesthesia:

• *Adult <55 yr:* Unpremedicated patients–IV 0.2-0.35 mg/kg over 30 sec, wait 2 min, follow with 25% of initial dose if needed; premedicated patients–0.15-0.35 mg/kg over 20-30 sec, allow 2 min for effect

• *Adult >55 yr:* ASA I or II, unpremedicated–IV 0.15-0.3 mg/kg administered over 20-30 sec; for ASA III or ASA IV, 0.15-0.25 mg/kg over 20-30 sec

Conscious sedation (use 1 mg/ml formulation):

• *Adult <60 yr:* Unpremedicated–IV titrate dose slowly, wait at least 2 min for response, titrate in small increments; doses of more than 5 mg are seldom required; dose may be as low as 1 mg but should not exceed 2.5 mg/min in the average healthy adult; allow at least 2 min to evaluate response; use of the more dilute solution, 1 mg/ml, allows for slower injection control; solutions can be diluted with 0.9% normal saline or dextrose 5% in water; avoid bolus doses; total dose of 5 mg is usually not necessary; patients with narcotic premedication or other CNS depressants: reduce midazolam dose by 30%

• *Adult >60 yr, debilitated:* Unpremedicated–IV (titrate doses) 1 mg or less slowly, wait at least 2 min; total dose of 3.5 mg usually unnecessary; doses must be carefully adjusted for this patient group; patients with other CNS depressant medication: reduce dose by 50%

IV sedation in children:

• *Child 6 mo-5 yr:* Caution–IV administer dose over 2-3 min and allow an additional 2-3 min before treatment or giving an additional dose; titrate with small incremental doses; reduce dose if other CNS depressants are used; initial dose 0.05-0.1 mg/kg; do not exceed 6 mg total

• *Child 6-12 yr:* Follow same cautions as for younger children–IV initial dose 0.025-0.05 mg/kg, total dose up to 0.4 mg/kg may be required; do not exceed 10 mg

• *Child 12-16 yr:* IV same as adult dose

Available forms include: Vials 1, 5 mg/ml in 1, 2, 5, 10 ml; 1 mg/ml in 2, 5, 10 ml; syr 2 mg/ml in 118 ml

Side effects/adverse reactions:

▼ *ORAL:* Increased salivation (because drugs with anticholinergic action are often used in general anesthesia techniques, salivation is usually not observed), acidic taste

CNS: Retrograde amnesia, headache, oversedation, euphoria, confusion, anxiety, insomnia, slurred speech, paresthesia, weakness, chills, agitation

CV: ***Hypotension, cardiac arrest,*** PVCs, tachycardia, bigeminy, nodal rhythm

GI: Nausea, vomiting, hiccups, increased salivation

RESP: ***Apnea, bronchospasm, respiratory depression, laryngospasm,*** coughing, dyspnea

EENT: Blurred vision, nystagmus, diplopia, blocked ears, loss of balance

INTEG: Pain, urticaria, swelling at injection site, rash, pruritus, phlebitis

MS: Involuntary movement, tremor

Contraindications: Hypersensitivity to benzodiazepines, shock, coma, alcohol intoxication, acute narrow-angle glaucoma, ritonavir, nelfinavir, indinavir, saquinavir

Precautions: COPD, CHF, chronic renal failure, chills, elderly, debilitated, pregnancy category D, children <18 yr; to be used only by health care professionals skilled in airway maintenance and ventilation and resuscitation techniques

Pharmacokinetics:

IM: Onset 15 min, peak 0.5-1 hr

IV: Onset 3-5 min, onset of anesthesia 1.5-2.5 min, half-life 1.2-12.3 hr; protein binding 97%; metabolized in liver; metabolites excreted in urine; crosses placenta, blood-brain barrier

Drug interactions of concern to dentistry:

• Prolonged respiratory depression: all CNS depressants, including alcohol, barbiturates, narcotics. All doses of midazolam must be reduced when used in combination with any CNS depressant. Serious respiratory and cardiovascular depression, including death, has occurred when midazolam is used in combination with other CNS depressants or given too rapidly. Medically compromised and elderly patients are at greater risk.

• Increased serum levels and prolonged effect of benzodiazepines: erythromycin, ketoconazole, itraconazole, fluconazole, miconazole (systemic), diltiazem, fluvoxamine

• Contraindicated with nelfinavir, ritonavir, indinavir, saquinavir

• Possible increase in CNS side effects: kava (herb)

• Suspected increase in midazolam

M

effects when used in general anesthesia: atorvastatin (*Anesthesia* 58: 899-904, 2003)

DENTAL CONSIDERATIONS

General:

• Monitor vital signs every 5 min during general anesthesia because of cardiovascular and respiratory side effects. Monitor vital signs at regular intervals during recovery.

• Degree of CNS depression is dose dependent; titrate all doses.

• Drug produces amnesia, especially in the elderly patient.

• A longer recovery period could be observed in an obese patient because half-life may be extended.

• Assist patient with ambulation until drowsy period has passed.

Teach patient/family:

• That drug may impair reaction time; avoid driving or potentially hazardous activities until drowsiness or weakness subsides

• That amnesia occurs; events may not be remembered

Treatment of overdose:

• O_2, vasopressors, flumazenil, resuscitation measures as required

---

miglitol

(mig'li-tol)

Glyset

Drug class.: Oligosaccharide, glucosidase enzyme inhibitor

Action: Inhibits α-glucosidase enzyme in GI tract to slow breakdown of carbohydrates to glucose, which results in reduced plasma glucose levels

Uses: Type 2 diabetes when diet control is ineffective in controlling blood glucose levels, used as single agent or in combination with other oral hypoglycemics

Dosage and routes:

• *Adult:* PO individualize doses; initial dose 25 mg tid with first bite of each meal; max recommended dose 100 mg tid; increase initial dose based on side effects and postprandial plasma glucose; usual maintenance dose 50 mg tid

Available forms include: Tabs 25, 50, 100 mg

Side effects/adverse reactions:

GI: Diarrhea, flatulence, abdominal pain, soft stools

INTEG: Rash

MISC: Low serum iron

Contraindications: Hypersensitivity, diabetic ketoacidosis, inflammatory bowel disease, colonic ulceration, partial intestinal obstruction, chronic intestinal diseases associated with disorders of absorption and digestion

Precautions: Renal impairment, hypoglycemia, pregnancy category B, lactation, children

Pharmacokinetics:

PO: Peak plasma levels 2-3 hr; negligible plasma protein binding, not metabolized, urinary excretion

Drug interactions of concern to dentistry:

• None reported with dental drugs

DENTAL CONSIDERATIONS

General:

• Ensure that patient is following prescribed diet and regularly takes medication.

• Type 2 patients may also be using insulin. Should symptomatic hypoglycemia occur while taking this drug, use dextrose rather than sucrose because of interference with sucrose metabolism.

• Place on frequent recall to evaluate healing response.

• Short appointments and a stress reduction protocol may be required for anxious patients.
• Diabetics may be more susceptible to infection and have delayed wound healing.
• Consider semisupine chair position for patient comfort if GI side effects occur.
• Question patient about self-monitoring of drug's antidiabetic effect, including blood glucose values or finger-stick records.
• Examine for oral manifestation of opportunistic infection.

Consultations:
• Medical consultation may be required to assess disease control and patient's ability to tolerate stress.
• Medical consultation may include data from patient's blood glucose monitoring, including glycosylated hemoglobin or HbA_{1c} testing.

Teach patient/family:
• Importance of updating health and drug history if physician makes any changes in evaluation or drug regimens
• Importance of good oral hygiene to prevent soft tissue inflammation

miglustat

(mi-gloo'stat)
Zavesca

Drug class.: Enzyme inhibitor

Action: A competitive and reversible inhibitor of glucosylceramide synthase leading to a reduced rate of synthesis of most glycosphingolipids

Uses: Treatment of adult patients with mild to moderate type 1 Gaucher disease for whom enzyme replacement therapy is not an option

Dosage and routes:
• *Adult:* PO 100 mg tid, may reduce to 100 mg bid to reduce side effects

Available forms include: Caps 100 mg

Side effects/adverse reactions:
ORAL: Dry mouth
CNS: Tremor, headache, paresthesia, dizziness, memory loss
GI: Diarrhea, flatulence, abdominal pain, nausea, anorexia, dyspepsia
HEMA: Thrombocytopenia
GU: Risk of infertility in males
META: Weight loss
MS: Leg cramps, generalized weakness, back pain
MISC: Peripheral neuropathy, numbness, tingling

Contraindications: Hypersensitivity, pregnancy, severe renal impairment

Precautions: Pregnancy category X, efficacy and safety not evaluated in patients <18 yr or >65 yr, renal impairment, women of reproductive age, provide pretreatment neurologic evaluation, lactation

Pharmacokinetics:
PO: Maximum plasma levels 2-2.5 hr, half-life ≈6-7 hr; oral bioavailability 97%, no plasma protein binding, excreted unchanged in urine

Drug interactions of concern to dentistry:
• None reported

DENTAL CONSIDERATIONS

General:
• Ask patient about disease control.
• Question patient about nosebleeds or other bleeding events.
• Short appointments and a stress reduction protocol may be required for anxious patients.

M

• Avoid products that affect platelet function, such as aspirin and NSAIDs.
• Patients on chronic drug therapy may rarely have symptoms of blood dyscrasias, which can include infection, bleeding, and poor healing.
• Assess salivary flow as a factor in caries, periodontal disease, and candidiasis.
• Consider semisupine chair position as needed.
• Place on frequent recall to evaluate healing response.

Consultations:

• Medical consultation may be required to assess disease control and patient's ability to tolerate stress.
• Medical consultation should include routine blood counts, including platelet counts and bleeding time.
• In a patient with symptoms of blood dyscrasias, request a medical consultation for blood studies and postpone treatment until normal values are reestablished.

Teach patient/family:

• To inform dentist of unusual bleeding episodes following dental treatment
• Importance of good oral hygiene to prevent soft tissue inflammation/infection
• Use of electric toothbrush if patient has difficulty holding conventional devices

minocycline HCl

(mi-noe-sye'kleen)

Dyancin, Minocin

Drug class.: Tetracycline antiinfective

Action: Inhibits protein synthesis, phosphorylation in microorganisms by binding to 30S ribosomal subunits, reversibly binding to 50S ribosomal subunits; bacteriostatic

Uses: Syphilis, *C. trachomatis* infection, gonorrhea, lymphogranuloma venereum, rickettsial infections, inflammatory acne, *M. marinum, Neisseria* meningitis carriers, actinomycosis, anthrax, ANUG, AA-induced periodontitis, and other susceptible infections; dental product is an adjunct to scaling and root planing in adult periodontitis

Dosage and routes:

• *Adult:* PO/IV 200 mg first day, then 100 mg q12h or 50 mg q6h, not to exceed 400 mg/24 hr IV
• *Child >8 yr, <45 kg:* PO/IV 4 mg/kg first day, then 2 mg/kg/day PO in divided doses q12h

Available forms include: Caps 50, 75, 100 mg; caps pellet filled 50, 100 mg; oral susp 50 mg/5 ml in 60 ml; powder for inj IV 100 mg/vial

Side effects/adverse reactions:

▼ *ORAL:* Candidiasis, tooth staining, discolored mucous membranes, discolored tongue, lichenoid reaction

CNS: Dizziness, fever, light-headedness, vertigo

CV: Pericarditis

GI: Nausea, abdominal pain, vomiting, diarrhea, ***hepatotoxicity,*** anorexia, enterocolitis, flatulence, abdominal cramps, epigastric burning

HEMA: ***Eosinophilia, neutropenia, thrombocytopenia, hemolytic anemia***

GU: Increased BUN, ***renal failure, nephrotoxicity,*** polyuria, polydipsia

EENT: Dysphagia

INTEG: Rash, urticaria, photosensitivity, increased pigmentation,

exfoliative dermatitis, pruritus, angioedema, bluish-gray color of skin

Contraindications: Hypersensitivity to tetracyclines, children <8 yr, pregnancy category D, isotretinoin

Precautions: Hepatic disease, lactation

Pharmacokinetics:

PO: Peak 2-3 hr, half-life 11-17 hr; 55%-88% protein bound; excreted in urine, feces, breast milk; crosses placenta

Drug interactions of concern to dentistry:

- Decreased effect: antacids, milk, or other calcium- and aluminum-containing products
- Decreased effect of penicillins
- Oral contraceptives: advise patient of a potential risk for decreased contraceptive action, to maintain compliance with oral contraceptive use while using antibiotics, and to consider the use of additional nonhormonal contraception
- Contraindicated with isotretinoin (Accutane)

DENTAL CONSIDERATIONS

General:

- This drug is reported to cause intrinsic staining in erupted permanent teeth not associated with the calcification stage.
- The drug readily distributes to gingival crevicular fluid.
- Do not prescribe drug during pregnancy or <8 yr because of tooth discoloration.
- Caution patients about driving or performing other tasks requiring alertness.
- Advise patient if dental drugs prescribed have a potential for photosensitivity.
- Do not use ingestible sodium bicarbonate products such as the air polishing system Prophy
- Jet at the same time dose is taken; take minocycline 2 hr later.
- Determine why the patient is taking the drug.

Consultations:

- Medical consultation may be required to assess disease control.

Teach patient/family:

- Importance of good oral hygiene to prevent soft tissue inflammation
- Caution to prevent injury when using oral hygiene aids
- To avoid mouth rinses with high alcohol content because of drying effects

When used for dental infection, advise patient:

- To report sore throat, oral burning sensation, fever, fatigue, any of which could indicate superinfection
- To take at prescribed intervals and complete dosage regimen
- To immediately notify the dentist if signs or symptoms of infection increase

minocycline HCl (microspheres)

(mi-noe-sye'kleen)

Arestin

Drug class.: Tetracycline antiinfective

Action: Inhibits protein synthesis, phosphorylation in microorganisms by binding to 30S ribosomal subunits, bacteriostatic

Uses: Adjunctive therapy to scaling and root planning procedures for reduction of pocket depth in adult periodontitis; also used as part of a periodontal maintenance

M

program, which includes good oral hygiene, scaling, and root planing

Dosage and routes:

• *Adult:* Connect cartridge to handle, remove tip and insert to base of periodontal pocket, express the powder while gradually withdrawing tip from pocket base

Available forms include: Box of 2 trays, each containing 12 cartridges (1 mg minocycline)

Side effects/adverse reactions:

▼ *ORAL: Dental pain,* stomatitis, ulceration

CNS: Headache

GI: Dyspepsia

RESP: Pharyngitis

MISC: Flulike syndrome, infection

Contraindications: Hypersensitivity

Precautions: Use in acute periodontal abscess has not been studied, has not been tested in immunocompromised patients, pregnant women, or patients with implants, overgrowth of opportunistic organisms, predisposition to candidiasis, pregnancy category D, lactation, efficacy in children unknown

Pharmacokinetics: With exposure to crevicular fluid, minocycline is released from channels in the microspheres, therapeutic levels are said to last for 14 days, data not available on systemic absorption

Drug interactions of concern to dentistry:

• No dental drug interactions reported with this product

DENTAL CONSIDERATIONS

General:

• Follow all general precautions when using tetracyclines.

Teach patient/family:

• To avoid eating hard, crunchy foods for 1 wk

• To postpone toothbrushing for 12 hr

• To postpone use of interproximal cleaning devices for 10 days

• To notify dentist immediately if pain, swelling, or other unexpected symptoms occur

minoxidil

(mi-nox'i-dil)

Systemic: Loniten

Topical: Rogaine, Rogaine for Men

♣ Apo-gain, Gen-Minoxidil, Minoxigaine

Drug class.: Antihypertensive

Action: Directly relaxes arteriolar smooth muscle, reducing peripheral resistance; alopecia action unclear

Uses: Severe hypertension not responsive to other therapy (used with a diuretic and α-adrenergic antagonist); topically to treat androgenic alopecia

Dosage and routes:

• *Adult:* PO 5 mg/day, not to exceed 100 mg daily; usual range 10-40 mg/day in single doses

• *Child <12 yr:* Initial 0.2 mg/kg/day; effective range 0.25-1 mg/kg/day; max 50 mg/day

Alopecia:

• *Adult:* Apply topically; rub 1 ml into scalp bid

Available forms include: Tabs 2.5, 10 mg; top 2%, 5%

Side effects/adverse reactions:

CNS: Drowsiness, dizziness, sedation, headache, depression, fatigue

CV: Severe rebound hypertension on withdrawal, ***CHF, pulmonary edema, pericardial effusion,*** tachycardia, angina, increased T wave, edema, sodium/water retention

GI: Nausea, vomiting

HEMA: Hct, Hgb, erythrocyte count may decrease initially

GU: Gynecomastia, breast tenderness

INTEG: ***Stevens-Johnson syndrome,*** pruritus, rash, hirsutism

Contraindications: Acute MI, dissecting aortic aneurysm, hypersensitivity, pheochromocytoma

Precautions: Pregnancy category C, lactation, children, renal disease, CAD, CHF

Pharmacokinetics:

PO: Onset 30 min, peak 2-3 hr, duration 75 hr, half-life 4.2 hr; metabolized in liver; metabolites excreted in urine, feces

Drug interactions of concern to dentistry:

- Decreased effects: NSAIDs, indomethacin, sympathomimetics
- Increased hypotension: CNS depressant drug used in conscious sedation technique may also lower blood pressure

DENTAL CONSIDERATIONS

General:

- Monitor vital signs at every appointment because of cardiovascular side effects.
- Patients on chronic drug therapy may rarely have symptoms of blood dyscrasias, which can include infection, bleeding, and poor healing.
- Limit use of sodium-containing products, such as saline IV fluids, for patients with a dietary salt restriction.
- Short appointments and a stress reduction protocol may be required for anxious patients.
- After supine positioning, have patient sit upright for at least 2 min before standing to avoid orthostatic hypotension.

Consultations:

- In a patient with symptoms of blood dyscrasias, request a medical consultation for blood studies and postpone dental treatment until normal values are reestablished.
- Medical consultation may be required to assess disease control and stress tolerance.

mirtazapine

(mir-taz'a-peen)

Remeron, Remeron SolTab

Drug class.: Tetracyclic antidepressant

Action: Mechanism of antidepressant effect is unknown; acts in CNS as an antagonist for presynaptic α_2-adrenergic inhibitory receptors, antagonizes serotonin (5-HT_2 and 5-HT_3) receptors and histamine H_1 receptors

Uses: Depression

Dosage and routes:

- *Adult:* PO initial dose 15 mg qd in PM, effective dose range 15-45 mg/day, allow 1-2 wk between dose changes to evaluate response

Available forms include: Tabs 15, 30, 45 mg; tabs oral disintegrating 15, 30, 45 mg

Side effects/adverse reactions:

▼ *ORAL: Dry mouth (25%), thirst,* glossitis, gingival hemorrhage, stomatitis (rare), tongue discoloration, ulcerative stomatitis, salivary gland enlargement, increased salivation, aphthous stomatitis, candidiasis, tongue edema

CNS: Somnolence, dizziness, ab-

normal dreams, malaise, mania, hypomania, confusion, tremor, migraine
CV: Peripheral edema, hypertension, vasodilation, ***MI,*** angina pectoris, bradycardia, syncope, hypotension
GI: Nausea, constipation, vomiting, abdominal pain, anorexia, increased ALT
RESP: Cough, flulike syndrome, dyspnea
HEMA: ***Agranulocytosis, leukopenia, thrombocytopenia,*** lymphadenopathy, lymphocytosis, pancytopenia, petechia, anemia (all rare)
GU: Urinary frequency
EENT: Sinusitis, eye pain
INTEG: Rash, pruritus, dry skin, herpes simplex, herpes zoster, photosensitivity
MS: Asthenia, arthralgia, back pain, myalgia, neck pain, neck rigidity
MISC: Increased appetite, weight gain, increased cholesterol/triglycerides

Contraindications: Hypersensitivity, MAOIs

Precautions: Hepatic impairment, renal impairment, elderly, pregnancy category C, nursing, pediatric, suicidal ideation, cardiovascular or cerebrovascular disease aggravated by hypotension, avoid alcohol use

Pharmacokinetics:
PO: Rapid absorption, half-life 20-40 hr; peak levels 2 hr, liver metabolism, bioavailability 50%, urinary excretion, 85% plasma protein binding

Drug interactions of concern to dentistry:

- Impairment of cognitive and motor performance with diazepam or other drugs used in conscious sedation
- Use opioid analgesics with caution because of impairment of cognitive or motor performance; NSAIDs may be a more appropriate choice

DENTAL CONSIDERATIONS

General:

- Patients on chronic drug therapy may rarely have symptoms of blood dyscrasias, which can include infection, bleeding, and poor healing.
- Assess salivary flow as a factor in caries, periodontal disease, and candidiasis.
- Monitor vital signs at every appointment because of cardiovascular side effects.
- Consider semisupine chair position when GI or MS side effects occur.
- Place on frequent recall if oral side effects are a problem.

Consultations:

- In a patient with symptoms of blood dyscrasias, request a medical consultation for blood studies and postpone dental treatment until normal values are reestablished.
- Take precaution if dental surgery is anticipated and sedation or general anesthesia is required; there is risk of hypotensive episode.
- Medical consultation may be required to assess disease control.
- Physician should be informed if significant xerostomic side effects occur (e.g., increased caries, sore tongue, problems eating or swallowing, difficulty wearing prosthesis) so that a medication change can be considered.

Teach patient/family:

• Importance of good oral hygiene to prevent soft tissue inflammation
• Caution to prevent soft tissue trauma when using oral hygiene aids
• Importance of updating health history/drug record if physician makes any changes in evaluation or drug regimens
• Caution about driving or performing other tasks requiring alertness

When chronic dry mouth occurs, advise patient:

• To avoid mouth rinses with high alcohol content because of drying effects
• To use daily home fluoride products for anticaries effect
• To use sugarless gum, frequent sips of water, or saliva substitutes

misoprostol

(mye-soe-prost'ole)

Cytotec

Drug class.: Gastric mucosa protectant

Action: A prostaglandin E_1 analog that inhibits gastric acid secretion, may protect gastric mucosa; can increase bicarbonate, mucus production

Uses: Prevention of NSAID-induced gastric ulcers; unapproved: duodenal ulcers

Dosage and routes:

• *Adult:* PO 200 μg qid with food for duration of NSAID therapy; if 200 μg is not tolerated, 100 μg may be given

Available forms include: Tabs 100, 200 μg

Side effects/adverse reactions:

GI: *Diarrhea,* nausea, vomiting, flatulence, constipation, dyspepsia, abdominal pain

GU: Spotting, cramps, hypermenorrhea, menstrual disorders

Contraindications: Hypersensitivity, contraindicated in women who are pregnant and using misoprostol to reduce risk of NSAID-induced stomach ulcers

Precautions: Lactation, children, elderly, renal disease

Pharmacokinetics:

PO: Peak 12 min; plasma steady state achieved within 2 days; excreted in urine

DENTAL CONSIDERATIONS

General:

• Avoid NSAIDs and salicylates in patients with upper active GI disease; acetaminophen/opioids are more appropriate for pain control in these patients.

Consultations:

• Medical consultation may be required to assess disease control.

mitotane

(mye'toe-tane)

Lysodren

Drug class.: Antineoplastic

Action: Acts on adrenal cortex to suppress activity and adrenal steroid production

Uses: Adrenocortical carcinoma; unapproved: Cushing's syndrome

Dosage and routes:

• *Adult:* PO 2-6 g/day in divided doses tid or qid; can increase to 10 g; may need to decrease dose if severe reactions occur

Available forms include: Tabs 500 mg

M

Side effects/adverse reactions:
CNS: Lethargy, somnolence, vertigo, dizziness, light-headedness, flushing, sedation
GI: Nausea, vomiting, anorexia, diarrhea
GU: ***Proteinuria, hematuria***
EENT: Blurring, retinopathy, double vision
INTEG: Rash
ENDO: ***Adrenal cortical insufficiency***
MS: Muscle ache
Contraindications: Hypersensitivity
Precautions: Lactation, hepatic disease, pregnancy category C, infection; caution: avoid use or discontinue if adrenal cortical suppression occurs
Pharmacokinetics: Adequately absorbed orally (40%), half-life 18-159 days; hepatic metabolism; excreted in urine, bile
Drug interactions of concern to dentistry:
• Increased CNS depression: all CNS depressants
• Decreased effects of corticosteroids; if glucocorticoid replacement is needed, use hydrocortisone
DENTAL CONSIDERATIONS
General:
• Evaluate respiration characteristics and rate.
• Drug may cause adrenal hypofunction, especially under conditions of stress such as surgery, trauma, or acute illness. Patients should be carefully monitored and given hydrocortisone or mineralocorticoid as needed.
• Consider semisupine chair position for patient comfort if GI side effects occur.
• Patients taking opioids for acute or chronic pain should be given alternative analgesics for dental pain.
Consultations:
• Medical consultation may be required to assess disease control and patient's ability to tolerate stress.
Teach patient/family:
• That secondary oral infection may occur; must see dentist immediately if infection occurs
• To report oral lesions, soreness, or bleeding to dentist
• Importance of updating medical/drug records if physician makes any changes in evaluation or drug regimens

modafinil

(mo-daf'i-nil)
Provigil
Drug class.: CNS stimulant

Controlled Substance Schedule IV
Action: Mechanism of action remains uncertain; has wake-promoting actions similar to amphetamine and other sympathomimetics; may have CNS α_1-receptor agonist activity; enhancement of dopamine has also been observed in animals
Uses: Improve wakefulness in narcolepsy, obstructive sleep apnea, shift work sleep disorder
Dosage and routes:
• *Adult:* PO 200 mg qd, 400 mg/day doses have been used
Available forms include: Tabs 100, 200 mg
Side effects/adverse reactions:
ORAL: Orofacial dyskinesia, dry mouth
CNS: Headache, nervousness, anxiety, insomnia, depression, catoplexy, confusion, amnesia

CV: Hypertension, hypotension
GI: Nausea, diarrhea, anorexia
RESP: Rhinitis, pharyngitis
EENT: Blurred vision
INTEG: Dry skin
META: Abnormal liver function

Contraindications: Hypersensitivity

Precautions: Ischemic heart disease, left ventricular hypertrophy, mitral valve prolapse, recent MI, unstable angina, renal impairment, hepatic impairment, pregnancy category C, lactation, children <16 yr, drug abuse

Pharmacokinetics:
PO: Absorption delayed by food, peak plasma levels 2-4 hr, plasma protein binding (60%), hepatic metabolism, excreted mostly in urine (81%), produces hepatic cytochrome P-450 enzymes (CYP3A4)

Drug interactions of concern to dentistry:
- No documented dental drug interactions reported; however, because it induces cytochrome P-450 isoenzymes, other P-450 isoenzyme inducers or inhibitors (antifungal agents, erythromycin) could result in a drug interaction (see Appendix I)

DENTAL CONSIDERATIONS
General:
- Monitor vital signs at every appointment because of cardiovascular side effects.
- Assess salivary flow as a factor in caries, periodontal disease, and candidiasis.
- Consider semisupine chair position for patient comfort because of GI side effects of drug.
- Short appointments and a stress reduction protocol may be required for anxious patients.

Teach patient/family:
- To prevent trauma when using oral hygiene aids

When chronic dry mouth occurs, advise patient:
- To avoid mouth rinses with high alcohol content because of drying effects
- To use daily home fluoride products for anticaries effect
- To use sugarless gum, frequent sips of water, or saliva substitutes

moexipril hydrochloride

(moe'x-i-pril)
Univasc

Drug class.: Angiotensin-converting enzyme (ACE) inhibitor

Action: Selectively suppresses renin-angiotensin-aldosterone system; inhibits ACE; prevents conversion of angiotensin I to angiotensin II; results in dilation of arterial, venous vessels; decreased aldosterone secretion results in diuresis and natriuresis

Uses: Hypertension as a single drug or in combination with a thiazide diuretic

Dosage and routes:
As single drug (not taking diuretic):
- *Adult:* PO 7.5 mg 1 hr before meals once daily; range 7.5-30 mg/day in 1 or 2 divided doses 1 hr ac

With diuretic:
- *Adult:* PO as single drug, but discontinue diuretic 2-3 days to avoid symptomatic hypotension; then restart diuretic carefully, if required; otherwise start with 3.75 mg under medical supervision

Renal impairment:
• *Adult:* Dose limited to 15 mg/day
Available forms include: Tabs 7.5, 15 mg
Side effects/adverse reactions:
▼ *ORAL:* ***Angioedema,*** dry mouth (<1%)
CNS: Dizziness, fatigue
CV: Symptomatic hypotension, postural hypotension, hyperkalemia, peripheral edema, chest pain, palpitation
GI: Diarrhea, ***hepatic failure***
RESP: Cough, pharyngitis
HEMA: ***Neutropenia, agranulocytosis***
GU: ***Acute renal failure,*** oliguria, azotemia, urinary frequency
EENT: Tinnitus
INTEG: Flushing, rash, photosensitivity
MS: Myalgia
MISC: ***Anaphylactic reactions***
Contraindications: Hypersensitivity, pregnancy (second or third trimester), angioedema history with other ACE inhibitors
Precautions: Food retards absorption, renal or hepatic impairment, CHF, SLE, scleroderma, renal artery stenosis, lactation, children, pregnancy categories C (first trimester) and D (second and third trimesters)
Pharmacokinetics:
PO: Peak plasma levels 1.5 hr; converted to active metabolite (moexiprilat); 50% plasma protein bound; excreted in urine, feces
Drug interactions of concern to dentistry:
• IV fluids containing potassium: risk of hyperkalemia
• Increased hypotension: other hypotensive drugs, alcohol, phenothiazines
• Decreased hypotensive effects: indomethacin, possibly other NSAIDs, sympathomimetics
• Suspected reduction in the antihypertensive and vasodilator effects by salicylates; monitor blood pressure if used concurrently

DENTAL CONSIDERATIONS
General:
• Monitor vital signs at every appointment because of cardiovascular side effects.
• After supine positioning, have patient sit upright for at least 2 min before standing to avoid orthostatic hypotension.
• Take precautions if dental surgery is anticipated and general anesthesia is required.
• Patients on chronic drug therapy may rarely have symptoms of blood dyscrasias, which can include infection, bleeding, and poor healing.
• Stress from dental procedures may compromise cardiovascular function; determine patient risk.
• Assess salivary flow as a factor in caries, periodontal disease, and candidiasis.
• Short appointments and a stress reduction protocol may be required for anxious patients.
Consultations:
• Medical consultation may be required to assess disease control and patient's ability to tolerate stress.
• In a patient with symptoms of blood dyscrasias, request a medical consultation for blood studies and postpone dental treatment until normal values are reestablished.
Teach patient/family:
• Importance of good oral hygiene to prevent soft tissue inflammation

• Caution to prevent trauma when using oral hygiene aids
• To report oral lesions, soreness, or bleeding to dentist

When chronic dry mouth occurs, advise patient:
• To avoid mouth rinses with high alcohol content because of drying effects
• Of need for daily home fluoride use to prevent caries
• To use sugarless gum, frequent sips of water, or saliva substitutes

molindone HCl

(moe-lin'done)

Moban, Moban Concentrate

Drug class.: Antipsychotic

Action: Depresses cerebral cortex, hypothalamus, limbic system, which control activity, aggression; blocks neurotransmission produced by dopamine at synapse; exhibits strong α-adrenergic, anticholinergic blocking action; mechanism for antipsychotic effects is unclear

Uses: Psychotic disorders

Dosage and routes:
• *Adult:* PO 50-75 mg/day, increasing to 225 mg/day if needed

Available forms include: Tabs 5, 10, 25, 50 mg

Side effects/adverse reactions:

▼ *ORAL: Dry mouth*

CNS: Extrapyramidal symptoms: pseudoparkinsonism, akathisia, dystonia, tardive dyskinesia, drowsiness, headache, seizures

CV: Orthostatic hypotension, ***cardiac arrest, tachycardia,*** ECG changes, hypertension

GI: Nausea, vomiting, anorexia, constipation, diarrhea, jaundice, weight gain

RESP: ***Laryngospasm, respiratory depression,*** dyspnea

HEMA: ***Anemia, leukopenia, leukocytosis, agranulocytosis***

GU: Urinary retention, urinary frequency, enuresis, impotence, amenorrhea, gynecomastia, menstrual irregularities

EENT: Blurred vision, glaucoma

INTEG: Rash, photosensitivity, dermatitis

Contraindications: Hypersensitivity, coma, child

Precautions: Pregnancy category C, lactation, hypertension, hepatic disease, cardiac disease, Parkinson's disease, brain tumor, glaucoma, urinary retention, diabetes mellitus, respiratory disease, prostatic hypertrophy

Pharmacokinetics:

PO: Onset erratic, peak 1.5 hr, duration 24-36 hr, half-life 1.5 hr; metabolized by liver; excreted in urine, feces; may cross placenta; excreted in breast milk

Drug interactions of concern to dentistry:
• Increased sedation: alcohol, other CNS depressants
• Increased anticholinergic effect: anticholinergics, antihistamines

DENTAL CONSIDERATIONS

General:
• Patients on chronic drug therapy may rarely have symptoms of blood dyscrasias, which can include infection, bleeding, and poor healing.
• Assess salivary flow as a factor in caries, periodontal disease, and candidiasis.
• After supine positioning, have patient sit upright for at least 2 min before standing to avoid orthostatic hypotension.

• Assess for presence of extrapyramidal motor symptoms, such as tardive dyskinesia and akathisia. Extrapyramidal motor activity may complicate dental treatment.
• Geriatric patients are more susceptible to drug effects; use lower dose.
• Use vasoconstrictors with caution, in low doses, and with careful aspiration.

Consultations:
• In a patient with symptoms of blood dyscrasias, request a medical consultation for blood studies and postpone dental treatment until normal values are reestablished.
• Medical consultation may be required to assess disease control.

Teach patient/family:
• Importance of good oral hygiene to prevent soft tissue inflammation
• Caution to prevent injury when using oral hygiene aids

When chronic dry mouth occurs, advise patient:
• To avoid mouth rinses with high alcohol content because of drying effects
• To use sugarless gum, frequent sips of water, or saliva substitutes
• To use daily home fluoride products for anticaries effect

---

mometasone furoate monohydrate

(moe-met'a-sone)

Nasonex

Drug class.: Synthetic corticosteroid

Action: Glucocorticoids have multiple actions that include anti-inflammatory and immunosuppressant effects. They inhibit phospholipase A_2 interfering with or reducing the synthesis of prostaglandins and leukotrienes. They also bind to cytoplasmic GRs and enter the cell nucleus to bind with DNA. This results in the synthesis of various enzymes such as collagenase, elastase, and cytokines that play important roles in inflammation and immunosuppression. They also suppress the production of lymphocytes, monocytes, and eosinophils.

Uses: Treatment of nasal symptoms of seasonal and perennial allergic rhinitis; prophylaxis of nasal symptoms of seasonal allergic rhinitis

Dosage and routes:
• *Adult and child >11 yr:* TOP (nasal) 2 sprays in each nostril daily
• *Children 2-11 yr:* TOP (nasal) 1 spray in each nostril daily

Available forms include: Nasal spray 50 µg each actuation (120 sprays in bottle)

Side effects/adverse reactions:
CNS: Headache
RESP: Pharyngitis, coughing, URI
GU: Dysmenorrhea
EENT: Epistaxis, sinusitis
MS: Pain
MISC: Viral infection

Contraindications: Hypersensitivity

Precautions: Caution in transferring patient from systemic to inhalation steroids; active or quiescent tuberculosis, untreated fungal, bacterial, or viral infections, pregnancy category C, lactation, safety and efficacy in child <12 yr not established

Pharmacokinetics:
INH: Virtually undetectable in plasma; if absorbed see extensive metabolism, any metabolites excreted in bile

Drug interactions of concern to dentistry:

• None reported

DENTAL CONSIDERATIONS

General:

• Allergic rhinitis may be a factor in mouth breathing and drying of oral tissues.

• Examine for oral manifestation of opportunistic infection.

Teach patient/family:

• Importance of gargling, rinsing mouth with water, and expectorating after each aerosol dose

montelukast sodium

(mon-te-loo'kast)

Singulair

Drug class.: Selective leukotriene receptor antagonist

Action: Competitive and selective antagonist for cysteinyl leukotriene receptor (Cys LT_1)

Uses: Prophylaxis and chronic treatment of asthma, seasonal allergic rhinitis

Dosage and routes:

Allergic rhinitis/asthma:

• *Adult and child >15 yr:* PO 10 mg hs

• *Child 6-14 yr:* PO 5 mg chewable tabs hs

• *Child 2-5 yr:* PO 4 mg chewable tabs or 1 packet daily (4 mg) hs

• *Child 12-23 mo:* PO 1 packet daily (4 mg) hs

Available forms include: Chew tabs 4, 5 mg; tab 10 mg; oral granules 4 mg/packet

Side effects/adverse reactions:

▼ *ORAL:* Unspecified dental pain

CNS: Dizziness, headache

GI: Abdominal pain, dyspepsia, gastroenteritis

RESP: Cough

EENT: Nasal congestion

META: Increased ALT and AST

MS: Asthenia

MISC: Fatigue, influenza, fever

Contraindications: Hypersensitivity

Precautions: Not for acute asthma attacks, not for treatment of exercise-induced bronchospasm or ASA-induced bronchospasm, chewable tablets contain aspartame, pregnancy category B, lactation; monitor patients when potent CYP3A4 isoenzyme inducers are used

Pharmacokinetics:

PO: Rapidly absorbed, peak levels 3-4 hr, bioavailability 64%-73%, highly plasma protein bound (99%), extensive hepatic metabolism by CYP3A4 and CYP2C9 isoenzymes, excretion in bile

Drug interactions of concern to dentistry:

• None reported; however, monitor patients when strong inhibitors of CYP 3A4 or CYP 2C9 are prescribed (see Appendix I)

DENTAL CONSIDERATIONS

General:

• Midday appointments and a stress reduction protocol may be required for anxious patients.

• Avoid prescribing aspirin-containing products.

• Acute asthmatic episodes may be precipitated in the dental office. Rapid-acting sympathomimetic inhalants should be available for emergency use. A stress reduction protocol may be required.

• Be aware that aspirin or sulfite preservatives in vasoconstrictor-containing products can exacerbate asthma.

• Consider semisupine chair position for patients with respiratory disease and when GI side effects are a problem.

Consultations:

• Medical consultation may be required to assess disease control.

Teach patient/family:

• Importance of updating health and drug history if physician makes any changes in evaluation or drug regimens

---

moricizine

(mor-i'siz-een)

Ethmozine

Drug class.: Antidysrhythmic, type I

Action: Decreased rate of rise of action potential, which prolongs the refractory period and shortens the action potential duration; depression of inward influx if sodium mediates the effects; drug may slow atrial and AV nodal conduction

Uses: Documented life-threatening dysrhythmias

Dosage and routes:

• *Adult:* PO 600-900 mg/day in 3 divided doses; dose must be individualized

Available forms include: Film-coated tabs 200, 250, 300 mg

Side effects/adverse reactions:

▼ *ORAL:* Dry mouth, altered taste, stomatitis, swelling of lips and tongue

CNS: Dizziness, headache, fatigue, perioral numbness, euphoria, nervousness, sleep disorders, depression, tinnitus, fatigue

CV: ***MI,*** palpitation, chest pain, CHF, hypertension, syncope, dysrhythmias, bradycardia, thrombophlebitis

GI: Nausea, abdominal pain, vomiting, diarrhea

RESP: ***Apnea,*** dyspnea, hyperventilation, asthma, pharyngitis, cough

GU: Sexual dysfunction, difficult urination, dysuria, incontinence

MISC: Sweating, musculoskeletal pain

Contraindications: Second- and third-degree heart block, right bundle branch block, cardiogenic shock, hypersensitivity

Precautions: CHF, hypokalemia, hyperkalemia, sick sinus syndrome, pregnancy category B, lactation, children, impaired hepatic and renal function, cardiac dysfunction

Pharmacokinetics: Peak 0.5-2.2 hr, half-life 1.5-3.5 hr; protein binding >90%; metabolized by the liver; metabolites excreted in feces, urine

Drug interactions of concern to dentistry:

• No specific interactions are reported with dental drugs; however, any drug that could affect the cardiac action of moricizine (e.g., other local anesthetics, vasoconstrictors, anticholinergics) should be used in the lowest effective dose

DENTAL CONSIDERATIONS

General:

• Monitor vital signs at every appointment because of cardiovascular side effects.

• Assess salivary flow as a factor in caries, periodontal disease, and candidiasis.

• Stress from dental procedures may compromise cardiovascular function; determine patient risk.

Consultations:

• Medical consultation should be made to assess disease control and patient's ability to tolerate stress.

Teach patient/family:

- Importance of good oral hygiene to prevent soft tissue inflammation
- Caution to prevent injury when using oral hygiene aids

When chronic dry mouth occurs, advise patient:

- To avoid mouth rinses with high alcohol content because of drying effects
- To use sugarless gum, frequent sips of water, or saliva substitutes
- To use daily home fluoride products for anticaries effect

---

morphine sulfate

(mor'feen)

Astramorph PF, Duramorph, Infumorph 200, Infumorph 500, Kadian, MS Contin, MSIR, Oramorph SR, RMS, Roxanol, Roxanol 100, Roxanol SR, Roxanol T

♣ MOS

Drug class.: Narcotic analgesic

Controlled Substance Schedule II, Canada N

Action: Depresses pain impulse transmission at the CNS by interacting with opioid receptors

Uses: Severe pain

Dosage and routes:

- *Adult:* SC/IM 4-15 mg q4h prn; PO 5-30 mg q4h prn; ext rel q12-24h; rec 10-20 mg q4h prn; IV 4-10 mg diluted in 4-5 ml of water for injection, over 5 min
- *Child:* SC 0.1-0.2 mg/kg, not to exceed 15 mg

Available forms include: Inj SC/IM/IV 0.5, 1, 2, 4, 5, 8, 10, 15, 25, 50 mg/ml; tabs 15, 30 mg; con rel tabs 15, 30, 60, 100, 200 mg; ext rel tabs 15, 30, 60, 100 mg; soluble tabs 10, 15, 30 mg; caps 15, 30 mg; sus rel caps 20, 30, 50, 60, 100 mg; oral sol 10, 20 mg/5 ml, 20 mg/ml, 100 mg/5 ml; rec supp 5, 10, 20, 30 mg

Side effects/adverse reactions:

▼ *ORAL:* Dry mouth

CNS: Drowsiness, dizziness, confusion, headache, sedation, euphoria

CV: Palpitation, bradycardia, change in BP

GI: Nausea, vomiting, anorexia, constipation, cramps, biliary tract pressure

RESP: ***Respiratory depression***

GU: Increased urinary output, dysuria, urinary retention

EENT: Tinnitus, blurred vision, miosis, diplopia

INTEG: Rash, urticaria, bruising, flushing, diaphoresis, pruritus

Contraindications: Hypersensitivity, addiction (narcotic), hemorrhage, bronchial asthma, increased intracranial pressure, MAOIs

Precautions: Addictive personality, pregnancy category C, lactation, MI (acute), severe heart disease, elderly, respiratory depression, hepatic disease, renal disease, child <18 yr

Pharmacokinetics:

PO: Onset variable, peak variable, duration variable

SC: Onset 15-30 min, peak 50-90 min, duration 3-5 hr

IV: Peak 20 min

Half-life 2.5-3 hr; metabolized by liver; excreted by kidneys; crosses placenta; excreted in breast milk

Drug interactions of concern to dentistry:

- Increased CNS depression: alcohol, all CNS depressants
- Contraindication: MAOIs
- Increased effects of anticholinergics

M

DENTAL CONSIDERATIONS

General:

• Monitor vital signs at every appointment because of cardiovascular and respiratory side effects.
• Assess salivary flow as a factor in caries, periodontal disease, and candidiasis.
• After supine positioning, have patient sit upright for at least 2 min before standing to avoid orthostatic hypotension.
• Psychologic and physical dependence may occur with chronic administration.
• Determine why the patient is taking the drug.
• Consider the use of NSAIDs when additional analgesia is required.

Teach patient/family:

When chronic dry mouth occurs, advise patient:

• To use daily home fluoride products for anticaries effect
• To avoid mouth rinses with high alcohol content because of drying effects
• To use sugarless gum, frequent sips of water, or saliva substitutes

---

moxifloxacin HCl

(mox-i-flox'a-sin)

Avelox, Avelox IV

Drug class.: Fluoroquinolone anti-infective

Action: A broad-spectrum bactericidal agent that inhibits the enzymes topoisomerase II (DNA gyrase) and topoisomerase IV required for bacterial DNA replication, transcription repair, and recombination

Uses: Acute bacterial sinusitis (*S. pneumoniae, H. influenzae,* or *M. catarrhalis*); acute bacterial exacerbation of chronic bronchitis (*S. pneumoniae, H. influenzae, H. parainfluenzae, K. pneumoniae, M. catarrhalis,* or *S. aureus*); community-acquired pneumonia (*S. pneumoniae, H. influenzae, M. catarrhalis, M. pneumoniae,* or *C. pneumoniae*)

Dosage and routes:

• *Adult and child >18 yr:* PO/IV 400 mg qd, duration varies from 5-10 days depending on type of infection; take at least 4 hr before or 8 hr after antacids (Mg^{2+}, Al^{3+}), sucralfate, metal cations (Fe^{2+}, Zn^{2+}), or didanosine
• *Adult:* IV inf >60 min, 400 mg qd for 5-14 days depending on the infection

Available forms include: Tabs 400 mg

Side effects/adverse reactions:

▼ *ORAL: Taste perversion,* candidiasis, dry mouth, stomatitis (infrequent)

CNS: Dizziness, light-headedness, headache, ***prolonged QT interval,*** risk of seizures, malaise, insomnia, confusion, tremor, vertigo

CV: Palpitation, tachycardia, hypertension, vasodilation

GI: Nausea, diarrhea, vomiting, abdominal pain, dyspepsia, pseudomembranous colitis

RESP: Asthma, dyspnea

HEMA: ***Thrombocytopenia, eosinophilia, leukopenia***

GU: Vaginal candidiasis, vaginitis

EENT: Pharyngitis, rhinitis, coughing, sinusitis, tinnitus, amblyopia

INTEG: Photosensitivity (has not been shown with this drug), skin rash, pruritus, urticaria

META: Abnormal liver function tests, GGTP elevated, hyperlipidemia, hyperglycemia

MS: Tendon rupture, cartilage damage, leg pain, arthralgia, myalgia
MISC: ***Anaphylaxis*** (rare), allergic reactions

Contraindications: Hypersensitivity to fluoroquinolones

Precautions: Divalent cations, retard absorption, not for use with class 1A and III antiarrhythmics, use in children not studied, cross resistance with other fluoroquinolones, may prolong QT interval in some patients, seizures, use with NSAIDs, pregnancy category C, children <18 yr, lactation

Pharmacokinetics:
PO: Well absorbed, bioavailability 90%, steady state plasma levels in 3 days, plasma protein binding 50%, widely distributed even to saliva, hepatic metabolism, sulfate conjugates excreted in feces, glucuronide conjugates excreted in urine

Drug interactions of concern to dentistry:
- Increased risk of CNS stimulation and seizures: NSAIDs
- Decreased absorption: divalent and trivalent antacids, iron and zinc salts
- Caution when using erythromycin, tricyclic antidepressants (no data, risk of ↑ QT interval)
- Increased risk of life-threatening arrhythmias: procainamide

DENTAL CONSIDERATIONS
General:
- Determine why patient is taking the drug.
- Examine for oral manifestation of opportunistic infection.
- Advise patient if dental drugs prescribed have a potential for photosensitivity.
- Ruptures of the shoulder, hand, and Achilles tendons that required surgical repair or resulted in prolonged disability have been reported with the use of fluoroquinolones. Question patient about history of side effects associated with fluoroquinolone use.
- Monitor vital signs at every appointment because of cardiovascular side effects.
- Patients on chronic drug therapy may rarely have symptoms of blood dyscrasias, which can include infection, bleeding, and poor healing.
- Consider semisupine chair position for patient comfort if GI side effects occur.

Consultations:
- In a patient with symptoms of blood dyscrasias, request a medical consultation for blood studies and postpone treatment until normal values are reestablished.
- Physician consultation is advised in the presence of an acute dental infection requiring another antibiotic.

Teach patient/family:
- *If used for dental infection:*
- To minimize exposure to sunlight and wear sunscreen if sun exposure is planned
- To discontinue treatment and inform dentist immediately if patient experiences pain or inflammation of a tendon, and to rest and refrain from exercise

moxifloxacin HCl

(mox-i-flox'a-sin)
Vigamox

Drug class.: Fluoroquinolone anti-infective

Action: A broad-spectrum bactericidal agent that inhibits the en-

zymes topoisomerase II DNA gyrase and topoisomerase IV required for bacterial DNA replication, transcription repair, and recombination
Uses: Bacterial conjunctivitis caused by susceptible bacterial strains including selected aerobic gram-positive species, selected aerobic gram-negative species, and *C. trachomatis*
Dosage and routes:
• *Adult:* TOP instill 1 drop in affected eye(s) tid × 7 days
Available forms include: Opth sol 0.5% in 3ml
Side effects/adverse reactions:
RESP: Cough
EENT: Decreased visual acuity, dry eyes, keratitis, ocular discomfort and pain, ocular pruritus, pharyngitis, rhinitis
INTEG: Rash
MISC: Serious allergic reactions
Contraindications: Hypersensitivity to this drug or other fluoroquinolones
Precautions: Prolonged use–risk of superinfections, do not wear contact lens if eye infection is present, use clean technique to avoid solution contamination, pregnancy category C, efficacy and safety in nursing mother or pediatric patient <1 yr have not been established, risk of tendon or cartilage damage unknown
Pharmacokinetics:
TOP: Extremely low systemic absorption, half-life 13 hr
Drug interactions of concern to dentistry:
• No data reported
DENTAL CONSIDERATIONS
General:
• Avoid dental light in patient's eyes.
• Protect patient's eyes from accidental spatter during dental treatment.

mupirocin/mupirocin calcium

(myoo-peer'o-sin)
Bactroban Ointment, Bactroban Cream, Bactroban Nasal 2%
Drug class.: Topical antiinfective, pseudomonic acid A

Action: Inhibits bacterial protein synthesis
Uses: Impetigo caused by *S. aureus,* β-hemolytic streptococci, *S. pyogenes;* nasal membranes: *S. aureus*
Dosage and routes:
• *TOP:* Apply small amount to affected area tid
• *CREAM:* For secondary infected, traumatic skin lesions; apply small amount to affected area tid × 10 days
• *Child >11 yr:* NASAL divide one half of the ointment from the single-use tube between the nostrils and apply bid for 5 days
Available forms include: Oint 2% (20 mg/g), 15, 30 g; nasal oint 2% single-use tube 1 g; cream 2% in 1 g
Side effects/adverse reactions:
INTEG: Burning, stinging, itching, rash, dry skin, swelling, contact dermatitis, erythema, tenderness, increased exudate
Contraindications: Hypersensitivity
Precautions: Pregnancy category B, lactation
DENTAL CONSIDERATIONS
General:
• The dentist may choose to avoid elective dental treatment if the

infected site may be affected by dental treatment.

mycophenolate mofetil

(mye-koe-fen'oh-late moe'fe-til)
CellCept

Drug class.: Immunosuppressant

Action: Selective inhibitor of inosine monophosphate dehydrogenase, thereby preventing the synthesis of guanosine nucleotide and resulting in cytostatic effects on T and B lymphocytes

Uses: Prophylaxis of organ rejection in patients receiving allogenic renal or hepatic transplants, cardiac transplants (in combination with cyclosporine and corticosteroids)

Dosage and routes:

• *Adult:* PO/IV 1 g bid in combination with corticosteroids and cyclosporine in renal transplant (within 72 hr of transplant); 1.5 g bid for cardiac transplant; 1 g bid for hepatic transplant

Available forms include: Tabs 500 mg; caps 250 mg; powder for inj 500 mg; powder oral susp 200 mg/ml in 225 ml

Side effects/adverse reactions:

▼ *ORAL: Candidiasis*

CNS: Fever, headache, tremor, insomnia, dizziness

CV: Hypertension, chest pain, peripheral edema

GI: Diarrhea, abdominal pain, nausea, dyspepsia, vomiting, ***ischemic colitis,*** GI bleeding

RESP: Infection, dyspnea, cough, pharyngitis

HEMA: ***Leukopenia, sepsis, anemia, thrombocytopenia***

GU: Infection, hematuria, ***renal tubular necrosis***

INTEG: Acne, rash

MS: Back pain, asthenia

Contraindications: Hypersensitivity

Precautions: Active GI diseases, pregnancy category C, lactation, reduce dose in severe chronic renal impairment, increased risk of development of lymphomas or other malignancies and susceptibility to infection

Pharmacokinetics:

PO: Rapidly absorbed; highly plasma bound (97%); metabolized to mycophenolic acid (MPA), the active form of the drug; primary excretion in urine (93%)

Drug interactions of concern to dentistry:

• Increased plasma concentration: acyclovir, ganciclovir

• Decreased availability of MPA: drugs that alter the GI flora

DENTAL CONSIDERATIONS

General:

• Determine why the patient is taking the drug.

• Short appointments and a stress reduction protocol may be required for anxious patients.

• Patients who have been or are currently on chronic steroid therapy (>2 wk) may require supplemental steroids for dental treatment.

• Patients on chronic drug therapy may rarely have symptoms of blood dyscrasias, which can include infection, bleeding, and poor healing.

• Place on frequent recall because of oral side effects.

• Determine dose and duration of steroid for patient to assess risk for stress tolerance and immunosuppression.

• Examine for oral manifestation of opportunistic infections.

M

• Monitor vital signs at every appointment because of cardiovascular and respiratory side effects.
• Consider semisupine chair position for patient comfort if GI side effects occur.
• Antibiotic prophylaxis is usually recommended in patients with organ transplants and immunosuppression.
• Monitor time since organ/tissue transplant; note duration of transplant and status of renal function.
• Place on frequent recall because of possible blood dyscrasias and oral side effects.

Consultations:

• Medical consultation may be required to assess disease control and patient's ability to tolerate stress.
• In a patient with symptoms of blood dyscrasias, request a medical consultation for blood studies and postpone dental treatment until normal values are reestablished.
• Request baseline blood pressure in renal transplant patients for patient evaluation before dental treatment.

Teach patient/family:

• That secondary oral infection may occur; must see dentist immediately if infection occurs
• Importance of good oral hygiene to prevent soft tissue inflammation
• Need for frequent recall because of possible blood dyscrasias and oral side effects
• To report oral lesions, soreness, or bleeding to dentist

nabumetone

(na-byoo'me-tone)
Relafen

Drug class.: Nonsteroidal antiinflammatory

Action: Inhibits prostaglandin synthesis by interfering with cyclooxygenase needed for biosynthesis; possesses analgesic, antiinflammatory, antipyretic properties

Uses: Osteoarthritis, rheumatoid arthritis, acute or chronic treatment

Dosage and routes:

• *Adult:* PO 1000 mg as a single dose; may increase to 1500-2000 mg/day if needed; may give qd or bid

Available forms include: Tabs 500, 750 mg

Side effects/adverse reactions:

▼ *ORAL:* Dry mouth, bleeding, stomatitis, lichenoid reactions

CNS: Dizziness, headache, drowsiness, fatigue, tremors, confusion, insomnia, anxiety, depression, nervousness

CV: Tachycardia, peripheral edema, palpitation, dysrhythmias, CHF

GI: ***Cholestatic hepatitis,*** constipation, flatulence, cramps, peptic ulcer, gastritis, nausea, anorexia, vomiting, diarrhea, jaundice

RESP: ***Bronchospasm,*** dyspnea, pharyngitis

HEMA: ***Blood dyscrasias***

GU: ***Nephrotoxicity, dysuria, hematuria, oliguria, azotemia,*** cystitis

EENT: Tinnitus, hearing loss, blurred vision

INTEG: Purpura, rash, pruritus, sweating, photosensitivity

Contraindications: Hypersensitivity to this drug or aspirin, iodides, NSAIDs, asthma, severe renal disease

Precautions: Pregnancy category C, lactation, children, bleeding disorders, GI disorders, cardiac disorders, renal disorders, hepatic dysfunction, elderly

Pharmacokinetics:

PO: Peak 2.5-4 hr, half-life 22-30 hr; plasma protein binding >90%; metabolized in liver to active metabolite; excreted in urine (metabolites), breast milk

Drug interactions of concern to dentistry:

- GI ulceration, bleeding: aspirin, alcohol, corticosteroids
- May decrease effects of nabumetone: salicylates
- Nephrotoxicity: acetaminophen (prolonged use and high doses)
- Possible risk of decreased renal function: cyclosporine
- First-time users of SSRIs also taking NSAIDs may have a higher risk of GI side effects; until more data are available, it may be advisable to avoid use of NSAIDs in these patients (*Br J Clin Pharmacol* 55:591-595, 2003)

DENTAL CONSIDERATIONS

General:

- Patients on chronic drug therapy may rarely have symptoms of blood dyscrasias, which can include infection, bleeding, and poor healing.
- Assess salivary flow as a factor in caries, periodontal disease, and candidiasis.
- Avoid prescribing for dental use in last trimester of pregnancy.
- Avoid prescribing aspirin-containing products.
- Consider semisupine chair position for patients with arthritic disease.

Consultations:

- In a patient with symptoms of blood dyscrasias, request a medical consultation for blood studies and postpone dental treatment until normal values are reestablished.
- Medical consultation may be required to assess disease control.

Teach patient/family:

- Importance of good oral hygiene to prevent soft tissue inflammation
- Caution to prevent injury when using oral hygiene aids

When chronic dry mouth occurs, advise patient:

- To avoid mouth rinses with high alcohol content because of drying effects
- Of need for daily use of home fluoride
- To use sugarless gum, frequent sips of water, or saliva substitutes

N

nadolol

(nay-doe'lole)

Corgard

♣ Syn-Nadolo

Drug class.: Nonselective β-adrenergic blocker

Action: This is a nonselective β_1- and β_2-adrenergic antagonist. The antihypertensive mechanism of action is unclear, but it may include a reduction in cardiac output and inhibition of renin release by the renal juxtaglomerular apparatus. Peripheral resistance decreases with long-term use. The antianginal action (when indicated for this use) may be related to a decrease in myocardial oxygen demand and negative chronotropic and inotro-

pic effects. The antiarrhythmic action (when indicated for this use) has been related to a reduction in spontaneous pacemaker firing and slowing of AV nodal conduction.
Uses: Chronic stable angina pectoris, mild-to-moderate hypertension; unapproved: dysrhythmias, MI prophylaxis, vascular headache
Dosage and routes:
Hypertension:
• *Adult:* PO 40 mg qd, increase by 40-80 mg q3-7d; dose range 40-320 mg/day
Angina:
• *Adult:* PO 40 mg/day, can increase dose over 3-7 day intervals until desired clinical response or pronounced slowing of heart; maintenance dose 40-80 mg/day; upper dose 240 mg/day
Available forms include: Oral tabs 20, 40, 80, 120, 160 mg
Side effects/adverse reactions:
▼ *ORAL:* Dry mouth, taste disturbances
CNS: Depression, hallucinations, dizziness, fatigue, lethargy, paresthesia, headache
CV: Bradycardia, hypotension, ***CHF,*** palpitation, AV block
GI: Nausea, vomiting, diarrhea, colitis, constipation, cramps, flatulence, hepatomegaly, pancreatitis
RESP: ***Laryngospasm, bronchospasm,*** dyspnea, respiratory dysfunction, cough, wheezing, nasal stuffiness, pharyngitis
HEMA: ***Agranulocytosis, thrombocytopenia,*** chest pain, peripheral ischemia, flushing, edema, vasodilation, conduction disturbances
EENT: Sore throat
INTEG: Rash, pruritus, fever
Contraindications: Hypersensitivity to this drug, cardiac failure, cardiogenic shock, second- or third-degree heart block, bronchospastic disease, sinus bradycardia, CHF, COPD
Precautions: Diabetes mellitus, pregnancy category C, renal disease, lactation, hyperthyroidism, peripheral vascular disease, myasthenia gravis
Pharmacokinetics:
PO: Onset variable, peak 3-4 hr, duration 17-24 hr, half-life 16-20 hr; not metabolized; excreted in urine (unchanged), bile, breast milk
Drug interactions of concern to dentistry:
• Decreased effects: sympathomimetics (epinephrine, norepinephrine, isoproterenol)
• Slows metabolism of nadolol: lidocaine
• Increased hypotension, myocardial depression: fentanyl derivatives, hydrocarbon inhalation anesthetics
• Decreased hypotensive effect: indomethacin and other NSAIDs

DENTAL CONSIDERATIONS
General:
• Monitor vital signs at every appointment because of cardiovascular side effects.
• Patients on chronic drug therapy may rarely have symptoms of blood dyscrasias, which can include infection, bleeding, and poor healing.
• After supine positioning, have patient sit upright for at least 2 min before standing to avoid orthostatic hypotension.
• Limit use of sodium-containing products, such as saline IV fluids, for patients with a dietary salt restriction.

• Assess salivary flow as a factor in caries, periodontal disease, and candidiasis.
• Stress from dental procedures may compromise cardiovascular function; determine patient risk.
• Short appointments and a stress reduction protocol may be required for anxious patients.
• Consider semisupine chair position for patients with respiratory distress.

Consultations:
• In a patient with symptoms of blood dyscrasias, request a medical consultation for blood studies and postpone dental treatment until normal values are reestablished.
• Take precautions if dental surgery is anticipated and anesthesia is required.
• Medical consultation may be required to assess disease control and patient's ability to tolerate stress.

Teach patient/family:
• Importance of good oral hygiene to prevent soft tissue inflammation
• Caution to prevent injury when using oral hygiene aids

When chronic dry mouth occurs, advise patient:
• To avoid mouth rinses with high alcohol content because of drying effects
• Of need for daily home fluoride use to prevent caries
• To use sugarless gum, frequent sips of water, or saliva substitutes

naftifine HCl

(naf'ti-fin)

Naftin

Drug class.: Topical antifungal

Action: Interferes with cell membrane permeability in fungi such as *T. rubrum, T. mentagrophytes, T. tonsurans, E. floccosum, M. canis, M. audouinii, M. gypseum, Candida;* broad-spectrum antifungal

Uses: Tinea cruris, tinea corporis, tinea pedis

Dosage and routes:
• Massage small amount into affected area, surrounding area bid; continue for 7-14 days

Available forms include: Cream 1%; gel 1%

Side effects/adverse reactions:
INTEG: Burning, stinging, dryness, itching, local irritation

Contraindications: Hypersensitivity

Precautions: Pregnancy category B, lactation, children

nalmefene HCl

(nal'me-feen)

Revex

Drug class.: Opioid antagonist

Action: Reverses the effects of opioids by competitive antagonism of opioid receptors

Uses: Management of opioid overdose and complete or partial reversal of opioid drug effects, including respiratory depression

Dosage and routes:

Reversal of opioid depression:
• *Adult:* IV (100 μg/ml strength) initial dose 0.25 μg/kg followed by 0.25 μg/kg, incremental dose at 2-5 min intervals; cumulative

N

doses over 1.0 μg/kg do not provide additional therapeutic effect; titrate all doses

Body weight (kg)	ml of 100 μg/ml solution
50	0.125
60	0.150
70	0.175
80	0.200
90	0.225
100	0.250

Known or suspected opioid overdose:

• *Adult:* IV (1 mg/ml strength) initial 0.5 mg/70 kg; if needed, a second dose of 1.0 mg/70 kg, 2-5 min later; doses over 1.5 mg/70 kg are unlikely to be beneficial

Available forms include: Ampule 100 μg/ml in 1 ml ampule; 1 mg/ml in 2 ml ampule

Side effects/adverse reactions:

▼ *ORAL:* Dry mouth (<1%)

CNS: Dizziness, headache, dysphoria, perception of pain, nervousness

CV: Tachycardia, hypertension, dysrhythmia, hypotension

GI: Nausea, abdominal cramps, vomiting, diarrhea

RESP: Pharyngitis, pulmonary edema

GU: Urinary retention

INTEG: Pruritus

MS: Myalgia, joint pain

MISC: Chills

Contraindications: Hypersensitivity

Precautions: Pregnancy category B, nursing, children, withdrawal symptoms in opioid addicts, renal impairment

Pharmacokinetics:

IV: Onset 2 min, peak plasma conc 1.1-2.3 hr; can also be given IM or SC; hepatic metabolism; excreted in urine

Drug interactions of concern to dentistry:

• None reported

DENTAL CONSIDERATIONS

General:

• This drug is intended for acute use only, but listed side effects can sometimes be seen.

• There is a risk of seizures reported in animal studies; be aware of this potential.

• Serious cardiovascular events have been associated with opioid reversal in postoperative patients; doses should be carefully titrated to reduce these events.

• Buprenorphine depression may not be completely reversed.

• In all cases, the establishment of a patent airway, ventilatory assistance, oxygen administration, and circulatory access should complement or precede opioid antagonist use.

• Significant opioid depression occurring in the dental office may require relocation of the patient to a medical facility for comprehensive management.

• Patients discharged from the office/emergency facility should be carefully observed for the return of opioid-induced depression.

naloxone HCl

(nal-ox'one)

Narcan

Drug class.: Narcotic antagonist

Action: Competes with narcotics at narcotic receptor sites

Uses: Respiratory depression induced by narcotics, to reverse postoperative opioid depression

Dosage and routes:

Narcotic-induced respiratory depression:

• *Adult and adolescent:* IV/SC/IM 0.4-2 mg; repeat q2-3 min, if needed

Postoperative respiratory depression:

• *Adult:* IV 0.1-0.2 mg q2-3min prn to desired level of response

• *Child:* IV/IM/SC 0.01 mg/kg q2-3min prn to desired level of response

Asphyxia neonatorum:

• *Neonates:* IV/IM/SC 0.01 mg/kg given into umbilical vein after delivery; may repeat in q2-3min × 3 doses

Available forms include: Inj IV/IM/SC 0.02, 0.4 mg/ml in 1, 2 ml ampules

Side effects/adverse reactions:

CNS: Drowsiness, nervousness, restlessness, excitement

CV: Rapid pulse, increased or decreased systolic BP high doses

GI: Nausea, vomiting

RESP: Hyperpnea

MISC: Sweating

Contraindications: Hypersensitivity, cardiac irritability

Precautions: Pregnancy category B, opioid dependence

Pharmacokinetics: Onset 1-2 min (IV), 2-5 min (IM), peak effect 5-15 min, duration variable up to 45 min, half-life 60-90 min; metabolized by liver; excreted by kidneys; crosses placenta; excreted in breast milk

Drug interactions of concern to dentistry:

• Antagonizes effects of opioid agonists and mixed agonist/antagonists

DENTAL CONSIDERATIONS

General:

• This drug is intended for acute use only, but listed side effects can sometimes be seen.

• There is a risk of seizures reported in animal studies; be aware of this potential.

• Serious cardiovascular events have been associated with opioid reversal in postoperative patients; doses should be carefully titrated to reduce these events.

• Buprenorphine depression may not be completely reversed.

• In all cases, the establishment of a patent airway, ventilatory assistance, oxygen administration, and circulatory access should complement or precede opioid antagonist use.

• Significant opioid depression occurring in the dental office may require relocation of the patient to a medical facility for comprehensive management.

• Patients discharged from the office/emergency facility should be carefully observed for the return of opioid-induced depression.

N

naltrexone HCl

(nal-trex'one)

Depade, ReVia, Trexan

Drug class.: Narcotic antagonist

Action: Competes with opioids at opioid receptor sites

Uses: Used in treatment of opioid addiction following detoxification, alcoholism

Dosage and routes:

Use after patient is opioid free for at least 7-10 days:

• *Adult:* PO 25 mg, may give 25 mg after 1 hr if there are no withdrawal symptoms; 50-150 mg may be given qd depending on patient need; maintenance 50 mg q24h

Alcoholism:

• *Adult:* PO 50 mg/day

Available forms include: Tabs 50 mg

Side effects/adverse reactions:

▼ *ORAL:* Increased thirst

CNS: Stimulation, drowsiness, dizziness, confusion, convulsion, headache, flushing, hallucinations

CV: Rapid pulse, pulmonary edema, hypertension

GI: Nausea, vomiting, diarrhea, heartburn, ***hepatitis,*** anorexia

RESP: Wheezing, hyperpnea

HEMA: ***Thrombocytopenia, agranulocytosis, leukopenia, neutropenia, hemolytic anemia,*** increased pro-time

EENT: Tinnitus, hearing loss

INTEG: Rash, urticaria, bruising

Contraindications: Hypersensitivity, opioid dependence, hepatic failure, hepatitis

Precautions: Pregnancy category C

Pharmacokinetics:

PO: Onset 15-30 min, peak 1-2 hr, duration is dose dependent, half-life 4 hr; extensive first-pass metabolism; metabolized by liver; excreted by kidneys; crosses placenta; excreted in breast milk

Drug interactions of concern to dentistry:

• Decreased effects of opioid narcotics

DENTAL CONSIDERATIONS

General:

• Monitor vital signs at every appointment because of cardiovascular and respiratory side effects.

• Patients on chronic drug therapy may rarely have symptoms of blood dyscrasias, which can include infection, bleeding, and poor healing.

• Patients should not be given opioid analgesics for dental pain management. Substitute with NSAID and long-acting local anesthetics.

• The dental professional must be aware of the patient's disease, and the patient must be active in treatment for chemical dependency.

Consultations:

• In a patient with symptoms of blood dyscrasias, request a medical consultation for blood studies and postpone dental treatment until normal values are reestablished.

• Medical consultation may be required to assess disease control.

• Inform aftercare provider or counselor if sedative medications are required for proper management.

Teach patient/family:

• Importance of good oral hygiene to prevent soft tissue inflammation

• Caution to prevent injury when using oral hygiene aids

naphazoline HCl

(naf-az'oh-leen)

AK-Con Ophthalmic, Albalon, Allerest Eye Drops, Allergy Drops, Clear Eyes ACR, Comfort Eye Drops, Digest 2, 20/20 Eye Drops, Maximum Strength Allergy Drops, Nafazair, Naphcon, Naphcon Forte, VasoClear, Vasocon

Drug class.: Ophthalmic vasoconstrictor

Action: Vasoconstriction of eye arterioles; decreases eye engorgement by stimulation of α-adrenergic receptors

Uses: Relieves hyperemia, irritation in superficial corneal vascularity

Dosage and routes:

• *Adult:* Instill 1-2 gtt up to tid or qid as needed

Available forms include: Sol 0.012, 0.02, 0.03, 0.1%

Side effects/adverse reactions:

CNS: Headache, dizziness, sedation, anxiety, weakness, sweating (systemic absorption)

CV: ***CV collapse (systemic absorption),*** hypertension, dysrhythmias, tachycardia

EENT: Pupil dilation, increased intraocular pressure, photophobia

Contraindications: Hypersensitivity, glaucoma (narrow-angle)

Precautions: Hypertension, hyperthyroidism, elderly, severe arteriosclerosis, cardiac disease, pregnancy category C

Pharmacokinetics:

INSTILL: Duration 2-3 hr

Drug interactions of concern to dentistry:

• Increased pressor effects: tricyclic antidepressants

DENTAL CONSIDERATIONS

General:

• Monitor vital signs at every appointment because of cardiovascular side effects.

• Avoid dental light in patient's eyes; offer dark glasses for patient comfort.

• Protect patient's eyes from accidental spatter during dental treatment.

naproxen/naproxen sodium

(na-prox'en)

Naproxen: EC Naprosyn, Naprosyn, Naprosyn Oral Suspension

♣ Apo-Naproxen, Naprosyn-E, Naprosyn SR, Naxen, Novo-Naprox, Nu-Prox

Naproxen sodium: Anaprox, Anaprox DS; *OTC:* Aleve

♣ Apo-Napro-Na, Apo-Napro-Na DS, Novo-Naprox Sodium, Novo-Naprox Sodium DS, Synflex, Synflex DS

Drug class.: Nonsteroidal antiinflammatory

Action: Inhibits prostaglandin synthesis by interfering with cyclooxygenase needed for biosynthesis; possesses analgesic, antiinflammatory, antipyretic properties

Uses: Mild-to-moderate pain, osteoarthritis, rheumatoid, juvenile, gouty arthritis, ankylosing spondylitis, primary dysmenorrhea; unapproved: migraine, PMS, fever

Dosage and routes:

Mild-to-moderate pain:

• *Adult:* PO 500 mg q12h or 250 mg q6-8 hr, not to exceed 1 g/day (base); 550 mg, then 275 mg q6-8h

N

prn, not to exceed 1475 mg (sodium); sus rel: 1000 mg once daily

Rheumatoid arthritis, osteoarthritis, dysmenorrhea, ankylosing spondylitis, tendinitis:

• *Adult:* PO tabs 250-500 mg bid, max dose 1.5 g/day; del rel tab 375-500 mg bid; con rel tab 750-1000 mg/day; naproxen sodium tab 275-550 mg bid

Juvenile arthritis:

• *Adult:* PO susp (naproxen only) 10 mg/kg/d in two divided doses

Available forms include: Tabs 200 mg (OTC), 250, 275, 375, 500, 550 mg; del rel tabs 375, 500 mg; con rel 375, 500 mg; susp 125 mg/5 ml

Side effects/adverse reactions:

▼ *ORAL:* Stomatitis, bleeding, dry mouth, lichenoid reactions

CNS: Dizziness, drowsiness, fatigue, tremors, confusion, insomnia, anxiety, depression

CV: Tachycardia, peripheral edema, palpitation, dysrhythmias

GI: ***Cholestatic hepatitis,*** nausea, anorexia, vomiting, diarrhea, jaundice, constipation, flatulence, cramps, peptic ulcer

HEMA: ***Blood dyscrasias***

GU: ***Nephrotoxicity: dysuria, hematuria, oliguria, azotemia***

EENT: Tinnitus, hearing loss, blurred vision

INTEG: Purpura, rash, pruritus, sweating

Contraindications: Hypersensitivity, asthma, severe renal disease, severe hepatic disease

Precautions: Pregnancy category B, lactation, children, bleeding disorders, GI disorders, cardiac disorders, hypersensitivity to other anti-inflammatory agents, elderly, >2 alcohol drinks daily

Pharmacokinetics:

PO: Peak 2-4 hr, half-life 3-3.5 hr; 99% protein binding; metabolized in liver; excreted in urine (metabolites), breast milk

Drug interactions of concern to dentistry:

• GI ulceration, bleeding: aspirin, alcohol, corticosteroids

• Nephrotoxicity: acetaminophen (chronic use and high doses)

• Possible risk of decreased renal function: cyclosporine

• Increased photosensitization: tetracycline

• Increased plasma levels: probenecid

• First-time users of SSRIs also taking NSAIDs may have a higher risk of GI side effects; until more data are available, it may be advisable to avoid use of NSAIDs in these patients (*Br J Clin Pharmacol* 55:591-595, 2003)

When prescribed for dental pain:

• Risk of increased effects: oral anticoagulants, oral antidiabetics, lithium, methotrexate

• Decreased antihypertensive effects of diuretics, β-adrenergic blockers, and ACE inhibitors

DENTAL CONSIDERATIONS

General:

• Patients on chronic drug therapy may rarely have symptoms of blood dyscrasias, which can include infection, bleeding, and poor healing.

• Assess salivary flow as a factor in caries, periodontal disease, and candidiasis.

• Avoid prescribing for dental use in last trimester of pregnancy.

• Avoid prescribing aspirin-containing products.

• Consider semisupine chair position for patients with arthritic disease.

Consultations:

• In a patient with symptoms of blood dyscrasias, request a medical consultation for blood studies and postpone dental treatment until normal values are reestablished.

• Medical consultation may be required to assess disease control.

Teach patient/family:

• Importance of good oral hygiene to prevent soft tissue inflammation

• Caution to prevent injury when using oral hygiene aids

When chronic dry mouth occurs, advise patient:

• To avoid mouth rinses with high alcohol content because of drying effects

• Of need for daily use of home fluoride products to prevent caries

• To use sugarless gum, frequent sips of water, or saliva substitutes

naratriptan HCl

(nar'a-trip-tan)

Amerge

Drug class.: Serotonin agonist

Action: A selective agonist for 5-HT_{1D} and 5-HT_{1B} receptors located on intracranial blood vessels leading to vasoconstriction and possibly inhibition of proinflammatory neuropeptide release

Uses: Acute treatment of migraine attacks with or without aura in adults

Dosage and routes:

• *Adult:* PO 1-2.5 mg with fluids; dose can be repeated once after 4 hr; max dose 5 mg/24 hr

Available forms include: Tabs 1, 2.5 mg

Side effects/adverse reactions:

▼ *ORAL:* Dry mouth

CNS: Paresthesias, dizziness, drowsiness, malaise, fatigue

CV: Palpitation, hypertension, tachyarrhythmias

GI: Nausea, vomiting, discomfort, dyspepsia

RESP: Bronchitis, cough

HEMA: Leukocytosis

GU: Bladder inflammation, polyuria

EENT: Throat/neck symptoms, photophobia, sinusitis, tinnitus, blurred vision, vertigo

INTEG: Sweating, rash

ENDO: Polydipsia, thirst

MS: Muscle pain, arthralgia

Contraindications: Hypersensitivity, ischemic heart disease, vasospastic coronary artery disease, cerebrovascular or periperipheral vascular disease, uncontrolled hypertension, severe renal or hepatic impairment, hemiplegic or basilar migraine, ergot-containing drugs, sibutramine

Precautions: Risk of serious cardiovascular events, including ischemia and MI; renal/hepatic dysfunction, SSRI antidepressants, pregnancy category C, lactation, use in children not established, not recommended in elderly

Pharmacokinetics:

PO: Bioavailability 70%, peak levels 2-3 hr, protein binding 28%-31%, metabolized by cytochrome P-450 enzymes; 50% of dose excreted in urine unchanged; 30% as metabolite

Drug interactions of concern to dentistry:

• No specific interactions with dental drugs reported

• Should not be used within 24 hr of another 5HT_1 agonist

N

DENTAL CONSIDERATIONS

General:

• This is an acute-use drug; it is doubtful that patients will come to the office if acute migraine is present.

• Be aware of patient's disease, its severity, and its frequency when known.

Consultations:

• If treating chronic orofacial pain, consult with physician of record.

• Medical consultation may be required to assess disease control and patient's ability to tolerate stress.

Teach patient/family:

• Importance of updating health and drug history if physician makes any changes in evaluation or drug regimens

• That dryness of the mouth may occur when taking this drug; avoid mouth rinses with high alcohol content because of additional drying effects.

nateglinide

(na-teg'lin-ide)

Starlix

Drug class.: Oral antidiabetic, meglitinide class

Action: Lowers blood glucose by stimulation of insulin release from the pancreatic β-cells; binds to ATP-dependent potassium channels in functioning β-cells with opening of calcium channels and subsequent insulin release

Uses: Type 2 diabetes mellitus when hyperglycemia cannot be controlled by diet and exercise, can be used in combination with metformin, not for patients who have been chronically treated with other antidiabetic drugs

Dosage and routes:

• *Adult:* PO 120 mg tid before meals as a single drug or in combination with metformin

Patients near HbA_{1C} goal:

• *Adult:* PO treatment can be initiated with 60 mg dose as a single drug or in combination with metformin

Available forms include: Tabs 60, 120 mg

Side effects/adverse reactions:

CNS: Dizziness, tremor

GI: Diarrhea, upset stomach

RESP: URI, flu symptoms, bronchitis, coughing

INTEG: Increased sweating

Contraindications: Hypersensitivity, type 1 diabetes, diabetic ketoacidosis

Precautions: Hypoglycemia (geriatric, malnourished, adrenal insufficiency or pituitary insufficiency more susceptible to hypoglycemia), β-blocker may mask hypoglycemia, administer before meals, infection, hepatic dysfunction, pregnancy category C, lactation, children

Pharmacokinetics:

PO: Rapid absorption, peak plasma levels 1 hr, bioavailability 73%, plasma protein binding 98%, hepatic metabolism (CYP450 2C9 isoenzyme [70%] and CYP450 3A4 isoenzyme [30%]); excretion renal (83%), feces (10%)

Drug interactions of concern to dentistry:

• Most drug interactions not clearly identified; may act as an inhibitor of CYP450 2C9 enzymes but not

CYP450 3A4 (see Appendix I) Does not appear to interact with highly protein bound drugs

• Potential potentiation of hypoglycemic effects: NSAIDs, salicylates, nonselective β-blockers

DENTAL CONSIDERATIONS

General:

• If dentist prescribes any of the drugs listed in the drug interaction section, monitor patient's blood sugar levels.

• Consider semisupine chair position for patient comfort if GI side effects occur.

• Ensure that patient is following prescribed diet and regularly takes medication.

• Place on frequent recall to evaluate healing response.

• Short appointments and a stress reduction protocol may be required.

• Diabetics may be more susceptible to infection and have delayed wound healing.

Consultations:

• Medical consultation may include data from patient's blood glucose monitoring, including glycosylated hemoglobin or HbA_{1c} testing.

• Medical consultation may be required to assess disease control and patient's ability to tolerate stress.

Teach patient/family:

• To prevent trauma when using oral hygiene aids

• Importance of updating health and drug history if physician makes any changes in evaluation or drug regimens

nedocromil sodium

(ne-doe-kroe'mil)

Tilade (inhalation)

♣ Alocril (ophthalmic solution)

Drug class.: Antiasthmatic, mast cell stabilizer

Action: Stabilizes the membrane of the sensitized mast cell, preventing release of chemical mediators after an antigen-Ig E interaction

Uses: Maintenance therapy in mild to moderate asthma; ophthalmic solution for allergic conjunctivitis

Dosage and routes:

• *Adult and child >6 yr:* Inh 4 mg bid-qid

Allergic conjunctivitis:

• *Adult:* Ophth 1 or 2 drops in each eye bid

Available forms include: Inhaler spray unit 1.75 mg per actuation; ophthalmic sol 2%

Side effects/adverse reactions:

▼ *ORAL:* Dry/burning mouth, bitter taste (aerosol)

CNS: Headache, dizziness, neuritis

GI: Nausea, vomiting, anorexia

GU: Frequency, dysuria

EENT: Throat irritation, cough, nasal congestion, burning eyes

INTEG: Rash, urticaria, angioedema

MS: Joint pain/swelling

Contraindications: Hypersensitivity to this drug or lactose, status asthmaticus

Precautions: Pregnancy category B, lactation, renal disease, hepatic disease, safety and efficacy in child <6 yr (INH) or ophthalmic sol <3 yr not established

Pharmacokinetics:
INH: Peak 15 min, duration 4-6 hr, half-life 80 min; excreted unchanged in feces

DENTAL CONSIDERATIONS

General:
• Assess salivary flow as a factor in caries, periodontal disease, and candidiasis.
• Consider semisupine chair position for patients with respiratory disease.
• Short appointments and a stress reduction protocol may be required for anxious patients.
• Be aware that aspirin or sulfite preservatives in vasoconstrictor-containing products can exacerbate asthma.

Consultations:
• Medical consultation may be required to assess disease control.

Teach patient/family:
• To avoid mouth rinses with high alcohol content because of drying effects
• For inhalation dosage forms, rinse mouth with water after each dose to prevent dryness

---

nefazodone HCl

(nef-ay'zoe-done)
Serzone
Drug class.: Antidepressant

Action: Inhibits neuronal uptake of serotonin and norepinephrine; the exact mechanism of antidepressant activity remains unknown

Uses: Major depressive disorders

Dosage and routes:
• *Adult:* PO initial dose 200 mg/day in 2 divided doses bid; gradually increase dose in increments of 100-200 mg/day, depending on response and need (all doses are given bid); dose range in clinical trials was 300-600 mg/day; initial doses in elderly should be reduced by one half

Available forms include: Tabs 50, 100, 150, 200, 250 mg

Side effects/adverse reactions:
▼ *ORAL: Dry mouth,* taste alteration, candidiasis (rare), stomatitis
CNS: Somnolence, dizziness, insomnia, confusion, light-headedness, headache, memory impairment, abnormal dreams, mania
CV: Postural hypotension, hypotension, dysrhythmias (rare), peripheral edema
GI: Constipation, nausea, dyspepsia, diarrhea, increased appetite, gastroenteritis, ***life-threatening liver failure, hepatic cirrhosis***
RESP: Pharyngitis, cough, bronchitis
GU: Urinary frequency, UTI, vaginitis, urinary retention, impotence, priapism
EENT: Blurred vision, abnormal vision, visual field defect, eye pain, tinnitus
INTEG: Rash, pruritus, dry skin, urticaria, photosensitivity
MS: Neck rigidity
MISC: Flulike syndrome, chills, fever

Contraindications: Hypersensitivity, coadministration of MAOIs

Precautions: Mania, hypomania, suicidal tendencies, seizures, history of MI or unstable heart conditions, hepatic impairment, pregnancy category C, lactation, child <18 yr, elderly (requires dose adjustment), priapism history, alcohol use; risk in operating auto or hazardous machinery

Pharmacokinetics: Bioavailability 20% with PO doses, peak plasma levels 1 hr, half-life 2-4 hr;

highly protein bound 99%; extensive hepatic metabolism; metabolites excreted in urine

Drug interactions of concern to dentistry:

• Must *not* be used concurrently with or within 14 days of discontinuing MAOI

• Risk of significant adverse drug interaction with triazolam, alprazolam, alcohol-containing products

• Increased sedation: St. John's wort (herb)

• Acts as an inhibitor of CYP3A4 isoenzymes: risk of interaction with drugs metabolized by CYP3A4 (see Appendix I)

• NOTE: No information is available on use of this drug in patients who are candidates for conscious sedation or general anesthesia.

DENTAL CONSIDERATIONS

General:

• Assess salivary flow as a factor in caries, periodontal disease, and candidiasis.

• Take vital signs at every appointment because of cardiovascular side effects.

• After supine positioning, have patient sit upright for at least 2 min before standing to avoid postural hypotension.

• There is no information concerning the use of vasoconstrictors in patients taking this drug.

• Advise patient if dental drugs prescribed have a potential for photosensitivity.

Consultations:

• Medical consultation may be required to assess disease control.

• Physician should be informed if significant xerostomic side effects occur (e.g., increased caries, sore tongue, problems eating or swallowing, difficulty wearing prosthesis) so that a medication change can be considered.

• Because there is no experience with the use of conscious sedation or general anesthesia in patients taking this drug, a medical consultation is recommended for risk evaluation.

• Patients showing anorexia, jaundice, GI complaints, or malaise should be referred for medical evaluation before treatment.

Teach patient/family:

When chronic dry mouth occurs, advise patient:

• To avoid mouth rinses with high alcohol content because of drying effects

• Of need for daily use of home fluoride products to prevent caries

• To use sugarless gum, frequent sips of water, or saliva substitutes

nelfinavir mesylate

(nel-fin'a-veer)

Viracept

Drug class.: Antiviral

Action: Inhibits HIV-I protease enzymes leading to the production of immature, noninfectious virus

Uses: HIV infection when indicated by surrogate marker changes in patients receiving nelfinavir in combination with nucleoside analogues or alone for up to 24 wk

Dosage and routes:

• *Adult:* PO tabs 750 mg tid or 1250 mg bid with meals or light snack

• *Child 2-13 yr:* PO 20-30 mg/kg per dose tid with meals or light snack; oral powder may be used for children unable to take tablets; oral powder can be mixed with a small amount of water, milk formula, soy formula, soy milk, or dietary supplement; do not use acidic juices or applesauce

Available forms include: Tabs 250, 625 mg; oral powder 50 mg/g (as free base nelfinavir)

Side effects/adverse reactions:

▼ *ORAL:* Oral ulceration (<2%)

CNS: Anxiety, depression, dizziness, sleep disorder, migraine, insomnia

GI: Diarrhea, nausea, anorexia, dyspepsia, vomiting, hepatitis, pancreatitis, GI bleeding

RESP: Pharyngitis, dyspnea, sinusitis

HEMA: Anemia, leukopenia, thrombocytopenia, abnormal laboratory values

GU: Kidney calculus, sexual dysfunction

EENT: Rhinitis

INTEG: Rash, pruritus, urticaria

META: Increased alk phosphatase, creatine phosphokinase, hyperlipidemia, abnormal liver function tests

MS: Arthralgia, asthenia, myalgia, myopathy, cramps

Contraindications: Hypersensitivity, concurrent use with triazolam, midazolam, ergot derivatives, rifampin, amiodarone, or quinidine

Precautions: Pediatric use, phenylketonuria (powder contains phenylalanine), diabetes mellitus, hyperglycemia, hepatic impairment, development of resistance, hemophilia, pregnancy category B, lactation, child <2 yr, an inhibitor of CYP3A4 isoenzymes; use with caution with drugs that are inducers of CYP3A4 or CYP2C19 isoenzymes

Pharmacokinetics:

PO: Peak plasma levels 2-4 hr with food; peak plasma levels 3-4 μg/ml, plasma protein bound (98%), hepatic metabolism (CYP3A4, CYP2C19 isoenzymes), active metabolite, excreted mostly in feces (87%), minor urinary excretion (1%-2%)

Drug interactions of concern to dentistry:

• Contraindicated with triazolam, midazolam, and other drugs dependent on CYP3A4 for metabolism (see Appendix I)

• Increased plasma levels: azithromycin, ketoconazole

• Increased plasma concentrations of fentanyl

DENTAL CONSIDERATIONS

General:

• Examine for oral manifestation of opportunistic infection.

• Patients on chronic drug therapy may rarely have symptoms of blood dyscrasias, which can include infection, bleeding, and poor healing.

• Palliative medication may be required for management of oral side effects.

Consultations:

• In a patient with symptoms of blood dyscrasias, request a medical consultation for blood studies and postpone treatment until normal values are reestablished.

• Medical consultation may be required to assess disease control.

Teach patient/family:

• Importance of good oral hygiene to prevent soft tissue inflammation

• Caution to prevent trauma when using oral hygiene aids

• Importance of updating health

and drug history if physician makes any changes in evaluation or drug regimens

• That secondary oral infection may occur; must see dentist immediately if infection occurs

neostigmine bromide/ neostigmine methylsulfate

(nee-oh-stig'meen)

Prostigmin Bromide/Prostigmin

Drug class.: Cholinesterase inhibitor

Action: Inhibits destruction of acetylcholine, increasing its concentration at sites where acetylcholine is released; this facilitates transmission of impulses across myoneural junction

Uses: Myasthenia gravis, nondepolarizing neuromuscular blocker, antagonist, bladder distention, postoperative ileus

Dosage and routes:

Myasthenia gravis:

• *Adult:* PO 15-375 mg/day; IM/IV 0.5-2 mg q1-3h

• *Child:* PO 2 mg/kg/day q3-4h

Tubocurarine antagonist:

• *Adult:* IV 0.5-2 mg slowly, may repeat if needed (give 0.6-1.2 mg atropine before this drug)

Prevention of abdominal distention/postoperative ileus:

• *Adult:* IM/SC 0.25-1 mg q4-6h, depending on condition

Available forms include: Tabs 15 mg; inj IM/SC/IV 1:1000, 1:2000, 1:4000

Side effects/adverse reactions:

▼ *ORAL: Increased salivation*

CNS: ***Paralysis, convulsions,*** dizziness, headache, sweating, confusion, weakness, incoordination

CV: ***Cardiac arrest,*** tachycardia, dysrhythmias, bradycardia, hypotension, AV block, ECG changes

GI: Nausea, diarrhea, vomiting, cramps, increased secretions

RESP: ***Respiratory depression, bronchospasm, constriction, laryngospasm, respiratory arrest***

GU: Frequency, incontinence

EENT: Miosis, blurred vision, lacrimation

INTEG: Rash, urticaria, flushing

Contraindications: Obstruction of intestine, renal system, pregnancy category C, bromide sensitivity

Precautions: Bradycardia, hypotension, seizure disorders, bronchial asthma, coronary occlusion, hyperthyroidism, dysrhythmias, peptic ulcer, megacolon, poor GI motility, lactation, children

Pharmacokinetics:

PO: Onset 45-75 min, duration 2.5-4 hr

IM/SC: Onset 10-30 min, duration 2.5-4 hr

IV: Onset 4-8 min, duration 2-4 hr

Metabolized in liver, excreted in urine

Drug interactions of concern to dentistry:

• Decreased action: hydrocarbon inhalation anesthetics, corticosteroids

• Decreased action of anticholinergics (may be contraindicated)

• Increased action of succinylcholine

• Increased toxicity of ester-type local anesthetics

DENTAL CONSIDERATIONS

General:

• Monitor vital signs at every appointment because of cardiovascular and respiratory side effects.

N

• Use amide-type local anesthetic agent.
• Early-morning and brief appointments are preferred because of effects of disease on oral musculature.

Consultations:
• Take precautions if dental surgery is anticipated and anesthesia is required.
• Medical consultation may be required to assess disease control and patient's tolerance for stress.

nevirapine (NVP)

(ne-vye'ra-peen)
Viramune
Drug class.: Antiviral

Action: A nonnucleoside reverse transcriptase inhibitor for HIV-1, results in blockade of RNA-dependent and DNA-dependent polymerase

Uses: Used in combination with nucleoside analogs for HIV-1 infection in adults who have demonstrated clinical or immunologic deterioration

Dosage and routes:
• *Adult:* PO 200 mg qd × 14 days; then 200 mg bid in combination with nucleoside analog retroviral agent

Available forms include: Tabs 200 mg

Side effects/adverse reactions:
▼ *ORAL:* Oral ulceration (Stevens-Johnson syndrome)
CNS: Headache, fever, fatigue, somnolence
GI: Nausea, diarrhea
INTEG: Rash (Stevens-Johnson syndrome)
ENDO: Hepatitis
MS: Myalgias, paresthesia
META: Abnormal liver function tests

Contraindications: Hypersensitivity, protease inhibitors

Precautions: Severe life-threatening skin reactions (Stevens-Johnson syndrome), fatal hepatotoxicity has occurred, renal dysfunction, pregnancy category C, lactation, children

Pharmacokinetics:
PO: Absorption 90%, peak plasma levels 4 hr, plasma protein binding 60%, hepatic metabolism, fecal excretion mainly, urinary excretion also

Drug interactions of concern to dentistry:
• Should not be given with ketoconazole; monitor patients when other CYP3A4 isoenzyme inhibitors are used (see Appendix I)

DENTAL CONSIDERATIONS

General:
• Determine why patient is taking the drug.
• Examine for oral manifestation of opportunistic infection.

Consultations:
• Medical consultation may be required to assess disease control.

Teach patient/family:
• Importance of good oral hygiene to prevent soft tissue inflammation
• To report oral lesions, soreness, or bleeding to dentist
• Importance of updating health history/drug record if physician makes any changes in evaluation or drug regimens
• That secondary oral infection may occur; must see dentist immediately if infection occurs

niacin (vitamin B_3/ nicotinic acid)/ niacinamide (nicotinamide)

(nye'a-sin) (nye-a-sin'a-mide)

Niacin (nicotinic acid): generic, Niacor, Nicotinex, Slo-Niacin

♣ Novo-Niacin

Niacinamide: Generic

Drug class.: Vitamin B_3

Action: Needed for conversion of fats, protein, carbohydrates by oxidation-reduction; acts directly on vascular smooth muscle, causing vasodilation; high doses decrease serum lipids

Uses: Pellagra, hyperlipidemias (niacin), peripheral vascular disease (niacin)

Dosage and routes:

Adjunct in hyperlipidemia:

• *Adult:* PO 1.5-3 g qd in 3 divided doses after meals, may be increased to 6 g/day; ext rel 500 or 1000 mg for 1 mo, increasing to 1.5 or 2 g hs if inadequate response, daily dose should not be increased >500 mg in 4 wk period

Pellagra:

• *Adult:* IM/SC/PO/IV inf 10-20 mg, not to exceed 500 mg total dose

• *Child:* IM/SC/PO/IV inf 300 mg until desired response

Peripheral vascular disease:

• *Adult:* PO 250-800 mg qd in divided doses

Available forms include: Nicotinic acid–tabs 50, 100, 250, 500 mg; con rel tabs 250, 500, 750 mg; sus rel tab 500 mg; time rel caps 250, 500 mg; ext rel caps 250, 400 mg; sus rel caps 125, 250 mg; elix 50 mg/5 ml; niacinamide–tabs 100, 500 mg

Side effects/adverse reactions:

▼ *ORAL:* Dry mouth

CNS: Paresthesia, headache, dizziness, anxiety

CV: Postural hypotension, vasovagal attacks, dysrhythmias, vasodilation

GI: ***Jaundice,*** nausea, vomiting, anorexia, flatulence, diarrhea, peptic ulcer

RESP: Wheezing

GU: ***Glycosuria, hypoalbuminemia,*** hyperuricemia

EENT: Blurred vision, ptosis

INTEG: Flushing, dry skin, rash, pruritus

Contraindications: Hypersensitivity, peptic ulcer, hepatic disease, lactation, hemorrhage, severe hypotension

Precautions: Glaucoma, cardiovascular disease, CAD, diabetes mellitus, gout, schizophrenia, pregnancy category A

Pharmacokinetics:

PO: Peak 30-70 min, half-life 45 min; metabolized in liver; 30% excreted unchanged in urine

Drug interactions of concern to dentistry:

• None reported

DENTAL CONSIDERATIONS

General:

• Take vital signs at every appointment because of cardiovascular side effects.

• After supine positioning, have patient sit upright for at least 2 min before standing to avoid postural hypotension.

• Assess salivary flow as a factor in caries, periodontal disease, and candidiasis.

N

Teach patient/family:

When chronic dry mouth occurs, advise patient:

- To avoid mouth rinses with high alcohol content because of drying effects
- Of need for daily use of home fluoride products to prevent caries
- To use sugarless gum, frequent sips of water, or saliva substitutes

nicardipine HCl

(nye-kar'de-peen)

Cardene, Cardene IV, Cardene SR

Drug class.: Calcium channel blocker

Action: Inhibits calcium ion influx across cell membrane during cardiac depolarization; produces relaxation of coronary vascular smooth muscle, peripheral vascular smooth muscle; dilates coronary vascular arteries; decreases SA/AV node conduction

Uses: Chronic stable angina pectoris, hypertension

Dosage and routes:

Angina pectoris:

- *Adult:* PO 20 mg tid initially; may increase after 3 days (range 20-40 mg tid)

Hypertension:

- *Adult:* PO 20 mg tid initially, then increase after 3 days (range 20-40 mg tid); timed rel caps start with 30 mg bid; dose range up to 60 mg bid

Available forms include: Caps 20, 30 mg; sus rel caps 30, 45, 60 mg; IV 2.5 mg/ml in 10 ml amps

Side effects/adverse reactions:

▼ *ORAL:* Dry mouth, sore throat (gingival overgrowth has been reported with other calcium channel blockers)

CNS: Headache, fatigue, drowsiness, dizziness, anxiety, depression, weakness, insomnia, confusion, paresthesia, somnolence

CV: ***MI, pulmonary edema,*** dysrhythmia, edema, CHF, bradycardia, hypotension, palpitation

GI: ***Hepatitis,*** nausea, vomiting, diarrhea, gastric upset, constipation, abdominal cramps

GU: ***Acute renal failure,*** nocturia, polyuria

INTEG: Rash, pruritus, urticaria, photosensitivity, hair loss

MISC: Blurred vision, flushing, nasal congestion, sweating, shortness of breath, gynecomastia, hyperglycemia, sexual difficulties

Contraindications: Sick sinus syndrome, second- or third-degree heart block, hypotension <90 mm Hg systolic, hypersensitivity

Precautions: CHF, hypotension, hepatic injury, pregnancy category C, lactation, children, renal disease, elderly

Pharmacokinetics:

PO: Onset 10 min, peak 1-2 hr, half-life 2-5 hr; metabolized by liver (CYP3A4 isoenzymes); excreted in urine (98% as metabolites)

Drug interactions of concern to dentistry:

- Decreased effect: indomethacin, possibly other NSAIDs, phenobarbital, St. John's wort (herb)
- Increased effect: parenteral and inhalational general anesthetics or other drugs with hypotensive actions
- Possible risk of increased plasma level, monitor patient: erythromycin, ketoconazole, other CYP3A4 inhibitors (see Appendix I)
- Increased effects of nondepolarizing muscle relaxants

• Increased effects of carbamazepine

DENTAL CONSIDERATIONS

General:

• Monitor cardiac status; take vital signs at each appointment because of CV side effects. Consider a stress reduction protocol to prevent stress-induced angina during the dental appointment.

• After supine positioning, have patient sit upright for at least 2 min to avoid orthostatic hypotension.

• Place on frequent recall to monitor gingival condition.

• Limit use of sodium-containing products, such as saline IV fluids, for patients with a dietary salt restriction.

• Assess salivary flow as a factor in caries, periodontal disease, and candidiasis.

• Use vasoconstrictors with caution, in low doses, and with careful aspiration. Avoid use of gingival retraction cord with epinephrine.

Consultations:

• Medical consultation may be required to assess disease control and tolerance for stress.

Teach patient/family:

• Importance of good oral hygiene to prevent soft tissue inflammation and minimize gingival overgrowth

• Need for frequent oral prophylaxis if hyperplasia occurs

When chronic dry mouth occurs, advise patient:

• To avoid mouth rinses with high alcohol content because of drying effects

• Of need for daily use of home fluoride products to prevent caries

• To use sugarless gum, frequent sips of water, or saliva substitutes

nicotine inhalation/ nicotine spray/nicotine transdermal system

(nik'oh-teen)

Inhalation: Nicotrol Inhaler

♣ *Spray:* Nicotrol NS

♣ *Transdermal:* Nicoderm CQ Step 1, Step 2, Step 3; Nicotrol Step 1, Step 2, Step 3

Drug class.: Smoking deterrent

Action: Binds to acetylcholine receptors at autonomic ganglia in the adrenal medulla, at neuromuscular junctions, and in the brain

Uses: Cigarette smoking cessation program

Dosage and routes:

• *Inhalation:* Individualize dose, range 6-16 cartridges/day for 3 mo; individual use will vary, gradually reduce dose over time

• *Nasal spray:* One spray in each nostril (1 mg total); adjust dose to individual of 1 or 2 doses/hr not to exceed 5 doses/hr or 40 doses/day and for no longer than 3 mo

• *Adult:* TRANS dose varies with 24 or 16 hr system selected; one example is 21 mg/day for 6 wk, then 14 mg/day for 2 wk, then 7 mg/day for 2 wk; for 16 hr system: 15 mg per 16 hr day for 6 wk

Available forms include: Transderm patch delivering 7, 14, 21 mg/day for 24 hr system and 15 mg for 16 hr system; spray pump 0.5 mg of nicotine per actuation; INH 4 mg per actuation in cartridges

Side effects/adverse reactions:

▼ *ORAL:* Dry mouth

CNS: Abnormal dreams, insomnia, nervousness, headache, dizziness, paresthesia

GI: Diarrhea, dyspepsia, constipa-

N

tion, nausea, abdominal pain, vomiting

INTEG: Erythema, pruritus, rash, burning at application site, cutaneous hypersensitivity, sweating

MS: Arthralgia, myalgia

Contraindications: Hypersensitivity, children, pregnancy, lactation, nonsmokers, during immediate post-MI period, life-threatening dysrhythmias, severe or worsening angina pectoris, hypertension

Precautions: Skin disease, angina pectoris, MI, renal or hepatic insufficiency, peptic ulcer, serious cardiac dysrhythmias, hyperthyroidism, pheochromocytoma, insulin-dependent diabetes, elderly, pregnancy category D

Pharmacokinetics:

TRANS: Half-life 3-4 hr; protein binding <5%; 30% is excreted unchanged in urine

Drug interactions of concern to dentistry:

- Decreased dose at cessation of smoking: acetaminophen, caffeine, oxazepam, pentazocine
- Decreased metabolism of propoxyphene

DENTAL CONSIDERATIONS

General:

- Assess salivary flow as a factor in caries, periodontal disease, and candidiasis.

Teach patient/family:

When chronic dry mouth occurs, advise patient:

- To avoid mouth rinses with high alcohol content because of drying effects
- Of need for daily use of home fluoride products to prevent caries
- To use sugarless gum, frequent sips of water, or saliva substitutes

When used in conjunction with a smoking cessation program in the dental office, teach:

- All aspects of product drug; give package insert to patient and explain
- That patch is to be used only to deter smoking
- Not to use during pregnancy; birth defects may occur
- To keep used and unused system out of reach of children and pets; potentially toxic if chewed or swallowed
- To apply once a day to a nonhairy, clean, dry area of skin on upper body or upper outer arm
- To stop smoking immediately when beginning treatment with patch
- To apply promptly after removing from protective covering; system may lose strength

nicotine polacrilex

(nik'o-teen)

Nicorette, Commit

✦ Nicorette Plus

Drug class.: Smoking deterrent

Action: Agonist at nicotinic receptors in the peripheral and central nervous systems; acts at sympathetic ganglia; on chemoreceptors of the aorta and carotid bodies; also affects adrenal-releasing catecholamines

Uses: Deters cigarette smoking when combined with a program of smoking cessation

Dosage and routes:

- *Adult (<25 cigarettes/day):* Gum initial start with 2 mg gum; slowly chew gum until it tingles; place gum between cheek and gum;

when tingle is gone chew again; use up to 9 pieces/day but no more than 24 pieces/day
• *Adult (>25 cigarettes/day):* Wk 1-6, chew 1 piece q1-2h; wk 7-9, chew 1 piece q2-4h; wk 10-12, chew 1 piece q4-8h
Available forms include: Gum 2, 4 mg/piece of gum
Side effects/adverse reactions:
▼ *ORAL:* Burning in mucosa, occlusal stress, unpleasant taste, increased salivation, dry mouth (rare), sore throat
CNS: Dizziness, vertigo, insomnia, headache, confusion, convulsions, depression, euphoria, numbness, tinnitus
CV: Dysrhythmias, tachycardia, palpitation
GI: Nausea, vomiting, anorexia, indigestion, diarrhea, abdominal pain, constipation, eructation
RESP: Breathing difficulty, cough, hoarseness, sneezing, wheezing
Contraindications: Hypersensitivity, immediate post-MI recovery period, severe angina pectoris, pregnancy category X, nicotine patch therapy
Precautions: Vasospastic disease, dysrhythmias, uncontrolled hypertension, diabetes mellitus, pregnancy, children, hyperthyroidism, pheochromocytoma, coronary disease, esophagitis, peptic ulcer, insulin or prescription medications for asthma or depression
Pharmacokinetics:
PO: Onset 15-30 min, half-life 2-3 hr, 30-120 hr (terminal); metabolized in liver; excreted in urine
Drug interactions of concern to dentistry:
• Increased blood levels with cessation of smoking: propoxyphene

DENTAL CONSIDERATIONS
General:
• Take vital signs at every appointment because of cardiovascular side effects.
• TMJ disorder may be aggravated by chewing because of heavier viscosity of gum.
Teach patient/family:
• Need for good oral hygiene to prevent periodontal inflammation
When chronic dry mouth occurs, advise patient:
• To avoid mouth rinses with high alcohol content because of drying effects
• Of need for daily use of home fluoride products to prevent caries
• To use sugarless gum, frequent sips of water, or saliva substitutes
When used in conjunction with a smoking cessation program in the dental office, teach:
• All aspects of product use; give package insert to patient and explain
• That gum is to be used only to deter smoking
• To avoid use in pregnancy; birth defects may occur
• To stop smoking when beginning treatment with gum
• To dispose of gum carefully because nicotine will still be present; to protect from children

N

nifedipine

(nye-fed'i-peen)

Adalat CC, Nifedical XL, Procardia, Procardia XL

🍁 Adalat XL, Adalat PA, Apo-Nifed, Novo-Nifedin, Nu-Nifed

Drug class.: Calcium channel blocker

Action: Inhibits calcium ion influx across cell membrane during cardiac depolarization; produces relaxation of coronary vascular smooth muscle, dilates coronary arteries; increases myocardial oxygen delivery in patients with vasospastic angina; dilates peripheral arteries

Uses: Chronic stable angina pectoris, vasospastic angina, hypertension (sustained release only)

Dosage and routes:

• *Adult:* PO (immed rel) 10 mg tid, increase in 10 mg increments q4-6h, not to exceed 180 mg or single dose of 30 mg; PO (sus rel) 30-60 mg qd, may increase q7-14 d, doses >120 mg not recommended

Available forms include: Caps 10, 20 mg; sus rel tabs 30, 60, 90 mg

Side effects/adverse reactions:

▼ *ORAL: Gingival overgrowth,* dry mouth

CNS: Giddiness, headache, fatigue, drowsiness, dizziness, anxiety, depression, weakness, insomnia, light-headedness, paresthesia, tinnitus, blurred vision

CV: Dysrhythmia, edema, CHF, ***MI,*** hypotension, palpitation, pulmonary edema, tachycardia

GI: Nausea, vomiting, diarrhea, gastric upset, constipation, increased liver function studies

GU: Nocturia, polyuria

INTEG: Rash, pruritus, flushing, photosensitivity, hair loss

MISC: Flushing, sexual difficulties, cough, fever, chills

Contraindications: Hypersensitivity

Precautions: CHF, hypotension, sick sinus syndrome, second- or third-degree heart block, hypotension <90 mm Hg systolic, hepatic injury, pregnancy category C, lactation, children, renal disease

Pharmacokinetics:

PO: Onset 20 min, peak 0.5-6 hr, half-life 2-5 hr; metabolized by liver (CYP3A4 isoenzymes); excreted in urine (98% as metabolites)

Drug interactions of concern to dentistry:

• Decreased effect: indomethacin, possibly other NSAIDs, phenobarbital

• Increased effect: parenteral and inhalational general anesthetics or other drugs with hypotensive actions

• Possible increase in effects, monitor patients: inhibitors of CYP3A4 isoenzyme (see Appendix I)

• Increased effects of nondepolarizing muscle relaxants

• Increased effects of carbamazepine

DENTAL CONSIDERATIONS

General:

• Monitor cardiac status; take vital signs at each appointment because of CV side effects. Consider a stress reduction protocol to prevent stress-induced angina during the dental appointment.

• After supine positioning, have patient sit upright for at least 2 min before standing to avoid orthostatic hypotension at dismissal.

• Place on frequent recall to monitor gingival condition.
• Limit use of sodium-containing products, such as saline IV fluids, for patients with a dietary salt restriction.
• Assess salivary flow as a factor in caries, periodontal disease, and candidiasis.
• Use vasoconstrictors with caution, in low doses, and with careful aspiration. Avoid use of gingival retraction cord with epinephrine.

Consultations:
• Medical consultation may be required to assess disease control and stress tolerance.

Teach patient/family:
• Importance of good oral hygiene to prevent soft tissue inflammation and minimize gingival overgrowth
• Need for frequent oral prophylaxis if hyperplasia occurs

When chronic dry mouth occurs, advise patient:
• To avoid mouth rinses with high alcohol content because of drying effects
• Of need for daily use of home fluoride products to prevent caries
• To use sugarless gum, frequent sips of water, or saliva substitutes

---

nisoldipine

(nye'sol-di-peen)
Sular

Drug class.: Calcium channel antagonist (dihydropyridine group)

Action: Inhibits calcium ion influx across cell membrane during cardiac depolarization; produces relaxation of coronary vascular smooth muscle; dilates coronary arteries; decreases SA/AV node conduction; dilates peripheral vessels

Uses: Hypertension as a single agent or in combination with other antihypertensive medications

Dosage and routes:
• *Adult <65 yr:* PO initial dose 20 mg daily; can increase dose by 10 mg weekly or at longer intervals depending on patient response and blood pressure control
• *Maintenance dose:* 20-40 mg daily; doses above 60 mg daily are not recommended; do not take with high-fat meals
• *Adult >65 yr or in renal impairment:* PO reduce initial dose to 10 mg daily

Available forms include: Tabs 10, 20, 30, 40 mg

Side effects/adverse reactions:
▼ *ORAL:* Dry mouth, facial edema, gingival overgrowth, glossitis, mouth ulcers
CNS: Headache, dizziness, migraine, abnormal dreams
CV: Peripheral edema, vasodilation, palpitation, CHF, CVA, chest pain, postural hypotension
GI: Anorexia, diarrhea, colitis, dyspepsia, flatulence
HEMA: Anemia, ecchymosis, leukopenia, petechiae
GU: Dysuria, impotence, urinary frequency
EENT: Pharyngitis, sinusitis, abnormal vision, watery eyes
INTEG: Rash, dry skin, pruritus
MS: Arthralgia, leg cramps, myalgia
MISC: Flulike syndrome, malaise

Contraindications: Hypersensitivity

Precautions: Avoid high-fat meals, severe coronary artery disease, monitor blood pressure, CHF, severe hepatic impairment, do not break or crush tablets, pregnancy category C, lactation, geriatric patients

Pharmacokinetics:

PO: Low bioavailability 5%, presystemic metabolism in intestinal wall, peak plasma levels 6-12 hr, highly metabolized (CYP3A4 isoenzymes), urinary excretion 60%-90%

Drug interactions of concern to dentistry:

• Possible increase in serum levels: fluconazole, ketoconazole, itraconazole, and other CYP3A4 isoenzyme inhibitors (see Appendix I)

• Decreased antihypertensive effect: indomethacin, possibly other NSAIDs, phenobarbital

• Increased effect: parenteral and inhalational general anesthetics or other drugs with hypotensive actions

• Increased effects of carbamazepine

DENTAL CONSIDERATIONS

General:

• Stress from dental procedures may compromise cardiovascular function; determine patient risk.

• Monitor vital signs at every appointment because of cardiovascular side effects.

• Short appointments and a stress reduction protocol may be required for anxious patients.

• When taken with grapefruit juice may see increased plasma levels.

• Limit use of sodium-containing products such as saline IV fluids for those patients with a dietary salt restriction.

• After supine positioning, have patient sit upright for at least 2 min before standing to avoid orthostatic hypotension.

• Assess salivary flow as a factor in caries, periodontal disease, and candidiasis.

Consultations:

• Medical consultation may be required to assess disease control and patient's ability to tolerate stress.

Teach patient/family:

• Need for frequent oral prophylaxis if gingival overgrowth should occur

When chronic dry mouth occurs, advise patient:

• To avoid mouth rinses with high alcohol content because of drying effects

• To use daily home fluoride products for anticaries effect

• To use sugarless gum, frequent sips of water, or saliva substitutes

---

nitrofurantoin/ nitrofurantoin macrocrystals

(nye-troe-fyoor'an-toyn)

Furadantin, Macrobid, Macrodantin

🍁 Apo-Nitrofurantoin, Novo-Furantoin

Drug class.: Urinary tract antiinfective

Action: Appears to inhibit bacterial enzymes, interfering with synthesis of essential cell activity including synthesis of DNA, RNA, cell wall, and proteins

Uses: UTIs caused by *E. coli, Klebsiella, Pseudomonas, P. vulgaris, P. morganii, Serratia, Citrobacter, S. aureus*

Dosage and routes:

• *Adult and child >12 yr:* PO 50-

100 mg qid pc or 50-100 mg hs for long-term treatment

• *Child 1 mo-3 yr:* PO 5-7 mg/kg/day in 4 divided doses; 1-3 mg/kg/day for long-term treatment

Available forms include: Caps 25, 50, 100 mg; susp 25 mg/5 ml

Side effects/adverse reactions:

▼ *ORAL:* Angioedema, brown discoloration of saliva, tooth staining, tingling or burning of mouth

CNS: Dizziness, headache, drowsiness, peripheral neuropathy

GI: Nausea, vomiting, abdominal pain, diarrhea, ***cholestatic jaundice***

INTEG: Pruritus, rash, urticaria, angioedema, alopecia, tooth staining

Contraindications: Hypersensitivity, anuria, severe renal disease

Precautions: Pregnancy category not listed (pregnant women at term), lactation

Pharmacokinetics:

PO: Half-life 20-60 min; crosses blood-brain barrier, placenta; excreted in breast milk; excreted as inactive metabolites in liver

Drug interactions of concern to dentistry:

• Increased effects: anticholinergic drugs

DENTAL CONSIDERATIONS

General:

• Determine why the patient is taking the drug.

Consultations:

• Medical consultation may be required to assess disease control and to select an antiinfective if a dental infection is diagnosed.

nitroglycerin

(nye-troe-gli'ser-in)

Nitroglycerin transmucosal tab: Nitrogard

Nitroglycerin sublingual spray: Nitrolingual

Nitroglycerin sustained release cap: Nitroglyn, Nitro-Time

Nitroglycerin sustained release tab: Nitrong, Nitrong SR

Nitroglycerin injection: Nitro-Bid IV, Tridil

Nitroglycerin sublingual tab: NitroQuick, Nitrostat

Topical dose forms: Nitro-Bid, Nitrol

Nitroglycerin transdermal patch: Deponit, Minitran, Nitrek, Nitrodisc, Nitro-Dur, Transderm-Nitro

Nitroglycerin buccal tablets: Nitrogard

Drug class.: Inorganic nitrate, vasodilator

Action: Decreases preload/afterload, decreasing left ventricular end-diastolic pressure, systemic vascular resistance; arterial and venous dilation

Uses: Chronic stable angina pectoris, prophylaxis of angina pain, CHF associated with acute MI, controlled hypotension in surgical procedures

Dosage and routes:

• *Adult:* SL dissolve tablet under tongue when pain begins; may repeat q5min until relief occurs; take no more than 3 tabs/15 min; use 1 tab prophylactically 5-10 min before activities; sus rel caps q6-12h on empty stomach; top 1-2 q8h, increase to 4 q4h as needed;

N

IV 5 µg/min, then increase by 5 µg/min q3-5min, if no response after 20 µg/min, increase by 10-20 µg/min until desired response; trans apply 1 pad qd to a hair-free site

Available forms include: Buccal tabs 2, 3 mg; spray 0.4 mg/meter spray; sus rel caps 2.5, 6.5, 9, 13 mg; sus rel tabs 2.6, 6.5, 9 mg; inj 0.5, 5 mg/ml; SL tabs 0.3, 0.4, 0.6 mg; top oint 2%; trans derm syst 0.1, 0.2, 0.3, 0.4, 0.6, 0.8 mg/hr

Side effects/adverse reactions:

▼ *ORAL:* Dry mouth, burning sensation

CNS: Headache, flushing, dizziness

CV: Postural hypotension, ***collapse,*** tachycardia, syncope

GI: Nausea, vomiting

INTEG: Pallor, sweating, rash

Contraindications: Hypersensitivity to this drug or nitrites, severe anemia, increased intracranial pressure, cerebral hemorrhage

Precautions: Postural hypotension, pregnancy category C, lactation

Pharmacokinetics:

SUS REL: Onset 20-45 min, duration 3-8 hr

SL: Onset 1-3 min, duration 30 min

TRANSDERM: Onset 0.5-1 hr, duration 12-24 hr

IV: Onset immediate, duration variable

TRANSMUC: Onset 3 min, duration 10-30 min

AEROSOL: Onset 2 min, duration 30-60 min

TOP OINT: Onset 30-60 min, duration 2-12 hr

Metabolized by liver, excreted in urine

Drug interactions of concern to dentistry:

• Increased hypotensive effects: alcohol, opioids, benzodiazepines, phenothiazines, and other drugs used in conscious sedation techniques

DENTAL CONSIDERATIONS

General:

• Take vital signs at every appointment because of cardiovascular side effects.

• After supine positioning, have patient sit upright for at least 2 min before standing to avoid orthostatic hypotension.

• Assess salivary flow as a factor in caries, periodontal disease, and candidiasis.

• Ensure that patient's drug is easily available if angina occurs.

• A benzodiazepine or nitrous oxide/oxygen may be prescribed to allay anxiety.

• Check expiration date on prescription to ensure drug activity. If bottle has been opened, there is a 3-month shelf life.

• Stress from dental procedures may compromise cardiovascular function; determine patient risk.

• Talk with patient about disease control (frequency of angina episodes).

• Use vasoconstrictors with caution, in low doses, and with careful aspiration. Avoid gingival retraction cord with epinephrine.

• Short appointments and a stress reduction protocol may be required for anxious patients.

• Consider semisupine chair position for patients with cardiovascular disease.

Consultations:

• Medical consultation may be re-

quired to assess disease control and patient's ability to tolerate stress.

Teach patient/family:

• Importance of good oral hygiene to prevent soft tissue inflammation

• Caution to prevent injury when using oral hygiene aids

When chronic dry mouth occurs, advise patient:

• To avoid mouth rinses with high alcohol content because of drying effects

• Of need for daily use of home fluoride products to prevent caries

• To use sugarless gum, frequent sips of water, or saliva substitutes

nizatidine

(ni-za'ti-deen)

Axid OTC: Axid AR

✤ Apo-Nizatidine

Drug class.: Histamine H_2-receptor antagonist

Action: Inhibits histamine at H_2-receptor site in parietal cells, inhibiting gastric acid secretion

Uses: Duodenal ulcer, Zollinger-Ellison syndrome, gastric ulcers, hypersecretory conditions, gastroesophageal reflux disease, stress ulcers; unapproved: GI symptoms associated with NSAID use in rheumatoid arthritis

Dosage and routes:

Duodenal ulcer:

• *Adult:* PO 300 mg daily hs or 150 mg bid

Maintenance:

• *Adult:* PO 150 mg daily hs; gastroesophageal reflux 150 mg bid

Available forms include: Caps 150, 300 mg; OTC tabs 75 mg

Side effects/adverse reactions:

CNS: Somnolence, fatigue, insomnia, headache

GI: Nausea, vomiting, abdominal discomfort, diarrhea, constipation

GU: Impotence, decreased libido

INTEG: Pruritus, urticaria, rash, increased sweating

Contraindications: Hypersensitivity

Precautions: Pregnancy category B, hepatic disease, renal disease, lactation, children <16 yr

Pharmacokinetics: Peak plasma levels 0.5-3 hr, half-life 2.5-3.5 hr, duration up to 12 hr; primary renal excretion

Drug interactions of concern to dentistry:

• Increased serum salicylate when administered with high doses of aspirin

• Decreased absorption of ketoconazole (take doses 2 hr apart)

DENTAL CONSIDERATIONS

General:

• Avoid prescribing aspirin-containing products in patients with active GI disease.

Teach patient/family:

• To avoid mouth rinses with high alcohol content because of drying effects

norethindrone acetate

(nor-eth-in'drone)

Aygestin

✤ Norulate

Drug class.: Progesterone derivative

Action: Inhibits secretion of pituitary gonadotropins, preventing follicular maturation, ovulation

N

Uses: Uterine bleeding (abnormal), amenorrhea, endometriosis

Dosage and routes:

Amenorrhea:

• *Adult:* PO 2.5-10 mg qd × 5-10 days, during second half of cycle

Endometriosis:

• *Adult:* PO 5 mg qd × 2 wk, then increased by 2.5 mg qd × 2 wk, up to 15 mg qd

Available forms include: Tabs 5 mg

Side effects/adverse reactions:

▼ *ORAL:* Gingival bleeding, gingival overgrowth

CNS: Dizziness, headache, migraines, depression, fatigue

CV: ***Thromboembolism, stroke, pulmonary embolism, MI,*** hypotension, thrombophlebitis, edema

GI: Nausea, ***cholestatic jaundice,*** vomiting, anorexia, cramps, increased weight

GU: Gynecomastia, testicular atrophy, impotence, ***spontaneous abortion,*** amenorrhea, endometriosis, cervical erosion, breakthrough bleeding, dysmenorrhea, vaginal candidiasis, breast changes

EENT: Diplopia

INTEG: Rash, urticaria, acne, hirsutism, alopecia, oily skin, seborrhea, purpura, melasma

META: Hyperglycemia

Contraindications: Breast cancer, hypersensitivity, thromboembolic disorders, reproductive cancer, genital bleeding (abnormal, undiagnosed), cerebral hemorrhage, pregnancy category X

Precautions: Lactation, hypertension, asthma, blood dyscrasias, gallbladder disease, CHF, diabetes mellitus, bone disease, depression, migraine headache, convulsive disorders, hepatic disease, renal disease, family history of breast or reproductive tract cancer

Pharmacokinetics:

PO: Duration 24 hr; metabolized in liver; excreted in urine, feces

Drug interactions of concern to dentistry:

• Decreased effectiveness of oral contraceptives: antibiotics, barbiturates

DENTAL CONSIDERATIONS

General:

• Place on frequent recall to evaluate gingival inflammation, if present.

• An increased incidence of dry socket has been reported after extraction.

• Monitor vital signs at each appointment.

Teach patient/family:

• Need for good oral hygiene to prevent periodontal inflammation

• That smoking cessation decreases risk of serious adverse cardiovascular effects

• Need for additional method of birth control while undergoing antibiotic therapy

---

norfloxacin

(nor-flox'-a-sin)

Noroxin

Drug class.: Fluoroquinolone anti-infective

Action: A broad-spectrum bactericidal agent that inhibits the enzymes topoisomerase II (DNA gyrase) and topoisomerase IV required for bacterial DNA replication, transcription repair, and recombination

Uses: Adult UTIs (including complicated) caused by *E. coli, E. cloacae, P. mirabilis, K. pneumo-*

niae, group D strep, indole-positive *Proteus, C. freundii, S. aureus;* sexually transmitted disease caused by *N. gonorrhoeae;* prostatitis caused by *E. coli*

Dosage and routes:

Uncomplicated UTI:

• *Adult:* PO 400 mg bid × 3-10 days 1 hr before or 2 hr after meals, for prostatitis give for 28 days

Complicated UTI:

• *Adult:* PO 400 mg bid × 10-21 days; 400 mg qd × 7-10 days in impaired renal function

Gonorrhea, uncomplicated:

• *Adult:* PO 800 mg single dose

Available forms include: Tabs 400 mg

Side effects/adverse reactions:

▼ *ORAL:* Dry mouth, stomatitis

CNS: Headache, dizziness, fatigue, somnolence, depression, insomnia

GI: Nausea, constipation, increased ALT/AST, flatulence, heartburn, vomiting, diarrhea

EENT: Visual disturbances, phototoxicity

INTEG: Rash, blue-black discoloration

MS: Tendinitis, tendon rupture

Contraindications: Hypersensitivity to quinolones

Precautions: Pregnancy category C, lactation, children, renal disease, seizure disorders, tendon rupture in shoulder, hand, and Achilles tendons

Pharmacokinetics:

PO: Peak 1 hr, steady state 2 days, half-life 3-4 hr; excreted in urine as active drug, metabolites

Drug interactions of concern to dentistry:

• Decreased absorption: sodium bicarbonate

DENTAL CONSIDERATIONS

General:

• Assess salivary flow as a factor in caries, periodontal disease, and candidiasis.

• Determine why the patient is taking the drug.

• Because of drug interaction, do not use ingestible sodium bicarbonate products such as the air polishing system Prophy

• Jet unless at least 2 hr have passed since norfloxacin was taken.

• Avoid dental light in patient's eyes; offer dark glasses for patient comfort.

• Ruptures of the shoulder, hand, and Achilles tendons that required surgical repair or resulted in prolonged disability have been reported with this drug.

Consultations:

• Consult with patient's physician if an acute dental infection occurs and another antiinfective is required.

Teach patient/family:

• To avoid mouth rinses with high alcohol content because of drying effects

• To discontinue treatment and inform dentist immediately if patient experiences pain or inflammation of a tendon, and to rest and refrain from exercise

---

norgestrel

(nor-jess'trel)

Ovrette

Drug class.: Progesterone derivative

Action: Inhibits secretion of pituitary gonadotropins, preventing follicular maturation, ovulation

Uses: Oral contraception

Dosage and routes:

• *Adult:* PO 1 tablet qd beginning on day 1 of cycle and continuing

Available forms include: Tabs 0.075 mg

Side effects/adverse reactions:

▼ *ORAL:* Gingival bleeding, dry socket

CNS: Dizziness, headache, migraines, depression, fatigue

CV: ***Thromboembolism, stroke, pulmonary embolism, MI,*** hypotension, thrombophlebitis, edema

GI: Nausea, ***cholestatic jaundice,*** vomiting, anorexia, cramps, increased weight

GU: Gynecomastia, testicular atrophy, impotence, endometriosis, ***spontaneous abortion,*** amenorrhea, cervical erosion, breakthrough bleeding, dysmenorrhea, vaginal candidiasis, breast changes

EENT: Diplopia

INTEG: Rash, urticaria, acne, hirsutism, alopecia, oily skin, seborrhea, purpura, melasma

META: Hyperglycemia

Contraindications: Breast cancer, hypersensitivity, thromboembolic disorders, reproductive cancer, genital bleeding (abnormal, undiagnosed), cerebral hemorrhage, pregnancy category X

Precautions: Lactation, hypertension, asthma, blood dyscrasias, gallbladder disease, CHF, diabetes mellitus, bone disease, depression, migraine headache, convulsive disorders, hepatic disease, renal disease, family history of breast or reproductive tract cancer

Pharmacokinetics:

PO: Duration 24 hr, excreted in urine and feces, metabolized in liver

Drug interactions of concern to dentistry:

• Decreased effectiveness of oral contraceptives: antibiotics, barbiturates

DENTAL CONSIDERATIONS

General:

• Place on frequent recall to evaluate gingival inflammation, if present.

• An increased incidence of dry socket has been reported after extraction.

• Monitor vital signs at each appointment.

Teach patient/family:

• Need for good oral hygiene to prevent periodontal inflammation

• That smoking cessation decreases risk of serious and adverse cardiovascular side effects

• Need for additional method of birth control while undergoing antibiotic therapy

nortriptyline HCl

(nor-trip'ti-leen)

Aventyl, Pamelor

Drug class.: Antidepressant–tricyclic

Action: Blocks reuptake of norepinephrine, serotonin into nerve endings, increasing action of norepinephrine, serotonin in nerve cells

Uses: Major depression

Dosage and routes:

• *Adult:* PO 25 mg tid or qid; may increase to max of 150 mg/day; may give daily dose hs

Available forms include: Caps 10, 25, 75 mg; sol 10 mg/5 ml

Side effects/adverse reactions:

▼ *ORAL: Dry mouth, unpleasant taste,* bleeding, sublingual adenitis

CNS: Dizziness, drowsiness, confusion, headache, anxiety, tremors, stimulation, weakness, insomnia, nightmares, EPS (elderly), increased psychiatric symptoms

CV: Orthostatic hypotension, ECG changes, tachycardia, ***hypertension,*** palpitation

GI: Constipation, ***hepatitis, paralytic ileus,*** increased appetite, nausea, vomiting, cramps, epigastric distress, jaundice

HEMA: ***Agranulocytosis, thrombocytopenia, eosinophilia, leukopenia***

GU: Retention, ***acute renal failure***

EENT: Blurred vision, tinnitus, mydriasis

INTEG: Rash, urticaria, sweating, pruritus, photosensitivity

Contraindications: Hypersensitivity to tricyclic antidepressants, recovery phase of MI, convulsive disorders, prostatic hypertrophy

Precautions: Suicidal patients, severe depression, increased intraocular pressure, narrow-angle glaucoma, urinary retention, cardiac disease, hepatic disease, hyperthyroidism, electroshock therapy, elective surgery, pregnancy category C, MAOIs

Pharmacokinetics:

PO: Steady state 4-19 days, half-life 18-28 hr; metabolized by liver; excreted by kidneys; crosses placenta; excreted in breast milk

Drug interactions of concern to dentistry:

- Increased anticholinergic effects: muscarinic blockers, antihistamines, phenothiazines
- Increased effects of direct-acting sympathomimetics (epinephrine, levonordefrin)
- Potential risk of increased CNS depression: alcohol, barbiturates, benzodiazepines, and other CNS depressants
- Decreased antihypertensive effect: clonidine, guanadrel, guanethidine
- Avoid concurrent use with St. John's wort

DENTAL CONSIDERATIONS

General:

- Take vital signs at every appointment because of cardiovascular side effects.
- Assess salivary flow as a factor in caries, periodontal disease, and candidiasis.
- Patients on chronic drug therapy may rarely have symptoms of blood dyscrasias, which can include infection, bleeding, and poor healing.
- After supine positioning, have patient sit upright for at least 2 min before standing to avoid orthostatic hypotension.
- Use vasoconstrictors with caution, in low doses, and with careful aspiration. Avoid use of gingival retraction cord with epinephrine.
- Place on frequent recall because of oral side effects.

Consultations:

- In a patient with symptoms of blood dyscrasias, request a medical consultation for blood studies and postpone dental treatment until normal values are reestablished.
- Medical consultation may be required to assess disease control.
- Physician should be informed if significant xerostomic side effects occur (e.g., increased caries, sore tongue, problems eating or swallowing, difficulty wearing prosthesis) so that a medication change can be considered.

Teach patient/family:
- Importance of good oral hygiene to prevent soft tissue inflammation
- Caution to prevent injury when using oral hygiene aids

When chronic dry mouth occurs, advise patient:
- To avoid mouth rinses with high alcohol content because of drying effects
- Of need for daily use of home fluoride products to prevent caries
- To use sugarless gum, frequent sips of water, or saliva substitutes

---

nystatin

(nye-sta'tin)

Mycostatin, Nilstat, Nystex, Pedi-Dri

♣ Nadostine, Nyaderm

Drug class.: Antifungal

Action: Interferes with fungal DNA replication; binds sterols in fungal cell membrane, increasing permeability and leaking of cell nutrients

Uses: *Candida* species causing oral, vaginal, intestinal infections

Dosage and routes:

Oral candidiasis:
- *Adult:* SUSP rinse 400,000-600,000 U qid × 14 days
- *Adult and child:* TOP apply to affected area bid-tid × 14 days; loz 200,000 up to 400,000 U, dissolve slowly in mouth 4-5 ×/day up to 14 days
- *Child and infant >3 mo:* SUSP rinse 250,000-500,000 U qid
- *Newborn and premature infant:* SUSP apply oral sol 100,000 U qid

Extemporaneous powder: 1/8 tsp powder (500,000 units) in 1/2 cup of water (120 ml); use as an oral rinse tid or qid

GI infection:
- *Adult:* PO (tabs or oral susp) 500,000-1,000,000 U tid

Vaginal infection:
- *Adult:* Vag tabs 100,000 U inserted high into vagina qd × 2 wk

Available forms include: Tabs 500,000 U; vag tabs 100,000 U; powder 50 million, 150 million, 500 million, 1 billion, 2 billion, 5 billion U; susp 100,000 U in 60 ml and 473 ml units; top cream, oint, powder 100,000 U/g in 15 mg and 60 g units; loz 200,000 U

Side effects/adverse reactions:

GI: Nausea, vomiting, anorexia, diarrhea, cramps

INTEG: Rash, urticaria (rare)

Contraindications: Hypersensitivity

Precautions: Pregnancy category not listed

Pharmacokinetics:

PO: Little absorption, excreted in feces

DENTAL CONSIDERATIONS

General:
- Determine why the patient is taking the drug.
- Broad-spectrum antibiotic may contribute to oral *Candida* infections.

Teach patient/family:
- That long-term therapy may be needed to clear infection; to complete entire course of medication
- Not to use commercial mouthwashes for mouth infection unless prescribed by dentist
- To soak full or partial dentures in a suitable antifungal solution nightly
- To prevent reinoculation of *Candida* infection by disposing of toothbrush or other contaminated oral hygiene devices used during period of infection

ofloxacin

(oh-flocks'a-sin)

Floxin, Floxin IV

Drug class.: Fluoroquinolone anti-infective

Action: A broad-spectrum bactericidal agent that inhibits the enzymes topoisomerase II (DNA gyrase) and topoisomerase IV required for bacterial DNA replication, transcription repair, and recombination

Uses: Treatment of lower respiratory tract infections (pneumonia, bronchitis), genitourinary infections (prostatitis, UTIs) caused by *E. coli, K. pneumoniae, C. trachomatis, N. gonorrhoeae;* skin and skin structure infections

Dosage and routes:

Lower respiratory tract infections/ skin and skin structure infections:

- *Adult:* PO 400 mg q12h × 10 days

Cervicitis, urethritis:

- *Adult:* PO 300 mg q12h × 7 days

Prostatitis:

- *Adult:* PO 300 mg q12h × 6 wk

Acute, uncomplicated gonorrhea:

- *Adult:* PO 400 mg as a single dose

Pneumonia:

- *Adult:* 400 mg by IV infusion given over 60 min q12h × 10 days

Available forms include: Tabs 200, 300, 400 mg; inj 200 mg/50 ml D_5W, 400 mg in 10, 20 ml vials or 100 ml (D_5W) bottles

Side effects/adverse reactions:

▼ *ORAL:* Candidiasis, dry mouth, dysgeusia

CNS: Dizziness, headache, fatigue, somnolence, depression, insomnia, lethargy, malaise, nervousness, anxiety

GI: Diarrhea, nausea, vomiting, anorexia, flatulence, heartburn, increased AST/ALT, abdominal pain/ cramps, constipation, decreased appetite, dyspepsia

EENT: Visual disturbances, phototoxicity

INTEG: Rash, pruritus

MS: Tendinitis, tendon rupture

Contraindications: Hypersensitivity to quinolones

Precautions: Pregnancy category C, lactation, children <18 yr, elderly, renal disease, seizure disorders, excessive sunlight, tendon rupture in shoulder, hand, and Achilles tendons

Pharmacokinetics:

PO: Peak 1-2 hr, steady state 2 days, half-life 9 hr; excreted in urine as active drug, metabolites; 0.9% bioavailability

Drug interactions of concern to dentistry:

- Decreased effects: antacids
- Possible increased risk of life-threatening arrhythmias: procainamide

DENTAL CONSIDERATIONS

General:

- Because of drug interaction, do not use ingestible sodium bicarbonate products such as the air polishing system ProphyJet unless 2 hr have passed since ofloxacin was taken.
- Examine for oral manifestation of opportunistic infections.
- Avoid dental light in patient's eyes; offer dark glasses for patient comfort.
- Minimize exposure to sunlight and wear sunscreen if sun exposure is planned.
- Ruptures of the shoulder, hand, and Achilles tendons that required

surgical repair or resulted in prolonged disability have been reported with this drug.

Consultations:

• Consult with patient's physician if an acute dental infection occurs and another antiinfective is required.

Teach patient/family:

• Importance of good oral hygiene to prevent soft tissue inflammation

• To avoid mouth rinses with high alcohol content because of drying effects

• To discontinue treatment and inform dentist immediately if patient experiences pain or inflammation of a tendon, and to rest and refrain from exercise

ofloxacin (optic)

(oh-flocks'a-sin)

Ocuflox Ophthalmic Solution

Drug class.: Fluoroquinolone antiinfective, topical

Action: A broad-spectrum bactericidal agent that inhibits the enzyme DNA gyrase needed for the replication of DNA

Uses: Treatment of bacterial conjunctivitis caused by susceptible organisms, corneal ulcers

Dosage and routes:

• *Adult and child:* TOP instill 1 drop in each eye q2-4h × 2 days; then 1 gtt qid up to 5 days

Bacterial corneal ulcer

• *Adult and child:* TOP instill 1-2 drops into affected eye q30min on days 1 and 2 while awake, afterward awaken at 4 hr and at 6 hr and instill 1-2 drops; on days 3-7 instill 1-2 drops hourly while awake; days 7-9 instill 1-2 drops qid

Available forms include: Sol 0.3% in 5 ml

Side effects/adverse reactions:

CNS: Dizziness

EENT: Burning sensation in eye, photophobia, redness

Contraindications: Hypersensitivity

Precautions: Pregnancy category C, children <1 yr

Pharmacokinetics:

TOP: Low systemic absorption, renal excretion of metabolites

DENTAL CONSIDERATIONS

General:

• Avoid dental light in patient's eyes; offer dark glasses for patient comfort and safety protection during dental treatment.

ofloxacin otic solution

(oh-flocks'a-sin)

Floxin Otic

Drug class.: Fluoroquinolone antiinfective

Action: A broad-spectrum bactericidal agent that inhibits the enzymes topoisomerase II (DNA gyrase) and topoisomerase IV required for bacterial DNA replication, transcription repair, and recombination

Uses: Otitis externa caused by *E. coli, P. aeruginosa, S. aureus;* acute otitis media caused by *H. influenzae, M. catarrhalis, P. aeruginosa, S. aureus, S. pneumoniae;* chronic suppurative otitis media caused by *P. mirabilis, P. aeruginosa, S. aureus*

Dosage and routes:

Otitis externa:

• *Child 6 mo-13 yr:* TOP instill 5 drops in affected ear once daily × 7 days

• *Child 13 yr and older:* TOP instill 10 drops in affected ear once daily × 7 days

Acute otitis media (with tympanostomy tubes):

• *Child 1-12 yr:* TOP instill 5 drops in affected ear bid × 10 days

Chronic suppurative otitis media (with perforated tympanic membrane):

• *Child 12 yr and older:* TOP instill 10 drops in affected ear bid × 14 days

Available forms include: 0.3% in 5, 10 ml

Side effects/adverse reactions:

▼ *ORAL: Taste perversion,* dry mouth

CNS: Dizziness, headache, paresthesia, vertigo, transient neuropyschiatric disturbances

CV: Hot flushes

GI: Dyspepsia, nausea, diarrhea, vomiting

EENT: Application site reactions: *pruritus, earache,* loss of hearing, tinnitus, fungal infection

INTEG: Dermatitis, eczema, erythematous rash

MISC: Fever

Contraindications: Hypersensitivity to this drug or other fluoroquinolones

Precautions: Use in ear only; risk of severe allergic reactions, avoid prolonged use, erosion of cartilage in weight-bearing joints, avoid contaminating tip of drug dispenser, pregnancy category C, lactation, safety and efficacy in child <6 mo not established

Pharmacokinetics:

TOP: Low serum levels detected; no other data provided about systemic effects

Drug interactions of concern to dentistry:

• Studies have not been conducted for this product

DENTAL CONSIDERATIONS

General:

• Determine why the patient is taking the drug.

• Severity or discomfort of infection may require postponing elective dental treatment

Consultations:

• Consult with patient's physician if an acute dental infection occurs and another antiinfective is required.

• Medical consultation may be required to assess disease control in the patient.

Teach patient/family:

When chronic dry mouth occurs, advise patient:

• To avoid mouth rinses with high alcohol content because of drying effects

• To use daily home fluoride products for anticaries effect

• To use sugarless gum, frequent sips of water, or saliva substitutes

---

olanzapine

(oh-lan'za-peen)

Zyprexa, Zyprexa Zydis

Drug class.: Antipsychotic

Action: Antipsychotic mechanism is unknown; acts as an antagonist for serotonin, dopamine, muscarinic, histamine, and α_1-adrenergic receptors

Uses: Psychotic disorders, schizophrenia, bipolar disorder; acute manic episode in bipolar 1 disorder in combination with lithium or valproate

O

Dosage and routes:

• *Adult:* PO initial dose 5-10 mg qd, target dose is 10 mg/day; use 5 mg dose for patients at higher risk for orthostatic hypotension and nonsmoking women >65 yr

Bipolar mania:

• *Adult:* PO 10-15 mg/day; can adjust dose in 5 mg increments q24h up to 20 mg/day

Available forms include: Tabs 2.5, 5, 7.5, 10, 15, 20 mg, orally disintegrating tabs 5, 10, 15, 20 mg

Side effects/adverse reactions:

▼ *ORAL: Dry mouth (7%)*

CNS: Extrapyramidal events, somnolence, agitation, dizziness, personality disorder, insomnia, nervousness, hostility, headache, anxiety

CV: Orthostatic hypotension, tachycardia

GI: Constipation, increased appetite, abdominal pain

RESP: Rhinitis, cough, pharyngitis

GU: Premenstrual syndrome

INTEG: Vesiculobullous rash

MS: Joint pain, extremity pain, twitching

META: Weight gain, edema, fever

Contraindications: Hypersensitivity

Precautions: Pregnancy category C, lactation, paralytic ileus, elderly; combination of age, smoking, and gender (female) may increase clearance rate; neuroleptic malignant syndrome, CV disease, cerebrovascular disease, seizures, orthostatic hypotension, Alzheimer's dementia, prostate hypertrophy, glaucoma; patients should be monitored for signs and symptoms of diabetes mellitus.

Pharmacokinetics:

PO: Well absorbed, peak plasma levels 6 hr, hepatic metabolism (CYP1A2 isoenzymes), half-life 21-54 hr; renal and fecal excretion

Drug interactions of concern to dentistry:

• Potentiation of orthostatic hypotension: diazepam, alcohol, other CNS depressants

• Increased anticholinergic affects: anticholinergic drugs

• Suspected reduction of plasma levels: carbamazepine

DENTAL CONSIDERATIONS

General:

• Consider semisupine chair position for patient comfort because of GI effects of drug.

• Assess salivary flow as factor in caries, periodontal disease, and candidiasis.

• Monitor vital signs at every appointment because of cardiovascular side effects.

• After supine positioning have patient sit upright for at least 2 min to avoid orthostatic hypotension.

• Patients on chronic drug therapy may rarely have symptoms of blood dyscrasias, which can include infection, bleeding, and poor healing.

• Assess for presence of extrapyramidal motor symptoms, such as tardive dyskinesia and akathisia. Extrapyramidal motor activity may complicate dental treatment.

Consultations:

• In a patient with symptoms of blood dyscrasias, request a medical consultation for blood studies and postpone dental treatment until normal values are reestablished.

• Medical consultation may be required to assess disease control.

• Physician should be informed if significant xerostomic side effects occur (e.g., increased caries, sore tongue, problems eating or swal-

lowing, difficulty wearing prosthesis) so that a medication change can be considered.

Teach patient/family:

• Importance of good oral hygiene to prevent soft tissue inflammation

• Use of electric toothbrush if patient has difficulty holding conventional devices

• Use caution when driving or performing other tasks requiring alertness

When chronic dry mouth occurs, advise patient:

• To avoid mouth rinses with high alcohol content because of drying effects

• To use daily home fluoride products for anticaries effect

• To use sugarless gum, frequent sips of water, or saliva substitutes

olmesartan medoxomil

(ol-me-sar'tan)

Benicar

Drug class.: Angiotensin II (AT_1) receptor antagonist

Action: Blocks the vasoconstrictor and aldosterone-releasing effects of angiotensin II

Uses: Hypertension, as a single drug or in combination with other antihypertensives

Dosage and routes:

• *Adult:* PO 20 mg/day as monotherapy in patients who are not volume contracted; after 2 wk the dose may be increased to 40 mg/day; for patients with volume depletion (taking diuretics or impaired renal function) use lower starting dose

Available forms include: Tabs 5, 20, 40 mg

Side effects/adverse reactions:

▼ *ORAL:* Facial edema (angioedema)

CNS: Dizziness, vertigo, insomnia

CV: Tachycardia

GI: Diarrhea, headache, dyspepsia, abdominal pain, nausea

RESP: Bronchitis, URT infection, cough

GU: Hematuria, UTI

EENT: Pharyngitis, rhinitis, sinusitis

INTEG: Rash

META: Increased creatine phosphokinase, increased bilirubin, hyperlipidemia, hyperuricemia, hypercholesterolemia, hyperglycemia, hypertriglyceridemia

MS: Back pain, arthralgia, myalgia

MISC: Flulike symptoms, fatigue

Contraindications: Hypersensitivity

Precautions: Discontinue drug if pregnancy occurs, pregnancy category C, use in volume- or salt-depleted patients, use in nursing mothers or pediatric patients has not been established, impaired renal function, CHF, renal artery stenosis.

Pharmacokinetics:

PO: Absolute bioavailability ~26%, steady state levels are achieved in 3-5 days, peak plasma levels 1-2 hr, ester hydrolysis occurs on absorption with no further metabolism of olmesartan, highly bound to plasma proteins (99%), excreted in urine and feces

Drug interactions of concern to dentistry:

• No significant drug interactions have been reported, but there is always a chance of increased hypotensive effects when used with other antihypertensives or sedatives

DENTAL CONSIDERATIONS
General:

• Monitor vital signs at every appointment because of cardiovascular side effects.

• Consider semisupine chair position for patient comfort if GI side effects occur.

• Limit use of sodium-containing products such as saline IV fluids for those patients with a dietary salt restriction.

• Stress from dental procedures may compromise cardiovascular function, determine patient risk.

• Patients with hypertensive disease may be taking more than one drug to control blood pressure; although not specifically noted for this drug, postural hypotension is always a possibility. After supine positioning, have patient sit upright for at least 2 min to avoid orthostatic hypotension.

• Short appointments and a stress reduction protocol may be required for anxious patients.

• Use precaution if sedation or general anesthesia is required; risk of hypotensive episode.

Consultations:

• Medical consultation may be required to assess disease control and patient's ability to tolerate stress.

Teach patient/family:

• Importance of updating health and drug history if physician makes any changes in evaluation/ drug regimens

olopatadine HCl

(oh-loe-pa-ta'deen)

Patanol

Drug class.: Ophthalmic antihistamine

Action: Selective H_1-receptor antagonist and inhibitor of histamine release from mast cells

Uses: Temporary prevention of itching of eye caused by allergic conjunctivitis

Dosage and routes:

• *Adult:* TOP 1 or 2 drops in each affected eye bid at 6 to 8 hr intervals

Available forms include: Sol 0.1% in 5 ml drop dispenser

Side effects/adverse reactions:

▼ *ORAL: Taste alteration*

EENT: Burning, dry eye, keratitis, lid edema, pruritus, foreign body reaction

MISC: Cold syndrome

Contraindications: Hypersensitivity

Precautions: Topical use only, do not use while wearing contact lenses, pregnancy category C, lactation, children <3 yr

Pharmacokinetics:

TOP: Low to nondetectable plasma levels, peak in 2 hr, renal excretion

Drug interactions of concern to dentistry:

• None reported

DENTAL CONSIDERATIONS
General:

• Protect patient's eyes from accidental spatter during dental treatment.

olsalazine sodium

(ole-sal'a-zeen)

Dipentum

Drug class.: Antiinflammatory, salicylate derivative

Action: Bioconverted to 5-aminosalicylic acid, which decreases inflammation in the colon

Uses: Maintenance of remission of ulcerative colitis in patients intolerant to sulfasalazine

Dosage and routes:

• *Adult:* PO 1 g/day in 2 divided doses with meals

Available forms include: Caps 250 mg

Side effects/adverse reactions:

▼ *ORAL:* Stomatitis

CNS: Headache, insomnia, hallucinations, depression, vertigo, fatigue, drug fever, chills, dizziness, drowsiness, tremors

CV: Allergic myocarditis, second-degree heart block, hypertension, peripheral edema, chest pain, palpitation

GI: Nausea, vomiting, abdominal pain, hepatitis, pancreatitis, diarrhea, bloating

RESP: ***Bronchospasm,*** shortness of breath

HEMA: ***Leukopenia, neutropenia, thrombocytopenia, agranulocytosis, anemia***

GU: Frequency, dysuria, hematuria, impotence

INTEG: ***Stevens-Johnson syndrome,*** erythema, photosensitivity, rash, dermatitis, urticaria, alopecia

SYST: ***Anaphylaxis***

Contraindications: Hypersensitivity to salicylates, child <14 yr

Precautions: Pregnancy category C, lactation, impaired hepatic function, severe allergy, bronchial asthma, renal disease

Pharmacokinetics:

PO: Partially absorbed, peak 1.5 hr, half-life 5-10 hr; excreted in urine as 5-aminosalicylic acid and metabolites; crosses placenta

DENTAL CONSIDERATIONS

General:

• Consider semisupine chair position for patient comfort because of GI effects of disease.

Consultations:

• Avoid drugs that could aggravate an inflammatory colon disease; consultation is recommended before selection of an antibiotic.

Teach patient/family:

• Importance of good oral hygiene to prevent soft tissue inflammation

• Caution to prevent injury when using oral hygiene aids

• To avoid mouth rinses with high alcohol content because of drying effects

omalizumab

(oh-mah-lye-zoo'mab)

Xolair

Drug class.: Anti-Ig E monoclonal antibody

Action: Inhibits binding of Ig E to the high-affinity Ig E receptor on mast cells and basophil surfaces, reducing the release of mediators of the allergic response

Uses: Reduction of asthma exacerbation in patients with moderate to severe asthma who have a positive skin test or in vitro reactivity to a perennial aeroallergen not adequately controlled by inhaled glucocorticoids

Dosage and routes:

• *Adult and child 12 yr and older:* SC 150-375 mg q2-4wk; doses and dose frequency are determined by body weight and serum IgE level before treatment; limit 150 mg per injection site

Available forms include: Sterile pwd for inj 150 mg/vial

Side effects/adverse reactions:

CNS: Headache, fatigue, dizziness

RESP: URI

EENT: Sinusitis, pharyngitis, earache

INTEG: Injection site pain, dermatitis, pruritus

MS: Arthralgia, leg pain, arm pain

MISC: ***Malignancies, anaphylaxis,*** *viral infections,* pain

Contraindications: Hypersensitivity

Precautions: Possible risk of malignancy, anaphylactic reactions, not for acute asthma or status asthmaticus, do not abruptly discontinue glucocorticoid therapy, pregnancy category B, use in nursing mothers or children <12 yr has not been established

Pharmacokinetics: *SC:* Absolute bioavailability 62%, slowly absorbed, peak serum levels 7-8 days, clearance involves Ig G clearance processes, excretion via bile

Drug interactions of concern to dentistry:

• None reported

DENTAL CONSIDERATIONS

General:

• Determine why patient is taking the drug.

• Be aware of patient's disease, its severity, and its frequency, when known.

• Question patient about other medications used for asthma or to prevent bronchoconstriction.

• Avoid drugs that may aggravate asthma.

• Short appointments and a stress reduction protocol may be required for anxious patients.

• Have patient bring personal short-acting bronchodilator to appointment for use in emergency.

• Acute asthmatic episodes may be precipitated in the dental office. Rapid-acting sympathomimetic inhalants should be available for emergency use. A stress reduction protocol may be required.

Consultations:

• Consultation with physician may be needed if sedation or general anesthesia is required.

• Medical consultation may be required to assess disease control and patient's ability to tolerate stress.

Teach patient/family:

• Importance of good oral hygiene to prevent soft tissue inflammation/infection

• Importance of updating health and drug history and reporting changes in health status, drug regimen, or disease/treatment status

omeprazole

(oh-me′pray-zol)

Prilosec, Prilosec OTC

♣ Losec

Drug class.: Antisecretory, proton pump inhibitor

Action: Suppresses gastric acid production by binding to the hydrogen/potassium ATPase enzyme system to inhibit the final step in gastric acid production

Uses: Gastroesophageal reflux disease (GERD), severe erosive esophagitis, poorly responsive systemic GERD, pathologic hypersecretory conditions (Zollinger-Ellison syndrome, systemic mastocytosis, multiple endocrine adenomas), with clarithromycin, short-term treatment of gastric ulcers; not approved for long-term ulcer maintenance therapy

Dosage and routes:

Severe erosive esophagitis/poorly responsive gastroesophageal reflux disease:

• *Adult:* PO 20 mg qd × 4-8 wk; take before eating

Gastric ulcers:

• *Adult:* PO 40 mg qd × 2 wk, then 20 mg qd × 2 wk

Duodenal ulcers:

• *Adult:* PO 20 mg/day × 4-8 wk

Duodenal ulcer (H. pylori):

• *Adult:* PO 40 mg in AM × 14 days with clarithromycin 500 mg tid; on days 15-28, 20 mg day; 20 mg with clarithromycin 500 mg and amoxicillin 1000 mg each bid × 10 days

Pathologic hypersecretory conditions:

• *Adult:* PO 60 mg/day; may increase to 120 mg tid; daily doses >80 mg in divided doses

Available forms include: Caps (del rel) 10, 20, 40 mg

Side effects/adverse reactions:

▼ *ORAL:* Dry mouth, mucosal atrophy of tongue, taste perversion, candidiasis

CNS: Headache, dizziness, asthenia, nervousness, anxiety disorders

CV: Chest pain, angina, tachycardia, bradycardia, palpitation, peripheral edema

GI: Diarrhea, abdominal pain, vomiting, nausea, constipation, flatulence, acid regurgitation, abdominal swelling, anorexia, irritable colon, esophageal candidiasis

RESP: Upper respiratory infections, cough, epistaxis

HEMA: ***Pancytopenia, thrombocytopenia, neutropenia, leukocytosis,*** anemia

GU: ***Proteinuria, hematuria,*** UTI, frequency, increased creatinine, testicular pain, glycosuria

EENT: Tinnitus

INTEG: Rash, dry skin, urticaria, pruritus, alopecia

META: Hypoglycemia, increased hepatic enzymes, weight gain

MISC: Back pain, fever, fatigue, malaise

Contraindications: Hypersensitivity

Precautions: Pregnancy category C, lactation, children

Pharmacokinetics:

PO: Peak 30 min-3.5 hr, half-life 30 min-1 hr; protein binding 95%; eliminated in urine as metabolites and in feces; in the elderly the elimination rate is decreased, bioavailability is increased

Drug interactions of concern to dentistry:

• Increased serum levels: diazepam

DENTAL CONSIDERATIONS

General:

• Question the patient about tolerance of NSAIDs or aspirin related to GI problem.

• Consider semisupine chair position for patient comfort because of GI effects of disease.

• Assess salivary flow as a factor in caries, periodontal disease, and candidiasis.

Teach patient/family:

• Caution to prevent injury when using oral hygiene aids

When chronic dry mouth occurs, advise patient:

• To avoid mouth rinses with high alcohol content because of drying effects

• Of need for daily use of home fluoride products to prevent caries
• To use sugarless gum, frequent sips of water, or saliva substitutes

ondansetron HCl

(on-dan-see'tron)

Zofran, Zofran ODT

Drug class.: Antiemetic

Action: A selective 5-HT_3 antagonist; antiemetic effect may be mediated centrally, peripherally, or both

Uses: Prevention of nausea/vomiting associated with cancer chemotherapy, radiotherapy, and postoperative nausea and vomiting

Dosage and routes:

• *Adult and child >4 yr:* PO 8 mg tid, administer first dose 30 min before chemotherapy and then at 4 hr and 8 hr intervals, continue 1-2 days after chemotherapy; IV 0.15 mg/kg, give first dose over 15 min beginning 30 min before chemotherapy and at 4 hr and 8 hr intervals

Prevention of nausea/vomiting caused by radiotherapy:

• *Adult:* PO 8 mg 1-2 hr before each fraction of radiotherapy each day

Prevention of postoperative nausea/vomiting:

• *Adult:* IV before or after surgery 4 mg over 2-5 min or IM 4 mg; PO 16 mg 1 hr before induction of anesthesia

Available forms include: Tabs 4, 8, 24 mg; oral disintegrating tabs 4, 8 mg; IV 2 mg/ml, 32 mg/50 ml in 20 ml vials; sol 4 mg/5 ml in 50 ml

Side effects/adverse reactions:

▼ *ORAL:* Dry mouth (1%-2%)
CNS: Headache, weakness, possible EPS, grand mal seizures
CV: Hypokalemia, ECG alterations, vascular occlusive events
GI: Constipation, abdominal pain
RESP: ***Bronchospasm***
EENT: Transient blurred vision
INTEG: Rash
MISC: ***Anaphylaxis***

Contraindications: Hypersensitivity

Precautions: Pregnancy category B, lactation, children <12 yr, elderly

Pharmacokinetics:

PO: Well absorbed, peak plasma levels 1.9 hr, food increases absorption; extensive metabolism
IV: Rapid peak levels; protein binding 70%-76%; extensively metabolized

Drug interactions of concern to dentistry:

• None reported

DENTAL CONSIDERATIONS

General:

• Be aware that patient is receiving active chemotherapy.
• Avoid procedures or drugs that could promote nausea/vomiting.
• Patients with cancer may be taking chronic opioids for pain. Consider NSAID for dental pain management.
• Patients receiving chemotherapy may require palliative therapy for stomatitis.
• An increased gag reflex may make dental procedures, such as obtaining radiographs or impressions, difficult.

Consultations:

• Medical consultation may be required to assess disease control.

Teach patient/family:
When chronic dry mouth occurs, advise patient:
• To avoid mouth rinses with high alcohol content because of drying effects
• Of need for daily use of home fluoride products to prevent caries
• To use sugarless gum, frequent sips of water, or saliva substitutes

oral contraceptives

Estrogens: ethinyl estradiol, mestranol
Progestins: desogestrel, drospirenone, ethynodiol diacetate, etonorgestrel, levonorgestrel, norethindrone, norgestimate, norgestrel
Many products are available. Examples:
Monophasic products: Alesse, Apri, Aviane, Brevicon, Cyselle, Demulen 1/35, Demulen 1/50, Desogen, Kriva, Lessina, Levilite, Levlen, Levora, Loestrin 21, Loestrin Fe, LoOgestrel, Lo/Ovral, Micette, Modicon, Mononssea, Necon 0.5/35, Necon 1/50, Nelova 0.5/35E, Nordette, Norethin 1/35E, Norinyl 1+50, Noripyl 1+35, Nortrel 1/35, Nortrel 0.5/35, Ogestrel 0.5/50, OrthoCept, Ortho-Cyclen, Ortho-Novum 1/35, Ortho-Novum 1/50, Ovcon 35, Ovcon-50, Ovral, Ovral-28, Portia, Sprintic, Zovia 1/35E, Zovia 1/50E, Yasmin, others
Biphasic products: Necon 10/11, Ortho-Novum 10/11
Triphasic products: Cyclessa, Enpress, Estrostep-21, Estrostep Fe, Neocon 7/7/7, Ortho-Novum 7/7/7, Ortho Tri-Cyclen, Tri-Levlen, Tri-Norinyl, Triphasil, Trivora
Progestin only: Camila, Errin, Nor-CD, Nora-BE, Ortho Micronor, Ovrette
Injectable once monthly: Lunelle
Patch: OrthoEvra Patch
Vaginal ring: Nuva Ring (etonorgestrel and ethinyl estradiol)
Progestin intrauterine device: Progestasert, Mirena
Emergency contraceptive–progestin only: Plan B
Emergency contraceptive–estrogen/progestin: Preven
Drug class.: Estrogen/progestin combinations

Action: Prevents ovulation by suppressing follicle-stimulating hormone, luteinizing hormone
Uses: To prevent pregnancy, endometriosis, hypermenorrhea, hypogonadism; acne (Tri-Cyclen)
Dosage and routes:
• *Adult:* PO 1 qd starting on day 5 of menstrual cycle (day 1 is first day of period)
• *INJ:* 0.5 ml IM inj every month, not to exceed 33 days
• *PATCH:* Wear 1 patch each week (7 days) × 3 wk; skip week 4
20/21-tablet packs
• *Adult:* PO 1 qd starting on day 7 of menstrual cycle (day 1 is first day of period); then on for 20 or 21 days, off 7 days
28-tablet packs
• *Adult:* PO 1 qd continuously
Biphasic
• *Adult:* PO 1 qd × 10 days, then next color 1 qd × 11 days
Triphasic
• *Adult:* PO 1 qd; check package insert for each new brand
Transdermal patch
• *Adult:* TOP apply one patch each week × 3 wk, skip week 4

Vaginal ring
• *Adult:* TOP insert ring in vagina for 3 continuous weeks, then remove; skip wk 4
Intrauterine devices
• *Adult:* TOP insert once yearly; Mirena system only: replace or remove by end of 5 yr

Available forms include: Check specific brand

Side effects/adverse reactions:
▼ *ORAL:* Gingival bleeding, dry socket
CNS: Depression, fatigue, dizziness, nervousness, anxiety, headache
CV: Increased BP, thromboembolic conditions, fluid retention, edema
GI: Nausea, vomiting, cramps, diarrhea, bloating, constipation, change in appetite, ***cholestatic jaundice***
HEMA: Increased fibrinogen, clotting factor
GU: Breakthrough bleeding, amenorrhea, spotting, dysmenorrhea, galactorrhea, endocervical hyperplasia, vaginitis, cystitis-like syndrome, breast change
EENT: Optic neuritis, retinal thrombosis, cataracts
INTEG: Melasma, acne, rash, urticaria, erythema multiforme or nodosum, pruritus, hirsutism, alopecia, photosensitivity
ENDO: Decreased glucose tolerance, increased TBG, PBI, T_4, T_3

Contraindications: Pregnancy category X, lactation, reproductive cancer, thrombophlebitis, MI, hepatic tumors, hepatic disease, CAD, women 40 yr and over, CVA

Precautions: Depression, hypertension, renal disease, seizure disorders, lupus erythematosus, rheumatic disease, migraine headache, amenorrhea, irregular menses, breast cancer (fibrocystic), gallbladder disease, diabetes mellitus, heavy smoking, acute mononucleosis, sickle cell disease; smoking increases risk of serious CV side effects

Pharmacokinetics:
PO: Excreted in breast milk

Drug interactions of concern to dentistry:
• Decreased effectiveness of oral contraceptives: rifampin, barbiturates, St. John's wort (herb)
• Antibiotics: advise patient of a potential risk for decreased contraceptive action, to maintain compliance with oral contraceptive use while using antiinfectives, and to consider the use of additional nonhormonal contraception
• Possible risk of contraceptive failure: itraconazole, ketoconazole, and fluconazole, additional contraception may be desirable

DENTAL CONSIDERATIONS

General:
• Monitor vital signs at every appointment because of cardiovascular side effects.
• Place on frequent recall to evaluate gingival inflammation, if present.
• An increased incidence of dry socket has been reported after extraction.
• Consider semisupine chair position for patient comfort if GI side effects occur.

Teach patient/family:
• Need for good oral hygiene to prevent periodontal inflammation
• That smoking cessation decreases risk of serious adverse cardiovascular effects

orlistat

(or'li-stat)

Xenical

Drug class.: Antiobesity

Action: A reversible inhibitor of lipases; acts in the intestinal lumen to inhibit both gastric and pancreatic lipases, thereby preventing the metabolism of fats into absorbable fatty acids

Uses: Obesity management, including weight loss and maintenance in conjunction with a reduced-calorie diet; used in patients with a defined body mass index with other risk factors for cardiovascular disease

Dosage and routes:

• *Adult:* PO 120 mg tid with each meal containing fat; give during meal or up to 1 hr after meal

Available forms include: Caps 120 mg

Side effects/adverse reactions:

▼ *ORAL:* Gingiva and tooth disorder (not defined)

CNS: Headache, dizziness, sleep disruption, anxiety

GI: Oily spotting, flatus with discharge, fecal urgency, oily or fatty stool, increased defecation, fecal incontinence, abdominal pain, ***liver failure,*** vomiting

RESP: Influenza, URI, LRI

GU: Menstrual irregularity, UTI

EENT: Otitis

INTEG: Rash, dry skin

MS: Back pain, myalgia, joint discomfort

MISC: Fatigue

Contraindications: Chronic malabsorption syndrome, cholestasis or hypersensitivity reactions to this product, lactation; organic causes of obesity should first be identified

Precautions: Adherence to dietary guidelines, supplemental fat-soluble vitamins may be required along with betacarotene, nephrolithiasis, pregnancy category B, use in children not established

Pharmacokinetics:

PO: Poor oral absorption (minimal), low plasma levels, highly plasma protein bound (99%), metabolized in intestinal wall, majority of dose passes through GI tract for fecal excretion

Drug interactions of concern to dentistry:

• None reported

DENTAL CONSIDERATIONS

General:

• Although no dental drug interactions are reported, observe expected outcomes of systemically administered drugs.

• Severely obese patients may have type 2 diabetes or cardiovascular diseases.

• Consider semisupine chair position for patient comfort if GI side effects occur.

• Ensure that patient is following prescribed diet and regularly takes medication.

Consultations:

• Medical consultation may be required to assess disease control.

Teach patient/family:

• Importance of updating health and drug history if physician makes any changes in evaluation or drug regimens

O

orphenadrine citrate

(or-fen'a-dreen)

Norflex, Banflex, Flexoject, Flexon

♣ Disipal

Drug class.: Skeletal muscle relaxant

Action: Acts centrally in brainstem, has anticholinergic, analgesic effects; may not have direct muscle relaxing effects

Uses: Pain in musculoskeletal conditions

Dosage and routes:

• *Adult:* PO 100 mg bid; IM/IV 60 mg q12h

Available forms include: Tabs 100 mg; sus rel tabs 100 mg; inj IM/IV 30 mg/ml, OTC tab 50 mg (Canada only)

Side effects/adverse reactions:

▼ *ORAL:* Dry mouth

CNS: Dizziness, weakness, drowsiness, headache, disorientation, insomnia, stimulation, hallucination, agitation, syncope

CV: Tachycardia, palpitation

GI: Nausea, vomiting, constipation

HEMA: ***Aplastic anemia***

GU: Urinary hesitancy, retention

EENT: Pupil dilation, blurred vision, increased intraocular pressure, mydriasis

INTEG: Rash, pruritus, urticaria

Contraindications: Hypersensitivity, narrow-angle glaucoma, GI obstruction, myasthenia gravis, stenosing peptic ulcer, bladder neck obstruction, cardiospasm

Precautions: Pregnancy category not listed, children, cardiac disease, tachycardia, caution in lactation

Pharmacokinetics:

PO: Peak 2 hr, duration 4-6 hr, half-life 14 hr; metabolized in liver; excreted in urine (unchanged)

Drug interactions of concern to dentistry:

• Increased CNS effects: propoxyphene, CNS depressants, alcohol

• Increased anticholinergic effect: other anticholinergics

DENTAL CONSIDERATIONS

General:

• Consider semisupine chair position for patients with back pain.

• Patients on chronic drug therapy may rarely have symptoms of blood dyscrasias, which can include infection, bleeding, and poor healing.

• Assess salivary flow as a factor in caries, periodontal disease, and candidiasis.

Consultations:

• In a patient with symptoms of blood dyscrasias, request a medical consultation for blood studies and postpone dental treatment until normal values are reestablished.

• Medical consultation may be required to assess disease control.

Teach patient/family:

• Importance of good oral hygiene to prevent soft tissue inflammation

• Caution to prevent injury when using oral hygiene aids

• Caution when driving or operating equipment because of risk of dizziness

When chronic dry mouth occurs, advise patient:

• To avoid mouth rinses with high alcohol content because of drying effects

• Of need for daily use of home fluoride products to prevent caries

• To use sugarless gum, frequent sips of water, or saliva substitutes

oseltamivir phosphate

(oh-sel'ta-me-veer)

Tamiflu

Drug class.: Antiviral

Action: Inhibits neuraminidase, which is essential for replication of influenza type A and B viruses

Uses: Uncomplicated acute illness caused by influenza infection in adults who have been symptomatic for no more than 2 days; more effective against influenza type A virus; prophylaxis for adults and child >13 yr

Dosage and routes:

Treatment:

• *Adult and child >13 yr:* PO 75 mg bid × 5 days; initiate treatment within 2 days of onset of symptoms

• *Child >1 yr:* PO oral susp 30 mg bid if <15 kg (33 lb); 45 mg bid if >15 kg to 23 kg (>31 to 51 lb); 60 mg bid if >23 kg to 40 kg (>57 to 88 lb); 75 mg bid if >40 kg (>88 lb)

Prophylaxis (after exposure or close contact to flu):

• *Adult and child >13 yr:* PO 75 mg/day × 7 days (no doses approved for <13 yr)

Available forms include: Caps 75 mg; powder for oral susp 12 mg/ml in 100 ml

Side effects/adverse reactions:

CNS: Insomnia, vertigo, headache

GI: Nausea, vomiting, abdominal pain

RESP: Bronchitis, cough

MISC: Fatigue

Contraindications: Hypersensitivity

Precautions: Renal impairment, pregnancy category C, lactation

Pharmacokinetics:

PO: Readily absorbed, hepatic conversion to oseltamivir carboxylate, low plasma protein binding (3%), half-life 1-3 hr, excreted in urine (99%)

Drug interactions of concern to dentistry:

• None reported

DENTAL CONSIDERATIONS

General:

• Acute influenza patients are unlikely to be seen in the dental office except for dental emergencies.

• Consider semisupine chair position for patient comfort because of respiratory effects of disease.

oxandrolone

(ox-an'droe-lone)

Oxandrin

Drug class.: Androgenic anabolic steroid

Controlled Substance Schedule III

Action: Reverses catabolic tissue processes; promotes buildup of protein; increases erythropoietin production

Uses: To promote weight gain in catabolic or tissue wasting processes, such as extensive surgery, burns, infection, or trauma; HIV wasting syndrome; Turner's syndrome

Dosage and routes:

• *Adult:* PO 2.5 mg bid-qid, not to exceed 20 mg qd × 2-3 wk

• *Child:* PO 0.25 mg/kg/day × 2-4 wk, not to exceed 3 mo

Available forms include: Tabs 2.5 mg

Side effects/adverse reactions:
CNS: Dizziness, headache, fatigue, tremors, paresthesia, flushing, sweating, anxiety, lability, insomnia
CV: Increased BP, ***edema (in cardiac patients)***
GI: ***Cholestatic jaundice, peliosis hepatitis, liver cell tumors,*** nausea, vomiting, constipation, weight gain
HEMA: ***Increased prothrombin time, iron deficiency anemia***
GU: ***Hematuria,*** amenorrhea, vaginitis, decreased libido, decreased breast size, clitoral hypertrophy, testicular atrophy, gynecomastia (males), priapism
EENT: Conjunctional edema, nasal congestion
INTEG: Rash, acneiform lesions, oily hair/skin, flushing, sweating, acne vulgaris, alopecia, hirsutism
ENDO: Abnormal GTT, decreased glucose tolerance, increased LDL
MS: Cramps, spasms

Contraindications: Severe renal disease, severe cardiac disease, severe hepatic disease, hypersensitivity, pregnancy category X, lactation, genital bleeding (abnormal), prostate or breast carcinoma in males, breast cancer in females with hypercalcemia

Precautions: Diabetes mellitus, CV disease, MI, increased risk of prostatic hypertrophy, prostatic carcinoma, virilization (women), increased prothrombin time

Pharmacokinetics:
PO: Metabolized in liver; excreted in urine; crosses placenta; excreted in breast milk

Drug interactions of concern to dentistry:
- Increased risk of bleeding: aspirin
- Edema: ACTH, adrenal steroids

DENTAL CONSIDERATIONS

General:
- Monitor vital signs at every appointment because of cardiovascular side effects.
- Determine why the patient is taking the drug.
- Consider local hemostasis measures to prevent excessive bleeding.
- Short appointments and a stress reduction protocol may be required for anxious patients.
- Avoid prescribing aspirin-containing products.

Consultations:
- If signs of anemia are observed in oral tissues, physician consultation may be required.
- Medical consultation may be required to assess disease control and patient's ability to tolerate stress.
- Medical consultation should include partial prothrombin time or prothrombin time.

Teach patient/family:
- Importance of good oral hygiene to prevent soft tissue inflammation
- That secondary oral infection may occur; must see dentist immediately if infection occurs

oxaprozin

(ox'a-proe-zin)

Daypro

Drug class.: Nonsteroidal antiinflammatory

Action: Inhibits prostaglandin synthesis by interfering with cyclooxygenase needed for biosynthesis; possesses analgesic, antiinflammatory, antipyretic properties

Uses: Rheumatoid arthritis, osteoarthritis, and ankylosing spondylitis

Dosage and routes:

• *Adult:* PO 600-1200 mg daily; max dose 1800 mg/day

Available forms include: Tabs 600 mg

Side effects/adverse reactions:

▼ *ORAL:* Dry mouth, stomatitis, lichenoid reaction, oral ulceration

CNS: Dizziness, drowsiness, fatigue, tremors, confusion, insomnia, anxiety, depression

CV: Tachycardia, peripheral edema, palpitation, dysrhythmias

GI: ***Cholestatic hepatitis,*** nausea, anorexia, vomiting, diarrhea, jaundice, constipation, flatulence, cramps, peptic ulcer

HEMA: ***Blood dyscrasias***

GU: ***Nephrotoxicity: dysuria, hematuria, oliguria, azotemia***

EENT: Tinnitus, hearing loss, blurred vision

INTEG: Purpura, rash, pruritus, sweating, photosensitivity

Contraindications: Hypersensitivity, asthma, severe renal disease, severe hepatic disease

Precautions: Pregnancy category not established, lactation, children, bleeding disorders, GI disorders, cardiac disorders, hypersensitivity to other antiinflammatory agents, diabetes

Pharmacokinetics:

PO: Peak 1-2 hr, half-life 2-4 hr; 90%-99% plasma protein binding; metabolized in liver (inactive metabolites); excreted in urine (inactive metabolites)

Drug interactions of concern to dentistry:

• GI ulceration, bleeding: aspirin, alcohol, corticosteroids

• Decreased action: salicylates

• Nephrotoxicity: acetaminophen (prolonged use and high doses)

• Possible risk of decreased renal function: cyclosporine

• First-time users of SSRIs also taking NSAIDs may have a higher risk of GI side effects; until more data are available, it may be advisable to avoid use of NSAIDs in these patients (*Br J Clin Pharmacol* 55:591-595, 2003)

When prescribed for dental pain:

• Risk of increased effects: oral anticoagulants, oral antidiabetics, lithium, methotrexate

• Decreased antihypertensive effects of diuretics, β-adrenergic blockers, and ACE inhibitors

DENTAL CONSIDERATIONS

General:

• Patients on chronic drug therapy may rarely have symptoms of blood dyscrasias, which can include infection, bleeding, and poor healing.

• Assess salivary flow as a factor in caries, periodontal disease, and candidiasis.

• Avoid prescribing for dental use in pregnancy.

• Consider semisupine chair position for patients with arthritic disease.

Consultations:

• Medical consultation may be required to assess disease control.

• In a patient with symptoms of blood dyscrasias, request a medical consultation for blood studies and postpone dental treatment until normal values are reestablished.

Teach patient/family:

• Importance of good oral hygiene to prevent soft tissue inflammation

• Caution to prevent injury when using oral hygiene aids

O

When chronic dry mouth occurs, advise patient:
• To avoid mouth rinses with high alcohol content because of drying effects
• Of need for daily use of home fluoride products to prevent caries
• To use sugarless gum, frequent sips of water, or saliva substitutes

---

oxazepam

(ox-a'ze-pam)
Serax
♣ Apo-Oxazepam, Novoxapam
Drug class.: Benzodiazepine

Controlled Substance Schedule IV
Action: Produces CNS depression by interacting with a benzodiazepine receptor to facilitate the action of the inhibitory neurotransmitter γ-aminobutyric acid (GABA)
Uses: Anxiety, alcohol withdrawal
Dosage and routes:
Anxiety:
• *Adult:* PO 10-30 mg tid-qid
Alcohol withdrawal:
• *Adult:* PO 15-30 mg tid-qid
Available forms include: Caps 10, 15, 30 mg; tabs 15 mg
Side effects/adverse reactions:
▼ *ORAL:* Dry mouth
CNS: Dizziness, drowsiness, confusion, headache, anxiety, tremors, fatigue, depression, insomnia, hallucinations, paradoxic excitement, transient amnesia, syncope, hangover
CV: Orthostatic hypotension, ***ECG changes, tachycardia,*** hypotension
GI: Nausea, vomiting, anorexia, abdominal discomfort
EENT: Blurred vision, tinnitus, mydriasis
INTEG: Rash, dermatitis, itching
Contraindications: Hypersensitivity to benzodiazepines, narrow-angle glaucoma, psychosis, pregnancy category D, child <12 yr
Precautions: Elderly, debilitated, hepatic disease, renal disease
Pharmacokinetics:
PO: Peak 2-4 hr, half-life 5-15 hr; metabolized by liver; excreted by kidneys
Drug interactions of concern to dentistry:
• Increased effects: CNS depressants, alcohol, and anticonvulsant medications
• Possible increase in CNS side effects of kava (herb)

DENTAL CONSIDERATIONS
General:
• Monitor vital signs at every appointment because of cardiovascular side effects.
• Psychologic and physical dependence may occur with chronic administration.
• Geriatric patients are more susceptible to drug effects; use lower dose.
• Assess salivary flow as a factor in caries, periodontal disease, and candidiasis.
Consultations:
• Medical consultation may be required to assess disease control.
Teach patient/family:
• To avoid mouth rinses with high alcohol content because of drying effects

---

oxcarbazepine

(ox-carb'az-e-peen)
Trileptal
Drug class.: Anticonvulsant

Action: Mechanism of antiseizure effect is unknown; the 10-monohydroxy-carbamazepine metabolite accounts for pharmacologic activity; may block sodium channels; inhibits seizure propagation and affects potassium conductance and calcium channels

Uses: Monotherapy or adjunctive therapy of partial seizures in adults with epilepsy; monotherapy or adjunctive therapy for partial seizures in children (4-16 yr) with epilepsy

Dosage and routes:

• *Adult:* PO initial 600 mg/day using bid regimen, doses may be increased to max of 1200 mg/day; patients taking other anticonvulsant drugs must be observed and plasma levels of other anticonvulsants must be monitored; patients should also be observed closely when switching to monotherapy

• *Child 4-16 yr:* PO initial dose 8-10 mg/kg, not to exceed 600 mg/day; give doses in bid regimen; target maintenance dose over 2 wk; final dose depends on patient's weight.

Available forms include: Tabs 150, 300, 600 mg; oral sus 300 mg/5 ml

Side effects/adverse reactions:

▼ *ORAL:* Dry mouth (high doses), gingival overgrowth (infrequent), taste alterations, stomatitis

CNS: Dizziness, headache, somnolence, fatigue, insomnia, tremor, nervousness, altered thinking (high dose)

CV: Hypotension (high dose), bradycardia, palpitation, syncope

GI: Nausea, vomiting, abdominal pain, diarrhea, dyspepsia, constipation, gastritis

RESP: UTI, coughing, bronchitis

HEMA: Purpura (high doses), ***leukopenia, thrombocytopenia***

GU: UTI, urination frequency

EENT: Diplopia, nystagmus, rhinitis, vertigo, pharyngitis

INTEG: Rash, ***SLE, Stevens-Johnson syndrome, toxic epidermal necrolysis,*** erythema multiforme, acne, dermatitis

META: Weight increase, hyponatremia, hypocalcemia, hyperglycemia, elevated liver enzymes

MS: Muscle weakness

MISC: Ataxia, leg edema

Contraindications: Hypersensitivity to this drug or carbamazepine

Precautions: Development of hyponatremia, withdraw drug slowly to avoid seizures, cognitive CNS adverse effects, decreases effect of oral contraceptives, caution when used with other anticonvulsants, renal impairment, pregnancy category C, lactation

Pharmacokinetics:

PO: Complete absorption, extensive hepatic metabolism to the 10-monohydroxy metabolite, may induce CYP450 3A4/5 enzymes, $T_{1/2}$ of parent drug and metabolite is 9 hr; plasma protein binding 40%, renal excretion

Drug interactions of concern to dentistry:

• Possible increase in CNS depression: all CNS depressants, alcohol

• No dental drug interactions reported; CYP450 3A4/5 enzyme inducers may decrease plasma levels

DENTAL CONSIDERATIONS

General:

• Monitor vital signs at every appointment because of cardiovascular side effects.

• Patients on chronic drug therapy may rarely have symptoms of blood dyscrasias, which can include infection, bleeding, and poor healing.

O

• Assess salivary flow as a factor in caries, periodontal disease, and candidiasis
• Consider semisupine chair position for patient comfort if GI side effects occur.
• Short appointments and a stress reduction protocol may be required for anxious patients.
• Determine type of epilepsy, seizure frequency, and quality of seizure control.

Consultations:
• In a patient with symptoms of blood dyscrasias, request a medical consultation for blood studies and postpone treatment until normal values are reestablished.
• Medical consultation may be required to assess disease control and patient's ability to tolerate stress.

Teach patient/family:
• Importance of good oral hygiene to prevent soft tissue inflammation
• To prevent trauma when using oral hygiene aids

When chronic dry mouth occurs, advise patient:
• To avoid mouth rinses with high alcohol content because of drying effects
• To use daily home fluoride products for anticaries effect
• To use sugarless gum, frequent sips of water, or saliva substitutes

---

oxidized cellulose

Oxycel, Surgicel

Drug class.: Cellulose hemostatic

Action: Mechanism unclear; may act physically to absorb blood and promote an artificial clot

Uses: Hemostasis in surgery, oral surgery, exodontia

Dosage and routes:
• *Adult and child:* TOP apply using sterile technique as needed; remove after bleeding stops, if possible, or leave in place if needed

Available forms include: TOP knitted fabric in pads, pledgets, and strips of various sizes

Side effects/adverse reactions:
CNS: Headache in epistaxis
EENT: Sneezing, burning in epistaxis
INTEG: Burning, stinging, encapsulation of fluid, foreign bodies

Contraindications: Hypersensitivity, large artery hemorrhage, oozing surfaces, implantation in bone deficit, placement around optic nerve and optic chiasm

Precautions: Do not autoclave; inactivation of topical thrombin

DENTAL CONSIDERATIONS

General:
• Apply dry; use only amount needed to control bleeding.
• Place loosely and avoid packing; remove excess before closure in surgery; irrigate first, then remove using sterile technique.
• Ensure therapeutic response: decreased bleeding in surgery.
• Can be left in situ when necessary, but should be removed once bleeding is controlled.
• Application of topical thrombin solution to the cellulose gauze will inactivate thrombin because of acidity.

oxtriphylline

(ox-trye'fi-lin)

Choledyl SA

✤ Apo-Oxitriphylline, PMS-Oxtriphylline

Drug class.: Choline salt of theophylline, bronchodilator

Action: Relaxes smooth muscle of respiratory system by blocking phosphodiesterase, increasing cAMP

Uses: Acute bronchial asthma, reversible bronchospasm in chronic bronchitis and COPD

Dosage and routes:

• *Adult and child >17 yr:* PO 4.7 mg/kg q8h; usually 300 mg/day, can be increased to 600 mg/day

• *Child 6-16 yr:* PO 4 mg/kg q6h; may be increased to desired response, therapeutic level

Available forms include: Elix 100 mg/5 ml; syr 50 mg/5 ml; tabs 100, 200; sus rel tabs 400, 600 mg

Side effects/adverse reactions:

▼ *ORAL:* Bitter taste

CNS: Anxiety, restlessness, insomnia, dizziness, ***convulsions,*** headache, light-headedness, muscle twitching

CV: Palpitation, sinus tachycardia, hypotension

GI: Nausea, vomiting, anorexia, diarrhea, dyspepsia

RESP: Increased rate

INTEG: Flushing, urticaria

Contraindications: Hypersensitivity to xanthines, tachydysrhythmias

Precautions: Elderly, CHF, cor pulmonale, hepatic disease, active peptic ulcer disease, diabetes mellitus, hyperthyroidism, hypertension, children, pregnancy category C, glaucoma, prostatic hypertrophy

Pharmacokinetics:

PO: Peak 1 hr; metabolized in liver; excreted in urine, breast milk; crosses placenta

Drug interactions of concern to dentistry:

• Increased action: erythromycin (macrolides), ephedrine, xanthines, fluoroquinolones

• Decreased therapeutic effects: barbiturates, β-adrenergic blockers, nicotine

DENTAL CONSIDERATIONS

General:

• Evaluate respiration characteristics and rate.

• Consider semisupine chair position for patient comfort because of GI effects of disease.

• Short appointments and a stress reduction protocol may be required for anxious patients.

• Be aware that aspirin or sulfite preservatives in vasoconstrictor-containing products can exacerbate asthma.

• Acute asthmatic episodes may be precipitated in the dental office. Sympathomimetic inhalants should be available for emergency use.

• Discuss tobacco cessation for patients using tobacco.

oxybutynin chloride

(ox-i-byoo'ti-nin)

Ditropan, Ditropan XL, Oxytrol Transdermal System

Drug class.: Antispasmodic

Action: Relaxes smooth muscles in urinary tract

Uses: Antispasmodic for neurogenic bladder, overactive bladder

Dosage and routes:

• *Adult:* PO 5 mg bid-tid, not to exceed 5 mg qid; XL formulation once-daily dosage

• *Child >5 yr:* PO 5 mg bid, not to exceed 5 mg tid

Transdermal:

• *Adult:* TOP 1 patch applied bid q3-4d

Available forms include: Syr 5 mg/5 ml; tabs 5 mg; ext rel tabs 5, 10 mg; transdermal patch 36 mg

Side effects/adverse reactions:

▼ *ORAL: Dry mouth*

CNS: Restlessness, dizziness, drowsiness, ***convulsions,*** confusion, insomnia, weakness, hallucinations

CV: Palpitation, tachycardia, hypotension

GI: Nausea, vomiting, anorexia, abdominal pain, constipation

GU: Dysuria, retention, hesitancy

EENT: Blurred vision, increased intraocular tension

INTEG: Urticaria, dermatitis

Contraindications: Hypersensitivity, GI obstruction, GI hemorrhage, GU obstruction, glaucoma, severe colitis, myasthenia gravis, unstable CV status in acute hemorrhage

Precautions: Pregnancy category C, lactation, suspected glaucoma, children <12 yr, hiatal hernia, esophageal reflux, coronary heart disease, CHF, hypertension

Pharmacokinetics:

PO: Onset 0.5-1 hr, peak 3-4 hr, duration 6-10 hr; metabolized by liver; excreted in urine

Drug interactions of concern to dentistry:

• Increased anticholinergic effect: anticholinergic drugs

• Increased depressant effect of both drugs: CNS depressants, alcohol

DENTAL CONSIDERATIONS

General:

• Assess salivary flow as a factor in caries, periodontal disease, and candidiasis.

• Monitor vital signs at every appointment because of cardiovascular side effects.

• Avoid dental light in patient's eyes; offer dark glasses for patient comfort.

• Consider semisupine chair position for patient comfort if GI side effects occur.

Consultations:

• Physician should be informed if significant xerostomic side effects occur (e.g, increased caries, sore tongue, problems eating or swallowing, difficulty wearing prosthesis) so that a medication change can be considered.

Teach patient/family:

• Importance of good oral hygiene to prevent soft tissue inflammation

When chronic dry mouth occurs, advise patient:

• To avoid mouth rinses with high alcohol content because of drying effects

• Of need for daily use of home fluoride products to prevent caries

• To use sugarless gum, frequent sips of water, or saliva substitutes

oxycodone HCl

(ox-i-koe'done)

Endocodone, M-Oxy, OxyContin, OxyFast, OxyIR, Oxydose, Percolone, Roxicodone, Roxicodone Intensol

♣ Supeudol

Combinations: Codoxy, Percocet-Demi, Percodan, Tylox

♣ Endodan, Percocet, Roxiprin

Drug class.: Synthetic opioid analgesic

Controlled Substance Schedule II, Canada N

Action: Interacts with opioid receptors in the CNS to alter pain perception

Uses: Moderate-to-severe pain, normally used in combination with aspirin or acetaminophen; combination products (see Appendix F)

Dosage and routes:

Acute pain:

• *Adult:* PO 5 mg q6h

Moderate-to-severe pain (around-the-clock analgesia):

• *Adult:* PO immed release 10-30 mg q4h; con rel tabs (80 and 160 mg) are for use only in opioid-tolerant patients; these doses are generally intended for cancer patients and not for use in general dental pain management

Available forms include: Tabs 5 mg; oral sol 5 mg/5 ml; oral sol concentrate 20 mg/ml, con rel tabs 10, 20, 40, 80, 160 mg; caps immed rel 5 mg; tabs immed rel 15, 30 mg

CAUTION: Controlled release dose forms are for moderate-to-severe pain for continous pain control over an extended time period; they are not for prn pain relief.

Side effects/adverse reactions:

▼ *ORAL:* Dry mouth

CNS: Drowsiness, dizziness, confusion, headache, sedation, euphoria

CV: Palpitation, bradycardia, tachycardia

GI: Nausea, vomiting, anorexia, constipation, cramps

RESP: ***Respiratory depression***

GU: Decreased urinary output, oliguria, dysuria, urinary retention

EENT: Tinnitus, blurred vision, miosis, diplopia

INTEG: Rash, urticaria, bruising, flushing, diaphoresis, pruritus

Contraindications: Hypersensitivity, addiction (narcotic)

Precautions: Addictive personality, pregnancy category B, lactation, increased intracranial pressure, MI (acute), severe heart disease, respiratory depression, hepatic disease, renal disease, child <18 yr, physical dependence

Pharmacokinetics:

PO: Onset 10-15 min, peak 0.5-1 hr, duration 4-5 hr; detoxified by liver; excreted in urine, breast milk; crosses placenta

Drug interactions of concern to dentistry:

• Increased effects with other CNS depressants: alcohol, other narcotics, sedative-hypnotics, skeletal muscle relaxants, phenothiazines, benzodiazepines

• Contraindication: MAOIs

• Increased effects of anticholinergics

DENTAL CONSIDERATIONS

General:

• Monitor vital signs at every ap-

O

pointment because of cardiovascular and respiratory side effects.
• Assess salivary flow as a factor in caries, periodontal disease, and candidiasis.
• Psychologic and physical dependence may occur with chronic administration.
• Determine why the patient is taking the drug.
Teach patient/family:
• To avoid mouth rinses with high alcohol content because of drying effects

oxymetazoline HCl (nasal)

(ox-i-met-az'oh-leen)
Afrin No-Drip 12 hour, Afrin 12-hour Original, Duramist Plus 12H, Neo-Synephrine 12 Hour, Nostrilla 12 Hour, and many others

Drug class.: Nasal decongestant, sympathomimetic amine

Action: Produces vasoconstriction (rapid, long acting) of arterioles, thereby decreasing fluid exudation, mucosal engorgement
Uses: Nasal congestion
Dosage and routes:
• *Adult and child >6 yr:* Instill 2-3 drops or sprays to each nostril bid
Available forms include: Sol 0.05%
Side effects/adverse reactions:
CNS: Anxiety, restlessness, tremors, weakness, insomnia, dizziness, fever, headache
GI: Nausea, vomiting, anorexia
EENT: Irritation, burning, sneezing, stinging, dryness, rebound congestion
INTEG: Contact dermatitis

Contraindications: Hypersensitivity to sympathomimetic amines
Precautions: Child <6 yr, elderly, diabetes, cardiovascular disease, hypertension, hyperthyroidism, increased ICP, prostatic hypertrophy, pregnancy category C, glaucoma
Drug interactions of concern to dentistry:
• Increased risk of hypertension: tricyclic antidepressants, but it requires adequate systemic absorption of oxymetazoline

DENTAL CONSIDERATIONS
General:
• Excessive use can lead to rebound congestion and cardiovascular side effects; follow recommended dosing intervals.
• Extensive nasal swelling and congestion may interfere with optimal use of nitrous oxide/oxygen sedation.

oxymetholone

(ox-i-meth'oh-lone)
Anadrol-50
✤ Anapolon 50

Drug class.: Androgenic anabolic steroid

Controlled Substance Schedule III
Action: Reverses catabolic tissue processes; promotes buildup of protein; increases erythropoietin production
Uses: Anemia associated with bone marrow failure and red cell production deficiencies; aplastic anemia, myelofibrosis, and anemia caused by myelotoxic drugs
Dosage and routes:
Aplastic anemia:
• *Adult and child:* PO 1-5 mg/kg/day, titrated to patient response,

with minimum trial period of 3-6 mo

Available forms include: Tabs 50 mg

Side effects/adverse reactions:

CNS: Dizziness, headache, fatigue, tremors, paresthesia, flushing, sweating, anxiety, lability, insomnia

CV: ***Edema (in cardiac patients),*** increased BP

GI: ***Peliosis hepatitis, liver cell tumors, cholestatic jaundice,*** nausea, vomiting, constipation, weight gain

HEMA: ***Increased prothrombin time, iron deficiency anemia***

GU: ***Hematuria,*** amenorrhea, vaginitis, decreased libido, decreased breast size, clitoral hypertrophy, testicular atrophy, gynecomastia (male), priapism

EENT: Conjunctival edema, nasal congestion

INTEG: Rash, acneiform lesions, oily hair/skin, flushing, sweating, acne vulgaris, alopecia, hirsutism

ENDO: Abnormal GTT, decreased glucose tolerance, increased LDL

MS: Cramps, spasms

Contraindications: Severe renal disease, severe cardiac disease, severe hepatic disease, hypersensitivity, pregnancy category X, lactation, genital bleeding (abnormal), prostate or breast carcinoma (males), breast cancer in females with hypercalcemia

Precautions: Diabetes mellitus, CV disease, MI, increased risk of prostatic hypertrophy, prostatic carcinoma, virilization (women), increased prothrombin time

Pharmacokinetics:

PO: Metabolized in liver, excreted in urine, crosses placenta, excreted in breast milk

Drug interactions of concern to dentistry:

- Increased risk of bleeding: aspirin
- Edema: ACTH, adrenal steroids

DENTAL CONSIDERATIONS

General:

- Monitor vital signs at every appointment because of cardiovascular side effects.
- Determine why the patient is taking the drug.
- Consider local hemostasis measures to prevent excessive bleeding.
- Short appointments and a stress reduction protocol may be required for anxious patients.
- Avoid prescribing aspirin-containing products.

Consultations:

- Physician consultation may be required if signs of anemia are observed in oral tissues.
- Medical consultation may be required to assess disease control and patient's ability to tolerate stress.
- Medical consultation should include partial prothrombin time or prothrombin time.

Teach patient/family:

- Importance of good oral hygiene to prevent soft tissue inflammation
- That secondary oral infection may occur; must see dentist immediately if infection occurs

paclitaxel

(pac-li-tax'el)

Onxol, Taxol

Drug class.: Antineoplastic

Action: Obtained from the Western yew tree; unique action inhibits microtubule network reorganization essential for cell division

Uses: Metastatic ovarian cancer,

P

non–small cell lung cancer; second-line treatment for AIDS-related Kaposi's sarcoma; adjuvant treatment of node-positive breast cancer sequential to a course of standard doxorubicin-containing combination chemotherapy

Dosage and routes:

• *Adult:* IV only, after oral premedication with PO dexamethasone, diphenhydramine, and H_2 antagonist, 135 mg/m^2 over 24 hr q3wk, depending on development of neutropenia; or IV 175 mg/m^2 over 3 hr q3wk

Available forms include: Inj 6 mg/ml in multiple-dose vials

Side effects/adverse reactions:

▼ *ORAL: Mucositis*

CV: Bradycardia, hypotension, abnormal ECG

GI: Nausea, vomiting, diarrhea, hepatic function impairment, ischemic colitis

RESP: Allergic dyspnea, infection

HEMA: Bone marrow depression, thrombocytopenia, anemia, bleeding

GU: UTIs

INTEG: Flushing, rash

METAB: Increased bilirubin, increased alk phosphatase, AST

MS: Myalgia, arthralgia

MISC: Alopecia, peripheral neuropathy, ***severe allergic reactions,*** fever

Contraindications: Hypersensitivity, other products containing polyethylated castor oil, neutropenia <1500/mm^3

Precautions: Pregnancy category D, bone marrow depression, AV block, hepatic impairment, lactation, children, recent MI, angina pectoris, CHF history, current use of drug with effect on cardiac conduction system

Pharmacokinetics:

IV: Terminal half-life 5-17 hr; plasma protein binding 88%-98%, hepatic metabolism mainly by CYP2C8 and lesser amount by CYP3A4 isoenzymes; excreted in bile

Drug interactions of concern to dentistry:

• Possible (not demonstrated) increase in action by strong inhibitiors of CYP2C8 and CYP3A4 isoenzymes: diazepam, ketoconazole, midazolam (monitor patient if prescribed)

DENTAL CONSIDERATIONS

General:

• Consider semisupine chair position for patient comfort if GI side effects occur.

• Patients receiving chemotherapy may require palliative therapy for stomatitis.

• Patients on chronic drug therapy may rarely have symptoms of blood dyscrasias, which can include infection, bleeding, and poor healing.

Consultations:

• Medical consultation may be required to assess disease control.

Teach patient/family:

• Importance of good oral hygiene to prevent soft tissue inflammation

• Caution to prevent trauma when using oral hygiene aids

pancrelipase

(pan-kre-li'pase)

Cotazym, Cotazym-S, Creon-10, Creon-20, Creon-25, Ku-Zyme HP, Lipram, Pancrease, Pancrease MT 4, Ultrase MT, Viokase, Zymase

Drug class.: Digestant

Action: Pancreatic enzyme needed for proper pancreatic functioning in metabolizing lipids, proteins, and carbohydrates

Uses: Exocrine pancreatic secretion insufficiency, cystic fibrosis (digestive aid), steatorrhea, pancreatic enzyme deficiency, chronic pancreatitis

Dosage and routes:

• *Adult and child:* PO 1-3 caps/tabs ac or with meals, or 1 cap/tab with snack or 1-2 pdr pkt ac

Available forms include: Tabs 8000, 11,000, 30,000 U; caps 8000, 10,000, 12,000, 16,000 U; enteric-coated caps 4000, 4500, 5000, 10,000, 20,000, 25,000 U; powder 16,800 U

Side effects/adverse reactions:

▼ *ORAL:* Irritation to mucous membranes

GI: Anorexia, nausea, vomiting, diarrhea, cramps

RESP: Asthma attack

GU: Hyperuricuria, hyperuricemia

Contraindications: Allergy to pork

Precautions: Pregnancy category C

DENTAL CONSIDERATIONS

General:

• Consider semisupine chair position for patient comfort because of GI effects of disease.

• To avoid oral irritation, mouth should be rinsed or drug taken with liquid.

pantoprazole sodium

(pan-toe′pra-zole)

Protonix, Protonix IV

Drug class.: Antisecretory, proton pump inhibitor

Action: Suppresses gastric acid production by binding to the hydrogen/potassium ATPase enzyme system to inhibit the final step in gastric acid production

Uses: Short-term treatment of erosive esophagitis associated with gastroesophageal reflux disease (GERD), pathologic hypersecretory disorders

Dosage and routes:

• *Adult:* PO 40 mg/day for up to 8 wk; for patients who have not healed, an additional 8 wk may be considered; maintenance 40 mg/day

Hypersecretory disorders:

• *Adult:* PO 40 mg bid, adjust dose as required

• *Adult:* IV infusion 80 mg q12h, adjust dose as required

GERD:

• *Adult:* IV infusion 40 mg/day, up to 7-10 day

Available forms include: Del rel tabs 20, 40 mg; powder for inj 40 mg vial

Side effects/adverse reactions:

▼ *ORAL:* Aphthous stomatitis, candidiasis, dry mouth, dysphagia (all <1%)

CNS: Headache, migraine, anxiety

CV: Arrhythmias, chest pain, palpitation (all <1%)

GI: Diarrhea, flatulence, abdominal pain, constipation, dyspepsia, gastroenteritis, nausea

RESP: Bronchitis, cough, URI

GU: Urinary frequency, UTI

EENT: Rhinitis, sinusitis

INTEG: Rash

META: Hyperglycemia, hyperlipidemia, abnormal liver function tests

MS: Back pain, asthenia, neck pain

MISC: Flu syndrome

Contraindications: Hypersensitivity

Precautions: Do not split, crush, or chew tablets; no data on children

P

<18 yr, severe hepatic impairment, pregnancy category B, lactation

Pharmacokinetics: *PO (enteric coated tab):* Peak plasma levels 2.5 hr, bioavailability ~77%, plasma protein binding 98%, extensive hepatic metabolism (CYP450 2C19 enzyme system), excreted mainly in urine 71%, feces 18%

Drug interactions of concern to dentistry:

• No relevant drug interactions with other drugs metabolized by CYP450 2C19 enzymes

• No dental drug interactions reported; however, with profound inhibition of gastric acid production, absorption of ketoconazole and amoxicillin could be affected

DENTAL CONSIDERATIONS

General:

• Consider semisupine chair position for patient comfort because of GI effects of disease.

• Question the patient about tolerance of NSAIDs or aspirin related to GI problem.

• Patients with gastroesophageal reflux disease may have oral symptoms, including burning mouth, secondary candidiasis, and signs of enamel erosion.

• Assess salivary flow as factor in caries, periodontal disease, and candidiasis.

Teach patient/family:

When chronic dry mouth occurs, advise patient:

• To avoid mouth rinses with high alcohol content because of drying effects

• To use sugarless gum, frequent sips of water, or saliva substitutes

• To use daily home fluoride products for anticaries effect

papaverine HCl

(pa-pav'er-een)

Pavabid, Pavagen

Drug class.: Peripheral vasodilator

Action: Relaxes all smooth muscle, inhibits cyclic nucleotide phosphodiesterase, increasing intracellular cAMP and causing vasodilation

Uses: Arterial spasm resulting in cerebral and peripheral ischemia; myocardial ischemia associated with vascular spasm or dysrhythmias; angina pectoris; peripheral pulmonary embolism; visceral spasm as in ureteral, biliary, GI colic PVD; unapproved: with phentolamine or alprostadil for intracavernous injection for impotence

Dosage and routes:

• *Adult:* PO sus rel 150-300 mg q8-12h; IM/IV 30-120 mg q3h prn

Available forms include: Time rel caps 150 mg; inj IM/IV 30 mg/ml

Side effects/adverse reactions:

CNS: Headache, dizziness, drowsiness, sedation, vertigo, malaise, depression

CV: ***Tachycardia,*** increased BP

GI: ***Hepatotoxicity,*** nausea, anorexia, abdominal pain, constipation, diarrhea, jaundice, altered liver enzymes

RESP: Increased depth of respirations

INTEG: Flushing, sweating, rash, pruritus

Contraindications: Hypersensitivity, complete AV heart block

Precautions: Cardiac dysrhythmias, glaucoma, pregnancy category C, lactation, drug dependency, children, hepatic hypersensitivity, Parkinson's disease

Pharmacokinetics:
PO: Onset 30 sec, peak 1-2 hr, duration 3-4 hr
SUS REL: Onset erratic; 90% bound to plasma proteins; metabolized in liver; excreted in urine (inactive metabolites)

Drug interactions of concern to dentistry:
- Increased hypotension: alcohol, other drugs that may also lower blood pressure

DENTAL CONSIDERATIONS

General:
- Monitor vital signs at every appointment because of cardiovascular and respiratory side effects.
- Short appointments and a stress reduction protocol may be required for anxious patients.

Consultations:
- Stress from dental procedures may compromise cardiovascular function; determine patient risk.
- Medical consultation may be required to assess disease control.

Teach patient/family:
- To avoid mouth rinses with high alcohol content
- Importance of good oral hygiene to prevent soft tissue inflammation

paregoric

(par-e-gor′ik)

Drug class.: Antidiarrheal

Controlled Substance Schedule III, Canada N

Action: Antiperistaltic and analgesic with activity related to morphine content

Uses: Diarrhea

Dosage and routes:
- *Adult:* PO 5-10 ml qd-qid
- *Child:* PO 0.25-0.5 ml/kg qd-qid

Available forms include: Liq 2 mg morphine equivalent per 5 ml in pints

Side effects/adverse reactions:
▼ *ORAL:* Dry mouth
*CNS: **CNS depression,*** dizziness, drowsiness, fainting, flushing, physical dependency
GI: Nausea, vomiting, constipation, abdominal pain

Contraindications: Hypersensitivity, severe ulcerative colitis, pseudomembranous colitis

Precautions: Liver disease, addiction-prone individuals, prostatic hypertrophy (severe), pregnancy category B, caution in lactation, safety and efficacy in pediatric patients not established

Pharmacokinetics:
PO: Duration 4 hr, half-life 2-3 hr; metabolized in liver; excreted in urine

Drug interactions of concern to dentistry:
- Increased action of both drugs: alcohol, all other CNS depressants
- Decreased peristalsis: anticholinergic drugs

DENTAL CONSIDERATIONS

General:
- Psychologic and physical dependence may occur with chronic administration.
- Determine why the patient is taking the drug.

Teach patient/family:
- To avoid mouth rinses with high alcohol content because of drying effects

P

paroxetine HCl

(pa-rox'e-teen)

Paxil, Paxil CR

Drug class.: Antidepressant

Action: Selectively inhibits the uptake of serotonin in the brain

Uses: Depression, panic disorder, obsessive compulsive disorder, social anxiety disorder; generalized anxiety disorder, posttraumatic stress disorder; premenstrual dysphoric disorder

Dosage and routes:

Depression:

• *Adult:* PO initially 20 mg/day, increase 10 mg/wk to effect, usual dose range 25-62.5 mg/day or 25 mg/day (con rel tab)

Panic disorder:

• *Adult:* PO 10 mg qd (con rel tabs 12.5 mg/day)

Obsessive compulsive disorder:

• *Adult:* PO initial dose 20 mg/day, titrate upward if needed to 60 mg/day (maximum dose)

Social anxiety disorder:

• *Adult:* PO initial dose 20 mg/day; titrate upward if needed, max 60 mg/day

Posttraumatic stress disorder:

• *Adult:* PO initial dose 20 mg/day; titrate upward if needed, max 50 mg/day

Available forms include: Tabs 10, 20, 30, 40 mg; con rel tabs 12.5, 25, 37.5 mg; oral susp 10 mg/5 ml

Side effects/adverse reactions:

▼ *ORAL: Dry mouth,* glossitis, aphthous stomatitis, (<0.1%), salivary gland enlargement (<0.1%), taste perversion

CNS: Somnolence, tremor, sweating, asthenia, insomnia, dizziness

CV: Palpitation, vasodilation, postural hypotension, syncope, tachycardia

GI: Constipation, nausea, diarrhea, anorexia, vomiting, flatulence, weight gain

RESP: Pharyngitis, yawning, respiratory complaints, coughing, rhinitis

GU: Decreased libido, sexual dysfunction, urinary frequency

EENT: Blurred vision, photophobia

SYST: Headache, myopathy, malaise, fever

METAB: Increased serum albumin, blood glucose, alk phosphatase

Contraindications: Hypersensitivity, MAOIs

Precautions: Pregnancy category B, lactation, elderly, oral anticoagulants, renal or hepatic impairment, children with suspected higher risk of suicide ideation, other serotonergic drugs

Pharmacokinetics:

PO: Peak plasma levels 5 hr (0.5-11 hr range), half-life 21 hr; highly protein bound; extensive first-pass metabolism; renal excretion

Drug interactions of concern to dentistry:

• Possible increased side effects: highly protein-bound drugs (aspirin), other antidepressants, alcohol

• Possible inhibition of fluoxetine metabolism: erythromycin, clarithromycin

• Increased half-life of diazepam

• First-time users of SSRIs also taking NSAIDs may have a higher risk of GI side effects; until more data are available, it may be advisable to avoid use of NSAIDs in these patients (*Br J Clin Pharmacol* 55:591-595, 2003)

DENTAL CONSIDERATIONS

General:

• After supine positioning, have patient sit upright for at least 2 min to avoid orthostatic hypotension.
• Assess salivary flow as a factor in caries, periodontal disease, and candidiasis.
• Avoid dental light in patient's eyes; offer dark glasses for patient comfort.

Consultations:

• Medical consultation may be required to assess disease control and patient's ability to tolerate stress.
• Physician should be informed if significant xerostomic side effects occur (e.g., increased caries, sore tongue, problems eating or swallowing, difficulty wearing prosthesis) so that a medication change can be considered.

Teach patient/family:

When chronic dry mouth occurs, advise patient:

• To avoid mouth rinses with high alcohol content because of drying effects
• Of need for daily use of home fluoride products to prevent caries
• To use sugarless gum, frequent sips of water, or saliva substitutes

---

peginterferon alfa-2a/ peginterferon alfa-2b

(peg-in-ter-feer'on)
alfa-2a: Pegasys
alfa-2b: PEG-Intron, Peg-Intron Redipen

Drug class.: Biologic response modifier

Action: In vitro studies indicate that interferons bind to specific cell surface receptors resulting in a variety of protein-protein interactions. This in turn leads to rapid activation of gene transcription. The overall response includes inhibition of viral replication in infected cells, inhibition of cell proliferation, and immunomodulation.

Uses: Treatment of adults with chronic hepatitis C with compensated liver disease who have not been previously treated with interferon-alfa; peginterferon alfa-2b can be used with ribavirin

Dosage and routes:

• *Adult:* SC 180 μg once weekly × 48 wk (peginterferon alfa-2a)
• *Adult >18 yr:* SC as a single drug 1 μg/kg/wk × 12 mo (peginterferon alfa-2b)

Peginterferon alfa-2b with ribavirin:

• *Adult >18 yr:* SC 1.5 μg/kg/wk

Available forms include:

Vial 180 μg/1.0 ml (store vials in refrigerator; do not freeze or shake)

Side effects/adverse reactions:

▼ *ORAL: Dry mouth*
CNS: Insomnia, dizziness, depression, fatigue, anorexia, headache, irritability, memory impairment, anxiety, ***psychiatric reactions***
GI: Nausea, diarrhea, abdominal pain, vomiting, ***colitis, pancreatitis***
RESP: Pulmonary disorders
HEMA: ***Neutropenia, thrombocytopenia, aplastic anemia***
EENT: Visual disturbances
INTEG: Injection-site reaction, alopecia, pruritus, dermatitis, rash
ENDO: Abnormal thyroid values
MS: Rigors, asthenia, myalgia, arthralgia, back pain
MISC: Flulike symptoms, fever

Contraindications: Hypersensitivity, autoimmune hepatitis, decompensated hepatic disease, neonates and infants

P

Precautions: Preexisting cardiac disease, may aggravate hypothyroidism, hyperthyroidism, hyperglycemia, hypoglycemia, diabetes, ophthalmologic disorders, pregnancy category C, lactation, children; closely monitor patients, severe life-threatening neuropsychiatric, autoimmune, ischemic, or infectious disorders may cause or aggravate these conditions

Pharmacokinetics: *SC:* Peak serum levels 72-96 hr; cleared from the body at 94 ml/hr; no data in children, pharmacokinetic data are limited

Drug interactions of concern to dentistry:

• Risk of hepatotoxicity in severe liver disease: acetaminophen

DENTAL CONSIDERATIONS

General:

• Determine why patient is taking the drug.

• Assess salivary flow as a factor in caries, periodontal disease, and candidiasis.

• Consider semisupine chair position for patient comfort if GI side effects occur.

• Question patient about tolerance of NSAIDs or aspirin related to GI disease.

• Patients on chronic drug therapy may rarely have symptoms of blood dyscrasias, which can include infection, bleeding, and poor healing.

• Avoid elective dental procedures if severe neutropenia (<500 cells/mm^3) or thrombocytopenia (<50,000 cell/mm^3) is present.

• Severe side effects may require deferring elective dental procedures until drug therapy is completed.

Consultations:

• Medical consultation may be required to assess disease control in the patient.

• In a patient with symptoms of blood dyscrasias, request a medical consultation for blood studies and postpone treatment until normal values are reestablished

• Liver function tests may be required to determine chronic liver disease.

Teach patient/family:

• Importance of good oral hygiene to prevent soft tissue inflammation/infection

• To evaluate efficacy of oral hygiene home care; preventive appointments may be necessary

• To prevent trauma when using oral hygiene aids

When chronic dry mouth occurs, advise patient:

• To avoid mouth rinses with high alcohol content because of drying effects

• To use daily home fluoride products for anticarics effect

• To use sugarless gum, frequent sips of water, or saliva substitutes

---

pemirolast potassium

(pe-mir'oh-last)

Alamast

Drug class.: Mast cell stabilizer

Action: Prevents release of mediators of inflammation from mast cells involved with type 1 immediate hypersensitivity reactions

Uses: Symptomatic treatment of ocular itching in allergic conjunctivitis

Dosage and routes:

• *Adult:* TOP 1-2 gtt in affected eye(s) qid

Available forms include: Sol 0.1%

Side effects/adverse reactions:

CNS: Headache

RESP: Bronchitis, cough

EENT: Rhinitis, burning eyes, dry eyes, ocular pain, sneezing, sinusitis, nasal congestion

ENDO: Dysmenorrhea

META: Increase in aminotransferases

MS: Back pain

MISC: Cold and flu symptoms

Contraindications: Hypersensitivity

Precautions: Pregnancy category C, lactation, children, do not wear contact lens if eyes are red, may affect soft contact lens, if no red eyes wait 10 min after using to place soft contacts

Pharmacokinetics:

TOP: Some systemic absorption occurs, detectable plasma levels noted, $T_{1/2}$ = 4.5 hr, hepatic metabolism, excreted in urine

Drug interactions of concern to dentistry:

• No dental drug interactions reported

DENTAL CONSIDERATIONS

General:

• Question patient about history of allergies to avoid using other potential allergens.

• Avoid dental light in patient's eyes; offer dark glasses for patient comfort.

• Protect patient's eyes from accidental spatter during dental treatment.

pemoline

(pem'oh-leen)

Cylert, Cylert Chewable, Pem-ADD CT

Drug class.: CNS stimulant

Controlled Substance Schedule IV

Action: Exact mechanism unknown; may act through dopaminergic mechanisms

Uses: Attention deficit disorder with hyperactivity

Dosage and routes:

• *Child >6 yr:* 37.5 mg in AM, increasing by 18.75 mg/wk, not to exceed 112.5 mg/day

Available forms include: Tabs 18.75, 37.5, 75 mg; chew tabs 37.5 mg

Side effects/adverse reactions:

CNS: Hyperactivity, insomnia, restlessness, dizziness, mild depression, headache, stimulation, irritability, aggressiveness, hallucinations, seizures, Tourette's syndrome, drowsiness, dyskinetic movements, fatigue, malaise

*GI: **Hepatic failure,*** nausea, anorexia, diarrhea, abdominal pain

MISC: Rashes, growth suppression in children, increased liver enzymes, hepatitis, jaundice

Contraindications: Hypersensitivity, hepatic insufficiency

Precautions: Renal disease, pregnancy category B, lactation, drug abuse, child <6 yr; liver function monitoring recommended

Pharmacokinetics:

PO: Peak 2-4 hr, duration 8 hr, half-life 12 hr; metabolized (50%) by liver; excreted (40%) by kidneys

Drug interactions of concern to dentistry:

• Increased irritability, stimulation: caffeine-containing products and food

DENTAL CONSIDERATIONS

General:

• Keep dental appointments short because of effects of disease.

Teach patient/family:

• Use of electric toothbrush for effective plaque control

penbutolol

(pen-byoo'toe-lole)

Levatol

Drug class.: Nonselective β-adrenergic blocker

Action: This is a nonselective β_1- and β_2-adrenergic antagonist. The antihypertensive mechanism of action is unclear, but it may include a reduction in cardiac output and inhibition of renin release by the renal juxtaglomerular apparatus. Peripheral resistance decreases with long-term use. The antianginal action (when indicated for this use) may be related to a decrease in myocardial oxygen demand and negative chronotropic and inotropic effects. The antiarrhythmic action (when indicated for this use) has been related to a reduction in spontaneous pacemaker firing and slowing of AV nodal conduction.

Uses: Hypertension alone or with other antihypertensive drugs

Dosage and routes:

• *Adult:* PO 20 mg qd, dose can be increased to 40-80 mg

Available forms include: Tabs 20 mg

Side effects/adverse reactions:

▼ *ORAL:* Dry mouth, taste alteration

CNS: Depression, hallucinations, dizziness, fatigue, lethargy, paresthesia, bizarre dreams, disorientation, syncope, vertigo, headache, sleep disturbances, nervousness, lethargy, behavior change, memory loss

CV: *Bradycardia, hypotension,* ***CHF,*** palpitation, AV block intensification, peripheral vascular insufficiency, vasodilation, chest pain, tachycardia

GI: Nausea, vomiting, diarrhea, colitis, constipation, cramps, hepatomegaly, gastric pain, acute pancreatitis, heartburn, anorexia

RESP: Dyspnea, respiratory dysfunction, *bronchospasm,* laryngospasm

HEMA: ***Agranulocytosis, thrombocytopenia,*** eosinophilia, leukopenia, pulmonary emboli, hyperlipidemia

GU: Impotence, decreased libido, UTIs, renal failure, urinary frequency or retention, dysuria, nocturia

EENT: Sore throat, ***laryngospasm,*** blurred vision, dry eyes

INTEG: Rash, pruritus, fever, photosensitivity

MS: Joint pain, arthralgia, muscle cramps, pain

META: Hyperglycemia, hypoglycemia

MISC: Facial swelling, weight change, Raynaud's phenomenon, lupus syndrome

Contraindications: Hypersensitivity to this drug, cardiac failure, cardiogenic shock, second- or third-degree heart block, bronchospastic disease, sinus bradycardia, CHF

Precautions: Diabetes mellitus, pregnancy category C, renal disease, lactation, hyperthyroidism, COPD, hepatic disease, children, myasthenia gravis, peripheral vascular disease, hypotension

Pharmacokinetics:

PO: Peak levels 1-1.5, half-life 3-5 hr; highly protein bound; hepatic metabolism

Drug interactions of concern to dentistry:

- Decreased hypotensive effect: indomethacin, NSAIDs
- Increased hypotension, myocardial depression: hydrocarbon inhalation anesthetics
- Hypertension, bradycardia: sympathomimetics (epinephrine, ephedrine)
- Slow metabolism of lidocaine

DENTAL CONSIDERATIONS

General:

- Monitor vital signs at every appointment because of cardiovascular side effects.
- Patients on chronic drug therapy may rarely have symptoms of blood dyscrasias, which can include infection, bleeding, and poor healing.
- Limit use of sodium-containing products, such as saline IV fluids, for patients with a dietary salt restriction.
- Assess salivary flow as a factor in caries, periodontal disease, and candidiasis.
- After supine positioning, have patient sit upright for at least 2 min before standing to avoid orthostatic hypotension.
- Stress from dental procedures may compromise cardiovascular function; determine patient risk.
- Short appointments and a stress reduction protocol may be required for anxious patients.
- Use vasoconstrictor with caution, in low doses, and with careful aspiration.
- Avoid using gingival retraction cord containing epinephrine.

Consultations:

- In a patient with symptoms of blood dyscrasias, request a medical consultation for blood studies and postpone dental treatment until normal values are reestablished.
- Medical consultation may be required to assess disease control and patient's ability to tolerate stress.

Teach patient/family:

- Caution to prevent injury when using oral hygiene aids
- Importance of good oral hygiene to prevent soft tissue inflammation
- If taste alterations occur, consider drug effects

When chronic dry mouth occurs, advise patient:

- To avoid mouth rinses with high alcohol content because of drying effects
- Of need for daily use of home fluoride products to prevent caries
- To use sugarless gum, frequent sips of water, or saliva substitutes

---

penciclovir cream

(pen-sye'kloe-veer)

Denavir

Drug class.: Antiviral

Action: Inhibits viral DNA synthesis needed for viral replication in herpes simplex virus (HSV-1,

P

HSV-2) following cellular kinase conversion to penciclovir triphosphate

Uses: Recurrent herpes labialis (cold sores)

Dosage and routes:

• *Adult:* TOP apply q2h while awake × 4 days; start treatment early in prodrome or when lesions first appear

Available forms include: Cream 1%, 1.5 g tube

Side effects/adverse reactions:

▼ *ORAL:* Taste alteration

CNS: Headache

INTEG: Hyperesthesia, local anesthesia, pruritus, rash

MISC: Allergic reaction, pain

Contraindications: Hypersensitivity

Precautions: Acyclovir-resistant herpes viruses, patients <18 yr, use on mucous membranes not recommended, avoid applications near the eye, pregnancy category B, lactation

Pharmacokinetics:

TOP: Not detected in plasma or urine

DENTAL CONSIDERATIONS

General:

• Use in immunocompromised patients not established.

• Postpone dental treatment when oral herpetic lesions are present.

Teach patient/family:

• To dispose of toothbrush or other contaminated oral hygiene devices used during period of infection to prevent reinoculation of herpetic infection

• To apply with a finger cot or latex glove to prevent herpes infection on fingers

penicillin G benzathine

(pen-i-sill'in)

Bicillin L-A, Permapen

Drug class.: Benzathine salt of natural penicillin G

Action: Interferes with cell wall replication of susceptible organisms; osmotically unstable cell wall swells and bursts from osmotic pressure

Uses: Respiratory infections, scarlet fever, erysipelas, otitis media, pneumonia, skin and soft tissue infections, bejel, pinta, yaws; effective for gram-positive cocci *(Staphylococcus, S. pyogenes, S. viridans, S. faecalis, S. bovis, S. pneumoniae),* gram-negative cocci *(N. gonorrhoeae),* gram-positive bacilli *(B. anthracis, C. perfringens, C. tetani, C. diphtheriae, L. monocytogenes),* gram-negative bacilli *(E. coli, P. mirabilis, Salmonella, Shigella, Enterobacter, S. moniliformis),* spirochetes *(T. pallidum), Actinomyces*

Dosage and routes:

Early syphilis:

• *Adult:* IM 2.4 million U in single dose

Prophylaxis of rheumatic fever, glomerulonephritis:

• *Adult and child >60 lb:* IM 1.2 million U in single dose once monthly

Upper respiratory infections (group A streptococcal):

• *Adult:* IM 1.2 million U in single dose

• *Child:* IM 50,000 U/kg in single dose, not to exceed adult dose

Available forms include: Inj IM

600,000 U/ml; 1,200,000, 2,400,000 U/dose

Side effects/adverse reactions:
▼ *ORAL: Candidiasis,* glossitis
*CNS: **Coma, convulsions,*** lethargy, hallucinations, anxiety, depression, twitching
GI: Nausea, vomiting, diarrhea, increased AST/ALT, abdominal pain, colitis
*HEMA: **Bone marrow depression, granulocytopenia,*** anemia, increased bleeding time
*GU: **Oliguria, proteinuria, hematuria, vaginal moniliasis, glomerulonephritis***
*INTEG: **Exfoliative dermatitis,*** rash, urticaria, hives
META: Hyperkalemia, hypokalemia, alkalosis, hypernatremia
*MISC: **Anaphylaxis***

Contraindications: Hypersensitivity to penicillins; neonates

Precautions: Hypersensitivity to cephalosporins, pregnancy category B

Pharmacokinetics:
IM: Very slow absorption, hydrolyzed to penicillin G, duration 21-28 days, half-life 30-60 min; excreted in urine, breast milk; crosses placenta

Drug interactions of concern to dentistry:
• Decreased antimicrobial effect of penicillin: tetracyclines, erythromycins, lincomycins
• Increased penicillin concentrations: aspirin, probenecid
• Suspected increased risk of methotrexate toxicity
• Oral contraceptives: advise patient of a potential risk for decreased contraceptive action, to maintain compliance with oral contraceptive use while using antibiotics, and to consider the use of additional nonhormonal contraception

DENTAL CONSIDERATIONS
General:
• Take precautions regarding allergy to medication.
• Determine why the patient is taking the drug.
• Place on frequent recall to evaluate healing response.

Consultations:
• Medical consultation may be required to assess disease control.

Teach patient/family:
When used for dental infection, advise patient:
• To report sore throat, oral burning sensation, fever, fatigue, any of which could indicate superinfection
• To take at prescribed intervals and complete dosage regimen
• To immediately notify the dentist if signs or symptoms of infection increase

---

penicillin V potassium/ penicillin V

Veetids

🍁 Apo-Pen-VK, Apo-Pen, Nadopen-V, Nadopen-V400, NovoPen-VK, Nu-Pen-VK, Pen-Vee K, PVFK

Drug class.: Semisynthetic penicillin

Action: Interferes with cell wall replication of susceptible organisms; the cell wall, rendered osmotically unstable, swells and bursts from osmotic pressure

Uses: Effective for gram-positive cocci *(S. aureus, S. viridans, S. faecalis, S. bovis, S. pneumoniae),*

P

gram-negative cocci *(N. gonorrhoeae, N. meningitidis)*, gram-positive bacilli *(B. anthracis, C. perfringens, C. tetani, C. diphtheriae)*, gram-negative bacilli *(S. moniliformis)*, spirochetes *(T. pallidum), Actinomyces, Peptococcus,* and *Peptostreptococcus* species

Dosage and routes:

Pneumococcal/staphylococcal infections:

• *Adult:* PO 250-500 mg q6-8h

• *Child <12 yr:* PO 25,000-90,000 U/kg/day in 3-6 divided doses (125 mg = 200,000 U)

Streptococcal infections:

• *Adult:* PO 250-500 mg q6-8h × 10 days

Prevention of recurrence of rheumatic fever/chorea:

• *Adult:* PO 125-250 mg bid continuously

Vincent's infection of oropharynx:

• *Adult:* PO 250-500 mg q6-8h

Anthrax (postexposure prophylaxis):

• *Adult:* PO 7.5 mg/kg qid

• *Child <9 yr:* PO 50 mg/kg in equally divided doses qid

Available forms include: Tabs 250, 500 mg; powder for oral susp 125, 250 mg/5 ml

Side effects/adverse reactions:

▼*ORAL:* Candidiasis, glossitis, stomatitis, black hairy tongue, dry mouth, altered taste

CNS: ***Depression, coma, convulsions,*** lethargy, hallucinations, anxiety, twitching

GI: Nausea, vomiting, diarrhea, abdominal pain, colitis, anorexia

HEMA: ***Bone marrow depression, granulocytopenia,*** eosinophilia, anemia, increased bleeding time

GU: ***Oliguria, proteinuria, hematuria, vaginitis, moniliasis, glomerulonephritis***

META: Hyperkalemia, hypokalemia, alkalosis; allergy symptoms: pruritus, urticaria, angioedema, bronchospasm, anaphylaxis

Contraindications: Hypersensitivity to penicillins; neonates

Precautions: Hypersensitivity to cephalosporins, pregnancy category B, lactation

Pharmacokinetics:

PO: Peak 30-60 min, duration 6-8 hr, half-life 30 min; excreted in urine, breast milk

Drug interactions of concern to dentistry:

• Decreased antimicrobial effectiveness of penicillin: tetracyclines, erythromycins, lincomycins

• Increased penicillin concentrations: probenecid

• Oral contraceptives: advise patient of a potential risk for decreased contraceptive action, to maintain compliance with oral contraceptive use while using antibiotics, and to consider the use of additional nonhormonal contraception

DENTAL CONSIDERATIONS

General:

• Take precautions regarding allergy to medication.

• Determine why the patient is taking the drug.

• If used for dental infection, place on frequent recall to evaluate healing response.

Consultations:

• Medical consultation may be required to assess disease control.

Teach patient/family:

When used for dental infection, advise patient:

• To report sore throat, oral burning

sensation, fever, fatigue, any of which could indicate superinfection
• To take at prescribed intervals and complete dosage regimen
• To immediately notify the dentist if signs or symptoms of infection increase

pentamidine isethionate

(pen-tam'i-deen)

NebuPent, Pentam 300

♣ Pentacarinat, Pneumopent

Drug class.: Antiprotozoal

Action: Interferes with DNA/RNA, phospholipids, and protein synthesis in protozoa

Uses: Treatment of *P. carinii* infections in immunocompromised patients (injection); prevention in high-risk HIV-infected patients (INH)

Dosage and routes:
• *Adult and child:* IV/IM 4 mg/kg/day × 2 wk; nebulize 300 mg via specific nebulizer once q4wk

Available forms include: Inj IV/IM 300 mg/vial; aerosol 300 mg/vial

Side effects/adverse reactions:

▼ *ORAL:* Bad taste (metallic), dry mouth, gingivitis, ulcerations or abscess, hypersalivation

CNS: Disorientation, hallucinations, dizziness

CV: Hypotension, ventricular tachycardia, ECG abnormalities

GI: Nausea, vomiting, anorexia, ***acute pancreatitis,*** increased AST/ALT

HEMA: ***Leukopenia, thrombocytopenia,*** anemia

GU: ***Acute renal failure***

INTEG: Sterile abscess, pain at injection site, pruritus, urticaria, rash

META: Hyperkalemia, hypocalcemia, hypoglycemia

Precautions: Blood dyscrasias, hepatic disease, renal disease, diabetes mellitus, cardiac disease, hypocalcemia, pregnancy category C

Pharmacokinetics:

IV/IM: Excreted unchanged in urine (66%)

Drug interactions of concern to dentistry:
• None reported

DENTAL CONSIDERATIONS

General:
• Monitor vital signs at every appointment because of cardiovascular side effects.
• Patients on chronic drug therapy may rarely have symptoms of blood dyscrasias, which can include infection, bleeding, and poor healing.
• Place on frequent recall to evaluate healing response.
• Assess salivary flow as a factor in caries, periodontal disease, and candidiasis.
• Consider semisupine chair position for patients with respiratory disease.
• For inhalation dosage forms, rinse mouth with water after each dose to prevent dryness.
• Place on frequent recall because of oral side effects.

Consultations:
• In a patient with symptoms of blood dyscrasias, request a medical consultation for blood studies and postpone dental treatment until normal values are reestablished.
• Medical consultation may be required to assess disease control.

bold italic = life-threatening conditions

Teach patient/family:

- That secondary oral infection may occur; must see dentist immediately if infection occurs
- Importance of good oral hygiene to prevent soft tissue inflammation
- Caution to prevent injury when using oral hygiene aids
- Importance of dietary suggestions to maintain oral and systemic health

When chronic dry mouth occurs, advise patient:

- To avoid mouth rinses with high alcohol content because of drying effects
- Of need for daily use of home fluoride products to prevent caries
- To use sugarless gum, frequent sips of water, or saliva substitutes

---

pentazocine HCl/ pentazocine lactate

(pen-taz'oh-seen)

Talwin, Talwin NX

Drug class.: Synthetic opioid/ mixed agonist/antagonist

Controlled Substance Schedule IV

Action: Interacts with opioid receptors in the CNS to alter pain perception

Uses: Moderate-to-severe pain alone or in combination with aspirin or acetaminophen

Dosage and routes:

- *Adult:* PO 50-100 mg q3-4h prn, not to exceed 600 mg/day; IV/ IM/SC 30 mg q3-4h prn, not to exceed 360 mg/day

Available forms include: SC/IM/ IV 30 mg/ml; tabs (NX) 50 mg in combination with 0.5 mg naloxone

Side effects/adverse reactions:

▼ *ORAL:* Dry mouth

CNS: Drowsiness, dizziness, confusion, headache, sedation, euphoria, hallucinations

CV: Palpitation, bradycardia, tachycardia, decreased BP (high doses)

GI: Nausea, vomiting, anorexia, constipation, cramps

RESP: ***Respiratory depression***

GU: Increased urinary output, dysuria

EENT: Tinnitus, blurred vision, miosis, diplopia

INTEG: Rash, urticaria, bruising, flushing, diaphoresis, pruritus

Contraindications: Hypersensitivity, addiction (narcotic)

Precautions: Addictive personality, pregnancy category C, lactation, increased intracranial pressure, head injury, MI (acute), severe heart disease, respiratory depression, hepatic disease, renal disease, children <12 yr, acute abdominal conditions, Addison's disease, prostatic hypertrophy, patients taking other narcotics

Pharmacokinetics:

SC/IM: Onset 15-30 min, peak 1-2 hr, duration 2-4 hr

IV: Onset 2-3 min, duration 4-6 hr

Half-life 2-3 hr; extensive first-pass metabolism with less than 20% entering circulation; metabolized by liver; excreted by kidneys; crosses placenta

Drug interactions of concern to dentistry:

- Increased effects: all CNS depressants, alcohol
- Contraindication: MAOIs
- Do not mix in solutions or syringe with barbiturates

• Additive side effects of opioid agonists
• Increased effects of anticholinergics
• Decreased effects of opioid agonists

DENTAL CONSIDERATIONS

General:

• Monitor vital signs at every appointment because of cardiovascular and respiratory side effects.
• Assess salivary flow as a factor in caries, periodontal disease, and candidiasis.
• Consider semisupine chair position for patient comfort if GI side effects occur.
• Psychologic and physical dependence may occur with chronic administration.

Teach patient/family:

When chronic dry mouth occurs, advise patient:

• To avoid mouth rinses with high alcohol content because of drying effects
• Of need for daily use of home fluoride products to prevent caries
• To use sugarless gum, frequent sips of water, or saliva substitutes

pentobarbital sodium

(pen-toe-bar'bi-tal)

Nembutal Sodium

♣ Nova-Rectal, Novopentobarb

Drug class.: Sedative-hypnotic barbiturate

Controlled Substance Schedule II, Canada C

Action: Depresses activity in brain cells, primarily in reticular activating system in brainstem; selectively depresses neurons in posterior hypothalamus, limbic structures; some actions may be related to enhancing the effect of the inhibitory neurotransmitter GABA

Uses: Insomnia, sedation, preoperative medication, increased intracranial pressure, dental anesthetic

Dosage and routes:

• *Adult:* PO 100-200 mg hs; IM 150-200 mg hs; IV 100 mg initially, then up to 500 mg; rec 120-200 mg hs
• *Child:* IM 3-5 mg/kg, not to exceed 100 mg
• *Child 2 mo-1 yr:* Rec 30 mg
• *Child 1-4 yr:* Rec 30-60 mg
• *Child 5-12 yr:* Rec 60 mg
• *Child 12-14 yr:* Rec 60-120 mg

Available forms include: Caps 50, 100 mg; elix 20 mg/5 ml; powder, rec supp 30, 60, 120, 200 mg; inj IM/IV 50 mg/ml

Side effects/adverse reactions:

CNS: Lethargy, drowsiness, hangover, ***CNS depression,*** dizziness, paradoxic stimulation in elderly and children, light-headedness, dependence, mental depression, slurred speech

CV: Hypotension, bradycardia, syncope

GI: Nausea, vomiting, diarrhea, constipation, epigastric pain, liver damage (long-term use)

RESP: ***Depression, apnea, laryngospasm, bronchospasm,*** circulatory collapse, hypoventilation

HEMA: ***Agranulocytosis, thrombocytopenia, megaloblastic anemia*** (long-term treatment)

INTEG: Rash, ***Stevens-Johnson syndrome,*** urticaria, pain, abscesses at injection site, angioedema, thrombophlebitis

Contraindications: Hypersensitivity to barbiturates, respiratory depression, addiction to barbitu-

P

rates, severe liver/renal impairment, porphyria, uncontrolled pain
Precautions: Anemia, pregnancy category D, lactation, hepatic disease, renal disease, hypertension, elderly, acute/chronic pain
Pharmacokinetics:
PO: Onset 15-30 min, duration 4-6 hr
REC: Onset slow, duration 4-6 hr
Half-life 15-48 hr; metabolized by liver; excreted by kidneys (metabolites)
Drug interactions of concern to dentistry:
• Hepatotoxicity: halogenated-hydrocarbon anesthetics
• Increased CNS depression: alcohol, all other CNS depressants
• Increased metabolism of carbamazepine, tricyclic antidepressants, corticosteroids
• Decreased half-life of doxycycline
DENTAL CONSIDERATIONS
General:
• Determine why the patient is taking the drug.
• Monitor vital signs at every appointment because of cardiovascular side effects. Evaluate respiration characteristics and rate.
• Patients on chronic drug therapy may rarely have symptoms of blood dyscrasias, which can include infection, bleeding, and poor healing.
When used for sedation in dentistry:
• Assess vital signs before use and q30min after use as sedative.
• Observe respiratory dysfunction: respiratory depression, character, rate, rhythm; hold drug if respirations are <10/min or if pupils are dilated.
• After supine positioning, have patient sit upright for at least 2 min before standing to avoid orthostatic hypotension.
• Have someone drive patient to and from dental office when used for conscious sedation.
• Barbiturates induce liver microsomal enzymes, which alter the metabolism of other drugs.
• Geriatric patients are more susceptible to drug effects; use lower dose.
Consultations:
• In a patient with symptoms of blood dyscrasias, request a medical consultation for blood studies and postpone dental treatment until normal values are reestablished.
Teach patient/family:
• To avoid driving or other activities requiring alertness
• To avoid alcohol ingestion or CNS depressants; serious CNS depression may result
• To avoid OTC preparations (antihistamines, cold remedies) that contain CNS depressants

pentoxifylline

(pen-tox-i'fi-leen)
Trental
Drug class.: Hemorrheologic agent

Action: Decreases blood viscosity, increases blood flow to affected microcirculation, and enhances tissue oxygenation in chronic peripheral arterial disease
Uses: Intermittent claudication related to chronic occlusive arterial disease of the limbs
Dosage and routes:
• *Adult:* PO 400 mg tid with meals
Available forms include: Con rel tabs 400 mg; tabs 400 mg, ext rel tab 400 mg

Side effects/adverse reactions:
▼*ORAL:* Dry mouth, thirst, bad taste
CNS: Headache, anxiety, tremors, confusion, dizziness, drowsiness, nervousness, agitation, seizures
CV: Angina, dysrhythmias, palpitation, hypotension, chest pain, dyspnea, edema
GI: Nausea, vomiting, anorexia, bloating, belching, constipation, dyspepsia, cholecystitis
EENT: Blurred vision, earache, sore throat, conjunctivitis
INTEG: Rash, pruritus, urticaria, brittle fingernails
MISC: Epistaxis, flulike symptoms: laryngitis, nasal congestion, leukopenia, malaise, weight changes, lymphedema
Contraindications: Hypersensitivity to this drug or xanthines
Precautions: Pregnancy category C, angina pectoris, cardiac disease, lactation, children, impaired renal function
Pharmacokinetics:
PO: Peak 1 hr, half-life 0.5-1 hr; degradation in liver; excreted in urine

DENTAL CONSIDERATIONS
General:
• Monitor vital signs at every appointment because of cardiovascular side effects.
• Assess salivary flow as a factor in caries, periodontal disease, and candidiasis.
• Stress from dental procedures may compromise cardiovascular function; determine patient risk.
• Short appointments and a stress reduction protocol may be required for anxious patients.
• Talk with patient about potential systemic diseases (e.g., diabetes, CV disease) that may be associated with claudication.
Consultations:
• Medical consultation may be required to assess disease control and patient's ability to tolerate stress.
Teach patient/family:
• Importance of good oral hygiene to prevent soft tissue inflammation
• Caution to prevent injury when using oral hygiene aids
When chronic dry mouth occurs, advise patient:
• To avoid mouth rinses with high alcohol content because of drying effects
• Of need for daily use of home fluoride products to prevent caries
• To use sugarless gum, frequent sips of water, or saliva substitutes

pergolide mesylate
(per'go-lide)
Permax
Drug class.: Antiparkinson agent

Action: Dopamine receptor agonist for D_1 and D_2 receptors
Uses: Adjunctive treatment of Parkinson's disease
Dosage and routes:
• *Adult:* PO initial 0.05 mg × 2 days; gradually increase by 0.1-0.15 mg/day q3days over next 12 days; doses can then be increased by 0.25 mg/day q3days; average dose 3 mg/day; max dose 5 mg/day usually in 3 divided doses/day
Available forms include: Tabs 0.05, 0.25, 1 mg
Side effects/adverse reactions:
▼*ORAL: Dry mouth,* sialadenitis, aphthous stomatitis
CNS: Dyskinesia, hallucinations, somnolence, confusion, dizziness,

headache, insomnia, tremor, extrapyramidal syndrome, anxiety, psychosis
CV: Postural hypotension, syncope, palpitation, vasodilation
GI: Nausea, constipation, diarrhea, abdominal pain, dyspepsia
RESP: Dyspnea
HEMA: Anemia
GU: Frequency, UTI
EENT: Rhinitis, diplopia
INTEG: Sweating, rash
MS: Back pain, neck pain, myalgia, twitching, arthralgia
MISC: Flulike syndrome, fever, peripheral edema

Contraindications: Hypersensitivity to this drug or ergot derivatives

Precautions: Symptomatic hypotension, cardiac dysrhythmias, dose adjustment for patients on levodopa, discontinue drug slowly, pregnancy category B, lactation, children

Pharmacokinetics:
PO: Plasma protein binding 90%, metabolized, urinary excretion, half-life 27 hr

Drug interactions of concern to dentistry:
- Decreased action: phenothiazines, haloperidol, droperidol, thiothixenes, and metoclopramide

DENTAL CONSIDERATIONS

General:
- Monitor vital signs at every appointment because of cardiovascular side effects.
- Short appointments may be required because of disease effects on musculature.
- Use precaution if sedation or general anesthesia is required; risk of hypotensive episode.
- After supine positioning have patient sit upright for at least 2 min before standing to avoid orthostatic hypotension.
- Assess salivary flow as a factor in caries, periodontal disease, and candidiasis.
- Assess for presence of extrapyramidal motor symptoms, such as tardive dyskinesia and akathisia. Extrapyramidal motor activity may complicate dental treatment.
- Consider semisupine chair position for patient comfort because of GI effects of drug.

Consultations:
- Medical consultation may be required to assess disease control.

Teach patient/family:
- Use of electric toothbrush if patient has difficulty holding conventional devices
- Importance of updating health history/drug record if physician makes any changes in evaluation or drug regimens

When chronic dry mouth occurs, advise patient:
- To avoid mouth rinses with high alcohol content because of drying effects
- Of need for daily use of home fluoride products to prevent caries
- To use sugarless gum, frequent sips of water, or saliva substitutes

perindopril erbumine

(per-in'doe-pril)
Aceon
✦ Coversyl

Drug class.: Angiotensin-converting enzyme (ACE) inhibitor

Action: Selectively suppresses renin-angiotensin-aldosterone system; inhibits ACE; prevents conversion of angiotensin I to angiotensin II; results in dilation of arterial and venous vessels

Uses: Essential hypertension as monotherapy or in combination with other antihypertensive medication

Dosage and routes:

Hypertension:

• *Adult:* PO 4 mg qd; can be titrated upward to max of 16 mg/day; doses can be given bid if needed

• *Adult >65 yr:* PO 4 mg in 1 or 2 divided doses; daily dose limit 8 mg

NOTE: This drug may have less efficacy in African-American patients.

Available forms include: Tabs 2, 4, 8 mg

Side effects/adverse reactions:

▼ *ORAL:* ***Angioedema (lips, tongue, mucous membranes),*** dry mouth, taste disturbances

CNS: *Orthostatic hypotension, headache, light-headedness, dizziness,* nervousness

CV: *Palpitation,* edema

GI: *Dyspepsia, nausea,* diarrhea, abdominal pain, vomiting

RESP: *Cough,* URI

HEMA: ***Agranulocytosis, neutropenia***

GU: Proteinuria, UTI, male sexual dysfunction

EENT: *Sinusitis, ear infection,* rhinitis, pharyngitis, tinnitus

INTEG: Rash

META: *Hyperkalemia,* ALT increase, triglyceride increase

MS: *Asthenia, back pain,* hypertonia, myalgia

MISC: ***Anaphylaxis,*** fever, upper extremity pain

Contraindications: Hypersensitivity to this drug or other ACE inhibitors, patients with a history of angioedema to other ACE inhibitors, pregnancy (second and third trimesters)

Precautions: Renal insufficiency, hypertension with CHF, severe CHF, renal artery stenosis, autoimmune disease, collagen vascular disease, pregnancy category C (first trimester); pregnancy category D (second and third trimesters), lactation

Pharmacokinetics:

PO: Absolute bioavailability 20%-30%, metabolized to active metabolite, perindoprilat, peak plasma levels 1 hr, active metabolite 3-4 hr; protein binding 10%-20%, hepatic metabolism, excreted mostly in urine (75%)

Drug interactions of concern to dentistry:

• Decreased hypotensive effects: NSAIDs, aspirin

• Increased hypotension: caution in use of other drugs that have hypotensive effects

• Suspected reduction in the antihypertensive and vasodilator effects by salicylates; monitor blood pressure if used concurrently

DENTAL CONSIDERATIONS

General:

• Monitor vital signs at every appointment because of cardiovascular side effects.

• Limit use of sodium-containing products such as saline IV fluids for those patients with a dietary salt restriction.

• Short appointments and a stress reduction protocol may be required for anxious patients.

• Stress from dental procedures may compromise cardiovascular function; determine patient risk.

• After supine positioning, have

P

patient sit upright for at least 2 min to avoid orthostatic hypotension.
• Use precaution if sedation or general anesthesia is required; risk of hypotensive episode.
• Assess salivary flow as a factor in caries, periodontal disease, and candidiasis.
• Consider semisupine chair position for patient comfort if GI or respiratory side effects occur.
• Patients on chronic drug therapy may rarely have symptoms of blood dyscrasias, which can include infection, bleeding, and poor healing.

Consultations:
• In a patient with symptoms of blood dyscrasias, request a medical consultation for blood studies and postpone treatment until normal values are reestablished.
• Medical consultation may be required to assess disease control and patient's ability to tolerate stress.

Teach patient/family:
• Importance of updating health and drug history if physician makes any changes in evaluation or drug regimens
• Importance of good oral hygiene to prevent soft tissue inflammation
• To prevent trauma when using oral hygiene aids

When chronic dry mouth occurs, advise patient:
• To avoid mouth rinses with high alcohol content because of drying effects
• To use daily home fluoride products for anticaries effect
• To use sugarless gum, frequent sips of water, or saliva substitutes

---

perphenazine

(per-fen'a-zeen)
Trilafon
🍁 APO-Perphenazine, PMS Perphenazine
Drug class.: Phenothiazine antipsychotic

Action: Blocks neurotransmission at dopaminergic synapses in the cerebral cortex, hypothalamus, and limbic system; exhibits strong peripheral α-adrenergic, anticholinergic blocking action; mechanism for antipsychotic effects is unclear

Uses: Psychotic disorders, schizophrenia, alcoholism, nausea, vomiting

Dosage and routes:

Nausea/vomiting/alcoholism/intractable hiccups:
• *Adult:* IM 5 mg q6h, max 15 mg in ambulatory patients, 30 mg in hospitalized patients; PO 8-16 mg/day in divided doses, up to 24 mg; IV not to exceed 5 mg, give diluted or slow IV drip

Psychiatric use in hospitalized patients:
• *Adult:* PO 8-16 mg bid-qid, gradually increased to desired dose, not to exceed 64 mg/day; IM 5 mg q6h, not to exceed 30 mg/day
• *Child >12 yr:* PO 6-12 mg in divided doses

Nonhospitalized patients:
• *Adult:* PO 4-8 mg tid; IM 5 mg q6h

Available forms include: Tabs 2, 4, 8, 16 mg; sol 16 mg/5 ml; inj IM 5 mg/ml

Side effects/adverse reactions:
▼ *ORAL: Dry mouth,* enlarged parotid glands, lichenoid reaction
CNS: Extrapyramidal symptoms: pseudoparkinsonism, akathisia,

dystonia, tardive dyskinesia, ***seizures,*** headache
CV: Orthostatic hypotension, ***cardiac arrest, tachycardia,*** ECG changes, syncope
GI: Nausea, vomiting, anorexia, constipation, diarrhea, jaundice, weight gain
RESP: ***Laryngospasm, respiratory depression,*** dyspnea
HEMA: ***Leukopenia, leukocytosis, agranulocytosis,*** anemia
GU: Urinary retention, urinary frequency, enuresis, impotence, amenorrhea, gynecomastia
EENT: Blurred vision, glaucoma
INTEG: Rash, photosensitivity, dermatitis

Contraindications: Hypersensitivity, blood dyscrasias, coma, child <12 yr, brain damage, bone marrow depression

Precautions: Pregnancy category C, lactation, seizure disorders, hypertension, hepatic disease, cardiac disease

Pharmacokinetics:
PO: Onset erratic, peak 2-4 hr
IM: Onset 10 min, peak 1-2 hr, duration 6 hr, occasionally 12-24 hr
Metabolized by liver, excreted in urine, crosses placenta, excreted in breast milk

Drug interactions of concern to dentistry:
- Increased sedation: other CNS depressants, alcohol, barbiturate anesthetics, opioid analgesics
- Hypotension, tachycardia: epinephrine
- Increased extrapyramidal effects: phenothiazines and related drugs (haloperidol, droperidol), metoclopramide
- Additive photosensitization: tetracyclines, fluoroquinolones
- Increased anticholinergic effects: anticholinergics

DENTAL CONSIDERATIONS

General:
- Monitor vital signs at every appointment because of cardiovascular side effects.
- Patients on chronic drug therapy may rarely have symptoms of blood dyscrasias, which can include infection, bleeding, and poor healing.
- After supine positioning, have patient sit upright for at least 2 min before standing to avoid orthostatic hypotension.
- Assess salivary flow as a factor in caries, periodontal disease, and candidiasis.
- Avoid dental light in patient's eyes; offer dark glasses for patient comfort.
- Assess for presence of extrapyramidal motor symptoms, such as tardive dyskinesia and akathisia. Extrapyramidal motor activity may complicate dental treatment.
- Geriatric patients are more susceptible to drug effects; use lower dose.
- Use vasoconstrictors with caution, in low doses, and with careful aspiration. Avoid use of gingival retraction cord with epinephrine.

Consultations:
- In a patient with symptoms of blood dyscrasias, request a medical consultation for blood studies and postpone dental treatment until normal values are reestablished.
- Take precautions if dental surgery is anticipated and anesthesia is required.
- If signs of tardive dyskinesia or akathisia are present, refer to physician.
- Physician should be informed if

significant xerostomic side effects occur (e.g., increased caries, sore tongue, problems eating or swallowing, difficulty wearing prosthesis) so that a medication change can be considered.

Teach patient/family:

• Importance of good oral hygiene to prevent soft tissue inflammation

• Caution to prevent injury when using oral hygiene aids

• To use electric toothbrush if patient has difficulty holding conventional devices

When chronic dry mouth occurs, advise patient:

• To avoid mouth rinses with high alcohol content because of drying effects

• Of need for daily use of home fluoride products to prevent caries

• To use sugarless gum, frequent sips of water, or saliva substitutes

phenazopyridine HCl

(fen-az-oh-peer'i-deen)

Geridium, Pyridate, Pyridium, Pyridium Plus, Urodine, Urogesic, UTI Relief

🍁 Phenazo

OTC: Azo-Standard, Baridium, Prodium

Drug class.: Urinary tract analgesic

Action: Exerts analgesic, anesthetic action on the urinary tract mucosa; exact mechanism of action unknown

Uses: Urinary tract irritation/infection

Dosage and routes:

• *Adult:* PO 200 mg tid

• *Child 6-12 yr:* PO 12 mg/kg/24 hr in 3 divided doses

Available forms include: Tabs 95, 97.2, 100, 150, 200 mg; OTC tabs 95 mg

Side effects/adverse reactions:

CNS: Headache, vertigo

GI: Nausea, vomiting, GI bleeding, diarrhea, heartburn, ***hepatic toxicity***

HEMA: ***Hemolytic anemia, methemoglobinemia (with overdose)***

GU: ***Renal toxicity, orange-red urine***

INTEG: Rash, urticaria, skin pigmentation

Contraindications: Hypersensitivity, hepatic disease

Precautions: Pregnancy category B, renal disease

Pharmacokinetics:

PO: Metabolized by liver, excreted by kidneys, crosses placenta, duration 6-8 hr

DENTAL CONSIDERATIONS

General:

• Consider semisupine chair position for patient comfort if GI side effects occur.

• Patients on chronic drug therapy may rarely have symptoms of blood dyscrasias, which can include infection, bleeding, and poor healing.

• Be aware that patient might have UTI; question if antiinfectives are also being used.

phendimetrazine tartrate

(fen-dye-me'tra-zeen)

Bontril PDM, Melfiat-105, Prelu-2

Drug class.: Anorexiant, amphetamine-like

Controlled Substance Schedule III

Action: Exact mechanism of action of appetite suppression unknown, but effects are similar to the amphetamines promoting release of norepinephrine and dopamine

Uses: Exogenous obesity

Dosage and routes:

• *Adult:* PO 35 mg bid-tid 1 hr ac, not to exceed 70 mg tid; sus rel 105 mg qd 30-60 min before breakfast

Available forms include: Tabs 35 mg; caps 35 mg; sus rel caps 105 mg

Side effects/adverse reactions:

▼ *ORAL:* Dry mouth, unpleasant taste

CNS: Hyperactivity, insomnia, restlessness, dizziness, tremors, headache

CV: Palpitation, tachycardia, hypertension

GI: Nausea, anorexia, diarrhea, constipation, cramps

HEMA: ***Bone marrow depression, leukopenia, agranulocytosis***

GU: Dysuria

EENT: Blurred vision

INTEG: Urticaria

Contraindications: Hypersensitivity, hyperthyroidism, hypertension, glaucoma, severe arteriosclerosis, severe cardiovascular disease, children <12 yr, agitated states, MAOIs

Precautions: Drug abuse, anxiety, pregnancy category C, lactation

Pharmacokinetics:

PO: Onset 30 min, peak 1-3 hr, duration 4-20 hr, half-life 2-10 hr; metabolized by liver; excreted by kidneys; crosses placenta; excreted in breast milk

Drug interactions of concern to dentistry:

• Hypertensive crisis: MAOIs or within 14 days of MAOIs

• Increased risk of dysrhythmia: hydrocarbon inhalation general anesthetics

• Decreased effect: tricyclic antidepressants, ascorbic acid, phenothiazines

• Caffeine or caffeine-containing products: may increase risk of insomnia and dry mouth

DENTAL CONSIDERATIONS

General:

• Monitor vital signs at every appointment because of cardiovascular side effects.

• Assess salivary flow as a factor in caries, periodontal disease, and candidiasis.

• Determine why the patient is taking the drug.

• Psychologic and physical dependence may occur with chronic administration.

• Patients on chronic drug therapy may rarely have symptoms of blood dyscrasias, which can include infection, bleeding, and poor healing.

Consultations:

• In a patient with symptoms of blood dyscrasias, request a medical consultation for blood studies and postpone dental treatment until normal values are reestablished.

Teach patient/family:

• Importance of good oral hygiene to prevent soft tissue inflammation

• To report oral lesions, soreness, or bleeding to dentist

• Caution to prevent injury when using oral hygiene aids

When chronic dry mouth occurs, advise patient:

• To avoid mouth rinses with high alcohol content because of drying effects

• Of need for daily use of home fluoride products to prevent caries

• To use sugarless gum, frequent sips of water, or saliva substitutes

P

phenelzine sulfate

(fen'el-zeen)
Nardil

Drug class.: Antidepressant, MAOI

Action: Increases concentrations of endogenous epinephrine, norepinephrine, serotonin, dopamine in storage sites in CNS by inhibition of MAO; antidepressant mechanism uncertain

Uses: Depression when uncontrolled by other means

Dosage and routes:

• *Adult:* PO 45 mg/day in 3 divided doses; may increase to 60 mg/day; dose should be reduced to 15 mg/day for maintenance; not to exceed 90 mg/day

Available forms include: Tabs 15 mg

Side effects/adverse reactions:

▼ *ORAL:* Dry mouth

CNS: Dizziness, drowsiness, confusion, headache, anxiety, tremors, stimulation, weakness, hyperreflexia, mania, insomnia, fatigue, weight gain

CV: Orthostatic hypotension, hypertension, dysrhythmias, hypertensive crisis, peripheral edema

GI: Constipation, nausea, vomiting, *anorexia,* diarrhea, weight changes, abdominal pain

HEMA: Anemia

GU: Change in libido, frequency

EENT: Blurred vision

INTEG: Rash, flushing, increased perspiration

ENDO: ***SIADH-like syndrome***

Contraindications: Hypersensitivity to MAOIs, elderly, hypertension, CHF, severe hepatic disease, pheochromocytoma, severe renal disease, severe cardiac disease, fluoxetine, meperidine

Precautions: Suicidal patients, convulsive disorders, severe depression, schizophrenia, hyperactivity, diabetes mellitus, pregnancy category C

Pharmacokinetics: Metabolized by liver, excreted by kidneys

Drug interactions of concern to dentistry:

• Increased anticholinergic effect: anticholinergics, haloperidol, phenothiazines, antihistamines

• Hyperpyretic crisis, convulsions, hypertensive episode: meperidine, carbamazepine, cyclobenzaprine

• Cardiac dysrhythmia: caffeine-containing medications

• Increased risk of serotonin syndrome: tricyclic antidepressants, other serotonin reuptake inhibitors

• Increased sedative effects of alcohol, barbiturates, benzodiazepines, CNS depressants

• Increased pressor effects: indirect-acting sympathomimetics such as ephedrine, amphetamine

DENTAL CONSIDERATIONS

General:

• Monitor vital signs at every appointment because of cardiovascular side effects.

• Assess salivary flow as a factor in caries, periodontal disease, and candidiasis.

• After supine positioning, have patient sit upright for at least 2 min before standing to avoid orthostatic hypotension.

• Hypertensive episodes are possible even though there are no specific contraindications to vasoconstrictor use in local anesthetics.

• Avoid prescribing caffeine-containing products.

• Take precautions if dental surgery is anticipated and general anesthesia is required.

Consultations:

• Medical consultation may be required to assess disease control and patient's ability to tolerate stress.

Teach patient/family:

• To use electric toothbrush if patient has difficulty holding conventional devices

When chronic dry mouth occurs, advise patient:

• To avoid mouth rinses with high alcohol content because of drying effects

• Of need for daily use of home fluoride products to prevent caries

• To use sugarless gum, frequent sips of water, or saliva substitutes

phenobarbital/ phenobarbital sodium

(fee-noe-bar'bi-tal)

Bellatal, Luminal Sodium, Solfoton

Drug class.: Barbiturate anticonvulsant

Controlled Substance Schedule IV

Action: A nonspecific depressant of the CNS; may enhance GABA activity in the brain

Uses: All forms of epilepsy, status epilepticus, febrile seizures in children, sedation, insomnia; unapproved: hyperbilirubinemia, chronic cholestasis

Dosage and routes:

Seizures:

• *Adult:* PO 100-200 mg/day in divided doses tid or total dose hs

• *Child:* PO 3-6 mg/kg/day in divided doses q12h; may be given as single dose hs

Status epilepticus:

• *Adult:* IV inf 10 mg/kg; run no faster than 50 mg/min; may give up to 20 mg/kg

• *Child:* IV inf 5-10 mg/kg; may repeat q10-15min, up to 20 mg/kg; run no faster than 50 mg/min

Sedation:

• *Adult:* PO 30-120 mg/day in 2-3 divided doses

• *Child:* PO 6 mg/kg/day in 3 divided doses

Preoperative sedation:

• *Adult:* IM 100-200 mg 1-1.5 hr before surgery

• *Child:* IM 1-3 mg/kg, 1-1.5 hr before surgery

Hyperbilirubinemia:

• *Neonate:* PO 7 mg/kg/day from days 1-5 after birth; IM 5 mg/kg/day on day 1, then PO on days 2-7 after birth

Chronic cholestasis:

• *Adult:* PO 90-180 mg/day in 2-3 divided doses

• *Child <12 yr:* PO 3-12 mg/kg/day in 2-3 divided doses

Available forms include: Caps 16 mg; elix 15, 20 mg/5 ml; tabs 15, 16, 16.2, 30, 60, 90, 100 mg; inj 30, 60, 65, 130 mg/ml

Side effects/adverse reactions:

CNS: Drowsiness, somnolence, paradoxic excitement (elderly), lethargy, hangover headache, flushing, hallucinations, coma, agitation, confusion, vertigo, insomnia, fever

CV: Bradycardia, hypotension, syncope

GI: Nausea, vomiting, diarrhea, constipation, liver damage (with chronic use)

RESP: Hypoventilation, apnea, respiratory depression, laryngospasm, bronchospasm, circulatory collapse

INTEG: ***Stevens-Johnson syndrome, angioedema,*** rash, urticaria, local pain, swelling, necrosis, thrombophlebitis, pemphigus-like reaction

Contraindications: Hypersensitivity to barbiturates, porphyria, hepatic disease, respiratory disease, nephritis, hyperthyroidism, diabetes mellitus, elderly, lactation, pregnancy category D

Precautions: Anemia

Pharmacokinetics:

PO: Onset 2-60 min, peak 8-12 hr, duration 6-10 hr, half-life 53-118 hr; metabolized by liver; excreted by kidneys; crosses placenta; excreted in breast milk

Drug interactions of concern to dentistry:

- Increased effects: alcohol, all CNS depressants, saquinavir
- Decreased effects of corticosteroids, doxycycline, carbamazepine

DENTAL CONSIDERATIONS

General:

- Determine why the patient is taking the drug.
- Monitor vital signs at every appointment because of cardiovascular side effects. Evaluate respiration characteristics and rate.
- Patients on chronic drug therapy may rarely have symptoms of blood dyscrasias, which can include infection, bleeding, and poor healing.

When used for sedation in dentistry:

- Assess vital signs before use and q30min after use as sedative.
- Observe respiratory dysfunction: respiratory depression, character, rate, rhythm; hold drug if respirations are <10/min or if pupils are dilated.
- After supine positioning, have patient sit upright for at least 2 min to avoid orthostatic hypotension.
- Have someone drive patient to and from dental office when used for conscious sedation.
- Barbiturates induce liver microsomal enzymes, which alter the metabolism of other drugs.
- Geriatric patients are more susceptible to drug effects; use lower dose.

Consultations:

- In a patient with symptoms of blood dyscrasias, request a medical consultation for blood studies and postpone dental treatment until normal values are reestablished.

Teach patient/family:

- To avoid driving or other activities requiring alertness
- To avoid alcohol ingestion or CNS depressants; serious CNS depression may result
- To use OTC preparations with caution because they may contain other CNS depressants (e.g., antihistamines, cold remedies)

phentermine HCl/ phentermine resin

(fen'ter-meen)

Adipex-P, Ionamin, Pro-Fast SA, Pro-Fast HS

Drug class.: Sympathomimetic, anorexiant

Controlled Substance Schedule IV, Canada C

Action: Exact mechanism of action of appetite suppression unknown, but effects are similar to the amphetamines promoting release of norepinephrine and dopamine

Uses: Exogenous obesity

Dosage and routes:
• *Adult:* PO 8 mg tid 30 min before meals or 15-37.5 mg qd before breakfast
Available forms include: Tabs 8, 30, 37.5 mg; caps 15, 18.75, 30, 37.5 mg
Side effects/adverse reactions:
▼ *ORAL:* Dry mouth, unpleasant taste
CNS: Insomnia, restlessness, agitation, hyperactivity, dizziness, tremor, headache, anxiety, agitation, euphoria, dyskinesia
CV: Palpitation, tachycardia, hypertension, ECG changes, dysrhythmias
GI: Nausea, anorexia, constipation, diarrhea
HEMA: ***Bone marrow depression, agranulocytosis, leukopenia***
GU: Impotence, change in libido, dysuria, urinary frequency
EENT: Blurred vision, mydriasis
INTEG: Urticaria, rash
Contraindications: Hypersensitivity, hyperthyroidism, hypertension, glaucoma, severe arteriosclerosis, angina pectoris, cardiovascular disease, child <12 yr, MAOI-type medications
Precautions: Pregnancy category C, lactation, drug abuse, anxiety, tolerance
Pharmacokinetics:
SUS REL: Duration 10-14 hr; metabolized by liver; excreted by kidneys
PO (NOT CON REL DOSE FORMS): Rapid onset, duration 4 hr
Drug interactions of concern to dentistry:
• Hypertensive crisis: MAOIs or within 14 days of MAOIs
• Increased risk of dysrhythmia: hydrocarbon inhalation general anesthetics
• Decreased effect: tricyclic antidepressants, ascorbic acid, phenothiazines
• Caffeine or caffeine-containing products may increase risk of insomnia

DENTAL CONSIDERATIONS
General:
• Monitor vital signs at every appointment because of cardiovascular side effects.
• Assess salivary flow as a factor in caries, periodontal disease, and candidiasis.
• Determine why the patient is taking the drug.
• Psychologic and physical dependence may occur with chronic administration.
• Patients on chronic drug therapy may rarely have symptoms of blood dyscrasias, which can include infection, bleeding, and poor healing.
Consultations:
• In a patient with symptoms of blood dyscrasias, request a medical consultation for blood studies and postpone dental treatment until normal values are reestablished.
Teach patient/family:
• Importance of good oral hygiene to prevent soft tissue inflammation
• To prevent injury when using oral hygiene aids
• To report oral lesions, soreness, or bleeding to dentist
When chronic dry mouth occurs, advise patient:
• To avoid mouth rinses with high alcohol content because of drying effects
• Of need for daily use of home fluoride products to prevent caries
• To use sugarless gum, frequent sips of water, or saliva substitutes

P

phentolamine mesylate

(fen-tole'a-meen)

Regitine

♣ Rogitine

Drug class.: Antihypertensive

Action: α-adrenergic blocker; binds to α-adrenergic receptors, dilating peripheral blood vessels, lowering peripheral resistances, and lowering blood pressure

Uses: Hypertension, pheochromocytoma, prevention and treatment of dermal necrosis following extravasation of norepinephrine or dopamine; unapproved: with papaverine for intracavernous injection for impotence

Dosage and routes:

Treatment of hypertensive episodes in pheochromocytoma:

- *Adult:* IV/IM 5 mg 1-2 hr before surgery; repeat if necessary
- *Child:* IV/IM 1 mg 1-2 hr before surgery; repeat if necessary

Prevention/treatment of necrosis:

- *Adult:* 5-10 mg/10 ml NS injected into area of norepinephrine extravasation within 12 hr; preventive dose 10 mg to each 1000 ml norepinephrine solution

Available forms include: Inj IM/IV 5 mg/ml

Side effects/adverse reactions:

▼ *ORAL: Dry mouth*

CNS: Dizziness, flushing, weakness

CV: Hypotension, tachycardia, angina, dysrhythmias, ***MI***

GI: Nausea, vomiting, diarrhea, abdominal pain

EENT: Nasal congestion

Contraindications: Hypersensitivity, MI, coronary insufficiency, angina, peptic ulcer

Precautions: Pregnancy category C, lactation

Pharmacokinetics:

IV: Peak 2 min, duration 10-15 min

IM: Peak 15-20 min, duration 3-4 hr

Metabolized in liver, excreted in urine

Drug interactions of concern to dentistry:

- Hypotension, tachycardia: epinephrine
- Decreased pressor effects of epinephrine, ephedrine

DENTAL CONSIDERATIONS

General:

- This is an acute-use drug; hypertension and pheochromocytoma are the immediate concerns.
- Patients with untreated pheochromocytoma or with extreme, uncontrolled hypertension are not candidates for elective dental treatment. Physician consultation is required.
- Short appointments and a stress reduction protocol may be required for anxious patients.
- Stress from dental procedures may compromise cardiovascular function; determine patient risk.
- Use vasoconstrictors with caution, in low doses, and with careful aspiration. Avoid use of gingival retraction cord with epinephrine.
- Assess vital signs at each appointment because of nature of disease.

Consultations:

- Medical consultation may be required to assess disease control and patient's ability to tolerate stress.

phenylephrine HCl (nasal)

(fen-ill-ef'rin)

Ah Chew D, Afrin Children's Pump, Neo-Synephrine, Little Noses Gentle, Rhinall, 4-Way Fast Acting, Vick's Sinex Ultra

Drug class.: Nasal decongestant, sympathomimetic

Action: Produces rapid and long-acting vasoconstriction of arterioles, thereby decreasing fluid exudation, mucosal engorgement

Uses: Nasal congestion (temporary relief)

Dosage and routes:

• *Adult:* Instill 2-3 drops to nasal mucosa bid (0.25%-1%) q3-4h

• *Child 6-12 yr:* Instill 1-2 drops (0.25%) q3-4h

• *Child <6 yr:* Instill 2-3 drops (0.125%) q3-4h

Available forms include: Sol 0.125%, 0.25%, 0.5%, 1%; chew tabs 10 mg

Side effects/adverse reactions:

▼ *ORAL: Dry mouth,* bitter taste

CNS: Anxiety, restlessness, tremors, weakness, insomnia, dizziness, fever, headache

GI: Nausea, vomiting, anorexia

EENT: Irritation, burning, sneezing, stinging, dryness, rebound congestion

INTEG: Contact dermatitis

Contraindications: Hypersensitivity to sympathomimetic amines, MAOIs

Precautions: Child <6 yr, elderly, diabetes, cardiovascular disease, hypertension, hyperthyroidism, increased IOP, prostatic hypertrophy, pregnancy category C, glaucoma, ischemic heart disease, excessive use

Drug interactions of concern to dentistry:

• None reported with normal topical use

• *With systemic absorption, risk* of:

• Bradycardia: β-adrenergic blockers

• Increased dysrhythmias and hypertension: tricyclic antidepressants

DENTAL CONSIDERATIONS

General:

• Consider semisupine chair position for patient comfort because of respiratory effects of disease.

• Assess salivary flow as a factor in caries, periodontal disease, and candidiasis.

• Patients with significant nasal congestion may complicate nasal administration of nitrous oxide/oxygen sedation.

Teach patient/family:

• That this product is not indicated for prolonged use because of congestion rebound; however, this may not always be the case

P

phenytoin sodium/ phenytoin sodium extended/phenytoin sodium prompt

(fen'i-toyn)

Dilantin, Dilantin Infatabs, Dilantin Kapseals, Dilantin-125

Drug class.: Hydantoin anticonvulsant

Action: Inhibits spread of seizure activity in motor cortex

Uses: Generalized tonic-clonic

(grand mal) seizures, status epilepticus, nonepileptic seizures, trigeminal neuralgia, cardiac dysrhythmias (class Ib) caused by digitalis-type drugs

Dosage and routes:

Seizures:

• *Adult:* IV loading dose 900 mg–1.5 g run at 50 mg/min; if patient has received phenytoin, 100-300 mg run at 50 mg/min; PO loading dose 900 mg-1.5 g divided tid, then 300 mg/day (extended) or divided tid (extended/prompt)

• *Child:* IV loading dose 15 mg/kg run at 50 mg/min; if patient has received phenytoin, 5-7 mg/kg run at 50 mg/min, may repeat in 30 min; PO loading dose 15 mg/kg divided q8-12h, then 5-7 mg/kg in divided doses q12h

Ventricular dysrhythmias:

• *Adult:* PO loading dose 1 g divided over 24 hr, then 500 mg/day for 2 days, maintenance 300 mg PO daily; IV 250 mg given over 5 min until dysrhythmias subside or 1 g is given, or 100 mg q15min until dysrhythmias subside or 1 g is given

• *Child:* PO 3-8 mg/kg or 250 mg/m^2/day as single dose or divided in 2 doses; IV 3-8 mg/kg given over several min, or 250 mg/m^2/day as single dose or divided in 2 doses

Available forms include: Susp 125 mg/5 ml; chew tabs 50 mg; inj 50 mg/ml; caps 30, 100 mg; caps prompt rel 100 mg

Side effects/adverse reactions:

▼ *ORAL: Gingival overgrowth,* oral ulceration (Stevens-Johnson syndrome), taste loss

CNS: Drowsiness, dizziness, insomnia, paresthesia, depression, headache, confusion, slurred speech, ataxia, numbness

CV: Hypotension, ventricular fibrillation

GI: Nausea, vomiting, constipation, ***hepatitis,*** anorexia, weight loss, jaundice, epigastric pain

HEMA: ***Agranulocytosis, leukopenia, aplastic anemia, thrombocytopenia, megaloblastic anemia***

GU: Nephritis, albuminuria

EENT: Nystagmus, diplopia, blurred vision

INTEG: Rash, ***Stevens-Johnson syndrome,*** lupus erythematosus, hirsutism

MISC: Lymphadenopathy, hyperglycemia

Contraindications: Hypersensitivity, psychiatric condition, pregnancy category D, bradycardia, SA and AV block, Stokes-Adams syndrome

Precautions: Allergies, hepatic disease, renal disease

Pharmacokinetics:

PO: Duration 5 hr; metabolized by liver; excreted by kidneys

Drug interactions of concern to dentistry:

• Increased serum levels: ketoconazole, fluconazole, fluoxetine, metronidazole

• Decreased effects: barbiturates, carbamazepine, chloral hydrate

• Hepatotoxicity: acetaminophen (chronic use and high doses only)

• Decreased effects of corticosteroids, doxycycline

DENTAL CONSIDERATIONS

General:

• Patients on chronic drug therapy may rarely have symptoms of blood dyscrasias, which can include infection, bleeding, and poor healing.

• Place on frequent recall to evaluate gingival condition and self-care.
• Short appointments and a stress reduction protocol may be required for anxious patients.
• Ask about type of epilepsy, seizure frequency, and quality of seizure control.

Consultations:

• In a patient with symptoms of blood dyscrasias, request a medical consultation for blood studies and postpone dental treatment until normal values are reestablished.
• Medical consultation may be required to assess disease control and the patient's ability to tolerate stress.

Teach patient/family:

• Importance of good oral hygiene to prevent soft tissue inflammation and minimize gingival overgrowth
• Caution to prevent injury when using oral hygiene aids

---

phytonadione (vitamin K_1)

(fye-toe-na-dye'one)

Aqua Mephyton, Mephyton

Drug class.: Vitamin K_1, fat-soluble vitamin

Action: Needed for adequate blood clotting (factors II, VII, IX, X)

Uses: Vitamin K malabsorption, hypoprothrombinemia, prevention of hypoprothrombinemia caused by oral anticoagulants

Dosage and routes:

Hypoprothrombinemia caused by vitamin K malabsorption:

• *Adult:* PO/IM 2-25 mg; may repeat or increase to 50 mg
• *Child:* PO/IM 5-10 mg
• *Infants:* PO/IM 2 mg

Prevention of hemorrhagic disease of the newborn:

• *Neonate:* SC/IM 0.5-1 mg after birth; repeat in 6-8 hr if required

Hypoprothrombinemia caused by oral anticoagulants:

• *Adult:* PO/SC/IM 2.5-10 mg; may repeat 12-48 hr after PO dose or 6-8 hr after SC/IM dose, based on PT

Available forms include: Tabs 5 mg; inj aqueous colloidal IM/IV 2 mg/ml; inj aqueous dispersion 10 mg/ml (IM only)

Side effects/adverse reactions:

▼ *ORAL:* Unusual taste
CNS: *Headache,* ***brain damage (large doses)***
CV: Cardiac irregularities
GI: Nausea, vomiting
HEMA: ***Hemolytic anemia, hemoglobinuria, hyperbilirubinemia***
INTEG: Rash, urticaria, flushing, erythema, sweating
MISC: Bronchospasms, dyspnea, cramplike pain

Contraindications: Hypersensitivity, severe hepatic disease, last few weeks of pregnancy

Precautions: Pregnancy category C

Pharmacokinetics: *PO/INJ:* Readily absorbed from duodenum and requires bile salts, rapid hepatic metabolism, onset of action 6-12 hr, normal PT in 12-24 hr, crosses placenta, renal and biliary excretion; because of severe side effects, restrict IV route when other administration routes are not available

Drug interactions of concern to dentistry:

• Decreased action: broad-spectrum antibiotics, salicylates (high doses)

P

• Antagonist to oral anticoagulants

DENTAL CONSIDERATIONS

General:

• Determine why the patient is taking this drug. Medical consultation should be made before dental treatment.

• Patients on chronic drug therapy may rarely have symptoms of blood dyscrasias, which can include infection, bleeding, and poor healing.

Consultations:

• Medical consultation to determine coagulation stability.

---

pilocarpine HCl

(pye-loe-kar'peen)

Adsorbocarpine, Akarpine, Isopto Carpine, Pilocar, Piloptic, Pilostat

♣ Miocarpine

Drug class.: Miotic, cholinergic agonist

Action: Acts directly on cholinergic receptor sites; induces miosis, spasm of accommodation, fall in intraocular pressure caused by stimulation of ciliary, pupillary sphincter muscles, leading to pulling of iris from filtration angle and resulting in increased outflow of aqueous humor

Uses: Primary glaucoma, early stages of wide-angle glaucoma (less useful in advanced stages), chronic open-angle glaucoma, acute narrow-angle glaucoma before emergency surgery; also used to neutralize mydriatics used during eye exam; may be used alternately with mydriatics to break adhesions between iris and lens

Dosage and routes:

• *Adult and child:* Instill sol 1-2 gtt of 1% or 2% solution in eye q6-8h; instill 20-40 μg/hr (Ocusert Pilo) in cul-de-sac of eye

Available forms include: Sol 0.25%, 0.5%, 1%, 2%, 3%, 4%, 5%, 6%, 8%, 10%; gel 4%

Side effects/adverse reactions:

▼ *ORAL:* Excessive salivation

CV: Hypotension, tachycardia

GI: Nausea, vomiting, abdominal cramps, diarrhea

RESP: ***Bronchospasm***

EENT: Blurred vision, brow ache, twitching of eyelids, eye pain with change in focus

Contraindications: Bradycardia, hyperthyroidism, coronary artery disease, hypertension, obstruction of GI/urinary tracts, epilepsy, parkinsonism, asthma

Precautions: Bronchial asthma, hypertension, pregnancy category C

DENTAL CONSIDERATIONS

General:

• Avoid drugs with anticholinergic activity, such as antihistamines, opioids, benzodiazepines, propantheline, atropine, and scopolamine.

• Avoid dental light in patient's eyes; offer dark glasses for patient comfort.

• Monitor vital signs at every appointment because of cardiovascular and respiratory side effects.

Consultations:

• Medical consultation may be required to assess disease control.

---

pilocarpine HCl (oral)

(pye-loe-kar'peen)

Salagen

Drug class.: Cholinergic agonist (parasympathomimetic)

Action: Mimics the action of acetylcholine on muscarinic receptors

Uses: Treatment of symptoms of xerostomia from salivary gland hypofunction caused by radiotherapy for cancer of the head and neck and Sjögren's syndrome

Dosage and routes:

• *Adult:* PO initially 5 mg tid; 10 mg tid may be considered for patients who are not responding adequately and who can tolerate the lower doses; with moderate hepatic impairment limit dose to 5 mg bid

Available forms include: Tabs 5 mg

Side effects/adverse reactions:

▼ *ORAL:* Taste alteration

CNS: Dizziness, headache, nervousness, anxiety

CV: Flushing, edema, tachycardia, palpitation, hypotension, hypertension, bradycardia

GI: Nausea, dyspepsia, diarrhea, abdominal pain, vomiting, diarrhea

HEMA: Leukopenia, lymphadenopathy

GU: Urinary frequency

EENT: Rhinitis, lacrimation, pharyngitis, amblyopia, conjunctivitis, sinusitis, visual distrubances

INTEG: Rash

MS: Asthenia

MISC: Sweating (high doses)

Contraindications: Uncontrolled asthma, hypersensitivity, when miosis is undesirable (acute iritis, narrow-angle glaucoma)

Precautions: Pregnancy category C, children, lactation, cardiovascular disease, retinal diseases, pulmonary diseases (asthma, chronic bronchitis, COPD), biliary tract disease, history of renal colic, psychiatric disorders, hepatic dysfunction

Pharmacokinetics:

PO: Onset 20 min, peak effect 1 hr, duration 3-5 hr; renal excretion

Drug interactions of concern to dentistry: With β-adrenergic agonists: use with caution; possibility of conduction disturbances Reduced effect: anticholinergic drugs Enhanced effects: other cholinergic agonists

DENTAL CONSIDERATIONS

General:

• Patients receiving chemotherapy may require palliative treatment for stomatitis.

• Assess salivary flow as a factor in caries, periodontal disease, and candidiasis.

• Monitor vital signs at every appointment because of cardiovascular side effects.

• Place on frequent recall because of oral effects of head and neck radiation.

Consultations:

• Medical consultation may be required to assess disease control.

• Medical consultation may be necessary before prescribing for those patients with cardiovascular, retinal, or respiratory disease.

Teach patient/family:

• To use caution when driving at night or performing hazardous activities in reduced lighting (visual blurring)

• That sweating can become extensive with high dose; have patient take plenty of fluids, observe for dehydration, or discontinue drug

When chronic dry mouth occurs, advise patient:

• To avoid mouth rinses with high alcohol content because of drying effects

• Of need for daily use of home fluoride products to prevent caries

• To use sugarless gum, frequent sips of water, or saliva substitutes

pimecrolimus

(pim-e-koe'li-mus)

Elidel

Drug class.: Topical antiinflammatory

Action: Mechanism in atopic dermatitis is unknown; however, it inhibits calcineurin and inflammatory cytokine release

Uses: Short-term and intermittent long-term treatment of mild to moderate atopic dermatitis in nonimmunocompromised patients age 2 yr and older in whom conventional therapies cannot be used because of potential risks; in patients with an inadequate response; or in patients who are not responsive to conventional therapies

Dosage and routes:

• *Adult and child >2 yr:* TOP apply thin layer to affected area bid, rub in gently and completely; reevaluate after 6 wk if symptoms persist

Available forms include: Cream 1% in 15, 30, and 100 g tubes

Side effects/adverse reactions:

CNS: Headache

EENT: Nasopharyngitis, pharyngitis, cough

INTEG: Burning, cutaneous infection, folliculitis, other localized symptoms

MISC: Influenza, viral infections, fever

NOTE: In clinical trials, other side effects reported were not distinguished from placebo or vehicle. No long-term trials have been reported.

Contraindications: Hypersensitivity to drug or vehicle components, Netherton's syndrome

Precautions: Do not use for active cutaneous viral infections, infected dermatitis, natural or artificial sunlight exposure, pregnancy category C, no data on excretion in human milk, child <2 yr

Pharmacokinetics:

TOP: Low levels of absorption (below assay limits), any absorbed drug is metabolized by CYP3A4 isoenzymes, excreted in feces (81%) as metabolites

Drug interactions of concern to dentistry:

• Drug interactions have not been evaluated. Low blood levels were measured in some patients. Use drugs that inhibit CYP3A4 isoenzymes with caution in patients with widespread and erythrodermic disease.

DENTAL CONSIDERATIONS

General:

• Determine why the patient is taking this drug.

pimozide

(pi'moe-zide)

Orap

Drug class.: Antipsychotic, antidyskinetic

Action: Blocks dopamine effects in the CNS

Uses: Motor and phonic tics in Gilles de la Tourette's syndrome; unapproved: psychotic disorders

Dosage and routes:

• *Adult and child >12 yr:* PO 1-2 mg qd in divided doses, usual dose 10 mg/day

Available forms include: Tabs 1, 2 mg

Side effects/adverse reactions:
▼ *ORAL: Dry mouth,* thirst, altered taste
CNS: Extrapyramidal symptoms: pseudoparkinsonism, akathisia, dystonia, tardive dyskinesia, drowsiness, headache, neuroleptic malignant syndrome, seizures, lethargy, sedation, muscle tightness
CV: Orthostatic hypotension, ***cardiac arrest, tachycardia,*** hypertension, ECG changes
GI: Nausea, vomiting, anorexia, constipation, diarrhea, jaundice, weight gain
GU: Urinary retention, urinary frequency, enuresis, impotence, amenorrhea, gynecomastia
EENT: Blurred vision, cataracts
INTEG: Rash, photosensitivity, dermatitis, hyperpyrexia
Contraindications: Hypersensitivity, CNS depression/coma, parkinsonism, liver disease, blood dyscrasias, renal disease, tics other than syndrome, cardiac dysrhythmias, macrolide antiinfectives, itraconazole
Precautions: Child <12 yr, pregnancy category C, lactation, hypertension, hepatic disease, cardiac disease, renal disease, breast cancer, hypokalemia
Pharmacokinetics:
PO: Onset erratic, peak 6-8 hr, half-life 50-55 hr; metabolized by liver; excreted in urine, feces
Drug interactions of concern to dentistry:
- Increased CNS depression: alcohol, CNS depressants
- Increased effects of both drugs: phenothiazines
- Increased effects of anticholinergic drugs
- Prolonged QT interval, fatal cardiac arrhythmia, contraindicated: clarithromycin, erythromycin, azithromycin, dirithromycin, itraconazole

DENTAL CONSIDERATIONS
General:
- Assess salivary flow as a factor in caries, periodontal disease, and candidiasis.
- Monitor vital signs at every appointment because of cardiovascular side effects.
- Assess for presence of extrapyramidal motor symptoms, such as tardive dyskinesia and akathisia. Extrapyramidal motor activity may complicate dental treatment.
- After supine positioning, have patient sit upright for at least 2 min to avoid orthostatic hypotension.
- Consider action of drug in assessment of altered taste.

Consultations:
- Medical consultation may be required to assess disease control.
- If signs of tardive dyskinesia or akathisia are present, refer to physician.

Teach patient/family:
- Importance of good oral hygiene to prevent soft tissue inflammation
- Caution to prevent injury when using oral hygiene aids

When chronic dry mouth occurs, advise patient:
- To avoid mouth rinses with high alcohol content because of drying effects
- Of need for daily use of home fluoride products to prevent caries
- To use sugarless gum, frequent sips of water, or saliva substitutes

P

pindolol

(pin'doe-lole)

Visken

♣ Novo-Pindol, Syn-Pindolol

Drug class.: Nonselective β-adrenergic blocker

Action: This is a nonselective β_1- and β_2-adrenergic antagonist. The antihypertensive mechanism of action is unclear, but it may include a reduction in cardiac output and inhibition of renin release by the renal juxtaglomerular apparatus. Peripheral resistance decreases with long-term use. The antianginal action (when indicated for this use) may be related to a decrease in myocardial oxygen demand and negative chronotropic and inotropic effects. The antiarrhythmic action (when indicated for this use) has been related to a reduction in spontaneous pacemaker firing and slowing of AV nodal conduction.

Uses: Mild-to-moderate hypertension

Dosage and routes:

• *Adult:* PO 5 mg bid, usual dose 15 mg/day (5 mg tid); may increase by 10 mg/day q3-4wk to a max of 60 mg/day

Available forms include: Tabs 5, 10 mg

Side effects/adverse reactions:

▼ *ORAL:* Dry mouth, taste changes

CNS: Insomnia, dizziness, hallucinations, anxiety, fatigue

CV: ***CHF, AV block,*** edema, chest pain, palpitation, claudication, tachycardia, ***cardiac arrest,*** hypertension, syncope

GI: Nausea, abdominal pain, ***mesenteric arterial thrombosis, ischemic colitis,*** vomiting, diarrhea

RESP: Dyspnea, ***bronchospasm,*** cough, rales

HEMA: ***Agranulocytosis, thrombocytopenia, purpura***

GU: Impotence, pollakiuria

EENT: Visual changes, double vision, sore throat, dry burning eyes

INTEG: Rash, alopecia, pruritus, fever

MISC: Joint pain, muscle pain, hypoglycemia

Contraindications: Hypersensitivity to β-blockers, cardiogenic shock, heart block (second or third degree), sinus bradycardia, CHF, cardiac failure, bronchial asthma, lactation

Precautions: Major surgery, pregnancy category B, diabetes mellitus, renal disease, thyroid disease, COPD, well-compensated heart failure, CAD, nonallergic bronchospasm, impaired hepatic function, children

Pharmacokinetics:

PO: Peak 1-2 hr, half-life 3-4 hr; 60%-65% is metabolized by liver; excreted 35%-50% unchanged; excreted in breast milk

Drug interactions of concern to dentistry:

• Increased hypotension, bradycardia: anticholinergics, hydrocarbon inhalation anesthetics, fentanyl derivatives

• Decreased antihypertensive effects: indomethacin, sympathomimetics

• Increased effect of both drugs: phenothiazines, xanthines

• Decreased bronchodilation: theophyllines

• Hypertension, bradycardia: epinephrine, ephedrine

• Slow metabolism of drug: lidocaine

DENTAL CONSIDERATIONS

General:

• Monitor vital signs at every appointment because of cardiovascular side effects.

• Patients on chronic drug therapy may rarely have symptoms of blood dyscrasias, which can include infection, bleeding, and poor healing.

• Stress from dental procedures may compromise cardiovascular function; determine patient risk.

• Use vasoconstrictors with caution, in low doses, and with careful aspiration. Avoid use of gingival retraction cord with epinephrine.

• Consider semisupine chair position for patient comfort if GI side effects occur.

• Assess salivary flow as a factor in caries, periodontal disease, and candidiasis.

• Consider drug effects if taste alteration occurs.

Consultations:

• In a patient with symptoms of blood dyscrasias, request a medical consultation for blood studies and postpone dental treatment until normal values are reestablished.

• Medical consultation may be required to assess disease control and patient's ability to tolerate stress.

Teach patient/family:

• Of need for good oral hygiene to prevent soft tissue inflammation

• Caution to prevent injury when using oral hygiene aids

When chronic dry mouth occurs, advise patient:

• To avoid mouth rinses with high alcohol content because of drying effects

• Of need for daily use of home fluoride products to prevent caries

• To use sugarless gum, frequent sips of water, or saliva substitutes

---

pioglitazone

(pye-oh-gli'ta-zone)

Actos

Drug class.: Antidiabetic, oral

Action: An agonist for peroxisome proliferator-activated receptor gamma (PPAR-γ); improves target cell response to insulin without increasing insulin secretion; insulin must be present for this drug to act

Uses: Monotherapy, as an adjunct to diet and exercise in patients with type 2 diabetes mellitus; may also be used with metformin when metformin, diet, and exercise are not adequate for control

Dosage and routes:

• *Adult (monotherapy):* PO 15-30 mg qd, if response is inadequate can increase to 45 mg in increments

• *Adult (in combination/sulfonylurea, metformin):* PO 15-30 mg qd, adjust dose of sulfonylurea downward as required; max dose 45 mg/day

Available forms include: Tabs 15, 30, 45 mg

Side effects/adverse reactions:

▼ *ORAL:* Undefined tooth disorder

CNS: Paresthesias, headache

CV: Edema

GI: Abdominal pain

RESP: URI

EENT: Sinusitis, pharyngitis

HEMA: Anemia

ENDO: Hypoglycemia, ↑ LDL cholesterol, ↑ CPK, ↑ ALT

P

MISC: Weight gain, myalgia, fluid retention

Contraindications: Hypersensitivity to pioglitazone or hypersensitivity to other glitazone oral antidiabetics

Precautions: Hepatic dysfunction (reduce dose), renal impairment, pregnancy category C, lactation, children <18 yr

Pharmacokinetics:

PO: Data lacking; some metabolism by cytochrome P-450 3A4 enzymes; highly plasma protein bound (98%), hepatic metabolism, some renal excretion

Drug interactions of concern to dentistry:

• None reported

DENTAL CONSIDERATIONS

General:

• Ensure that patient is following prescribed diet and regularly takes medication.

• Place on frequent recall to evaluate healing response.

• Short appointments and a stress reduction protocol may be required for anxious patients.

• Diabetics may be more susceptible to infection and have delayed wound healing.

• Question patient about self-monitoring of drug's antidiabetic effect, including blood glucose values or finger-stick records.

• Consider semisupine chair position for patient comfort if GI side effects occur.

Consultations:

• Medical consultation may be required to assess disease control and patient's ability to tolerate stress.

• Medical consultation may include data from patient's blood glucose monitoring, including glycosylated hemoglobin or HbA_{1c} testing.

Teach patient/family:

• To prevent trauma when using oral hygiene aids

• Importance of updating health and drug history if physician makes any changes in evaluation or drug regimens

pirbuterol acetate

(perr-byoo'ter-ole)

Maxair

Drug class.: Bronchodilator

Action: Causes bronchodilation with little effect on heart rate by acting on β-receptors, causing increased cAMP and relaxation of smooth muscle

Uses: Reversible bronchospasm (prevention, treatment), including asthma; may be given with theophylline or steroids

Dosage and routes:

• *Adult and child >12 yr:* Aerosol 1-2 inh (0.4 mg) q4-6h; do not exceed 12 inh/day

Available forms include: Aerosol delivers 0.2 mg pirbuterol/actuation

Side effects/adverse reactions:

▼ *ORAL:* Taste changes, dry mouth

CNS: Tremors, anxiety, insomnia, headache, dizziness, stimulation, restlessness, hallucinations, drowsiness, irritability

CV: Palpitation, tachycardia, hypertension, angina, hypotension, dysrhythmias

GI: Heartburn, nausea, vomiting, anorexia

RESP: ***Bronchospasm,*** dyspnea, coughing

EENT: Dry nose, irritation of nose/throat

MS: Muscle cramps

Contraindications: Hypersensitivity to sympathomimetics, tachycardia

Precautions: Lactation, pregnancy category C, cardiac disorders, hyperthyroidism, diabetes mellitus, prostatic hypertrophy

Pharmacokinetics:

INH: Onset 3 min, peak 0.5-1 hr, duration 5 hr

DENTAL CONSIDERATIONS

General:

• Acute asthmatic episodes may be precipitated in the dental office. Sympathomimetic inhalants should be available for emergency use.

• Be aware that aspirin or sulfite preservatives in vasoconstrictor-containing products can exacerbate asthma.

• Monitor vital signs at every appointment because of cardiovascular and respiratory side effects.

• Assess salivary flow as a factor in caries, periodontal disease, and candidiasis.

• Consider semisupine chair position for patients with respiratory disease.

• Short appointments and a stress reduction protocol may be required for anxious patients.

Consultations:

• Medical consultation may be required to assess disease control and patient's ability to tolerate stress.

Teach patient/family:

• To rinse mouth with water after each dose to prevent dryness (for inhalation dosage forms)

When chronic dry mouth occurs, advise patient:

• To avoid mouth rinses with high alcohol content because of drying effects

• Of need for daily use of home fluoride products to prevent caries

• To use sugarless gum, frequent sips of water, or saliva substitutes

piroxicam

(peer-ox'i-kam)

Feldene

♣ Apo-Piroxicam, Novo-Pirocam, Nu-Pirox, PMS-Piroxicam

Drug class.: Nonsteroidal antiinflammatory

Action: Inhibits prostaglandin synthesis by interfering with cyclooxygenase needed for biosynthesis; possesses analgesic, antiinflammatory, antipyretic properties

Uses: Osteoarthritis, rheumatoid arthritis; unapproved: gouty arthritis

Dosage and routes:

• *Adult:* PO 20 mg qd or 10 mg bid

Available forms include: Caps 10, 20 mg; supp 10, 20 mg

Side effects/adverse reactions:

▼ *ORAL:* Stomatitis, bleeding, dry mouth, lichenoid reaction

CNS: Dizziness, drowsiness, headache, insomnia, depression, malaise, somnolence, nervousness, vertigo

CV: Peripheral edema

GI: Nausea, anorexia, vomiting, diarrhea, ***cholestatic hepatitis,*** jaundice, constipation, flatulence, cramps, peptic ulcer, epigastric distress, bleeding

HEMA: ***Blood dyscrasias***

GU: ***Nephrotoxicity: hematuria, oliguria, azotemia***

EENT: Tinnitus, hearing loss, blurred vision

INTEG: Purpura, rash, pruritus, sweating, photosensitivity, pemphigus-like reaction

META: Elevated ALT/AST, hypoglycemia
Contraindications: Hypersensitivity, asthma, severe renal disease, severe hepatic disease, ritonavir
Precautions: Pregnancy category C, lactation, children, bleeding disorders, GI disorders, cardiac disorders, hypersensitivity to other antiinflammatory agents, hypertension
Pharmacokinetics:
PO: Peak 2 hr, half-life 3-3.5 hr; 99% protein binding; metabolized in liver; excreted in urine (metabolites), breast milk
Drug interactions of concern to dentistry:
• GI ulceration, bleeding: aspirin, alcohol, corticosteroids
• Nephrotoxicity: acetaminophen (prolonged use and high doses)
• Possible risk of decreased renal function: cyclosporine
• Decreased action: salicylates
• First-time users of SSRIs also taking NSAIDs may have a higher risk of GI side effects; until more data are available, it may be advisable to avoid use of NSAIDs in these patients (*Br J Clin Pharmacol* 55:591-595, 2003)
When prescribed for dental pain:
• Risk of increased effects of oral anticoagulants, oral antidiabetics, lithium, methotrexate
• Decreased antihypertensive effects of diuretics, β-adrenergic blockers, ACE inhibitors
DENTAL CONSIDERATIONS
General:
• Patients on chronic drug therapy may rarely have symptoms of blood dyscrasias, which can include infection, bleeding, and poor healing.
• Assess salivary flow as a factor in caries, periodontal disease, and candidiasis.
• Avoid prescribing for dental use during pregnancy.
• Minimize use of aspirin-containing products.
• Consider semisupine chair position for patients with arthritic disease or if GI side effects occur.
Consultations:
• In a patient with symptoms of blood dyscrasias, request a medical consultation for blood studies and postpone dental treatment until normal values are reestablished.
• Medical consultation may be required to assess disease control.
Teach patient/family:
• Importance of good oral hygiene to prevent soft tissue inflammation
• Caution to prevent injury when using oral hygiene aids
• To report oral lesions, soreness, or bleeding to dentist
When chronic dry mouth occurs, advise patient:
• To avoid mouth rinses with high alcohol content because of drying effects
• Of need for daily use of home fluoride products to prevent caries
• To use sugarless gum, frequent sips of water, or saliva substitutes

polymyxin B sulfate (ophthalmic)

(pol-i-mix'in)

Drug class.: Antiinfective (ophthalmic)

Action: Inhibits cell wall permeability in susceptible organism
Uses: Superficial external ocular infections

Dosage and routes:
• *Adult and child:* Instill 1-2 drops of 0.1%-0.25% sol bid-qid × 7-10 days
Available forms include: Powder for sol 500,000 U
Side effects/adverse reactions:
EENT: Poor corneal wound healing, temporary visual haze, overgrowth of nonsusceptible organisms, photosensitivity
Contraindications: Hypersensitivity; viral, mycobacterial, or fungal ocular infection
Precautions: Antibiotic hypersensitivity, pregnancy category B
DENTAL CONSIDERATIONS
General:
• Avoid dental light in patient's eyes; offer dark glasses for patient comfort and safety during dental treatment.

---

polythiazide

(pol-i-thye'azide)
Renese
Drug class.: Thiazide diuretic

Action: Acts on distal tubule by increasing excretion of water, sodium, chloride, potassium
Uses: Edema, hypertension, diuresis
Dosage and routes:
• *Adult:* PO 1-4 mg/day
Available forms include: Tabs 1, 2, 4 mg
Side effects/adverse reactions:
▼ *ORAL:* Dry mouth, increased thirst, bitter taste, lichenoid reaction
CNS: Drowsiness, paresthesia, anxiety, depression, headache, dizziness, fatigue, weakness, restlessness, syncope
CV: Irregular pulse, orthostatic hypotension, palpitation, volume depletion, dehydration
GI: Nausea, vomiting, anorexia, constipation, diarrhea, cramps, pancreatitis, GI irritation, hepatitis
HEMA: ***Aplastic anemia, hemolytic anemia, leukopenia, agranulocytosis, thrombocytopenia,*** neutropenia
GU: Frequency, polyuria, uremia, glucosuria, impotence, reduced libido
EENT: Blurred vision
INTEG: Rash, urticaria, purpura, photosensitivity, fever
META: Hyperglycemia, hyperuricemia, increased creatinine, BUN
ELECT: Hypokalemia, hypercalcemia, hyponatremia, hypochloremia
Contraindications: Hypersensitivity to thiazides or sulfonamides, anuria, renal decompensation, pregnancy category D
Precautions: Hypokalemia, renal disease, hepatic disease, gout, COPD, lupus erythematosus, diabetes mellitus
Pharmacokinetics:
PO: Onset 2 hr, peak 6 hr, duration 24-48 hr, half-life 26 hr; excreted unchanged by kidneys; crosses placenta; excreted in breast milk
Drug interactions of concern to dentistry:
• Decreased hypotensive response: indomethacin, NSAIDs, sympathomimetics
• Increased toxicity of nondepolarizing skeletal muscle relaxants
DENTAL CONSIDERATIONS
General:
• Monitor vital signs at every appointment because of cardiovascular side effects.
• Patients on chronic drug therapy may rarely have symptoms of blood dyscrasias, which can in-

P

clude infection, bleeding, and poor healing.

• After supine positioning, have patient sit upright for at least 2 min before standing to avoid orthostatic hypotension.

• Assess salivary flow as a factor in caries, periodontal disease, and candidiasis.

Consultations:

• In a patient with symptoms of blood dyscrasias, request a medical consultation for blood studies and postpone dental treatment until normal values are reestablished.

• Medical consultation may be required to assess disease control.

Teach patient/family:

• Need for good oral hygiene to prevent periodontal inflammation

• Caution to prevent injury when using oral hygiene aids

When chronic dry mouth occurs, advise patient:

• To avoid mouth rinses with high alcohol content because of drying effects

• Of need for daily use of home fluoride products to prevent caries

• To use sugarless gum, frequent sips of water, or saliva substitutes

potassium acetate/ potassium bicarbonate/ potassium chloride/ potassium gluconate/ potassium phosphate

Potassium bicarbonate effervescent: Effer-K, K^+ Care ET, K-Electrolyte, K-Ide, Klor-Con/EF, Klorvess, K-Lyte, Vesant

Potassium chloride: Cena-K, Effer-K, K-8, K^+10, Kaochlor, Kaochlor-SF, Kaon-Cl, KayCiel, K-Dur, K-Lease, K-Lor, Klor-Con 8, Klor-Con 10, Klorvess, Klotrix, K-Lyte, K-Norm, K-Tab, Micro-K, Rum-K, Slow-K, Ten-K, Tri-K

🍁 Apo-K, Kalium, Novolente-K

Potassium gluconate: Kaon, Kayelixir, K-G Elixir

Drug class.: Potassium electrolyte

Action: Needed for adequate transmission of nerve impulses and cardiac contraction, renal function, intracellular ion maintenance

Uses: Prevention and treatment of hypokalemia

Dosage and routes:

Potassium bicarbonate:

• *Adult:* PO dissolve 25-50 mEq in water qd-qid

Potassium acetate–hypokalemia:

• *Adult and child:* PO 40-100 mEq/day in divided doses 2-4 days

Hypokalemia (prevention):

• *Adult and child:* PO 20 mEq/day in 2-4 divided doses

Potassium chloride:

• *Adult:* PO 40-100 mEq in divided doses tid-qid; IV 20 mEq/hr when diluted as 40 mEq/1000 ml, not to exceed 150 mEq/day

Potassium gluconate:

• *Adult:* PO 40-100 mEq in divided doses tid-qid

Potassium phosphate:

• *Adult:* IV 1 mEq/hr in sol of 60 mEq/L, not to exceed 150 mEq/day; PO 40-100 mEq/day in divided doses

Available forms include: Liq 20, 30, 40, 45 mEq per 15 ml; powder 15, 20, 25 mEq per packet; effervescent tabs 20, 25, 50 mEq per tablet; con rel tabs 6.7, 8.0, 10 mEq per tab; ext rel tabs 10, 20 mEq per tab; con rel caps 8, 10 mEq per capsule; IV preps 10 mEq/g, 40 mEq/ml in 10, 20 ml vials

Side effects/adverse reactions:

CNS: Confusion, hyperkalemia

CV: ***Cardiac depression, dysrhythmias, arrest, peaking T waves, lowered R and depressed RST, prolonged P-R interval, widened QRS complex,*** bradycardia

GI: Nausea, vomiting, cramps, pain, diarrhea, ulceration of small bowel

GU: Oliguria

INTEG: Cold extremities, rash

Contraindications: Renal disease (severe), severe hemolytic disease, Addison's disease, hyperkalemia, acute dehydration, extensive tissue breakdown

Precautions: Cardiac disease, potassium-sparing diuretic therapy, systemic acidosis, pregnancy category A, renal impairment

Pharmacokinetics:

PO: Excreted by kidneys and in feces

IV: Immediate onset of action

Drug interactions of concern to dentistry:

• Decreased potassium requirement: corticosteroids

• Increased GI side effects: anticholinergic drugs, NSAIDs

• Increased serum potassium: NSAIDs, cyclosporine

DENTAL CONSIDERATIONS

General:

• Patients taking potassium supplements will normally be taking a diuretic. Compliance with potassium supplements can be a problem. Verify serum potassium levels as required.

• Consider semisupine chair position for patient comfort if GI side effects occur.

---

povidone iodine

(poe'vi-done)

ACU-dyne, Aerodine, Betadine, Betagen, Biodine, Efodine, Iodex-P, Mallisol, Minidyne, Operand, Polydine

♣ Proviodine

Drug class.: Iodophor disinfectant

Action: Destroys a wide variety of microorganisms by local irritation, germicidal action

Uses: Cleansing wounds, disinfection, preoperative skin preparation removal

Dosage and routes:

• *Adult and child:* Sol use as needed, topical only

Available forms include:

TOP: A variety of solutions, ointments, aerosols, foams, creams, gels, and pads

Side effects/adverse reactions:

GU: ***Renal damage***

META: Metabolic acidosis

INTEG: Irritation

Contraindications: Hypersensitivity to iodine, pregnancy category D (vaginal antiseptic)

Precautions: Extensive burns

Drug interactions of concern to dentistry:

• Do not use with alcohol or hydrogen peroxide

DENTAL CONSIDERATIONS
General:
• Assess for allergies to seafood; if present, drug should not be used.
• Store in tight, light-resistant container.
• Evaluate area of the body involved for irritation, rash, breaks, dryness, and scales.
Teach patient/family:
• To discontinue use if rash, irritation, or redness occurs

pramipexole dihydrochloride

(pra-mi-pex'ole)
Mirapex
Drug class.: Antiparkinson agent

Action: Acts as a dopamine agonist at D_2 receptor sites
Uses: Idiopathic Parkinson's disease
Dosage and routes:
• *Adult:* PO all doses should be titrated gradually beginning with an initial dose of 0.125 mg tid for 5-7 days; doses can be increased by increments each week to a tolerated range of 1.5-4.5 mg/day in 3 divided doses; dose must be reduced in renal impairment
Available forms include: Tabs 0.125, 0.25, 1, 1.5 mg
Side effects/adverse reactions:
▼ *ORAL:* Dry mouth, taste perversion
CNS: Hallucinations, dizziness, somnolence, insomnia, headache, malaise
CV: Postural hypotension, edema
GI: Nausea, constipation, dyspepsia, anorexia
GU: Impotence, urinary frequency
EENT: Vision abnormalities
INTEG: Rash
MS: Extrapyramidal syndrome
MISC: Asthenia, accidental injury
Contraindications: Hypersensitivity
Precautions: Orthostatic hypotension, hallucination risk higher >65 yr, renal insufficiency, caution in driving a car (somnolence), risk of falling asleep while performing daily activities, pregnancy category C, lactation, use not established in children
Pharmacokinetics:
PO: Rapid absorption, peak levels in 2 hr, bioavailability 90%, low plasma protein binding (15%), 90% of dose excreted unchanged in urine
Drug interactions of concern to dentistry:
• Increased CNS depression: all CNS depressants
• Possible decreased effects: dopamine antagonists (phenothiazines, butyrophenones, or thioxanthenes) and metoclopramide
DENTAL CONSIDERATIONS
General:
• Monitor vital signs at every appointment because of cardiovascular side effects.
• Assess salivary flow as factor in caries, periodontal disease, and candidiasis.
• Consider semisupine chair position for patient comfort if GI side effects occur.
• After supine positioning, have patient sit upright for at least 2 min to avoid orthostatic hypotension.
Consultations:
• Medical consultation may be required to assess disease control and patient's ability to tolerate stress.

Teach patient/family:
• Importance of good oral hygiene to prevent soft tissue inflammation
• Caution to prevent trauma when using oral hygiene aids
• Use of electric toothbrush if patient has difficulty holding conventional devices
• Importance of updating health and drug history if physician makes any changes in evaluation or drug regimens
When chronic dry mouth occurs, advise patient:
• To avoid mouth rinses with high alcohol content because of drying effects
• To use daily home fluoride products for anticaries effect
• To use sugarless gum, frequent sips of water, or saliva substitutes

pravastatin sodium

(pra'va-sta-tin)
Pravachol
Drug class.: Antihyperlipidemic

Action: Inhibits HMG-Co A reductase enzyme, reducing cholesterol synthesis; reduced synthesis of VLDL; plasma triglyceride levels may also be decreased
Uses: As an adjunct in homozygous or heterozygous familial hypercholesterolemia, mixed hyperlipidemia, elevated serum triglyceride levels and type IV hyperproteinemia, also reduces total cholesterol LDL-C, apo B, and triglyceride levels; patient should first be placed on cholesterol-lowering diet; primary prevention of coronary events, secondary prevention of CV events

Dosage and routes:
• *Adult:* PO initial dose 40 mg/day; max dose 80 mg/day
Heterozygous familial hypercholesterolemia:
• *Child 8-13 yr:* PO 20 mg/day
• *Adolescent 14-18 yr:* PO 40 mg/day
Available forms include: Tabs 10, 20, 40, 80 mg
Side effects/adverse reactions:
CNS: Headache, dizziness, psychic disturbances, fatigue
CV: Chest pain
GI: ***Liver dysfunction, hepatitis,*** pancreatitis, nausea, constipation, diarrhea, dyspepsia, flatus, abdominal pain, heartburn, vomiting
GU: Gynecomastia, libido loss
EENT: Lens opacities, common cold, rhinitis, cough, cataracts
INTEG: Rash, pruritus
MS: ***Myositis, rhabdomyolysis,*** muscle cramps, myalgia
MISC: Alopecia, edema
Contraindications: Hypersensitivity, pregnancy category X, lactation, active liver disease
Precautions: Past liver disease, alcoholics, severe acute infections, trauma, hypotension, uncontrolled seizure disorders, severe metabolic disorders, electrolyte imbalances
Pharmacokinetics:
PO: Peak 1-1.5 hr; highly protein bound; metabolized by liver; excreted in urine, feces, breast milk; crosses placenta
Drug interactions of concern to dentistry:
• Increased risk of myopathy or rhabdomyolysis: erythromycin, itraconazole
DENTAL CONSIDERATIONS
General:
• Monitor vital signs at every ap-

P

pointment because of possible cardiovascular disease.

• Consider semisupine chair position for patient comfort if GI side effects occur.

prazosin HCl

(pra'zoe-sin)

Minipress

Drug class.: Antihypertensive, α-adrenergic antagonist

Action: Reduction in blood pressure results from blockage of α-adrenergic receptors and reduced peripheral resistance

Uses: Hypertension; unapproved: CHF, urinary retention in prostatic hypertrophy, pheochromocytoma

Dosage and routes:

• *Adult:* PO 1 mg bid or tid, increasing to 20 mg qd in divided doses if required; usual range 6-15 mg/day, not to exceed 1 mg initially

Available forms include: Caps 1, 2, 5 mg; tabs 1, 2, 5 mg

Side effects/adverse reactions:

▼ *ORAL:* Dry mouth, lichenoid drug reaction

CNS: Dizziness, headache, drowsiness, anxiety, depression, vertigo, weakness, fatigue, light-headedness, lethargy, syncope

CV: Palpitation, orthostatic hypotension, tachycardia, edema, dyspnea, angina

GI: Nausea, vomiting, diarrhea, constipation, abdominal pain

GU: Urinary frequency, incontinence, impotence, priapism

EENT: Blurred vision, epistaxis, tinnitus, red sclera

Contraindications: Hypersensitivity, severe CHF

Precautions: Pregnancy category C, children

Pharmacokinetics:

PO: Onset 2 hr, peak 1-3 hr, duration 6-12 hr, half-life 2-4 hr; metabolized in liver; excreted via bile, feces (>90%), in urine (<10%)

Drug interactions of concern to dentistry:

• Increased effects: epinephrine

• Decreased effect: indomethacin, NSAIDs

DENTAL CONSIDERATIONS

General:

• Monitor vital signs at every appointment because of cardiovascular side effects.

• After supine positioning, have patient sit upright for at least 2 min before standing to avoid orthostatic hypotension.

• Assess salivary flow as a factor in caries, periodontal disease, and candidiasis.

• Limit use of sodium-containing products, such as saline IV fluids, for patients with a dietary salt restriction.

• Stress from dental procedures may compromise cardiovascular function; determine patient risk.

• Short appointments and a stress reduction protocol may be required for anxious patients.

Consultations:

• Medical consultation may be required to assess disease control.

Teach patient/family:

When chronic dry mouth occurs, advise patient:

• To avoid mouth rinses with high alcohol content because of drying effects

• Of need for daily use of home fluoride products to prevent caries

• To use sugarless gum, frequent sips of water, or saliva substitutes

prednicarbate

(pred'ni-kar-bate)

Dermatop Emollient Cream

Drug class.: Topical corticosteroid, group III potency

Action: Glucocorticoids have multiple actions that include antiinflammatory and immunosuppressant effects. They inhibit phospholipase A_2, interfering with or reducing the synthesis of prostaglandins and leukotrienes. They also bind to cytoplasmic GRs and enter the cell nucleus to bind with DNA. This results in the synthesis of various enzymes such as collagenase, elastase, and cytokines that play important roles in inflammation and immunosuppression. They also suppress the production of lymphocytes, monocytes, and eosinophils.

Uses: Relief of inflammatory and pruritic manifestations of corticosteroid-responsive dermatoses

Dosage and routes:

• *Adult:* TOP apply a thin film to affected area bid

Available forms include: Cream 0.1% in 15, 60 g

Side effects/adverse reactions:

INTEG: Skin atrophy, pruritus, burning, urticaria, edema, rash

Contraindications: Hypersensitivity

Precautions: Pregnancy category C, lactation, children <18 yr, occlusive dressings; bacterial, viral, or fungal skin infections

Drug interactions of concern to dentistry:

• None reported

DENTAL CONSIDERATIONS

General:

• Determine why the patient is taking the drug.

• Use on oral herpetic ulcerations is contraindicated.

prednisolone/ prednisolone acetate/ prednisolone phosphate/ prednisolone tebutate

(pred-niss'oh-lone)

Prednisolone: Delta-Cortef, Prelone

Prednisolone acetate (not for IV use): Key-Pred 25 and 50, Predalone-50, Predcor-50

Prednisolone tebutate: Prednisol TBA

Prednisolone sodium phosphate: Hydeltrasol, Key-Pred-SP, Pediapred

Drug class.: Glucocorticoid, immediate acting

Action: Glucocorticoids have multiple actions that include antiinflammatory and immunosuppressant effects. They inhibit phospholipase A_2, interfering with or reducing the synthesis of prostaglandins and leukotrienes. They also bind to cytoplasmic GRs and enter the cell nucleus to bind with DNA. This results in the synthesis of various enzymes such as collagenase, elastase, and cytokines that play important roles in inflammation and immunosuppression. They also suppress the production of lymphocytes, monocytes, and eosinophils.

Uses: Severe inflammation, immunosuppression, neoplasms, adrenal insufficiency, acute exacerbation of multiple sclerosis

Dosage and routes:

• *Adult:* PO 5-60 mg/day; IM 4-60 mg/day (acetate, phosphate); IV

P

4-60 mg (phosphate); 4-5 mg in small joints, 10-20 mg in large joints (phosphate); 8-20 mg in joint lesion (tebutate); 40 mg intralesional (acetate); 10-30 mg soft tissue (phosphate); syr 15 mg/5 ml

Multiple sclerosis (acute exacerbation):

• *Adult:* PO 200 mg/day × 1 wk, then 80 mg qod × 1 mo

Available forms include: Tabs 5 mg; syr 5 mg/5 ml and 15 mg/5 ml; inj 25, 50 mg/ml (acetate); inj 20 mg/ml (terbutate); inj 20 mg/ml (phosphate); PO liq 5 mg/5 ml

Side effects/adverse reactions:

▼ *ORAL: Candidiasis,* dry mouth, delayed wound healing, petechiae

CNS: Depression, flushing, sweating, headache, mood changes

CV: Hypertension, ***circulatory collapse, thrombophlebitis, embolism,*** tachycardia

GI: Diarrhea, nausea, abdominal distention, ***GI hemorrhage, pancreatitis,*** increased appetite

HEMA: ***Thrombocytopenia***

EENT: Fungal infections, increased intraocular pressure, blurred vision

INTEG: Acne, delayed wound healing, ecchymosis, petechiae, striae

MS: Fractures, osteoporosis, muscle weakness

Contraindications: Psychosis, hypersensitivity, idiopathic thrombocytopenia, acute glomerulonephritis, amebiasis, fungal infections, nonasthmatic bronchial disease, child <2 yr

Precautions: Pregnancy category C, diabetes mellitus, glaucoma, osteoporosis, seizure disorders, ulcerative colitis, CHF, myasthenia gravis, ulcerative GI disease, rifampin

Pharmacokinetics:

PO: Peak 1-2 hr, duration 2 days

IM: Peak 3-45 hr

Drug interactions of concern to dentistry:

• Decreased action: barbiturates, rifampin, rifabutin

• Increased side effects: alcohol, salicylates, NSAIDs

• Increased action: ketoconazole, macrolide antibiotics (erythromycin, clarithromycin, azithromycin)

• Hepatotoxicity: acetaminophen (chronic use, high doses)

DENTAL CONSIDERATIONS

General:

• Monitor vital signs at every appointment because of cardiovascular side effects.

• Patients on chronic drug therapy may rarely have symptoms of blood dyscrasias, which can include infection, bleeding, and poor healing.

• Assess salivary flow as a factor in caries, periodontal disease, and candidiasis.

• Avoid prescribing aspirin-containing products.

• Place on frequent recall to evaluate healing response.

• Prophylactic antibiotics may be indicated to prevent infection if surgery or deep scaling is planned.

• Symptoms of oral infections may be masked.

• Determine dose and duration of steroid therapy for each patient to assess risk for stress tolerance and immunosuppression.

• Patients who have been or are currently on chronic steroid therapy (>2 wk) require supplemental steroids for dental treatment.

• Determine why the patient is taking the drug.

Consultations:

• In a patient with symptoms of blood dyscrasias, request a medical consultation for blood studies and postpone dental treatment until normal values are reestablished.

• Medical consultation may be required to assess disease control.

• Consultation may be required to confirm steroid dose and duration of use.

Teach patient/family:

• Importance of good oral hygiene to prevent soft tissue inflammation

• Caution to prevent injury when using oral hygiene aids

When chronic dry mouth occurs, advise patient:

• To avoid mouth rinses with high alcohol content because of drying effects

• Of need for daily use of home fluoride products to prevent caries

• To use sugarless gum, frequent sips of water, or saliva substitutes

prednisone

(pred'ni-sone)

Deltasone, Liquid Pred, Meticorten, Orasone, Panasol-S, Prednicen-M, Prednisone Intensol, Sterapred-DS

♣ Apo-Prednisone, Winpred

Drug class.: Glucocorticoid, intermediate acting

Action: Glucocorticoids have multiple actions that include antiinflammatory and immunosuppressant effects. They inhibit phospholipase A_2, interfering with or reducing the synthesis of prostaglandins and leukotrienes. They also bind to cytoplasmic GRs and enter the cell nucleus to bind with DNA. This results in the synthesis of various enzymes such as collagenase, elastase, and cytokines that play important roles in inflammation and immunosuppression. They also suppress the production of lymphocytes, monocytes, and eosinophils.

Uses: Severe inflammation, immunosuppression, neoplasms, multiple sclerosis, collagen disorders, dermatologic disorders, acute exacerbation of multiple sclerosis

Dosage and routes:

• *Adult:* PO 5 to 60 mg/day

Multiple sclerosis (acute exacerbation):

• *Adult:* PO 200 mg/day × 1 wk, then 80 mg qod × 1 mo

Available forms include:

Tabs 1, 2.5, 5, 10, 20, 50 mg; oral sol 5 mg/ml, 5 mg/5 ml; syr 5 mg/5 ml

Side effects/adverse reactions:

▼ *ORAL: Candidiasis,* dry mouth, poor wound healing, petechiae

CNS: Depression, flushing, sweating, headache, mood changes

CV: Hypertension, ***circulatory collapse, thrombophlebitis, embolism,*** tachycardia

GI: Diarrhea, nausea, abdominal distention, ***GI hemorrhage, pancreatitis,*** increased appetite

HEMA: ***Thrombocytopenia***

EENT: Fungal infections, increased intraocular pressure, blurred vision

INTEG: Acne, poor wound healing, ecchymosis, petechiae

MS: Fractures, osteoporosis, weakness

Contraindications: Psychosis, hypersensitivity, idiopathic thrombocytopenia, acute glomerulonephritis, amebiasis, fungal infections, nonasthmatic bronchial disease, child <2 yr, AIDS, TB

Precautions: Pregnancy category C, diabetes mellitus, glaucoma, osteoporosis, seizure disorders, ulcerative colitis, CHF, myasthenia gravis, renal disease, esophagitis, peptic ulcer, rifampin

Pharmacokinetics:

PO: Peak 1-2 hr, duration 1-1.5 days, half-life 3.5-4 hr

Drug interactions of concern to dentistry:

- Decreased action: barbiturates, rifampin, rifabutin
- Increased side effects: alcohol, salicylates, NSAIDs
- Increased action: ketoconazole, macrolide antibiotics
- Hepatotoxicity: acetaminophen (chronic, high doses)

DENTAL CONSIDERATIONS

General:

- Monitor vital signs at every appointment because of cardiovascular side effects.
- Patients on chronic drug therapy may rarely have symptoms of blood dyscrasias, which can include infection, bleeding, and poor healing.
- Avoid aspirin-containing products.
- Assess salivary flow as a factor in caries, periodontal disease, and candidiasis.
- Symptoms of oral infections may be masked.
- Place on frequent recall to evaluate healing response.
- Prophylactic antibiotics may be indicated to prevent infection if surgery or deep scaling is planned.
- Determine dose and duration of steroid therapy for each patient to assess risk for stress tolerance and immunosuppression.
- Patients who have been or are currently on chronic steroid therapy (>2 wk) may require supplemental steroids for dental treatment.
- Determine why the patient is taking the drug.

Consultations:

- In a patient with symptoms of blood dyscrasias, request a medical consultation for blood studies and postpone dental treatment until normal values are reestablished.
- Medical consultation may be required to assess disease control.
- Consultation may be required to confirm steroid dose and duration of use.

Teach patient/family:

- Importance of good oral hygiene to prevent soft tissue inflammation
- Caution to prevent injury when using oral hygiene aids

When chronic dry mouth occurs, advise patient:

- To avoid mouth rinses with high alcohol content because of drying effects
- Of need for daily use of home fluoride products to prevent caries
- To use sugarless gum, frequent sips of water, or saliva substitutes

prilocaine hydrochloride (local)

(pry'lo-kane)

Citanest

With vasoconstrictor: Citanest Forte with epinephrine

Drug class.: Amide local anesthetic

Action: Inhibits ion fluxes across membranes, particularly sodium transport across cell membrane; decreases rise of depolarization phase of action potential; blocks nerve action potential

Uses: Local dental anesthesia

Dosage and routes:

Dental injection: infiltration or conduction block:

• *Prilocaine 4% without vasoconstrictor:* Max dose of 400 mg over a 2 hr period per dental appointment for healthy adult patient*; doses must be adjusted for medically compromised, debilitated, or elderly and for each individual patient. Doses in excess of 400 mg have caused methemoglobinemia. **Always use the lowest effective dose, a slow injection rate, and a careful aspiration technique.** In considering the dose of local anesthesia with vasoconstrictor, the dose of epinephrine must also be considered. The recommended dose of epinephrine in a local anesthetic solution is 3 μg/kg, not to exceed a total dose of 0.2 mg per appointment for a healthy adult. For adult patients with clinically significant CV disease, the dose limit of epinephrine is 0.04 mg per appointment. The dose limits of epinephrine will affect the amount of local anesthetic allowable in a given appointment.

Example calculations illustrating amount of drug administered per dental cartridge(s):

# of dental cartridges (1.8 ml)	mg of prilocaine (4%)
1	72
2	144
3	216
4	288

*Max dose cited from *Handbook of local anesthesia,* ed 5, 2004, Mosby, as well as manufacturer's package insert. Doses may differ in other published reference resources.

• *Prilocaine 4% with epinephrine 1:200,000:* Recommended doses are the same; adjust doses for each individual as previously indicated

Example calculations illustrating amount of drug administered per dental cartridge(s):

# of cartridges (1.8 ml)	mg of prilocaine (4%)	mg (μg) vasoconstrictor (1:200,000)
1	72	0.009 (9)
2	144	0.018 (18)
4	288	0.036 (36)

Available forms include: 4% sol, 4% sol with epinephrine 1:200,000

Side effects/adverse reactions:

▼ *ORAL: Numbness, tingling,* trismus

CNS: ***Convulsions, loss of consciousness,*** drowsiness, disorientation, tremors, shivering, anxiety, restlessness

CV: ***Myocardial depression, cardiac arrest, dysrhythmias,*** bradycardia, hypotension, hypertension

GI: Nausea, vomiting

P

RESP: ***Status asthmaticus, respiratory arrest, anaphylaxis***
HEMA: ***Methemoglobinemia***
INTEG: Rash, urticaria, allergic reactions

Contraindications: Hypersensitivity, cross-sensitivity among amides (rare), severe liver disease

Precautions: Elderly, pregnancy category B, large doses of local anesthetic in myasthenia gravis, risk of methemoglobinemia

Pharmacokinetics: *INJ:* Onset 2-10 min, duration 2-4 hr; metabolized in liver; excreted in urine

Drug interactions of concern to dentistry:

• CNS depressants: increased risk of CNS depression with all CNS depressants, especially in children and when larger doses are used

• Avoid placing dental cartridges in disinfection solutions with heavy metals or surface-active agents; may see release of ions into local anesthetic solutions with tissue irritation following injection

• Avoid excessive exposure of dental cartridges to light or heat; hastens deterioration of vasoconstrictor; observe for color change in local anesthetic solution

• Risk of cardiovascular side effects; rapid intravascular administration of local anesthetic containing vasoconstrictor, either alone or in patients taking tricyclic antidepressants, MAOIs, digitalis drugs, cocaine, phenothiazines, β-blockers, and in the presence of halogenated-hydrocarbon general anesthetics; use smallest effective vasoconstrictor dose and careful aspiration technique

• Avoid use of vasoconstrictors in patients with uncontrolled hyperthyroidism, diabetes, angina, or hypertension; refer these patients for medical treatment before elective dental treatment

DENTAL CONSIDERATIONS

General:

• Monitor vital signs at every appointment because of cardiovascular side effects.

• Often used with vasoconstrictor for increased duration of action.

• Lubricate dry lips before injection or dental treatment as required.

Teach patient/family:

• To use care to prevent injury while numbness exists and to refrain from chewing gum and eating following dental anesthesia

• To report any signs of infection, muscle pain, or fever to dentist when feeling returns

• To report any unusual soft tissue reactions

primaquine phosphate

(prim'a-kween)

generic

Drug class.: Antiprotozoal

Action: Action is unknown; thought to destroy exoerythrocytic forms by gametocidal action

Uses: Malaria caused by *P. vivax;* unapproved: with clindamycin in the treatment of *P. carinii* in AIDS

Dosage and routes:

• *Adult:* PO 15 mg base qd × 2 wk

• *Child:* PO 0.3 mg/kg base daily × 2 wk

Available forms include: Tabs 26.3 mg (equivalent to 15 mg base)

Side effects/adverse reactions:

CNS: Headache
CV: Hypertension

GI: Nausea, vomiting, anorexia, cramps
HEMA: ***Agranulocytosis, granulocytopenia, leukopenia, hemolytic anemia, leukocytosis,*** mild anemia, ***methemoglobinemia***
EENT: Blurred vision, difficulty focusing
INTEG: Pruritus, skin eruptions

Contraindications: Hypersensitivity, anemia, lupus erythematosus, methemoglobinemia, porphyria, rheumatoid arthritis, methemoglobin reductase deficiency, G6PD deficiency

Precautions: Pregnancy category C

Pharmacokinetics:
PO: Half-life 3.7-9.6 hr; metabolized by liver (metabolites)

Drug interactions of concern to dentistry:
• None

DENTAL CONSIDERATIONS

General:
• Patients on chronic drug therapy may rarely have symptoms of blood dyscrasias, which can include infection, bleeding, and poor healing.
• Avoid dental light in patient's eyes; offer dark glasses for patient comfort.

Consultations:
• In a patient with symptoms of blood dyscrasias, request a medical consultation for blood studies and postpone dental treatment until normal values are reestablished.

Teach patient/family:
• Importance of good oral hygiene to prevent soft tissue inflammation
• Caution to prevent injury when using oral hygiene aids

primidone

(pri'mi-done)
Mysoline
✤ APO-Primidone, PMS-Primidone, Sertan
Drug class.: Anticonvulsant, barbiturate derivative

Action: Raises seizure threshold by unknown mechanism; may be related to facilitation of GABA; metabolized to phenobarbital

Uses: Generalized tonic-clonic (grand mal), complex-partial psychomotor seizures

Dosage and routes:
• *Adult and child >8 yr (no prior treatment):* PO 100-125 mg hs, days 1-3; 100-125 mg bid, days 4-6; 100-125 mg tid, days 7-9; then 250 mg tid to qid, not to exceed 500 mg qid
• *Adult and child >8 yr (taking other anticonvulsants):* PO 100-125 mg hs, increase gradually as other drug is decreased
• *Child <8 yr (no prior treatment):* PO 50 mg hs, days 1-3; 50 mg bid, days 4-6; 100 mg bid, days 7-9; then maintenance dose of 125-250 mg tid

Available forms include: Tabs 50, 250 mg; susp 250 mg/5 ml

Side effects/adverse reactions:
CNS: Stimulation, drowsiness, dizziness, confusion, sedation, headache, flushing, hallucinations, coma, psychosis, ataxia, vertigo
GI: Nausea, vomiting, anorexia
HEMA: ***Thrombocytopenia, leukopenia, neutropenia, eosinophilia, megaloblastic anemia,*** reduces serum folate level, lymphadenopathy
GU: Impotence, polyuria

P

EENT: Diplopia, nystagmus, edema of eyelids
INTEG: *Rash,* edema, alopecia, lupus-like syndrome
Contraindications: Hypersensitivity, hypersensitivity to phenobarbital, porphyria
Precautions: COPD, hepatic disease, renal disease, abrupt withdrawal, lactation, hyperactive children, pregnancy category D
Pharmacokinetics:
PO: Peak 4 hr, half-life 3-24 hr; excreted by kidneys, in breast milk
Drug interactions of concern to dentistry:
• Increased CNS depression: alcohol, other CNS depressants
• Increased metabolism/hepatotoxicity: halothane, halogenated-hydrocarbon inhalation anesthetics
• Increased seizure threshold: haloperidol, phenothiazines
• Decreased effects of acetaminophen, corticosteroids, doxycycline, fenoprofen
• Lower blood concentrations: carbamazepine
DENTAL CONSIDERATIONS
General:
• Ask about type of epilepsy, seizure frequency, and quality of seizure control.
• After supine positioning, have patient sit upright for at least 2 min before standing to avoid orthostatic hypotension.
• Patients on chronic drug therapy may rarely have symptoms of blood dyscrasias, which can include infection, bleeding, and poor healing.
• Short appointments and a stress reduction protocol may be required for anxious patients.
Consultations:
• Medical consultation may be required to assess disease control and patient's ability to tolerate stress.
• In a patient with symptoms of blood dyscrasias, request a medical consultation for blood studies and postpone dental treatment until normal values are reestablished.
Teach patient/family:
• Importance of good oral hygiene to prevent soft tissue inflammation
• Caution to prevent injury when using oral hygiene aids
• To avoid mouth rinses with high alcohol content because of drying effects

---

probenecid

(proe-ben'e-sid)
generic
Drug class.: Uricosuric

Action: Inhibits tubular reabsorption of urates, with increased excretion of uric acids
Uses: Hyperuricemia in gout, gouty arthritis, adjunct to cephalosporin or penicillin treatment by reducing excretion and maintaining high blood levels
Dosage and routes:
Gout/gouty arthritis:
• *Adult:* PO 250 mg bid for 1 wk, then 500 mg bid, not to exceed 2 g/day; maintenance 500 mg/day for 6 mo
Adjunct in penicillin/cephalosporin treatment:
• *Adult and child >50 kg:* PO 500 mg qid with antibiotic
• *Child 2-14 yr, <50 kg:* PO 25 mg/kg, then 40 mg/kg in divided doses qid
Available forms include: Tabs 500 mg

Side effects/adverse reactions:
▼ *ORAL:* Painful gingivae, increased thirst
CNS: Drowsiness, headache
CV: Bradycardia
GI: Gastric irritation, nausea, vomiting, anorexia, ***hepatic necrosis***
RESP: ***Apnea,*** irregular respirations
GU: ***Nephrotic syndrome,*** glycosuria, frequency
INTEG: Rash, dermatitis, pruritus, fever
META: Acidosis, hypokalemia, hyperchloremia, hyperglycemia
Contraindications: Hypersensitivity, severe hepatic disease, blood dyscrasias, severe renal disease, CrCl <50 mg/min, history of uric acid calculus, ketorolac, child <2 yr
Precautions: Pregnancy category B, severe respiratory disease, lactation, cardiac edema
Pharmacokinetics:
PO: Peak 2-4 hr, duration 8 hr, half-life 8-10 hr; metabolized by liver; excreted in urine; crosses placenta
Drug interactions of concern to dentistry:
- Increased toxicity: dapsone, indomethacin, other NSAIDs, acyclovir
- Increased sedation: benzodiazepines
- Decreased action: alcohol, salicylates
- Increased duration of action: penicillins, cephalosporins
- Contraindicated: ketorolac

DENTAL CONSIDERATIONS
General:
- Avoid prescribing aspirin-containing products.

Teach patient/family:
- Importance of good oral hygiene to prevent soft tissue inflammation
- Caution to prevent injury when using oral hygiene aids
- To avoid mouth rinses with high alcohol content because of drying effects

procainamide HCl

(proe-kane-a'mide)
Procanbid, Pronestyl, Pronestyl SR
🍁 Procan SR
Drug class.: Antidysrhythmic (class Ia)

Action: Depresses excitability of cardiac muscle to electrical stimulation and slows conduction in atrium, bundle of His, and ventricle
Uses: PVCs, atrial fibrillation, PAT, atrial dysrhythmias, ventricular tachycardia
Dosage and routes:
Atrial fibrillation/PAT:
- *Adult:* PO 1-1.25 g, may give another 750 mg if needed; if no response then 500 mg-1 g q2h until desired response; maintenance 50 mg/kg in divided doses q6h

Ventricular tachycardia:
- *Adult:* PO 1 g; maintenance 50 mg/kg/day given in 3 hr intervals; sus rel tabs 500 mg-1.25 g q6h

Other dysrhythmias:
- *Adult:* IV bol 100 mg q5min, given 25-50 mg/min, not to exceed 500 mg; then IV inf 2-6 mg/min

Available forms include: Caps 250, 375, 500 mg; ext rel tabs 250, 500, 750, 1000 mg; inj IV 100, 500 mg/ml

P

Side effects/adverse reactions:
▼ *ORAL:* Dry mouth
CNS: Headache, dizziness, confusion, psychosis, restlessness, irritability, weakness
CV: Hypotension, ***heart block, cardiovascular collapse, arrest***
GI: Nausea, vomiting, anorexia, diarrhea, hepatomegaly
HEMA: ***Agranulocytosis, thrombocytopenia, neutropenia, hemolytic anemia,*** SLE syndrome
INTEG: Rash, urticaria, edema, swelling, pruritus

Contraindications: Hypersensitivity, myasthenia gravis, severe heart block

Precautions: Prolonged use leads to development of positive ANA, renal disease, liver disease, CHF, respiratory depression, elderly, pregnancy category C, lactation, children

Pharmacokinetics:
PO: Peak 1-2 hr, duration 3 hr (8 hr extended)
IM: Peak 10-60 min, duration 3 hr
Half-life 3 hr; metabolized in liver to active metabolites; excreted unchanged by kidneys (60%)

Drug interactions of concern to dentistry:
- Decreased effects: barbiturates
- Increased effects of neuromuscular blockers, anticholinergics, antiarrhythmics
- Increased risk of life-threatening arrhythmias: sparfloxacin, gatifloxacin, moxifloxacin, possibly ofloxacin

DENTAL CONSIDERATIONS

General:
- Monitor vital signs at every appointment because of cardiovascular side effects.
- Patients on chronic drug therapy may rarely have symptoms of blood dyscrasias, which can include infection, bleeding, and poor healing.
- After supine positioning, have patient sit upright for at least 2 min before standing to avoid orthostatic hypotension.
- Assess salivary flow as a factor in caries, periodontal disease, and candidiasis.
- Stress from dental procedures may compromise cardiovascular function; determine patient risk.

Consultations:
- In a patient with symptoms of blood dyscrasias, request a medical consultation for blood studies and postpone dental treatment until normal values are reestablished.
- Medical consultation may be required to assess disease control and patient's ability to tolerate stress.

Teach patient/family:
- Importance of good oral hygiene to prevent soft tissue inflammation
- Caution to prevent injury when using oral hygiene aids

When chronic dry mouth occurs, advise patient:
- To avoid mouth rinses with high alcohol content because of drying effects
- Of need for daily use of home fluoride products to prevent caries
- To use sugarless gum, frequent sips of water, or saliva substitutes

---

procarbazine HCl

(proe-kar'ba-zeen)
Matulane
🍁 Natulan

Drug class.: Antineoplastic, miscellaneous

Action: Inhibits DNA, RNA, protein synthesis; has multiple sites of action; a nonvesicant, also inhibits monoamine oxidase enzymes

Uses: Lymphoma, Hodgkin's disease, cancers resistant to other therapy

Dosage and routes:

• *Adult:* PO 2-4 mg/kg/day for first week; maintain dosage of 4-6 mg/kg/day until platelets and WBC count fall; after recovery: 1-2 mg/kg/day

• *Child:* PO 50 mg/day for 7 days, then 100 mg/m^2 until desired response, leukopenia, or thrombocytopenia occurs; 50 mg/day is maintenance after bone marrow recovery

Available forms include: Caps 50 mg

Side effects/adverse reactions:

▼ *ORAL:* Petechiae, bleeding, dry mouth, stomatitis

CNS: Headache, dizziness, insomnia, hallucinations, confusion, coma, pain, chills, fever, sweating, paresthesia

CV: Orthostatic hypotension, fast or slow heartbeat

GI: Nausea, vomiting, anorexia, diarrhea, constipation

RESP: Cough, pneumonitis

HEMA: ***Thrombocytopenia, anemia, leukopenia, myelosuppression, bleeding tendencies,*** purpura, petechiae, epistaxis

GU: Azoospermia, cessation of menses

EENT: Retinal hemorrhage, nystagmus, photophobia, diplopia

INTEG: Rash, pruritus, dermatitis, alopecia, herpes, hyperpigmentation

Contraindications: Hypersensitivity, thrombocytopenia, bone marrow depression

Precautions: Renal disease, hepatic disease, pregnancy category D, radiation therapy

Pharmacokinetics:

PO: Peak levels 1 hr; concentrates in liver, kidney, skin; metabolized in liver, excreted in urine

Drug interactions of concern to dentistry:

• Increased CNS depression: barbiturates, antihistamines, narcotics

• Disulfiram-like reaction: ethyl alcohol

• Hypertension: indirect-acting sympathomimetics

• Increased anticholinergic effect: anticholinergic drugs, antihistamines

• Increased risk of severe toxic reactions: tricyclic antidepressants, meperidine and other opioids, tyramine-containing foods and other MAOIs; may also include cyclobenzaprine and carbamazepine

DENTAL CONSIDERATIONS

General:

• Patients on chronic drug therapy may rarely have symptoms of blood dyscrasias, which can include infection, bleeding, and poor healing.

• Monitor vital signs at every appointment because of cardiovascular side effects.

• Consider semisupine chair position when GI side effects occur.

• Assess salivary flow as a factor in caries, periodontal disease, and candidiasis.

• After supine positioning, have patient sit upright for at least 2 min before standing to avoid orthostatic hypotension.

• Avoid dental light in patient's eyes; offer dark glasses for patient comfort.

• Avoid aspirin-containing products because of bleeding risk.
• Avoid use of gingival retraction cord with epinephrine.
• Patients receiving chemotherapy may require palliative treatment for stomatitis.

Consultations:
• In a patient with symptoms of blood dyscrasias, request a medical consultation for blood studies and postpone dental treatment until normal values are reestablished.
• Take precautions if dental surgery is anticipated and sedation or general anesthesia is required; there is risk of hypotensive episode.

Teach patient/family:
• Importance of good oral hygiene to prevent soft tissue inflammation
• Caution to prevent injury when using oral hygiene aids
• To report oral lesions, soreness, or bleeding to dentist

When chronic dry mouth occurs, advise patient:
• To avoid mouth rinses with high alcohol content because of drying effects
• Of need for daily use of home fluoride products to prevent caries
• To use sugarless gum, frequent sips of water, or saliva substitutes

prochlorperazine edisylate/ prochlorperazine maleate

(proe-klor-per'a-zeen)

Compazine

🍁 Nu-Prochlor, PMS Prochlorperazine, Prorazin, Stemetil

Drug class.: Phenothiazine antipsychotic

Action: Blocks neurotransmission at dopaminergic synapses in the cerebral cortex, hypothalamus, and limbic system; exhibits strong peripheral α-adrenergic, anticholinergic blocking action; mechanism for antipsychotic effects is unclear

Uses: Antipsychotic; for nausea, vomiting

Dosage and routes:

Psychiatry:
• *Adult:* PO 5-10 mg tid-qid, increasing dosage every 2-3 days; more severe cases start 10 mg tid-qid; patients may tolerate 100-150 mg/day
• *Child 2-12 yr:* PO/RECT initial doses 2.5 mg bid or tid, no more than 10 mg on first day; adjust dose according to patient response

Postoperative nausea/vomiting:
• *Adult:* IM 5-10 mg 1-2 hr before anesthesia, may repeat in 30 min; IV 5-10 mg 15-30 min before anesthesia; IV inf 20 mg/L D_5W or NS 15-30 min before anesthesia, not to exceed 40 mg/day

Severe nausea/vomiting:
• *Adult:* PO 5-10 mg tid-qid; sus rel 15 mg qd in AM or 10 mg q12h; rec 25 mg/bid; IM 5-10 mg; may repeat q4h, not to exceed 40 mg/day

• *Child 18-39 kg:* PO 2.5 mg tid or 5 mg bid, not to exceed 15 mg/day; IM 0.132 mg/kg
• *Child 14-17 kg:* PO/rec 2.5 mg bid-tid, not to exceed 10 mg/day; IM 0.132 mg/kg
• *Child 9-13 kg:* PO/rec 2.5 mg qd-bid, not to exceed 7.5 mg/day; IM 0.132 mg/kg

Available forms include: Oral syr 5 mg/ml; inj 5 mg/ml; tabs 5, 10, 25 mg; sus rel caps 10, 15, 30 mg; supp 2.5, 5, 25 mg

Side effects/adverse reactions:
▼ *ORAL:* Dry mouth, metallic taste, lichenoid reaction
CNS: *Euphoria,* ***depression, extrapyramidal symptoms,*** restlessness, tremor, dizziness
CV: ***Circulatory failure, tachycardia***
GI: Nausea, vomiting, anorexia, diarrhea, constipation, weight loss, cramps
RESP: ***Respiratory depression***

Contraindications: Hypersensitivity to phenothiazines, coma, seizure, encephalopathy, bone marrow depression

Precautions: Children <2 yr, pregnancy category C, elderly

Pharmacokinetics:
PO: Onset 30-40 min, duration 3-4 hr
SUS REL: Onset 30-40 min, duration 10-12 hr
REC: Onset 60 min, duration 3-4 hr
IM: Onset 10-20 min, duration 12 hr
Metabolized by liver, excreted by kidneys, crosses placenta, excreted in breast milk

Drug interactions of concern to dentistry:
• Increased sedation: other CNS depressants, alcohol, barbiturate anesthetics, opioid analgesics
• Hypotension, tachycardia: epinephrine
• Increased extrapyramidal effects: phenothiazines and related drugs (haloperidol, droperidol), metoclopramide
• Additive photosensitization: tetracyclines
• Increased anticholinergic effects: anticholinergics

DENTAL CONSIDERATIONS

General:
• Monitor vital signs at every appointment because of cardiovascular side effects.
• Patients on chronic drug therapy may rarely have symptoms of blood dyscrasias, which can include infection, bleeding, and poor healing.
• After supine positioning, have patient sit upright for at least 2 min before standing to avoid orthostatic hypotension.
• Assess salivary flow as a factor in caries, periodontal disease, and candidiasis.
• Avoid dental light in patient's eyes; offer dark glasses for patient comfort.
• Assess for presence of extrapyramidal motor symptoms, such as tardive dyskinesia and akathisia. Extrapyramidal motor activity may complicate dental treatment.
• Geriatric patients are more susceptible to drug effects; use lower dose.
• Use vasoconstrictors with caution, in low doses, and with careful aspiration.

Consultations:
• In a patient with symptoms of blood dyscrasias, request a medical consultation for blood studies and postpone dental treatment until normal values are reestablished.

• Take precautions if dental surgery is anticipated and anesthesia is required.
• If signs of tardive dyskinesia or akathisia are present, refer to physician.

Teach patient/family:
• Importance of good oral hygiene to prevent soft tissue inflammation
• Caution to prevent injury when using oral hygiene aids
• To use electric toothbrush if patient has difficulty holding conventional devices

When chronic dry mouth occurs, advise patient:
• To avoid mouth rinses with high alcohol content because of drying effects
• Of need for daily use of home fluoride products to prevent caries
• To use sugarless gum, frequent sips of water, or saliva substitutes

procyclidine HCl

(proe-sye'kli-deen)
Kemadrin
♣ PMS-Procyclidine, Procyclid
Drug class.: Anticholinergic, antidyskinetic

Action: Blockade of central acetylcholine receptors
Uses: Parkinson symptoms, extrapyramidal symptoms associated with neuroleptic drugs
Dosage and routes:
• *Adult:* PO 2.5 mg tid pc, titrated to patient response up to 5 mg tid
Available forms include: Tabs 5 mg; elixir 2.5 mg/5 ml
Side effects/adverse reactions:
▼ *ORAL: Dry mouth,* glossitis
CNS: Confusion, anxiety, restlessness, irritability, delusions, hallucinations, headache, sedation, depression, incoherence, dizziness, light-headedness, memory loss
CV: Palpitation, tachycardia, postural hypotension, bradycardia
GI: Constipation, nausea, vomiting, abdominal distress, paralytic ileus, ***epigastric distress***
GU: Hesitancy, retention
EENT: Blurred vision, photophobia, dilated pupils, difficulty swallowing, mydriasis
INTEG: Rash, urticaria, dermatoses
MS: Weakness, cramping
MISC: Increased temperature, flushing, decreased sweating, hyperthermia, heatstroke, numbness of fingers
Contraindications: Hypersensitivity, narrow-angle glaucoma, myasthenia gravis, GI/GU obstruction, child <3 yr, megacolon, stenosing peptic ulcer
Precautions: Pregnancy category C, elderly, lactation, tachycardia, prostatic hypertrophy, children, kidney or liver disease, drug abuse, hypotension, hypertension, psychiatric patients
Pharmacokinetics:
PO: Onset 30-45 min, duration 4-6 hr

Drug interactions of concern to dentistry:
• Increased anticholinergic effect: antihistamines, anticholinergics, meperidine
• Increased CNS depression: alcohol, CNS depressants

DENTAL CONSIDERATIONS
General:
• Monitor vital signs at every appointment because of cardiovascular side effects.
• Assess salivary flow as a factor in caries, periodontal disease, and candidiasis.
• After supine positioning, have

patient sit upright for at least 2 min before standing to avoid orthostatic hypotension.

• Avoid dental light in patient's eyes; offer dark glasses for patient comfort.

• Do not ingest sodium bicarbonate products, such as the air polishing system ProphyJet, within 1 hr of taking procyclidine.

• Place on frequent recall because of oral side effects.

Consultations:

• Medical consultation may be required to assess disease control.

• Medical consultation may be required to assess patient's ability to tolerate stress.

Teach patient/family:

• Use of electric toothbrush if patient has difficulty holding conventional devices

• Importance of good oral hygiene to prevent soft tissue inflammation

• Caution to prevent injury when using oral hygiene aids

When chronic dry mouth occurs, advise patient:

• To avoid mouth rinses with high alcohol content because of drying effects

• To use daily home fluoride products for anticaries effect

• To use sugarless gum, frequent sips of water, or saliva substitutes

---

promethazine HCl

(proe-meth'a-zeen)

Phenergan

✤ Histanil

Drug class.: Antihistamine, H_1-receptor antagonist

Action: Acts on blood vessels, GI, respiratory system by competing with histamine for H_1-receptor site; decreases allergic response by blocking histamine

Uses: Motion sickness, rhinitis, allergy symptoms, sedation, nausea, preoperative or postoperative sedation

Dosage and routes:

Nausea:

• *Adult:* PO/IM 25 mg, may repeat 12.5-25 mg q4-6h; rec 12.5-25 mg q4-6h

• *Child >2 yr:* PO/IM/rec 0.5 mg/lb q4-6h not to exceed adult dose

Motion sickness:

• *Adult:* PO 12.5-25 mg bid, may repeat tid or qid

• *Child >2 yr:* PO/IM/rec 12.5-25 mg bid not to exceed adult dose

Allergy/rhinitis:

• *Adult:* PO 12.5 mg qid or 25 mg hs

• *Child >2 yr:* PO 6.25-12.5 mg tid or 25 mg hs not to exceed adult dose

Sedation:

• *Adult:* PO/IM 25-50 mg hs

• *Child >2 yr:* PO/IM/rec 12.5-25 mg hs not to exceed adult dose

Sedation (preoperative/postoperative):

• *Adult:* PO/IM/IV 25-50 mg

• *Child >2 yr:* PO/IM/IV 12.5-25 mg not to exceed adult dose

Available forms include: Tabs 12.5, 25, 50 mg; syr 6.25, 25 mg/5 ml; supp 12.5, 25, 50 mg; inj 25, 50 mg/ml

Side effects/adverse reactions:

▼ *ORAL:* Dry mouth

CNS: Dizziness, drowsiness, poor coordination, fatigue, anxiety, euphoria, confusion, paresthesia, neuritis

CV: Hypotension, palpitation, tachycardia

GI: Constipation, nausea, vomiting, anorexia, diarrhea
RESP: Increased thick secretions, wheezing, chest tightness
HEMA: ***Thrombocytopenia, agranulocytosis, hemolytic anemia***
GU: Retention, dysuria, frequency
EENT: Blurred vision, dilated pupils, tinnitus, nasal stuffiness, dry nose/throat, photosensitivity
INTEG: Rash, urticaria, photosensitivity

Contraindications: Hypersensitivity to H_1-receptor antagonist, acute asthma attack, lower respiratory tract disease

Precautions: Increased intraocular pressure, renal disease, cardiac disease, hypertension, bronchial asthma, seizure disorder, stenosed peptic ulcers, hyperthyroidism, prostatic hypertrophy, bladder neck obstruction, pregnancy category C

Pharmacokinetics:
PO: Onset 20 min, duration 4-6 hr; metabolized in liver; excreted by kidneys, GI tract (inactive metabolites)

Drug interactions of concern to dentistry:
- Increased CNS depression: alcohol, all CNS depressants
- Hypotension: general anesthetics
- Increased effect of anticholinergic drugs

DENTAL CONSIDERATIONS
General:
- Determine why the patient is taking the drug.
- Patients on chronic drug therapy may rarely have symptoms of blood dyscrasias, which can include infection, bleeding, and poor healing.
- Monitor vital signs at every appointment because of cardiovascular side effects.
- Assess salivary flow as a factor in caries, periodontal disease, and candidiasis.
- Assess vital signs q30min after use as sedative.

Teach patient/family:
When chronic dry mouth occurs, advise patient:
- To avoid mouth rinses with high alcohol content because of drying effects
- Of need for daily use of home fluoride products to prevent caries
- To use sugarless gum, frequent sips of water, or saliva substitutes

propafenone
(proe-pa-fen′one)
Rythmol

Drug class.: Antidysrhythmic (class Ic)

Action: Able to slow conduction velocity; reduces cardiac muscle membrane responsiveness; inhibits automaticity; increases ratio of effective refractory period to action potential duration; β-blocking activity

Uses: Documented life-threatening dysrhythmias; unapproved: sustained ventricular tachycardia

Dosage and routes:
- *Adult:* PO initial doses 150 mg q8h; allow a 3-4 day interval before increasing dose; 900 mg max daily dose

Available forms include: Tabs 150, 225, 300 mg

Side effects/adverse reactions:
▼ *ORAL:* Dry mouth, altered taste, stomatitis
CNS: ***Seizures,*** headache, dizzi-

ness, abnormal dreams, syncope, confusion

CV: ***Sudden death,*** dysrhythmias, palpitation, AV block, intraventricular conduction delay, AV dissociation, CHF, atrial flutter

GI: Nausea, vomiting, ***hepatitis,*** constipation, dyspepsia, cholestasis, abnormal liver function studies

RESP: Dyspnea

HEMA: ***Leukopenia, agranulocytosis, granulocytopenia, thrombocytopenia,*** anemia

EENT: Blurred vision, tinnitus

INTEG: Rash

Contraindications: Second- and third-degree heart block, right bundle branch block, cardiogenic shock, hypersensitivity, bradycardia, uncontrolled CHF, sick sinus node syndrome, marked hypotension, bronchospastic disorders

Precautions: CHF, hypokalemia, hyperkalemia, recent MI, nonallergic bronchospasm, pregnancy category C, lactation, children, hepatic or renal disease

Pharmacokinetics: Peak 3-5 hr, half-life 2-10 hr; metabolized in liver; excreted in urine (metabolite)

Drug interactions of concern to dentistry:

• No specific interactions are reported; however, any drug that could affect the cardiac action of propafenone (other local anesthetics, vasoconstrictors, anticholinergics) should be used in the lowest effective dose

DENTAL CONSIDERATIONS

General:

• Monitor vital signs at every appointment because of cardiovascular side effects.

• Patients on chronic drug therapy may rarely have symptoms of blood dyscrasias, which can include infection, bleeding, and poor healing.

• Assess salivary flow as a factor in caries, periodontal disease, and candidiasis.

• Stress from dental procedures may compromise cardiovascular function; determine patient risk.

• Consider semisupine chair position for patients with respiratory distress.

Consultations:

• In a patient with symptoms of blood dyscrasias, request a medical consultation for blood studies and postpone dental treatment until normal values are reestablished.

• Medical consultation may be required to assess disease control and patient's ability to tolerate stress.

Teach patient/family:

• Importance of good oral hygiene to prevent soft tissue inflammation

• Caution to prevent injury when using oral hygiene aids

When chronic dry mouth occurs, advise patient:

• To avoid mouth rinses with high alcohol content because of drying effects

• Of need for daily use of home fluoride products to prevent caries

• To use sugarless gum, frequent sips of water, or saliva substitutes

propantheline bromide

(proe-pan'the-leen)

Pro-Banthine

Propanthel

Drug class.: Anticholinergic

Action: Inhibits muscarinic actions of acetylcholine at postganglionic parasympathetic neuroeffector sites

P

Uses: Treatment of peptic ulcer disease, irritable bowel syndrome, duodenography, urinary incontinence; unapproved: reduction in salivary flow

Dosage and routes:

• *Adult:* PO 15 mg tid ac, 30 mg hs

• *Elderly:* PO 7.5 mg tid ac

Antisialagogue:

• *Adult:* 7.5-15 mg 45-60 min before dental appointment

Available forms include: Tabs 7.5, 15 mg

Side effects/adverse reactions:

▼ *ORAL: Dry mouth,* absence of taste

CNS: Confusion, stimulation in elderly, headache, insomnia, dizziness, drowsiness, anxiety, weakness, hallucinations

CV: Palpitation, tachycardia

GI: Constipation, ***paralytic ileus,*** heartburn, nausea, vomiting, dysphagia

GU: Hesitancy, retention, impotence

EENT: Blurred vision, photophobia, mydriasis, cycloplegia, increased ocular tension

INTEG: Urticaria, rash, pruritus, anhidrosis, fever, allergic reactions

Contraindications: Hypersensitivity to anticholinergics, narrow-angle glaucoma, GI obstruction, myasthenia gravis, paralytic ileus, GI atony, toxic megacolon

Precautions: Hyperthyroidism, CAD, dysrhythmias, CHF, ulcerative colitis, hypertension, hiatal hernia, hepatic disease, renal disease, pregnancy category C, urinary retention, prostatic hypertrophy

Pharmacokinetics:

PO: Onset 30-45 min, duration 6 hr; metabolized by liver, GI system; excreted in urine, bile

Drug interactions of concern to dentistry:

• Increased anticholinergic effect: other anticholinergic drugs

• Constipation, urinary retention: opioid analgesics

• Decreased absorption of ketoconazole; take doses 2 hr apart

DENTAL CONSIDERATIONS

General:

• Assess salivary flow as a factor in caries, periodontal disease, and candidiasis.

• Avoid dental light in patient's eyes; offer dark glasses for patient comfort.

• Place on frequent recall because of oral side effects.

• Avoid prescribing aspirin-containing products.

• Consider semisupine chair position for patient comfort because of GI effects of disease.

Consultations:

• Physician should be informed if significant xerostomic side effects occur (e.g., increased caries, sore tongue, problems eating or swallowing, difficulty wearing prosthesis) so that a medication change can be considered.

Teach patient/family:

When chronic dry mouth occurs, advise patient:

• To avoid mouth rinses with high alcohol content because of drying effects

• Of need for daily use of home fluoride products to prevent caries

• To use sugarless gum, frequent sips of water, or saliva substitutes

propofol

(proe-po'fole)

Diprivan

Drug class.: General anesthetic

Action: Produces dose-dependent CNS depression; mechanism of action is unknown

Uses: Induction or maintenance of anesthesia as part of balanced anesthetic technique, ICU sedation

Dosage and routes:

WARNING: Propofol should be administered by persons trained in the administration of general anesthesia. Patients must be continuously monitored, and facilities for maintenance of a patent airway, ventilatory support, oxygen supplementation, and circulatory resuscitation must be immediately available. Strict aseptic technique must be followed in handling propofol.

Induction of general anesthesia:

- *Adult <55 yr ASA I or II:* IV 2-2.5 mg/kg, approximately 40 mg q10sec until induction onset
- *Child >3 yr:* IV 2.5-3.5 mg/kg over 20-30 sec
- *Elderly or ASA III or IV patients:* IV 1-1.5 mg/kg, approximately 20 mg q10sec until induction onset

Maintenance:

- *Adult <55 yr:* IV 0.1-0.2 mg/kg/min (6-12 mg/kg/hr)
- *Child >3 yr:* IV 125-300 μg/kg/min (7.5-18 mg/kg/hr)
- *Elderly or ASA III or IV patients:* IV 0.05-0.1 mg/kg/min (3-6 mg/kg/hr)

Intermittent bolus (maintenance):

- *Adult:* IV increments of 25-50 mg as needed with nitrous oxide/oxygen

NOTE: Only general dose information is listed because all doses should be individualized and carefully adjusted for each patient.

Available forms include: Inj 10 mg/ml in 20 ml amp, 50, 100 ml inf vials

Side effects/adverse reactions:

▼ *ORAL:* Dry mouth, strange taste

CNS: Movement, headache, jerking, fever, dizziness, shivering, tremor, confusion, somnolence, paresthesia, agitation, abnormal dreams, euphoria, fatigue, dystonia

CV: Bradycardia, hypotension, hypertension, PVC, PAC, tachycardia, abnormal ECG, ST segment depression

GI: Nausea, vomiting, abdominal cramping, swallowing

RESP: ***Apnea, cough, hiccups,*** dyspnea, hypoventilation, sneezing, wheezing, tachypnea, hypoxia

GU: Urine retention, green urine

EENT: Blurred vision, tinnitus, eye pain

INTEG: Flushing, phlebitis, hives, burning/stinging at injection site

MS: Myalgia

META: Hyperlipidemia

MISC: Anaphylaxis

Contraindications: Hypersensitivity

Precautions: Elderly, debilitated, respiratory depression, severe respiratory disorders, cardiac dysrhythmias, pregnancy category B, labor and delivery, lactation, children <3 yr, epilepsy

Pharmacokinetics:

IV: Onset 40 sec, rapid distribution, half-life 1-8 min, terminal elimination half-life 5-10 hr; metabolized in liver by conjugation to inactivate metabolites; 70% excreted in urine

Drug interactions of concern to dentistry:
• Increased CNS depression: alcohol, narcotics, sedative-hypnotics, antipsychotics, skeletal muscle relaxants, inhalational anesthetics

DENTAL CONSIDERATIONS
General:
• Monitor vital signs at regular intervals during recovery after use as anesthetic.
• Have someone drive patient to and from dental office if used for general anesthesia.
• Geriatric patients are more susceptible to drug effects; use lower dose.
• Use only with resuscitative equipment available and only by qualified persons trained in anesthesia.

Monitor:
• Injection site: phlebitis, burning/stinging
• ECG for changes: PVC, PAC, ST segment changes
• Allergic reactions: hives

Administer:
• After diluting with D_5W, use only glass containers when mixing; not stable in plastic
• By injection (IV only)
• Alone; do not mix with other agents before using

Perform/provide:
• Storage in light-resistant area at room temperature
• Coughing, turning, deep breathing for postoperative patients
• Safety measures: side rails, night light, call bell within reach

Evaluate:
• CNS changes: movement, jerking, tremors, dizziness, LOC, pupil reaction
• Respiratory dysfunction: respiratory depression, character, rate, rhythm; notify physician if respirations are <10/min

Treatment of overdose:
• Discontinue drug, artificial ventilation, administer vasopressor agents or anticholinergics

---

propoxyphene HCl/ propoxyphene napsylate

(proe-pox'i-feen)

Darvon-N, Darvon Pulvules

Drug class.: Synthetic opioid narcotic analgesic

Controlled Substance Schedule IV

Action: Depresses pain impulse transmission in the CNS by interacting with opioid receptors

Uses: Mild-to-moderate pain

Dosage and routes:
• *Adult:* PO 65 mg q4h prn (HCl); PO 100 mg q4h prn (napsylate); commonly used in combination products with ASA or APAP (see Appendix F)

Available forms include: HCl–caps 65 mg; napsylate–tabs 100 mg

Side effects/adverse reactions:

▼ *ORAL:* Dry mouth

CNS: Drowsiness, dizziness, confusion, headache, sedation, ***convulsions, hyperthermia,*** euphoria

CV: ***Dysrhythmias,*** palpitation, bradycardia, change in BP

GI: Nausea, vomiting, anorexia, constipation, cramps

RESP: ***Respiratory depression***

GU: Increased urinary output, dysuria

EENT: Tinnitus, blurred vision, miosis, diplopia

INTEG: ***Rash,*** urticaria, bruising, flushing, diaphoresis, pruritus

Contraindications: Hypersensitivity to ASA products (some preparations), addiction (narcotic), ritonavir, suicidal patient
Precautions: Addictive personality, pregnancy category C, lactation, increased intracranial pressure, MI (acute), severe heart disease, respiratory depression, hepatic disease, renal disease, child <18 yr, alcoholism
Pharmacokinetics:
PO: Onset 15-30 min, peak 2-3 hr, duration 4-6 hr; metabolized by liver; half-life 6-12 hr; excreted by kidneys (as metabolites); equimolar doses of HCl or napsylate provide similar plasma levels
Drug interactions of concern to dentistry:
- Increased effects with other CNS depressants: alcohol, narcotics, sedative-hypnotics, skeletal muscle relaxants
- Contraindication: MAOIs
- Increased effects of anticholinergics, antihypertensives, carbamazepine

DENTAL CONSIDERATIONS
General:
- Monitor vital signs because of cardiovascular and respiratory side effects.
- Consider semisupine chair position for patient comfort if GI side effects occur.
- Assess salivary flow as a factor in caries, periodontal disease, and candidiasis.
- Psychologic and physical dependence may occur with chronic administration.
- When combined with nonopioid analgesics (aspirin, NSAIDs, acetaminophen), permits better-quality pain relief.

Teach patient/family:
When chronic dry mouth occurs, advise patient:
- To avoid mouth rinses with high alcohol content because of drying effects
- Of need for daily use of home fluoride products to prevent caries
- To use sugarless gum, frequent sips of water, or artificial saliva substitutes

propranolol HCl

(proe-pran'oh-lole)
Inderal, Inderal LA, InnoPran XL
♣ Apo-Propranolol, Detensol, Novo-Pranol, PMS-Propranolol
Drug class.: Nonselective β-adrenergic blocker

Action: This is a nonselective β_1- and β_2-adrenergic antagonist. The antihypertensive mechanism of action is unclear, but it may include a reduction in cardiac output and inhibition of renin release by the renal juxtaglomerular apparatus. Peripheral resistance decreases with long-term use. The antianginal action (when indicated for this use) may be related to a decrease in myocardial oxygen demand and negative chronotropic and inotropic effects. The antiarrhythmic action (when indicated for this use) has been related to a reduction in spontaneous pacemaker firing and slowing of AV nodal conduction.
Uses: Chronic stable angina pectoris, hypertension, supraventricular dysrhythmias (class II), migraine, MI prophylaxis, pheochromocytoma, essential tremor, hypertrophic cardiomyopathy, anxiety

P

Dosage and routes:
Dysrhythmias:
• *Adult:* PO 10-30 mg tid-qid; IV bol 0.5-3 mg over 1 mg/min; may repeat in 2 min
Hypertension:
• *Adult:* PO sus rel 40 mg bid or 80 mg qd initially; usual dose 120-240 mg/day bid-tid or 120-160 mg qd
Angina:
• *Adult:* PO sus rel 80-320 mg in divided doses bid-qid or 80 mg qd; usual dose 160 mg qd
MI:
• *Adult:* PO 180-240 mg/day tid-qid
Migraine:
• *Adult:* PO sus rel 80 mg/day or in divided doses; may increase to 160-240 mg/day in divided doses
Available forms include: Sus rel caps 60, 80, 120, 160 mg; tabs 10, 20, 40, 60, 80, 90 mg; inj 1 mg/ml; oral sol 4 mg, 8 mg/ml; conc oral sol 80 mg/ml
Side effects/adverse reactions:
▼ *ORAL:* Dry mouth, lichenoid reaction
CNS: Depression, hallucinations, dizziness, fatigue, lethargy, paresthesias, bizarre dreams, disorientation
CV: Bradycardia, hypotension, ***CHF,*** palpitation, AV block, peripheral vascular insufficiency, vasodilation
GI: Nausea, vomiting, diarrhea, colitis, constipation, cramps, hepatomegaly, gastric pain, acute pancreatitis
RESP: Bronchospasm, dyspnea, respiratory dysfunction
HEMA: ***Agranulocytosis, thrombocytopenia***
GU: Impotence, decreased libido, UTIs
EENT: ***Laryngospasm,*** blurred vision, sore throat, dry eyes
INTEG: Rash, pruritus, fever
MS: Joint pain, arthralgia, muscle cramps, pain
META: Hypoglycemia
MISC: Facial swelling, weight change, Raynaud's disease
Contraindications: Hypersensitivity to this drug, cardiac failure, cardiogenic shock, second- and third-degree heart block, bronchospastic disease, sinus bradycardia, CHF
Precautions: Diabetes mellitus, pregnancy category C, renal disease, lactation, hyperthyroidism, COPD, hepatic disease, children, myasthenia gravis, peripheral vascular disease, hypotension
Pharmacokinetics:
PO: Onset 30 min, peak 1-1.5 hr
IV: Onset 2 min, peak 15 min, duration 3-6 hr, half-life 3-5 hr (immed rel), 8-11 hr (sus rel); metabolized by liver; crosses placenta, blood-brain barrier; excreted in breast milk
Drug interactions of concern to dentistry:
• Decreased hypotensive effect: indomethacin, NSAIDs
• Increased hypotension, myocardial depression: hydrocarbon inhalation anesthetics
• Hypertension, bradycardia: sympathomimetics (epinephrine, ephedrine)
• Suspected increase in plasma levels: diphenhydramine
• Slow metabolism of lidocaine
• Decreased effects: didanosine (take 2 hr before didanosine tabs)
DENTAL CONSIDERATIONS
General:
• Monitor vital signs at every ap-

pointment because of cardiovascular side effects.

• Patients on chronic drug therapy may rarely have symptoms of blood dyscrasias, which can include infection, bleeding, and poor healing.

• Limit use of sodium-containing products, such as saline IV fluids, for patients with a dietary salt restriction.

• Assess salivary flow as a factor in caries, periodontal disease, and candidiasis.

• After supine positioning, have patient sit upright for at least 2 min before standing to avoid orthostatic hypotension.

• Stress from dental procedures may compromise cardiovascular function; determine patient risk.

• Short appointments and a stress reduction protocol may be required for anxious patients.

• Consider semisupine chair position for patients with respiratory distress.

• Use vasoconstrictors with caution, in low doses, and with careful aspiration. Avoid use of gingival retraction cord with epinephrine.

Consultations:

• In a patient with symptoms of blood dyscrasias, request a medical consultation for blood studies and postpone dental treatment until normal values are reestablished.

• Medical consultation may be required to assess disease control and patient's ability to tolerate stress.

Teach patient/family:

• Caution to prevent injury when using oral hygiene aids

• Importance of good oral hygiene to prevent soft tissue inflammation

When chronic dry mouth occurs, advise patient:

• To avoid mouth rinses with high alcohol content because of drying effects

• Of need for daily use of home fluoride products to prevent caries

• To use sugarless gum, frequent sips of water, or saliva substitutes

---

propylthiouracil (ptu)

(proe-pil-thye-oh-yoor'a-sil)

generic

✱ Propyl-Thyracil

Drug class.: Thyroid hormone antagonist

Action: Blocks synthesis of thyroid hormones T_3, T_4 (triiodothyronine), and T_4 (thyroxine)

Uses: Preparation for thyroidectomy, thyrotoxic crisis, hyperthyroidism, thyroid storm

Dosage and routes:

Hyperthyroidism:

• *Adult:* PO 100 mg tid, increasing to 300 mg q8h if condition is severe; continue to euthyroid state, then 100 mg qd-tid

• *Child >10 yr:* PO 100 mg tid; continue to euthyroid state, then 25 mg tid to 100 mg bid

• *Child 6-10 yr:* PO 50-150 mg in divided doses q8h

Available forms include: Tabs 50 mg

Side effects/adverse reactions:

▼ *ORAL:* Loss of taste, bleeding (rare)

CNS: Drowsiness, headache, vertigo, fever, paresthesias, neuritis

GI: Nausea, diarrhea, vomiting, ***jaundice, hepatitis***

HEMA: ***Agranulocytosis, leukopenia, thrombocytopenia, hypothrombinemia, lymphadenopathy,*** bleeding, vasculitis, periarteritis

P

GU: ***Nephritis***
INTEG: Rash, urticaria, pruritus, alopecia, hyperpigmentation, lupus-like syndrome
MS: Myalgia, arthralgia, nocturnal muscle cramps
Contraindications: Hypersensitivity, pregnancy category D, lactation
Precautions: Infection, bone marrow depression, hepatic disease
Pharmacokinetics:
PO: Onset 30-40 min, duration 2-4 hr, half-life 1-2 hr; excreted in urine, bile, breast milk; crosses placenta
Drug interactions of concern to dentistry:
- Increased CV side effects in uncontrolled patients: anticholinergics and sympathomimetics
- Patients with uncontrolled hyperthyroidism are at risk when vasoconstrictors are used
- Patients with uncontrolled hypothyroidism may be more responsive to CNS depressants

DENTAL CONSIDERATIONS
General:
- Patients on chronic drug therapy may rarely have symptoms of blood dyscrasias, which can include infection, bleeding, and poor healing.
- Patients with uncontrolled hyperthyroidism should not be treated in the dental office until thyroid values are normalized.
- Uncontrolled patients should be referred for medical evaluation and treatment.
- Monitor vital signs at every appointment because of cardiovascular side effects.
- Consider semisupine chair position for patient comfort if GI side effects occur.

Consultations:
- Medical consultation may be required to assess disease control and patient's ability to tolerate stress.

protriptyline HCl

(proe-trip'te-leen)
Vivactil
Triptil
Drug class.: Tricyclic antidepressant

Action: Inhibits both norepinephrine and serotonin (5-HT) uptake in the brain, although the precise antidepressant mechanism remains unclear
Uses: Depression; unapproved use: adjunctive use in narcolepsy and attention-deficit disorders
Dosage and routes:
- *Adult:* PO 15-40 mg/day in divided doses; may increase to 60 mg/day
- *Adolescent and elderly:* PO 5 mg tid

Available forms include: Tabs 5, 10 mg
Side effects/adverse reactions:
ORAL: Dry mouth, unpleasant taste, bleeding, stomatitis
CNS: Dizziness, drowsiness, confusion, headache, anxiety, tremors, stimulation, weakness, insomnia, nightmares, EPS (elderly), increased psychiatric symptoms, paresthesia
CV: Orthostatic hypotension, ECG changes, tachycardia, ***hypertension,*** palpitation
GI: Diarrhea, ***paralytic ileus, hepatitis,*** increased appetite, nausea, vomiting, cramps, epigastric distress, jaundice
HEMA: ***Agranulocytosis, thrombo-***

cytopenia, eosinophilia, leukopenia

GU: Retention, ***acute renal failure***

EENT: Blurred vision, tinnitus, mydriasis

INTEG: Rash, urticaria, sweating, pruritus, photosensitivity

Contraindications: Hypersensitivity to tricyclic antidepressants, recovery phase of MI, convulsive disorders, prostatic hypertrophy

Precautions: Suicidal patients, severe depression, increased intraocular pressure, narrow-angle glaucoma, urinary retention, cardiac disease, hepatic disease, hyperthyroidism, electroshock therapy, elective surgery, pregnancy category not established, MAOIs

Pharmacokinetics:

PO: Onset 15-30 min, peak 24-30 hr, duration 4-6 hr, therapeutic effect 2-3 wk, half-life 67-89 hr; metabolized by liver; excreted by kidneys; crosses placenta

Drug interactions of concern to dentistry:

• Increased anticholinergic effects: muscarinic blockers, antihistamines, phenothiazines

• Increased effects of direct-acting sympathomimetics (epinephrine, levonordefrin)

• Possible risk of increased CNS depression: alcohol, barbiturates, benzodiazepines, and other CNS depressants

• Decreased antihypertensive effects of: clonidine, guanadrel, guanethidine

• Avoid concurrent use with St. John's wort

DENTAL CONSIDERATIONS

General:

• Monitor vital signs at every appointment because of cardiovascular side effects.

• Assess salivary flow as a factor in caries, periodontal disease, and candidiasis.

• Patients on chronic drug therapy may rarely have symptoms of blood dyscrasias, which can include infection, bleeding, and poor healing.

• After supine positioning, have patient sit upright for at least 2 min before standing to avoid orthostatic hypotension.

• Use vasoconstrictors with caution, in low doses, and with careful aspiration. Avoid use of gingival retraction cord with epinephrine.

• Place on frequent recall because of oral side effects.

Consultations:

• In a patient with symptoms of blood dyscrasias, request a medical consultation for blood studies and postpone dental treatment until normal values are reestablished.

• Medical consultation may be required to assess disease control.

• Physician should be informed if significant xerostomic side effects occur (e.g., increased caries, sore tongue, problems eating or swallowing, difficulty wearing prosthesis) so that a medication change can be considered.

Teach patient/family:

• Importance of good oral hygiene to prevent soft tissue inflammation

• Caution to prevent injury when using oral hygiene aids

When chronic dry mouth occurs, advise patient:

• To avoid mouth rinses with high alcohol content because of drying effects

• Of need for daily use of home fluoride products to prevent caries

• To use sugarless gum, frequent sips of water, or saliva substitutes

P

pseudoephedrine HCl/ pseudoephedrine sulfate

(soo-doe-e-fed'rin)

pseudoephedrine HCl: Cenafed, Decofed, Diametapp Maximum, Effidac24, Genaphed, Medi-Fast Sinus, Sudafed, Sudafed 12 Hour, Sinustop, Sudodrin, Simply Stuffy, Triaminic Allergy, and others

♣ Eltor 120, Robidrine

pseudoephedrine sulfate: Drixoral 12-Hour Non-Drowsy

Drug class.: α-adrenergic agonist

Action: Acts primarily on α-receptors, causing vasoconstriction in blood vessels; has some beta activity and to a lesser degree CNS stimulant effects

Uses: Decongestant, nasal congestion

Dosage and routes:

- *Adult:* PO 60 mg q6h; ext rel 60-120 mg q12h
- *Child 6-12 yr:* PO 30 mg q6h, not to exceed 120 mg/day
- *Child 2-6 yr:* PO 15 mg q6h, not to exceed 60 mg/day

Available forms include: Caps 30, 60 mg; ext rel caps 120 mg; sol 15 mg, 30 mg/5 ml drops; 7.5 mg/0.8 ml drops; tabs 30, 60 mg; ext rel tabs 120, 240 mg; con rel tabs 240 mg; chew tabs 15 mg

Side effects/adverse reactions:

▼ *ORAL:* Dry mouth

CNS: Tremors, anxiety, ***seizures,*** insomnia, headache, dizziness, anxiety, hallucinations

CV: ***Dysrhythmias,*** palpitation, tachycardia, hypertension, chest pain

GI: Anorexia, nausea, vomiting

GU: Dysuria

EENT: Dry nose, irritation of nose and throat

Contraindications: Hypersensitivity to sympathomimetics, narrow-angle glaucoma, lactation

Precautions: Pregnancy category B, cardiac disorders, hyperthyroidism, diabetes mellitus, prostatic hypertrophy

Pharmacokinetics:

PO: Onset 15-30 min, duration 4-6 hr, 8-12 hr (ext rel); metabolized in liver; excreted in feces, breast milk

Drug interactions of concern to dentistry:

- Dysrhythmia: hydrocarbon inhalation anesthetics
- Increased CNS, CV effects: sympathomimetics

DENTAL CONSIDERATIONS

General:

- Assess salivary flow as a factor in caries, periodontal disease, and candidiasis.
- Monitor vital signs at every appointment because of cardiovascular side effects.
- Consider semisupine chair position for patient comfort if GI side effects occur.

Teach patient/family:

- Use of electric toothbrush if patient has difficulty holding conventional devices

When chronic dry mouth occurs, advise patient:

- To avoid mouth rinses with high alcohol content because of drying effects
- Of need for daily use of home fluoride products to prevent caries
- To use sugarless gum, frequent sips of water, or saliva substitutes

pyrazinamide

(peer-a-zin'a-mide)
generic
✦ PMS-Pyrazinamide, Tebrazid
Drug class.: Antitubercular

Action: Bactericidal interference with lipid, nucleic acid biosynthesis
Uses: TB, as an adjunct with other drugs
Dosage and routes:
• *Adult:* PO 15-30 mg/kg/day in 3-4 divided doses, not to exceed 2 g/day
Available forms include: Tabs 500 mg
Side effects/adverse reactions:
CNS: Headache
GI: ***Hepatotoxicity,*** abnormal liver function tests, peptic ulcer
HEMA: ***Hemolytic anemia***
GU: Urinary difficulty, increased uric acid
INTEG: Photosensitivity, urticaria
Contraindications: Hypersensitivity
Precautions: Pregnancy category C, child <13 yr
Pharmacokinetics:
PO: Peak 2 hr, half-life 9-10 hr; metabolized in liver, excreted in urine (metabolites/unchanged drug)
DENTAL CONSIDERATIONS
General:
• Determine why the patient is taking the drug (for prophylaxis or active therapy).
• Determine that noninfectious status exists by ensuring that (1) anti-TB drugs have been taken >3 wk, (2) culture has confirmed TB susceptibility to antiinfectives, (3) patient has had three consecutive negative sputum smears, and (4) patient is not in the coughing stage.
Consultations:
• Medical consultation may be required to assess disease control.
Teach patient/family:
• Importance of taking medications for full length of regimen to ensure effectiveness of treatment and to prevent the emergence of resistant strains

pyridostigmine bromide

(peer-id-oh-stig'meen)
Mestinon
Drug class.: Cholinergic

Action: Inhibits destruction of acetylcholine, increasing its concentration at sites where acetylcholine is released; this facilitates transmission of impulses across myoneural junction
Uses: Nondepolarizing muscle relaxant antagonist, myasthenia gravis
Dosage and routes:
Myasthenia gravis:
• *Adult:* PO initial 30-60 mg q3-4h, titrate as required, not to exceed 1.5 g/day; IM/IV 1/30 of PO dose q2-3h; sus rel 180-540 mg 1-2 × daily at intervals of at least 6 hr
Tubocurarine antagonist:
• *Adult:* 0.6-1.2 mg IV atropine, then 10-20 mg
Available forms include: Tabs 60 mg; ext rel tabs 180 mg; syr 60 mg/5 ml; inj IM/IV 5 mg/ml
Side effects/adverse reactions:
▼ *ORAL: Salivation, tongue weakness*

P

CNS: ***Convulsions,*** dizziness, headache, sweating, confusion, incoordination, paralysis
CV: Bradycardia, ***cardiac arrest,*** tachycardia, dysrhythmias, AV block, hypotension, ECG changes
GI: Nausea, diarrhea, vomiting, cramps
RESP: Increased bronchial secretions, ***respiratory depression, bronchospasm, constriction, laryngospasm, respiratory arrest,*** SOB
GU: Frequency, incontinence
EENT: Miosis, blurred vision, lacrimation
INTEG: Rash, urticaria, flushing
MS: Weakness (arms, neck), cramps, twitching

Contraindications: Bradycardia, hypotension, obstruction of intestine, renal system, sensitivity to bromides

Precautions: Seizure disorders, bronchial asthma, coronary occlusion, hyperthyroidism, dysrhythmias, peptic ulcer, megacolon, poor GI motility, pregnancy category C, elderly, lactation

Pharmacokinetics:
PO: Onset 20-30 min, duration 3-6 hr
IM/IV/SC: Onset 2-15 min, duration 2.5-4 hr; metabolized in liver, excreted in urine

Drug interactions of concern to dentistry:
- Decreased effects: atropine, scopolamine, and other anticholinergic drugs; methocarbamol
- Reduced rate of metabolism of ester local anesthetics
- Avoid anticholinergic drugs to control excessive salivation

DENTAL CONSIDERATIONS

General:
- Monitor vital signs at every appointment because of cardiovascular and respiratory side effects.
- After supine positioning, have patient sit upright for at least 2 min before standing to avoid orthostatic hypotension.
- Schedule short appointments because of effects of disease on oral musculature.
- Avoid dental light in patient's eyes; offer dark glasses for patient comfort.
- Place on frequent recall because of oral side effects.
- Consider semisupine chair position if GI side effects occur.

Consultations:
- Medical consultation may be required to assess disease control.
- Consult with physician about adjusting dose if excessive salivation becomes a problem.

Teach patient/family:
- Use of electric toothbrush or other oral hygiene aids if patient has difficulty in maintaining oral hygiene
- Importance of good oral hygiene to prevent soft tissue inflammation
- To prevent injury when using oral hygiene aids

---

pyridoxine HCl/ vitamin B_6

(peer-i-dox'een)

Aminolin, generic, Nestrex

Drug class.: Vitamin B_6, water soluble

Action: Needed for fat, protein, and carbohydrate metabolism as a coenzyme

Uses: Vitamin B_6 deficiency associated with inborn errors of metabolism, inadequate diet; unapproved: drug-induced deficiencies

Dosage and routes:
Vitamin B_6 deficiency (dietary deficiency):
• *Adult:* PO 10-20 mg qd × 3 wk, then 2-5 mg qd (large doses ranging from 50-200 mg daily are usually required for drug-induced deficiency)
• *Child:* PO 2-10 mg qd × 3 wk, then 2-5 mg qd
Available forms include: Tabs 25, 50, 100, 250, 500 mg; enteric coat tabs 20 mg; inj IM/IV 100 mg/ml
Side effects/adverse reactions:
CNS: Paresthesia, flushing, warmth, lethargy, ataxia (rare with normal renal function)
INTEG: Pain at injection site
Contraindications: Hypersensitivity
Precautions: Pregnancy category A, lactation, children, Parkinson's disease
Pharmacokinetics: *PO/INJ:* Half-life 2-3 wk; metabolized in liver; excreted in urine
Drug interactions of concern to dentistry:
• Decreased effectiveness: levodopa
• Decreased serum levels of phenytoin, phenobarbital
DENTAL CONSIDERATIONS
General:
• Vitamin B deficiency and peripheral neuropathy may manifest with oral symptoms of glossitis and cheilosis.

quazepam

(kway'ze-pam)
Doral
Drug class.: Benzodiazepine, sedative-hypnotic

Controlled Substance Schedule IV
Action: Produces CNS depression by interacting with a benzodiazepine receptor to facilitate the action of the inhibitory neurotransmitter γ-aminobutyric acid (GABA)
Uses: Insomnia
Dosage and routes:
• *Adult:* PO 15 mg hs; may decrease if needed
Available forms include: Tabs 7.5, 15 mg
Side effects/adverse reactions:
▼ *ORAL:* Dry mouth, taste alteration
CNS: Lethargy, drowsiness, daytime sedation, dizziness, confusion, light-headedness, headache, anxiety, irritability, weakness, tremor, depression
CV: Chest pain, pulse changes, palpitation, tachycardia
GI: Nausea, vomiting, diarrhea, heartburn, abdominal pain, constipation, anorexia
HEMA: ***Leukopenia, granulocytopenia (rare)***
MISC: Joint pain, congestion, dermatitis, sweating
Contraindications: Hypersensitivity to benzodiazepines, pregnancy category X, lactation, ritonavir, saquinavir
Precautions: Hepatic disease, renal disease, suicidal individuals, drug abuse, elderly, psychosis, child <18 yr, lactation, depression, pulmonary insufficiency

Pharmacokinetics:
PO: Onset 15-45 min, duration 7-8 hr; metabolized by liver; excreted by kidneys (inactive/active metabolites); crosses placenta; excreted in breast milk

Drug interactions of concern to dentistry:
- Increased effects: CNS depressants, alcohol
- Delayed elimination: erythromycin
- Contraindicated with saquinavir, ritonavir
- Possible increase in CNS side effects: kava (herb)
- Increased serum levels and prolonged effect of benzodiazepines: erythromycin, ketoconazole, itraconazole, fluconazole, miconazole (systemic)

DENTAL CONSIDERATIONS
General:
- Assess salivary flow as a factor in caries, periodontal disease, and candidiasis.
- Psychologic and physical dependence may occur with chronic administration.
- Geriatric patients are more susceptible to drug effects; use a lower dose.
- Avoid using this drug in a patient with a history of drug abuse or alcoholism.

Consultations:
- Medical consultation may be required to assess disease control.

Teach patient/family:
When chronic dry mouth occurs, advise patient:
- To avoid mouth rinses with high alcohol content because of drying effects
- Of need for daily use of home fluoride products to prevent caries
- To use sugarless gum, frequent sips of water, or saliva substitutes

quetiapine fumarate

(kwe-tye'a-peen)
Seroquel
Drug class.: Antipsychotic, atypical

Action: Acts as an agonist at serotonin ($5\text{-}HT_2$) receptors and to a lesser extent at dopamine (D_2) receptors
Uses: Schizophrenia
Dosage and routes:
- *Adult:* PO initial dose 25 mg bid, on second day increase dose by 25 mg bid or tid, as tolerated, to target range of 300-400 mg daily by the fourth day; doses of 75 mg daily have been used

Available forms include: Tabs 25, 100, 200, 300 mg
Side effects/adverse reactions:
▼ *ORAL: Dry mouth (8%-17%),* taste perversion
CNS: Somnolence, headache, agitation, insomnia, dizziness, extrapyramidal symptoms, anorexia
CV: Orthostatic hypotension, tachycardia, palpitation, peripheral edema
GI: Abdominal pain, constipation, dyspepsia
RESP: Cough, dyspnea
HEMA: Leukopenia
EENT: Rhinitis, ear pain, pharyngitis, dry eyes, conjunctivitis
INTEG: Rash, sweating, pruritus
META: Elevation of liver enzymes, cholesterol, triglycerides
MS: Asthenia, dysarthia, hypertonia
MISC: Weight gain, flulike syndrome

Contraindications: Hypersensitivity, severe CNS depression

Precautions: Renal impairment, hepatic impairment, CV disease, thyroid disease, hyperprolactinemia, neuromalignant syndrome, tardive dyskinesia, seizure disorders, cataracts, dementia, suicide tendency, pregnancy category C, lactation; patients should be monitored for signs and symptoms of diabetes mellitus

Pharmacokinetics:

PO: Peak serum levels 1.5 hr; hepatic metabolism, renal excretion (70% as unchanged drug)

Drug interactions of concern to dentistry:

- Risk of increased CNS depression: CNS depressants

DENTAL CONSIDERATIONS

General:

- Monitor vital signs at every appointment because of cardiovascular and respiratory side effects.
- Assess salivary flow as factor in caries, periodontal disease, and candidiasis.
- Assess for presence of extrapyramidal motor symptoms, such as tardive dyskinesia and akathisia. Extrapyramidal motor activity may complicate dental treatment.
- After supine positioning, have patient sit upright for at least 2 min before standing to avoid orthostatic hypotension.
- Consider semisupine chair position for patient comfort if GI side effects occur.
- Patients on chronic drug therapy may rarely have symptoms of blood dyscrasias, which can include infection, bleeding, and poor healing.
- Place on frequent recall because of oral side effects.

Consultations:

- In a patient with symptoms of blood dyscrasias, request a medical consultation for blood studies and postpone treatment until normal values are reestablished.
- Medical consultation may be required to assess disease control and patient's ability to tolerate stress.
- If signs of tardive dyskinesia or akathisia are present, refer to physician.
- Consultation with physician may be needed if sedation or general anesthesia is required.
- Physician should be informed if significant xerostomic side effects occur (e.g., increased caries, sore tongue, problems eating or swallowing, difficulty wearing prosthesis) so that a medication change can be considered.

Teach patient/family:

- Caution to prevent trauma when using oral hygiene aids
- Use of electric toothbrush if patient has difficulty holding conventional devices
- Importance of good oral hygiene to prevent soft tissue inflammation
- Importance of updating health and drug history if physician makes any changes in evaluation or drug regimens
- To be aware of oral side effects and potential sequelae

When chronic dry mouth occurs, advise patient:

- To avoid mouth rinses with high alcohol content because of drying effects
- To use daily home fluoride products for anticaries effect

Q

• To use sugarless gum, frequent sips of water, or saliva substitutes

quinapril

(kwyn'a-pril)

Accupril

Drug class.: Angiotension-converting enzyme (ACE) inhibitor

Action: Selectively suppresses renin-angiotensin-aldosterone system; inhibits ACE; prevents conversion of angiotensin I to angiotensin II; results in dilation of arterial, venous vessels

Uses: Hypertension, alone or in combination with thiazide diuretics, heart failure

Dosage and routes:

• *Adult:* PO 10 mg qd initially, then 20-80 mg/day divided bid or qd

• *Elderly >65 yr:* PO initial 10 mg qd, then titration to optimal response

Heart failure (in combination with other measures):

• *Adult:* PO 5 mg bid, titrate upward to 20-40 mg/day

Available forms include: Tabs 5, 10, 20, 40 mg

Side effects/adverse reactions:

▼ *ORAL:* Dry mouth

CNS: Headache, dizziness, fatigue, somnolence, depression, malaise, nervousness, vertigo

CV: Hypotension, postural hypotension, syncope, palpitation, angina pectoris, MI, tachycardia, vasodilation

GI: Nausea, constipation, vomiting, gastritis, GI hemorrhage

RESP: Cough, bronchitis

HEMA: ***Thrombocytopenia, agranulocytosis***

GU: Increased BUN, creatinine, decreased libido, impotence

INTEG: ***Angioedema,*** rash, sweating, photosensitivity, pruritus

MS: Arthralgia, arthritis, myalgia, back pain

META: Hyperkalemia

MISC: Amblyopia

Contraindications: Hypersensitivity, children

Precautions: Pregnancy category D, impaired renal/liver function, dialysis patients, hypovolemia, blood dyscrasias, CHF, COPD, asthma, elderly, lactation

Pharmacokinetics:

PO: Peak 0.5-1 hr, half-life 2 hr; serum protein binding 97%; metabolized by liver (metabolites); metabolites excreted in urine

Drug interactions of concern to dentistry:

• Increased hypotension: alcohol, phenothiazines

• Decreased hypotensive effects: indomethacin and possibly other NSAIDs, sympathomimetics

• Suspected reduction in the antihypertensive and vasodilator effects by salicylates; monitor blood pressure if used concurrently

DENTAL CONSIDERATIONS

General:

• Monitor vital signs at every appointment because of cardiovascular side effects.

• After supine positioning, have patient sit upright for at least 2 min before standing to avoid orthostatic hypotension.

• Patients on chronic drug therapy may rarely have symptoms of blood dyscrasias, which can include infection, bleeding, and poor healing.

• Assess salivary flow as a factor in caries, periodontal disease, and candidiasis.

• Limit use of sodium-containing products, such as saline IV fluids, for patients with a dietary salt restriction.
• Use vasoconstrictors with caution, in low doses, and with careful aspiration.
• Stress from dental procedures may compromise cardiovascular function; determine patient risk.
• Short appointments and a stress reduction protocol may be required for anxious patients.

Consultations:
• Medical consultation may be required to assess disease control and patient's ability to tolerate stress.
• In a patient with symptoms of blood dyscrasias, request a medical consultation for blood studies and postpone dental treatment until normal values are reestablished.
• Take precautions if dental surgery is anticipated and sedation or general anesthesia is required; there is risk of a hypotensive episode.

Teach patient/family:
• Importance of good oral hygiene to prevent soft tissue inflammation
• Caution to prevent injury when using oral hygiene aids

When chronic dry mouth occurs, advise patient:
• To avoid mouth rinses with high alcohol content because of drying effects
• Of need for daily use of home fluoride products to prevent caries
• To use sugarless gum, frequent sips of water, or saliva substitutes

quinidine gluconate/ quinidine sulfate

(kwin'i-deen)

Quinaglute, Quinidex Extentabs
🍁 Apo-Quinidine, Novoquindin, Quinate

Drug class.: Antidysrhythmic (class Ia)

Action: Prolongs effective refractory period; decreases myocardial excitability, conduction velocity, and contractility; indirect anticholinergic properties

Uses: PVCs, atrial flutter and fibrillation, PAT, ventricular tachycardia

Dosage and routes:

Atrial fibrillation/flutter:
• *Adult:* PO 200 mg q2-3h × 5-8 doses; may increase qd until sinus rhythm is restored; max 4 g/day given only after digitalization

Paroxysmal supraventricular tachycardia:
• *Adult:* PO 400-600 mg q2-3h

All other dysrhythmias:
• *Adult:* PO 50-200 mg as a test dose, then 200-400 mg q4-6h

Available forms include: Gluconate–sus rel tabs 324 mg; inj 80 mg/ml in 10 ml vials; sulfate–tabs 200, 300 mg; sus rel tabs 300 mg

Side effects/adverse reactions:

▼ *ORAL: Bitter taste, lichenoid drug reaction,* pigmentation

CNS: Headache, dizziness, involuntary movement, confusion, psychosis, restlessness, irritability, syncope, excitement

CV: Hypotension, bradycardia, ***heart block, cardiovascular collapse, arrest,*** PVCs

GI: Diarrhea, ***hepatotoxicity,*** nausea, vomiting, anorexia

RESP: Dyspnea, ***respiratory depression***
HEMA: ***Thrombocytopenia,*** hemolytic anemia, agranulocytosis, hypoprothrombinemia
EENT: Cinchonism: tinnitus, blurred vision, hearing loss, mydriasis, disturbed color vision
INTEG: Rash, urticaria, angioedema, swelling, photosensitivity

Contraindications: Hypersensitivity, blood dyscrasias, severe heart block, myasthenia gravis, itraconazole

Precautions: Pregnancy category C, lactation, children, renal disease, potassium imbalance, liver disease, CHF, respiratory depression

Pharmacokinetics:
PO: Peak 0.5-6 hr (depending on form given), duration 6-8 hr, half-life 6-7 hr; metabolized in liver; excreted unchanged by kidneys

Drug interactions of concern to dentistry:
- May decrease effects of quinidine: barbiturates
- Increased anticholinergic effect: anticholinergic drugs
- Increased effects of neuromuscular blockers, tricyclic antidepressants
- Contraindicated with itraconazole
- Prevention of action: cholinergics

DENTAL CONSIDERATIONS

General:
- Monitor vital signs at every appointment because of cardiovascular and respiratory side effects.
- Patients on chronic drug therapy may rarely have symptoms of blood dyscrasias, which can include infection, bleeding, and poor healing.
- After supine positioning, have patient sit upright for at least 2 min before standing to avoid orthostatic hypotension.
- Use vasoconstrictors with caution, in low doses, and with careful aspiration. Avoid use of gingival retraction cord with epinephrine.
- Consider semisupine chair position for patient comfort if GI side effects occur.

Consultations:
- In a patient with symptoms of blood dyscrasias, request a medical consultation for blood studies and postpone dental treatment until normal values are reestablished.
- Medical consultation may be required to assess patient's ability to tolerate stress.

Teach patient/family:
- Importance of good oral hygiene to prevent soft tissue inflammation

quinine sulfate

(kwye'nine)

generic

Drug class.: Antimalarial

Action: Schizonticidal, but mechanism is unclear; increases refractory period in skeletal muscle

Uses: *P. falciparum* malaria, nocturnal leg cramps

Dosage and routes:
- *Adult:* PO 260-650 mg q8h over 3-7 days, given with concurrent antiinfective drugs
- *Child:* PO 10 mg/kg q8h for 5-7/day

Available forms include: Caps 200, 260, 325 mg; tabs 260

Side effects/adverse reactions:
▼ *ORAL:* Lichenoid drug reaction
CNS: ***Convulsion,*** headache, stimulation, fatigue, irritability, bad dreams, dizziness, fever, confusion, anxiety

CV: ***Acute circulatory failure,*** angina, dysrhythmias, tachycardia, hypotension
GI: *Nausea, vomiting, anorexia,* diarrhea, epigastric pain
HEMA: ***Thrombocytopenia, purpura, hypothrombinemia, hemolysis***
GU: Dysuria
EENT: *Blurred vision, corneal changes, retinal changes, difficulty focusing,* tinnitus, vertigo, deafness, photophobia, diplopia, night blindness
INTEG: Pruritus, pigment changes, skin eruptions, lichen planus-like eruptions, flushing, facial edema, sweating
ENDO: Hypoglycemia

Contraindications: Hypersensitivity, G6PD deficiency, retinal field changes, pregnancy category X

Precautions: Blood dyscrasias, severe GI disease, neurologic disease, severe hepatic disease, psoriasis, cardiac dysrhythmias, tinnitus

Pharmacokinetics:
PO: Peak 1-3 hr, half-life 4-5 hr; metabolized in liver; excreted in urine

Drug interactions of concern to dentistry:
• Decreased absorption: magnesium or aluminum salts
• Prolonged duration of neuromuscular blocking drugs

DENTAL CONSIDERATIONS
General:
• Patients on chronic drug therapy may rarely have symptoms of blood dyscrasias, which can include infection, bleeding, and poor healing.
• Avoid dental light in patient's eyes; offer dark glasses for patient comfort.
• Monitor vital signs at every appointment because of cardiovascular side effects.
• Consider semisupine chair position for patient comfort if GI side effects occur.

Consultations:
• Medical consultation may be required to assess disease control.
• In a patient with symptoms of blood dyscrasias, request a medical consultation for blood studies and postpone dental treatment until normal values are reestablished.

Teach patient/family:
• Importance of good oral hygiene to prevent soft tissue inflammation

---

quinupristin/ dalfopristin

(qwen'nyoo-pris-ten) (dal'foe-pristen)
Synercid I.V.
Drug class.: Antiinfective, a streptogramin antibacterial

Action: Combination of quinupristin (30%) with dalfopristin (70%); inhibition of the synthesis of bacterial protein by irreversible binding to 50S ribosomal subunits

Uses: Serious or life-threatening infections caused by vancomycin-resistant *Enterococcus faecium;* complicated skin and skin structure infections caused by *Streptococcus pyogenes* or methicillin-susceptible *Staphylococcus aureus*

Dosage and routes:
• *Adult:* IV inf in D_5W over 60 min; for vancomycin-resistant *E. faecium,* 7.5 mg/kg q8h; for complicated skin and skin structure infections, 7.5 mg/kg q12h with minimum dose duration of 7 days

R

• *Child <16 yr:* Limited data available; no dose adjustment required
Available forms include: Single-dose vial: quinupristin 150 mg and dalfopristin 350 mg/10 ml vials
Side effects/adverse reactions:
▼ *ORAL:* Candidiasis
CNS: Headache, chest pain
CV: Infusion site reactions (pain, inflammation), peripheral edema
GI: Nausea, vomiting, ***pseudomembranous colitis,*** diarrhea, abdominal pain, dyspepsia, pancreatitis
GU: UTI
INTEG: Rash, pruritus
META: Hyperbilirubinemia, elevation of ALT, AST
MS: Arthralgia, myalgia, leg cramps
MISC: Asthenia, allergic reaction
Contraindications: Known hypersensitivity or prior hypersensitivity to other streptogramins, heparin flush
Precautions: Venous irritation, inhibits cytochrome P-450 3A4 isoenzymes, pregnancy category B, lactation; hepatic impairment, safety and efficacy in children <12 yr not established
Pharmacokinetics:
IV: Both constituents are converted to active metabolites, short half-life but prolonged postantibiotic effect on *S. aureus* and *S. pneumoniae,* peak concentration 1 hr, protein-binding quinupristin (55%-78%), dalfopristin (11%-26%), extensive metabolism in liver and blood, renal excretion 20%, mostly fecal excretion
Drug interactions of concern to dentistry:
• Patients with serious, life-threatening systemic infections will not be candidates for dental care except for extreme emergencies
• Use with caution; monitor drugs metabolized by CYP3A4 isoenzymes (see Appendix I)
DENTAL CONSIDERATIONS
General:
• Examine for oral manifestation of opportunistic candida infection.

---

rabeprazole sodium

(ra-be′pray-zole)
Aciphex
Drug class.: Antisecretory, proton pump inhibitor

Action: Suppresses gastric acid production by binding to the hydrogen/potassium ATPase enzyme system to inhibit the final step in gastric acid production
Uses: Gastroesophageal reflux disease (GERD), duodenal ulcers, and hypersecretory conditions (Zollinger-Ellison disease); eradication of *Helicobacter pylori* infection (with amoxicillin and clarithromycin), *H. pylori* eradication to reduce risk of duodenal ulcer
Dosage and routes:
GERD and duodenal ulcer:
• *Adult:* PO 20 mg qd × 4-8 wk; if healing is not evident can continue 8 wk more, maintenance 80 mg/day
Hypersecretory conditions:
• *Adult:* PO 60 mg qd
H. pylori eradication:
• *Adult:* PO 20 mg bid; amoxicillin 1000 mg bid and clarithromycin 500 mg bid × 7 days
Available forms include: Del rel tabs 20 mg

Side effects/adverse reactions:
ORAL: Dry mouth, mouth ulceration
CNS: Headache, insomnia, anxiety, abnormal dreams
CV: Hypertension, ECG abnormalities, syncope, palpitation, bundle branch block
GI: Diarrhea, nausea, abdominal pain
RESP: Dyspnea, asthma, hiccups
HEMA: Anemia, abnormal blood cell counts
EENT: Dry eyes, eye pain
INTEG: Photosensitivity, rash, pruritus, sweating
ENDO: Alteration in thyroid function
META: Weight gain, gout, abnormal liver function tests
MS: Asthenia, chest pain, neck rigidity, myalgia
MISC: Fever

Contraindications: Hypersensitivity

Precautions: Do not break, crush, or chew tablets, pregnancy category B, avoid nursing, pediatric use not studied

Pharmacokinetics:
PO: Del rel tabs: bioavailability 52%, peak plasma levels 2-5 hr, half-life 1-2 hr, highly plasma protein bound (96.3%), extensive hepatic metabolism (CYP450 3A), about 90% excreted in urine

Drug interactions of concern to dentistry:
- None documented

DENTAL CONSIDERATIONS
General:
- Assess salivary flow as a factor in caries, periodontal disease, and candidiasis.
- Consider semisupine chair position for patient comfort because of GI side effects of disease.
- Patients with gastroesophageal reflux may have oral symptoms including burning mouth, secondary candidiasis, and signs of tooth erosion.
- Question the patient about tolerance of NSAIDs or aspirin related to GI problems.

Teach patient/family:
- To prevent trauma when using oral hygiene aids

When chronic dry mouth occurs, advise patient:
- To avoid mouth rinses with high alcohol content because of drying effects
- To use daily home fluoride products for anticaries effect
- To use sugarless gum, frequent sips of water, or saliva substitutes

---

raloxifene hydrochloride
(ral-ox'i-feen)
Evista

Drug class.: Synthetic estrogen

Action: Acts as a selective estrogen receptor modulator (SERM) to reduce resorption of bone and decrease overall bone turnover; may act as an estrogen antagonist in uterine and breast tissues

Uses: Prevention and treatment of osteoporosis in postmenopausal women, supplemented with calcium as based on need

Dosages and routes:
- *Adult:* PO 60 mg daily

Available forms include: Tabs 60 mg

Side effects/adverse reactions:
CNS: Insomnia, depression
CV: Chest pain, *hot flashes*
GI: Nausea, vomiting, dyspepsia, flatulence

RESP: Cough
GU: Vaginitis, UTI, cystitis, leukorrhea, vaginal bleeding
EENT: Sinusitis, pharyngitis
INTEG: Rash, sweating
ENDO: Weight gain
*MS: Leg cramps, arthralgia, m*yalgia
MISC: Flulike syndrome, infection
Contraindications: Hypersensitivity, pregnancy, prior history of venous thromboembolic events, premenopausal use, lactation, children
Precautions: Hepatic impairment, risk of thromboembolitic events, pregnancy category X, lactation
Pharmacokinetics:
PO: Rapidly absorbed, bioavailability 2%, plasma levels depend on systemic interconversion and enterohepatic cycling, highly bound to plasma proteins, extensive first-pass metabolism, glucuronide metabolites, mainly excreted in feces, urinary excretion is minor

Drug interactions of concern to dentistry:

• Reduced absorption: ampicillin
• Risk of potential drug interactions with other highly plasma protein–bound drugs is unknown, such as NSAIDs, aspirin, and diazepam

DENTAL CONSIDERATIONS

General:

• This drug should be discontinued 72 hr before prolonged immobilization such as hospitalization, postsurgical recovery, and bed rest.
• Consider short appointments and dental chair position if needed for patient comfort.

Consultations:

• Medical consultation may be required to assess disease control and patient's ability to tolerate stress.

---

ramipril

(ra-mi'pril)
Altace
Drug class.: Angiotensin-converting enzyme (ACE) inhibitor

Action: Selectively suppresses renin-angiotensin-aldosterone system; inhibits ACE; prevents conversion of angiotensin I to angiotensin II; results in dilation of arterial, venous vessels
Uses: Hypertension; alone or in combination with thiazide diuretics; CHF immediately after MI; reduce risk of MI, stroke, and death from cardiovascular causes
Dosage and routes:
• *Adult:* PO 2.5 mg qd initially, then 2.5-20 mg/day divided bid or qd; renal impairment: 1.25 mg qd with CrCl <40 ml/min/1.73 m^2, increase as needed to max of 5 mg/day
Reduction in risk of MI, stroke, and death from CV causes
• *Adult:* PO 2.5 mg/day × 1 wk initially; 5 mg/day × 3 wk, then increase dose as tolerated to 10 mg/day
Available forms include: Caps 1.25, 2.5, 5, 10 mg
Side effects/adverse reactions:
▼ *ORAL:* Angioedema (lips, tongue, mucous membranes), dry mouth
CNS: Headache, dizziness, ***convulsions,*** anxiety, insomnia, paresthesia, fatigue, depression, malaise, vertigo, hearing loss
CV: Hypotension, chest pain, palpitation, angina, syncope, dysrhythmia

GI: Nausea, constipation, vomiting, dyspepsia, dysphagia, anorexia, diarrhea, abdominal pain
RESP: Cough, dyspnea
HEMA: ***Eosinophilia, leukopenia,*** decreased Hct/Hgb
GU: ***Proteinuria,*** increased BUN, creatinine, impotence
INTEG: ***Angioedema,*** rash, sweating, photosensitivity, pruritus
MS: Arthralgia, arthritis, myalgia
META: Hyperkalemia

Contraindications: Hypersensitivity to ACE inhibitors, pregnancy category D, lactation, children

Precautions: Impaired renal/liver function, dialysis patients, hypovolemia, blood dyscrasias, CHF, COPD, asthma, elderly

Pharmacokinetics:
PO: Peak 1 hr, half-life 5 hr, duration 24 hr; high serum protein binding; metabolized by liver; metabolites excreted in urine, feces

Drug interactions of concern to dentistry:
- Increased hypotension: alcohol, phenothiazines
- Decreased hypotensive effects: indomethacin and possibly other NSAIDs, sympathomimetics
- Suspected reduction in the antihypertensive and vasodilator effects by salicylates; monitor blood pressure if used concurrently

DENTAL CONSIDERATIONS

General:
- Monitor vital signs at every appointment because of cardiovascular and respiratory side effects.
- After supine positioning, have patient sit upright for at least 2 min before standing to avoid orthostatic hypotension.
- Patients on chronic drug therapy may rarely have symptoms of blood dyscrasias, which can include infection, bleeding, and poor healing.
- Assess salivary flow as a factor in caries, periodontal disease, and candidiasis.
- Limit use of sodium-containing products, such as saline IV fluids, for patients with a dietary salt restriction.
- Use vasoconstrictors with caution, in low doses, and with careful aspiration.
- Stress from dental procedures may compromise cardiovascular function; determine patient risk.
- Short appointments and a stress reduction protocol may be required for anxious patients.

Consultations:
- Medical consultation may be required to assess patient's ability to tolerate stress.
- In a patient with symptoms of blood dyscrasias, request a medical consultation for blood studies and postpone dental treatment until normal values are reestablished.
- Take precautions if dental surgery is anticipated and sedation or general anesthesia is required; there is risk of a hypotensive episode.

Teach patient/family:
- Importance of good oral hygiene to prevent soft tissue inflammation
- Caution to prevent injury when using oral hygiene aids

When chronic dry mouth occurs, advise patient:
- To avoid mouth rinses with high alcohol content because of drying effects
- Of need for daily use of home fluoride products to prevent caries
- To use sugarless gum, frequent sips of water, or saliva substitutes

R

ranitidine

(ra-nye'te-deen)

Zantac, Zantac EFFERdose, Zantac GELdose; *OTC:* Zantac 75

🍁 Alti-Ranitidine, Apo-Ranitidine, Gen-Ranitidine, Novo-Ranitidine, Nu-Ranit

Drug class.: H_2 histamine receptor antagonist

Action: Inhibits histamine at H_2-receptor site in parietal cells, thus inhibiting gastric acid secretion

Uses: Duodenal ulcer, Zollinger-Ellison syndrome, benign gastric ulcers, hypersecretory conditions, gastroesophageal reflux disease, erosive esophagitis, stress ulcers; unapproved: GI symptoms associated with NSAID use in rheumatoid arthritis

Dosage and routes:

• *Adult:* PO 150 mg bid or 300 mg hs; IM 50 mg q6-8h; IV bol 50 mg diluted to 20 ml over 5 min q6-8h; IV int inf 50 mg/100 ml D_5 over 15-20 min q6-8h; PO (OTC dose) 75 mg qd-bid

Available forms include: Tabs (OTC) 75 mg; tabs 150, 300 mg; syr 15 mg/ml; inj IM/IV 1.0, 25 mg/ml; effervescent tabs 150 mg; effervescent granules 150 mg

Side effects/adverse reactions:

CNS: Headache, sleeplessness, dizziness, confusion, agitation, depression, hallucination

CV: Tachycardia, bradycardia, PVCs

GI: ***Hepatotoxicity,*** constipation, abdominal pain, diarrhea, nausea, vomiting

GU: Impotence, gynecomastia

EENT: Blurred vision, increased intraocular pressure

INTEG: Urticaria, rash, fever

Contraindications: Hypersensitivity

Precautions: Pregnancy category B, lactation, child <12 yr, hepatic disease, renal disease

Pharmacokinetics:

PO: Peak 2-3 hr, duration 8-12 hr, half-life 2-3 hr; less than 10% metabolized by liver; excreted in urine, breast milk

Drug interactions of concern to dentistry:

• Decreased absorption of diazepam, anticholinergics, ketoconazole (take doses 2 hr apart)

DENTAL CONSIDERATIONS

General:

• Avoid prescribing aspirin-containing products in patients with active GI disease.

• Consider semisupine chair position for patient comfort because of GI effects of disease.

repaglinide

(re-pag'lin-ide)

Prandin

Drug class.: Oral antidiabetic, meglitinide class

Action: Lowers blood glucose by stimulation of insulin release from the pancreatic β-cells; binds to ATP-dependent potassium channels in functioning β-cells with opening of calcium channels and subsequent insulin release

Uses: Type 2 diabetes mellitus when hyperglycemia cannot be controlled by diet and exercise; may also be used in combination with metformin, rosiglitazone maleate, or pioglitazone HCl

Dosage and routes:

Adult not previously treated or whose HbA$_{1c}$ is <8%:

• *Adult:* PO initial dose 0.5 mg before meals; doses can be given 2, 3, or 4 times/day depending on blood glucose control; dose range 0.5-4.0 mg with limit of 16 mg/day

Adult previously treated with blood glucose–lowering drugs and whose HbA$_{1c}$ is ≥8%:

• *Adult:* PO initial dose 1 or 2 mg before meals

Available forms include: Tabs 0.5, 1, 2 mg

Side effects/adverse reactions:

CNS: Headache, paresthesia

CV: Chest pain, angina, palpitation, hypertension, ECG changes

GI: Diarrhea, nausea, vomiting, constipation, dyspepsia

RESP: URI, bronchitis

EENT: Sinusitis, rhinitis

META: Hypoglycemia

MS: Arthralgia, back pain

Contraindications: Hypersensitivity, diabetic ketoacidosis, type 1 diabetes

Precautions: Increased cardiac mortality risk, hypoglycemia, hypoglycemia in patients taking β-adrenergic blockers, monitor laboratory values, pregnancy category C, lactation, pediatric patients

Pharmacokinetics:

PO: Rapid absorption, bioavailability 56%, peak plasma levels 1 hr; half-life 1 hr; plasma protein binding 98%, hepatic metabolism, metabolites excreted mainly in feces, small amount in urine

Drug interactions of concern to dentistry:

• Clinical studies have not been completed; metabolism may be inhibited by ketoconazole, miconazole, erythromycin

• Risk of increased hypoglycemia: NSAIDs, salicylates

• Suspected increase in plasma levels: clarithromycin, erythromycin

DENTAL CONSIDERATIONS

General:

• If dentist prescribes any of the drugs listed in the drug interactions section, monitor patient blood sugar levels.

• Consider semisupine chair position for patient comfort because of GI side effects of drug.

• Ensure that patient is following prescribed diet and regularly takes medication.

• Place on frequent recall to evaluate healing response.

• Short appointments and a stress reduction protocol may be required.

• Diabetics may be more susceptible to infection and have delayed wound healing.

Consultations:

• Medical consultation may include data from patient's blood glucose monitoring, including glycosylated hemoglobin or HbA$_{1c}$ testing.

• Medical consultation may be required to assess disease control and patient's ability to tolerate stress.

Teach patient/family:

• To prevent trauma when using oral hygiene aids

• Importance of updating health and drug history if physician makes any changes in evaluation or drug regimens

R

reserpine

(re-ser'peen)

♣ Novoreserpine, Reserfia

Drug class.: Antiadrenergic agent, antihypertensive

Action: Depletes catecholamine stores in CNS and in adrenergic nerve endings

Uses: Hypertension

Dosage and routes:

Hypertension:

• *Adult:* PO 0.25-0.5 mg qd for 1-2 wk, then 0.1-0.25 mg qd maintenance

Available forms include: Tabs 0.1, 0.25, 1 mg

Side effects/adverse reactions:

▼ *ORAL: Dry mouth,* bleeding

CNS: Drowsiness, fatigue, lethargy, dizziness, depression, anxiety, headache, increased dreaming, nightmares, convulsions, parkinsonism, EPS (high doses)

CV: ***Thrombocytopenic purpura,*** bradycardia, chest pain, dysrhythmias, prolonged bleeding time

GI: Nausea, vomiting, cramps, peptic ulcer, increased appetite, anorexia

RESP: Bronchospasm, dyspnea, cough, rales

GU: Impotence, dysuria, nocturia, sodium, water retention, edema, breast engorgement, galactorrhea, gynecomastia

EENT: Lacrimation, miosis, blurred vision, ptosis, epistaxis

INTEG: Rash, purpura, alopecia, flushing, warm feeling, pruritus, ecchymosis

Contraindications: Hypersensitivity, depression, suicidal patients, active peptic ulcer disease, ulcerative colitis, concurrently with or within 14 days of discontinuing MAOIs

Precautions: Pregnancy category C, lactation, seizure disorders, renal disease

Pharmacokinetics:

PO: Peak 4 hr, duration 2-6 wk, half-life 50-100 hr; metabolized by liver; excreted in urine, feces, breast milk; crosses placenta, blood-brain barrier

Drug interactions of concern to dentistry:

• Increased CNS depression: barbiturates, alcohol, opioids

• Increased pressor effects: epinephrine

• Decreased pressor effects: ephedrine, tricyclic antidepressants

• Decreased hypotensive effect: indomethacin and possibly other NSAIDs

DENTAL CONSIDERATIONS

General:

• Monitor vital signs at every appointment because of cardiovascular side effects.

• Patients on chronic drug therapy may rarely have symptoms of blood dyscrasias, which can include infection, bleeding, and poor healing.

• Assess salivary flow as a factor in caries, periodontal disease, and candidiasis.

• After supine positioning, have patient sit upright for at least 2 min before standing to avoid orthostatic hypotension.

• Limit use of sodium-containing products, such as saline IV fluids, for patients with a dietary salt restriction.

Consultations:

• Medical consultation may be required to assess disease control.

Teach patient/family:
• Importance of good oral hygiene to prevent soft tissue inflammation
When chronic dry mouth occurs, advise patient:
• To avoid mouth rinses with high alcohol content because of drying effects
• Of need for daily use of home fluoride products to prevent caries
• To use sugarless gum, frequent sips of water, or saliva substitutes

---

ribavirin

(rye-ba-vye'rin)
Copegus, Rebetol, Virazole
Drug class.: Antiviral

Action: The precise mechanism of action is unknown but has a wide antiviral spectrum of activity; after transport into cells it is converted to monophosphate, diphosphate, and triphosphate forms that inhibit selective viral enzymes

Uses: Treatment of adults and children with chronic hepatitis C but only in combination with interferon alfa-2b or peginterferon alfa-2a; patients must have compensated liver disease and not previously been treated with interferons; respiratory syncytial virus (RSV) in hospitalized infants and young children, unapproved use in influenza A or B or in lower respiratory tract pneumonia associated with an adenovirus

Dosage and routes:

Chronic hepatitis C:
• *Adult (for Copegus only):* PO 800-1200 mg/day divided into 2 equal doses with food; dose must be individualized for each patient depending on baseline disease characteristics (gene type), preexisting cardiac disease, response to therapy, regimen tolerability, and hemoglobin values; take with food; must be used in combination with peginterferon alfa-2a; duration 24-48 wk
• *Adult (for Rebetol only):* PO for body weight <75 kg 400 mg in AM and 600 mg in PM; for body weight >75 kg 600 mg in AM and 600 mg in PM; in combination with peginterferon alfa-2a or interferon alfa-2b the dose is 800 mg/day in 2 equally divided doses; all doses are taken with food; dose modifications are required in preexisting cardiac disease, creatine clearance, hemoglobin levels, and other factors
• *Child (for Rebetol only):* PO: 25-36 kg 200 mg in AM and PM daily; 37-49 kg 200 mg in AM and 400 mg daily in PM; 50-61 kg 400 mg in AM and PM daily; over 61 kg use adult dose; used in combination with interferon alfa-2b; duration up to 48 wk; child <25 kg, recommended dose is 15 mg/kg per day in equally divided doses AM and PM; use oral concentrate for child who cannot take capsules

RSV infections:
• *Child:* INH aerosol 20 mg/ml solution for use in a SPAG-2 unit, apply treatment for 12-18 hr/day for 3-7 days

Available forms include: Tabs 200 mg; caps 200 mg; oral sol 40 mg/ml in 120 ml, powder for aerosol preparation 6 g/100 ml vial

Side effects/adverse reactions:
NOTE: Side effects may reflect interferon use as well.
▼ *ORAL: Dry mouth*
CNS: Depression, psychiatric reactions, insomnia, anxiety, anorexia, headache, dizziness, ***suicide,*** fatigue, anorexia

CV: ***Myocardial infarction***
GI: Nausea, vomiting, abdominal pain, dyspepsia
RESP: Dyspnea, cough
HEMA: Neutropenia, thrombocytopenia, anemia, lymphopenia, ***hemolytic anemia***
EENT: Blurred vision
INTEG: Alopecia, pruritus, dermatitis, dry skin, rash, eczema, sweating
ENDO: Hypothyroidism
META: Weight loss
MS: Myalgia, arthralgia, back pain
MISC: Relapse of drug abuse, bacterial infections, flulike symptoms

Contraindications: Concurrent use with didanosine, stavudine, zidovudine; unstable cardiac disease; hypersensitivity, pregnancy, men with pregnant female partners, hemoglobinopathies (thalassemia major, sickle cell anemia), creatinine clearance <50 ml/min, autoimmune hepatitis, hepatic decompensation (Child-Pugh class B and C)

Precautions: Must not be used alone for hepatitis C, severe side effects occur, pregnancy category X, aggravation of sarcoidosis, stop therapy if pancreatitis occurs, use aerosol only for RSV, extra contraception required to prevent pregnancy during use and for up to 6 mo after discontinuing use

Pharmacokinetics:
PO: Bioavailability increased by high-fat meal, absolute bioavailability 64%, peak plasma levels 1-1.6 hr, half-life 298 hr, metabolism and excretion mechanisms unknown

Drug interactions of concern to dentistry:
- None reported

DENTAL CONSIDERATIONS

General:
- Patients taking this drug will also be taking an interferon drug; be sure to conduct a thorough drug history.
- Assess salivary flow as a factor in caries, periodontal disease, and candidiasis.
- Patients on chronic drug therapy may rarely have symptoms of blood dyscrasias, which can include infection, bleeding, and poor healing.
- Consider semisupine chair position for patient comfort if GI side effects occur.
- Examine for oral manifestation of opportunistic infection.
- Take precautions if dental surgery is anticipated and general anesthesia is required.
- Monitor vital signs at every appointment because of cardiovascular side effects.

Consultations:
- In a patient with symptoms of blood dyscrasias, request a medical consultation for blood studies and postpone treatment until normal values are reestablished.
- Medical consultation may be required to assess disease control and patient's ability to tolerate stress.
- Consultation with physician may be needed if sedation or general anesthesia is required.

Teach patient/family:
- Importance of updating health and drug history if physician makes any changes in evaluation/drug regimens
- Importance of good oral hygiene to prevent soft tissue inflammation
- To prevent trauma when using oral hygiene aids

When chronic dry mouth occurs, advise patient:

• To avoid mouth rinses with high alcohol content because of drying effects

• To use daily home fluoride products for anticaries effect

• To use sugarless gum, frequent sips of water, or saliva substitutes

riboflavin (vitamin B_2)

(rey'boo-flay-vin)

Various generic sources

Drug class.: Vitamin B_2, water soluble

Action: Needed for normal tissue respiratory reactions; functions as a coenzyme

Uses: Vitamin B_2 deficiency

Dosage and routes:

• *Adult and child >12 yr:* PO 5-50 mg qd

• *Child <12 yr:* PO 2-10 mg qd

Available forms include: Tabs 50, 100 mg

Side effects/adverse reactions:

GU: Yellow discoloration of urine (large doses)

Contraindications: Child <12 yr

Precautions: Pregnancy category A, lactation

Pharmacokinetics:

PO: Readily absorbed, half-life 65-85 min; 60% protein bound; unused amounts excreted in urine (unchanged)

Drug interactions of concern to dentistry:

• Chronic alcohol use impairs absorption

• Patients taking tricyclic antidepressants or phenothiazines may require supplement

DENTAL CONSIDERATIONS

General:

• Patients deficient in B vitamins, including riboflavin, may have cheilosis, bald tongue, beefy red tongue, glossitis, or anemia.

• Determine why the patient is taking the drug.

Teach patient/family:

• About addition of needed foods that are rich in riboflavin

rifabutin

(rif'a-byoo-ten)

Mycobutin

Drug class.: Antimycobacterial agent

Action: Inhibits DNA-dependent RNA polymerase synthesis of bacterial RNA

Uses: Prevention of disseminated *M. avium* complex (MAC) disease with advanced HIV infection

Dosage and routes:

• *Adult:* PO 300 mg qd

Available forms include: Caps 150 mg

Side effects/adverse reactions:

▼ *ORAL:* Altered taste, colored saliva (brownish-orange)

CNS: Asthenia, headache, anorexia, insomnia

GI: Abdominal pain, flatulence, nausea, vomiting, diarrhea

HEMA: ***Leukopenia, neutropenia, thrombocytopenia***

GU: Discolored urine

INTEG: Rash

MS: Myalgia

MISC: Fever

Contraindications: Hypersensitivity, active TB

Precautions: Pregnancy category B, lactation, concurrent corticosteroid therapy

Pharmacokinetics:
PO: Peak 2-4 hr, terminal half-life average 45 hr; moderately protein bound; hepatic metabolism; both renal and fecal excretion

Drug interactions of concern to dentistry:
• Decreases plasma concentrations of corticosteriods; may be significant
• May induce CYP3A4 isoenzymes, possible reduction in action of ketoconazole, itraconazole, benzodiazepines, doxycycline, erythromycin, clarithromycin (see Appendix I)

DENTAL CONSIDERATIONS
General:
• Examine for evidence of oral signs of opportunistic disease.
• Determine why the patient is taking the drug.
• Patients on chronic drug therapy may rarely have symptoms of blood dyscrasias, which can include infection, bleeding, and poor healing.

Consultations:
• Medical consultation may be required to assess patient's ability to tolerate stress.
• In a patient with symptoms of blood dyscrasias, request a medical consultation for blood studies and postpone dental treatment until normal values are reestablished.

Teach patient/family:
• To avoid mouth rinses with high alcohol content because of drying effects
• Importance of good oral hygiene to prevent soft tissue inflammation

rifampin
(rif'am-pin)
Rifadin, Rifadin IV, Rimactane
✤ Rofact
Drug class.: Antitubercular antiinfective

Action: Inhibits DNA-dependent RNA polymerase synthesis of bacterial RNA
Uses: Pulmonary TB, meningococcal carriers (prevention); unapproved: leprosy and atypical mycobacterial infections
Dosage and routes:
• *Adult:* PO 10 mg/kg/day as single dose 1 hr ac or 2 hr pc; not to exceed 600 mg/day
• *Child >5 yr:* PO 10-20 mg/kg/day as single dose 1 hr ac or 2 hr pc; not to exceed 600 mg/day, with other antituberculars
Meningococcal carriers:
• *Adult:* PO 600 mg bid × 2 days
• *Child >5 yr:* PO 10 mg/kg bid × 2 days, not to exceed 600 mg/dose
Available forms include: Caps 150, 300 mg; powder for inj 600 mg
Side effects/adverse reactions:
▼ *ORAL:* Stomatitis, glossitis, candidiasis, bleeding, discolored saliva
CNS: Headache, fatigue, anxiety, drowsiness, confusion
GI: ***Pseudomembranous colitis,*** nausea, vomiting, anorexia, diarrhea, heartburn, pancreatitis
HEMA: ***Hemolytic anemia, eosinophilia, thrombocytopenia, leukopenia***
GU: ***Hematuria, acute renal failure, hemoglobinuria***
EENT: Visual disturbances

INTEG: Rash, pruritus, urticaria, pemphigus-like reaction
MS: Ataxia, weakness
MISC: Flulike symptoms, menstrual disturbances, edema, shortness of breath
Contraindications: Hypersensitivity
Precautions: Pregnancy category C, lactation, hepatic disease, blood dyscrasias, concurrent therapy with corticosteroids
Pharmacokinetics:
PO: Peak 2-3 hr, duration >24 hr, half-life 3 hr; metabolized in liver (active/inactive metabolites); excreted in urine as free drug (30% crosses placenta); excreted in breast milk
Drug interactions of concern to dentistry:
- Increased risk of hepatotoxicity: acetaminophen (chronic use and high doses), alcohol, hydrocarbon inhalation anesthetics (except isoflurane)
- Decreased effects of corticosteroids, dapsone, ketoconazole, fluconazole, itraconazole, oral contraceptives, benzodiazepines, doxycycline, erythromycin, clarithromycin, opioid analgesics
- Suspected decrease in fexofenadine effects
- Induces CYP450 isoenzymes (see Appendix I)

DENTAL CONSIDERATIONS
General:
- Examine for oral manifestation of opportunistic infections.
- Patients on chronic drug therapy may rarely have symptoms of blood dyscrasias, which can include infection, bleeding, and poor healing.
- Determine why the patient is taking the drug (prophylaxis or active therapy).
- Determine that noninfectious status exists by ensuring that (1) anti-TB drugs have been taken >3 wk, (2) culture has confirmed TB susceptibility to antiinfectives, (3) patient has had three consecutive negative sputum smears, and (4) patient is not in the coughing stage.

Consultations:
- Medical consultation may be required to assess patient's ability to tolerate stress.
- In a patient with symptoms of blood dyscrasias, request a medical consultation for blood studies and postpone dental treatment until normal values are reestablished.

Teach patient/family:
- To avoid mouth rinses with high alcohol content because of drying effects
- Importance of good oral hygiene to prevent soft tissue inflammation
- Importance of taking medications for full length of regimen to ensure effectiveness of treatment and to prevent the emergence of resistant strains

R

rifapentine

(rif'a-pen-teen)
Priftin

Drug class.: Antimycobacterial agent

Action: Inhibits DNA-dependent RNA polymerase; bactericidal for *Mycobacterium tuberculosis*
Uses: Pulmonary tuberculosis in combination with other antituberculosis drugs; unlabeled use includes prophylaxis of *Mycobacte-*

rium avium complex in patients with AIDS

Dosage and routes:

• *Adult:* PO in combination with other anti-TB drugs; intensive phase 600 mg twice weekly at an interval of not less than 3 days for 2 mo, then continue once weekly for 4 mo in combination with another anti-TB drug; concomitant use of pyridoxine (B_6) is recommended for malnourished patients, patients predisposed to neuropathy, and adolescents; can give with food

Available forms include: Tabs 150 mg

Side effects/adverse reactions:

NOTE: Adverse effects are reported for combination drug therapy only and may or may not be due solely to rifapentine.

▼ *ORAL:* Reddish discoloration of saliva

CNS: Anorexia, headache, dizziness

CV: Hypertension

GI: Nausea, vomiting, dyspepsia, diarrhea, ***pseudomembranous colitis,*** hyperbilirubinemia

HEMA: Anemia, lymphopenia, thrombocytosis, ***leukopenia, neutropenia***

GU: Hyperuricemia, pyuria, proteinuria, hematuria

EENT: Hemoptysis

INTEG: Rash, pruritus, acne, urticaria

META: Increased ALT, AST

MS: Arthralgia, gout

MISC: Fatigue, reddish discoloration of urine, sweat, tears

Contraindications: Hypersensitivity to rifampin, rifabutin

Precautions: Significant hepatic dysfunction, induces hepatic microsomal enzymes, pregnancy category C, lactation, children <12 yr

Pharmacokinetics:

PO: Slow absorption, peak levels 5-6 hr, highly plasma protein bound (97%-93%), hepatic metabolism, 25-desacetylrifapentine is active metabolite, hepatic metabolism, excreted in feces (70%) and urine (17%)

Drug interactions of concern to dentistry:

• May accelerate metabolism of clarithromycin, doxycycline, ciprofloxacin, fluconazole, ketoconazole, itraconazole, diazepam, barbiturates, corticosteroids, opioids, zolpidem, sildenafil, tricyclic antidepressants

• Inducer of CYP3A4 and CYP2C8/9 isoenzymes may cause drug interactions (see Appendix I)

DENTAL CONSIDERATIONS

General:

• Determine why patient is taking the drug (prophylaxis or active therapy).

• Examine for oral manifestation of opportunistic infections.

• Patients on chronic drug therapy may rarely have symptoms of blood dyscrasias, which can include infection, bleeding, and poor healing.

• Determine that noninfectious status exists by ensuring that (1) anti-TB drugs have been taken >3 wk, (2) culture has confirmed TB susceptibility to antiinfectives, (3) patient has had three consecutive negative sputum smears, and (4) patient is not in the coughing stage.

• Consider semisupine chair position for patient comfort because of GI side effects of drug.

Consultations:

• Medical consultation may be required to assess disease control and patient's ability to tolerate stress.

• In a patient with symptoms of blood dyscrasias, request a medical consultation for blood studies and postpone treatment until normal values are reestablished.

Teach patient/family:

• To avoid mouth rinses with high alcohol content because of drying effects

• To prevent trauma when using oral hygiene aids

• Importance of good oral hygiene to prevent soft tissue inflammation

• Importance of taking medication for full length of regimen to ensure effectiveness of treatment and prevent emergence of resistant strains

• Of potential for extrinsic oral staining side effect

---

riluzole

(ril'yoo-zole)

Rilutek

Drug class.: Glutamate antagonist

Action: Inhibits presynaptic release of glutamate in CNS; may also interfere with effects of excitatory amino acids and inactivation of voltage-dependent sodium channels

Uses: Treatment of amyotrophic lateral sclerosis (Lou Gehrig's disease)

Dosage and routes:

• *Adult:* PO 50 mg bid 1 hr before morning and evening meals or 2 hr after meals

Available forms include: Tabs 50 mg

Side effects/adverse reactions:

▼ *ORAL: Dry mouth (3%),* stomatitis (1%), candidiasis (0.5%), circumoral paresthesia (1.3%), glossitis

CNS: Asthenia, dizziness, depression, headache, hypertonia, insomnia, incoordination, anorexia

CV: Hypertension, peripheral edema, tachycardia, palpitation, postural hypotension

GI: Nausea, vomiting, dyspepsia, anorexia, diarrhea, flatulence

RESP: Cough, sinusitis

HEMA: ***Neutropenia***

GU: UTI

EENT: Rhinitis

INTEG: Pruritus, eczema

META: Weight loss, liver enzyme abnormalities

MS: Stiffness, worsening of spasticity, fasciculation

Contraindications: Hypersensitivity

Precautions: Hepatic impairment, renal impairment, hypertension, other CNS disorders, pregnancy category C, lactation, children

Pharmacokinetics:

PO: Well absorbed, extensively metabolized by liver (CYP1A2 isoenzymes), excreted in urine/feces

Drug interactions of concern to dentistry:

• No data reported with dental drugs, but use with caution when given with inducers or inhibitors of CYP1A2 isoenzymes (see Appendix I)

DENTAL CONSIDERATIONS

General:

• Short appointments may be required because of nature of disease process.

• Monitor vital signs at every appointment because of cardiovascular and respiratory side effects.
• Consider semisupine chair position for patient comfort.
• Assess salivary flow as factor in caries, periodontal disease, and candidiasis.
• Examine for oral manifestation of opportunistic infection.
• Patients on chronic drug therapy may rarely have symptoms of blood dyscrasias, which can include infection, bleeding, and poor healing.
• After supine positioning, have patient sit upright for at least 2 min before standing to avoid orthostatic hypotension.

Consultations:
• Medical consultation may be required to assess disease control.
• In a patient with symptoms of blood dyscrasias, request a medical consultation for blood studies and postpone treatment until normal values are reestablished.

Teach patient/family:
• Instructions for management of oral hygiene, including use of electric toothbrush or directions to caregiver
• That professional oral hygiene home care may be needed
• Caution to prevent trauma when using oral hygiene aids

When chronic dry mouth occurs, advise patient:
• To avoid mouth rinses with high alcohol content because of drying effects
• To use daily home fluoride products for anticaries effect
• To use sugarless gum, frequent sips of water, or saliva substitutes

rimantadine HCl

(ri-man'ta-deen)
Flumadine
Drug class.: Antiviral

Action: May inhibit viral uncoating

Uses: Adult–prophylaxis and treatment of illnesses caused by strains of influenza A virus; child–prophylaxis against influenza A virus

Dosage and routes

Prophylaxis:
• *Adult and child >10 yr:* PO 100 mg bid; patients with severe hepatic dysfunction, renal failure, and elderly nursing home patients 100 mg/day
• *Child <10 yr:* PO 5 mg/kg once daily, not to exceed 150 mg

Treatment:
• *Adult:* PO 100 mg bid; 100 mg/day recommended for patients with severe hepatic dysfunction, patients with renal failure, and elderly nursing home patients; continue therapy for 7 days from initial onset of symptoms

Available forms include: Tabs 100 mg; syr 50 mg/5 ml in 240 ml

Side effects/adverse reactions:
▼ *ORAL: Dry mouth,* stomatitis, altered taste
CNS: Insomnia, dizziness, headache, fatigue, nervousness, anorexia, depression
CV: Palpitation, hypertension, tachycardia, syncope
GI: Nausea, vomiting, diarrhea, dyspepsia
RESP: Dyspnea
EENT: Tinnitus, eye pain
INTEG: Rash
MS: Asthenia

Contraindications: Hypersensi-

tivity, hypersensitivity to amantadine, nursing mothers, children <1 yr

Precautions: Pregnancy category C, elderly, epilepsy, hepatic or renal impairment, emergence of resistant viral strains

Pharmacokinetics:

PO: Peak plasma levels 6 hr; 40% plasma protein binding; hepatic metabolism; renal excretion

Drug interactions of concern to dentistry:

• Reduced peak plasma levels: aspirin, acetaminophen

DENTAL CONSIDERATIONS

General:

• Monitor vital signs at each appointment because of cardiovascular side effects.

• Determine why the patient is taking the drug (will probably be used only during peak seasons for influenza).

• Assess salivary flow as a factor in caries, periodontal disease, and candidiasis.

Teach patient/family:

• Importance of good oral hygiene to prevent soft tissue inflammation

When chronic dry mouth occurs, advise patient:

• To avoid mouth rinses with high alcohol content because of drying effects

• Of need for daily use of home fluoride products to prevent caries

• To use sugarless gum, frequent sips of water, or saliva substitutes

rimexolone

(re-mex'oh-lone)

Vexol

Drug class.: Corticosteroid

Action: Glucocorticoids have multiple actions that include antiinflammatory and immunosuppressant effects. They inhibit phospholipase A_2, interfering with or reducing the synthesis of prostaglandins and leukotrienes. They also bind to cytoplasmic GRs and enter the cell nucleus to bind with DNA. This results in the synthesis of various enzymes such as collagenase, elastase, and cytokines that play important roles in inflammation and immunosuppression. They also suppress the production of lymphocytes, monocytes, and eosinophils.

Uses: Inflammation of the eye associated with ocular surgery and uveitis

Dosage and routes:

Ocular surgery:

• *Adult:* Ophth top after postoperative inflammation, instill 1 or 2 gtt qid beginning 24 hr after surgery; continue up to 2 wk

Uveitis:

• *Adult:* Ophth top use 1 or 2 gtt in affected eye qh while awake × 1 wk; then 1 or 2 gtt q2h while awake × 1 wk; then reduce dose according to need

Available forms include: Susp 1% in 2.5, 5, 10 ml droptainers

Side effects/adverse reactions:

▼ *ORAL:* Alteration of taste (rare)

CNS: Headache (rare)

CV: Hypotension (rare)

EENT: Blurred vision, ocular pain, corneal edema, ulceration, increased ocular pressure

INTEG: Pruritus

Contraindications: Hypersensitivity, fungal or herpetic infections of eye

Precautions: Increased intraocular

pressure, pregnancy category C, lactation, children, secondary ocular infections

Pharmacokinetics:

OPHTH TOP: Immediate onset, systemic absorption, extensive metabolism, excretion in feces

Drug interactions of concern to dentistry:

- None reported

DENTAL CONSIDERATIONS

General:

- Determine why the patient is taking the drug.
- Protect patient's eyes from accidental spatter during dental treatment.
- Avoid dental light in patient's eyes; offer dark glasses for patient comfort.

---

risedronate sodium

(ris-ed'roe-nate)

Actonel

Drug class.: Bisphosphonate

Action: Binds to bone hydroxyapatite, inhibits osteoclast-mediated bone resorption, and modulates bone metabolism

Uses: Paget's disease of bone; treatment and prevention of osteoporosis in postmenopausal women and glucocorticoid-induced osteoporosis

Dosage and routes:

Paget's disease:

- *Adult:* PO 30 mg daily × 2 mo, take at least 30 min before first food or drink of the day (other than water), take in upright position with 6-8 oz water, avoid lying down for 30 min after dose is taken; patient should also take supplemental calcium and vitamin D if dietary intake is inadequate

Prevention/treatment of osteoporosis:

- *Adult:* PO 5 mg/day or 35 mg once weekly

Available forms include: Tabs 5, 30, 35 mg

Side effects/adverse reactions:

CNS: Headache, dizziness

CV: Chest pain, peripheral edema

GI: Diarrhea, abdominal pain, nausea, constipation, belching, colic

RESP: Bronchitis, sinusitis

EENT: Amblyopia, tinnitus, dryness

INTEG: Rash

MS: Asthenia, arthralgia, bone pain, leg cramps, myasthenia

MISC: Flulike symptoms

Contraindications: Hypersensitivity, hypocalcemia

Precautions: Upper GI disease, avoid use in significant renal impairment, pregnancy category C, lactation, pediatric patients

Pharmacokinetics:

PO: Rapid oral absorption, food decreases bioavailability, bisphosphonates are not metabolized, renal excretion, unabsorbed drug excreted in feces

Drug interactions of concern to dentistry:

- Retarded absorption: calcium, antacids, medications with divalent cations
- Increased GI side effects: NSAIDs, aspirin

DENTAL CONSIDERATIONS

General:

- Be aware of the oral manifestations of Paget's disease (macrognathia, alveolar pain).
- Consider semisupine chair position for patient comfort because of GI side effects of drug.
- Short appointments may be required for patient comfort.

Consultations:

• Medical consultation may be required to assess disease control.

Teach patient/family:

• Use of electric toothbrush if patient has difficulty holding conventional devices

risperidone

(ris-per'i-done)

Risperdal

Drug class.: Antipsychotic (benzisoxazole derivative)

Action: Unclear, but may be related to antagonism for dopamine (DA_2) and serotonin ($5\text{-}HT_2$) receptors; also has affinity for alpha receptors and histamine (H_1) receptors

Uses: Schizophrenia

Dosage and routes:

• *Adult:* PO initial 1 mg bid; increase by 1 mg bid on second and third day to 3 mg bid (target dose); further dose increase at 1 wk intervals; dose range 4-16 mg/day; reduce doses for elderly or debilitated patients or for those with severe renal or hepatic impairment (limit 3 mg/day)

Available forms include: Tabs 0.25, 0.5, 1, 2, 3, 4 mg; oral sol 1 mg/ml, tabs orally disintegrating 0.5, 1, 2 mg

Side effects/adverse reactions:

▼ *ORAL: Dry mouth,* stomatitis, taste alteration (rare)

CNS: Anxiety, ***neuromalignant syndrome,*** *EPS, dystonia, somnolence, hyperkinesia, dizziness,* tardive dyskinesia, syncope, motor impairment, insomnia

CV: Dysrhythmias, orthostatic hypotension, *tachycardia,* ***stroke (elderly patient with dementia)***

GI: Nausea, constipation, dyspepsia

RESP: Cough, dyspnea

HEMA: ***Thrombocytopenia,*** purpura, anemia, leukocytosis, leukopenia (all rare)

GU: Decreased libido, sexual dysfunction (male), menorrhagia, priapism, amenorrhea

EENT: Rhinitis, sinusitis, visual changes

INTEG: Rash, dry skin, photosensitivity

MS: Arthralgia

MISC: Hyperprolactinemia, akathisia

Contraindications: Hypersensitivity

Precautions: Pregnancy category C, lactation, seizures, suicidal patients, cardiac diseases, renal or hepatic impairment, elderly; patients should be monitored for signs and symptoms of diabetes mellitus

Pharmacokinetics:

PO: Good absorption, peak plasma levels 1-2 hr; high plasma protein binding; extensive hepatic metabolism (active metabolite); renal excretion

Drug interactions of concern to dentistry:

• Increased excretion: chronic use of carbamazepine

• Increased sedation: other CNS depressants, alcohol, barbiturate anesthesia, opioid analgesics

• Increased extrapyramidal effects: phenothiazines and related drugs (haloperidol, droperidol), metoclopramide

• Additive photosensitization: tetracyclines

• Increased anticholinergic effects: anticholinergics such as atropine and scopolamine

DENTAL CONSIDERATIONS

General:

• Monitor vital signs at every appointment because of cardiovascular side effects.

• Patients on chronic drug therapy may rarely have symptoms of blood dyscrasias, which can include infection, bleeding, and poor healing.

• After supine positioning, have patient sit upright for at least 2 min before standing to avoid orthostatic hypotension.

• Assess salivary flow as a factor in caries, periodontal disease, and candidiasis.

• Consider semisupine chair position for patient comfort because of GI effects of drug.

• Assess for presence of extrapyramidal motor symptoms, such as tardive dyskinesia and akathisia. Extrapyramidal motor activity may complicate dental treatment.

• Use vasoconstrictors with caution, in low doses, and with careful aspiration; avoid use of gingival retraction cord with epinephrine.

Consultations:

• In a patient with symptoms of blood dyscrasias, request a medical consultation for blood studies and postpone dental treatment until normal values are reestablished.

• Take precautions if dental surgery is anticipated and anesthesia is required.

• If signs of tardive dyskinesia or other extrapyramidal symptoms are present, refer to physician.

• Physician should be informed if significant xerostomic side effects occur (e.g., increased caries, sore tongue, problems eating or swallowing, difficulty wearing prosthesis) so that a medication change can be considered.

Teach patient/family:

• Importance of good oral hygiene to prevent soft tissue inflammation

• Caution to prevent injury when using oral hygiene aids

• Use of electric toothbrush if patient has difficulty holding conventional devices

When chronic dry mouth occurs, advise patient:

• To avoid mouth rinses with high alcohol content because of drying effects

• To use daily home fluoride products for anticaries effect

• To use sugarless gum, frequent sips of water, or saliva substitutes

ritonavir

(ri-toe'na-veer)

Norvir

Drug class.: Antiviral, protease inhibitor

Action: Inhibits HIV-1 and HIV-2 proteases essential for production of HIV virion particles

Uses: Treatment of HIV infection in adults and children as single-drug therapy or in combination with nucleoside analogues

Dosage and routes:

• *Adult:* PO 600 mg bid with food; start with lower doses if nausea is a problem at outset

• *Children:* PO give with another antiretroviral agent initial dose 250 mg/m^2, increase at 2-3 day intervals by 50 mg/m^2 bid, max dose 400 mg/m^2 bid; dose range from 62.5-600 mg bid

Available forms include: Caps 100 mg; oral sol 80 mg/ml in 240 ml

Side effects/adverse reactions:
▼ *ORAL: Circumoral paresthesia,* taste alteration, dry mouth
CNS: Headache, dizziness, somnolence, insomnia, anorexia
CV: Hypotension, palpitation, syncope
GI: Nausea, vomiting, abdominal pain, diarrhea
RESP: Cough, asthma, hiccough
HEMA: Anemia
GU: Dysuria
EENT: Pharyngitis
INTEG: Rash, urticaria, acne
MS: Asthenia, arthralgia, weakness
MISC: Peripheral paresthesia, weight loss

Contraindications: Hypersensitivity; **note multiple drug interactions with potential adverse effects**

Precautions: Hepatic impairment, pregnancy category B, lactation, children <12 yr, alters lab chemistry values (triglycerides, ALT, AST, GGT, CPK, uric acid)

Pharmacokinetics:
PO: Peak plasma levels with food 2 hr, hepatic metabolism, active metabolite excreted in feces, highly plasma protein bound (98%), half-life 3-5 hr

Drug interactions of concern to dentistry:
- Contraindicated with alprazolam, clorazepate, diazepam, bupropion, estazolam, flurazepam, midazolam, triazolam, zolpidem, meperidine, piroxicam, propoxyphene, chlordiazepoxide, halazepam, quazepam
- Increased plasma levels: clarithromycin, fluconazole, fluoxetine, desipramine, theophylline
- Possible alcohol-disulfiram reaction: metronidazole, disulfiram
- Decreased plasma levels with carbamazepine, dexamethasone, phenobarbital, St. John's wort
- Increased plasma levels of fentanyl

NOTE: Multiple drug interactions are reported; check before prescribing dental drugs. This drug is a potent inhibitor of CYP3A4, CYP2D6 isoenzymes (see Appendix I).

DENTAL CONSIDERATIONS

General:
- Monitor vital signs at every appointment because of cardiovascular side effects.
- Examine for oral manifestation of opportunistic infection.
- Place on frequent recall to evaluate healing response.
- Assess salivary flow as a factor in caries, periodontal disease, and candidiasis.
- Consider semisupine chair position for patient comfort because of GI effects of drug.

Consultations:
- Medical consultation may be required to assess disease control.

Teach patient/family:
- Importance of good oral hygiene to prevent soft tissue inflammation
- That secondary oral infection may occur; must see dentist immediately if infection occurs

When chronic dry mouth occurs, advise patient:
- To avoid mouth rinses with high alcohol content because of drying effects
- To use daily home fluoride products for anticaries effect
- To use sugarless gum, frequent sips of water, or saliva substitutes

R

rivastigmine tartrate

(riv-a-stig'meen)

Exelon

Drug class.: Reversible cholinesterase inhibitor

Action: Inhibits destruction of acetylcholine; its role in Alzheimer's dementia is unknown, but may enhance cholinergic function

Uses: Mild to moderate Alzheimer's-type dementia

Dosage and routes:

• *Adult:* PO initial 1.5 mg bid; after 2 wk if this dose is tolerated increase to 3 mg bid; with 2 wk intervals between dose increases 4.5 mg bid then 6.0 mg bid may be attempted; max dose is 6 mg bid

Available forms include: Caps 1.5, 3.0, 4.5, 6 mg

Side effects/adverse reactions:

▼ *ORAL:* Dry mouth, alteration of taste, ulcerative stomatitis, increased salivation, facial edema (infrequent)

CNS: Dizziness, syncope, fatigue, malaise, headache, somnolence, tremor

CV: Hypertension, bradycardia, palpitation

GI: Nausea, vomiting, anorexia, dyspepsia, abdominal pain, flatulence

HEMA: (rare) ***Thrombocytopenic purpura,*** anemia, leukocytosis, hematoma

GU: UTI, impotence, atrophic vaginitis, hematuria

EENT: Rhinitis, tinnitus, epistaxis, diplopia

INTEG: Sweating

META: Weight loss, dehydration, hypokalemia

MS: Asthenia, myalgia, leg cramps

MISC: Accidental trauma, flulike syndrome

Contraindications: Hypersensitivity to this drug or other carbamate derivatives

Precautions: Significant GI reactions, nausea, vomiting, and weight-loss occur; history of GI ulcers or GI bleeding, patients taking NSAIDs, seizures, asthma, COPD, pregnancy category B, lactation, pediatric patients (no studies); smoking increases renal clearance

Pharmacokinetics:

PO: Well absorbed, bioavailability 40%, peak plasma levels 1 hr, widely distributed, plasma protein binding 40%, metabolized by cholinesterases, renal excretion

Drug interactions of concern to dentistry:

• Caution in use of NSAIDs if GI side effects are significant

• Decreased response to neuromuscular blocking agents used in general anesthesia

• Increased cholinergic response: other cholinergic drugs

• Decreased cholinergic response: anticholinergics or other drugs with anticholinergic actions

DENTAL CONSIDERATIONS

General:

• Determine why patient is taking the drug.

• Monitor vital signs at every appointment because of cardiovascular side effects.

• Drug is used early in the disease; ensure that patient or care giver understands informed consent.

• Place on frequent recall because early attention to dental health is important for Alzheimer's patients.

• Assess salivary flow as a factor in caries, periodontal disease, and candidiasis.
• Use precaution if sedation or general anesthesia is required; risk of hypotensive episode.
• Consider semisupine chair position for patient comfort if GI side effects occur.
• Patients on chronic drug therapy may rarely have symptoms of blood dyscrasias, which can include infection, bleeding, and poor healing.

Consultations:
• Consultation with physician may be needed if sedation or general anesthesia is required.
• In a patient with symptoms of blood dyscrasias, request a medical consultation for blood studies and postpone treatment until normal values are reestablished.
• Medical consultation may be required to assess disease control and patient's ability to tolerate stress.

Teach patient/family:
• Use of electric toothbrush if patient has difficulty holding conventional devices
• To prevent trauma when using oral hygiene aids
• Importance of good oral hygiene to prevent soft tissue inflammation

rizatriptan benzoate

(rye-za-trip'tan)
Maxalt, Maxalt-MLT
Drug class.: Serotonin agonist

Action: A selective agonist for 5-HT_{1D} and 5-HT_{1B} receptors on intracranial vessels leading to vasoconstriction and possibly inhibition of proinflammatory neuropeptide release

Uses: Acute treatment of migraine attacks with or without aura

Dosage and routes:
• *Adult:* PO initial dose 5-10 mg, can repeat dose in 2 hr, limit 30 mg/24 hr

Orally disintegrating tablet (MLT):
• *Adult:* PO remove tablet from sealed pouch immediately before use; place tablet on tongue, allow it to dissolve, and swallow with saliva; 5-10 mg initial dose, can repeat in 2 hr, limit 30 mg/24 hr

Available forms include: Tabs 5, 10 mg; orally disintegrating tabs 5, 10 mg

Side effects/adverse reactions:
▼ *ORAL:* Dry mouth
CNS: Fatigue, somnolence, dizziness, paresthesia, euphoria
CV: Palpitation, syncope, orthostatic hypotension
GI: Nausea, diarrhea, vomiting
RESP: Dyspnea, URI
GU: Hot flashes
EENT: Dry throat, nasal congestion, blurred vision, eye dryness
INTEG: Flushing
MS: Muscle weakness, arthralgia
MISC: Asthenia, pain or pressure (chest, neck, throat)

Contraindications: Hypersensitivity, MAOIs, uncontrolled hypertension, ischemic heart disease, cerebrovascular or peripheral vascular disease, ergot-type drugs

Precautions: Risk of serious cardiovascular events, renal/hepatic impairment, SSRI antidepressants, pregnancy category C, lactation, use in children not established, orally disintegrating tabs contain aspartame

Pharmacokinetics:
PO: Bioavailability 45%, mean peak plasma levels 1-1.5 hr for oral

tablet, MLT tablets slower rate of absorption, peak levels 1.6-2.5 hr, metabolized by MAO type A, metabolites excreted in urine (82%) and feces (12%), plasma protein binding (14%)

Drug interactions of concern to dentistry:

- Increased plasma levels: propranolol
- No specific interactions with dental drugs reported
- Should not be used within 24 hr of another 5-HT agonist

DENTAL CONSIDERATIONS

General:

- This is an acute-use drug; it is doubtful that patients will be treated in the office if acute migraine is present.
- Be aware of patient's disease, its severity, and its frequency, when known.
- Avoid dental light in patient's eyes; offer dark glasses for patient comfort.
- Short appointments and a stress reduction protocol may be required for anxious patients.
- After supine positioning, have patient sit upright for at least 2 min to avoid orthostatic hypotension.

Consultations:

- If treating chronic orofacial pain, consult with physician of record.
- Medical consultation may be required to assess disease control and patient's ability to tolerate stress.

Teach patient/family:

- Importance of updating health and drug history if physician makes any changes in evaluation or drug regimens

rofecoxib

(ro-fe-kox'ib)

Vioxx

Drug class.: Nonsteroidal antiinflammatory analgesic

Action: May be related to a selective inhibition of inducible cyclooxygenase 2 (COX 2) enzymes preventing the synthesis of prostaglandins

Uses: Relief of signs and symptoms of osteoarthritis, rheumatoid arthritis; acute pain in adults, including dental pain; and primary dysmenorrhea

Dosage and routes:

Osteoarthritis:

- *Adult:* PO initial dose 12.5 mg daily; max recommended dose 25 mg daily

Acute pain and primary dysmenorrhea:

- *Adult:* PO 50 mg qd; use for more than 5 days for acute pain has not been studied

Rheumatoid arthritis:

- *Adult:* PO 25 mg qd

Available forms include: Tabs 12.5, 25, 50 mg; oral susp 12.5 mg/5 ml and 25 mg/5 ml in 150 ml volumes

Side effects/adverse reactions:

▼ *ORAL:* Dry mouth, aphthous stomatitis (low incidence)

CNS: Dizziness, fatigue, headache, ***aseptic meningitis***

CV: Hypertension (high dose), edema, PVC, tachycardia, palpitation

GI: Abdominal pain, diarrhea, dyspepsia, heartburn, epigastric discomfort, nausea

RESP: URI, bronchitis

HEMA: Anemia

GU: UTI
EENT: Sinusitis
INTEG: Rash, urticaria
MS: Back pain
MISC: Asthenia, influenza-like disease

Contraindications: Hypersensitivity; patients who have experienced asthma, urticaria, or allergic-type reactions to aspirin or other NSAIDs

Precautions: Serious GI toxicity including ulceration and bleeding; prior history of GI disease (ulcer or bleeding); preexisting asthma, severe renal impairment, severe hepatic impairment, dehydrated patients, fluid retention, CHF, hypertension, pregnancy category C, lactation, children <18 yr; patients should be made aware of potential GI and hepatic side effects; risk of serious cardiovascular thromboembolic events

Pharmacokinetics:
PO: Bioavailability 93%, peak plasma levels 2-3 hr; high-fat meal delays peak plasma time; highly plasma protein bound (87%), hepatic metabolism, renal excretion (72%), minor fecal excretion

Drug interactions of concern to dentistry:
- Possible increased GI symptoms: aspirin
- As with other NSAIDs: reduced effectiveness of diuretics, ACE inhibitors
- Decreased plasma levels: rifampin
- Increased plasma levels of lithium, methotrexate, warfarin
- Monitor INR, small risk of bleeding: warfarin
- First-time users of SSRIs also taking NSAIDs may have a higher risk of GI side effects; until more data are available, it may be advisable to avoid use of NSAIDs in these patients (*Br J Clin Pharmacol* 55:591-595, 2003)

DENTAL CONSIDERATIONS
General:
- Assess salivary flow as a factor in caries, periodontal disease, and candidiasis.
- Update health and drug history if physician makes changes in evaluation or drug regimens.
- Monitor vital signs at every appointment because of cardiovascular side effects.
- Consider semisupine chair position for patient comfort if GI side effects occur.

Teach patient/family:
- Importance of good oral hygiene to prevent soft tissue inflammation
- Use of electric toothbrush if patient has difficulty holding conventional devices

When chronic dry mouth occurs, advise patient:
- To avoid mouth rinses with high alcohol content because of drying effects
- To use daily home fluoride products for anticaries effect
- To use sugarless gum, frequent sips of water, or saliva substitutes

ropinirole HCl
(roe-pin'i-role)
ReQuip
Drug class.: Antiparkinson agent

Action: Acts as a dopamine (D_2 and D_3) receptor agonist in the caudate-putamen region of the brain

Uses: Parkinson's disease

R

Dosage and routes:

• *Adult:* PO initial 0.25 mg tid with weekly incremental dose increase based on patient response

Dose schedule:

Week	Dose	Total daily dose
1	0.25 mg tid	0.75 mg
2	0.5 mg tid	1.5 mg
3	0.75 mg tid	2.25 mg
4	1.0 mg tid	3.0 mg

Available forms include: Tabs 0.25, 0.5, 1, 2, 5 mg

Side effects/adverse reactions:

▼ *ORAL: Dry mouth*

CNS: Confusion, hallucination, drowsiness, somnolence, euphoria, dyskinesia, dizziness, headache

CV: Supraventricular ectopy, postural hypotension, syncope, fatigue, bradycardia

GI: Nausea, vomiting, dyspepsia, constipation

RESP: Bronchitis, URI

HEMA: ***Thrombocytopenia*** (rare), vitamin B_{12} deficiency, hypochromic anemia

GU: UTI

EENT: Pharyngitis, blurred vision, rhinitis

INTEG: Sweating

ENDO: Decrease in prolactin levels

META: Increased alk phosphatase, increased BUN

MS: Asthenia, leg cramps

MISC: Viral infection

Contraindications: Hypersensitivity

Precautions: Cardiovascular disease, severely impaired renal or hepatic function, lactation, pregnancy category C, syncope, hypotension

Pharmacokinetics:

PO: Peak plasma levels 1-2 hr, good oral absorption, bioavailability 55%, hepatic metabolism, 40% plasma protein binding, urinary excretion of metabolites

Drug interactions of concern to dentistry:

• Possible increase in sedation with all CNS depressants

• Possible diminished effects: dopamine antagonists, phenothiazines, haloperidol, droperidol, and metoclopramide

DENTAL CONSIDERATIONS

General:

• Monitor vital signs at every appointment because of cardiovascular side effects.

• Assess salivary flow as factor in caries, periodontal disease, and candidiasis.

• After supine positioning, have patient sit upright for at least 2 min before standing to avoid orthostatic hypotension.

• Patients on chronic drug therapy may rarely have symptoms of blood dyscrasias, which can include infection, bleeding, and poor healing.

• Consider semisupine chair position for patient comfort if GI side effects occur.

Consultations:

• In a patient with symptoms of blood dyscrasias, request a medical consultation for blood studies and postpone treatment until normal values are reestablished.

• Medical consultation may be required to assess disease control and patient's ability to tolerate stress.

Teach patient/family:

• Caution to prevent trauma when using oral hygiene aids

• Use of electric toothbrush if patient has difficulty holding conventional devices
• Importance of good oral hygiene to prevent soft tissue inflammation
• Importance of updating health and drug history if physician makes any changes in evaluation or drug regimens

When chronic dry mouth occurs, advise patient:

• To avoid mouth rinses with high alcohol content because of drying effects
• To use daily home fluoride products for anticaries effect
• To use sugarless gum, frequent sips of water, or saliva substitutes

---

rosiglitazone maleate

(ros-i-gli'ta-zone)
Avandia

Drug class.: Oral antidiabetic

Action: An agonist for peroxisome proliferator-activated receptor gamma (PPAR-γ); improves target cell response to insulin without increasing insulin secretion; insulin must be present for this drug to act

Uses: Monotherapy, as an adjunct to diet and exercise in patients with type 2 diabetes mellitus; may also be used with metformin when metformin, diet, and exercise are not adequate for control

Dosage and routes:

• *Adult:* PO initial dose 4 mg in a single dose or 2 equal doses daily; after evaluation (12 wk) can increase to 8 mg daily

With metformin:

• *Adult:* PO 4 mg daily as a single dose or 2 equal doses; after evaluation (12 wk) can increase dose to 8 mg daily

Available forms include: Tabs 2, 4, 8 mg

Side effects/adverse reactions:

CNS: Headache
CV: Edema
GI: Diarrhea
RESP: URI
HEMA: Anemia, decreased hemoglobin/hematocrit
EENT: Sinusitis
META: Hyperglycemia, hypoglycemia, hyperbilirubinemia
MISC: Fatigue, fluid retention

Contraindications: Hypersensitivity, patients with jaundice associated with use of troglitazone, type 1 diabetes

Precautions: May cause resumption of ovulation in premenopausal anovulatory women (risk of pregnancy), patients with edema, advanced heart failure, hepatic impairment, monitor liver enzymes, pregnancy category C, lactation

Pharmacokinetics:

PO: Absolute bioavailability 99%, peak plasma levels approximately 1 hr, half-life 3-4 hr; highly bound to plasma proteins (99.8%), extensive metabolism (CYP450 2C8), excreted mostly in urine (64%)

Drug interactions of concern to dentistry:

• None reported

DENTAL CONSIDERATIONS

General:

• Ensure that patient is following prescribed diet and regularly takes medication.
• Place on frequent recall to evaluate healing response.
• Short appointments and a stress reduction protocol may be required for anxious patients.
• Diabetics may be more susceptible to infection and have delayed wound healing.

• Question patient about self-monitoring of drug's antidiabetic effect, including blood glucose values or finger-stick records.

Consultations:

• Medical consultation may include data from patient's blood glucose monitoring, including glycosylated hemoglobin or HbA_{1c} testing.

• Medical consultation may be required to assess disease control and patient's ability to tolerate stress.

Teach patient/family:

• To prevent trauma when using oral hygiene aids

• Importance of updating health and drug history if physician makes any changes in evaluation or drug regimens

---

rosuvastatin calcium

(roe-soo'va-sta-tin)

Crestor

Drug class.: Antihyperlipidemic

Action: Inhibits HMG-Co A reductase enzyme, thus reducing cholesterol synthesis; reduces LDL, VLDL, Apo B, non-HDL cholesterol and triglycerides; increase in hepatic LDL receptors

Uses: As an adjunct to diet in primary hypercholesterolemia, mixed lipidemia (Fredricksen types II_a and II_b), and homogygous familial hypercholesterolemia and to lower triglycerides in Fredrickson type IV hyperlipidemia

Dosage and routes:

Hypercholesterolemia (heterozygous familial and nonfamilial) and mixed dyslipidemia:

• *Adult:* PO 5-40 mg/day; initial starting dose 10 mg

Homozygous familial hypercholesterolemia:

• *Adult:* PO initial dose 20 mg/day; limit 40 mg/day

NOTE: Doses must be reduced in patients taking cyclosporine or gemfibrozil or in patients with severe renal impairment.

Available forms include: Tabs 5, 10, 20, 40 mg

Side effects/adverse reactions:

CNS: Asthenia, headache

CV: Chest pain, hypertension

GI: Abdominal pain, nausea, constipation, diarrhea, gastritis, dyspepsia

RESP: Pharyngitis

GU: UTI, pelvic pain

EENT: Rhinitis, sinusitis

INTEG: Rash, pruritus

META: Elevated creatine phosphokinase, hyperglycemia, ALT, AST, bilirubin; abnormal thyroid function

MS: Myalgia, ***rhabdomyolysis,*** back pain, neck pain

MISC: Flulike syndrome, hypersensitivity reactions

Contraindications: Hypersensitivity, active liver disease, pregnancy, nursing

Precautions: Severe renal impairment, hepatic impairment, pregnancy category X, liver function test recommended, alcoholics, efficacy and safety in pediatric patients unknown

Pharmacokinetics:

PO: Absolute bioavailability ≈20%, peak plasma levels 3-5 hr, plasma protein binding 88%, not extensively metabolized, but CYP2C9 is involved; excreted primarily in feces (90%)

Drug interactions of concern to dentistry:
- Does not inhibit CYP3A4
- No dental drug interactions reported; however, interactions with cyclosporine, warfarin, and gemfibrozil are noted

DENTAL CONSIDERATIONS
General:
- Monitor vital signs because patients with high cholesterol levels are predisposed to cardiovascular disease.
- Consider semisupine chair position for patient comfort if GI side effects occur.

salmeterol xinafoate

(sal-me'te-role)
Serevent Diskus

Drug class.: Long-acting selective β_2-adrenergic receptor agonist

Action: Relaxes bronchial smooth muscle by directly acting on β_2-adrenergic receptors; also inhibits release of mast cell mediators

Uses: Bronchospasm associated with COPD, maintenance treatment of bronchospasm associated with COPD, asthma, and exercise-induced bronchospasm

Dosage and routes:
Bronchospasm and asthma:
- *Adult and child >12 yr:* INH aerosol 2 puffs bid (12 hr apart); avoid higher doses and more frequent use
- *Adult and child >4 yr:* INH powder 1 inhalation of 50 µg bid

Exercise-induced bronchospasm (prevention):
- *Adult and child >12 yr:* INH aerosol 2 puffs 30-60 min before exercise, not more than once q12h and not in patients using the drug on a regular basis

COPD:
- *Adult:* INH aerosol 2 puffs bid (12 hr apart)
- *Adult:* INH powder 1 puff (50 µg) bid (12 hr apart)

Available forms include: Canisters 13 g containing 120 actuations, 6.5 g containing 60 actuations; inh powder 50 µg/disk

Side effects/adverse reactions:
▼ *ORAL: Dry throat,* dental pain (1%-3%, type or origin not defined)
CNS: Headache, tremors, anxiety, dizziness, vertigo, nervousness, fatigue
CV: Tachycardia, palpitation
GI: Stomachache, nausea, vomiting, diarrhea
RESP: Upper/lower respiratory infections, cough, **bronchospasm**
GU: Dysmenorrhea
EENT: Ear/nose/throat infections, nasopharyngitis, sinus headache
INTEG: Rash, urticaria
MS: Tremor, joint pain, muscular soreness, myalgia, back pain, muscle cramps, myositis
MISC: Immediate hypersensitivity reactions

Contraindications: Hypersensitivity

Precautions: Pregnancy category C, lactation, children <12 yr, hepatic impairment, coronary insufficiency, dysrhythmias, hypertension, convulsive disorders; ***not for acute symptoms,*** not to exceed recommended dose, paradoxic bronchospasm may occur with use; not recommended for use with a spacer or other aerosol device

Pharmacokinetics:
PO/INH: Rapid onset 5-15 min, peak 4 hr, duration 12 hr; plasma levels are not used to predict local effects in the lung; 94%-98% plasma protein bound; metabolized in liver; excreted mainly in feces, to a lesser degree in urine

Drug interactions of concern to dentistry:
- Increased cardiovascular effects: tricyclic antidepressants

DENTAL CONSIDERATIONS
General:
- Monitor vital signs at every appointment because of cardiovascular and respiratory side effects.
- Be aware that aspirin or sulfite preservatives in vasoconstrictor-containing products can exacerbate asthma.
- Acute asthmatic episodes may be precipitated in the dental office. Rapid-acting sympathomimetic inhalants should be available for emergency use. Salmeterol is not a rapid-acting drug and is not intended for use in acute asthmatic attacks.
- Consider semisupine chair position for patients with respiratory disease.
- Midmorning appointments and a stress reduction protocol may be required for anxious patients.

Consultations:
- Medical consultation may be required to assess disease control and stress tolerance.

Teach patient/family:
- Importance of good oral hygiene to prevent soft tissue inflammation

salsalate
(sal'sa-late)
Amigesic, Argesic-SA, Artha-G, Disalcid, Marthritic, Mono-Gesic, Salflex, Salsitab

Drug class.: Salicylate, nonnarcotic analgesic

Action: Blocks formation of peripheral prostaglandins, which cause pain and inflammation; antipyretic action results from inhibition of hypothalamic heat-regulating center; does not inhibit platelet aggregation

Uses: Mild-to-moderate pain or fever, including arthritis, juvenile rheumatoid arthritis

Dosage and routes:
- *Adult:* PO 500-1000 mg in 2 or 3 doses/day

Available forms include: Caps 500 mg; tabs 500, 750 mg

Side effects/adverse reactions:
CNS: Stimulation, drowsiness, dizziness, confusion, ***convulsions,*** headache, flushing, hallucinations, coma
CV: Rapid pulse, ***pulmonary edema***
GI: Nausea, vomiting, GI bleeding, diarrhea, heartburn, anorexia, ***hepatotoxicity***
RESP: Wheezing, hyperpnea
HEMA: ***Thrombocytopenia, agranulocytosis, leukopenia, neutropenia, hemolytic anemia,*** increased prothrombin time
EENT: Tinnitus, hearing loss
INTEG: *Rash,* urticaria, bruising
ENDO: Hypoglycemia, hyponatremia, hypokalemia, alteration in acid-base balance

Contraindications: Hypersensitivity to salicylates, NSAIDs, GI

bleeding, bleeding disorders, children <3 yr, vitamin K deficiency
Precautions: Anemia, hepatic disease, renal disease, Hodgkin's disease, pregnancy category C, lactation
Pharmacokinetics:
PO: Half-life 1 hr; highly protein bound; metabolized by liver; excreted by kidneys; slowly crosses blood-brain barrier and placenta
Drug interactions of concern to dentistry:
• Increased risk of GI complaints and occult blood loss: alcohol, NSAIDs, corticosteroids
• Increased risk of bleeding: oral anticoagulants, valproic acid, dipyridamole
• Avoid prolonged or concurrent use with NSAIDs, corticosteroids, acetaminophen
• Increased risk of hypoglycemia: oral antidiabetics
• Increased risk of toxicity: methotrexate, lithium, zidovudine
• Decreased effects of probenecid, sulfinpyrazone
• Suspected reduction in the antihypertensive and vasodilator effects of ACE inhibitors; monitor blood pressure if used concurrently
DENTAL CONSIDERATIONS
General:
• Patients on chronic drug therapy rarely have symptoms of blood dyscrasias, which can include infection, bleeding, and poor healing.
• Potential cross-allergies with other salicylates such as aspirin.
• Consider semisupine chair position for patients with inflammatory joint diseases.
• Avoid prescribing aspirin-containing products because this drug is a salicylate.
• If used for dental patients, take with food or milk to decrease GI complaints; give 30 min before meals or 2 hr after meals; take with a full glass of water.
Consultations:
• In a patient with symptoms of blood dyscrasias, request a medical consultation for blood studies and postpone dental treatment until normal values are reestablished.
• Medical consultation may be required to assess disease control.
Teach patient/family:
• That salicylates should not be placed directly on a tooth or oral mucosa because of risk of chemical burns
• Not to exceed recommended dosage; acute toxicity may result
• To read label on other OTC drugs; many contain aspirin
• To avoid alcohol ingestion; GI bleeding may occur
• Importance of good oral hygiene to prevent soft tissue inflammation
• Caution to prevent injury when using oral hygiene aids

saquinavir mesylate/ saquinavir

(sa-kwin'a-veer)
Saquinavir mesylate: Fotovase
Saquinavir: Invirase
Drug class.: Antiviral

Action: Inhibits HIV protease important for viral replication
Uses: Used in combination with nucleoside analogs, zidovudine, or zalcitabine in the treatment of AIDS
Dosage and routes:
Invirase:
• *Adult:* PO 200 mg tid; take within 2 hr after eating with a nucleoside analog

Fotovase:
• *Adult:* PO 1200 mg tid; take within 2 hr after eating with a nucleoside analog

Available forms include: Caps 200 mg; Fotovase and Invirase caps are not interchangeable

Side effects/adverse reactions:
▼ *ORAL:* Buccal mucosal ulceration (<2%), dry mouth, taste alteration, stomatitis
CNS: Headache, paresthesia, extremity numbness, dizziness, peripheral neuropathy
CV: Hypotension, syncope (infrequent)
GI: Diarrhea, abdominal discomfort, nausea, dyspepsia
RESP: Cough, dyspnea, pharyngitis, rhinitis, sinusitis
HEMA: Anemia, ***thrombocytopenia, pancytopenia***
GU: UTI
EENT: Blepharitis, earache, eye irritation, tinnitus
INTEG: Rash, pruritus, photosensitivity
ENDO: Dry eyes
MS: Musculoskeletal pain, myalgia

Contraindications: Hypersensitivity, rifampin

Precautions: Hepatic impairment, child <16 yr, pregnancy category B, lactation (unknown), bone marrow suppression, renal impairment

Pharmacokinetics:
PO: Peak serum levels 3 hr, serum levels decrease by 8 hr; hepatic metabolism; renal excretion

Drug interactions of concern to dentistry:
• Increased plasma levels of clindamycin, troleandomycin, ketoconazole, itraconazole, fentanyl, clarithromycin, midazolam, triazolam
• Increased metabolism of carbamazepine, dexamethasone, phenobarbital
• Inhibits CYP3A4 isoenzymes: use with caution or avoid use with drugs metabolized by these enzymes (see Appendix I)

DENTAL CONSIDERATIONS

General:
• Examine for oral manifestations of opportunistic infections.
• Patients on chronic drug therapy may rarely have symptoms of blood dyscrasias, which can include infection, bleeding, and poor healing.
• Palliative medication may be required for management of oral side effects.

Consultations:
• Medical consultation may be required to assess disease control.
• In a patient with symptoms of blood dyscrasias, request a medical consultation for blood studies and postpone dental treatment until normal values are reestablished.

Teach patient/family:
• Importance of good oral hygiene to prevent soft tissue inflammation
• Caution to prevent trauma when using oral hygiene aids
• That secondary oral infection may occur; must see dentist immediately if infection occurs
• Importance of updating medical/drug history if physician makes any changes in evaluation or drug regimen

scopolamine (transdermal)

(skoe-pol'a-meen)
Transderm Scop
🍁 Transderm-V

Drug class.: Antiemetic, anticholinergic

Action: Competitive antagonism of acetylcholine at receptor sites in the eye, smooth muscle, cardiac muscle, glandular cells; inhibition of vestibular input to the CNS, resulting in inhibition of vomiting reflex

Uses: Prevention of motion sickness; prevent nausea, vomiting associated with anesthesia or opiate analgesia

Dosage and routes:

• *Adult:* Patch 1.5 mg placed behind ear 4-5 hr before travel; replace after 3 days if continued use is required

Not recommended for children

Available forms include: Patch 1.5 mg

Side effects/adverse reactions:

▼ *ORAL: Dry mouth*

CNS: Dizziness, drowsiness, confusion, disorientation, memory disturbances, hallucinations

GU: Difficult urination

EENT: Blurred vision, dilated pupils, altered depth perception, photophobia, dry/itchy/red eyes, acute narrow-angle glaucoma

INTEG: Rash, erythema

Contraindications: Hypersensitivity, glaucoma

Precautions: Children, elderly, pregnancy category C; pyloric, urinary, bladder neck, intestinal obstruction; liver, kidney disease

Pharmacokinetics: *PATCH:* Onset 4-5 hr, duration 72 hr

Drug interactions of concern to dentistry:

• Increased anticholinergic effects: propantheline and other anticholinergic drugs

• Increased risk of CNS depression: alcohol, all CNS depressants

DENTAL CONSIDERATIONS

General:

• Avoid dental light in patient's eyes; offer dark glasses for patient comfort.

• Caution patients about driving or performing other tasks requiring alertness

Teach patient/family:

• To avoid mouth rinses with high alcohol content because of drying effects

secobarbital/ secobarbital sodium

(see-koe-bar'bi-tal)
Seconal
🍁 Novosecobarb

Drug class.: Sedative-hypnotic barbiturate

Controlled Substance Schedule II, Canada G

Action: Nonselective depression of the CNS, ranging from sedation to hypnosis to anesthesia to coma, depending on the dose administered

Uses: Insomnia, sedation, preoperative medication, status epilepticus, acute tetanus convulsions

Dosage and routes:

Insomnia:

• *Adult:* PO 100 mg hs

Sedation (preoperatively):
• *Adult:* PO 100-200 mg 1-2 hr preoperatively
• *Child:* PO 2-6 mg/kg 1-2 hr preoperatively; rectal up to a max of 100 mg

Available forms include: Caps 100 mg

Side effects/adverse reactions:

▼ *ORAL:* Oral ulcerations (rare), bleeding (rare)

CNS: Lethargy, drowsiness, hangover, dizziness, paradoxic stimulation in the elderly and children, light-headedness, dependence, CNS depression, mental depression, slurred speech

CV: Hypotension, bradycardia

GI: Nausea, vomiting, diarrhea, constipation

RESP: ***Apnea, laryngospasm, bronchospasm,*** depression

HEMA: ***Agranulocytosis, thrombocytopenia, megaloblastic anemia*** (long-term treatment)

INTEG: Rash, ***Stevens-Johnson syndrome,*** urticaria, pain, abscesses at injection site, angioedema, thrombophlebitis

Contraindications: Hypersensitivity to barbiturates, respiratory depression, addiction to barbiturates, severe liver impairment, porphyria, uncontrolled severe pain

Precautions: Anemia, pregnancy category D, lactation, hepatic disease, renal disease, hypertension, elderly, acute/chronic pain

Pharmacokinetics:

IM: Onset 10-15 min, duration 3-6 hr

REC: Onset slow, duration 3-6 hr Half-life 15-40 hr; metabolized by liver; excreted by kidneys (metabolites)

Drug interactions of concern to dentistry:
• Hepatotoxicity: halogenated hydrocarbon anesthetics
• Increased CNS depression: alcohol, all CNS depressants
• Increased metabolism of carbamazepine, tricyclic antidepressants, corticosteroids
• Decreased half-life of doxycycline

DENTAL CONSIDERATIONS

General:
• Determine why the patient is taking the drug.
• Monitor vital signs at every appointment because of cardiovascular side effects. Evaluate respiration characteristics and rate.
• Patients on chronic drug therapy may rarely have symptoms of blood dyscrasias, which can include infection, bleeding, and poor healing.

When used for sedation in dentistry:
• Assess vital signs before and q30min after use as sedative.
• Observe respiratory dysfunction: respiratory depression, character, rate, rhythm; hold drug if respirations are <10/min or if pupils are dilated.
• After supine positioning, have patient sit upright for at least 2 min before standing to avoid orthostatic hypotension.
• Have someone drive patient to and from dental office when used for conscious sedation.
• Barbiturates induce liver microsomal enzymes, which alter the metabolism of other drugs.
• Geriatric patients are more susceptible to drug effects; use a lower dose.

Consultations:
• In a patient with symptoms of blood dyscrasias, request a medical consultation for blood studies and postpone dental treatment until normal values are reestablished.
Teach patient/family:
• To avoid driving or other activities requiring alertness
• To avoid alcohol ingestion and CNS depressants; serious CNS depression may result
• Caution when using OTC preparations (antihistamines, cold remedies) that contain CNS depressants

selegiline HCl (l-deprenyl)

(se-le'ji-leen)
Carbex, Eldepryl
✤ Apo-Selegiline, Gen-Selegiline, Novo-Selegiline, Nu-Selegiline, SD Deprenyl, Selegiline-5
Drug class.: Antiparkinson agent

Action: Increased dopaminergic activity by irreversibly inhibiting MAO type B activity
Uses: Adjunct management of Parkinson's disease in patients being treated with levodopa/carbidopa
Dosage and routes:
• *Adult:* PO 10 mg/day in divided doses of 5 mg at breakfast and lunch; doses of 20 mg/day increase the risk of side effects/drug interactions but provide no additional therapeutic benefits
Available forms include: Tabs 5 mg, caps 5 mg
Side effects/adverse reactions:
▼ *ORAL:* Dry mouth
CNS: Increased tremors, chorea, restlessness, blepharospasm, increased bradykinesia, grimacing, tardive dyskinesia, dystonic symptoms, involuntary movements, increased apraxia, hallucinations, dizziness, mood changes, nightmares, delusions, lethargy, apathy, overstimulation, sleep disturbances, headache, migraine, numbness, muscle cramps, confusion, anxiety, tiredness, vertigo, personality change, back/leg pain
CV: Orthostatic hypotension, hypertension, dysrhythmia, palpitation, angina pectoris, hypotension, tachycardia, edema, sinus bradycardia, syncope
GI: Nausea, vomiting, constipation, weight loss, anorexia, diarrhea, heartburn, rectal bleeding, poor appetite, dysphagia
RESP: Asthma, shortness of breath
GU: Slow urination, nocturia, prostatic hypertrophy, hesitation, retention, frequency, sexual dysfunction
EENT: Diplopia, blurred vision, tinnitus
INTEG: Increased sweating, alopecia, hematoma, rash, photosensitivity, facial hair
Contraindications: Hypersensitivity; fluoxetine, meperidine
Precautions: Pregnancy category C, lactation, children
Pharmacokinetics:
PO: Rapidly absorbed, peak 0.5-2 hr; rapidly metabolized (active metabolites: *N*-desmethyldeprenyl, l-amphetamine, l-methamphetamine); metabolites excreted in urine
Drug interactions of concern to dentistry:
• ***Fatal interaction:*** opioids (especially meperidine); do not administer together
• Risk of serotonin syndrome: serotonin uptake inhibitors (fluoxetine, sertraline, paroxetine)

S

DENTAL CONSIDERATIONS
General:
• Monitor vital signs at every appointment because of cardiovascular side effects.
• After supine positioning, have patient sit upright for at least 2 min before standing to avoid orthostatic hypotension.
• Assess for presence of extrapyramidal motor symptoms, such as tardive dyskinesia and akathisia. Extrapyramidal motor activity may complicate dental treatment.
• Assess salivary flow as a factor in caries, periodontal disease, and candidiasis.
Consultations:
• Medical consultation may be required to assess disease control and patient's ability to tolerate stress.
• If signs of tardive dyskinesia or akathisia are present, refer to physician.
Teach patient/family:
• To use electric toothbrush if patient has difficulty holding conventional devices
When chronic dry mouth occurs, advise patient:
• To avoid mouth rinses with high alcohol content because of drying effects
• Of need for daily use of home fluoride products to prevent caries
• To use sugarless gum, frequent sips of water, or saliva substitutes

---

sertraline HCl

(ser'tra-leen)
Zoloft
Drug class.: Antidepressant

Action: Selectively inhibits the uptake of serotonin in the brain

Uses: Major depression, obsessive-compulsive disorder (OCD), panic disorder; posttraumatic stress disorder, premenstrual dysphoric mood disorder; social anxiety disorder

Dosage and routes:
Depression and OCD:
• *Adult:* PO 50 mg qd; may increase to a max of 200 mg/day; do not change dose at intervals of <1 wk; administer qd in AM or PM
Posttraumatic stress disorder/panic disorder:
• *Adult:* PO 25 mg/day; can increase to 50 mg/day after 1 wk
Premenstrual dysphoric disorder:
• *Adult:* PO 50 mg/day throughout cycle, or less as determined by physician
Available forms include: Tabs 25, 50, 100 mg; oral conc 20 mg/ml in 60 ml; (Canada) caps 25, 50, 100, 150, 200 mg

Side effects/adverse reactions:
▼ *ORAL: Dry mouth,* aphthous stomatitis (<0.1%), taste alteration, lichenoid reaction
CNS: Insomnia, headache, dizziness, somnolence, tremor, fatigue, twitching, confusion
CV: Palpitation, chest pain, postural hypotension, syncope
GI: Diarrhea, nausea, dyspepsia, constipation, anorexia, vomiting, flatulence
RESP: Rhinitis, pharyngitis, coughing
GU: Male sexual dysfunction, micturition disorder
EENT: Vision abnormalities, tinnitus
INTEG: Sweating, rash
MS: Myalgia

Contraindications: Hypersensitivity, MAOIs, fluvoxamine

Precautions: Pregnancy category C, lactation, elderly, hepatic/renal disease, epilepsy

Pharmacokinetics:

PO: Peak 6-10 hr, elimination half-life 25 hr; plasma protein binding 99%; extensively metabolized; metabolites excreted in urine

Drug interactions of concern to dentistry:

• Increased CNS depression: alcohol, CNS depressants, St. John's wort (herb)

• Increased side effects: highly protein-bound drugs (aspirin), tricyclic antidepressants

• Increased half-life of diazepam

• Possible inhibition of sertraline metabolism: erythromycin, clarithromycin

• A potent inhibitor of CYP2D6 isoenzymes; use drugs metabolized by the enzyme only with caution (see Appendix I)

• Possible risk of serotonin syndrome with tramadol, oxycodone

• Decreased effects: carbamazepine

• First-time users of SSRIs also taking NSAIDs may have a higher risk of GI side effects; until more data are available, it may be advisable to avoid use of NSAIDs in these patients (*Br J Clin Pharmacol* 55:591-595, 2003)

DENTAL CONSIDERATIONS

General:

• Monitor vital signs at every appointment because of cardiovascular side effects.

• After supine positioning, have patient sit upright for at least 2 min to avoid orthostatic hypotension.

• Assess salivary flow as a factor in caries, periodontal disease, and candidiasis.

• Avoid dental light in patient's eyes; offer dark glasses for patient comfort.

• Consider semisupine chair position for patient comfort if GI side effects occur.

Consultations:

• Medical consultation may be required to assess patient's ability to tolerate stress.

• Physician should be informed if significant xerostomic side effects occur (e.g., increased caries, sore tongue, problems eating or swallowing, difficulty wearing prosthesis) so that a medication change can be considered.

Teach patient/family:

• To use electric toothbrush if patient has difficulty holding conventional devices

When chronic dry mouth occurs, advise patient:

• To avoid mouth rinses with high alcohol content because of drying effects

• Of need for daily use of home fluoride products to prevent caries

• To use sugarless gum, frequent sips of water, or saliva substitutes

---

sibutramine

(si-byoo'tra-meen)

Meridia

Drug class.: Amphetamine analog anorexiant

Controlled Substance Schedule IV

Action: Anoretic action unclear, blocks the reuptake of norepinephrine, serotonin, and dopamine; action depends on formation of two active metabolites, M_1 and M_2

Uses: Obesity

Dosage and routes:

• *Adult:* PO initial dose 10 mg/day; after 4 wk can titrate dose to 15 mg/day; doses >15 mg/day are not recommended

Available forms include: Caps 5, 10, 15 mg

Side effects/adverse reactions:

▼ *ORAL: Dry mouth,* taste prevention

CNS: Headache, insomnia, irritability, asthenia, migraine

CV: Tachycardia, hypertension, palpitation

GI: Abdominal pain, dyspepsia, nausea

GU: Dysmenorrhea, UTI

EENT: Rhinitis, pharyngitis

MS: Back pain, arthralgia

MISC: Flulike syndrome

INTEG: Skin rash, dry skin

META: Elevated ALT, AST, alk phosphatase

Contraindications: Hypersensitivity, MAOI, anorexia nervosa, severe hepatic or renal impairment, CAD, CHF, arrhythmias, stroke, other CNS appetite suppressants, meperidine

Precautions: Requires monitoring of BP, risk of serotonin syndrome with other serotonin reuptake inhibitors, glaucoma, pregnancy category C, lactation, children <16 yr, elderly, seizures

Pharmacokinetics:

PO: Rapid absorption, extensive first-pass metabolism, two active metabolites (M_1 and M_2), highly protein bound (94%-97%), hepatic metabolism; excreted mostly in urine, less in feces

Drug interactions of concern to dentistry:

• Avoid use of meperidine: risk of serotonin syndrome

DENTAL CONSIDERATIONS

General:

• Monitor vital signs at every appointment because of cardiovascular side effects.

• Assess salivary flow as factor in caries, periodontal disease, and candidiasis.

• Information on any abuse liability is unknown.

• Determine why patient is taking the drug.

Teach patient/family:

When chronic dry mouth occurs, advise patient:

• To avoid mouth rinses with high alcohol content because of drying effects

• Of need for daily use of home fluoride products to prevent caries

• To use sugarless gum, frequent sips of water, or saliva substitutes

sildenafil citrate

(sil-den'a-fil)

Viagra

Drug class.: Impotence therapy

Action: A selective inhibitor of cyclic guanosine monophosphate (cGMP)–specific phosphodiesterase type 5 (PDE5). It enhances the effect of nitric oxide (produced by sexual stimulation) that is involved in increased production of cGMP, both of which are involved in the physiologic processes leading to penile erection. cGMP is required for smooth muscle relaxation in the corpus cavernosum that allows inflow of blood.

Uses: Male erectile dysfunction

Dosage and routes:

• *Adult:* PO (male only) 50 mg taken as needed approximately 1 hr before sexual activity with once-a-

day dosing at a maximum. The dosage range is 25-100 mg based on tolerance and effectiveness. It can be taken anywhere from 0.5-4 hr before sexual activity. Sexual activity is required for effective response.
WARNINGS: Concurrent use with a protease inhibitor–do not exceed 25 mg in a 48 hr period. Concurrent use with α-adrenergic blockers do not take 50 mg or 100 mg doses within 4 hr of taking α-adrenergic blocker.
Available forms include: Tabs 25, 50, 100 mg
Side effects/adverse reactions:
▼ *ORAL:* Dry mouth, glossitis (very low incidence)
CNS: Headache, dizziness, insomnia, somnolence, abnormal dreams
CV: Flushing, syncope, palpitation, hemorrhoidal hemorrhage
GI: Dyspepsia, diarrhea, vomiting, dysphagia, gastritis
RESP: Dyspnea, increased cough, asthma
GU: UTI, cystitis, nocturia, urinary frequency, abnormal ejaculation
EENT: Nasal congestion, sinusitis
INTEG: Rash, urticaria, pruritus, contact dermatitis
MS: Musculoskeletal pain, synovitis
Contraindications: Hypersensitivity, patients who are currently using organic nitrates
Precautions: Complete medical and physical exam to determine cause of erectile dysfunction; because of cardiac risk associated with sexual activity, cardiovascular status should be evaluated; anatomic deformation of penis, conditions predisposing to priapism (sickle cell anemia, anemia, multiple myeloma, leukemia), retinitis pigmentosa, not indicated for women, children, or newborns, pregnancy category B; hepatic or renal impairment, men >65 yr
Pharmacokinetics:
PO: Rapid oral absorption, bioavailability 40%, peak plasma levels 30 min-2 hr, hepatic metabolism by CYP3A4 (major) and CYP2C9 (minor) isoenzymes, active metabolite, highly plasma protein bound (96%), major excretion route in feces, lesser route in urine
Drug interactions of concern to dentistry:
- Avoid use of nitroglycerin within 24 hr
- Increased plasma levels caused by interference with metabolism: cimetidine, erythromycin, ketoconazole, itraconazole
- Strong inhibitors of CYP3A4 or CYP2C9 isoenzymes: should be used with caution (see Appendix I)

DENTAL CONSIDERATIONS
General:
- This is an acute-use drug intended to be taken just before sexual activity, and the reported incidence of oral side effects does not differ from a placebo. However, the potential interacting drugs should be avoided.

S

simvastatin

(sim′va-sta-tin)
Zocor
Drug class.: Antihyperlipidemic

Action: Inhibits HMG-Co A reductase enzyme, thus reducing cholesterol synthesis; reduced synthesis of VLDL; plasma triglyceride levels may also be decreased
Uses: As an adjunct in homozygous familial hypercholesterol-

emia, mixed hyperlipidemia, elevated serum triglyceride levels, and type IV hyperproteinemia; also reduces total cholesterol LDL-C, apo B, and triglyceride levels; patient should first be placed on cholesterol-lowering diet; effective in reducing risk of heart attacks and strokes

Dosage and routes:

• *Adult:* PO initial 20 mg/day with evening meal; may increase to 5-40 mg/day in single or divided doses; not to exceed 80 mg/day; dosage adjustments should be made qmo

Available forms include: Tabs 5, 10, 20, 40, 80 mg

Side effects/adverse reactions:

CNS: Dizziness, headache

GI: Nausea, constipation, diarrhea, dyspepsia, flatulence, abdominal pain, heartburn, ***liver dysfunction***

EENT: Blurred vision, dysgeusia, lens opacities

INTEG: Rash, pruritus

MS: Muscle cramps, myalgia, ***myositis, rhabdomyolysis***

Contraindications: Pregnancy category X, lactation, active liver disease

Precautions: Past liver disease, alcoholics (first-pass metabolism with CYP3A4 isoenzymes); severe acute infections, trauma, hypotension, uncontrolled seizure disorders, severe metabolic disorders, electrolyte imbalances

Pharmacokinetics:

PO: Peak 1-2.5 hr; highly protein bound; metabolized in liver (active metabolites); excreted in bile, feces

Drug interactions of concern to dentistry:

• Increased myalgia, myositis: erythromycin, cyclosporin, itraconazole, ketoconazole

• Caution with use of drugs that are strong inhibitors of CYP3A4 isoenzymes (see Appendix I)

DENTAL CONSIDERATIONS

General:

• Consider semisupine chair position for patient comfort because of GI side effects.

---

sodium fluoride

Fluoritabs, Flura-Drops, Fluor-a-day, fluotic, Flurodex Karidium, Luride Lozi-Tabs, Pediaflor, Pedi-Dent, Solu-Flur; also found in pediatric vitamin formulas

Fluor-A-Day, Fluotic

Drug class.: Fluoride ion

Action: Interacts with tooth structure to increase resistance to acid dissolution; promotes enamel remineralization and inhibits dental plaque microorganisms

Uses: Prevention of dental caries

Dosage and routes:

• *Adult and child >12 yr:* TOP 10 ml 0.2% sol qd after brushing teeth; rinse mouth for >1 min with sol

• *Child 6-12 yr:* TOP 5 ml 0.2% sol

Revised fluoride supplement schedules (infants and children–ADA, American Academy of Pediatric Dentistry, American Academy of Pediatrics)

• Must ascertain fluoride concentration in patient's drinking water before prescribing, as shown in the following tables:

USA–fluoride supplementation schedule

Child's age	<0.3 ppm	0.3-0.6 ppm	>0.6 ppm
birth-6 mo	0.0	0.0	0.0
6 mo-3 yr	0.25 mg/day	0.0	0.0
3-6 yr	0.50 mg/day	0.25 mg/day	0.0
6-16 yr	1.0 mg/day	0.50 mg/day	0.0

Canada–fluoride supplementation schedule

Age	Canadian Paediatric Society (applies to all children)	Canadian Dental Association (applies to children with high risk of caries)
6 mo-2 yr	0.25 mg/day	0
3-5 yr	0.50 mg/day	0.25 mg/day (0.5 mg/day if fluoridated toothpaste is not used regularly)
6-12 yr	Not applicable	1.00 mg/day
6-16 yr	1.0 mg/day	Not applicable

Reference: Kowalchuk I: *CMAJ* 154(7): 1007, 1996.

Available forms include: Chew tabs 0.25 mg; tabs 0.5, 1 mg, effervescent tabs 10 mg; drops 0.125, 0.25, 0.5 mg/ml; rinse supplements 0.2 mg/ml; rinse 0.01%, 0.02%, 0.09%; gel 0.1%, 0.5%, 1.23%

Side effects/adverse reactions:
▼ *ORAL:* Mottled enamel (chronic use), stomatitis
ACUTE OVERDOSE: ***Black tarry stools, bloody vomit, diarrhea, decreased respiration, increased salivation, watery eyes***
CHRONIC OVERDOSE: ***Hypocalcemia, tetany, respiratory arrest, constipation, loss of appetite, nausea, vomiting, weight loss***

Contraindications: Hypersensitivity, renal insufficiency, GI ulcerations

Precautions: Child <6 yr (must evaluate total fluoride ingestion), pregnancy category not established

Pharmacokinetics:
PO: Efficient oral absorption; distributed to calcified tissues (bones and teeth); excreted in urine, feces; crosses placenta, excreted in breast milk

Drug interactions of concern to dentistry:
- Avoid use with dairy products and gastric alkalinizers

DENTAL CONSIDERATIONS

General:
- Determine fluoride concentration in water supply, then calculate dosage.
- In the United States, the use of fluoride supplements is not recommended when community drinking water contains at least 0.6 ppm fluoride or after age 16.
- Recommended dose should not be exceeded or dental fluorosis and osseous changes may occur.
- To reduce risk of accidental ingestion and overdosage, ADA recommends that a limit of 264 mg sodium fluoride be dispensed in prepackaged containers.
- Give drops after meals with fluids

S

or undiluted tablets; may be chewed; do not swallow whole; may be given with water or juice; avoid milk.

• Systemic fluoride use during pregnancy has not been shown to prevent tooth decay in children.

Teach patient/family:

• To monitor children using gel or rinse; not to be swallowed

• Not to drink, eat, or rinse mouth for at least 0.5 hr after topical use

• To apply after brushing and flossing hs

• To store out of children's reach

Treatment of acute overdose:

• Gastric lavage with calcium chloride or calcium hydroxide solution to precipitate fluoride

• Maintenance of high urine output

• Refer to hospital emergency facility

sodium fluoride (topical)

Sodium fluoride (topical) nonabrasive: Karigel, Neutracare, Prevident

Sodium fluoride (topical) with abrasive: PreviDent 5000 Plus

Drug class.: Fluoride ion

Action: Interacts with enamel surface to increase resistance to acid dissolution; promotes enamel remineralization and inhibits dental plaque microorganisms

Uses: Prevention of dental caries, hypersensitive root surfaces

Dosage and routes:

• *Adult and child >6 yr:* Nonabrasive gels–use daily; apply thin ribbon to toothbrush for at least 1 min after regular brushing, preferably at bedtime; expectorate and refrain from eating, drinking, and rinsing; children should use under parental supervision.

Available forms include: Gel or cream 2 oz (56 g) squeeze tube 0.5% (as 1.1% sodium fluoride) with and without mild abrasive

Other fluoride topical products include the following daily-use gels: 1.1% APF (Thera-Flur); 0.4% Sn F_2 (Control, Easy-Gel, Flocare, Flo-Gel, Florentine, Gel-Kam, Gel-Pro, Gel-Tin, Perfect Choice, Quick-Gel, Stan-Gard, Stop Gel)

Rinses: 0.05% APF daily use (NaF-rinse, Phos-Flur) and 0.2% NaF weekly use (NaFrinse, Point-Two, Preventive, Prevident)

Product strength	F^- ion (%)	ppm F equivalence
1.1% NaF	0.5	4950
0.4% SnF_2	0.10	970
0.2% NaF	0.10	910
0.05% NaF	0.02	230

Contraindications: Hypersensitivity; may be used in areas of fluoridated drinking water

Precautions: Child <6 yr (repeated swallowing of agent could cause dental fluorosis); do not use in pediatric patients <6 yr, infants. Supervise children <6 yr. A 2-oz tube of 1.1% NaF contains 250 mg fluoride, more than twice the amount that the ADA recommends to be dispensed in 1 container. Ingestion of as little as 0.29 oz could cause acute toxicity in a 1-year-old child. Repeated swallowing could cause fluorosis.

DENTAL CONSIDERATIONS

General:

• Neutral sodium fluoride preparations are recommended for patients with exposed root surfaces, which may be hypersensitive.

Teach patient/family:

• To apply daily a thin ribbon of dental cream or gel to toothbrush and brush thoroughly for 2 min, preferably at bedtime

• To expectorate after use and not to eat, drink, or rinse for 30 min

• That children should use under parental supervision

sotalol HCl

(soe'ta-lole)

Betapace, Betapace AF

♣ Sotacor

Drug class.: Nonselective β-adrenergic blocker

Action: This is a nonselective β_1- and β_2-adrenergic antagonist. The antihypertensive mechanism of action is unclear, but it may include a reduction in cardiac output and inhibition of renin release by the renal juxtaglomerular apparatus. Peripheral resistance decreases with long-term use. The antianginal action (when indicated for this use) may be related to a decrease in myocardial oxygen demand and negative chronotropic and inotropic effects. The antiarrhythmic action (when indicated for this use) has been related to a reduction in spontaneous pacemaker firing and slowing of AV nodal conduction.

Uses: Life-threatening ventricular dysrhythmias (class II), atrial fibrillation (Betapace AF only)

Dosage and routes:

• *Adult:* PO initial 80 mg bid; may be increased gradually to 240 or 320 mg/day; some patients may require 480-640 mg/day

Available forms include: Tabs 80, 120, 160, 240 mg; AF tabs 80, 120, 160 mg

Side effects/adverse reactions:

CNS: Fatigue, dizziness, asthenia, light-headedness, headache, insomnia, sedation

CV: ***Bradycardia, dysrhythmia, hypotension, CHF, syncope,*** chest pain, palpitation

GI: Nausea, vomiting, dyspepsia

RESP: ***Asthma, dyspnea***

GU: Sexual dysfunction

EENT: Visual problems

INTEG: Rash

Contraindications: Hypersensitivity to this drug, cardiac failure, cardiogenic shock, second- or third-degree heart block, bronchospastic disease, sinus bradycardia, CHF

Precautions: Pregnancy category B, lactation, diabetes mellitus, renal disease, before initiating doses place patient in cardiac care facility to monitor for drug induced arrhythmia

Pharmacokinetics:

PO: Peak plasma levels 2.5-4 hr, half-life 12 hr; low protein binding; excreted in urine unchanged

Drug interactions of concern to dentistry:

• Decreased hypotensive effect: NSAIDs, indomethacin

• Increased hypotension, myocardial depression: hydrocarbon inhalation anesthetics

• Hypertension, bradycardia: sympathomimetics

• Slow metabolism of lidocaine

DENTAL CONSIDERATIONS

General:

• Monitor vital signs at every appointment because of cardiovascular side effects.

• After supine positioning, have

patient sit upright for at least 2 min before standing to avoid orthostatic hypotension.

• Stress from dental procedures may compromise cardiovascular function; determine patient risk.
• Use vasoconstrictors with caution, in low doses, and with careful aspiration. Avoid use of gingival retraction cord with epinephrine.
• Short appointments and a stress reduction protocol may be required for anxious patients.

Consultations:

• Medical consultation should be made to assess disease control and patient's ability to tolerate stress.

---

sparfloxacin

(spar-flox'a-sin)

Zagam

Drug class.: Fluoroquinolone anti-infective

Action: A broad-spectrum bactericidal agent that inhibits the enzymes topoisomerase II (DNA gyrase) and topoisomerase IV required for bacterial DNA replication, transcription repair, and recombination

Uses: Community-acquired pneumonia and acute bacterial exacerbations of chronic bronchitis caused by susceptible microorganisms *(C. pneumoniae, H. influenzae, M. pneumoniae, S. pneumoniae, K. pneumoniae, M. catarrhalis, S. aureus, E. cloacae)*

Dosage and routes:

• *Adult >18 yr:* PO 400 mg first day, then 200 mg qd for total of 10 days therapy (total 11 tabs)

Renal impairment:

• *Adult >18 yr:* PO 400 mg first day; then 200 mg q48h for total of 9 days therapy (6 tabs)

Available forms include: Tabs 200 mg

Side effects/adverse reactions:

▼ *ORAL: Taste alteration,* dry mouth

CNS: Headache, insomnia, convulsions, toxic psychoses, dizziness, light-headedness

CV: Prolonged QT interval, vasodilation, palpitation, postural hypotension

GI: Diarrhea, nausea, dyspepsia, abdominal pain, vomiting, flatulence, ***pseudomembranous colitis***

RESP: Pharyngitis, epistaxis, cough, sinusitis

HEMA: Cyanosis, ecchymosis

GU: Vaginitis, dysuria

EENT: Ear pain, tinnitus, diplopia, eye pain

INTEG: Photosensitization, pruritus

MS: Rupture of Achilles tendon, tendons in shoulder or hand

MISC: ***Anaphylaxis***

Contraindications: Hypersensitivity, photosensitivity, disopyramide, amiodarone, class Ia and III antiarrhythmics, bepridil; patients with prolonged QT_c interval, hypokalemia, significant bradycardia

Precautions: Antacids retard absorption, renal impairment, avoid exposure to sun, artificial ultraviolet light, patients <18 yr, seizures, CV arrhythmics, MI, congestive heart failure, pregnancy category C, lactation

Pharmacokinetics:

PO: Oral bioavailability 92%, peak plasma levels 3-6 hr, hepatic metabolism, equally excreted in urine and feces

Drug interactions of concern to dentistry:

• Avoid concurrent use with erythromycin, pentamidine, tricyclic antidepressants, phenothiazines

• Concurrent administration with antacids greatly reduces oral absorption, can increase warfarin levels

• Increased risk of life-threatening arrhythmias: procainamide

DENTAL CONSIDERATIONS

General:

• Contraindicated for patients whose lifestyle or employment will not permit compliance with photosensitivity precautions.

• Determine why patient is taking the drug.

• Assess salivary flow as factor in caries, periodontal disease, and candidiasis.

• Consider semisupine chair position for patient comfort if GI side effects occur.

• Avoid dental light in patient's eyes; offer dark glasses for patient comfort.

Consultations:

• Consult with patient's physician if an acute dental infection occurs and another antiinfective is required.

Teach patient/family:

• To avoid exposure to sunlight and wear sunscreen if sun exposure is planned during treatment and for 5 days after treatment is stopped

---

spironolactone

(speer-on-oh-lak'tone)

Aldactone

♣ Novospiroton

Drug class.: Potassium-sparing diuretic

Action: Competitive inhibitor of aldosterone at receptor sites in distal tubule, resulting in excretion of sodium chloride, water, retention of potassium and phosphate

Uses: Edema, hypertension, diuretic-induced hypokalemia, primary hyperaldosteronism (diagnosis, short-term treatment, long-term treatment), nephrotic syndrome, cirrhosis of the liver with ascites

Dosage and routes:

Edema/hypertension:

• *Adult:* PO 25-200 mg qd in single or divided doses

• *Child:* PO 3.3 mg/kg/day in single or divided doses

Hypokalemia:

• *Adult:* PO 25-100 mg/day; if PO, K supplements must not be used

Primary hyperaldosteronism diagnosis:

• *Adult:* PO 400 mg/day for 4 days or 4 wk depending on test, then 100-400 mg/day maintenance

Available forms include: Tabs 25, 50, 100 mg

Side effects/adverse reactions:

▼ *ORAL:* Gingival bleeding (rare); dry mouth may be a symptom of hyponatremia, lichenoid drug reaction

CNS: Headache, confusion, drowsiness, lethargy, ataxia

GI: Diarrhea, ***bleeding*** (rare), gastritis, cramps, vomiting

HEMA: Decreased WBCs, platelets

INTEG: Rash, pruritus, urticaria

ENDO: Impotence, gynecomastia, irregular menses, amenorrhea, postmenopausal bleeding, hirsutism, deepening voice

ELECT: ***Hyperkalemia,*** hyperchloremic metabolic acidosis, hyponatremia

Contraindications: Hypersensitivity, anuria, severe renal disease, hyperkalemia, pregnancy category not established

Precautions: Dehydration, hepatic disease, lactation, hyponatremia

Pharmacokinetics:

PO: Onset 24-48 hr, peak 48-72 hr; metabolized in liver; excreted in urine; crosses placenta

Drug interactions of concern to dentistry:

• Nephrotoxicity: indomethacin and possibly other NSAIDs

• Decreased antihypertensive effect: indomethacin and possibly other NSAIDs

DENTAL CONSIDERATIONS

General:

• Monitor vital signs at every appointment because of cardiovascular side effects.

• Assess salivary flow as a factor in caries, periodontal disease, and candidiasis.

• If dry mouth occurs, follow usual preventive and palliative measures, but consider hyponatremia as a contributing factor.

• Consider semisupine chair position for patient comfort if GI side effects occur.

Consultations:

• Medical consultation may be required to assess disease control and patient's ability to tolerate stress.

Teach patient/family:

When chronic dry mouth occurs, advise patient:

• To avoid mouth rinses with high alcohol content because of drying effects

• Of need for daily use of home fluoride products to prevent caries

• To use sugarless gum, frequent sips of water, or saliva substitutes

stanozolol

(stan-oh'zoe-lole)

Winstrol

Drug class.: Androgenic anabolic steroid

Controlled Substance Schedule III

Action: Reverses catabolic tissue processes; promotes buildup of protein; increases erythropoietin production

Uses: Hereditary angioedema prophylaxis

Dosage and routes:

Angioedema:

• *Adult:* PO 2 mg tid, then decrease q1-3mo, down to 2 mg qd or q2d

• *Child 6-12 yr:* PO up to 2 mg/day only during the attack

• *Child <6 yr:* PO 1 mg/day only during the attack

Available forms include: Tabs 2 mg

Side effects/adverse reactions:

CNS: Dizziness, headache, fatigue, tremors, paresthesia, flushing, sweating, anxiety, lability, insomnia

CV: ***Edema (in cardiac patients),*** increased BP

GI: ***Peliosis hepatitis, liver cell tumors, cholestatic jaundice,*** nausea, vomiting, constipation, weight gain

HEMA: Increased prothrombin time, iron deficiency anemia

GU: ***Hematuria,*** amenorrhea, vaginitis, decreased libido, decreased breast size, clitoral hypertrophy, testicular atrophy, gynecomastia (males), priapism

EENT: Conjunctival edema, nasal congestion

INTEG: Rash, acneiform lesions,

oily hair/skin, flushing, sweating, acne vulgaris, alopecia, hirsutism
ENDO: Abnormal GTT, decreased glucose tolerance, increased LDL
MS: Cramps, spasms
Contraindications: Severe renal disease, severe cardiac disease, severe hepatic disease, hypersensitivity, pregnancy category X, lactation, genital bleeding (abnormal), prostate or breast carcinoma in males, breast cancer in females with hypercalcemia, nephrosis
Precautions: Diabetes mellitus, CV disease, MI, increased risk of prostatic hypertrophy, prostatic carcinoma, virilization (women), increased prothrombin time
Pharmacokinetics:
PO: Metabolized in liver, excreted in urine, crosses placenta, excreted in breast milk
Drug interactions of concern to dentistry:
- Increased risk of bleeding: aspirin
- Edema: ACTH, adrenal steroids

DENTAL CONSIDERATIONS
General:
- Determine why the patient is taking the drug.
- Consider local hemostasis measures to prevent excessive bleeding.
- Psychologic and physical dependence may occur with chronic administration.
- Short appointments and a stress reduction protocol may be required for anxious patients.
- Monitor vital signs at every appointment because of cardiovascular side effects.
- Avoid prescribing aspirin-containing products.

Consultations:
- If signs of anemia are observed in oral tissues, physician consultation may be required.
- Medical consultation may be required to assess disease control and patient's ability to tolerate stress.
- Medical consultation should include partial prothrombin time, prothrombin time, or INR.

Teach patient/family:
- Importance of good oral hygiene to prevent soft tissue inflammation
- That secondary oral infection may occur; must see dentist immediately if infection occurs

stavudine (d4T)

(stav'yoo-deen)
Zerit, Zerit XR
Drug class.: Antiviral, nucleoside analog

Action: A nucleoside analog that undergoes phosphorylation by cellular enzymes and inhibits HIV replication by termination of DNA elongation and inhibition of HIV reverse transcriptase
Uses: Treatment of HIV infection in combination with other antiretroviral drugs
Dosage and routes:
Immediate release tab:
- *Adult:* PO 40 mg bid for patients >60 kg; 30 mg bid for patients <60 kg; dose interval 12 hr apart; doses must be adjusted to creatinine clearance and appearance of peripheral neuropathy
- *Child 14 days and older:* PO child <30 kg, 1 mg/kg/dose q12h; child >30 kg receives adult dose
- *Child birth to 13 days:* PO 0.5 mg/kg q12h

S

Extended release caps:
• *Adult:* PO 100 mg/day for patients >60 kg; 75 mg/day for patients <60 kg

Available forms include: Caps 15, 20, 30, 40 mg; caps ext rel 37.5, 50, 75, 100 mg; powder after reconstitution 1 mg/ml sol in 200 ml

Side effects/adverse reactions:
▼ *ORAL:* Ulcerative stomatitis, aphthous stomatitis
CNS: Headache, asthenia, malaise, anorexia, neuropathy, insomnia, anxiety, depression, nervousness
CV: Chest pain
GI: Abdominal pain, diarrhea, nausea, vomiting, ***pancreatitis, lactic acidosis, severe hepatomegaly with steatosis***
RESP: Dyspnea
HEMA: ***Neutropenia, thrombocytopenia,*** lymphadenopathy
GU: Dysuria
EENT: Conjunctivitis, abnormal vision
INTEG: Rash, pruritus
MS: Myalgia, arthralgia
MISC: Chills, fever, peripheral neurologic symptoms, sweating

Contraindications: Hypersensitivity

Precautions: Pregnancy category C, lactation, children, alcoholism, hepatic or renal impairment; monitor for peripheral neuropathy

Pharmacokinetics:
PO: Rapid absorption, peak plasma levels <1 hr; renal excretion

Drug interactions of concern to dentistry:
• None reported at this time

DENTAL CONSIDERATIONS

General:
• Examine for oral disease.
• Palliative treatment of oral ulcers may be required if they occur.
• Patients on chronic drug therapy may rarely have symptoms of blood dyscrasias, which can include infection, bleeding, and poor healing.
• Consider semisupine chair position for patient comfort because of GI effects of drug.
• Place on frequent recall because of oral side effects and immunocompromised condition.

Consultations:
• Refer to physician if signs of peripheral neuropathy occur.
• In a patient with symptoms of blood dyscrasias, request a medical consultation for blood studies and postpone dental treatment until normal values are reestablished.
• Medical consultation may be required to assess disease control.

Teach patient/family:
• Importance of good oral hygiene to prevent soft tissue inflammation
• To prevent injury when using oral hygiene aids
• To see dentist if secondary oral infection occurs
• To report oral lesions, soreness, or bleeding to dentist

---

sucralfate

(soo-kral′fate)
Carafate
♣ Apo-Sucralfate, Sulcrate
Drug class.: Protectant, aluminum salt of a sulfated sucrose

Action: Forms an ulcer-adherent complex that covers and protects the ulcer site

Uses: Duodenal ulcer

Dosage and routes:
• *Adult:* PO 1 g qid 1 hr ac, hs, maintenance 1 g bid

Available forms include: Tabs 1 g; susp 1 g/10 ml in 415 ml

Side effects/adverse reactions:
▼ *ORAL:* Metallic taste, dry mouth
CNS: Drowsiness, dizziness
GI: *Constipation,* nausea, gastric pain, vomiting
INTEG: Urticaria, rash, pruritus
Contraindications: Hypersensitivity
Precautions: Pregnancy category B, lactation, children
Pharmacokinetics:
PO: Duration up to 5 hr
Drug interactions of concern to dentistry:
- Gastric irritation: chloral hydrate
- Decreased absorption of tetracyclines, fluoroquinolones
- Decreased effects of diclofenac, ketoconazole

DENTAL CONSIDERATIONS
General:
- Prescribe acetaminophen for analgesia if needed. ASA and NSAIDs are contraindicated in active upper GI disease.
- Consider semisupine chair position for patient comfort because of GI effects of disease.
- Tetracycline doses should be given 2 hr before or after the sucralfate dose.

Teach patient/family:
- To avoid mouth rinses with high alcohol content because of drying effects

---

sulconazole nitrate

(sul-kon'a-zole)
Exelderm
Drug class.: Topical antifungal

Action: Interferes with fungal cell membrane, increasing permeability and leaking of nutrients
Uses: Treatment of tinea pedis, tinea corporis, tinea cruris, tinea versicolor; unapproved: cutaneous candidiasis
Dosage and routes:
- *Adult:* TOP apply once or twice daily × 3 wk, except tinea pedis use × 4 wk

Available forms include: Cream 1%; sol 1%
Side effects/adverse reactions:
INTEG: *Stinging,* burning, itching, redness
Contraindications: Hypersensitivity
Precautions: Pregnancy category C
DENTAL CONSIDERATIONS
General:
- There are no significant dental considerations. One possible concern will be those few patients with topical candidiasis, in whom broad-spectrum antiinfectives could potentially contribute to a superinfection.

---

sulfacetamide sodium (ophthalmic)

(sul-fa-see'ta-mide)
AK-Sulf, Bleph-10, Cetamide, Isopto Cetamide, Ocusulf-10, Sodium Sulamyd, Sulster, Storz Sulf, Sulf-10
♣ Sulfex
Drug class.: Antibacterial sulfonamide

Action: Inhibits folic acid synthesis by preventing PABA use, which is necessary for bacterial growth
Uses: Conjunctivitis, superficial eye infections, corneal ulcers, trachoma
Dosage and routes:
- *Adult and child:* INSTILL 1-2 drops q2-3h; top apply 0.5-1 inch

oint into conjunctival sac qid-tid and hs

Trachoma:

• *Adult and child:* TOP 2 drops q2h; concurrent with systemic sulfonamides

Available forms include: Sterile ophth sol 1%, 10%, 15%, 30%; sterile ophth oint 10%

Side effects/adverse reactions:

EENT: Burning, stinging, swelling

Contraindications: Hypersensitivity

Precautions: Cross-sensitivity with other sulfas; pregnancy category C

Drug interactions of concern to dentistry:

• No specific interactions listed

DENTAL CONSIDERATIONS

General:

• Protect patient's eye from accidental spatter during dental treatment.

• Avoid dental light in patient's eyes; offer dark glasses for patient comfort.

sulfamethoxazole/ trimethoprim (SMZ/ TMP) (co-trimoxazole)

(sulf-a-meth-ox'a-zole)/(tri-meth'o-prim)

Bactrim, Bactrim IV, Cofatrim Forte, Cotrim, Sulfatrim, Septra IV, Septra (also all DS and pediatric brands)

Apo-Sulfatrim, Novo-Trimel, Nu-Cotrimox, Roubac

Drug class.: Sulfonamide and folic acid antagonist

Action: Sulfamethoxazole interferes with bacterial biosynthesis of proteins by competitive antagonism of PABA when adequate levels are maintained; trimethoprim blocks synthesis of tetrahydrofolic acid; this combination blocks two consecutive steps in bacterial synthesis of essential nucleic acids/ protein

Uses: UTIs, otitis media, acute and chronic prostatitis, shigellosis, *P. carinii* pneumonitis, chronic bronchitis, chancroid

Dosage and routes:

Urinary tract infections:

• *Adult:* PO 160 mg TMP/800 mg SMZ q12h × 10-14 days

• *Child:* PO 8 mg/kg TMP/40 mg/kg SMZ qd in 2 divided doses q12h

Otitis media:

• *Child:* PO 8 mg/kg TMP/40 mg/kg SMZ qd in 2 divided doses q12h × 10 days

Chronic bronchitis:

• *Adult:* PO 160 mg TMP/800 mg SMZ q12h × 14 days

Pneumocystis carinii pneumonitis:

• *Adult and child:* PO 20 mg/kg TMP/100 mg/kg SMZ qd in 4 divided doses q6h × 14 days; IV 15-20 mg/kg/day (based on TMP) in 3-4 divided doses for up to 14 days

Traveler's diarrhea:

• *Adult:* PO 100 mg TMP/800 mg SMZ q12h × 5 days

WARNING: Dosage reduction is necessary in moderate-to-severe renal impairment (CrCl <30 ml/ min).

Available forms include: Tabs 80 mg TMP/400 mg SMZ; DS (double strength): 160 mg TMP/ 800 mg SMZ; susp 40 mg/200 mg/5 ml; IV inj 16 mg TMP/80 mg SMZ/ml, 80 mg TMP/400 mg SMZ/5 ml

Side effects/adverse reactions:
▼ *ORAL:* Candidiasis, glossitis, stomatitis (Stevens-Johnson syndrome), salivary gland pain
CNS: Headache, insomnia, hallucinations, depression, vertigo, fatigue, anxiety, convulsions, drug fever, chills, aseptic meningitis
CV: ***Allergic myocarditis***
GI: Nausea, vomiting, abdominal pain, ***hepatitis, enterocolitis,*** pancreatitis, diarrhea, anorexia
RESP: Cough, shortness of breath
HEMA: ***Leukopenia, neutropenia, thrombocytopenia, agranulocytosis, hemolytic anemia, hypoprothrombinemia, Henoch-Schönlein purpura, methemoglobinemia, eosinophilia***
GU: ***Renal failure, toxic nephrosis,*** increased BUN, creatinine, crystalluria
INTEG: ***Stevens-Johnson syndrome,*** rash, dermatitis, urticaria, erythema, photosensitivity, pain, inflammation at injection site
SYST: ***Anaphylaxis, SLE***

Contraindications: Hypersensitivity to trimethoprim or sulfonamides, pregnancy at term, megaloblastic anemia, infants <2 mo, CrCl <15 ml/min, lactation

Precautions: Pregnancy category C, renal disease, elderly, G6PD deficiency, impaired hepatic function, possible folate deficiency, severe allergy, bronchial asthma

Pharmacokinetics:
PO: Rapidly absorbed, peak 1-4 hr, half-life 8-13 hr; highly bound to plasma proteins; excreted in urine (metabolites and unchanged), breast milk; crosses placenta; TMP achieves high levels in prostatic tissue and fluid

Drug interactions of concern to dentistry:
- None identified

DENTAL CONSIDERATIONS

General:
- Determine why the patient is taking the drug.
- Patients on chronic drug therapy may rarely have symptoms of blood dyscrasias, which can include infection, bleeding, and poor healing.
- Ensure that dental therapy does not interfere with fluid intake.

Consultations:
- In a patient with symptoms of blood dyscrasias, request a medical consultation for blood studies and postpone dental treatment until normal values are reestablished.
- Inform physician if antibiotics are required for dental infection.

Teach patient/family:
- Importance of good oral hygiene to prevent soft tissue inflammation
- Caution to prevent injury when using oral hygiene aids

---

sulfasalazine

(sul-fa-sal'a-zeen)

Asulfidine-En-Tabs, Azulfidine
♣ Alti-Sulfasalazine, PMS-Sulfasalazine, Salazopyrin EN-Tab, SAS-500

Drug class.: Sulfonamide derivative with antiinflammatory action

Action: Acts as prodrug to deliver sulfapyridine and mesalamine (5-aminosalicylic acid) to the colon

Uses: Ulcerative colitis, Crohn's disease, rheumatoid arthritis, juvenile rheumatoid arthritis; unapproved: ankylosing spondylitis

Dosage and routes:

• *Adult:* PO 3-4 g/day in divided doses; maintenance 1.5-2 g/day in divided doses q6h

• *Child >2 yr:* PO 40-60 mg/kg/day in 4-6 divided doses, then 20-30 mg/kg/day in 4 doses; max 2 g/day

Available forms include: Tabs 500 mg; oral susp 250 mg/5 ml; del rel tabs 500 mg

Side effects/adverse reactions:

▼ *ORAL:* Stomatitis, glossitis, ulcers (Stevens-Johnson syndrome), bleeding, lichenoid reaction

CNS: Headache, ***convulsions,*** confusion, insomnia, hallucinations, depression, vertigo, fatigue, anxiety, drug fever, chills

CV: ***Allergic myocarditis***

GI: Nausea, vomiting, abdominal pain, anorexia, ***hepatitis,*** pancreatitis, diarrhea

HEMA: ***Leukopenia, neutropenia, thrombocytopenia, agranulocytosis, hemolytic anemia***

GU: Reversible low sperm count, ***renal failure, toxic nephrosis,*** increased BUN, creatinine, crystalluria

INTEG: ***Stevens-Johnson syndrome,*** rash, dermatitis, urticaria, erythema, photosensitivity

SYST: ***Anaphylaxis***

Contraindications: Hypersensitivity to sulfonamides or salicylates, pregnancy at term, child <2 yr, intestinal or urinary obstruction

Precautions: Pregnancy category B, lactation, impaired hepatic function, severe allergy, bronchial asthma, impaired renal function, intolerance to aspirin

Pharmacokinetics:

PO: Partially absorbed, peak 1.5-6 hr, half-life 5-10 hr; excreted in urine as sulfasalazine (15%), sulfapyridine (60%), 5-aminosalicylic acid, and metabolites (20%-33%); excreted in breast milk; crosses placenta

Drug interactions of concern to dentistry:

• Increased photosensitizing effects: tetracycline

• Decreased absorption: folic acid

DENTAL CONSIDERATIONS

General:

• Patients on chronic drug therapy may rarely have symptoms of blood dyscrasias, which can include infection, bleeding, and poor healing.

• Question patient about response to antibiotics to avoid responses that might provoke pseudomembranous colitis.

• Palliative medication may be required for management of oral side effects.

• Consider semisupine chair position for patient comfort because of GI effects of disease.

Consultations:

• Medical consultation may be required to assess disease control and patient's ability to tolerate stress.

• In a patient with symptoms of blood dyscrasias, request a medical consultation for blood studies and postpone dental treatment until normal values are reestablished.

Teach patient/family:

• Caution to prevent injury when using oral hygiene aids

sulfinpyrazone

(sul-fin-peer'a-zone)

Anturane

♣ Anturan, Apo-Sulfinpyrazone, Novopyrazone

Drug class.: Uricosuric

Action: Inhibits tubular reabsorption of urates and increases excretion of uric acid; inhibits prostaglandin synthesis, decreasing platelet aggregation

Uses: Chronic gouty arthritis

Dosage and routes:

Gout/gouty arthritis:

• *Adult:* PO 100-200 mg bid for 1 wk, then 200-400 mg bid, not to exceed 800 mg/day

Available forms include: Tabs 100 mg; caps 200 mg

Side effects/adverse reactions:

▼ *ORAL:* Bleeding (rare)

CNS: ***Convulsions, coma,*** dizziness

GI: Gastric irritation, nausea, vomiting, anorexia, ***hepatic necrosis,*** GI bleeding

RESP: ***Apnea,*** irregular respirations

HEMA: ***Agranulocytosis (rare)***

GU: Renal calculi, hypoglycemia

EENT: Tinnitus

INTEG: Rash, dermatitis, pruritus, fever, photosensitivity

Contraindications: Hypersensitivity to pyrazolone derivatives, severe hepatic disease, blood dyscrasias, severe renal disease, CrCl <50 mg/min, active peptic ulcer, GI inflammation, renal calculi

Precautions: Pregnancy category C, lactation

Pharmacokinetics:

PO: Peak 1-2 hr, duration 4-6 hr, half-life 3 hr; metabolized by liver, excreted in urine

Drug interactions of concern to dentistry:

• Increased bleeding: NSAIDs, aspirin

• Decreased effects of salicylates

DENTAL CONSIDERATIONS

General:

• Consider local hemostasis measures to prevent excessive bleeding.

• Avoid prescribing aspirin-containing products.

• Patients on chronic drug therapy may rarely have symptoms of blood dyscrasias, which can include infection, bleeding, and poor healing.

• Consider semisupine chair position for patient comfort if GI side effects occur.

• Evaluate respiration characteristics and rate.

Consultations:

• In a patient with symptoms of blood dyscrasias, request a medical consultation for blood studies and postpone dental treatment until normal values are reestablished.

Teach patient/family:

• Caution to prevent injury when using oral hygiene aids

sulfisoxazole

(sul-fi-sox'a-zole)

♣ Apo-Sulfisoxazole, Novo-Soxazole, Sulfizole

Drug class.: Sulfonamide, short acting; antiinfective

Action: Interferes with bacterial biosynthesis of proteins by competitive antagonism of PABA

Uses: Urinary tract, systemic infections; chancroid; trachoma; toxoplasmosis; acute otitis media; lymphogranuloma venereum; eye infections

Dosage and routes:

- *Adult:* PO 2-4 g loading dose, then 1-2 g qid × 7-10 days
- *Child >2 mo:* PO 75 mg/kg or 2 g/m^2 loading dose, then 120-150 mg/kg/day or 4 g/m^2/day in divided doses q6h, not to exceed 6 g/day

Available forms include: Tabs 500 mg; syr/pediatric susp 500 mg/5 ml

Side effects/adverse reactions:

▼ *ORAL:* Stomatitis, ulcers (Stevens-Johnson syndrome)

CNS: ***Convulsions,*** headache, insomnia, hallucinations, depression, vertigo, fatigue, anxiety, drug fever, chills, drowsiness

CV: ***Allergic myocarditis***

GI: Nausea, vomiting, abdominal pain, ***hepatitis, enterocolitis,*** pancreatitis, diarrhea, anorexia

HEMA: ***Leukopenia, thrombocytopenia, agranulocytosis, hemolytic anemia, aplastic anemia***

GU: ***Renal failure, toxic nephrosis,*** increased BUN, creatinine, crystalluria, hematuria, proteinuria

INTEG: ***Stevens-Johnson syndrome,*** rash, dermatitis, urticaria, erythema, photosensitivity, alopecia

SYST: ***Anaphylaxis***

Contraindications: Hypersensitivity to sulfonamides, sulfonylureas, thiazide, loop diuretics, salicylates, pregnancy at term

Precautions: Pregnancy category C, lactation, impaired hepatic function, severe allergy, bronchial asthma

Pharmacokinetics:

PO: Rapidly absorbed, peak 2-4 hr, half-life 4-7 hr; 85% protein bound; excreted in urine; crosses placenta

Drug interactions of concern to dentistry:

- Decreased effect: ester-type local anesthetics (procaine, tetracaine)
- Increased photosensitizing effect: tetracycline
- Decreased effect of penicillins, cephalosporins

DENTAL CONSIDERATIONS

General:

- Patients on chronic drug therapy may rarely have symptoms of blood dyscrasias, which can include infection, bleeding, and poor healing.
- Determine why the patient is taking the drug.
- Palliative medication may be required for management of oral side effects.
- Consider semisupine chair position for patient comfort if GI side effects occur.

Consultations:

- Medical consultation may be required to assess disease control.
- In a patient with symptoms of blood dyscrasias, request a medical consultation for blood studies and postpone dental treatment until normal values are reestablished.

Teach patient/family:

- Importance of good oral hygiene to prevent soft tissue inflammation

---

sulindac

(sul-in'dak)

Clinoril

✤ Apo-Sulin, Novo-Sundac

Drug class.: Nonsteroidal antiinflammatory

Action: Inhibits prostaglandin synthesis by interfering with cyclooxygenase, an enzyme needed for biosynthesis; possesses analgesic, antiinflammatory, antipyretic properties

Uses: Osteoarthritis, rheumatoid arthritis, acute gouty arthritis, tendinitis, bursitis, ankylosing spondylitis

Dosage and routes:

Arthritis:

• *Adult:* PO 150 mg bid with food, may increase to 200 mg bid; max dose 400 mg day

Bursitis/acute arthritis:

• *Adult:* PO 200 mg bid × 1-2 wk, then reduce dose

Available forms include: Tabs 150, 200 mg

Side effects/adverse reactions:

▼ *ORAL:* Dry mouth, gingival bleeding, mucosal ulceration and soreness, white spots in mouth or lips, aphthous stomatitis, bitter taste, glossitis, lichenoid reaction

CNS: Dizziness, drowsiness, fatigue, tremors, confusion, insomnia, anxiety, depression

CV: Tachycardia, peripheral edema, palpitations, dysrhythmias

GI: ***Cholestatic hepatitis,*** constipation, flatulence, cramps, peptic ulcer, nausea, anorexia, vomiting, diarrhea, jaundice

HEMA: ***Blood dyscrasias***

GU: ***Nephrotoxicity: dysuria, hematuria, oliguria, azotemia***

EENT: Tinnitus, hearing loss, blurred vision

INTEG: Purpura, rash, pruritus, sweating

Contraindications: Hypersensitivity, asthma (provoked by aspirin or NSAIDs), severe renal disease, severe hepatic disease, systemic lupus erythematosus

Precautions: Pregnancy category not established, lactation, children, bleeding disorders, GI disorders, cardiac disorders, hypersensitivity to other NSAIDs, geriatric patients

Pharmacokinetics:

PO: Peak 2 hr, half-life 3-3.5 hr; 93% protein binding; metabolized in liver; excreted in urine (metabolites), breast milk

Drug interactions of concern to dentistry:

• Increased bleeding, GI effects: alcohol, aspirin, steroids, other NSAIDs

• Renal toxicity: acetaminophen (prolonged use)

• Possible risk of decreased renal function: cyclosporine

• Increased photosensitizing effect: tetracycline

• Increased toxicity of methotrexate, cyclosporine

• Decreased plasma levels: diflunisal

• First-time users of SSRIs also taking NSAIDs may have a higher risk of GI side effects; until more data are available, it may be advisable to avoid use of NSAIDs in these patients (*Br J Clin Pharmacol* 55:591-595, 2003)

DENTAL CONSIDERATIONS

General:

• Patients on chronic drug therapy may rarely have symptoms of blood dyscrasias, which can include infection, bleeding, and poor healing.

• Assess salivary flow as a factor in caries, periodontal disease, and candidiasis.

• Avoid prescribing in last trimester of pregnancy.

• Should oral inflammation or lesions occur, refer to physician and consider palliative treatment for the lesions.

S

• Consider semisupine chair position because of GI side effects, if present.

Consultations:

• Medical consultation may be required to assess disease control.

• In a patient with symptoms of blood dyscrasias, request a medical consultation for blood studies and postpone dental treatment until normal values are reestablished.

Teach patient/family:

• To report oral lesions, soreness, or bleeding to dentist

• Caution to prevent injury in use of oral hygiene aids

• Importance of good oral hygiene to prevent soft tissue inflammation

When chronic dry mouth occurs, advise patient:

• To avoid mouth rinses with high alcohol content because of drying effects

• Of need for daily use of home fluoride products to prevent caries

• To use sugarless gum, frequent sips of water, or saliva substitutes

---

sumatriptan succinate

(soo-ma-trip'tan)

Imitrex

Drug class.: Serotonin agonist

Action: Selective agonist for the serotonin (5-HT) receptor in cranial blood vessels, causing vasoconstriction; may also decrease release of inflammatory neuropeptides or other inflammatory mediators; actual antimigraine action is not clear

Uses: Migraine headaches; cluster headaches

Dosage and routes:

All doses must be individualized:

• *Adult:* SC 6 mg; max 2 injections/24 hr; side effects may limit dose

• *Adult:* PO 25-100 mg as a single dose; then, if required, 100 mg q2h, not to exceed 300 mg/day; if migraine returns after injection, 1 tab q2h, not to exceed 200 mg/day; hepatic dysfunction dose limit 50 mg

• *Adult:* Intranasal 5, 10, or 20 mg as a single dose given in one nostril; dose may be repeated once after 2 hr with a daily limit of 40 mg

Available forms include: Tabs 25, 50, 100 mg; inj 12 mg/ml self-use syringes/vial; nasal spray 5 and 20 mg in 100 μl nasal spray device

Side effects/adverse reactions:

▼ *ORAL:* Discomfort in jaw/mouth/tongue

CNS: Dizziness, vertigo, drowsiness, sedation, headache, anxiety, fatigue

CV: Hypertension, hypotension, bradycardia, palpitation, dysrhythmias, coronary vasospasm

GI: Abdominal discomfort, dysphagia, diarrhea, reflux

RESP: Chest tightness, pressure in chest, dyspnea

GU: Dysuria

EENT: Discomfort in throat/sinuses/nasal cavity, photophobia

INTEG: Redness at injection site, sweating, rashes

MS: Weakness, neck pain, cramps, myalgia

MISC: Tingling, hot or burning sensation, numbness

Contraindications: IV use, ischemic heart disease, MI, uncontrolled hypertension and ergot-containing drugs, concurrent use with or within 14 days of discontinuing MAOIs

Precautions: Pregnancy category C, hepatic and renal impairment, elderly, lactation, children

Pharmacokinetics:

PO: Rapid onset, peak serum levels 5-20 min, terminal half-life 115 min

Drug interactions of concern to dentistry:

• None reported; avoid ergot-containing medications

DENTAL CONSIDERATIONS

General:

• Be aware of the patient's disease, its severity, and its frequency, when known.

• Monitor vital signs at every appointment because of cardiovascular side effects.

• Avoid dental light in patient's eyes; offer dark glasses for patient comfort.

Consultations:

• If treating chronic orofacial pain, consult with physician of record.

Teach patient/family:

• That oral symptoms uncommonly occur and will disappear when drug is discontinued

---

tacrine HCl

(tak'reen)

Cognex

Drug class.: Cholinesterase inhibitor

Action: A centrally acting, reversible inhibitor of cholinesterase enzyme

Uses: Treatment of mild-to-moderate cognitive defects associated with Alzheimer's disease

Dosage and routes:

• *Adult:* PO initially 10 mg qid × 4 wk min; after 4 wk titrate dose to 20 mg qid; higher doses up to 120-160 mg/day in 4 equal doses; monitored every 4 wk, all doses depend on transaminase levels and patient responses

Available forms include: Caps 10, 20, 30, 40 mg

Side effects/adverse reactions:

▼ *ORAL:* Glossitis, dry mouth, stomatitis, increased salivation (variable, low incidence)

CNS: Dizziness, confusion, ataxia, agitation, headache, paresthesia, nervousness, EPS, Bell's palsy (rare)

CV: Hypertension, peripheral edema, bradycardia, hypotension

GI: Increase in serum transaminase levels, nausea, vomiting, diarrhea, ***hepatotoxicity***

RESP: Dyspnea, upper respiratory infection, coughing

HEMA: ***Leukopenia, thrombocytopenia,*** lymphadenopathy, anemia

GU: Urinary frequency or incontinence, infection

EENT: Rhinitis, sinusitis

INTEG: ***Rash,*** flushing of skin

MS: Arthralgia, muscle hypertonia

Contraindications: Hypersensitivity; previously treated patients with jaundice associated with elevated total bilirubin >3 mg/dl

Precautions: Pregnancy category C, cardiovascular disease, GI ulcers, general anesthesia, smokers, liver disease, seizures, asthma, lactation, children, decrease in absolute neutrophil count; liver enzyme monitoring required

T

Pharmacokinetics:
PO: Peak plasma levels 1-2 hr; plasma levels are higher in females; hepatic metabolism (CYP1A2 isoenzymes); renal excretion

Drug interactions of concern to dentistry:
• Potential increase in GI complaints: NSAIDs
• Action inhibited by anticholinergic drugs
• Increased effects with succinylcholine and other cholinergic agonists

DENTAL CONSIDERATIONS
General:
• Patients on chronic drug therapy may rarely have symptoms of blood dyscrasias, which can include infection, bleeding, and poor healing.
• Monitor vital signs at every appointment because of cardiovascular and respiratory side effects.
• After supine positioning, have patient sit upright for at least 2 min before standing to avoid orthostatic hypotension.
• Assess salivary flow as a factor in caries, periodontal disease, and candidiasis.
• Take precautions if dental surgery is anticipated and anesthesia is required.
• Consider semisupine chair position for patient comfort because of GI effects of drug.
• Place on frequent recall because early attention to dental health is important for Alzheimer's patients.

Consultations:
• Medical consultation may be required to assess disease control in the patient.
• In a patient with symptoms of blood dyscrasias, request a medical consultation for blood studies and postpone dental treatment until normal values are reestablished.

Teach patient/family:
• Importance of good oral hygiene to prevent soft tissue inflammation
• To prevent injury when using oral hygiene aids
• Use of electric toothbrush if patient has difficulty holding conventional devices

When chronic dry mouth occurs, advise patient:
• To avoid mouth rinses with high alcohol content because of drying effects
• Of need for daily home fluoride use to prevent caries
• To use sugarless gum, frequent sips of water, or saliva substitutes

---

tacrolimus (topical)

(ta-kroe'li-mus)
Protopic

Drug class.: Immunosuppressant

Action: Mechanism of action unknown; however, it inhibits T-lymphocyte activation and also inhibits transcription of genes associated with cytokine production

Uses: Short-term and intermittent long-term treatment of moderate to severe atopic dermatitis in patients not able to use or who do not respond to alternative, conventional therapies

Dosage and routes:
• *Adult:* TOP apply thin layer of either strength to affected areas bid; rub in gently and completely; continue applications for 1 wk after clearing of signs and symptoms
• *Child 2-5 yr:* TOP use 0.03% strength only; apply thin layer to

affected area bid; rub in gently and completely; continue applications for 1 wk after clearing of signs and symptoms
Available forms include: Oint 0.03%, 0.1% in 30, 60 g
Side effects/adverse reactions:
▼ *ORAL:* Taste alteration
CV: Headache
INTEG: Skin burning, pruritus, rash, folliculitis, acne, contact allergy, varicella zoster lesion
EENT: Sinusitis
MS: Myalgia
MISC: Flulike symptoms, fever, alcohol intolerance
Contraindications: Hypersensitivity, Netherton's syndrome
Precautions: Infections at treatment site; lymphadenopathy, acute infections, mononucleosis, reduce exposure to sunlight or artificial sunlight, pregnancy category C, lactation, use has not been established in children <2 yr
Pharmacokinetics:
TOP: Some systemic absorption; low systemic levels
Drug interactions of concern to dentistry:
• Although no drug interactions are documented, use with caution in patients taking CYP3A4 isoenzyme inhibitors: erythromycin, itraconazole, ketoconazole, fluconazole (see Appendix I)

DENTAL CONSIDERATIONS
General:
• Advise patient if dental drugs prescribed have a potential for photosensitivity.

tacrolimus (FK506)

(ta-kroe'li-mus)
Prograf, Protopic
Drug class.: Immunosuppressant

Action: Inhibits T-lymphocyte activation, leading to immunosuppression
Uses: Prophylaxis of organ rejection in patients receiving allogeneic liver or kidney transplants; used in conjunction with steroids; moderate to severe eczema; unapproved uses: other transplant tissues, including bone marrow, pancreas, small bowel, also severe recalcitrant psoriasis
Dosage and routes:
• *Adult:* PO initial 0.15-0.2 mg/kg/day in 2 divided doses 12 hr apart no sooner than 6 hr after transplant and 8-12 hr after discontinuing IV infusion dose; IV (if patient cannot take PO) initial 0.03-0.05 mg/kg/day by infusion no sooner than 6 hr after graft
• *Pediatric:* IV 0.3 mg/kg/day; PO 0.15-0.2 mg/kg/day; show increased tolerance for doses at high end of adult schedules
Available forms include: Caps 0.5, 1, 5 mg; inj 5 mg/ml in 1 mg amp
Side effects/adverse reactions:
▼ *ORAL:* Candidiasis
CNS: Tremors, headache, insomnia, paresthesia, anorexia, neurotoxicity, seizures
CV: Hyperkalemia, hypertension
GI: Diarrhea, nausea, vomiting, constipation
RESP: Pleural effusion, dyspnea
HEMA: Anemia, leukocytosis, thrombocytopenia, lymphoproliferative disorders, lymphoma

T

GU: ***Nephrotoxicity,*** hyperuricemia, oliguria, UTI
INTEG: Rash, pruritus
MISC: Anaphylaxis, *hyperglycemia*
Contraindications: Hypersensitivity, simultaneous use with cyclosporine, castor oil derivative allergy, potassium-sparing diuretics, lactation
Precautions: Pregnancy category C, renal impairment, hepatic impairment; discontinue cyclosporine doses 24 hr before using this drug, increased susceptibility to infection and lymphoma
Pharmacokinetics:
PO: Peak levels 1.5-3.5 hr; highly bound to plasma proteins, erythrocytes; liver metabolism (CYP3A4 isoenzymes); urinary excretion of metabolites
Drug interactions of concern to dentistry:
• No confirmed studies to date: avoid drugs with potential for renal impairment
• Risk of increased blood levels with clotrimazole, fluconazole, ketoconazole, clarithromycin, erythromycin, and methylprednisolone (see Appendix I)
• Risk of decreased blood levels with carbamazepine, phenobarbital, St. John's wort (herb)
DENTAL CONSIDERATIONS
General:
• Patients on immunosuppressant therapy have an increased susceptibility to infection.
• Patients on chronic drug therapy may rarely have symptoms of blood dyscrasias, which can include infection, bleeding, and poor healing.
• Monitor vital signs at every appointment because of cardiovascular side effects.
• Prophylactic antibiotics may be indicated to prevent infection if surgery or deep scaling is planned.
• Examine for evidence of oral candidiasis. Topically acting antifungals may be preferred.
Consultations:
• Medical consultation may be required to assess disease control in the patient.
• In a patient with symptoms of blood dyscrasias, request a medical consultation for blood studies and postpone dental treatment until normal values are reestablished.
• Consult with patient's physician for recommendations for possible antibiotic prophylaxis before dental treatment or when considering the use of systemic antifungals.
Teach patient/family:
• Importance of good oral hygiene to prevent soft tissue inflammation
• Caution to prevent injury when using oral hygiene aids
• Use of electric toothbrush if patient has difficulty holding conventional devices
• That secondary oral infection may occur; must see dentist immediately if infection occurs
• To report oral lesions, soreness, or bleeding to dentist

tadalafil

(tah-da'la-fil)
Cialis
Drug class.: Impotence therapy

Action: A selective inhibitor of cyclic guanosine monophosphate (cGMP)–specific phosphodiesterace type 5 (PEDS). It enhances the effect of nitric oxide (produced by sexual stimulation) that is involved in increased production of cGMP, both of which are involved in the physiologic processes leading to penile erection. cGMP is required for the smooth muscle relaxation in the corpus cavernosum allowing for increase in blood flow.

Uses: Male erectile dysfunction

Dosages and routes:

• *Adult (male):* PO 10 mg before anticipated sexual activity; dose ranges from 5-20 mg depending on response

Available forms include: Tabs 5, 10, and 20 mg

Side effects/adverse reactions:

▼ *ORAL:* Dry mouth, facial edema

CNS: Headache, asthenia, dizziness, vertigo

CV: Flushing, angina pectoris, hypotension, hypertension, palpitation

GI: Dyspepsia, diarrhea, nausea

RESP: Dyspnea

GU: Prolonged erection

INTEG: Rash, pruritus

EENT: Nasal congestion, blurred vision

METAB: Abnormal liver function tests, elevated GGTP

MS: Back pain, myalgia, arthralgia

MISC: Limb pain

Contraindications: Hypersensitivity; patients currently using organic nitrates or α-adrenergic antagonists

Precautions: Renal impairment, hepatic dysfunction, risk of hypotension in CV disease, ischemic heart disease, patients at risk of priapism, penile deformities, safety and efficacy for use in women not established

Pharmacokinetics:

PO: Good oral absorption not affected by food, peak concentrations 2 hr, hepatic metabolism (CYP 3A4 isoenzymes), excretion not clear (low amounts excreted in urine)

Drug interactions of concern to dentistry:

• Maximum dose in patients taking CYP 3A4 isoenzyme inhibitors is 10 mg: includes ketoconazole, erythromycin, itraconazole, and other potent inhibitors of CYP 3A4

• Avoid use of nitroglycerin within 24-36 hr

DENTAL CONSIDERATIONS

General:

• This is an acute-use drug intended to be taken just before sexual activity. Be mindful of the drug interactions when prescribing potent inhibitors of CYP 3A4 isoenzymes and warn patient.

---

tamoxifen citrate

(ta-mox'i-fen)

Nolvadex

✤ Apo-Tamoxifen, Gen-Tamoxifen, Novo-Tamoxifen, Tamofen, Tamone, Tamoplex

Drug class.: Antineoplastic, antiestrogen hormone

Action: Inhibits cell division by binding to cytoplasmic receptors (estrogen receptors); resembles normal cell complex but inhibits DNA synthesis

Uses: Advanced breast carcinoma that has not responded to other therapy in estrogen receptor–positive patients (usually postmenopausal), to reduce the incidence of breast cancer in healthy women with high risk of developing the disease; ductal carcinoma in situ

Dosage and routes:

• *Adult:* PO 10-20 mg bid or 20 mg daily

Available forms include: Tabs 10, 20 mg
Side effects/adverse reactions:
▼ *ORAL:* Altered taste
CNS: Hot flashes, headache, lightheadedness, depression
CV: Chest pain
GI: Nausea, vomiting
HEMA: ***Thrombocytopenia, leukopenia***
GU: Vaginal bleeding, pruritus vulvae
EENT: Ocular lesions, retinopathy, corneal opacity, blurred vision (high doses)
INTEG: Rash, alopecia
META: Hypercalcemia
Contraindications: Hypersensitivity, pregnancy category D
Precautions: Leukopenia, thrombocytopenia, lactation, cataracts, risk of stroke, pulmonary emboli, and uterine malignancy
Pharmacokinetics:
PO: Peak 4-7 hr, half-life 7 days (1 wk terminal); excreted primarily in feces
Drug interactions of concern to dentistry:
• No dental drug interactions reported
DENTAL CONSIDERATIONS
General:
• Patients on chronic drug therapy may rarely have symptoms of blood dyscrasias, which can include infection, bleeding, and poor healing.
• Consider semisupine chair position for patient comfort if GI side effects occur.
Consultations:
• Medical consultation may be required to assess disease control in the patient.
• In a patient with symptoms of blood dyscrasias, request a medical consultation for blood studies and postpone dental treatment until normal values are reestablished.
Teach patient/family:
• Importance of good oral hygiene to prevent soft tissue inflammation

tamsulosin HCl

(tam-soo'loe-sin)
Flomax
Drug class.: Adrenoreceptor antagonist

Action: Acts as an antagonist for α-adrenoreceptors in the prostate
Uses: Benign prostatic hyperplasia (BPH)
Dosage and routes:
• *Adult:* PO 0.4 mg given 30 min after the same meal each day; patients failing to respond after 2-4 wk can be increased to 0.8 mg daily
Available forms include: Tabs 0.4 mg
Side effects/adverse reactions:
▼ *ORAL:* Tooth disorder (not defined)
CNS: Dizziness, vertigo, headache, somnolence, insomnia
CV: Orthostatic hypotension
GI: Nausea, diarrhea
RESP: Cough, pharyngitis
GU: Decreased libido, abnormal ejaculation
EENT: Rhinitis, amblyopia
MS: Asthenia, back pain, chest pain
MISC: Infection
Contraindications: Hypersensitivity
Precautions: Potential syncope risk caused by hypotension, vertigo, dizziness, carcinoma of prostate, avoid use with other α-adrenoreceptor antagonists, not for use

in women, pregnancy category B, lactation, children (not for use)

Pharmacokinetics:

PO: Good oral absorption, maximum plasma levels 4.5 hr (fasting), highly bound to plasma proteins (94%-99%), extensive liver metabolism, renal excretion

Drug interactions of concern to dentistry:

• No interactions reported with usual dental drugs; it is possible but not known that risk of orthostatic hypotension could be increased with conscious sedation techniques

• Opioids and anticholinergic drugs may enhance urinary retention; use alternative analgesics (NSAIDs)

• Caution in use or avoid concurrent use with other adrenergic antagonists

DENTAL CONSIDERATIONS

General:

• Monitor vital signs at every appointment because of cardiovascular and respiratory side effects.

• Consider semisupine chair position for patient comfort when GI side effects occur.

• After supine positioning, have patient sit upright for at least 2 min before standing to avoid orthostatic hypotension.

tazarotene topical

(taz-ar'oh-teen)

Tazorac

Drug class.: Topical retinoid

Action: Unclear; binds to retinoid receptors and inhibits mouse ornithine decarboxynase activity associated with cell proliferation and hyperplasia; also inhibits corneocyte accumulation in rhino mouse skin

Uses: Topical treatment in stable plaque psoriasis, mild to moderate facial acne vulgaris

Dosage and routes:

Psoriasis:

• *Adult:* TOP apply a thin film once daily in evening to psoriatic lesions to no more than 20% of body surface area; skin should be clean and dry before applying; avoid application to unaffected skin

Acne vulgaris:

• *Adult:* TOP apply a thin film once daily in evening to skin area where acne lesions appear; skin should be dry and clean (0.1% gel only)

Available forms include: Top gel 0.05, 0.1% in 30 g and 100 g sizes; top cream 0.05, 0.1% in 15, 30, and 60 g sizes

Side effects/adverse reactions:

INTEG: Pruritus, burning, stinging, erythema, worsening of psoriasis, rash, dermatitis, fissuring, dry skin, bleeding, desquamations

Contraindications: Pregnancy, hypersensitivity, eczematous skin

Precautions: Pregnancy category X, use birth control measures in women of childbearing age, avoid contact with eyes, eyelids, mouth; exposure to tanning (sun, sun lamps) or drugs that cause photosensitivity, lactation, children <12 yr

Pharmacokinetics:

TOP: After application converted to active metabolite by esterase hydrolysis, metabolite highly plasma protein bound (99%); half-life 18 hr; renal and fecal excretion; systemic absorption less than 1%, 4.5% found in stratum corneum layers of epidermis

Drug interactions of concern to dentistry:

- Increased risk of photosensitivity: tetracyclines, fluoroquinolones, phenothiazines
- Caution in use with systemic vitamin A

DENTAL CONSIDERATIONS

General:

- Apply lubricant to dry lips for patient comfort before dental procedures.
- Advise patient if dental drugs are prescribed that have a potential for photosensitivity.

Teach patient/family:

- Should not be used if pregnant
- To avoid application to oral mucous membranes or lips

---

tegaserod maleate

(teg-a-ser'od)

Zelnorm

Drug class.: Serotonin agonist, a prokinetic drug

Action: A partial agonist that binds to 5-HT_4 receptors resulting in stimulation of the peristaltic reflex and intestinal secretions

Uses: Short-term treatment of irritable bowel syndrome in women whose primary bowel symptom is constipation

Dosage and routes:

- *Adult:* PO (women only) 6 mg bid before meals × 4-6 wk; for patients who respond to therapy an additional 4-6 wk can be considered

Available forms include: Tabs 2, 6 mg

Side effects/adverse reactions:

▼ *ORAL:* Facial edema

CNS: Headache, dizziness, migraine, vertigo

CV: Flushing, hypotension, angina, syncope, arrhythmias

GI: Abdominal pain, diarrhea, nausea, flatulence, irritable colon, cholecystitis, appendicitis, subileus

RESP: Asthma

GU: Menorrhagia, albuminuria, polyuria, renal pain

INTEG: Pruritus, sweating

META: ↑ ALT, ↑ AST, bilirubinemia, ↑ creatine phosphokinase

MS: Back pain, arthropathy

MISC: Accidental trauma, leg pain

Contraindications: Hypersensitivity, severe renal impairment, moderate or severe hepatic impairment, history of bowel obstruction, gallbladder disease, suspected sphincter of Oddi obstruction or abdominal adhesions

Precautions: Avoid use in patients with diarrhea, pregnancy category B, lactation (discontinue drug or discontinue nursing), safety and usefulness in children <18 yr not established

Pharmacokinetics:

PO: Absolute bioavailability in fasting patients is ~10%, peak plasma levels ~1 hr; plasma protein binding 98%, undergoes presystemic acid hydrolysis in stomach, then oxidation and conjugation to inactive metabolites, excreted in feces (67%) and in urine (33%)

Drug interactions of concern to dentistry:

- No dental drug interactions reported; does not induce CYP450 isoenzymes
- Avoid use of drugs (opioids, anticholinergics) that could lead to risk of constipation
- Use NSAIDs or acetaminophen for mild or moderate pain

DENTAL CONSIDERATIONS
General:
• Monitor vital signs at every appointment because of cardiovascular side effects.
• Consider semisupine chair position for patient comfort if GI side effects occur.
• Short appointments and a stress reduction protocol may be required for anxious patients.
• Avoid drugs with anticholinergic activity, such as antihistamines, opioids, benzodiazepines, propantheline, atropine, and scopolomine.
• Question patient about tolerance of NSAIDs or aspirin related to GI disease.
Consultations:
• Consult with physician before prescribing drugs that can cause constipation (opioids).
• Consultation with physician may be needed if sedation or general anesthesia is required.
• Medical consultation may be required to assess disease control and patient's ability to tolerate stress.
Teach patient/family:
• Importance of updating health and drug history if physician makes any changes in evaluation/drug regimens

telmisartan

(tel-mi-sar'tan)
Micardis
Drug class.: Angiotensin II (AT_1) receptor antagonist

Action: Blocks the vasoconstrictor and aldosterone-releasing effects of angiotensin II
Uses: Hypertension, as a single drug or in combination with other antihypertensives
Dosage and routes:
• *Adult:* PO initial dose 40 mg qd, daily dosage range 20-80 mg
Available forms include: Tabs 40, 80 mg
Side effects/adverse reactions:
CNS: Headache, dizziness, fatigue
CV: Peripheral edema
GI: Diarrhea, dyspepsia, abdominal pain, nausea
RESP: URI, coughing
GU: UTI
EENT: Sinusitis, pharyngitis
MS: Myalgia
MISC: Back pain
Contraindications: Hypersensitivity
Precautions: Discontinue if pregnancy occurs, risk of fetal and neonatal injury, correct volume depletion if present, hepatic impairment, impaired renal function; pregnancy categories C (first trimester) and D (second, third trimesters), lactation
Pharmacokinetics:
PO: Peak levels 0.5-1 hr, bioavailability is dose dependent at 40 mg (42%), excreted in feces (97%), some hepatic metabolism, highly plasma protein bound
Drug interactions of concern to dentistry:
• None reported; CYP450 isoenzymes are not involved with metabolism of this drug
DENTAL CONSIDERATIONS
General:
• Monitor vital signs at every appointment because of cardiovascular side effects.
• Stress from dental procedures may compromise cardiovascular function; determine patient risk.
• Use precaution if sedation or general anesthesia is required; risk of hypotensive episode.

• Short appointments and a stress reduction protocol may be required for anxious patients.

• Limit use of sodium-containing products such as saline IV fluids for those patients with a dietary salt restriction.

Consultations:

• Medical consultation may be required to assess disease control and patient's ability to tolerate stress.

temazepam

(te-maz'e-pam)

Restoril Apo-Temazepam, Novo-Temazepam

Drug class.: Benzodiazepine, sedative-hypnotic

Controlled Substance Schedule IV, Canada F

Action: Produces CNS depression at limbic, thalamic, hypothalamic levels of the CNS; interacts with benzodiazepine receptors to facilitate action of the inhibitory neurotransmitter γ-aminobutyric acid (GABA)

Uses: Sedative and hypnotic for insomnia

Dosage and routes:

• *Adult:* PO 15-30 mg hs

Available forms include: Caps 7.5, 15, 30 mg

Side effects/adverse reactions:

CNS: Lethargy, drowsiness, daytime sedation, dizziness, confusion, light-headedness, headache, anxiety, irritability

CV: Chest pain, pulse changes

GI: Nausea, vomiting, diarrhea, heartburn, abdominal pain, constipation, anorexia

HEMA: ***Leukopenia, granulocytopenia*** (rare)

Contraindications: Hypersensitivity to benzodiazepines, pregnancy category X, lactation, intermittent porphyria

Precautions: Anemia, hepatic disease, renal disease, suicidal individuals, drug abuse, elderly, psychosis, child <18 yr, acute narrow-angle glaucoma

Pharmacokinetics:

PO: Onset 30-45 min, duration 6-8 hr, half-life 8-14 hr; metabolized by liver; excreted by kidneys; crosses placenta; excreted in breast milk

Drug interactions of concern to dentistry:

• Increased action of both drugs: alcohol, all CNS depressants

• Increased bioavailability: macrolide antibiotics

DENTAL CONSIDERATIONS

General:

• Psychologic and physical dependence may occur with chronic administration.

• Geriatric patients are more susceptible to drug effects; use lower dose.

Teach patient/family:

• Importance of good oral hygiene to prevent soft tissue inflammation

tenofovir disoproxil fumarate

(te-noe'fo-veer)

Viread

Drug class.: Antiviral

Action: Following metabolic conversion to tenofovir diphosphate, it inhibits the activity of HIV reverse transcriptase

Uses: HIV-1 infection, in combination with other antiretroviral drugs

Dosage and routes:
• *Adult:* PO 300 mg/day with a meal
Available forms include: Tabs 300 mg
Side effects/adverse reactions:
CNS: Headache
GI: Nausea, diarrhea, vomiting, flatulence, anorexia, abdominal pain
HEMA: Neutropenia
GU: Proteinuria
META: Elevation in creatine kinase, serum amylase, AST, ALT, serum glucose
MISC: Asthenia
Contraindications: Hypersensitivity; avoid breastfeeding
Precautions: Obesity and prolonged nucleoside use; risk of lactic acidosis/severe hepatomegaly with steatosis; no data on hepatic impairment; redistribution of body fat, pregnancy category B
Pharmacokinetics:
PO: Bioavailability 5% (improves with meal); maximum serum levels 0.6-1.4 hr; low plasma protein binding less than 7%; minimal systemic metabolism; excreted by glomerular filtration and active tubular secretion; use in children not evaluated
Drug interactions of concern to dentistry:
• Potential for competition for renal clearance: acyclovir, valacyclovir

DENTAL CONSIDERATIONS
General:
• Examine for oral manifestation of opportunistic infection.
Consultations:
• Medical consultation may be required to assess disease control and patient's ability to tolerate stress.
Teach patient/family:
• Importance of good oral hygiene to prevent soft tissue inflammation/infection

terazosin HCl
(ter-ay'zoe-sin)
Hytrin
Drug class.: Antihypertensive, antiadrenergic

Action: Reduction in blood pressure results from α-adrenergic receptor blockade and reduced peripheral resistance; also causes relaxation of smooth muscle in bladder neck and prostate capsule reducing uretheral resistance
Uses: Hypertension as a single agent or in combination with diuretics or β-blockers; benign prostatic hypertrophy
Dosage and routes:
• *Adult:* PO 1 mg hs; usual dose range 1-5 mg daily; may increase dose slowly to desired response; not to exceed 20 mg/day
Benign prostatic hypertrophy:
• *Adult:* PO initial dose 1 mg hs; increase dose by increasing daily to achieve the desired response; 10 mg/day may be required
Available forms include: Tabs 1, 2, 5, 10 mg; caps 1, 2, 5, 10 mg
Side effects/adverse reactions:
▼ *ORAL:* Dry mouth
CNS: Dizziness, headache, drowsiness, anxiety, depression, vertigo, weakness, fatigue
CV: Orthostatic hypotension, palpitation, tachycardia, edema, rebound hypertension
GI: Nausea, vomiting, diarrhea, constipation, abdominal pain
RESP: Dyspnea, pharyngitis, rhinitis

GU: Urinary urgency, incontinence, impotence
EENT: Epistaxis, tinnitus, red sclera, nasal congestion, sinusitis
Contraindications: Hypersensitivity
Precautions: Pregnancy category C, children, lactation
Pharmacokinetics:
PO: Peak 1 hr, half-life 9-12 hr; highly bound to plasma proteins; metabolized in liver; excreted in urine, feces
Drug interactions of concern to dentistry:
• Decreased antihypertensive effects: NSAIDs, indomethacin
DENTAL CONSIDERATIONS
General:
• Monitor vital signs at every appointment because of cardiovascular side effects.
• After supine positioning, have patient sit upright for at least 2 min before standing to avoid orthostatic hypotension.
• Assess salivary flow as a factor in caries, periodontal disease, and candidiasis.
• Limit use of sodium-containing products, such as saline IV fluids, for patients with a dietary salt restriction.
• Consider semisupine chair position for patient comfort if GI side effects occur.
Teach patient/family:
When chronic dry mouth occurs, advise patient:
• To avoid mouth rinses with high alcohol content because of drying effects
• Of need for daily home fluoride use to prevent caries
• To use sugarless gum, frequent sips of water, or saliva substitutes

terbinafine HCl

(ter-bin'a-feen)
Lamisil
Drug class.: Antifungal, systemic

Action: Inhibits key enzyme, squalene epoxidase, involved with sterol synthesis with resultant fungal cell death
Uses: Treatment of onychomycosis of the toenail or fingernail caused by dermatophytes (tinea unguium)
Dosage and routes:
Fingernail onychomycosis:
• *Adult:* PO 250 mg qd × 6 wk
Toenail onychomycosis:
• *Adult:* PO 250 mg qd × 12 wk
Available forms include: Tabs 250 mg
Side effects/adverse reactions:
▼ *ORAL: Taste disturbances*
GI: Diarrhea, dyspepsia, abdominal pain, nausea, flatulence, ***hepatic failure,*** cholestatic hepatitis (rare)
HEMA: ***Severe neutropenia*** (rare), transient decrease in absolute lymphocyte counts
INTEG: Rash, urticaria, pruritus
META: Abnormal liver tests
MS: Arthralgia, myalgia
MISC: Malaise, fatigue
Contraindications: Hypersensitivity
Precautions: Preexisting liver or renal disease, pregnancy category B, use not recommended during nursing, pediatric patients
Pharmacokinetics:
PO: Bioavailability 40%, peak plasma levels approximately 2 hr; highly plasma protein bound (99%), extensive metabolism, excreted in urine (70%)

Drug interactions of concern to dentistry:

• None reported

DENTAL CONSIDERATIONS

General:

• Determine why patient is taking the drug.

• Consider semisupine chair position for patient comfort if GI side effects occur.

• Patients on chronic drug therapy may rarely have symptoms of blood dyscrasias, which can include infection, bleeding, and poor healing.

Consultations:

• In a patient with symptoms of blood dyscrasias, request a medical consultation for blood studies and postpone treatment until normal values are reestablished.

Teach patient/family:

• Importance of good oral hygiene to prevent soft tissue inflammation

• To prevent trauma when using oral hygiene aids

---

terbinafine HCl (topical)

(ter-bin'a-feen)

Lamisil, Lamisil DermaGel

Drug class.: Antifungal

Action: Inhibits key enzyme, squalene epoxidase, involved with sterol synthesis with resultant fungal cell death

Uses: Tinea pedis, tinea cruris, tinea corporis; unapproved uses: cutaneous candidiasis, tinea versicolor

Dosage and routes:

• *Adult:* TOP apply to affected area bid until symptoms show significant improvement, usually 7-14 days; duration usually 7 days, but should not exceed 4 wk

Available forms include: Cream 1% in 15, 30 g containers, gel 1% in 5, 15, 30 g

Side effects/adverse reactions:

INTEG: Irritation, burning, drying, itching

Contraindications: Hypersensitivity

Precautions: Pregnancy category B, lactation, children <12 yr

Drug interactions of concern to dentistry:

• None reported

---

terbutaline sulfate

(ter-byoo'ta-leen)

Brethaire, Brethine, Bricanyl

Drug class.: Selective β_2-agonist

Action: Relaxes bronchial smooth muscle by direct action on β_2-adrenergic receptors

Uses: Bronchospasm, asthma prophylaxis

Dosage and routes:

Bronchospasm:

• *Adult and child >15 yr:* PO 5 mg q6h while awake, can reduce dose by 50% if required, limit 15 mg/day; SC 0.25 mg; if significant improvement does not occur in 15-30 min give second dose; limit 0.5 mg in 4 hr

• *Child 12-15 yr:* PO 2.5 mg tid, limit 7.5 mg/day

Available forms include: Tabs 2.5, 5 mg; inj 1 mg/ml in 2 ml ampules

Side effects/adverse reactions:

▼ *ORAL:* Dry mouth, unusual taste

CNS: Tremors, anxiety, insomnia, headache, dizziness, stimulation

T

CV: Palpitation, tachycardia, hypertension, ***cardiac arrest***
GI: Nausea, vomiting
Contraindications: Hypersensitivity to sympathomimetics, narrow-angle glaucoma, tachydysrhythmias
Precautions: Pregnancy category B, cardiac disorders, hyperthyroidism, diabetes mellitus, prostatic hypertrophy, lactation, elderly, hypertension, glaucoma, not for use in children <12 yr
Pharmacokinetics:
PO: Onset 0.5 hr, duration 4-8 hr
SC: Onset 6-15 min, duration 1.5 hr
INH: Onset 5-30 min, duration 3-6 hr
Drug interactions of concern to dentistry:
• Increased CNS side effects: other sympathomimetics
• Risk of dysrhythmias with halogenated-hydrocarbon anesthetics
• Increased vascular side effects: tricyclic antidepressants
DENTAL CONSIDERATIONS
General:
• Consider semisupine chair position for patients with respiratory disease.
• Monitor vital signs at every appointment because of cardiovascular side effects.
• Assess salivary flow as a factor in caries, periodontal disease, and candidiasis.
• Be aware that aspirin or sulfite preservatives in vasoconstrictor-containing products can exacerbate asthma.
• Acute asthmatic episodes may be precipitated in the dental office. Sympathomimetic inhalants should be available for emergency use.
• Midday appointments and a stress reduction protocol may be required for anxious patients.
Teach patient/family:
• For inhalation dosage forms: to rinse mouth with water after each dose to help prevent dryness
• Use of electric toothbrush if patient has difficulty holding conventional devices
When chronic dry mouth occurs, advise patient:
• To avoid mouth rinses with high alcohol content because of drying effects
• Of need for daily home fluoride use to prevent caries
• To use sugarless gum, frequent sips of water, or saliva substitutes

terconazole

(ter-kone'a-zole)
Terazol 3, Terazol 7
Drug class.: Local antifungal

Action: Interferes with fungal DNA replication; binds sterols in fungal cell membranes, which increases permeability, leaking of nutrients
Uses: Vaginal, vulval, vulvovaginal candidiasis (moniliasis)
Dosage and routes:
• *Adult:* Vag 5 g (1 applicator full) hs × 7 days (0.4%); vag 5 g (1 applicator full) hs × 3 days (0.8%); suppos 1 hs × 3 days
Available forms include: Vag cream 0.4%, 0.8%; vag suppos 80 mg
Side effects/adverse reactions:
GU: Vulvovaginal burning, itching, pelvic cramps
INTEG: Rash, urticaria, stinging, burning
MISC: Headache, body pain

Contraindications: Hypersensitivity

Precautions: Children <2 yr, pregnancy, lactation

DENTAL CONSIDERATIONS

General:

• Be aware that broad-spectrum antibiotics can exacerbate vaginal candidiasis.

---

teriparatide

(ter-i-par'a-tide)

Forteo

Drug class.: Bone resorption inhibitor (a synthetic polypeptide of rDNA origin, contains recombinant human parathyroid hormone [rhPTH(1-34)])

Action: Has the same action as the 34 *N*-terminal amino acids of parathyroid hormone, including regulation of bone metabolism, renal tubular reabsorption of calcium and phosphate, and intestinal calcium absorption

Uses: Treatment of postmenopausal women with osteoporosis at high risk for fracture; to increase bone mass in men with primary or hypogonadal osteoporosis at high risk for fracture

Dosage and routes:

• *Adult:* SC 20 μg/day (can be administered by patients or caregivers after proper training; orthostatic hypotension may follow after injection)

Available forms include: Prefilled pen delivery device (refrigeration required, do not freeze); cartridge system contains enough drug for 28 days of use

Side effects/adverse reactions:

CNS: Dizziness, headache, syncope, vertigo

CV: Hypertension, angina pectoris

GI: Nausea, constipation, diarrhea, dyspepsia, vomiting

RESP: Dyspnea, cough

EENT: Rhinitis

INTEG: Rash

MS: Leg cramps, arthralgia

MISC: Generalized pain, neck pain, sweating

Contraindications: Hypersensitivity, Paget's disease of bone, prior history of radiation therapy of the skeleton, metastatic bone lesions or skeletal malignancies, metabolic bone disease (other than osteoporosis), patients at increased risk for osteosarcoma, pediatric patients or young adults with open epiphyses, preexisting hypercalcemia

Precautions: Active or recent urolithiasis, use longer than 2 yr, postinjection orthostatic hypotension, symptoms of hypercalcemia, pregnancy category C, avoid in nursing mothers, not for use in children

Pharmacokinetics:

SC: Absolute bioavailability 95%, peak serum levels 30 min, half-life 1 hr, no excretion or metabolism studies have been done, may be the same as PTH with hepatic metabolism and renal excretion

Drug interactions of concern to dentistry:

• No dental drug interactions reported

DENTAL CONSIDERATIONS

General:

• Patients with osteoporosis and risk of fracture should be asked if they use this drug; otherwise some patients may not report its use.

• Patients may need special assistance in the dental office to avoid risk of falling.

Teach patient/family:

• Importance of updating health and drug history, reporting changes in health status, drug regimen, or disease/treatment status

• To contact physician if symptoms of hypercalcemia appear (nausea, vomiting, constipation, lethargy, muscle weakness)

testosterone/ testosterone cypionate/ testosterone enanthate

(tess-toss'ter-one)

Testosterone Pellets: Testopel

Testosterone cypionate (IM use only): Depo-Testosterone

Testosterone enanthate (IM use only): Delasteryl

♣ *Testosterone undecanoate:* Andriol

Testosterone transdermal: Testaderm, Testaderm TTS, Androderm

Testosterone gel: AndroGel

Testosterone Buccal: Striant

Drug class.: Androgen, anabolic steroid

Controlled Substance Schedule III

Action: In many tissues testosterone is converted to dihydrotestosterone, which interacts with cytoplasmic protein receptors to increase protein production; natural hormone that functions to regulate spermatogenesis and male secondary sex characteristics; also functions as an anabolic steroid

Uses: Treatment of androgen deficiency, delayed puberty, female breast cancer, certain anemias, gender changes, hypogonadism, cryptorchidism

Dosage and routes:

Replacement therapy:

• *Adult (male):* IM 50-400 mg q2-4wk (cypionate or enanthate)

• *Adult (male):* Scrotal patch 1 patch (4 or 6 mg) q22-24h

• *Adult (male):* Pellets SC 150-450 mg q3-6mo

• *Adult (male):* Buccal tablets: 1 buccal system (30 mg) applied to the gum region AM and PM (12 hr apart)

Hypogonadotropic hypogonadism:

• *Adult (gel):* TOP apply one 5 g packet (≈50 mg testosterone) to clean dry skin of shoulders or upper arms or abdomen (not to genitals) in AM; PELLETS dose varies from 150-400 mg q3-6mo

Breast cancer:

• *Adult (female):* IM 200-400 mg q2-4 wk (enanthate)

Delayed puberty:

• *Child (male):* IM 100 mg (max) per month up to 4-6 mo (all forms)

Available forms include: Enanthate inj IM 200 mg/ml; cypionate inj IM 100, 200 mg/ml; scrotal patch 2.5, 4, 6 mg; gel 1%, pellets 75 mg; buccal system 30 mg in pack of 10

Side effects/adverse reactions:

CNS: Dizziness, headache, fatigue, tremors, paresthesias, flushing, sweating, anxiety, lability, insomnia

CV: ***Edema (in cardiac patients),*** increased BP

GI: **Hepatic necrosis (rare), cholestatic jaundice,** nausea, vomiting, constipation, weight gain

HEMA: Increased prothrombin time, iron deficiency anemia

GU: Amenorrhea, gynecomastia (males), hematuria, priapism, vag-

initis, decreased libido, decreased breast size, clitoral hypertrophy, testicular atrophy
EENT: Conjunctival edema, nasal congestion
INTEG: Rash, acneiform lesions, oily hair/skin, flushing, sweating, acne vulgaris, alopecia, hirsutism
ENDO: Abnormal GTT
MS: Cramps, spasms, hypercalcification in breast

Contraindications: Severe renal disease, severe cardiac disease, severe hepatic disease, hypersensitivity, pregnancy category X, lactation, genital bleeding (abnormal), prostate or breast carcinoma (males), breast cancer in females with hypercalcemia

Precautions: Diabetes mellitus, CV disease, MI, increased risk of prostatic hypertrophy, prostatic carcinoma, virilization (women), increased prothrombin time

Pharmacokinetics:
IM: Highly protein bound, metabolized in liver, half-life 10-20 min; excreted in urine, breast milk; crosses placenta
PATCH: Absorption from scrotal skin much higher than other skin sites, half-life 10-100 min, peak levels 2-4 hr

Drug interactions of concern to dentistry:
- Increased risk of bleeding: aspirin
- Edema: ACTH, adrenal steroids

DENTAL CONSIDERATIONS

General:
- Avoid prescribing aspirin-containing products.
- Determine why the patient is taking the drug.
- Consider local hemostasis measures to prevent excessive bleeding.
- Short appointments and a stress reduction protocol may be required for anxious patients.
- Prophylactic antibiotics may be indicated to prevent infection if surgery or deep scaling is planned.

Consultations:
- Physician consultation may be required if signs of anemia are observed in oral tissues.
- Medical consultation may be required to assess disease control and patient's ability to tolerate stress.
- Medical consultation should include partial prothrombin time or prothrombin time.

Teach patient/family:
- Importance of good oral hygiene to prevent soft tissue inflammation
- To be aware of the possibility of secondary oral infection and the need to see dentist immediately if infection occurs

tetracaine/tetracaine HCl (topical)

(tet'ra-cane)
Pontocaine, Pontocaine Cream, Viractin
Drug class.: Topical anesthetic (ester group)

Action: Inhibits nerve impulses from sensory nerves, which produces anesthesia

Uses: Local anesthesia of mucous membranes, pruritus, sunburn, sore throat, cold sores, oral pain, rectal pain and irritation, control of gagging

Dosage and routes:
- *Adult:* TOP apply to affected area using smallest effective amount at point of needle insertion

Available forms include: Oint 1%; cream 2%; gel 2%; sol 2%

Side effects/adverse reactions:
INTEG: Rash, irritation, sensitization, dermatitis
MISC: Hypersensitivity reactions (systemic), angioedema
More severe systemic reactions can be observed if excessive absorption leads to toxic doses

Contraindications: Hypersensitivity, infants <1 yr, application to large areas, PABA allergies

Precautions: Child <12 yr, sepsis, pregnancy category C, lactation, local infection, geriatric, debilitated patient

Pharmacokinetics:
TOP: Onset 3-10 min, duration up to 60 min; metabolized in plasma when absorbed; excreted in urine

Drug interactions of concern to dentistry:
- Specific drug interactions are not listed; it would be wise to use with caution in patients taking tocainide, mexiletine; significant systemic absorption could lead to synergistic and potentially toxic effects

DENTAL CONSIDERATIONS

General:
- Apply smallest effective dose; apply to small area because significant absorption can occur, especially from denuded areas.
- Absorption of excessive amounts of drug may lead to signs of local anesthetic toxicity; with correct use, toxicity is a rare event.
- Use for topical anesthesia or temporary relief of symptoms; reevaluate if symptoms persist.
- Toxic amounts can be absorbed from denuded mucosa or skin.
- Apply with cotton-tipped applicator by pressing, not rubbing, paste on lesion.

Teach patient/family:
- How to apply
- Not to chew gum or eat while numbness is present after dental treatment
- Symptoms of systemic toxicity, which could include nervousness, nausea, excitement followed by drowsiness, convulsions, and cardiac and respiratory depression
- That symptoms may vary because they depend on the amount of drug actually absorbed

tetracycline/tetracycline HCl

(tet-ra-sye'kleen)

Helidac Therapy, Panmycin, Sumycin, Tetracyn, Tetralan Syrup, Tetracap

♣ Apo-Tetra, Novotetra, Nu-Tetra

Drug class.: Tetracycline, broad-spectrum antibiotic

Action: Inhibits protein synthesis and phosphorylation in microorganisms; bacteriostatic

Uses: Syphilis, *C. trachomatis,* gonorrhea, lymphogranuloma venereum, *M. pneumoniae,* rickettsial infections, acne, actinomycosis, anthrax, bronchitis, GU infections, sinusitis, and many other infections produced by susceptible organisms; *H. pylori*–associated duodenal ulcer

Dosage and routes:
- *Adult:* PO 250 mg q6h or 500 mg bid, 1 hr before or 2 hr after meals
- *Child >8 yr:* PO 25-50 mg/kg/day in divided doses q6h 1 hr before or 2 hr after meals

Gonorrhea:
- *Adult:* PO 500 mg qid for 7 days

Chlamydia trachomatis:
• *Adult:* PO 500 mg qid × 7 days
Syphilis:
• *Adult:* PO 500 mg qid × 14 days; must treat 28 days if syphilis duration >1 yr
Urethral syndrome in women:
• *Adult:* PO 500 mg qid × 7 days
H. pylori eradication:
• *Adult:* PO 500 mg tetracycline, 250 mg metronidazole, and 525 mg bismuth subsalicylate, plus an H_2 antagonist as directed, qid × 14 days
Acne:
• *Adult:* 1 g/day in divided doses; maintenance 125-500 mg/day
Available forms include: Oral susp 125 mg/5 ml; caps 250, 500 mg
Side effects/adverse reactions:
▼ *ORAL: Tooth discoloration in children <8 yr, candidiasis, tongue discoloration and hypertrophy of papilla,* enamel hypoplasia, bleeding (long-term use), stomatitis, lichenoid drug reaction, erythema multiforme
CNS: Fever, headache, paresthesia
CV: Pericarditis
GI: Nausea, abdominal pain, vomiting, diarrhea, anorexia, ***hepatotoxicity,*** enterocolitis, flatulence, abdominal cramps, epigastric burning
HEMA: ***Eosinophilia, neutropenia, thrombocytopenia, leukocytosis, hemolytic anemia***
GU: Increased BUN
EENT: Dysphagia
INTEG: Rash, urticaria, photosensitivity, increased pigmentation, ***exfoliative dermatitis, angioedema,*** pruritus
Contraindications: Hypersensitivity to tetracyclines, children <8 yr, pregnancy category D, lactation
Precautions: Renal disease, hepatic disease
Pharmacokinetics:
PO: Peak 2-3 hr, duration 6 hr, half-life 6-10 hr; 20%-60% protein bound; excreted in urine; crosses placenta; excreted in breast milk
Drug interactions of concern to dentistry:
• Decreased absorption: $NaHCO_3$, other antacids
• Decreased effect of penicillins, cephalosporins
• Possible increase in serum levels of methotrexate
• Suspected increase in effects of warfarin, theophylline

DENTAL CONSIDERATIONS
General:
• Determine why the patient is taking tetracycline.
• Broad-spectrum antibiotics may be a factor in oral or vaginal *Candida* infections.
• Advise patient if dental drugs prescribed have a potential for photosensitivity.
Consultations:
• Medical consultation may be required to assess disease control in the patient.
Teach patient/family:
• Importance of good oral hygiene to prevent soft tissue inflammation
• Caution to prevent injury when using oral hygiene aids
• To avoid milk products; to take with a full glass of water
• To take tetracycline doses 1 hr before or 2 hr after air polishing device (ProphyJet), if used
When used for dental infection, advise patient:
• Taking birth control pill to use

T

additional method of contraception for duration of cycle

• To report sore throat, oral burning sensation, fever, fatigue, any of which could indicate superinfection

• To take at prescribed intervals and complete dosage regimen

• To immediately notify the dentist if signs or symptoms of infection increase

tetracycline periodontal fiber

(tet-ra-sye'kleen)

Actisite

Drug class.: Tetracycline, broad-spectrum antiinfective

Action: Antimicrobial effect related to inhibition of protein synthesis; decreases incidence of post-surgical inflammation and edema; suppresses bacteria and acts as a barrier to bacterial entry; acts on cementum or fibroblasts to enhance periodontal ligament regeneration

Uses: Adjunctive treatment in adult periodontitis

Dosage and routes:

• *Fiber:* Adjust length to fit pocket depth and contour of teeth treated; fiber should contact base of pocket; apply cyanoacrylate adhesive to secure fiber for 10 days; replace if lost before 7 days; up to 11 teeth can be treated

Available forms include: Fiber supplied in boxes of 4 and 10 fibers, each 23 cm long and each with 12.7 mg tetracycline

Side effects/adverse reactions:

▼ *ORAL: Gingival inflammation and pain, glossitis,* local erythema, candidiasis, staining of tongue

EENT: Minor throat irritation

INTEG: Photosensitivity

Contraindications: Hypersensitivity, children <8 yr, acutely abscessed periodontal pocket

Precautions: Pregnancy category C, lactation, children, superinfection, patients with predisposition to candidiasis; must remove fibers after 10 days

Pharmacokinetics:

TOP: In vitro release rate 2 μg/cm/hr; gingival concentration maintained over 10 days; plasma levels below detectable limits

Drug interactions of concern to dentistry:

• It is not known if the tetracycline fiber will decrease the effectiveness of oral contraceptives; however, manufacturer recommends suggesting the use of an alternative form of contraception during the remaining cycle to female patients taking oral contraceptives

DENTAL CONSIDERATIONS

General:

• Take precautions regarding allergy to tetracyclines.

• Examine oral mucosa for candidiasis before placing fiber.

Teach patient/family:

• Not to chew hard, crusty, or sticky foods

• Not to brush or floss near treated area, but clean other teeth

• To avoid other oral hygienic practices that could dislodge fibers, such as the use of toothpicks

• Not to probe or pick at the treated area

• To notify dentist if fiber dislodges or falls out

• To notify dentist if pain, swelling, or other symptoms occur

theophylline

(thee-off'i-lin)

Accubron, Aquaphyllin, Asmalix, Broncodyl, Elixomin, Elixophyllin, Lanophyllin, Quibron-T, Respbid, Slo-Bid, Slo-Phyllin, Sustaire, T-Phyl, Theobid, Theoclear LA, Theolair, Theo-Dur, Theo-24, Theolair-24, Theochron, Theo-Sav, Theovent, , Theo-X, Uni-Dur, Uniphyl

♣ Apo-Theo-LA, PMS-Theophylline

Drug class.: Xanthine

Action: Relaxes smooth muscle of respiratory system by blocking phosphodiesterase, which increases cAMP

Uses: Bronchial asthma, bronchospasm of COPD, chronic bronchitis; unapproved use: apnea in the neonate

Dosage and routes:

Bronchospasm, bronchial asthma

- *Adult:* PO 100-200 mg q6h, dosage must be individualized
- *Child:* PO 50-100 mg q6h, not to exceed 12 mg/kg/24 hr

Available forms include: Tabs ext rel 100, 200, 300 mg; time rel tabs 100, 200, 250, 300, 400, 500, 600 mg; time rel caps 50, 75, 100, 125 mg; elix 80 mg/15 ml; sol 80 mg/15 ml; syr 150 mg/15 ml, 80 mg/15 ml

Side effects/adverse reactions:

▼ *ORAL:* Bitter taste, dry mouth

CNS: Anxiety, restlessness, insomnia, dizziness, convulsions, headache, light-headedness, muscle twitching

CV: Palpitation, sinus tachycardia, hypotension, other dysrhythmias

GI: Nausea, vomiting, anorexia, diarrhea, dyspepsia, gastric distress

RESP: Increased rate

INTEG: Flushing, urticaria

Contraindications: Hypersensitivity to xanthines, tachydysrhythmias

Precautions: Elderly, CHF, cor pulmonale, hepatic disease, active peptic ulcer disease, diabetes mellitus, hyperthyroidism, hypertension, children, pregnancy category C

Pharmacokinetics:

PO: Peak 1 hr; metabolized in liver; excreted in urine, breast milk; crosses placenta

Drug interactions of concern to dentistry:

- Increased action: erythromycin, ciprofloxacin, glucocorticoids
- Increased risk of cardiac dysrhythmia: halothane inhalation anesthesia, CNS stimulants
- Decreased effect: barbiturates, carbamazepine, ketoconazole
- May decrease sedative effects of benzodiazepines

DENTAL CONSIDERATIONS

General:

- Consider semisupine chair position for patients with respiratory disease.
- Monitor vital signs at every appointment because of cardiovascular side effects.
- Assess salivary flow as a factor in caries, periodontal disease, and candidiasis.
- Be aware that aspirin or sulfite preservatives in vasoconstrictor-containing products can exacerbate asthma.
- Acute asthmatic episodes may be

T

precipitated in the dental office. Sympathomimetic inhalants should be available for emergency use.
• Midday appointments and a stress reduction protocol may be required for anxious patients.

Consultations:
• Medical consultation may be required to assess disease control in the patient.

Teach patient/family:
When chronic dry mouth occurs, advise patient:
• To avoid mouth rinses with high alcohol content because of drying effects
• Of need for daily home fluoride use to prevent caries
• To use sugarless gum, frequent sips of water, or saliva substitutes

---

thiamin HCl (vitamin B_1)

(thye'a-min)
Thiamilate
♣ Betaxin

Drug class.: Vitamin B_1, water soluble

Action: Needed for carbohydrate metabolism

Uses: Vitamin B_1 deficiency or prophylaxis, beriberi, Wernicke-Korsakoff syndrome

Dosage and routes:
Recommended dietary allowance (RDA):
• *Adult:* PO men 1.2-1.5 mg; women 1.0-1.1 mg; pregnant women 1.5 mg; lactating women 1.6 mg
• *Child:* PO ages 1-3 yr, 0.7 mg; ages 4-6 yr, 0.9 mg; ages 7-10 yr, 1 mg

Beriberi:
• *Adult (critical):* IM or slow IV 5-100 mg tid; use injection only when necessary
• *Adult:* PO 5-10 mg tid with multivitamin, then RDA (dose recommendations are highly variable)
• *Infant (mild):* PO 10 mg qd

Alcohol-induced deficiency:
• *Adult:* PO 40 mg qd

Available forms include: Tabs 50, 100, 250 mg; enteric-coated tabs 20 mg; inj IM/IV 100 mg/ml

Side effects/adverse reactions:
NOTE: Parenteral doses are more likely to cause severe adverse reactions.
▼ *ORAL:* ***Angioedema***
CNS: Weakness, restlessness
CV: ***Collapse, pulmonary edema,*** hypotension
GI: Nausea, diarrhea, hemorrhage
EENT: Tightness of throat
INTEG: Cyanosis, sweating, warmth
SYST: ***Anaphylaxis*** (after parenteral doses)

Contraindications: None known

Precautions: Pregnancy category A, sensitivity to thiamin, Wernicke's encephalopathy

Pharmacokinetics:
PO/INJ: Unused amounts excreted in urine (unchanged)

DENTAL CONSIDERATIONS

General:
• Determine why the patient is taking this vitamin.

Teach patient/family:
• Food sources to be included in diet: yeast, whole grain, beef, liver, legumes

thiethylperazine maleate

(thye-eth-il-per'a-zeen)
Torecan

Drug class.: Phenothiazine-type, antiemetic

Action: Acts centrally by blocking chemoreceptor trigger zone, which in turn acts on vomiting center
Uses: Nausea, vomiting
Dosage and routes:
• *Adult:* PO/IM 10 mg qd-tid
Available forms include: Tabs 10 mg; inj 5 mg/ml
Side effects/adverse reactions:
▼ *ORAL:* Dry mouth, metallic taste
CNS: Euphoria, depression, ***convulsions,*** restlessness, tremor, EPS, drowsiness
CV: ***Circulatory failure, tachycardia,*** postural hypotension, ECG changes
GI: Nausea, vomiting, anorexia, diarrhea, constipation, weight loss, cramps
RESP: Respiratory depression
GU: Urinary retention, dark urine
Contraindications: Hypersensitivity to phenothiazines, coma, seizure, encephalopathy, bone marrow depression
Precautions: Children <12 yr, pregnancy category C, elderly
Pharmacokinetics:
PO: Onset 45-60 min
REC: Onset 45-60 min
Metabolized by liver; excreted by kidneys; crosses placenta; excreted in breast milk
Drug interactions of concern to dentistry:
• Increased anticholinergic action: anticholinergics
• Increased CNS depression, hypotension: alcohol, CNS depressants
DENTAL CONSIDERATIONS
General:
• Defer elective dental treatment when symptoms are present.
Consultations:
• Medical consultation may be required to assess disease control in the patient.

thioridazine HCl

(thye-oh-rid'a-zeen)
Mellaril
♣ Apo-Thioridazine, Novo-Ridazine

Drug class.: Phenothiazine antipsychotic

Action: Blocks neurotransmission at dopaminergic synapses in the cerebral cortex, hypothalamus, and limbic system; exhibits strong peripheral α-adrenergic, anticholinergic blocking action; mechanism for antipsychotic effects is unclear
Uses: Psychotic disorders, schizophrenia, behavioral problems in children, alcohol withdrawal as adjunct, anxiety, major depressive disorders, organic brain syndrome
Dosage and routes:
Psychosis:
• *Adult:* PO 50-100 mg tid; max dose 800 mg/day; dose is gradually increased to desired response, then reduced to minimum maintenance
• *Child unresponsive to other agents:* PO 0.5 mg/kg/day in divided doses; maximum dose 3 mg/kg/day
Available forms include: Tabs 10, 15, 25, 50, 100, 150, 200 mg; conc 30 mg/ml

T

Side effects/adverse reactions:
▼ *ORAL: Dry mouth,* movements of lips and tongue (tardive dyskinesia), erythema multiforme, lichenoid reaction
CNS: Extrapyramidal symptoms: pseudoparkinsonism, akathisia, dystonia, tardive dyskinesia, ***seizures, headache,*** confusion
CV: Orthostatic hypotension, ***cardiac arrest,*** ECG changes, ***tachycardia***
GI: Nausea, vomiting, anorexia, constipation, diarrhea, jaundice, weight gain
RESP: ***Laryngospasm,*** dyspnea, ***respiratory depression***
HEMA: Anemia, ***leukopenia, leukocytosis, agranulocytosis***
GU: Urinary retention, enuresis, impotence, amenorrhea, gynecomastia
EENT: Blurred vision, glaucoma, dry eyes
INTEG: Rash, photosensitivity, dermatitis

Contraindications: Hypersensitivity, blood dyscrasias, coma, child <2 yr, brain damage, bone marrow depression

Precautions: Pregnancy category C, lactation, seizure disorders, hypertension, hepatic disease, cardiac disease

Pharmacokinetics:
PO: Onset erratic, peak 2-4 hr, half-life 26-36 hr; metabolized by liver; excreted in urine; crosses placenta; excreted in breast milk

Drug interactions of concern to dentistry:
- Increased sedation: other CNS depressants, alcohol, barbiturate anesthetics, opioid analgesics
- Hypotension, tachycardia: epinephrine (systemic)
- Increased extrapyramidal effects: phenothiazines and related drugs (haloperidol, droperidol), metoclopramide
- Additive photosensitization: tetracyclines
- Increased anticholinergic effects: anticholinergics

DENTAL CONSIDERATIONS

General:
- Monitor vital signs at every appointment because of cardiovascular side effects.
- Patients on chronic drug therapy may rarely have symptoms of blood dyscrasias, which can include infection, bleeding, and poor healing.
- After supine positioning, have patient sit upright for at least 2 min before standing to avoid orthostatic hypotension.
- Assess salivary flow as a factor in caries, periodontal disease, and candidiasis.
- Avoid dental light in patient's eyes; offer dark glasses for patient comfort.
- Assess for presence of extrapyramidal motor symptoms, such as tardive dyskinesia and akathisia. Extrapyramidal motor activity may complicate dental treatment.
- Geriatric patients are more susceptible to drug effects; use lower dose.
- Use vasoconstrictors with caution, in low doses, and with careful aspiration.

Consultations:
- In a patient with symptoms of blood dyscrasias, request a medical consultation for blood studies and postpone dental treatment until normal values are reestablished.
- Take precautions if dental surgery is anticipated and anesthesia is required.

- Refer to physician if signs of tardive dyskinesia or akathisia are present.
- Physician should be informed if significant xerostomic side effects occur (e.g., increased caries, sore tongue, problems eating or swallowing, difficulty wearing prosthesis) so that a medication change can be considered.

Teach patient/family:

- Importance of good oral hygiene to prevent soft tissue inflammation
- Caution to prevent injury when using oral hygiene aids
- To use electric toothbrush if patient has difficulty holding conventional devices

When chronic dry mouth occurs, advise patient:

- To avoid mouth rinses with high alcohol content because of drying effects
- Of need for daily home fluoride use to prevent caries
- To use sugarless gum, frequent sips of water, or saliva substitutes

---

thiothixene

(thye-oh-thix'een)

Navane

Drug class.: Thioxanthene/antipsychotic

Action: Depresses cerebral cortex, hypothalamus, limbic system, which control activity, aggression; blocks neurotransmission produced by dopamine at the synapse; exhibits strong peripheral α-adrenergic blocking action; mechanism for antipsychotic effects is unclear

Uses: Psychotic disorders, schizophrenia, acute agitation

Dosage and routes:

- *Adult:* PO 2-5 mg bid-qid depending on severity of condition; dose is gradually increased to 15-30 mg/day if needed

Available forms include: Caps 1, 2, 5, 10, 20 mg

Side effects/adverse reactions:

▼ *ORAL: Dry mouth,* uncontrolled tongue and lip movements

CNS: Extrapyramidal symptoms: pseudoparkinsonism, akathisia, dystonia, tardive dyskinesia, headache, seizures

CV: Orthostatic hypotension, ***cardiac arrest, tachycardia,*** hypertension, ECG changes

GI: Nausea, vomiting, anorexia, constipation, diarrhea, jaundice, weight gain

RESP: ***Laryngospasm, respiratory depression,*** dyspnea

HEMA: ***Leukopenia, leukocytosis, agranulocytosis,*** anemia

GU: Urinary retention, enuresis, impotence, amenorrhea, gynecomastia

EENT: Blurred vision, glaucoma

INTEG: Rash, photosensitivity, dermatitis

Contraindications: Hypersensitivity, blood dyscrasias, child <12 yr, bone marrow depression, circulatory collapse, CNS depression, coma, alcoholism, CV disease, hepatic disease, Reye's syndrome, narrow-angle glaucoma

Precautions: Pregnancy category C, lactation, seizure disorders, hypertension, hepatic disease

Pharmacokinetics:

PO: Onset slow, peak 2-8 hr, duration up to 12 hr

IM: Onset 15-30 min, peak 1-6 hr, duration up to 12 hr

Half-life 34 hr; metabolized by

T

liver; excreted in urine; crosses placenta; excreted in breast milk

Drug interactions of concern to dentistry:

• Increased sedation: other CNS depressants, alcohol, barbiturate anesthetics, opioid analgesics

• Hypotension, tachycardia: epinephrine (systemic)

• Increased extrapyramidal effects: phenothiazines and related drugs (haloperidol, droperidol), metoclopramide

• Additive photosensitization: tetracyclines

• Increased anticholinergic effects: anticholinergics

DENTAL CONSIDERATIONS

General:

• Monitor vital signs at every appointment because of cardiovascular side effects.

• Patients on chronic drug therapy may rarely have symptoms of blood dyscrasias, which can include infection, bleeding, and poor healing.

• After supine positioning, have patient sit upright for at least 2 min before standing to avoid orthostatic hypotension.

• Assess salivary flow as a factor in caries, periodontal disease, and candidiasis.

• Assess for presence of extrapyramidal motor symptoms, such as tardive dyskinesia and akathisia. Extrapyramidal motor activity may complicate dental treatment.

• Use vasoconstrictors with caution, in low doses, and with careful aspiration.

• Avoid dental light in patient's eyes; offer dark glasses for patient comfort.

• Geriatric patients are more susceptible to drug effects; use lower dose.

Consultations:

• In a patient with symptoms of blood dyscrasias, request a medical consultation for blood studies and postpone dental treatment until normal values are reestablished.

• Take precautions if dental surgery is anticipated and anesthesia is required.

• If signs of tardive dyskinesia or akathisia are present, refer to physician.

Teach patient/family:

• Importance of good oral hygiene to prevent soft tissue inflammation

• Caution to prevent injury when using oral hygiene aids

• To use electric toothbrush if patient has difficulty holding conventional devices

When chronic dry mouth occurs, advise patient:

• To avoid mouth rinses with high alcohol content because of drying effects

• Of need for daily home fluoride use to prevent caries

• To use sugarless gum, frequent sips of water, or saliva substitutes

---

thyroid USP (desiccated)

(thye'roid)

Armour Thyroid, Bio-throid, Nature-Throid, Westthroid

♣ Cholaxin

Drug class.: Thyroid hormone

Action: Increases metabolic rates; increases cardiac output, O_2 consumption, body temperature, blood volume, growth/development at cellular level

Uses: Hypothyroidism, cretinism, myxedema

Dosage and routes:

Hypothyroidism:

• *Adult:* PO 65 mg qd, increased by 15 mg q3wk, until desired response; maintenance dose 65-195 mg qd

Congenital hypothyroidism:

• *Child 0-6 mo:* PO 7.5-30 mg/day
• *Child 6-12 mo:* PO 35-45 mg/day
• *Child 1-5 yr:* PO 45-60 mg/day
• *Child 6-12 yr:* PO 60-90 mg/day
• *Child >12 yr:* PO 90 mg/day, adjust dose as needed

Myxedema:

• *Adult:* PO 16 mg qd, double dose q2wk; maintenance 65-195 mg/day

Available forms include: Tabs 15, 30, 32.4, 32.5, 60, 64.8, 65, 90, 120, 129.6, 130, 180, 194.4, 195, 240, 300 mg; caps 7.5, 15, 30, 60, 90, 120, 150, 180, 240 mg

Side effects/adverse reactions:

CNS: Insomnia, tremors, headache, thyroid storm

CV: ***Cardiac arrest,*** tachycardia, palpitation, angina, dysrhythmias, hypertension

GI: Nausea, diarrhea, increased or decreased appetite, cramps

MISC: Menstrual irregularities, weight loss, sweating, heat intolerance, fever

Contraindications: Adrenal insufficiency, MI, thyrotoxicosis

Precautions: Elderly, angina pectoris, hypertension, ischemia, cardiac disease, pregnancy category A, lactation

Pharmacokinetics:

PO: Peak 12-48 hr, half-life 6-7 days

Drug interactions of concern to dentistry:

• Increased effects of sympathomimetics when thyroid doses are not carefully monitored or with coronary artery disease

DENTAL CONSIDERATIONS

General:

• Increased nervousness, excitability, sweating, or tachycardia may indicate uncontrolled hyperthyroidism or a dose of medication that is too high. Uncontrolled patients should be referred for medical treatment.

Consultations:

• Medical consultation may be required to assess disease control in the patient.

---

tiagabine HCl

(tye-ag'a-been)

Gabitril

Drug class.: Anticonvulsant

Action: Antiseizure mechanism unknown; acts as an antagonist for γ-aminobutyric acid (GABA) uptake and may enhance the activity of GABA

Uses: Adjunctive therapy for partial seizures

Dosage and routes:

• *Adult and child >18 yr:* PO initial dose 4 mg; increase dose by 4-8 mg increments at weekly intervals until response or up to 32 mg/day
• *Child 12-18 yr:* PO initial dose 4 mg/day; after 1 wk can increase dose 2-8 mg/day; thereafter can be increased by 4-8 mg at weekly intervals up to total dose of 32 mg/day

Available forms include: Tabs 4, 12, 16, 20 mg

Side effects/adverse reactions:

▼ *ORAL:* Dry mouth (1%), gingivitis, stomatitis, gingival hyperplasia (uncommon)

CNS: Sedation, dizziness, headache, memory impairment, emotional state, nervousness, tremor, depression, confusion
CV: Hypertension, palpitation, tachycardia, edema
GI: Abdominal pain, nausea, diarrhea, vomiting, constipation, dyspepsia
RESP: Cough, bronchitis, dyspnea
HEMA: Lymphadenopathy
GU: UTI
EENT: Pharyngitis, amblyopia, ear pain
INTEG: Pruritus, rash, dry skin
MS: Asthenia, myalgia
MISC: Flulike syndrome, pain

Contraindications: Hypersensitivity

Precautions: Hepatic disease, Alzheimer's disease, dementia, organic brain disease, stroke

Pharmacokinetics:
PO: Rapid absorption, peak plasma levels 0.5-1 hr; highly plasma protein bound (95%), hepatic metabolism (CYP 3A isoenzymes), some enterohepatic circulation

Drug interactions of concern to dentistry:
• Increased tiagabine clearance: carbamazepine, phenobarbital
• Use CNS depressants with caution because possible additional effects may occur

DENTAL CONSIDERATIONS

General:
• Monitor vital signs at every appointment because of cardiovascular and respiratory side effects.
• Consider semisupine chair position for patient comfort when GI side effects occur.
• Short appointments and a stress reduction protocol may be required for anxious patients.
• Determine type of epilepsy, seizure frequency, and quality of seizure control.
• Assess salivary flow as factor in caries, periodontal disease, and candidiasis.
• Place on frequent recall if oral side effects occur.

Consultations:
• Consultation with physician may be needed if sedation or general anesthesia is required.

Teach patient/family:
• Caution to prevent trauma when using oral hygiene aids
• Use of electric toothbrush if patient has difficulty holding conventional devices
• Importance of good oral hygiene to prevent soft tissue inflammation
• Importance of updating health and drug history if physician makes any changes in evaluation/drug regimens
• To be aware of oral side effects and potential sequelae

When chronic dry mouth occurs, advise patient:
• To avoid mouth rinses with high alcohol content because of drying effects
• To use daily home fluoride products for anticaries effect
• To use sugarless gum, frequent sips of water, or saliva substitutes

---

ticlopidine

(tye-chloe'pi-deen)
Ticlid

Drug class.: Platelet aggregation inhibitor

Action: Inhibits first and second phases of ADP-induced effects in platelet aggregation

Uses: Reducing the risk of stroke in high-risk patients

Dosage and routes:
• *Adult:* PO 250 mg bid with food
Available forms include: Tabs 250 mg
Side effects/adverse reactions:
GI: ***Cholestatic jaundice, hepatitis,*** increased cholesterol, LDL, VLDL, nausea, vomiting, diarrhea, GI discomfort
HEMA: ***Bleeding (epistaxis, hematuria, conjunctival hemorrhage, GI bleeding), agranulocytosis, neutropenia, thrombocytopenia, erythroleukemia, thrombotic thrombocytopenic purpura***
INTEG: Rash, pruritus
Contraindications: Hypersensitivity, active liver disease, blood dyscrasias
Precautions: Past liver disease, renal disease, elderly, pregnancy category B, lactation, children; increased bleeding risk requires hematologic monitoring every 2 wk for the first 3 mo of therapy
Pharmacokinetics: Peak 1-3 hr, half-life increases with repeated dosing; metabolized by the liver; excreted in urine, feces
Drug interactions of concern to dentistry:
• Increased bleeding tendencies: aspirin, NSAIDs
DENTAL CONSIDERATIONS
General:
• Patients on chronic drug therapy may rarely have symptoms of blood dyscrasias, which can include infection, bleeding, and poor healing.
• Consider local hemostatic measures to prevent excessive bleeding.
Consultations:
• Medical consultation may be required to assess disease control and patient's ability to tolerate stress. Consultation should include data on hematologic profile.
Teach patient/family:
• Caution to prevent injury when using oral hygiene aids

---

tiludronate disodium

(tye-loo'droe-nate)
Skelid
Drug class.: Biphosphonate derivative

Action: Acts to inhibit bone resorption by a mechanism that involves inhibition of osteoclastic activity
Uses: Paget's disease of bone in patients with twice normal upper limit values for serum alkaline phosphatase (SAP) and who are symptomatic and at risk for future complications
Dosage and routes:
• *Adult:* PO 400 mg/day taken with 6-8 oz of plain water only for 3 mo; do not take with other beverages; do not eat for 2 hr after dosing
Available forms include: Tabs 240 mg (equivalent to 200 mg tiludronic acid)
Side effects/adverse reactions:
ORAL: Tooth disorder (not specified), dry mouth (<1%)
CNS: *Headache,* dizziness, paresthesia, nervousness, anxiety
CV: Peripheral edema, hypertension
GI: *Nausea, diarrhea, dyspepsia,* vomiting
RESP: URI, cough, pharyngitis
EENT: *Rhinitis,* sinusitis, cataract, conjunctivitis, glaucoma
INTEG: Rash, pruritus
ENDO: Hyperparathyroidism
META: Vitamin D deficiency

T

MS: Back pain, chest pain, arthralgia
MISC: Flulike symptoms
Contraindications: Hypersensitivity, severe renal failure
Precautions: Pregnancy category C, lactation, safety in children <18 yr not established
Pharmacokinetics:
PO: Rapid but incomplete absorption, bioavailability 6% (fasted), peak plasma levels 2 hr, little or no metabolism, excreted in urine
Drug interactions of concern to dentistry:
• Bioavailability decreased by calcium, food, aluminum or magnesium antacids
• Do not take indomethacin, aspirin, or calcium supplements 2 hr before or after tiludronate
DENTAL CONSIDERATIONS
General:
• Be aware of oral manifestations of Paget's disease (macrognathia, alveolar pain).
• Consider semisupine chair position for patient comfort when GI side effects occur.
• Consider short appointments for patient comfort.
• Assess salivary flow as a factor in caries, periodontal disease, and candidiasis.
Consultations:
• Medical consultation may be required to assess disease control in the patient.
Teach patient/family:
• Caution to prevent trauma when using oral hygiene aids
• Importance of good oral hygiene to prevent soft tissue inflammation
• Importance of updating health and drug history if physician makes any changes in evaluation/drug regimens
When chronic dry mouth occurs, advise patient:
• To avoid mouth rinses with high alcohol content because of drying effects
• To use daily home fluoride products for anticaries effect
• To use sugarless gum, frequent sips of water, or saliva substitutes

---

timolol maleate

(tye'moe-lole)
Blocadren
Apo-Timol, Novo-Timol
Drug class.: Nonselective β-adrenergic blocker

Action: This is a nonselective β_1- and β_2-adrenergic antagonist. The antihypertensive mechanism of action is unclear, but it may include a reduction in cardiac output and inhibition of renin release by the renal juxtaglomerular apparatus. Peripheral resistance decreases with long-term use. The antianginal action (when indicated for this use) may be related to a decrease in myocardial oxygen demand and negative chronotropic and inotropic effects. The antiarrhythmic action (when indicated for this use) has been related to a reduction in spontaneous pacemaker firing and slowing of AV nodal conduction.
Uses: Mild-to-moderate hypertension, reduction of mortality risk after MI, migraine prophylaxis; unapproved uses: essential tremors, angina, cardiac dysrhythmias, anxiety
Dosage and routes:
Hypertension:
• *Adult:* PO 10 mg bid, may increase by 10 mg q2-3d, not to exceed 60 mg/day

Myocardial infarction:
• *Adult:* PO 10 mg bid
Migraine headache:
• *Adult:* PO initial 10 mg bid; maximum dose 30 mg/day
Available forms include: Tabs 5, 10, 20 mg
Side effects/adverse reactions:
▼ *ORAL:* Dry mouth
CNS: Insomnia, dizziness, hallucinations, anxiety
*CV: **CHF,*** hypotension, bradycardia, edema, chest pain, claudication
GI: Nausea, vomiting, abdominal pain, ***mesenteric arterial thrombosis, ischemic colitis,*** diarrhea
RESP: ***Bronchospasm, dyspnea,*** cough, rales
HEMA: ***Agranulocytosis, thrombocytopenia***
GU: Impotence, frequency
EENT: Visual changes, double vision, sore throat, dry/burning eyes
INTEG: Rash, alopecia, pruritus, fever
META: Hypoglycemia
MISC: Joint pain, muscle pain
Contraindications: Hypersensitivity to β-blockers, cardiogenic shock, second- or third-degree heart block, sinus bradycardia, CHF, cardiac failure
Precautions: Major surgery, pregnancy category C, lactation, diabetes mellitus, renal disease, thyroid disease, COPD, well-compensated heart failure, CAD, nonallergic bronchospasm
Pharmacokinetics:
PO: Peak 2-4 hr, half-life 3-4 hr; excreted 30%-45% unchanged; 60%-65% is metabolized by liver; excreted in breast milk
Drug interactions of concern to dentistry:
• Increased hypotension, bradycardia: anticholinergics, sympathomimetics (epinephrine)
• Decreased antihypertensive effects: indomethacin and other NSAIDs
• Suspected increase in plasma levels: diphendydramine
• May slow metabolism of lidocaine

DENTAL CONSIDERATIONS
General:
• Monitor vital signs at every appointment because of cardiovascular side effects.
• Patients on chronic drug therapy may rarely have symptoms of blood dyscrasias, which can include infection, bleeding, and poor healing.
• Assess salivary flow as a factor in caries, periodontal disease, and candidiasis.
• Limit use of sodium-containing products, such as saline IV fluids, for patients with a dietary salt restriction.
• After supine positioning, have patient sit upright for at least 2 min before standing to avoid orthostatic hypotension.
• Stress from dental procedures may compromise cardiovascular function; determine patient risk.
• Short appointments and a stress reduction protocol may be required for anxious patients.
• Consider semisupine chair position for patients with nausea or respiratory distress.
Consultations:
• In a patient with symptoms of blood dyscrasias, request a medical consultation for blood studies and postpone dental treatment until normal values are reestablished.
• Medical consultation may be re-

T

quired to assess disease control and patient's ability to tolerate stress.

Teach patient/family:

- Importance of good oral hygiene to prevent soft tissue inflammation
- Caution to prevent injury when using oral hygiene aids

When chronic dry mouth occurs, advise patient:

- To avoid mouth rinses with high alcohol content because of drying effects
- Of need for daily home fluoride use to prevent caries
- To use sugarless gum, frequent sips of water, or saliva substitutes

timolol maleate (optic)

(tye'moe-lole)

Betimol, Timoptic Solution, Timoptic-XE

Drug class.: β-adrenergic blocker

Action: Reduces production of aqueous humor by unknown mechanism

Uses: Ocular hypertension, chronic open-angle glaucoma, secondary glaucoma, aphakic glaucoma

Dosage and routes:

- *Adult:* Instill 1 drop of 0.25% sol in affected eye(s) bid, then 1 drop for maintenance; may increase to 1 drop of 0.5% sol bid if needed

Available forms include: Sol 0.25%, 0.5%, in 2.5, 5, 10, 15 ml; gel forming sol 0.25%, 0.5% in 2.5, 5 ml

Side effects/adverse reactions:

CNS: Weakness, fatigue, depression, anxiety, headache, confusion

CV: Bradycardia, hypotension, dysrhythmias

GI: Nausea

RESP: ***Bronchospasm***

EENT: Eye irritation, conjunctivitis, keratitis

INTEG: Rash, urticaria

Contraindications: Hypersensitivity, asthma, second- or third-degree heart block, right ventricular failure, congenital glaucoma (infants), COPD

Precautions: May be absorbed systemically, can mask hypoglycemia in patients with diabetes, pregnancy category C, lactation, children

Pharmacokinetics:

INSTILL: Onset 15-30 min, peak 1-2 hr, duration 24 hr

Drug interactions of concern to dentistry:

- Avoid use of anticholinergic drugs, atropine-like drugs, propantheline, and diazepam (benzodiazepines)

DENTAL CONSIDERATIONS

General:

- Check compliance of patient with prescribed drug regimen for glaucoma.
- Avoid dental light in patient's eyes; offer dark glasses for patient comfort.

Consultations:

- Consultation with physician may be needed if sedation or anesthesia is required.

tizanidine HCl

(tye-zan'i-deen)

Zanaflex

Drug class.: Centrally acting α_2-adrenergic agonist

Action: Acts as an agonist at α_2-adrenoreceptor sites; believed to reduce spasticity by increasing presynaptic inhibition on motor neurons

Uses: Treatment of acute and intermittent management of increased muscle tone caused by spasticity (multiple sclerosis, spinal cord injury)

Dosage and routes:

• *Adult:* PO initial 4 mg at 6-8 hr intervals; increase dose by 2-4 mg steps to satisfactory reduction of muscle tone; daily dose limit 36 mg

Available forms include: Tabs 4 mg

Side effects/adverse reactions:

▼ *ORAL: Dry mouth (3%-10%)*

CNS: Light-headedness, dizziness, sedation, hallucination, drowsiness, psychosis, nervousness

CV: Hypotension, bradycardia, orthostatic hypotension, syncope

GI: Abdominal pain, diarrhea, dyspepsia, constipation

GU: UTI, candidiasis

EENT: Blurred vision, rhinitis, pharyngitis, ear pain

INTEG: Skin rash

META: Liver injury, liver enzymes elevated

MS: Asthenia, increased spasm, myasthenia

Contraindications: Hypersensitivity

Precautions: Long-term use, concurrent hypotensive drugs, renal impairment, oral contraceptives, pregnancy category C, lactation, elderly, children

Pharmacokinetics:

PO: Half-life 2.5 hr, peak levels 1.5 hr, first-pass metabolism, extensively metabolized, 30% plasma protein bound, excretion in urine and feces

Drug interactions of concern to dentistry:

• Additive CNS side effects: ethanol and other CNS depressants

• Orthostatic hypotension: drugs that lower blood pressure

DENTAL CONSIDERATIONS

General:

• Monitor vital signs at every appointment because of cardiovascular side effects.

• Short appointments may be required because of effects of disease on musculature.

• Use precaution if sedation or general anesthesia is required; risk of hypotensive episode.

• Assess salivary flow as factor in caries, periodontal disease, and candidiasis.

• After supine positioning, have patient sit upright for at least 2 min before standing to avoid orthostatic hypotension.

Consultations:

• Medical consultation may be required to assess disease control and patient's ability to tolerate stress.

Teach patient/family:

• Not to drive or perform other tasks requiring alertness

• Use of electric toothbrush if patient has difficulty holding conventional devices

When chronic dry mouth occurs, advise patient:

• To avoid mouth rinses with high alcohol content because of drying effects

• To use daily home fluoride products for anticaries effect

• To use sugarless gum, frequent sips of water, or saliva substitutes

T

tobramycin (ophthalmic)

(toe-bra-mye'sin)
AKTob, Defy, Tobrex
Drug class.: Antiinfective

Action: Inhibits bacterial protein synthesis
Uses: Infection of eye
Dosage and routes:
• *Adult and child:* Instill 1-2 gtt q1-4h depending on infection; oint 1 cm bid-tid
Available forms include: Oint 0.3%; sol 0.3%
Side effects/adverse reactions:
EENT: Poor corneal wound healing, visual haze (temporary), overgrowth of nonsusceptible organisms
Contraindications: Hypersensitivity
Precautions: Antibiotic hypersensitivity, pregnancy category D
DENTAL CONSIDERATIONS
General:
• Avoid directing dental light into patient's eyes; provide dark glasses during treatment to avoid irritation.
• Protect patient's eyes from accidental spatter during dental treatment.

tocainide HCl

(toe-kay'nide)
Tonocard
Drug class.: Antidysrhythmic (class IB), lidocaine analog

Action: Decreases sodium and potassium conductance, which decreases myocardial excitability
Uses: Documented life-threatening ventricular dysrhythmias
Dosage and routes:
• *Adult:* PO 400 mg q8h; range 1200-1800 mg/day
Available forms include: Tabs 400, 600 mg
Side effects/adverse reactions:
▼ *ORAL:* Dry mouth, oral ulcerations, erythema multiforme (rare)
CNS: Headache, dizziness, ***seizures,*** involuntary movement, confusion, psychosis, restlessness, irritability, paresthesia, tremors
CV: Hypotension, bradycardia, ***heart block, cardiovascular collapse, arrest, CHF,*** chest pain, angina, PVCs, tachycardia
GI: Nausea, vomiting, anorexia, diarrhea, hepatitis
RESP: ***Respiratory depression, pulmonary fibrosis,*** dyspnea
HEMA: ***Blood dyscrasias: leukopenia, agranulocytosis, hypoplastic anemia, thrombocytopenia, aplastic anemia, bone marrow depression***
EENT: Tinnitus, blurred vision, hearing loss
INTEG: Rash, urticaria, edema, swelling
Contraindications: Hypersensitivity to amides, severe heart block
Precautions: Pregnancy category C, lactation, children, renal disease, liver disease, CHF, respiratory depression, myasthenia gravis, blood dyscrasias
Pharmacokinetics:
PO: Peak 0.5-3 hr; half-life 10-17 hr; metabolized by liver; excreted in urine
Drug interactions of concern to dentistry:
• No specific interactions are reported with dental drugs; however, any drug that could affect the cardiac action of tocainide (local

anesthetics, vasoconstrictors, and anticholinergics) should be used in the least effective dose

DENTAL CONSIDERATIONS

General:

• Monitor vital signs at every appointment because of cardiovascular and respiratory side effects.

• After supine positioning, have patient sit upright for at least 2 min before standing to avoid orthostatic hypotension.

• Patients on chronic drug therapy may rarely have symptoms of blood dyscrasias, which can include infection, bleeding, and poor healing.

• Assess salivary flow as a factor in caries, periodontal disease, and candidiasis.

• Stress from dental procedures may compromise cardiovascular function; determine patient risk.

Consultations:

• In a patient with symptoms of blood dyscrasias, request a medical consultation for blood studies and postpone dental treatment until normal values are reestablished.

• Medical consultation may be required to assess disease control and patient's ability to tolerate stress.

Teach patient/family:

• Importance of good oral hygiene to prevent soft tissue inflammation

• Caution to prevent injury when using oral hygiene aids

When chronic dry mouth occurs, advise patient:

• To avoid mouth rinses with high alcohol content because of drying effects

• Of need for daily home fluoride use to prevent caries

• To use sugarless gum, frequent sips of water, or saliva substitutes

tolazamide

(tole-az'a-mide)

Tolinase

Drug class.: Sulfonylurea (first-generation) oral antidiabetic

Action: Causes functioning β-cells in pancreas to release insulin, leading to drop in blood glucose levels; may improve binding to insulin receptors or increase the number of insulin receptors; this drug is not effective if patient lacks functioning β-cells

Uses: Type 2 diabetes mellitus (NIDDM)

Dosage and routes:

• *Adult:* PO 100 mg/day for FBS <200 mg/dl or 250 mg/day for FBS >200 mg/dl; dose should be titrated to patient response (1 g or less/day)

Available forms include: Tabs 100, 250, 500 mg

Side effects/adverse reactions:

▼ *ORAL:* Lichenoid reaction

CNS: Headache, weakness, fatigue, lethargy, dizziness, vertigo, tinnitus

GI: ***Hepatotoxicity, jaundice,*** heartburn, nausea, vomiting, diarrhea, constipation, gas

HEMA: ***Leukopenia, thrombocytopenia, agranulocytosis, aplastic anemia, pancytopenia, hemolytic anemia***

INTEG: Rash, allergic reactions, pruritus, urticaria, eczema, photosensitivity, erythema

ENDO: ***Hypoglycemia***

Contraindications: Hypersensitivity to sulfonylureas, juvenile or brittle diabetes

Precautions: Pregnancy category C, elderly, cardiac disease, thyroid disease, severe hypoglycemic reactions, renal disease, hepatic disease

Pharmacokinetics:
PO: Completely absorbed by GI route; onset 4-6 hr, peak 4-8 hr, duration 12-24 hr, half-life 7 hr; highly protein bound; metabolized in liver; excreted in urine (metabolites), breast milk

Drug interactions of concern to dentistry:
• Increased hypoglycemic reaction: NSAIDs, salicylates, ketoconazole, miconazole
• Decreased action of tolazamide: corticosteroids, sympathomimetics (epinephrine)

DENTAL CONSIDERATIONS
General:
• Patients on chronic drug therapy may rarely have symptoms of blood dyscrasias, which can include infection, bleeding, and poor healing.
• Place on frequent recall to evaluate healing response.
• Short appointments and a stress reduction protocol may be required for anxious patients.
• Patients with diabetes may be more susceptible to infection and have delayed wound healing.
• Ensure that patient is following prescribed diet and regularly takes medication.
• Question patient about self-monitoring of drug's antidiabetic effect.
• Avoid prescribing aspirin-containing products.

Consultations:
• In a patient with symptoms of blood dyscrasias, request a medical consultation for blood studies and postpone dental treatment until normal values are reestablished.
• Medical consultation may be required to assess disease control in the patient.

Teach patient/family:
• Importance of good oral hygiene to prevent soft tissue inflammation
• To avoid mouth rinses with high alcohol content because of drying effects

---

tolbutamide

(tole-byoo'ta-mide)
Orinase
✦ Apo-Tolbutamide, Mobenol, Novo-Butamide

Drug class.: Sulfonylurea (first-generation) oral antidiabetic

---

Action: Causes functioning β-cells in pancreas to release insulin, leading to drop in blood glucose levels; may improve binding to insulin receptors or increase the number of insulin receptors; this drug is not effective if patient lacks functioning β-cells

Uses: Type 2 diabetes mellitus

Dosage and routes:
• *Adult:* PO 1-2 g/day in divided doses, titrated to patient response

Available forms include: Tabs 500 mg

Side effects/adverse reactions:
▼ *ORAL:* Changes in taste sensation, lichenoid reaction
CNS: Headache, weakness, paresthesia, tinnitus, dizziness, vertigo
GI: ***Hepatotoxicity, cholestatic jaundice,*** nausea, fullness, heartburn, diarrhea
HEMA: ***Leukopenia, thrombocytopenia, agranulocytosis, aplastic anemia,*** increased AST/ALT, alk phosphatase
INTEG: Rash, allergic reactions, pruritus, urticaria, eczema, photosensitivity, erythema
ENDO: ***Hypoglycemia***
MS: Joint pain

Contraindications: Hypersensitivity to sulfonylureas, juvenile or brittle diabetes

Precautions: Pregnancy category C, elderly, cardiac disease, thyroid disease, severe hypoglycemic reactions, renal disease, hepatic disease

Pharmacokinetics:

PO: Completely absorbed by GI route, onset 30-60 min, peak 3-5 hr, duration 6-12 hr, half-life 4-5 hr; 90%-95% is plasma protein bound; metabolized in liver; excreted in urine (metabolites), breast milk

Drug interactions of concern to dentistry:

- Increased hypoglycemic reactions: NSAIDs, salicylates, ketoconazole, miconazole
- Decreased effects: corticosteroids, sympathomimetics

DENTAL CONSIDERATIONS

General:

- Patients on chronic drug therapy may rarely have symptoms of blood dyscrasias, which can include infection, bleeding, and poor healing.
- Ensure that patient is following prescribed diet and regularly takes medication.
- Question patient about self-monitoring of drug's antidiabetic effect, including blood glucose values or finger-stick records.
- Place on frequent recall to evaluate healing response.
- Short appointments and a stress reduction protocol may be required for anxious patients.
- Patients with diabetes may be more susceptible to infection and have delayed wound healing.
- Avoid prescribing aspirin-containing products.

Consultations:

- In a patient with symptoms of blood dyscrasias, request a medical consultation for blood studies and postpone dental treatment until normal values are reestablished.
- Medical consultation may be required to assess disease control in the patient.
- Medical consultation may include data from patient's blood glucose monitoring, including glycosylated hemoglobin or Hb
- A_{1c} testing.

Teach patient/family:

- Importance of good oral hygiene to prevent soft tissue inflammation
- To avoid mouth rinses with high alcohol content because of drying effects

---

tolcapone

(tole'ka-pone)

Tasmar

Drug class.: Antiparkinsonian

Action: Reversibly and selectively inhibits catechol-*O*-methyltransferase (COMT) and may alter the plasma pharmacokinetics of levodopa; levodopa (with carbidopa) plasma levels are more sustained

Uses: Adjunct to levodopa and carbidopa in the treatment of Parkinson's disease

Dosage and routes:

- *Adult:* PO initial 100 mg tid as an adjunct to levodopa/carbidopa therapy; use 200 mg tid with caution because of elevated ALT or AST

Available forms include: Tabs 100, 200 mg

Side effects/adverse reactions:

▼ *ORAL: Xerostomia (5%-6%)*

CNS: Hallucinations, dyskinesia, sleep disorders, dystonia, anorexia,

T

headache, dizziness, confusion, somnolence, excessive dreaming
CV: Orthostatic hypotension, chest pain
GI: ***Hepatocellular injury,*** diarrhea, nausea, anorexia, abdominal pain, constipation, vomiting
RESP: Pulmonary effusion, URI
GU: Hematuria, UTI, discolored urine
EENT: Sinus congestion
META: Elevation of SGT and AST
MS: Muscle cramps
MISC: Sweating, fatigue

Contraindications: Hypersensitivity, patients with SGPT/ALT and SGOT/AST exceeding upper limit of normal or other signs of hepatic impairment; informed consent required; history of nontraumatic rhabdomyolysis, hyperpyrexia, and confusion related to medication

Precautions: Discontinue drug with signs of hepatocellular injury, MAOIs, hypotension, dyskinesia, pregnancy category C, lactation

Pharmacokinetics:
PO: Rapidly absorbed, bioavailability 65%, highly plasma protein bound (99.9%), hepatic metabolism, 60% excreted in urine, 40% in feces

Drug interactions of concern to dentistry:
• Increased sedation: alcohol and all CNS depressants
• No other data for dental drugs reported

DENTAL CONSIDERATIONS
General:
• Notify physician immediately if symptoms of liver failure are observed (bleeding, jaundice, etc.).
• Assess salivary flow as a factor in caries, periodontal disease, and candidiasis.
• After supine positioning, have patient sit upright for at least 2 min to avoid orthostatic hypotension.
• Consider semisupine chair position for patient comfort because of GI side effects of drug.

Consultations:
• Medical consultation may be required to assess disease control in the patient.
• Take precaution if dental surgery is anticipated and general anesthesia is required.

Teach patient/family:
• Use of electric toothbrush if patient has difficulty holding conventional devices

When chronic dry mouth occurs, advise patient:
• To avoid mouth rinses with high alcohol content because of drying effects
• To use daily home fluoride products for anticaries effect
• To use sugarless gum, frequent sips of water, or saliva substitutes

---

tolmetin sodium

(tole'met-in)
Tolectin, Tolectin DS
Novo-Tolmetin

Drug class.: Nonsteroidal antiinflammatory

Action: Inhibits prostaglandin synthesis by interfering with cyclooxygenase needed for biosynthesis

Uses: Osteoarthritis, rheumatoid arthritis, juvenile rheumatoid arthritis

Dosage and routes:
• *Adult:* PO 400 mg tid, not to exceed 2 g/day
• *Child >2 yr:* PO 15-30 mg/kg/day in 3 or 4 divided doses

Available forms include: Tabs 200, 600 mg; caps 400 mg

Side effects/adverse reactions:

▼ *ORAL:* Dry mouth, gingival bleeding, mucosal ulceration, lichenoid reaction

CNS: Dizziness, drowsiness, fatigue, tremors, confusion, insomnia, anxiety, depression

CV: Tachycardia, peripheral edema, palpitation, dysrhythmias

GI: ***Cholestatic hepatitis,*** nausea, anorexia, vomiting, diarrhea, jaundice, constipation, flatulence, cramps, peptic ulcer

HEMA: ***Blood dyscrasias***

GU: ***Nephrotoxicity: dysuria, hematuria, oliguria, azotemia***

EENT: Tinnitus, hearing loss, blurred vision

INTEG: Purpura, rash, pruritus, sweating

Contraindications: Hypersensitivity, asthma, severe renal disease, severe hepatic disease

Precautions: Pregnancy category C, lactation, children, bleeding disorders, GI disorders, cardiac disorders, hypersensitivity to aspirin, NSAIDs, peptic ulcer disease, geriatric patients

Pharmacokinetics:

PO: Peak 2 hr, half-life 3-3.5 hr; 99% protein binding; metabolized in liver; excreted in urine (metabolites), breast milk

Drug interactions of concern to dentistry:

• Increased risk of GI side effects: ASA, NSAIDs, ethanol (alcohol)

• Nephrotoxicity: acetaminophen (prolonged use and high doses)

• Possible risk of decreased renal function: cyclosporine

• Decreased antihypertensive effect of diuretics, β-adrenergic blockers, and ACE inhibitors

• First-time users of SSRIs also taking NSAIDs may have a higher risk of GI side effects; until more data are available, it may be advisable to avoid use of NSAIDs in these patients (*Br J Clin Pharmacol* 55:591-595, 2003)

DENTAL CONSIDERATIONS

General:

• Patients on chronic drug therapy may rarely have symptoms of blood dyscrasias, which can include infection, bleeding, and poor healing.

• Monitor vital signs at every appointment because of cardiovascular side effects.

• Assess salivary flow as a factor in caries, periodontal disease, and candidiasis.

• Avoid prescribing for dental use in last trimester of pregnancy.

• Possibility of cross-allergenicity when patient is allergic to aspirin.

Consultations:

• Medical consultation may be required to assess disease control in the patient.

• In a patient with symptoms of blood dyscrasias, request a medical consultation for blood studies and postpone dental treatment until normal values are reestablished.

Teach patient/family:

• Importance of good oral hygiene to prevent soft tissue inflammation

• Caution to prevent injury when using oral hygiene aids

When chronic dry mouth occurs, advise patient:

• To avoid mouth rinses with high alcohol content because of drying effects

• Of need for daily home fluoride use to prevent caries

• To use sugarless gum, frequent sips of water, or saliva substitutes

tolterodine tartrate

(tole-ter'o-deen)

Detrol, Detrol LA

Drug class.: Antispasmodic

Action: Inhibits muscarinic actions of acetylcholine at postganglionic receptors

Uses: Overactive bladder, with symptoms of urinary frequency or incontinence

Dosage and routes:

• *Adult:* PO initial dose 2 mg bid; may be reduced to 1 mg bid based on individual response; ext rel 4 mg/day with liquids

With hepatic dysfunction or concurrent use with inhibitors of cytochrome P-450 3A4:

• *Adult:* PO 1 mg bid; 2 mg/day ext rel caps

Available forms include: Tabs 1, 2 mg; ext rel caps 2, 4 mg

Side effects/adverse reactions:

▼ *ORAL: Dry mouth (39.5%)*

CNS: Headache, dizziness, fatigue, vertigo, somnolence, paresthesia, nervousness

GI: Dyspepsia, constipation, abdominal pain, nausea, diarrhea

RESP: URI, bronchitis, coughing

GU: Urinary retention, dysuria, UTI

EENT: Xerophthalmia, blurred vision, rhinitis

INTEG: Rash, erythema, pruritus, dry skin

MS: Arthralgia, back pain

MISC: Weight gain, flulike symptoms

Contraindications: Hypersensitivity, urinary retention, gastric retention, uncontrolled narrow-angle glaucoma

Precautions: Bladder obstruction, pyloric stenosis, GI obstructive disorders, treated narrow-angle glaucoma, significant hepatic dysfunction, renal impairment, pregnancy category C, lactation, pediatric use

Pharmacokinetics:

PO: Onset 1 hr, peak serum levels 1-2 hr, highly plasma protein bound (96%), hepatic metabolism (CYP2D6 isoenzymes), active metabolite, urinary excretion (77%)

Drug interactions of concern to dentistry:

• Studies not available; however, drugs that inhibit cytochrome P-450 3A4 enzymes, such as erythromycin, clarithromycin, ketoconazole, itraconazole, and fluoxetine, require a dose reduction to 1 mg bid (see Appendix I)

• Increased anticholinergic effects: possibly with other anticholinergic drugs

DENTAL CONSIDERATIONS

General:

• Assess salivary flow as a factor in caries, periodontal disease, and candidiasis.

• Consider semisupine chair position for patient comfort because of GI side effects of drug.

• Avoid dental light in patient's eyes; offer dark glasses for patient comfort.

• Avoid drugs with anticholinergic activity, such as antihistamines, opioids, benzodiazepines, propantheline, atropine, and scopolamine.

Consultations:

• Physician should be informed if significant xerostomic side effects occur (e.g., increased caries, sore tongue, problems eating or swallowing, difficulty wearing prosthesis) so that a medication change can be considered.

Teach patient/family:

- Importance of good oral hygiene to prevent soft tissue inflammation

When chronic dry mouth occurs, advise patient:

- To avoid mouth rinses with high alcohol content because of drying effects
- To use daily home fluoride products for anticaries effect
- To use sugarless gum, frequent sips of water, or saliva substitutes

topiramate

(toe-pyre'a-mate)

Topamax

Drug class.: Anticonvulsant

Action: Anticonvulsant action is unclear; blocks repetitively elicited action potentials and enhances GABA activity along with antagonism of kainate activity on non-NMDA receptors

Uses: Adjunctive therapy for adult patients with partial-onset seizures or for primary generalized tonic-clonic seizures; Lennox-Gastaut syndrome

Dosage and routes:

- *Adult and child >17 yr:* PO 400 mg/day in 2 divided doses; initiate therapy at 50 mg/day and titrate to effective dose level
- *Children 2-16 yr:* PO total daily dose range 5-9 mg/kg/day in 2 equal doses; start at 25 mg hs × 1 wk, then increase at 1-2 wk intervals to achieve desired response

Available forms include: Tabs 25, 100, 200 mg; sprinkle caps 15, 25 mg

Side effects/adverse reactions:

▼ *ORAL:* Dry mouth (1.1%), gingival overgrowth (rare), taste alteration

CNS: Psychomotor slowing, somnolence, fatigue, ataxia, confusion, dizziness, memory problems, irritability, depression

CV: Palpitation, bradycardia

GI: Nausea, dyspepsia, abdominal pain

RESP: Coughing, bronchitis

HEMA: Epistaxis, ***leukopenia, purpura, thrombycytopenia***

GU: Hematuria, UTI

EENT: Decreased hearing, eye pain, photophobia, severe myopia, secondary angle-closure glaucoma

INTEG: Dermatitis, acne

MS: Back pain, asthenia, leg pain, myalgia

MISC: Paresthesia

Contraindications: Hypersensitivity

Precautions: Renal impairment, hepatic impairment, rapid drug withdrawal, kidney stones, pregnancy category C, lactation, children

Pharmacokinetics:

PO: Rapid oral absorption, peak plasma levels 2 hr, low protein binding (13%-17%), 70% excreted in urine unchanged, little metabolism

Drug interactions of concern to dentistry:

- Increased CNS depression: opioids, sedatives, ethanol, and other CNS depressants
- Decreased serum levels: carbamazepine

DENTAL CONSIDERATIONS

General:

- Patients on chronic drug therapy may rarely have symptoms of blood dyscrasias, which can include infection, bleeding, and poor healing.

• Short appointments and a stress reduction protocol may be required for anxious patients.
• Assess salivary flow as factor in caries, periodontal disease, and candidiasis.
• Avoid dental light in patient's eyes; offer dark glasses for patient comfort.
• Determine type of epilepsy, seizure frequency, and quality of seizure control. A stress reduction protocol may be required.

Consultations:

• In a patient with symptoms of blood dyscrasias, request a medical consultation for blood studies and postpone dental treatment until normal values are reestablished.
• Medical consultation may be required to assess disease control in the patient.

Teach patient/family:

• Importance of good oral hygiene to prevent soft tissue inflammation
• Caution to prevent trauma when using oral hygiene aids
• Use of electric toothbrush if patient has difficulty holding conventional devices
• Importance of updating health and drug history if physician makes any changes in evaluation/drug regimens

When chronic dry mouth occurs, advise patient:

• To avoid mouth rinses with high alcohol content because of drying effects
• To use daily home fluoride products for anticaries effect
• To use sugarless gum, frequent sips of water, or saliva substitutes

toremifene citrate

(tore'em-i-feen)
Fareston

Drug class.: Antineoplastic, antiestrogen agent

Action: Inhibits cell division by binding to cytoplasmic receptors (estrogen receptors); resembles normal cell complex but inhibits DNA synthesis

Uses: Metastatic breast cancer in postmenopausal women with estrogen receptor–positive or unknown tumors

Dosage and routes:

• *Adult:* PO 60 mg qd continued until disease progression is observed

Available forms include: Tabs 60 mg

Side effects/adverse reactions:

CNS: Dizziness
CV: Edema
GI: Nausea, vomiting
HEMA: Thrombophlebitis, thrombosis
GU: Vaginal discharge, vaginal bleeding
EENT: Cataracts, dry eyes, abnormal visual fields, glaucoma
INTEG: Sweating
ENDO: Hot flashes
META: Elevated SGOT, alkaline phosphatase, bilirubin, hypercalcemia

Contraindications: Hypersensitivity

Precautions: Thromboembolic diseases, endometrial hyperplasia, hypercalcemia with bone metastases, monitor leukocyte and platelet counts, pregnancy category D, tumor flare

Pharmacokinetics:
PO: Well absorbed, peak levels average 3 hr, extensive metabolism with active metabolite, enterohepatic circulation, highly protein bound (99.5%), excreted mainly in feces, 10% in urine

Drug interactions of concern to dentistry:
• None reported

DENTAL CONSIDERATIONS
General:
• Patients on chronic drug therapy may rarely have symptoms of blood dyscrasias, which can include infection, bleeding, and poor healing.
• Consider semisupine chair position for patient comfort because of GI side effects of drug.

Consultations:
• Medical consultation may be required to assess disease control in the patient.

Teach patient/family:
• Importance of good oral hygiene to prevent soft tissue inflammation

---

torsemide
(tore'se-mide)
Demadex
Drug class.: Loop diuretic

Action: Acts on loop of Henle to decrease the reabsorption of chloride, sodium, and potassium with resultant diuresis

Uses: Hypertension and edema associated with CHF, liver disease, chronic renal failure

Dosage and routes:
Hypertension:
• *Adult:* PO 5 mg/day; may increase to 10 mg after 4-6 wk if required
CHF, chronic renal failure:
• *Adult:* PO or IV, 10-20 mg/day; may increase if inadequate response; no data for doses >200 mg
Hepatic cirrhosis:
• *Adult:* PO or IV 5-10 mg/day

Available forms include: Tabs 5, 10, 20, 100 mg; inj IV 10 mg/ml in 2, 5 ml amps

Side effects/adverse reactions:
CNS: Dizziness, headache, fatigue, insomnia, nervousness, syncope
CV: Orthostatic hypotension, ECG abnormalities, chest pain, edema, dysrhythmias
GI: Diarrhea, nausea, dyspepsia, irritation, GI bleeding
RESP: Cough
GU: Excessive urination
EENT: Sore throat, rhinitis
INTEG: Rash, photosensitvity
MS: Asthenia, muscle cramps, arthralgia

Contraindications: Hypersensitivity, anuria, severe electrolyte depletion, hypersensitivity to sulfonylureas, hepatic coma, cisapride

Precautions: Pregnancy category B, lactation, children <18 yr, dehydration, systemic lupus erythematosus, ototoxicity, electrolyte imbalance

Pharmacokinetics:
PO: Onset 1 hr, peak effects 1-2 hr, duration 6-8 hr; liver metabolism; renal excretion
IV: Onset 10 min, peak effect 1 hr, duration 6-8 hr

Drug interactions of concern to dentistry:
• Increased electrolyte imbalance: systemic corticosteroids
• Masked ototoxicity: phenothiazines
• Decreased antihypertensive effects: NSAIDs, especially indomethacin

T

• Increased sweating, hot flashes, weakness, CV symptoms: chloral hydrate (rare)

DENTAL CONSIDERATIONS

General:

• Monitor vital signs at every appointment because of cardiovascular side effects.

• After supine positioning, have patient sit upright for at least 2 min before standing to avoid orthostatic hypotension.

• Patients on high-potency loop diuretics should be questioned about serum potassium levels or potassium supplement use.

• Short appointments and a stress reduction protocol may be required for anxious patients.

• Consider semisupine chair position if GI side effects occur.

Consultations:

• Medical consultation may be required to assess disease control and stress tolerance in the patient.

Teach patient/family:

• Importance of updating health history/drug record if physician makes any changes in evaluation/drug regimens

tramadol HCl

(tra'ma-dole)

Ultram

Drug class.: Synthetic opioid analgesic

Action: Unknown, but it has been shown to bind to opioid receptors and inhibit the reuptake of norepinephrine and serotonin

Uses: Moderate-to-severe pain

Dosage and routes:

• *Adult:* PO 50-100 mg q4-6h, limit 400 mg/day (do not exceed limit); for moderately severe pain, 100 mg initial dose may be required

Moderate chronic pain not requiring rapid analgesic onset:

• *Adult:* PO initial 25 mg/day, then titrate doses by 25 mg as separate doses q3d to maximum dose of 100 mg, then titrate doses by 50 mg q3d to max of 200 mg daily; max daily dose 400 mg

Renal/hepatic impairment or elderly 65 yr or older:

• *Adult:* PO limit dose to 200 mg/day

Cirrhosis:

• *Adult:* PO limit dose to 50 mg q12h

Available forms include: Tabs 50 mg

Side effects/adverse reactions:

▼ *ORAL:* Dry mouth (<5%), stomatitis

CNS: Dizziness, vertigo, headache, somnolence, seizures, anxiety, confusion, drug abuse risk

CV: Vasodilation, palpitation

GI: Constipation, vomiting, dyspepsia, diarrhea, flatulence

GU: Urinary retention, frequency

EENT: Visual disturbances

INTEG: Pruritus, sweating, rash

MS: Hypertonia

MISC: Malaise

Contraindications: Hypersensitivity to tramadol, codeine, or other opioids; acute alcohol, hypnotic, other opioid, or psychotropic drug intoxication, opioid addicts; pregnancy category C; lactation; child <16 yr; elderly; renal or hepatic impairment; risk of seizures in patients taking MAOIs, tricyclic antidepressants, or other drugs that reduce the seizure threshold; increased intracranial pressure caused by head injury

Precautions: Not a controlled substance, but dependence and abuse are possible

Pharmacokinetics:

PO: Rapid oral absorption, can be given with food, peak levels 2 hr, half-life 6-7 hr; hepatic metabolism (a portion of metabolism is by CYP2D6 isoenzyme); excreted in urine

Drug interactions of concern to dentistry:

• Increased risk of respiratory depression: anesthetics, alcohol
• Significant increase in metabolism: carbamazepine
• Increased serum concentrations: quinidine
• Increased risk of seizures: MAOIs, tricyclic antidepressants, selective serotonin reuptake inhibitors
• Increased risk of sedation: other CNS depressant drugs, alcohol

DENTAL CONSIDERATIONS

General:

• Determine why the patient is taking the drug.
• Patients taking opioids for acute or chronic pain should be given alternative analgesics for dental pain.
• Geriatric patients are more susceptible to drug effects; use lower dose.
• Assess salivary flow as a factor in caries, periodontal disease, and candidiasis.
• Take precautions if dental surgery is anticipated and general anesthesia is required.
• Risk of cross-hypersensitivity to other opioid analgesics.

Teach patient/family:

• Caution to prevent trauma when using oral hygiene aids
• That opioid drugs may alter reaction time; caution patient about driving or operating complex equipment

When chronic dry mouth occurs, advise patient:

• To avoid mouth rinses with high alcohol content because of drying effects
• To use daily home fluoride products for anticaries effect
• To use sugarless gum, frequent sips of water, or saliva substitutes

---

trandolapril

(tran'dole-a-pril)

Mavik

Drug class.: Angiotensin-converting enzyme (ACE) inhibitor

Action: Selectively suppresses renin-angiotensin-aldosterone system; inhibits ACE; prevents conversion of angiotension I to angiotensin II; results in reduced peripheral resistance, decreased aldosterone secretion, and increase in plasma renin

Uses: Hypertension alone or in combination with other antihypertensive medications; maintenance therapy to prevent CHF after MI; ventricular dysfunction after MI

Dosage and routes:

Not taking diuretic:

• *Adult:* PO initial dose 1 mg (non–African-American patient) and 2 mg (African-American patient) daily; adjust dose to BP response; usual dose 2-4 mg daily

Taking diuretic:

• *Adult:* Discontinue diuretic for 2-3 days before initiating trandolapril therapy, add diuretic if BP is not controlled

T

When diuretic cannot be discontinued:

• *Adult:* Initial dose is 0.5 mg with caution and medical supervision until BP is stabilized

Post-MI:

• *Adult:* PO initial dose 1 mg, then titrate slowly to 4 mg/day

Available forms include: Tabs 1 mg, 2 mg, and 4 mg

Side effects/adverse reactions:

▼ *ORAL:* ***Angioedema (lips, tongue, mucous membranes)***

CNS: Dizziness, drowsiness, insomnia, vertigo, headache, fatigue

CV: Hypotension, syncope, bradycardia, chest pain, palpitation, AV first-degree block, bradycardia, hyperkalemia

GI: Diarrhea, ***pancreatitis,*** cholestatic jaundice

RESP: Cough, URI, dyspnea

HEMA: ***Neutropenia, leukopenia***

GU: Impotence, decreased libido

EENT: Throat inflammation, epistaxis

INTEG: Pruritus, rash, pemphigus

MS: Cramps, gout, extremity pain

MISC: ***Anaphylactoid reactions***

Contraindications: Hypersensitivity or angioedema with prior use of ACE inhibitors, second or third trimester of pregnancy, lactation

Precautions: Angioedema (higher rate in African-American patients), congestive heart failure, ischemic heart disease, aortic stenosis, cerebrovascular disease, monitor WBC count in SLE or scleroderma, impaired renal function, hyperkalemia, pregnancy category C (first trimester), pregnancy category D (second, third trimester), pediatric patients, potassium-sparing diuretics

Pharmacokinetics:

PO: Active metabolite trandolaprilat, peak levels trandolapril 1 hr, trandolaprilat 4-10 hr, excreted 66% in feces, 33% in urine, protein binding 80%

Drug interactions of concern to dentistry:

• Decreased absorption of tetracycline

• Drugs that lower blood pressure could possibly exaggerate hypotensive effects

DENTAL CONSIDERATIONS

General:

• Monitor vital signs at every appointment because of cardiovascular disease.

• Limit use of sodium-containing products such as saline IV fluids for those patients with a dietary salt restriction.

• Stress from dental procedures may compromise cardiovascular function; determine patient risk.

• Short appointments and a stress reduction protocol may be required for anxious patients.

• Use precaution if sedation or general anesthesia is required; risk of hypotensive episode.

• After supine positioning, have patient sit upright for at least 2 min before standing to avoid orthostatic hypotension.

• Consider semisupine chair position for patient comfort because of respiratory side effects of drug.

• Patients on chronic drug therapy may rarely have symptoms of blood dyscrasias, which can include infection, bleeding, and poor healing.

Consultations:

• Medical consultation may be required to assess disease control and patient's ability to tolerate stress.

Teach patient/family:

- Importance of good oral hygiene to prevent soft tissue inflammation
- Caution to prevent trauma when using oral hygiene aids
- Importance of updating health and drug history if physician makes any changes in evaluation/ drug regimens

tranexamic acid

(tran-ex-am'ik)

Cyklokapron

Drug class.: Hemostatic, antithrombolytic

Action: Competitive inhibitor of plasminogen activation, decreases the conversion of plasminogen to plasmin; a much higher dose acts as a noncompetitive inhibitor of plasmin

Uses: Prophylaxis and treatment of hemophilia patients to reduce or prevent hemorrhage during and after extractions; unapproved uses: in hyperfibrinolysis-induced hemorrhage, angioedema; oral rinse (with systemic therapy) to reduce bleeding in oral surgery patients who are also taking anticoagulants

Dosage and routes:

Dental extraction in hemophilia patient:

- *Adult and adolescent:* IV immediately before surgery, 10 mg/kg; after surgery give 25 mg/kg tid or qid for 2-8 days
- *Adult and adolescent:* PO beginning day before surgery, 25 mg/kg tid or qid; after surgery give 25 mg/kg tid or qid for 2-8 days; patients unable to take PO meds—IV, 10 mg/kg tid-qid

NOTE: Reduce dose with moderate to severe renal impairment

Unlabeled use: Dental procedures producing bleeding in patients taking oral anticoagulants (rinse): Some reports suggest the use of tranexamic oral rinse for use in patients who cannot reduce their use of oral anticoagulants. One report (Ramstrom et al: *J Oral Maxillofac Surg* 51:1211-1216, 1963) used the following procedure:

- *Adult:* Before suturing, the area is irrigated with 10 ml of 4.8% tranexamic acid solution. Patients rinse for 2 min 4 times daily for the next 7 days. No food or drink is to be consumed within 1 hr of using mouthwash. Tranexamic acid mouthwash is not commercially available in Canada or the United States. It could be extemporaneously prepared using the commercial tablets or injection. Because stability data for aqueous solutions are lacking, extemporaneous solutions should be freshly prepared. In another report (Souto et al: *J Oral Maxillofac Surg* 54:27-32, 1996) a mouth rinse of 1 ampule of the antifibrinolytic agent for 2 min q6h for 2 days was used.

Available forms include: Tabs 500 mg; amps 100 mg/ml in 10 ml size

Side effects/adverse reactions:

CNS: Giddiness

CV: Hypotension (IV doses)

GI: Nausea, vomiting, diarrhea

EENT: Blurred vision

Contraindications: Patients with acquired defective color vision, subarachnoid hemorrhage

Precautions: Pregnancy category B, lactation, reduce dose in renal impairment, limited use experience in children

Pharmacokinetics:
PO: Bioavailability 30%-50%, low protein binding (<3%), peak plasma levels 3 hr, little metabolism, renal excretion

Drug interactions of concern to dentistry:
• Increased risk of bleeding: drugs that affect coagulation
• Factor IX complex: increased risk of thrombotic complications when used concurrently

DENTAL CONSIDERATIONS
General:
• Has been used as an antifibrinolytic mouthwash following oral surgery to prevent hemorrhage in patients taking oral anticoagulants.

Consultations:
• Hematologist consultation is strongly recommended.

Teach patient/family:
• Importance of updating health and drug history if physician makes any changes in evaluation/drug regimens
• To report hemorrhage or bleeding not responding to postsurgical hemostasis
• Caution to prevent trauma when using oral hygiene aids

---

tranylcypromine sulfate

(tran-il-sip′roe-meen)
Parnate

Drug class.: Antidepressant, MAO inhibitor

Action: Increases concentrations of endogenous norepinephrine, serotonin, and dopamine in CNS storage sites by inhibiting MAO; the precise antidepressant mechanism is unknown

Uses: Depression (when uncontrolled by other means)

Dosage and routes:
• *Adult:* PO 10 mg bid; may increase to 30 mg/day after 2 wk; max 60 mg/day

Available forms include: Tabs 10 mg

Side effects/adverse reactions:
▼ *ORAL:* Dry mouth
CNS: Dizziness, drowsiness, confusion, headache, anxiety, tremors, stimulation, weakness, hyperreflexia, mania, insomnia, fatigue, weight gain
CV: Orthostatic hypotension, hypertension, dysrhythmias, hypertensive crisis
GI: Anorexia, constipation, nausea, vomiting, diarrhea, weight gain
HEMA: Anemia
GU: Change in libido, urinary retention
EENT: Blurred vision
INTEG: Rash, flushing, increased perspiration
ENDO: ***SIADH-like syndrome***

Contraindications: Hypersensitivity to MAOIs, elderly, hypertension, CHF, severe hepatic disease, pheochromocytoma, severe renal disease, severe cardiac disease

Precautions: Suicidal patients, convulsive disorders, severe depression, schizophrenia, hyperactivity, diabetes mellitus, pregnancy category C

Pharmacokinetics:
PO: Metabolized in liver, excreted by kidneys, crosses placenta, excreted in breast milk

Drug interactions of concern to dentistry:
• Increased pressor effects: indirect-acting sympathomimetics (ephedrine)

• Hyperpyretic crisis, convulsions, hypertensive episode, and death: carbamazepine, meperidine, and possibly other opioids
• Increased anticholinergic effects: anticholinergics and antihistamines
• Increased effects of alcohol, barbiturates, benzodiazepines, CNS depressants, fluoxetine, tricyclic antidepressants

DENTAL CONSIDERATIONS

General:

• After supine positioning, have patient sit upright for at least 2 min before standing to avoid orthostatic hypotension.
• Monitor vital signs at every appointment because of cardiovascular side effects.
• Assess salivary flow as a factor in caries, periodontal disease, and candidiasis.
• Hypertensive episodes are possible even though there are no specific contraindications to vasoconstrictor use in local anesthetics.

Consultations:

• Medical consultation may be required to assess patient's ability to tolerate stress.

Teach patient/family:

• To use electric toothbrush if patient has difficulty holding conventional devices

When chronic dry mouth occurs, advise patient:

• To avoid mouth rinses with high alcohol content because of drying effects
• Of need for daily home fluoride use to prevent caries
• To use sugarless gum, frequent sips of water, or saliva substitutes

travoprost ophthalmic solution

(tra'voe-prost)

Travatan

Drug class.: Synthetic prostaglandin F_2-α analogue

Action: Rapidly hydrolyzed to the biologically active, travoprost free acid that is a selective FP prostanoid receptor agonist; reduces intraocular pressure (IOP) by increasing uveoscleral outflow

Uses: Reduction of elevated IOP in patients with open-angle glaucoma or ocular hypertension in patients intolerant to, or who show insufficient response to, other IOP-reducing drugs

Dosage and routes:

• *Adult:* TOP 1 drop in affected eye(s) qd in PM

Available forms include:

Sterile sol 0.004% in 2.5 ml

Side effects/adverse reactions:

CNS: Anxiety, depression, headache

CV: Angina pectoris, bradycardia, hypertension, hypotension

GI: Dyspepsia

RESP: Bronchitis, sinusitis

GU: UTI, incontinence

EENT: ***Ocular hyperemia, conjunctival hyperemia,*** decreased visual acuity, eye discomfort, pain, pruritus, dry eyes, iris discoloration, keratitis, photophobia

META: Hypercholesterolemia

MISC: Back pain, arthritis

Contraindications: Hypersensitivity to this drug or benzalkonium chloride, pregnancy

Precautions: May cause changes in pigmented tissues (iris, eyelid),

T

and growth of eyelashes (length, thickness, color); do not administer with contact lens in place; renal or hepatic impairment, pregnancy category C, lactation, pediatric use, macular edema

Pharmacokinetics:

TOP: Absorbed through cornea, peak plasma levels 30 min, free acid in cornea, free acid is further metabolized to inactive metabolite, rapid elimination

Drug interactions of concern to dentistry:

• None reported

DENTAL CONSIDERATIONS

General:

• Monitor vital signs at every appointment because of cardiovascular and respiratory side effects and question patient about occurrence of CV side effects.

• Avoid drugs with anticholinergic activity, such as antihistamines, opioids, benzodiazepines, propantheline, atropine, and scopolomine.

• Protect patient's eyes from accidental spatter during dental treatment.

• Avoid dental light in patient's eyes; offer dark glasses for patient comfort.

Consultations:

• Medical consultation may be required to assess disease control in the patient.

Teach patient/family:

• Importance of updating health and drug history if physician makes any changes in evaluation/ drug regimens

trazodone HCl

(traz'oh-done)

Desyrel

Drug class.: Antidepressant

Action: Selectively inhibits serotonin-specific reuptake in the brain

Uses: Depression; unapproved use: chronic pain, diabetes-associated painful neuropathy, burning mouth syndrome

Dosage and routes:

• *Adult:* PO 150 mg/day in divided doses; may be increased by 50 mg/day q3-4d, not to exceed 600 mg/day

Available forms include: Tabs 50, 100, 150, 300 mg

Side effects/adverse reactions:

ORAL: Dry mouth, stomatitis

CNS: Dizziness, drowsiness, confusion, headache, anxiety, tremors, stimulation, weakness, insomnia, nightmares, EPS (elderly), increase in psychiatric symptoms

CV: Orthostatic hypotension, ECG changes, tachycardia, ***hypertension,*** palpitations

GI: Diarrhea, ***paralytic ileus, hepatitis,*** increased appetite, nausea, vomiting, cramps, epigastric distress, jaundice

HEMA: ***Agranulocytosis, thrombocytopenia, eosinophilia, leukopenia***

GU: Retention, ***acute renal failure, priapism***

EENT: Blurred vision, tinnitus, mydriasis

INTEG: Rash, urticaria, sweating, pruritus, photosensitivity

Contraindications: Hypersensitivity to tricyclic antidepressants, recovery phase of myocardial infarction, convulsive disorders, prostatic hypertrophy

Precautions: Suicidal patients, severe depression, increased intraocular pressure, narrow-angle glaucoma, urinary retention, cardiac disease, hepatic disease, hyperthyroidism, electroshock therapy, elective surgery, pregnancy category C

Pharmacokinetics:

PO: Half-life 4.4-7.5 hr; metabolized by liver; excreted by kidneys, feces

Drug interactions of concern to dentistry:

- Increased anticholinergic effects: anticholinergic drugs
- Increased CNS depression: alcohol, all other CNS depressants

DENTAL CONSIDERATIONS

General:

- Monitor vital signs at every appointment because of cardiovascular side effects.
- Patients on chronic drug therapy may rarely have symptoms of blood dyscrasias, which can include infection, bleeding, and poor healing.
- Assess salivary flow as a factor in caries, periodontal disease, and candidiasis.
- After supine positioning, have patient sit upright for at least 2 min before standing to avoid orthostatic hypotension.

Consultations:

- In a patient with symptoms of blood dyscrasias, request a medical consultation for blood studies and postpone dental treatment until normal values are reestablished.
- Medical consultation may be required to assess disease control in the patient.
- Physician should be informed if significant xerostomic side effects occur (e.g., increased caries, sore tongue, problems eating or swallowing, difficulty wearing prosthesis) so that a medication change can be considered.

Teach patient/family:

- To report oral lesions, soreness, or bleeding to dentist

When chronic dry mouth occurs, advise patient:

- To avoid mouth rinses with high alcohol content because of drying effects
- Of need for daily home fluoride use to prevent caries
- To use sugarless gum, frequent sips of water, or saliva substitutes

tretinoin (vitamin A acid, retinoic acid)

(tre'ti-noyn)

Avita, Altinac, Retin-A, , Retin-A Micro, Renova

Stieva-A

Drug class.: Vitamin A acid

Action: Decreases cohesiveness of follicular epithelium, decreases microcomedone formation

Uses: Acne vulgaris, reducing fine facial wrinkles associated with sun exposure and aging; unlabeled uses: skin cancer, lichen planus (Renova: not for use in acne)

Dosage and routes:

- *Adult and child:* Topical; cleanse area, apply hs, cover lightly

Available forms include: TOP cream 0.025, 0.02%, 0.1%, 0.05%; gel 0.025%, 0.01%,0.04, 0.1%; liq 0.05%

Side effects/adverse reactions:

INTEG: Rash, stinging, warmth, redness, erythema, blistering,

T

crusting, peeling, contact dermatitis, hypopigmentation, hyperpigmentation

Contraindications: Hypersensitivity

Precautions: Pregnancy category C, lactation, eczema, sunburn

Pharmacokinetics:

TOP: Poor absorption, excreted in urine

Drug interactions of concern to dentistry:

- Increased peeling: medication-containing agents such as alcohol or astringents
- Avoid concurrent use with photosensitizing drugs: tetracycline, fluoroquinolones, sulfonamides

DENTAL CONSIDERATIONS

General:

- May cause dry, peeling skin if used around lips; provide lip lubricant for patient comfort during dental treatment.
- Advise patient if dental drugs prescribed have a potential for photosensitivity.

Teach patient/family:

- To avoid application on normal skin or getting cream in eyes, mouth, or other mucous membranes

triamcinolone acetonide

(trye-am-sin'oh-lone)

Azmacort Oral Inhaler

Drug class.: Glucocorticoid, intermediate acting

Action: Glucocorticoids have multiple actions that include antiinflammatory and immunosuppressant effects. They inhibit phospholipase A_2, interfering with or reducing the synthesis of prostaglandins and leukotrienes. They also bind to cytoplasmic GRs and enter the cell nucleus to bind with DNA. This results in the synthesis of various enzymes such as collagenase, elastase, and cytokines that play important roles in inflammation and immunosuppression. They also suppress the production of lymphocytes, monocytes, and eosinophils.

Uses: Maintenance treatment of chronic asthma

Dosage and routes:

- *Adult:* Oral inh 2 inhalations tid or qid or 4 inhalations bid
- *Child 6-12 yr:* Oral inh 1 or 2 inhalations tid or qid or 2-4 inhalations bid; max 12 inh/day

Available forms include: Oral inh 20 g inhaler 100 μg per actuation/240 metered dose container

Side effects/adverse reactions:

▼ *ORAL: Candidiasis*

EENT: Dry throat, hoarseness, irritation

Contraindications: Acute asthma, status asthmaticus, nonasthmatic bronchitis, hypersensitivity

Precautions: TB; untreated fungal, bacterial, or viral infections of respiratory tract; pregnancy category C, lactation, children <6 yr; different doses may be required for patients on systemic glucocorticoids or patients with chickenpox, measles; transfer from systemic glucocorticoid therapy to inhalation must be done cautiously to avoid adrenal insufficiency response

Pharmacokinetics:

INH ORAL: Little systemic absorption from lungs, hepatic metabolism

Drug interactions of concern to dentistry:

- None reported

DENTAL CONSIDERATIONS

General:

- Place on frequent recall because of oral side effects.
- Evaluate respiration characteristics, rate.
- Midday appointments and a stress reduction protocol may be required for anxious patients.
- Acute asthmatic episodes may be precipitated in the dental office. Rapid-acting sympathomimetic inhalants should be available for emergency use. Triamcinolone is not a rapid-acting drug and is not intended for use in acute asthmatic attacks.
- Be aware that aspirin or sulfite preservatives in vasoconstrictor-containing products can exacerbate asthma.
- Examine for oral manifestation of opportunistic infection.

Consultations:

- Medical consultation may be required to assess disease control in the patient.

Teach patient/family:

- Importance of good oral hygiene to prevent soft tissue inflammation
- Importance of gargling, rinsing mouth with water, and expectorating after each aerosol dose

triamcinolone/ triamcinolone acetonide/ triamcinolone diacetate/triamcinolone hexacetonide

(trye-am-sin'oh-lone)

Triamcinolone (oral): Aristocort, Atolone, Kenacort

Triamcinolone acetonide: Kenaject-40, Kenalog-10, Kenalog-40, Tac-3, Tac-40, Triam-A, Triamonide 40, Tri-Kort, Trilog

Triamcinolone diacetate (not for IV use): Amcort, Aristocort Forte, Clinacort, Triam Forte, Tristoject, Trilone

Triamcinolone diacetate syrup: Aristospan, Kenacort

Triamcinolone hexacetonide (not for IV use): Aristospan Intraarticular, Aristospan Intralesional

Drug class.: Glucocorticoid, intermediate acting

Action: Glucocorticoids have multiple actions that include antiinflammatory and immunosuppressant effects. They inhibit phospholipase A_2, interfering with or reducing the synthesis of prostaglandins and leukotrienes. They also bind to cytoplasmic GRs and enter the cell nucleus to bind with DNA. This results in the synthesis of various enzymes such as collagenase, elastase, and cytokines that play important roles in inflammation and immunosuppression. They also suppress the production of lymphocytes, monocytes, and eosinophils.

Uses: Severe inflammation; immunosuppression; neoplasms; asthma (steroid dependent); collagen, re-

T

spiratory, dermatologic disorders; seasonal and perennial allergic rhinitis

Dosage and routes:

- *Adult:* PO dose depends on disease to be treated with a range of 4-60 mg per day as a single dose or divided dose
- *Child:* PO dose depends on disease to be treated; suggested dose is 1.7 mg/kg as a single dose or divided dose

Parenteral doses:

- *Adult:* Triamcinolone acetonide—IM, 40-80 mg at 4 wk intervals; intraarticular, 2.5-15 mg; intralesional, up to 1 mg per injection site; triamcinolone diacetate—IM, 40 mg once weekly; intraarticular, intralesional, or soft tissue 3-48 mg repeated at 1-8 wk intervals; triamcinolone hexacetonide—intraarticular, 2-20 mg at 3-4 wk intervals; intralesional up to 0.5 mg per square inch of skin, repeat as needed

Available forms include: Tabs 4, 8 mg; syr 4 mg/5 ml; inj 25, 40 mg/ml diacetate; inj 3, 10, 40 mg/ml acetonide; inj 20, 5 mg/ml hexacetonide

Side effects/adverse reactions:

▼ *ORAL: Candidiasis,* poor wound healing, petechiae, dry mouth

CNS: Depression, flushing, sweating, headache, mood changes

CV: Hypertension, circulatory collapse, thrombophlebitis, embolism, tachycardia, edema

GI: Diarrhea, nausea, abdominal distention, ***GI hemorrhage, pancreatitis,*** increased appetite

HEMA: ***Thrombocytopenia***

EENT: Fungal infections, increased intraocular pressure, blurred vision

INTEG: Acne, poor wound healing, ecchymosis, petechiae

MS: Fractures, osteoporosis, weakness

Contraindications: Psychosis, hypersensitivity, idiopathic thrombocytopenia, acute glomerulonephritis, amebiasis, fungal and viral infections, nonasthmatic bronchial disease, child <2 yr, AIDS, TB

Precautions: Pregnancy category D, diabetes mellitus, glaucoma, osteoporosis, seizure disorders, ulcerative colitis, CHF, myasthenia gravis, renal disease, esophagitis, peptic ulcer, herpetic infections, rifampin

Pharmacokinetics:

PO/IM: Peak 1-2 hr, 2 days, 1-6 wk (IM), half-life 2-5 hr

Drug interactions of concern to dentistry:

- Decreased action: barbiturates, rifampin, rifabutin
- Increased GI side effects: alcohol, salicylates, NSAIDs
- Increased action: ketoconazole, macrolide antibiotics

DENTAL CONSIDERATIONS

General:

- Symptoms of oral infections may be masked.
- Examine for oral manifestation of opportunistic infections.
- Oral side effects may be more common with inhalation products; significant steroid side effects are more likely to occur with chronic systemic doses.
- Acute asthmatic episodes may be precipitated in the dental office. Rapid-acting sympathomimetic inhalants should be available for emergency use. A stress reduction protocol may be required.

• Monitor vital signs at every appointment because of cardiovascular side effects.
• Assess salivary flow as a factor in caries, periodontal disease, and candidiasis.
• Prophylactic antibiotics may be indicated to prevent infection.
• Place on frequent recall to monitor healing response.
• Determine dose and duration of steroid therapy for each patient to assess risk for stress tolerance and immunosuppression.
• Be aware that aspirin or sulfite preservatives in vasoconstrictor-containing products can exacerbate asthma.
• Patients who have been or are currently on chronic steroid therapy (>2 wk) may require supplemental steroids for dental treatment.

Consultations:

• Medical consultation may be required to assess disease control in the patient.
• Consultation may be required to confirm steroid dose and duration of use.

Teach patient/family:

• Importance of good oral hygiene to prevent soft tissue inflammation
• To report oral lesions, soreness, or bleeding to dentist

When chronic dry mouth occurs, advise patient:

• To avoid mouth rinses with high alcohol content because of drying effects
• To use daily home fluoride products for anticaries effect
• To use sugarless gum, frequent sips of water, or saliva substitutes

triamcinolone acetonide (topical)

(trye-am-sin'oh-lone)

Aristocort, Aristicort A, Delta-Tritex, Flutex, Kenalog, Kenalog-H, Kenonel, Triacet, Tri-derm

Dental products: Kenalog in Orabase, Oralone Dental

Drug class.: Topical corticosteroid, synthetic fluorinated agent, group II potency (0.5%), group III potency (0.1%), group IV potency (0.025%)

Action: Interacts with steroid cytoplasmic receptors to induce antiinflammatory effects; possesses antipruritic, antiinflammatory actions

Uses: Psoriasis, eczema, contact dermatitis, pruritus; topical dental paste used to treat nonviral inflammatory oral lesions, including aphthous stomatitis, lichen planus, and cicatricial pemphigoid

Dosage and routes:

• *Adult and child:* Apply to affected area bid-qid

Available forms include: Oint 0.025%, 0.1%, 0.5%; cream 0.025%, 0.1%, 0.5%; lotion 0.025%, 0.1%; aerosol 0.2 mg/2 sec; paste 0.1%, 0.5%

Side effects/adverse reactions:

▼ *ORAL:* Mucosal thinning and petechial hemorrhage (rare), stinging sensation (oral application)

INTEG: Burning, dryness, itching, irritation, acne, folliculitis, hypertrichosis, perioral dermatitis, hypopigmentation, atrophy, striae, allergic contact dermatitis, secondary infection

Contraindications: Hypersensi-

T

tivity to corticosteroids, fungal or viral (herpetic) infections

Precautions: Pregnancy category C, lactation, viral infections, bacterial infections, diabetes mellitus, TB

DENTAL CONSIDERATIONS

General:

• Apply approximately 0.25 inch; measure with cotton-tipped applicator; press on lesion, do not rub. Use after brushing and eating and at bedtime for optimal effect.

• When used for oral lesions, return for oral evaluation if response of oral tissues has not occurred in 7-14 days.

Teach patient/family:

• To avoid sunlight on affected area; burns may occur

• Not to use on herpetic lesions

triamterene

(trye-am'ter-een)

Dyrenium

Drug class.: Potassium-sparing diuretic

Action: Acts on distal tubule to inhibit reabsorption of sodium and chloride; increases potassium retention

Uses: Edema; hypertension; more commonly used in combination with a thiazide diuretic

Dosage and routes:

• *Adult:* PO 100 mg bid pc, not to exceed 300 mg

Available forms include: Cap 50, 100 mg

Side effects/adverse reactions:

▼ *ORAL:* Dry mouth

CNS: Confusion, nervousness, numbness in hands or feet, weakness, headache, dizziness

GI: Nausea, diarrhea, vomiting, jaundice, liver disease

HEMA: ***Thrombocytopenia, megaloblastic anemia,*** low folic acid levels

GU: ***Azotemia, interstitial nephritis,*** increased BUN, creatinine, renal stones

INTEG: Photosensitivity, rash

ELECT: Hyperkalemia, hyponatremia, hypochloremia

Contraindications: Hypersensitivity, anuria, severe renal disease, severe hepatic disease, hyperkalemia, pregnancy category D

Precautions: Dehydration, hepatic disease, lactation, CHF, renal disease, cirrhosis

Pharmacokinetics:

PO: Onset 2 hr, peak 6-8 hr, duration 12-16 hr, half-life 3 hr; metabolized in liver; excreted in bile, urine

Drug interactions of concern to dentistry:

• Nephrotoxicity: possible risk with indomethacin, NSAIDs

• Decreased antihypertensive effect: possible risk with NSAIDs, indomethacin

• Decreased effect of folic acid

DENTAL CONSIDERATIONS

General:

• Limit use of sodium-containing products, such as saline IV fluids, for those patients with a dietary salt restriction.

• Assess salivary flow as a factor in caries, periodontal disease, and candidiasis.

• Monitor vital signs at every appointment because of cardiovascular effects and possible hyperkalemia.

• Patients on chronic drug therapy may rarely have symptoms of

blood dyscrasias, which can include infection, bleeding, and poor healing.

Consultations:

• In a patient with symptoms of blood dyscrasias, request a medical consultation for blood studies and postpone dental treatment until normal values are reestablished.

• Medical consultation may be required to assess disease control in the patient.

Teach patient/family:

• Importance of good oral hygiene to prevent soft tissue inflammation

• Caution to prevent injury when using oral hygiene aids

• To report oral lesions, soreness, or bleeding to dentist

When chronic dry mouth occurs, advise patient:

• To avoid mouth rinses with high alcohol content because of drying effects

• Of need for daily home fluoride use to prevent caries

• To use sugarless gum, frequent sips of water, or saliva substitutes

---

triazolam

(trye-ay'zoe-lam)

Halcion

♣ Apo-Triazo, Gen-Triazolam, Novo-Triolam

Drug class.: Benzodiazepine, sedative-hypnotic

Controlled Substance Schedule IV, Canada F

Action: Produces CNS depression by interacting with a benzodiazepine receptor to facilitate the action of the inhibitory neurotransmitter γ-aminobutyric acid (GABA)

Uses: Insomnia; unlabeled use: oral sedation of anxious dental patients

Dosage and routes:

• *Adult:* PO 0.125-0.5 mg hs

• *Elderly:* PO 0.125-0.25 mg hs

Available forms include: Tabs 0.125, 0.25 mg

Side effects/adverse reactions:

▼ *ORAL:* Dry mouth

CNS: Headache, lethargy, drowsiness, daytime sedation, dizziness, confusion, light-headedness, anxiety, irritability, amnesia, poor coordination

CV: Chest pain, pulse changes

GI: Nausea, vomiting, diarrhea, heartburn, abdominal pain, constipation

HEMA: ***Leukopenia, granulocytopenia*** (rare)

Contraindications: Hypersensitivity to benzodiazepines, pregnancy category X, lactation, intermittent porphyria, ketoconazole, itraconazole, nefazodone, ritonavir, indinavir, nelfinavir

Precautions: Anemia, hepatic disease, renal disease, suicidal individuals, drug abuse, elderly, psychosis, child <15 yr, acute narrow-angle glaucoma, seizure disorders

Pharmacokinetics:

PO: Onset 30-45 min, duration 6-8 hr, half-life 2-3 hr; metabolized by liver (CYP3A4 isoenzymes); excreted by kidneys (inactive metabolites); crosses placenta; excreted in breast milk

Drug interactions of concern to dentistry:

• Increased effects: erythromycin, clarithromycin

• Increased sedation: alcohol, CNS depressants, opioid analgesics, diltiazem, anesthetics

• Avoid use with ketoconazole, itraconazole, ritonavir, indinavir, nelfinavir
• Caution if used with fluvoxamine, reduce dose by 50%
• Caution when used with drugs that are strong inhibitors of CYP3A4 isoenzymes (see Appendix I)

DENTAL CONSIDERATIONS
General:
• Assess salivary flow as a factor in caries, periodontal disease, and candidiasis.
• If dizziness occurs, provide assistance when escorting patient to and from dental chair.
• When used for conscious sedation, have someone drive patient to and from dental office.
• Avoid the use of this drug in a patient with a history of drug abuse or alcoholism.
• Geriatric patients are more susceptible to drug effects; use a lower dose.
• Psychologic and physical dependence may occur with chronic administration.
• Determine why the patient is taking the drug.
• Patients on chronic drug therapy may rarely have symptoms of blood dyscrasias, which can include infection, bleeding, and poor healing.

Teach patient/family:
When chronic dry mouth occurs, advise patient:
• To avoid mouth rinses with high alcohol content because of drying effects
• Of need for daily home fluoride use to prevent caries
• To use sugarless gum, frequent sips of water, or saliva substitutes

---

trifluoperazine HCl

(trye-floo-oh-per′a-zeen)
Generic
♣ Apo-Trifluoperazine, Novo-Flurazine

Drug class.: Phenothiazine antipsychotic

Action: Blocks neurotransmission at dopaminergic synapses in the cerebral cortex, hypothalamus, and limbic system; exhibits strong peripheral α-adrenergic, anticholinergic blocking action; mechanism for antipsychotic effects is unclear

Uses: Psychotic disorders, nonpsychotic anxiety, schizophrenia

Dosage and routes:
Psychotic disorders:
• *Adult:* PO 2-5 mg bid, usual range 15-20 mg/day, may require 40 mg/day or more; IM 1-2 mg q4-6h
• *Child >6 yr:* PO 1 mg qd or bid; IM not recommended for children, but 1 mg may be given qd or bid

Nonpsychotic anxiety:
• *Adult:* PO 1-2 mg bid, not to exceed 5 mg/day; do not give longer than 12 wk

Available forms include: Tabs 1, 2, 5, 10 mg

Side effects/adverse reactions:
▼ *ORAL: Dry mouth*
CNS: Extrapyramidal symptoms: pseudoparkinsonism, akathisia, dystonia, tardive dyskinesia, seizures, headache, lichenoid reaction
CV: Orthostatic hypotension, hypertension, ***cardiac arrest,*** ECG changes, ***tachycardia***
GI: Nausea, vomiting, anorexia, constipation, diarrhea, jaundice, weight gain

RESP: ***Laryngospasm,*** dyspnea, ***respiratory depression***
HEMA: Anemia, ***leukopenia, leukocytosis, agranulocytosis***
GU: Urinary retention, enuresis, impotence, amenorrhea, gynecomastia
EENT: Blurred vision, glaucoma, dry eyes
INTEG: Rash, photosensitivity, dermatitis

Contraindications: Hypersensitivity, cardiovascular disease, coma, blood dyscrasias, severe hepatic disease, child <6 yr, glaucoma

Precautions: Breast cancer, seizure disorders, pregnancy category C, lactation, diabetes mellitus, respiratory conditions, prostatic hypertrophy

Pharmacokinetics:
PO: Onset rapid, peak 2-3 hr, duration 12 hr
IM: Onset immediate, peak 1 hr, duration 12 hr
Metabolized by liver, excreted in urine, crosses placenta, excreted in breast milk

Drug interactions of concern to dentistry:
- Increased sedation: other CNS depressants, alcohol, barbiturate anesthetics, opioid analgesics
- Hypotension, tachycardia: epinephrine
- Increased extrapyramidal effects: phenothiazines and related drugs (haloperidol, droperidol), metoclopramide
- Additive photosensitization: tetracyclines
- Increased anticholinergic effects: anticholinergics

DENTAL CONSIDERATIONS
General:
- Monitor vital signs at every appointment because of cardiovascular side effects.
- Patients on chronic drug therapy may rarely have symptoms of blood dyscrasias, which can include infection, bleeding, and poor healing.
- After supine positioning, have patient sit upright for at least 2 min before standing to avoid orthostatic hypotension.
- Assess salivary flow as a factor in caries, periodontal disease, and candidiasis.
- Avoid dental light in patient's eyes; offer dark glasses for patient comfort.
- Assess for presence of extrapyramidal motor symptoms, such as tardive dyskinesia and akathisia. Extrapyramidal motor activity may complicate dental treatment.
- Geriatric patients are more susceptible to drug effects; use lower dose.
- Use vasoconstrictors with caution, in low doses, and with careful aspiration.

Consultations:
- In a patient with symptoms of blood dyscrasias, request a medical consultation for blood studies and postpone dental treatment until normal values are reestablished.
- Take precautions if dental surgery is anticipated and anesthesia is required.
- Physician should be informed if significant xerostomic side effects occur (e.g., increased caries, sore tongue, problems eating or swal-

T

lowing, difficulty wearing prosthesis) so that a medication change can be considered.

- If signs of tardive dyskinesia or akathisia are present, refer to physician.

Teach patient/family:

- Importance of good oral hygiene to prevent soft tissue inflammation
- Caution to prevent injury when using oral hygiene aids
- To use electric toothbrush if patient has difficulty holding conventional devices

When chronic dry mouth occurs, advise patient:

- To use daily home fluoride products for anticaries effect
- To avoid mouth rinses with high alcohol content because of drying effects
- To use sugarless gum, frequent sips of water, or saliva substitutes

trifluridine (ophthalmic)

(trye-flure'i-deen)

Viroptic Ophthalmic Solution

Drug class.: Antiviral

Action: Inhibits viral DNA synthesis and replication

Uses: Primary keratoconjunctivitis, recurring epithelial keratitis, keratitis associated with herpes simplex virus types 1 and 2, and vicciniavirus

Dosage and routes:

- *Adult and child >6 yr:* Instill 1 drop q2h while awake, not to exceed 9 drops/day, until corneal epithelium is regrown; then 1 drop q4h × 1 wk

Available forms include: Sol 1% in 7.5 ml container

Side effects/adverse reactions:

EENT: Burning, stinging, swelling, photophobia

Contraindications: Hypersensitivity

Precautions: Antibiotic hypersensitivity, pregnancy category C

Drug interactions of concern to dentistry:

- None reported

DENTAL CONSIDERATIONS

General:

- Protect patient's eyes from accidental spatter during dental treatment.
- Avoid dental light in patient's eyes; offer dark glasses for patient comfort.

Evaluate:

- Therapeutic response: absence of redness, inflammation, tearing
- Allergy: itching, lacrimation, redness, swelling

trihexyphenidyl HCl

(trye-hex-ee-fen'i-dil)

Artane, Trihexy-2, TriHexy-5

♣ Apo-Trihex, PMS-Trihexyphenidyl

Drug class.: Antiparkinsonian, anticholinergic

Action: Blocks central muscarinic receptors, which decreases the severity of involuntary movements

Uses: Parkinson symptoms

Dosage and routes:

Parkinson symptoms

- *Adult:* PO 1 mg, increased by 2 mg q3-5d to a total of 6-10 mg/day

Drug-induced extrapyramidal symptoms:

- *Adult:* PO 1 mg/day; usual dose 5-15 mg/day

Available forms include: Tabs 2, 5 mg; sus rel caps 5 mg; elix 2 mg/5 ml

Side effects/adverse reactions:

▼ *ORAL: Dry mouth,* soreness of mouth or tongue

CNS: Confusion, anxiety, restlessness, irritability, delusions, hallucinations, headache, sedation, depression, incoherence, dizziness, flushing, weakness

CV: Palpitation, tachycardia, postural hypotension

GI: Constipation, ***paralytic ileus,*** nausea, vomiting, abdominal distress

GU: Hesitancy, retention

EENT: Blurred vision, photophobia, dilated pupils, difficulty swallowing

INTEG: Urticaria, rash

MS: Weakness, cramping

MISC: Suppression of lactation, nasal congestion, decreased sweating, increased temperature

Contraindications: Hypersensitivity, narrow-angle glaucoma, myasthenia gravis, GI/GU obstruction, tachycardia, myocardial ischemia, unstable CV disease

Precautions: Pregnancy category C, children, gastric ulcer

Pharmacokinetics:

PO: Onset 1 hr, peak 2-3 hr, duration 6-12 hr; excreted in urine

Drug interactions of concern to dentistry:

- Increased anticholinergic effects: scopolamine, atropine, phenothiazines, antihistamines, and other anticholinergics
- Increased CNS depression: alcohol, CNS depressants
- Decreased effects of phenothiazines

DENTAL CONSIDERATIONS

General:

- Assess salivary flow as a factor in caries, periodontal disease, and candidiasis.
- Place on frequent recall because of oral side effects.
- After supine positioning, have patient sit upright for at least 2 min before standing to avoid orthostatic hypotension.
- Avoid dental light in patient's eyes; offer dark glasses for patient comfort.

Teach patient/family:

- Importance of good oral hygiene to prevent soft tissue inflammation
- To use electric toothbrush if patient has difficulty holding conventional devices

When chronic dry mouth occurs, advise patient:

- To avoid mouth rinses with high alcohol content because of drying effects
- Of need for daily home fluoride use to prevent caries
- To use sugarless gum, frequent sips of water, or saliva substitutes

trimethadione

(trye-meth-a-dye'one)

Tridione:

Drug class.: Anticonvulsant

Action: Increases the threshold for seizures initiated in the cortex, decreases CNS synaptic stimulation to low-frequency impulses

Uses: Refractory absence (petit mal) seizures

Dosage and routes:

- *Adult:* PO 300-600 mg tid; may increase by 300 mg/wk
- *Child >6 yr:* PO 0.9 g/day in divided doses tid or qid

T

• *Child 2-6 yr:* PO 0.6 g/day in divided doses tid or qid
• *Child <2 yr:* PO 0.3 g/day in divided doses tid or qid

Available forms include: Caps 300 mg; chew tabs 150 mg

Side effects/adverse reactions:

▼ *ORAL: Bleeding gums*

CNS: Drowsiness, dizziness, fatigue, paresthesia, irritability, headache, insomnia, myasthenia gravis syndrome

CV: Hypertension, hypotension

GI: Nausea, vomiting, abnormal liver function tests

HEMA: ***Thrombocytopenia, agranulocytosis, leukopenia, neutropenia, hemolytic anemia, eosinophilia, aplastic anemia,*** increased pro-time

GU: ***Fatal nephrosis,*** vaginal bleeding, albuminuria, nephrosis, abdominal pain, weight loss

EENT: Photophobia, diplopia, epistaxis, retinal hemorrhage, scotomata, hemeralopia

INTEG: ***Exfoliative dermatitis,*** rash, alopecia, petechiae, erythema

Contraindications: Hypersensitivity, blood dyscrasias, pregnancy category D

Precautions: Hepatic disease, renal disease, retinal disease, porphyria, lactation, systemic lupus erythematosus

Pharmacokinetics:

PO: Peak 30 min–2 hr, half-life 10 days; excreted by kidneys

Drug interactions of concern to dentistry:

• Increased CNS depression: all CNS depressants

DENTAL CONSIDERATIONS

General:

• Short appointments and a stress reduction protocol may be required for anxious patients.
• Determine type of epilepsy, seizure frequency, and quality of seizure control. A stress reduction protocol may be required.
• Patients on chronic drug therapy may rarely have symptoms of blood dyscrasias, which can include infection, bleeding, and poor healing.
• Avoid dental light in patient's eyes; offer dark glasses for patient comfort.
• Place on frequent recall because of oral side effects.
• Monitor vital signs at every appointment because of cardiovascular side effects.

Consultations:

• Obtain a medical consultation for blood studies (CBC) because leukopenic and thrombocytopenic effects of drug may result in infection, delayed healing, and excessive bleeding. Dental treatment should be postponed until normal values are maintained.
• Medical consultation may be required to assess disease control and patient's ability to tolerate stress.

Teach patient/family:

• Importance of good oral hygiene to prevent soft tissue inflammation
• To prevent trauma when using oral hygiene aids

trimethobenzamide

(trye-meth-oh-ben′za-mide)

Pediatric Triban, Tigan, T-Gen

Drug class.: Antiemetic

Action: Acts centrally by blocking chemoreceptor trigger zone, which in turn acts on vomiting center

Uses: Nausea, vomiting

Dosage and routes:
Nausea/vomiting:
• *Adult:* PO 250 mg tid-qid; IM/rec 200 mg tid-qid
Children 30-90 lb:
PO or rectal 100 mg to 200 mg tid or qid
Available forms include: Caps 100, 250 mg; supp 100, 200 mg; inj IM 100 mg/ml
Side effects/adverse reactions:
▼ *ORAL:* Dry mouth
CNS: Drowsiness, restlessness, headache, dizziness, insomnia, confusion, nervousness, tingling, *vertigo,* extrapyramidal symptoms
CV: Hypertension, hypotension, palpitation
GI: Nausea, anorexia, diarrhea, vomiting, constipation
EENT: Blurred vision, diplopia, nasal congestion, photosensitivity
INTEG: Rash, urticaria, fever, chills, flushing
Contraindications: Hypersensitivity, shock, children (parenterally)
Precautions: Children, cardiac dysrhythmias, elderly, asthma, pregnancy category C, prostatic hypertrophy, bladder neck obstruction, narrow-angle glaucoma, stenosing peptic ulcer, pyloroduodenal obstruction
Pharmacokinetics:
PO: Onset 20-40 min, duration 34 hr
IM: Onset 15 min, duration 2-3 hr
Metabolized by liver, excreted by kidneys
Drug interactions of concern to dentistry:
• Increased effect: CNS depressants
• May mask ototoxic symptoms associated with antibiotics or large doses of salicylates

DENTAL CONSIDERATIONS
General:
• Nausea and vomiting may be accompanied by dehydration and electrolyte imbalance and should be corrected as part of treatment.
• Defer elective dental treatment when symptoms are present.

trimetrexate glucuronate
(tri-me-trex'ate)
Neutrexin
Drug class.: Folate antagonist

Action: Inhibits the enzyme dihydrofolate reductase, which leads to interference with DNA, RNA, and protein synthesis in the *P. carinii* organism
Uses: Alternative therapy for *P. carinii* pneumonia in immunocompromised patients, including patients with AIDS; unapproved uses: lung, prostate, colon cancer
Dosage and routes:
Must be given concurrently with leucovorin:
• *Adult:* IV infusion 45 mg/m^2 once daily over 60-90 min; leucovorin is given IV 20 mg/m^2 over 5-10 min q6h for total dose of 80 mg/m^2; course of treatment is 21 days with trimetrexate and 24 days with leucovorin
Available forms include: IV 25 mg/5 ml vials with or without 50 mg leucovorin
Side effects/adverse reactions:
▼ *ORAL:* Oral ulceration if leucovorin is not used
GI: Nausea, vomiting, ***hepatotoxicity,*** mucosal ulceration
HEMA: Thrombocytopenia (<75,000/mm^3), anemia (Hgb <8 g/dl)

GU: Renal toxicity
INTEG: Rash, pruritus
MISC: Hyponatremia, hypocalcemia
Contraindications: Hypersensitivity to trimetrexate, methotrexate, or leucovorin
Precautions: Pregnancy category D, lactation, child <18 yr; impaired hematologic, renal, or hepatic function; serious bone marrow depression can occur if leucovorin is not used concurrently
Pharmacokinetics:
IV: Extended plasma levels up to 72 hr; highly plasma protein bound 95%-98%; hepatic metabolism (CYP450 isoenzymes); renal excretion
Drug interactions of concern to dentistry:
• Alteration of plasma levels: concurrent use with erythromycin, ketoconazole, and fluconazole
• Alteration in trimetrexate metabolites: acetaminophen
• Caution with use of drugs that are strong inhibitors of CYP3A4 isoenzymes (see Appendix I)
DENTAL CONSIDERATIONS
General:
• Examine for evidence of oral manifestations of blood dyscrasia (infection, bleeding, poor healing).
• Place on frequent recall because of oral side effects.
• Determine why the patient is taking the drug.
• Examine for oral manifestations of opportunistic infections.
• Consider local hemostasis measures to prevent excessive bleeding.
• Palliative treatment may be required for stomatitis.
• Refer to physician if oral ulcerative lesions occur.
• Consider semisupine chair position for patient comfort because of GI effects of disease.
Consultations:
• Obtain a medical consultation for blood studies (CBC) because leukopenic or thrombocytopenic side effects may result in infection, delayed healing, and excessive bleeding. Postpone elective dental treatment until normal values are maintained.
• Medical consultation may be required to assess disease control in the patient.
Teach patient/family:
• Importance of good oral hygiene to prevent soft tissue inflammation
• Caution to prevent injury when using oral hygiene aids
• That secondary oral infection may occur; must see dentist immediately if infection occurs

---

trimipramine maleate

(tri-mi'pra-meen)
Surmontil
Apo-Trimip, Novo-Trimipramine, Rhotrimine
Drug class.: Antidepressant–tricyclic

Action: Inhibits both norepinephrine and serotonin (5-HT) uptake in the brain, although the precise antidepressant mechanism remains unclear
Uses: Depression
Dosage and routes:
• *Adult:* PO 75 mg/day in divided doses; may be increased to 200 mg/day
• *Elderly and adolescent:* PO initial 50 mg/day; may be gradually increased to 100 mg/day

Available forms include: Caps 25, 50, 100 mg

Side effects/adverse reactions:

▼ *ORAL: Dry mouth,* unpleasant taste

CNS: Dizziness, drowsiness, confusion, headache, anxiety, tremors, stimulation, weakness, insomnia, nightmares, EPS (elderly), increase in psychiatric symptoms

CV: Orthostatic hypotension, ECG changes, tachycardia, ***hypertension,*** palpitation

GI: Diarrhea, ***paralytic ileus, hepatitis,*** increased appetite, nausea, vomiting, cramps, epigastric distress, jaundice

HEMA: ***Agranulocytosis, thrombocytopenia, eosinophilia, leukopenia***

GU: Retention, ***acute renal failure***

EENT: Blurred vision, tinnitus, mydriasis

INTEG: Rash, urticaria, sweating, pruritus, photosensitivity

Contraindications: Hypersensitivity to tricyclic antidepressants, recovery phase of MI, convulsive disorders, prostatic hypertrophy

Precautions: Suicidal patients, severe depression, increased intraocular pressure, narrow-angle glaucoma, urinary retention, cardiac disease, hepatic disease, hyperthyroidism, electroshock therapy, elective surgery, pregnancy category C, MAOIs

Pharmacokinetics:

PO: Steady state 2-6 days, half-life 7-30 hr; metabolized by liver; excreted by kidneys

Drug interactions of concern to dentistry:

• Increased anticholinergic effects: muscarinic blockers, antihistamines, phenothiazines

• Increased effects of direct-acting sympathomimetics (epinephrine, levonordefrin)

• Possible risk of increased CNS depression: alcohol, barbiturates, benzodiazepines, and other CNS depressants

• Decreased antihypertensive effects: clonidine, guamadrel, guanethidine

DENTAL CONSIDERATIONS

General:

• Monitor vital signs at every appointment because of cardiovascular side effects.

• Assess salivary flow as a factor in caries, periodontal disease, and candidiasis.

• Patients on chronic drug therapy may rarely have symptoms of blood dyscrasias, which can include infection, bleeding, and poor healing.

• After supine positioning, have patient sit upright for at least 2 min to avoid orthostatic hypotension.

• Use vasoconstrictors with caution, in low doses, and with careful aspiration. Avoid use of gingival retraction cord with epinephrine.

• Place on frequent recall because of oral side effects.

Consultations:

• In a patient with symptoms of blood dyscrasias, request a medical consultation for blood studies and postpone dental treatment until normal values are reestablished.

• Medical consultation may be required to assess disease control in the patient.

• Physician should be informed if significant xerostomic side effects occur (e.g., increased caries, sore tongue, problems eating or swallowing, difficulty wearing prosthesis) so that a medication change can be considered.

Teach patient/family:
- Importance of good oral hygiene to prevent soft tissue inflammation
- Caution to prevent injury when using oral hygiene aids

When chronic dry mouth occurs, advise patient:
- To avoid mouth rinses with high alcohol content because of drying effects
- Of need for daily home fluoride use to prevent caries
- To use sugarless gum, frequent sips of water, or saliva substitutes

---

trovafloxacin mesylate/ alatrofloxacin mesylate

(troe'va-flox-a-sin)/(ala-troe'flox-a-sin)

Trovafloxacin mesylate oral: Trovan

Alatrofloxacin mesylate injection: Trovan I.V.

Drug class.: A fluoronaphthyridone antiinfective (related to the fluoroquinolones)

Action: A broad-spectrum bactericidal agent that inhibits the enzymes topoisomerase II (DNA gyrase) and topoisomerase IV required for bacterial DNA replication, transcription repair, and recombination

Uses: For infections caused by susceptible microorganisms in nosocomial pneumonia, community-acquired pneumonia, acute bacterial exacerbated chronic bronchitis, acute sinusitis, abdominal infections, gynecologic infections, UTI, bacterial prostatitis, skin and skin structure infections, and selected STDs

Dosage and routes:
- *Adults >18 yr:* PO dose depends on type of infection; 200 mg daily for 1-14 days
- *Adults >18 yr:* IV dose depends on type of infection; range 300 mg daily; single IV doses can be followed by appropriate oral doses for 10-14 days

Available forms include: Tabs 100 and 200 mg; vials IV (alatrofloxacin for injection) 5 mg/ml in 40 and 60 ml

Side effects/adverse reactions:

▼ *ORAL:* Dry mouth, stomatitis, angular cheilitis

CNS: Dizziness, headache, lightheadedness, confusion, anxiety, hallucinations

CV: Hypotension, palpitation, flushing, peripheral edema, chest pain

GI: Vomiting, nausea, diarrhea, abdominal pain, flatulence, ***antibiotic-associated pseudomembranous colitis, hepatic toxicity***

RESP: Dyspnea, bronchospasm, coughing

HEMA: Anemia, leukopenia, thrombocytopenia

GU: Vaginitis, frequency of urination, abnormal renal function

EENT: Rhinitis, sinusitis

INTEG: Pruritus, rash, photosensitization

META: Increased liver enzymes

MS: Arthralgia, myalgia, muscle cramps

MISC: Pain on injection, increased sweating, fatigue, fever, ***anaphylaxis***

Contraindications: Hypersensitivity and allergy to the fluoroquinolones

Precautions: Children <18 yr, mild to moderate cirrhosis, potential for liver damage, exposure to sunlight, visible or ultraviolet radiation, seizure disorders, cerebral atherosclerosis, pregnancy category C, lactation, warning associated with possible serious hepatic injury leading to death or transplant

Pharmacokinetics:

PO: Good oral absorption, bioavailability 88%, can be administered with food, peak serum levels 1.7 hr, plasma protein binding 76%, wide tissue distribution, excreted in breast milk, hepatic metabolism, excretion in feces and urine, 50% of dose is excreted unchanged in feces

IV: Alatrofloxacin is a prodrug converted to trovafloxacin

Drug interactions of concern to dentistry:

• Reduction in absorption: magnesium or aluminum antacid products, iron salts, sucralfate, and morphine within 30 min of oral trovafloxacin; separate doses by at least 2 hr

• Increases serum levels of caffeine

DENTAL CONSIDERATIONS

General:

• Determine why patient is taking the drug; specific infection.

• Do not use ingestible sodium bicarbonate products, such as the air polishing system Prophy

• Jet, within 2 hr of drug use.

• Examine for oral manifestation of opportunistic infection.

• Avoid dental light in patient's eyes; offer dark glasses for patient comfort.

• Use caution in prescribing caffeine-containing analgesics.

Consultations:

• Medical consultation may be required to assess disease control in the patient.

• Consult with patient's physician if an acute dental infection occurs and another antiinfective is required.

Teach patient/family:

• To prevent trauma when using oral hygiene aids

• Importance of good oral hygiene to prevent soft tissue inflammation

• To avoid mouth rinses with high alcohol content because of drying effects

---

unoprostone isopropyl

(yoo-noe-pros'tone)

Rescula

Drug class.: Prostaglandin agonist

Action: Reduces elevated intraocular pressure by increasing the outflow of aqueous humor; the precise mechanism is unknown

Uses: Indicated for lowering IOP in patients with open-angle glaucoma or ocular hypertension who are intolerant to other medications or who failed to achieve a targeted IOP

Dosage and routes:

• *Adult:* TOP 1 gtt in affected eye(s) bid (caution with contact lens; may be inserted 15 min after applying drop)

Available forms include: Ophth sol 0.15% in 5 ml

Side effects/adverse reactions:

CNS: Dizziness, headache, insomnia

CV: Hypertension

RESP: Bronchitis, cough

EENT: Dry eyes, stinging, burning, itching, increased eyelash length, abnormal vision, lacrimation, foreign body sensation, rhinitis, sinusitis

MS: Back pain

MISC: Flulike syndrome, allergic reaction

Contraindications: Hypersensitivity to unoprostone isopropyl, benzalkonium chloride, or other ingredients contained in the solution

Precautions: Permanent changes in pigmented tissues of eye, bacterial keratitis, do not use while wearing contact lens, no data on use in renal or hepatic failure or pediatric patients, pregnancy category C

Pharmacokinetics:

TOP: Little systemic absorption is reported; plasma half-life 14 min, metabolites excreted in urine

Drug interactions of concern to dentistry:

• None reported; avoid use of anticholinergic drugs: atropine-like drugs, propantheline, diazepam, other benzodiazepines

DENTAL CONSIDERATIONS

General:

• Check compliance of patient with prescribed drug regimen for glaucoma.

• Protect patient's eyes from accidental spatter during dental treatment.

• Avoid dental light in patient's eyes; offer dark glasses for patient comfort.

Consultations:

• Medical consultation may be required to assess disease control.

ursodiol

(er'soe-dye-ole)

Actigall

Ursofalk

Drug class.: Gallstone solubilizing agent

Action: Suppresses hepatic synthesis, secretion of cholesterol; inhibits intestinal absorption of cholesterol

Uses: Dissolution of radiolucent, noncalcified gallbladder stones (<20 mm in diameter) in which surgery is not indicated; prevent gallstones in obese patients experiencing rapid weight loss

Dosage and routes:

• *Adult:* PO 8-10 mg/kg/day in 2-3 divided doses using gallbladder ultrasound q6mo; determine if stones have dissolved; if so, continue therapy and repeat ultrasound within 1-3 mo

Gallstone prevention:

• *Adult:* PO 300 mg bid for 4-6 mo

Available forms include: Caps 300 mg

Side effects/adverse reactions:

▼ *ORAL:* Metallic taste, stomatitis

CNS: Headache, anxiety, depression, insomnia, fatigue

GI: Diarrhea, nausea, vomiting, abdominal pain, constipation, flatulence, dyspepsia, biliary pain

RESP: Cough, rhinitis

INTEG: Pruritus, rash, urticaria, dry skin, sweating, alopecia

MS: Arthralgia, myalgia, back pain

Contraindications: Calcified cholesterol stones, radiopaque stones, radiolucent bile pigment stones, chronic liver disease, hypersensitivity

Precautions: Pregnancy category B, lactation, children

Pharmacokinetics:
PO: 80% excreted in feces, 20% metabolized, excreted into bile, lost in feces

Drug interactions of concern to dentistry:
• Reduced action: aluminum-based antacids

DENTAL CONSIDERATIONS
General:
• Consider semisupine chair position for patient comfort because of GI effects of disease.
• Some opioids can cause spasm of bile duct leading to epigastric distress. Use caution in use for sedation or pain control. NSAIDs may be better choice.
• Consider drug as a factor in the diagnosis of altered taste.

---

valacyclovir HCl

(val-ay-sye'kloe-veer)
Valtrex, Zelitrex (Europe)
Drug class.: Antiviral

Action: Converted to acyclovir, which interferes with DNA synthesis required for viral replication

Uses: Herpes zoster in immunocompetent patients, genital herpes, recurrent genital herpes; treatment of herpes labialis

Dosage and routes:
Initial herpes infection:
• *Adult:* PO 1 g tid × 7 days with or without meals
Genital herpes treatment:
• *Adult:* PO initial episode 500 mg bid × 10 days; recurrent episodes PO 500 mg × 3 days
Herpes labialis infection:
• *Adult:* PO 1 g q12h × 1 day; initiate therapy at earliest sign of symptoms; no clinical benefit beyond 1 day

Available forms include: Caps 500 mg, 1 g

Side effects/adverse reactions:
▼ *ORAL:* Glossitis, medication taste; although unknown for this drug, lichenoid drug reactions are reported with acyclovir
CNS: Headache, ***convulsions,*** tremors, confusion, lethargy, hallucinations, dizziness
GI: Nausea, vomiting, diarrhea, increased ALT/AST, abdominal pain, colitis
HEMA: ***Bone marrow depression, granulocytopenia, thrombocytopenia, leukopenia, megaloblastic anemia,*** anemia, increased bleeding time
GU: Vaginitis, candidiasis, ***glomerulonephritis, acute renal failure,*** oliguria, proteinuria, hematuria, changes in menses
INTEG: Rash, urticaria, pruritus
MS: Asthenia

Contraindications: Hypersensitivity to valacyclovir or acyclovir, avoid in patients with HIV or bone marrow or renal transplants because of risk of hemolytic uremic syndrome

Precautions: Pregnancy category B, renal impairment, lactation, children; reduce dose in renal impairment

Pharmacokinetics:
PO: Rapid absorption and conversion to acyclovir, renal excretion, extensive tissue distribution

Drug interactions of concern to dentistry:
• None reported in otherwise uncompromised patients

DENTAL CONSIDERATIONS
General:
• Determine why the patient is taking the drug.

• Be aware of general discomfort associated with shingles; acute symptoms may preclude patient's routine dental visit or mandate short appointments.
• Patients on chronic drug therapy may rarely have symptoms of blood dyscrasias, which can include infection, bleeding, and poor healing.

Consultations:

• Medical consultation may be required to assess disease control.
• In a patient with symptoms of blood dyscrasias, request a medical consultation for blood studies and postpone dental treatment until normal values are reestablished.

Teach patient/family:

• Importance of good oral hygiene to prevent soft tissue inflammation
• Caution to prevent trauma when using oral hygiene aids

valdecoxib

(val-de-kox'-ib)

Bextra

Drug class.: Nonsteroidal antiinflammatory analgesic

Action: Mechanism of action is thought to be related to the inhibition of cyclooxygenase-2 (COX-2); appears to have antiinflammatory, analgesic, and antipyretic activity

Uses: Relief of signs and symptoms of osteoarthritis and adult rheumatoid arthritis, treatment of primary dysmenorrhea

Dosage and routes:

Osteoarthritis and adult rheumatoid arthritis:

• *Adult:* PO 10 mg daily

Primary dysmenorrhea:

• *Adult:* PO 20 mg bid

Available forms include: Tabs 10, 20 mg

Side effects/adverse reactions:

▼ *ORAL:* Dry mouth, taste alteration

CNS: Dizziness, headache, neuralgia, tremor, vertigo

CV: Peripheral edema, hypertension, some irregularities in heart rate

GI: Abdominal pain, diarrhea, dyspepsia, flatulence, nausea, ***peptic ulcer bleed***

RESP: URI

HEMA: Anemia, thrombocytopenia

GU: Menstrual irregularities

EENT: Pharyngitis, sinusitis, earache

INTEG: Rash, dermatitis, pruritus

ENDO: Elevated liver enzymes, AST, ALT

MS: Back pain, myalgia

MISC: Flulike symptoms, allergic reactions

Contraindications: Hypersensitivity; patients who have experienced asthma, urticaria, or allergic reactions after taking aspirin or NSAIDs, advanced renal disease

Precautions: Hepatic impairment, renal impairment, presence or prior history of ulcers or GI bleeding; avoid in pregnancy; fluid retention, hypertension, CHF; asthma; may increase INR in patients taking warfarin; anaphylaxis and skin reactions that are life threatening have occurred; pregnancy category C, excreted in milk; no data to support use in lactating mothers or children <18 yr

Pharmacokinetics:

PO: Absolute bioavailability 83%; food does not appear to alter absorption; peak plasma levels in approximately 3 hr; half-life 8-11 hr; high plasma protein binding (98%); hepatic metabolism (CYP 3A4 and CYP 2C9); active metabolite; excreted as metabolites in urine

Drug interactions of concern to dentistry:

• Increased plasma levels: fluconazole, ketoconazole, probenecid
• Increased risk of GI side effects: aspirin, methotrexate
• Decreased antihypertensive effects: diuretics, calcium channel blockers, ACE inhibitors, β-blockers
• Decreased renal clearance of lithium
• Monitor PT time: anticoagulants
• Increased renal toxicity: cyclosporine
• First-time users of SSRIs also taking NSAIDs may have a higher risk of GI side effects; until more data are available, it may be advisable to avoid use of NSAIDs in these patients (*Br J Clin Pharmacol* 55:591-595, 2003)

DENTAL CONSIDERATIONS

General:

• Patients on chronic drug therapy may rarely have symptoms of blood dyscrasias, which can include infection, bleeding, and poor healing.
• Use aspirin or NSAIDs with caution.
• Consider altering chair position for comfort of arthritic patients.
• Assess salivary flow as a factor in caries, periodontal disease, and candidiasis.
• Monitor vital signs at each dental appointment because of cardiovascular side effects.

Consultations:

• In a patient with symptoms of blood dyscrasias, request a medical consultation for blood studies and postpone treatment until normal values are reestablished.

Teach patient/family:

• Importance of good oral hygiene to prevent soft tissue inflammation
• Importance of updating health and drug history if physician makes any changes in evaluation or drug regimens

When chronic dry mouth occurs, advise patient:

• To avoid mouth rinses with high alcohol content because of drying effects
• To use fluoride products for anticaries effects
• To use sugarless gum, frequent sips of water, or saliva substitutes

valganciclovir HCl

(val-gan-sye'kloh-veer)

Valcyte

Drug class.: Antiviral

Action: The L-valyl ester is a prodrug that is rapidly converted to ganciclovir; ganciclovir is initially phosphorylated by CMV protein kinase and further phosphorylated to ganciclovir triphosphate, which inhibits viral DNA synthesis

Uses: Treatment of cytomegalovirus (CMV) retinitis in patients with AIDS

Dosage and routes:

Active CMV retinitis:

• *Adult:* PO 900 mg bid for 21 days with food; dose modification required in patients with renal impairment; do not crush or break tablets

V

Maintenance:

• *Adult:* PO 900 mg qd with food; dose modification required in patients with renal impairment; do not crush or break tablets

Available forms include: Tabs 450 mg

Side effects/adverse reactions:

CNS: Headache, insomnia, convulsions, confusion, psychosis, hallucinations, sedation

GI: Diarrhea, nausea, hepatitis, liver function disorder, vomiting

HEMA: Anemia, pancytopenia, ***granulocytopenia, neutropenia, aplastic anemia, bone marrow depression, thrombocytopenia***

GU: Decreased creatinine clearance

EENT: Retinal detachment

MISC: Pyrexia, peripheral neuropathy, infections

Contraindications: Hypersensitivity to ganciclovir or acyclovir, low neutrophil, platelet, or hemoglobin, patients on hemodialysis, lactation

Precautions: Renal impairment (requires dose adjustment), preexisting cytopenias, cannot be substituted for ganciclovir capsules on a one-to-one basis, pregnancy category C, >65 yr, pediatric use

Pharmacokinetics:

PO: Well absorbed, absolute bioavailability (60%), prodrug rapidly converted by hepatic and intestinal esterases to ganciclovir, slowly metabolized intracellularly, excreted in the urine

Drug interactions of concern to dentistry:

• Increased risk of blood dyscrasias: dapsone, carbamazepine, phenothiazines

• Increased risk of seizures: imipenem/cilastatin (Primaxin)

• Low platelet counts may prevent the use of aspirin, NSAIDs

DENTAL CONSIDERATIONS

General:

• Patients on chronic drug therapy may rarely have symptoms of blood dyscrasias, which can include infection, bleeding, and poor healing.

• Examine for oral manifestation of opportunistic infection.

• Place on frequent recall to evaluate healing response.

• Consider local hemostasis measures to control excessive bleeding.

Consultations:

• Medical consultation for blood studies (CBC); leukopenic or thrombocytopenic side effects may result in infection, delayed healing, and excessive bleeding. Postpone elective dental treatment until normal values are maintained.

• Medical consultation may be required to assess disease control.

Teach patient/family:

• To prevent trauma when using oral hygiene aids

• About the possibility of secondary oral infection and the need to see dentist immediately if signs of infection occur

• Importance of good oral hygiene to prevent soft tissue inflammation

valproic acid/valproate sodium/divalproex sodium

(val-proe'ate)

Divalproex sodium: Depakote, Depakote ER, Depakote Sprinkle

♣ Epival

Valproate sodium: Depacon

Valproic acid: Depakene

♣ Alti-Valproic, Deproic, Dom-Valproic, MedValproic, Novo-Valproic, Nu-Valproic, Penta-Valproic, PMS-Valproic Acid

Drug class.: Anticonvulsant

Action: Increased levels of γ-aminobutyric acid (GABA) in the brain

Uses: Simple, complex (petit mal) absence, mixed seizures; divalproex for manic episodes in bipolar disorder, complex partial seizures, migraine prophylaxis; unapproved: tonic-clonic (grand mal) seizures

Dosage and routes:

• *Adult and child:* PO 15 mg/kg/day divided in 2-3 doses; may increase by 5-10 mg/kg/day qwk, not to exceed 30 mg/kg/day in 2-3 divided doses

Manic episodes in bipolar disorder:

• *Adult:* PO (divalproex del rel tabs only) initially 750 mg in divided doses; increase dose to desired effect with max dose 60 mg/kg/day

Migraine prophylaxis:

• *Adult and child >16 yr:* PO divalproex ext rel 250-500 mg bid, up to 1000 mg/day

Available forms include: Caps 250 mg; caps sprinkles 125 mg; delayed rel tabs 125, 250, 500 mg; ext rel tab 250, 500 mg; syr 250 mg/5 ml; inj single dose vial 5 ml, 100 mg/ml

Side effects/adverse reactions:

▼ *ORAL:* Prolonged bleeding, delayed healing, gingival enlargement (rare)

CNS: Sedation, drowsiness, dizziness, headache, incoordination, paresthesia, depression, hallucinations, behavioral changes, tremors, aggression, weakness

GI: Nausea, vomiting, abdominal pain, ***severe hepatic failure, pancreatitis, toxic hepatitis,*** anorexia, cramps, constipation, diarrhea, dyspepsia

HEMA: ***Thrombocytopenia, leukopenia, lymphocytosis,*** increased prothrombin time

GU: Enuresis, irregular menses

INTEG: Rash, alopecia, bruising

MISC: Asthenia

Contraindications: Hypersensitivity, hepatic disease or significant hepatic dysfunction

Precautions: MI (recovery phase), hepatic disease, renal disease, Addison's disease, pancreatitis, pregnancy category D, lactation, children <2yr have higher risk for hepatotoxicity, urea cycle disorders, thrombocytopenia, acute head injury

Pharmacokinetics:

PO: Onset 15-30 min, peak 1-4 hr, duration 4-6 hr

REC: Absorption of enteric coated divalproex is delayed 1 hr

Drug interactions of concern to dentistry:

• Increased effects: CNS depressants; carbamazepine, phenobarbital levels may be increased; phenothiazines can lower the seizure threshold

• Increased bleeding and toxicity: salicylates, NSAIDs

• Increased blood levels: erythromycin
• Increased serum levels of amitriptyline, nortriptyline (start with low dose and monitor)
• Decreased effects of diazepam

DENTAL CONSIDERATIONS

General:

• Patients on chronic drug therapy may rarely have symptoms of blood dyscrasias, which can include infection, bleeding, and poor healing.
• Evaluate for clotting ability during gingival instrumentation because inhibition of platelet aggregation may occur.
• Consider semisupine chair position for patient comfort if GI side effects occur.
• Place on frequent recall if gingival overgrowth occurs.
• Ask about type of epilepsy, seizure frequency, and quality of seizure control.

Consultations:

• In a patient with symptoms of blood dyscrasias, request a medical consultation for blood studies and postpone dental treatment until normal values are reestablished.
• Medical consultation may be required to assess disease control.

Teach patient/family:

• Importance of good oral hygiene to prevent soft tissue inflammation and minimize gingival overgrowth
• Caution to prevent injury when using oral hygiene aids
• To use electric toothbrush if patient has difficulty holding conventional devices
• Need for frequent oral prophylaxis if gingival overgrowth occurs
• To report oral lesions, soreness, or bleeding to dentist

valsartan

(val-sar'tan)

Diovan

Drug class.: Angiotensin II receptor (AT_1) antagonist

Action: Acts as a competitive antagonist for angiotensin II receptors, inhibiting both vasoconstrictor and aldosterone secreting effects

Uses: Hypertension as a single drug or in combination with other antihypertensive medications, heart failure

Dosage and routes:

• *Adult:* PO initial dose 80-160 mg/day; adjust initial dose upward or add a diuretic; dose range 80-320 mg qd

Heart failure:

• *Adult:* PO initial dose 40 mg bid; then titrate dose upward to 80-160 mg bid; maximum daily dose 320 mg

Available forms include: Caps 40, 80, 160, 320 mg

Side effects/adverse reactions:

▼ *ORAL:* Taste alterations

CNS: Insomnia, dizziness, fatigue, vertigo

CV: Edema, palpitation

RESP: Cough, URI

GI: Diarrhea, dyspepsia, nausea

GU: Impotence

MS: Arthralgia, back pain, leg pain, muscle cramp

Contraindications: Hypersensitivity, second and third trimesters of pregnancy

Precautions: Pregnancy category C (first trimester), pregnancy category D (second and third trimesters), volume depletion, less effect in African-Americans, liver impairment, lactation, children <18 yr, elevated labs for liver function, BUN, and potassium

Pharmacokinetics:

PO: Bioavailability 25%, highly plasma protein bound (95%), peak plasma levels 2-4 hr, limited metabolism; excreted in feces 83%, urine 13%

Drug interactions of concern to dentistry:

- Possible reduction in effect: ketoconazole

DENTAL CONSIDERATIONS

General:

- Monitor vital signs at every appointment because of cardiovascular side effects.
- Limit use of sodium-containing products such as saline IV fluids for those patients with a dietary salt restriction.
- Stress from dental procedures may compromise cardiovascular function; determine patient risk.
- Short appointments and a stress reduction protocol may be required for anxious patients.
- Use precaution if sedation or general anesthesia is required; risk of hypotensive episode.

Consultations:

- Medical consultation may be required to assess disease control and patient's ability to tolerate stress.

---

vancomycin HCl

(van-koe-mye'sin)

Vancocin

Drug class.: Glycopeptide-type antiinfective

Action: Inhibits bacterial cell wall synthesis

Uses: Resistant staphylococcal infections, pseudomembranous colitis, staphylococcal enterocolitis, endocarditis

Dosage and routes:

Serious staphylococcal infections:

- *Adult:* IV 500 mg q6h or 1 g q12h
- *Child:* IV 10 mg/kg dose q6h
- *Neonate:* IV 15 mg/kg initially followed by 10 mg/kg q8-12h

Pseudomembranous colitis/staphylococcal enterocolitis:

- *Adult:* PO 500 mg-2 g/day in 3-4 divided doses for 7-10 days
- *Child:* PO 40 mg/kg/day divided q6h, not to exceed 2 g/day

Available forms include: Pulvules 125, 250 mg; powder for oral sol 1, 10 g; powder for inj IV 500 mg, 1, 5, 10 g

Side effects/adverse reactions:

ORAL: Bitter taste sensation

CV: ***Cardiac arrest, vascular collapse***

GI: Nausea

RESP: Wheezing, dyspnea

HEMA: ***Leukopenia, eosinophilia, neutropenia***

GU: ***Nephrotoxicity, fatal uremia,*** increased BUN, creatinine, albumin

EENT: ***Ototoxicity, permanent deafness,*** tinnitus

INTEG: Chills, fever, rash, thrombophlebitis at injection site, urticaria, pruritus, necrosis

SYST: ***Anaphylaxis***

Contraindications: Hypersensitivity, decreased hearing

Precautions: Renal disease, pregnancy category C, lactation, elderly, neonates

Pharmacokinetics:

PO/IV: Oral absorption poor; rapid peak plasma levels with IV infusion of repeated doses; little metabolism because most of drug is excreted by kidney; delayed clearance occurs with renal dysfunction

V

Drug interactions of concern to dentistry:
• Ototoxicity or nephrotoxicity: aminoglycosides and high-dose salicylates
• Increased effects of nondepolarizing muscle relaxants

DENTAL CONSIDERATIONS

General:
• Monitor vital signs at every appointment because of cardiovascular side effects.
• Administer IV slowly over 1 hr; an administration that is too rapid can lead to a fall in blood pressure (monitor) and a red rash on the face, neck, and chest caused by local histamine release. No specific treatment is required for this reaction; evaluate recovery progress.
• Determine why the patient is taking the drug.

Consultations:
• Medical consultation may be required to assess disease control.

---

vardenafil HCl

(var-den'a-fil)

Levitra

Drug class.: Impotence therapy

Action: A selective inhibitor of cGMP-specific phosphodiesterase type 5 (PDE_5); it enhances the effect of nitric oxide (produced by sexual stimulation) that is involved in increased production of cGMP, both of which are involved in the physiologic processes lending to penile erection

Uses: Male erectile dysfunction

Dosage and routes:
• *Adult:* PO suggested starting dose is 10 mg taken 60 min before sexual activity; max dose 20 mg; take with or without food
• *Adult >65 yr:* 5 mg initially, adjust dose up or down based on response

Hepatic impairment:
• *Adult:* PO initial dose 5 mg; do not exceed 10 mg max dose

Available forms include: Tabs 2.5, 5, 10, 20 mg

Side effects/adverse reactions:
▼ *ORAL:* Facial edema
CNS: Headache, insomnia, vertigo, somnolence
CV: Flushing, dizziness, chest pain, angina pectoris, hypertension, hypotension, syncope, postural hypotension
GI: Dyspepsia, nausea
GU: Priapism, abnormal ejaculation
EENT: Rhinitis, sinusitis, tinnitus, abnormal vision, eye pain
INTEG: Photosensitivity, rash, pruritus, sweating
META: Increased creatine kinase, ↑ GGT
MS: Back pain, neck pain
MISC: Flulike syndrome, ***anaphylactic reaction***

Contraindications: Hypersensitivity, patients taking nitrates or α-adrenergic blockers, unstable CV disease, severe hepatic impairment, ESRD, degenerative retinal disorders

Precautions: Men with CV disease in whom sexual activity is not recommended, left ventricular outflow destruction, vasodilator effects on BP, strong inhibitors of CYP3A4 isoenzymes, anatomic deformation of penis, not approved for use in women or children, pregnancy category B

Pharmacokinetics:
PO: Absolute bioavailability 15%, peak plasma levels 30 min-2 hr; plasma protein binding 95%, me-

tabolized in liver by CYP3A4 and to a lesser extent by CYP2C isoenzymes, active metabolite, excreted primarily in feces (91%-95%) and some in urine (2%-6%)

Drug interactions of concern to dentistry:

• Dose adjustments caused by potential drug interactions—do not exceed the maximum single dose of 2.5 mg in a 72 hr period: ritonavir

• Do not exceed 2.5 mg in a 24 hr period: indinavir, ketoconazole (400 mg), itraconazole (400 mg)

• Do not exceed 5 mg in a 24 hr period: ketoconazole (200 mg), itraconazole (200 mg), erythromycin

• Increased plasma levels: drugs that are potent inhibitors of CYP3A4 isoenzymes (erythromycin, ketoconazole—see Appendix I)

• Avoid nitroglycerin within a 24 hour period

DENTAL CONSIDERATIONS

General:

• This is an acute-use drug intended to be taken just before sexual activity. Be sure to include drug use in medical history and avoid use of potentially interacting drugs or warn patient of the interaction when CYP3A4 isoenzyme inhibitors are required.

• If signs of angina pectoris occur during dental treatment, do not use sublingual nitroglycerin.

venlafaxine HCl

(ven'la-fax-een)

Effexor, Effexor XR

Drug class.: Bicyclic antidepressant

Action: Inhibits both norepinephrine and serotonin (5-HT) neuronal uptake and to a lesser extent uptake of dopamine, but the precise antidepressant mechanism remains unclear

Uses: Depression, prevention of major depressive disorder relapse; generalized anxiety disorder (XR product only)

Dosage and routes:

Depression:

• *Adult:* PO 75 mg/day in 2 or 3 divided doses; can increase dose 75 mg/day at no less than 4-day intervals; max dose 375 mg/day in 3 divided doses

Generalized anxiety disorder (XR product only):

• *Adult:* PO 75 mg/day in single dose; max daily dose 225 mg

Available forms include: Tabs 25, 37.5, 50, 75, 100 mg; ext rel caps 37.5, 75, 150 mg

Side effects/adverse reactions:

▼ *ORAL: Dry mouth,* glossitis (rare), cheilitis, gingivitis, candidiasis

CNS: Somnolence, dizziness, migraine, nervousness, anxiety, headache, anorexia, insomnia, mania, hypomania

CV: Hypertension, tachycardia, vasodilation, postural hypotension

GI: Nausea, constipation, vomiting, dyspepsia

RESP: Dyspnea, bronchitis, yawning

HEMA: Ecchymosis, anemia, thrombocytopenia, leukopenia

GU: Abnormal ejaculation (male), male impotence, painful urination, decreased libido

EENT: Blurred vision, ear pain, mydriasis

INTEG: Sweating, rash, pruritus

MS: Asthenia, tremor, trismus

MISC: General body discomfort, asthenia, hyponatremia

Contraindications: Hypersensitivity, concurrent use with or within 14 days of discontinuing MAOI

Precautions: Pregnancy category C, lactation, children <18 yr, sustained hypertension with use, renal or hepatic impairment, elderly, long-term use (>4-6 wk), history of seizures, suicidal patients, mania, hyperthyroidism, impairment of driving, avoid use of alcohol

Pharmacokinetics:

PO: Good bioavailability (92%), metabolized in liver (CYP2D6 isoenzymes), active metabolite, renal excretion, plasma protein binding is low (27%)

Drug interactions of concern to dentistry:

• None currently reported; however, because this drug is similar in action to other antidepressants, it would be wise to avoid excessive amounts of vasoconstrictors, especially in gingival retraction cords

• Increased CNS depression: all CNS depressants

• Risk of serotonin syndrome: St. John's wort

DENTAL CONSIDERATIONS

General:

• Monitor vital signs at every appointment because of cardiovascular side effects.

• After supine positioning, have patient sit upright for at least 2 min before standing to avoid orthostatic hypotension.

• Assess salivary flow as a factor in caries, periodontal disease, and candidiasis.

• Examine for evidence of oral manifestations of blood dyscrasias (infection, bleeding, poor healing).

• Place on frequent recall to evaluate healing response.

• Consider semisupine chair position for patient comfort because of GI effects of disease.

Consultations:

• Medical consultation may be required to assess disease control.

• Physician should be informed if significant xerostomic side effects occur (e.g., increased caries, sore tongue, problems eating or swallowing, difficulty wearing prosthesis) so that a medication change can be considered.

• Obtain a medical consultation for blood studies (CBC) because leukopenic or thrombocytopenic side effects may result in infection, delayed healing, and excessive bleeding. Postpone elective dental treatment until normal values are maintained.

Teach patient/family:

• Importance of good oral hygiene to prevent soft tissue inflammation

• Caution to prevent injury when using oral hygiene aids

When chronic dry mouth occurs, advise patient:

• To avoid mouth rinses with high alcohol content because of drying effects

• Of need for daily use of home fluoride products to prevent caries

• To use sugarless gum, frequent sips of water, or saliva substitutes

verapamil/verapamil HCl

(ver-ap'a-mil)

Calan, Calan SR, Covera HS, Isoptin, Isoptin SR, Verelan, Verelan PM

♣ Apo-Verap, Novo-Veramil, Nu-Verap

Drug class.: Calcium channel blocker

Action: Inhibits calcium ion influx across cell membrane during cardiac depolarization; produces relaxation of coronary vascular smooth muscle; dilates coronary arteries; decreases SA/AV node conduction; dilates peripheral arteries

Uses: Chronic stable angina pectoris, vasospastic angina, dysrhythmias (class IV), hypertension; unapproved: migraine headache, cardiomyopathy

Dosage and routes:

Angina pectoris:

- *Adult:* PO 80-120 mg tid

Arrhythmia/chronic atrial fibrillation:

- *Adult:* PO 240-320 mg/day

Hypertension:

- *Adult:* PO initial 80 mg tid; dose range 360-480 mg/day
- *Adult:* IV 5-10 mg as a bolus over 2 min or longer; may repeat 10 mg 30 min after first dose
- *Child 1-15 yr:* IV bolus 0.1-0.3 mg/kg over 2 min or longer with ECG monitoring
- *Child ≤1 yr:* IV bolus 0.1-0.2 mg/kg over 2 min or longer with ECG monitoring

Available forms include: Tabs 40, 80, 120; sus rel tabs 120, 180, 240 mg; ext rel caps 100, 120, 180, 200, 240, 300 mg; sus rel caps 120, 180, 240, 360 mg; inj 2.5 mg/ml

Side effects/adverse reactions:

▼ *ORAL: Gingival enlargement,* dry mouth, ulcers

CNS: Headache, drowsiness, dizziness, anxiety, depression, weakness, insomnia, confusion, lightheadedness

CV: Edema, ***CHF,*** bradycardia, hypotension, palpitation, AV block

GI: Nausea, diarrhea, gastric upset, constipation, increased liver function studies

GU: Nocturia, polyuria

Contraindications: Sick sinus syndrome, second- or third-degree heart block, hypotension <90 mm Hg systolic, cardiogenic shock, severe CHF

Precautions: CHF, hypotension, hepatic injury, pregnancy category C, lactation, children, renal disease, concomitant β-blocker therapy

Pharmacokinetics:

IV: Onset 3 min, peak 3-5 min, duration 10-20 min, hepatic metabolism (CYP3A4 isoenzymes)

PO: Onset variable, peak 3-4 hr, duration 17-24 hr

Half-life 4 min (biphasic), 3-7 hr (terminal); metabolized by liver; excreted in urine (96% as metabolites)

Drug interactions of concern to dentistry:

- Decreased effect: indomethacin, possibly other NSAIDs, phenobarbital
- Increased effect: parenteral and inhalation general anesthetics or other drugs with hypotensive actions, benzodiazepines
- Increased effects of nondepolarizing muscle relaxants
- Increased effects of carbamazepine

• Caution in use of strong inhibitors of CYP3A4 isoenzymes, itraconazole (see Appendix I)

DENTAL CONSIDERATIONS

General:

• Monitor cardiac status; take vital signs at each appointment because of CV side effects. Consider a stress reduction protocol to prevent stress-induced angina during the dental appointment.

• After supine positioning, have patient sit upright for at least 2 min before standing to avoid orthostatic hypotension.

• Place on frequent recall to monitor gingival condition.

• Limit use of sodium-containing products, such as saline IV fluids, for patients with a dietary salt restriction.

• Assess salivary flow as a factor in caries, periodontal disease, and candidiasis.

• Use vasoconstrictors with caution, in low doses, and with careful aspiration. Avoid use of gingival retraction cord with epinephrine.

Consultations:

• In a patient with symptoms of blood dyscrasias, request a medical consultation for blood studies and postpone dental treatment until normal values are reestablished.

• Medical consultation may be required to assess disease control and patient's tolerance for stress.

Teach patient/family:

• Importance of good oral hygiene to prevent soft tissue inflammation and minimize gingival overgrowth

• Need for frequent oral prophylaxis if gingival overgrowth occurs

When chronic dry mouth occurs, advise patient:

• To avoid mouth rinses with high alcohol content because of drying effects

• Of need for daily use of home fluoride products to prevent caries

• To use sugarless gum, frequent sips of water, or saliva substitutes

---

vidarabine (ophthalmic)

(vye-dare'a-been)

Vira-A Ophthalmic

Drug class.: Antiviral

Action: Inhibits viral DNA synthesis by blocking DNA polymerase

Uses: Keratoconjunctivitis caused by herpes simplex virus, recurrent epithelial keratitis

Dosage and routes:

• *Adult and child:* TOP 0.5 inch oint into conjunctival sac q3h 5× daily

Available forms include: Oint 3%

Side effects/adverse reactions:

EENT: Burning, stinging, photophobia, pain, temporary visual haze

Contraindications: Hypersensitivity

Precautions: Antibiotic hypersensitivity, pregnancy category C

DENTAL CONSIDERATIONS

General:

• Protect patient's eyes from spatter during dental procedures.

• Avoid dental light in patient's eyes; offer dark glasses for patient comfort.

---

vitamin A

Aquasol A, Palmitate-A 500

Drug class.: Fat-soluble vitamin

Action: Vitamin A (retinol) combines with opsin to form rhodopsin necessary for visual adaptation to darkness and normal function of the retina; it is required for normal bone development and epithelial tissue growth; probably acts as a cofactor in many metabolic reactions

Uses: Vitamin A deficiency

Dosage and routes:

Recommended dietary allowance:

• *Adult male:* PO 1000 μg retinol equivalent (RE)

• *Adult female:* PO 800 μg retinol equivalent (RE)

NOTE: 0.3 μg of retinol = 1 IU of vitamin A.

Treatment (Kwashiorkor deficiency state):

• *Child:* IM 30 μg retinol

Xerophthalmia:

• *Adult:* IM 100,000 IU qd × 3 days, then 50,000 IU/day × 14 days

• *Child 1-8 yr:* IM 17,500-35,000 IU qd × 10 days

• *Child <1 yr:* IM 7500-15,000 IU qd × 10 days

Available forms include: Caps 10,000, 15,000, 25,000 IU; tabs 5000 IU; inj 50,000 IU/ml

Side effects/adverse reactions:

▼ *ORAL: Gingival bleeding, dry/cracked lips*

CNS: Headache, increased intracranial pressure, intracranial hypertension, lethargy, malaise

GI: ***Jaundice,*** nausea, vomiting, anorexia, abdominal pain

EENT: Papilledema, exophthalmos

INTEG: Drying of skin, pruritus, increased pigmentation, night sweats, alopecia

MS: Arthralgia, retarded growth, hard areas on bone

META: Hypomenorrhea, hypercalcemia

Contraindications: Hypersensitivity to vitamin A, malabsorption syndrome (PO)

Precautions: Impaired renal function; pregnancy category A (RDA doses), otherwise pregnancy category C

Pharmacokinetics:

PO/INJ: Stored in liver, kidneys, fat; excreted (metabolites) in urine, feces

DENTAL CONSIDERATIONS

General:

• Oral manifestation of side effects could indicate hypervitaminosis.

• May cause dry/peeling skin around lips; provide lip lubricant for patient comfort during dental treatment.

---

vitamin D (calcifediol [D_3], calcitriol, ergocalciferol [D_2], dihydrotachysterol [vitamin D analog], and doxercalciferol)

Dihydrotachysterol (DHT): DHT, Hytakerol

Calcitriol (1α, 25-dihydrocalciferol): Calcijex, Rocaltrol

Calcifediol (25-hydroxycholecalciferol): Calderol

Ergocalciferol (D_2): Calciferol, Calciferol Drops, Disdol, Drisdol Drops

Cholecalciferol (D_3): Delta-D

♣ One-Alpha, Ostoforte, Radiostol Forte

Other vitamin D–related products: paricalcitrol (Zemplar); doxercalciferol (Hectoral)

Drug class.: Fat-soluble vitamin

Action: Needed for regulation of calcium phosphate levels, normal bone development, parathyroid activity, neuromuscular functioning

Uses: Varies with the type of vitamin D selected but generally includes vitamin D deficiency, rickets, renal osteodystrophy, tetany, hypoparathyroidism, and hypophosphatemia; doxercalciferol is indicated for reduction of elevated intact parathyroid hormone (iPTH) levels for secondary hyperparathyroidism in patients receiving chronic renal dialysis

Dosage and routes:

Dialysis (calcifediol):

• *Adult:* PO at dialysis 300-350 μg/wk

Hypoparathyroidism (vitamin D_2):

• *Adult:* PO (DHT) 0.75-2.5 mg/day; after several days establish maintenance dose 0.2-1.75 mg/day; supplement with oral calcium; calcitriol—initial dose 0.25 μg/day may increase after 2-3 wk if required, dose range for adults and children >6 yr 0.5-2 μg/day; (D_2) 50,000-200,000 IU/day, plus 500 mg calcium 6 ×/day

Available forms include: DHT tabs 0.125, 0.2, 0.4 mg; sol 0.2 mg/ml; caps 0.125 mg; calcitriol caps 0.25, 0.5 μg; oral sol 1 μg/ml; inj 1 and 2 μg/ml; calcifediol caps 20, 50 μg; D_2 caps 50,000 IU; liq 8000 IU/ml; inj 500,000 IU/ml; D_3 tabs 400, 1000 IU

Side effects/adverse reactions:

▼ *ORAL:* Metallic taste, dry mouth can be early signs of toxicity

CNS: ***Convulsions,*** fatigue, weakness, drowsiness, headache, psychosis

CV: Hypertension, dysrhythmias

GI: Nausea, vomiting, anorexia, cramps, diarrhea, constipation, decreased libido

GU: ***Hematuria, albuminuria, renal failure,*** polyuria, nocturia

INTEG: Pruritus, photophobia

MS: Decreased bone growth, early joint pain, early muscle pain

Contraindications: Hypersensitivity, hypercalcemia, renal dysfunction, hyperphosphatemia

Precautions: Cardiovascular disease, renal calculi, pregnancy category C, hyperphosphatemia

Pharmacokinetics:

PO/INJ: Half-life 7-12 hr, duration 2 mo; stored in liver; excreted in bile (metabolites), urine

Drug interactions of concern to dentistry:

• Reduction in calcitriol levels: ketoconazole

DENTAL CONSIDERATIONS

General:

• Sensitivity of eyes to dental light may indicate late toxicity.

• Monitor vital signs at every appointment because of cardiovascular side effects.

Teach patient/family:

• That oral side effects are associated with early symptoms of overdose

vitamin E (alpha tocopherol)

Aquavit-E, d'Alpha E, Dry E 400, Mixed E 400, Vita

✤ Plus E

Drug class.: Vitamin E (fat-soluble vitamin)

Action: Needed for digestion and metabolism of polyunsaturated fats, decreased platelet aggregation; decreases blood clot formation; promotes normal growth and development of muscle tissue, prostaglandin synthesis; antioxidant effect protects against free radicals

Uses: Vitamin E deficiency, hemolytic anemia in premature neonates, prevention of retrolental fibroplasia

Dosage and routes:

Recommended dietary allowance:

• *Adult male:* PO 15 IU qd

• *Adult female:* PO 12 IU qd

Prophylaxis:

• *Adult and adolescent:* PO 30 IU qd

Treatment:

• *Adult and adolescent:* PO 60-75 IU/day

• *Child:* PO 1 IU/kg/day or 4-5 times the RDA

Available forms include: Caps 100, 200, 400, 1000 IU; tabs 100, 200, 400, 500, 800 IU; drops 15 IU/0.3 ml; liquid 15 IU/0.3 ml

Side effects/adverse reactions:

CNS: Headache, fatigue

CV: Increased risk of thrombophlebitis

GI: Nausea, cramps, diarrhea

GU: Gonadal dysfunction

EENT: Blurred vision

INTEG: Sterile abscess, contact dermatitis

MS: Weakness

META: Altered metabolism of hormones (thyroid, pituitary, adrenal), altered immunity

Contraindications: None significant

Precautions: Pregnancy category A

Pharmacokinetics:

PO: Metabolized in liver, excreted in bile

Drug interactions of concern to dentistry:

• With doses >400 IU: increased action of oral anticoagulants

DENTAL CONSIDERATIONS

General:

• Determine why the patient is taking the drug.

warfarin sodium

(war'far-in)

Coumadin

Drug class.: Oral anticoagulant

Action: Interferes with blood clotting by indirect means; depresses hepatic synthesis of vitamin K–dependent coagulation factors (II, VII, IX, X) and the anticoagulant proteins C and S

Uses: Pulmonary emboli, deep vein thrombosis, MI, atrial dysrhythmias, to reduce risk of recurrent MI and thromboembolic events

Dosage and routes:

• *Adult:* PO/IV individualized for each patient depending on PT, doses can range from 1-10 mg; usual INR therapeutic ranges from 2 to 3.5

Available forms include: Tabs 1, 2, 2.5, 3, 4, 5, 6, 7.5, 10 mg; inj 2 mg/5 ml

Side effects/adverse reactions:

▼ *ORAL: Gingival bleeding,* stomatitis, salivary gland pain/swelling

CNS: Fever

GI: Diarrhea, ***hepatitis,*** nausea, vomiting, anorexia, cramps

HEMA: ***Hemorrhage, agranulocytosis, leukopenia, eosinophilia***

GU: ***Hematuria***

INTEG: Rash, dermatitis, urticaria, alopecia, pruritus

Contraindications: Hypersensitivity, hemophilia, leukemia with bleeding, peptic ulcer disease, thrombocytopenic purpura, hepatic disease (severe), severe hypertension, subacute bacterial endocarditis, acute nephritis, blood dys-

W

crasias, pregnancy category D, eclampsia, preeclampsia

Precautions: Alcoholism, elderly

Pharmacokinetics:

PO: Onset 12-24 hr, peak 1.5-3 days, duration 3-5 days, half-life 1.5-2.5 days; 99% bound to plasma proteins; metabolized in liver; excreted in urine, feces (active/inactive metabolites); crosses placenta

Drug interactions of concern to dentistry:

- Increased action: diflunisal, salicylates, propoxyphene, metronidazole, erythromycin, clarithromycin, ketoconazole, itraconazole, fluconazole, NSAIDs, indomethacin, chloral hydrate, tetracyclines, fluoroquinolones, acetaminophen, ciprofloxacin, levofloxacin
- If NSAIDs must be used, monitor patient
- Decreased action: barbiturates, carbamazepine
- Possible increase in anticoagulant effects with celecoxib, rofecoxib, acetaminophen (monitor INR levels)
- Herbal products with some anticoagulant activity: feverfew, garlic, ginger, ginkgo, ginseng

DENTAL CONSIDERATIONS

General:

- Reports regarding the concomitant use of acetaminophen and warfarin seem to suggest a possible increase in anticoagulant effects, especially in patients with other diseases or contributing factors (diarrhea, age, debilitation, etc.). Patients taking warfarin should be questioned about recent use of acetaminophen and current INR values. Acetaminophen has been shown to increase the INR depending on the amount of acetaminophen taken and duration of use. A new PT or INR value may be required if surgical procedures are planned. Data from one study indicated that use of four regular strength acetaminophen tablets (325 mg) qd for 1 wk can increase the INR values. Use of acetaminophen over a long duration and in higher doses suggests that it is important to closely monitor INR values (*JAMA* 279:657-662, 1998).
- Patients on chronic drug therapy may rarely have symptoms of blood dyscrasias, which can include infection, bleeding, and poor healing.
- Consider local hemostasis measures to prevent excessive bleeding.
- Increase in bleeding with IM injections may occur.

Consultations:

- Medical consultation should include partial prothrombin time, prothrombin time, or INR.
- For dental surgical procedures that may result in excessive bleeding, consider requesting dose reduction before dental treatment so that PT is no more than twice normal.
- In a patient with symptoms of blood dyscrasias, request a medical consultation for blood studies and postpone dental treatment until normal values are reestablished.

Teach patient/family:

- Importance of good oral hygiene to prevent soft tissue inflammation
- Caution to prevent injury when using oral hygiene aids
- To report oral lesions, soreness, or bleeding to dentist

zafirlukast

(za-fir'loo-kast)

Accolate

Drug class.: Selective leukotriene receptor antagonist

Action: Competitive and selective receptor antagonist of leukotriene LD_4 and LTE_3, resulting in inhibition of bronchospasm and airway edema

Uses: Prophylaxis and chronic treatment of asthma

Dosage and routes:

• *Adult and child >12 yr:* PO 20 mg bid at least 1 hr before or 2 hr after meals

• *Child 5-11 yr:* PO 10 mg bid

Available forms include: Tabs 10, 20 mg

Side effects/adverse reactions:

CNS: Headache, dizziness

GI: Nausea, diarrhea, abdominal pain, vomiting, dyspepsia

RESP: Infections

META: Elevation of ALT

MS: Asthenia, myalgia, back pain, arthralgia

MISC: Generalized pain, fever, accidental injury

Contraindications: Hypersensitivity, hepatic dysfunction with prior use of zafirlukast

Precautions: Not for acute bronchospasm, food decreases bioavailability, pregnancy category B, lactation, patients <7 yr, hepatic impairment, liver enzyme elevation, elderly (increased infection); if liver dysfunction suspected, discontinue use and measure liver enzymes, serum ALT

Pharmacokinetics:

PO: Rapid absorption, peak plasma levels 3 hr, extensively metabolized by CYP2C9 isoenzymes, 90% fecal excretion, 10% urinary excretion, 99% plasma protein bound

Drug interactions of concern to dentistry:

• Increased PT with concurrent use of warfarin

• Reduced plasma levels: erythromycin, terfenadine, theophylline

• Increased plasma levels with aspirin

• Inhibits CYP2C9 and CYP3A4 isoenzymes: use with caution when drugs metabolized by these enzymes are used (see Appendix I)

DENTAL CONSIDERATIONS

General:

• Midday appointments and a stress reduction protocol may be required for anxious patients.

• Avoid prescribing aspirin-containing products.

• Acute asthmatic episodes may be precipitated in the dental office. Sympathomimetic inhalants should be available for emergency use. A stress reduction protocol may be required.

• Be aware that aspirin or sulfite preservatives in vasoconstrictor-containing products can exacerbate asthma.

• Consider semisupine chair position for patients with respiratory disease and if GI side effects are a problem.

Consultations:

• Medical consultation may be required to assess disease control.

Teach patient/family:

• Use of electric toothbrush if patient has difficulty holding conventional devices

• Importance of updating health and drug history if physician makes any changes in evaluation or drug regimens

zalcitabine (ddC)

(zal-site'a-been)

Hivid

Drug class.: Synthetic pyrimidine antiviral

Action: Converted by cellular enzymes to active drug; functions as antimetabolite to inhibit replication of HIV in vitro

Uses: Used in combination with zidovudine in advanced HIV infection

Dosage and routes:

• *Adult:* PO 0.75 mg q8h in combination with other antiretroviral agents

Available forms include: Tabs 0.375, 0.75 mg

Side effects/adverse reactions:

▼ *ORAL: Oral ulcers, dry mouth, glossitis*

CNS: ***Peripheral neuropathy,*** headache, nervousness, fatigue, Bell's palsy

CV: ***Hypertension, syncope palpitation, tachycardia, CHF***

GI: ***Pancreatitis, lactic acidosis, severe hepatomegaly with steatosis,*** nausea, dysphagia, diarrhea, GI pain, anorexia, esophageal ulcers

HEMA: Epistaxis

GU: ***Renal failure,*** polyuria, renal calculus, abnormal renal function

EENT: Abnormal vision

INTEG: Rash, sweating, pruritus, dermatitis

MS: Muscle pain

MISC: ***Anaphylaxis***

Contraindications: Hypersensitivity

Precautions: Pregnancy category C, lactation, children <13 yr, renal impairment, hepatic impairment, risk of serious peripheral neuropathy, risk of severe hepatic impairment, CHF

Pharmacokinetics:

PO: Peak plasma levels following oral doses in 0.8-1.6 hr; phosphorylated form excreted in urine (70%); food decreases rate of oral absorption

Drug interactions of concern to dentistry:

• Increased peripheral neuropathy: metronidazole, dapsone, or other drugs associated with peripheral neuropathy

DENTAL CONSIDERATIONS

General:

• Examine oral cavity for side effects if on long-term drug therapy.

• Monitor vital signs at every appointment because of cardiovascular side effects.

• Palliative medication may be required for management of oral side effects.

• Assess salivary flow as a factor in caries, periodontal disease, and candidiasis.

• Prophylactic antibiotics may be indicated to prevent infection if surgery or deep scaling is planned.

• Patients may be more susceptible to infection and have delayed wound healing.

Consultations:

• Medical consultation may be required to assess disease control and patient's ability to tolerate stress.

Teach patient/family:

• Importance of good oral hygiene to prevent soft tissue inflammation

• Caution to prevent injury when using oral hygiene aids

• That secondary oral infection may occur; must see dentist immediately if infection occurs

When chronic dry mouth occurs, advise patient:

• To avoid mouth rinses with high alcohol content because of drying effects

• Of need for daily use of home fluoride products to prevent caries

• To use sugarless gum, frequent sips of water, or saliva substitutes

zaleplon

(zal'e-plon)

Sonata

Drug class.: Hypnotic

Controlled Substance Schedule IV

Action: Interacts with the GABA benzodiazepine receptor complex binding to the omega-1 receptor subunit

Uses: Short-term treatment of insomnia

Dosage and routes:

• *Adult:* PO 10 mg immediately before bedtime; dose should not exceed 20 mg

Elderly, debilitated, or smaller patient:

• *Adult:* PO 5 mg immediately before bedtime

Available forms include: Caps 5, 10 mg

Side effects/adverse reactions:

▼ *ORAL: Dry mouth*

CNS: Headache, dizziness, amnesia, anxiety, paresthesia, somnolence, depression, nervousness

CV: Palpitation, arrhythmia, tachycardia, syncope

GI: Nausea, constipation, abdominal pain, dyspepsia

RESP: Bronchitis

HEMA: Anemia

GU: Dysmenorrhea, bladder pain, dysuria

EENT: Abnormal vision, ear pain, eye pain, conjunctivitis, dry eyes

INTEG: Pruritus, rash

META: Weight gain, gout, hypercholesterolemia

MS: Myalgia, asthenia

Contraindications: Hypersensitivity

Precautions: Abuse potential similar to benzodiazepines, elderly, debilitated, smaller patients adjust dose downward; pregnancy category C, lactation, children

Pharmacokinetics:

PO: Rapid absorption, bioavailability 30%, peak plasma levels 1 hr, wide tissue distribution, rapid hepatic metabolism (CYP3A4 minor pathway), excretion in urine; heavy, high-fat meal significantly delays absorption

Drug interactions of concern to dentistry:

• Caution when using dental drugs that inhibit or induce cytochrome P-450 enzymes; this drug is a minor substrate for CYP3A4, however, use caution (see Appendix I)

• CNS depression: all CNS depressant drugs

DENTAL CONSIDERATIONS

General:

• Assess salivary flow as a factor in caries, periodontal disease, and candidiasis.

• Determine why patient is taking the drug.

• Consider semisupine chair position for patient comfort if GI side effects occur.

Consultations:

• Medical consultation may be required to assess disease control and patient's ability to tolerate stress.

Z

Teach patient/family:
When chronic dry mouth occurs, advise patient:
• To avoid mouth rinses with high alcohol content because of drying effects
• To use daily home fluoride products for anticaries effect
• To use sugarless gum, frequent sips of water, or saliva substitutes

zanamivir

(za-nam′a-veer)
Relenza
Drug class.: Antiviral

Action: Inhibits neuraminidase, which is essential for replication of influenza type A and B viruses
Uses: Uncomplicated influenza in adults and children >7 yr with symptoms of no more than 2 days; more effective against influenza type A virus
Dosage and routes:
• *Adult and child >7 yr:* Inh 2 inhalations by Diskhaler device (total amount 10 mg) twice daily, 12 hr apart × 5 days; 2 doses should be given on day 1 if at least 2 hr apart, then q12h thereafter; doses must be given not more than 2 days after onset of flu symptoms
Available forms include: Oral inh rotadisks 5 mg each, packaged as a unit with inhaler sufficient for 5-day therapy
Side effects/adverse reactions:
CNS: Headache, dizziness
GI: Diarrhea, nausea, vomiting
RESP: Bronchitis, cough, bronchospasm (asthmatics)
HEMA: Lymphopenia, neutropenia
EENT: Sinusitis; ear, nose, and throat infections
INTEG: Urticaria
META: Elevation of liver enzymes, CPK
MS: Myalgia, arthralgia
MISC: Fever, malaise, fatigue
Contraindications: Hypersensitivity
Precautions: Teach use of inhaler to patient; chronic obstructive pulmonary disease or asthma does not preclude influenza vaccine, safety in high-risk medical conditions is unknown, pregnancy category C, lactation, children <12 yr
Pharmacokinetics:
▼ *ORAL INH:* 4%-17% of inhaled dose is absorbed, peak serum levels 1-2 hr, low plasma protein binding (<10%), excreted unchanged in urine
Drug interactions of concern to dentistry:
• None reported
DENTAL CONSIDERATIONS
General:
• Acute influenza patients are unlikely to be seen in the dental office except for dental emergencies.

zidovudine (AZT)

(zye-doe′vyoo-deen)
Retrovir
✦ Apo-Zidovine, Novo-AZT
Drug class.: Antiviral thymidine analog

Action: Phosphorylated by viral thymidine kinase and competes with thymidine triphosphate inhibiting viral DNA replication
Uses: Symptomatic HIV infections (AIDS, ARC), confirmed *P. carinii* pneumonia, or absolute CD4 lymphocytes <200/mm^3; prevention of maternal-fetal transmission

Dosage and routes:

- *Adult:* PO 600 mg/day in divided doses with adjustment for severity; must stop treatment if severe bone marrow depression occurs; restart after bone marrow recovery; also given IV; 600 mg daily limit
- *Child 6 wk-12 yr:* PO 160 mg/m^2 q8h, up to maximum of 200 mg q8h

Maternal-fetal transmission >14 wk pregnancy:

- *Adult:* PO 100 mg 5 ×/day until onset of labor; IV during labor/delivery 2 mg/kg over 1 hr; then continuous IV infusion 1 mg/kg/hr until umbilical cord is clamped
- *Neonate:* PO 2 mg/kg q6h, begin 12 hr after birth and continue to 6 wk of age; IV infusion 1.5 mg/kg over 30 min and repeated q6h

Available forms include: Tabs 300 mg; caps 100 mg; syr 50 mg/5 ml; inj 10 mg/ml

Side effects/adverse reactions:

▼ *ORAL: Taste changes, gingival bleeding,* mucosal ulceration, swelling of lips or tongue, delayed healing, opportunistic infection

CNS: Fever, headache, malaise, diaphoresis, dizziness, insomnia, paresthesia, somnolence, chills, tremor, twitching, anxiety, confusion, depression, lability, vertigo, loss of mental acuity

GI: ***Lactic acidosis, severe hepatomegaly with steatosis,*** nausea, vomiting, diarrhea, anorexia, cramps, dyspepsia, constipation, dysphagia, flatulence, rectal bleeding

RESP: Dyspnea

HEMA: ***Granulocytopenia, anemia***

GU: Dysuria, polyuria, frequency, hesitancy

EENT: Hearing loss, photophobia

INTEG: Rash, acne, pruritus, urticaria

MS: Myalgia, arthralgia, muscle spasm

Contraindications: Hypersensitivity

Precautions: Granulocyte count <1000/mm^3 or Hgb <9.5 g/dl, pregnancy category C, lactation, children, severe renal disease, severe hepatic function, risk of severe neutropenia and anemia

Pharmacokinetics:

PO: Rapidly absorbed from GI tract, peak 0.5-1.5 hr; metabolized in liver (inactive metabolites); excreted by kidneys

Drug interactions of concern to dentistry:

- Decreased blood levels: acetaminophen, clarithromycin
- Increased serum levels: fluconazole

DENTAL CONSIDERATIONS

General:

- Examine for oral manifestations of opportunistic infections.
- Patients on chronic drug therapy may rarely have symptoms of blood dyscrasias, which can include infection, bleeding, and poor healing.
- Avoid dental light in patient's eyes; offer dark glasses for patient comfort.
- Place on frequent recall because of oral side effects.

Consultations:

- In a patient with symptoms of blood dyscrasias, request a medical consultation for blood studies and postpone dental treatment until normal values are reestablished.
- Medical consultation may be required to assess disease control.

Z

Teach patient/family:

• Importance of good oral hygiene to prevent soft tissue inflammation

• Caution to prevent injury when using oral hygiene aids

• That secondary oral infection may occur; must see dentist immediately if infection occurs

---

zileuton

(zye-loo'ton)

Zyflo Filmtab

Drug class.: Leukotriene pathway inhibitor

Action: Inhibits the enzyme 5-lipoxygenase, thus interfering with synthesis of leukotrienes (LTB_4, LTC_4, LTD_4, and LTE_4), which contribute to inflammation, edema, mucous secretion, and bronchoconstriction

Uses: Prophylaxis and chronic treatment of asthma

Dosage and routes:

• *Adult and child >12 yr:* PO 600 mg qid with meals and hs, daily dose 2400 mg

Available forms include: Tabs 600 mg

Side effects/adverse reactions:

CNS: Headache, dizziness, insomnia, somnolence, malaise

CV: Chest pain

GI: Abdominal pain, dyspepsia, nausea, constipation, flatulence, vomiting

HEMA: Lymphadenopathy, hyperbilirubinemia

GU: UTI, vaginitis

EENT: Conjunctivitis

INTEG: Pruritus

MS: Asthenia, myalgia, arthralgia, neck pain

MISC: Generalized pain, malaise, elevation liver enzymes, fever

Contraindications: Hypersensitivity; active liver disease or transaminase elevations greater than or equal to 3 times the upper limit

Precautions: Not for acute bronchospasm, status asthmaticus; theophylline, warfarin, propranolol; hepatic impairment, pregnancy category C, lactation, children <12 yr, monitor ALT levels

Pharmacokinetics:

PO: Rapid absorption, peak plasma levels 1.7 hr, 93% bound to plasma proteins, metabolized by CYP1A2, CYP2C9, CYP3A4 isoenzymes, 94.5% excreted in urine

Drug interactions of concern to dentistry:

• Increased plasma levels of theophylline, propranolol

• Significant increase in PT when taking warfarin

• Use caution when prescribing dental drugs that are strong inhibitors of CYP1A2 isoenzymes (see Appendix I)

DENTAL CONSIDERATIONS

General:

• Consider semisupine chair position for patient comfort because of GI side effects of disease.

• Acute asthmatic episodes may be precipitated in the dental office. Sympathomimetic inhalants should be available for emergency use.

• Midday appointments and a stress reduction protocol may be required for anxious patients.

• Be aware that aspirin or sulfite preservatives in vasoconstrictor-containing products can exacerbate asthma.

Consultations:

• Medical consultation may be required to assess disease control.

Teach patient/family:

• Importance of updating health

and drug history if physician makes any changes in evaluation or drug regimens

ziprasidone HCl

(zi-pray'si-done)

Geodon

Drug class.: Antipsychotic, atypical

Action: Unclear, but may be related to antagonism of dopamine (D_2) and serotonin (5-HT_2) receptors; also has affinity for D_3, 5-HT_{a2}, 5-HT_{2c}, 5-HT_{1d}, α_1-adrenergic receptors, and histamine H_1 receptors

Uses: Schizophrenia

Dosage and routes:

• *Adult:* PO initial daily dose 20 mg bid with food; dosage adjustments (if indicated) should occur at intervals of not less than 2 days (although several weeks are preferred); doses up to 80 mg bid have been used

Available forms include: Caps 20, 40, 60, 80 mg; inj 20 mg/ml in single-use vial

Side effects/adverse reactions:

▼ *ORAL: Dry mouth*

CNS: Dizziness, seizures, anorexia, extrapyramidal syndrome, somnolence, agitation, confusion

CV: Orthostatic hypotension, syncope, tachycardia, ***increased QT interval***

GI: Nausea, constipation, dyspepsia, diarrhea

RESP: URI, cold symptoms

HEMA: Anemia (infrequent), severe blood dyscrasias (rare)

GU: Impotence, urinary retention, priapism

EENT: Abnormal vision

INTEG: Rash, urticaria, fungal dermatitis

ENDO: Elevated prolactin levels

META: Increased transaminase, increased creatinine phosphokinase, hypercholesterolemia

MS: Myalgia, akathisia, dystonia, hypertonia

MISC: Asthenia, accidental injury, weight gain

Contraindications: Hypersensitivity, other drugs that prolong the QT interval (quinidine, pimozide, dofetilide, sotalol, thioridazine, moxifloxacin, and sparfloxacin), recent MI, congenital long QT syndrome, heart failure

Precautions: May antagonize levodopa, dopamine agonists; QT prolongation and risk of sudden death, bradycardia, hypokalemia, hypomagnesemia, electrolyte depletion caused by diarrhea, diuretics, or vomiting, neuromalignant syndrome, tardive dyskinesia, seizures, suicide, pregnancy category C, lactation, pediatric use

Pharmacokinetics:

PO: Absolute bioavailability 60%, steady state plasma levels 2-3 days, plasma protein building 99%, hepatic metabolism by aldehyde oxidase (major) and CYP450 3A4 (minor) enzymes, excreted mostly in feces (66%) and in urine (20%)

Drug interactions of concern to dentistry:

• Avoid use of any drug that prolongs the QT interval

• Caution in use of other CNS depressants: increased risk of CNS depressant effects

• Reduced plasma levels: carbamazepine

• Increased plasma levels: ketoconazole and other strong inhibitors of CYP3A4 isoenzymes (see Appendix I)

• Drugs that lower BP: increased risk of hypotension

• Increased extrapyramidal effects: phenothiazines and related drugs (haloperidol, droperidol), metoclopramide

DENTAL CONSIDERATIONS

General:

• Monitor vital signs at every appointment because of cardiovascular side effects.

• After supine positioning, have patient sit upright for at least 2 min to avoid orthostatic hypotension.

• Assess salivary flow as a factor in caries, periodontal disease, and candidiasis.

• Consider semisupine chair position for patient comfort if GI side effects occur.

• Assess for presence of extrapyramidal motor symptoms such as tardive dyskinesia and akathisia. Extrapyramidal motor activity may complicate dental treatment.

• Use vasoconstrictors with caution, in low doses, and with careful aspiration; avoid use of epinephrine-impregnated gingival retraction cord.

Consultations:

• Consultation with physician may be needed if sedation or general anesthesia is required.

• Physician should be informed if significant xerostomic side effects occur (e.g., increased caries, sore tongue, problems eating or swallowing, difficulty wearing prosthesis) so that a medication change can be considered.

• Medical consultation may be required to assess disease control and patient's ability to tolerate stress.

Teach patient/family:

• Importance of good oral hygiene to prevent soft tissue inflammation

• To prevent trauma when using oral hygiene aids

• Use of electric toothbrush if patient has difficulty holding conventional devices

When chronic dry mouth occurs, advise patient:

• To avoid mouth rinses with high alcohol content because of drying effects

• To use daily home fluoride products for anticaries effect

• To use sugarless gum, frequent sips of water, or saliva substitutes

zoledronic acid

(zoe'le-dron-ik)

Zometa

Drug class.: Osteoporosis therapy adjunct, bisphosphonate

Action: Inhibits bone resorption but exact mechanism unclear; inhibits osteoclastic activity, induces osteoclast apoptosis, blocks osteoclastic resorption of mineralized bone and cartilage

Uses: Treatment of hypercalcemia from malignancy, bone metastases associated with prostate and lung cancer; multiple myeloma, bone metastases from solid tumors

Dosage and routes:

• *Adult:* IV maximum recommended dose for IV infusion is 4 mg given over no less than 15 min; at least 7 days must lapse between doses if re-treatment is required

Multiple myeloma and bone metastases:

• *Adult:* IV 4 mg infused over 15 min q3-4wk; supplement with oral calcium 500 mg containing vitamin D 400 IU/day

Available forms include: Vial 4 mg

Side effects/adverse reactions:

▼ *ORAL:* Candidiasis

CNS: Insomnia, anxiety, confusion, fatigue, agitation

CV: Hypotension

GI: Nausea, constipation, diarrhea, abdominal pain

RESP: Dyspnea, coughing

HEMA: Anemia

GU: UTI

META: Hypophosphatemia, hypokalemia, hypomagnesemia

MISC: Fever, skeletal pain, flulike symptoms

Contraindications: Hypersensitivity, risk of renal failure if dose rate is exceeded

Precautions: Data for use in children not available, monitor hypercalemic parameters, ensure good hydration, renal impairment, bronchospasm in aspirin-sensitive asthmatics, hypocalcemia, hypoparathyroidism, pregnancy category C, lactation

Pharmacokinetics:

IV INF: Shows triphasic half-life; plasma protein binding 22%; little to no metabolism; excreted mainly in urine; a high percentage of the dose remains bound to bone

Drug interactions of concern to dentistry:

• None reported

DENTAL CONSIDERATIONS

General:

• This drug is used in oncology units or hospitals only.

• Examine for oral manifestation of opportunistic infection.

• Consider semisupine chair position for patient comfort if GI side effects occur.

• Short appointments may be required.

• If oral candidiasis occurs, treat with suitable antifungal drug.

Consultations:

• Medical consultation may be required to assess disease control.

zolmitriptan

(zole'my-trip-tan)

Zomig, Zomig ZMT

Drug class.: Serotonin agonist

Action: A selective serotonin agonist for $5\text{-}HT_{1D}$ and $5\text{-}HT_{1B}$ serotonin receptors on intracranial blood vessels, trigeminal sensory nerves (cranial vessel constriction), and inhibition of proinflammatory neuropeptide release

Uses: Acute treatment of migraine with or without aura in adults

Dosage and routes:

• *Adult:* PO initial 2.5 mg or lower; if headache returns repeat dose in 2 hr not to exceed 10 mg in 24 hr; lack of response to first dose requires physician consultation before taking second dose; safe use in treating more than 3 headaches in 30 days has not been established; doses of 5 mg cause an increase in side effects

Available forms include: Tabs 2.5, 5 mg; tabs oral disintegrating 2.5 mg

Side effects/adverse reactions:

▼ *ORAL: Dry mouth (5%)*

CNS: Dizziness, somnolence, warm sensation, hyperesthesia, paresthe-

sia, dizziness, vertigo, numbness
CV: Chest pain, chest tightness, palpitation, ***serious cardiac events may occur (coronary artery spasm, myocardial ischemia, MI, ventricular tachycardia, ventricular fibrillation)***
GI: Nausea, dyspepsia, dysphagia
RESP: Bronchitis, hiccups
HEMA: Ecchymosis
GU: Hematuria, cystitis, frequency
EENT: Sweating, photosensitivity, pruritus, rash, dry eyes
MS: Myalgia, leg cramps, back pain; neck, jaw, and throat pain
MISC: Asthenia, allergy reaction

Contraindications: Hypersensitivity, ischemic heart disease (angina, MI), Prinzmetal's variant angina, uncontrolled hypertension, within 24 hr of use of ergotamine or other $5HT_1$ agonist, hemiplegic or basilar migraine, prophylactic therapy of migraine, Wolff-Parkinson-White syndrome, accessory conduction arrhythmias, MAOIs

Precautions: Renal impairment, hepatic impairment, may cause coronary vasospasm, pregnancy category C, lactation, children, geriatric

Pharmacokinetics:
PO: Good absorption, peak plasma levels 2 hr; bioavailability 40%, metabolized to active *N*-desmethyl metabolite; half-life of metabolite 2-3 hr; plasma protein binding 25%; excreted mainly in urine (65%) and less in feces (30%)

Drug interactions of concern to dentistry:
• Potential serotonin crises: selective serotonin reuptake inhibitors, ergot-containing drugs (avoid use within 24 hr of taking this drug)
• Decreased plasma levels: cimetidine

DENTAL CONSIDERATIONS

General:
• This is an acute-use drug; thus it is doubtful that patients will come to the office if acute migraine is present.
• Be aware of patient's disease, its severity, and its frequency, when known.
• Advise patient if dental drugs prescribed have a potential for photosensitivity.

Consultations:
• If treating chronic orofacial pain, consult with physician of record.
• Medical consultation may be required to assess disease control and patient's ability to tolerate stress.

Teach patient/family:
• That dryness of the mouth may occur when taking this drug
• To avoid mouth rinses with high alcohol content because of drying effects
• Importance of updating health and drug history if physician makes any changes in evaluation or drug regimens

zolpidem tartrate

(zole-pi'dem)

Ambien

Drug class.: Nonbarbiturate, nonbenzodiazepine sedative-hypnotic

Controlled substance Schedule IV

Action: Presumed to interact with a subunit of the GABA-benzodiazepine receptor, binding only to the omega-1 subunit

Uses: Insomnia

Dosage and routes:
• *Adult:* PO 10 mg before bedtime
• *Elderly and debilitated:* PO 5 mg before bedtime
Available forms include: Tabs 5, 10 mg
Side effects/adverse reactions:
▼ *ORAL:* Dry mouth, taste alteration
CNS: Dizziness, daytime drowsiness, amnesia, headache
*CV: **Tachycardia, hypertension***
GI: Nausea, vomiting, dyspepsia
GU: Menstrual disorder, vaginitis, cystitis
EENT: Double vision, tinnitus
INTEG: Urticaria, acne
MS: Muscle pain
Contraindications: Hypersensitivity, ritonavir
Precautions: Pregnancy category B, lactation, altered reaction time, elderly, limit duration of use
Pharmacokinetics:
PO: Half-life 2.5 hr, peak plasma levels 1.6 hr; highly protein bound
Drug interactions of concern to dentistry:
• Increased CNS depression: alcohol, all CNS depressants, fluconazole, ketoconazole, itraconazole

DENTAL CONSIDERATIONS
General:
• Assess salivary flow as a factor in caries, periodontal disease, and candidiasis.
• Monitor vital signs at every appointment because of cardiovascular side effects.
Consultations:
• Medical consultation may be required to assess disease control.
Teach patient/family:
When chronic dry mouth occurs, advise patient:
• To avoid mouth rinses with high alcohol content because of drying effects
• Of need for daily use of home fluoride products to prevent caries
• To use sugarless gum, frequent sips of water, or saliva substitutes

---

zonisamide

(zoe-nis'a-mide)
Zonegran
Drug class.: Anticonvulsant (sulfonamide derivative)

Action: Mechanism of action is unknown; has been shown to block sodium and T-type calcium channels; suppresses electroshock-induced seizures in experimental models
Uses: Adjunctive therapy in partial seizures in adults with epilepsy
Dosage and routes:
• *Adult >16 yr:* PO initial dose 100 mg/day; after 2 wk may increase the dose to 200 mg/day for at least 2 wk; recommended limit 400 mg/day; 2 wk must be allowed between increases in doses
Available forms include: Caps 25, 50, 100 mg
Side effects/adverse reactions:
▼ *ORAL:* Taste perversion, gingival overgrowth, stomatitis
CNS: Difficulty concentrating, mental slowness, somnolence, fatigue, anorexia, dizziness, headache, agitation, irritability, depression, psychiatric symptoms, psychomotor slowness
CV: Palpitation, bradycardia, hypotension (all infrequent)
GI: Nausea, vomiting, abdominal pain, diarrhea, dyspepsia
RESP: Pharyngitis

HEMA: ***Aplastic anemia, agranulocytosis, leukopenia, thrombocytopenia,*** anemia (all rare)
GU: Kidney stones, urinary frequency
EENT: Diplopia, rhinitis, increased cough
INTEG: ***Stevens-Johnson syndrome, toxic epidermal necrolysis,*** rash
META: Increase in serum creatinine, BUN, serum alk phosphatase
MS: Leg cramps, myalgia

Contraindications: Hypersensitivity to this drug or sulfonamides

Precautions: Discontinue if skin rash occurs, pediatric patients at risk for oligohidrosis, hyperthermia; seizures with abrupt withdrawal; use contraception in women of childbearing age; pregnancy category C, hepatic or renal dysfunction; lactation, kidney stones

Pharmacokinetics:
PO: Peak plasma levels 2-6 hr, half-life >60 hr, steady state plasma levels reached in 14 days with stable doses, significant binding to erythrocytes, excreted unchanged or as metabolite in urine, metabolism involves CYP450 3A4 enzymes

Drug interactions of concern to dentistry:
- No dental drug interactions reported; it has been proposed that drugs which either induce or inhibit CYP 3A4 enzymes may not significantly alter serum levels
- Carbamazepine increases renal clearance

DENTAL CONSIDERATIONS

General:
- Determine type of epilepsy, seizure frequency, and quality of seizure control.
- Patients on chronic drug therapy may rarely have symptoms of blood dyscrasias, which can include infection, bleeding, and poor healing.
- Short appointments and a stress reduction protocol may be required for anxious patients.
- Place on frequent recall to evaluate gingival condition and self-care.
- Consider semisupine chair position for patient comfort if GI side effects occur.
- Warn patient of increased CNS side effects when sedation is used. Advise not to drive a car to and from dental appointment.

Consultations:
- Consultation with physician may be needed if sedation or general anesthesia is required.
- In a patient with symptoms of blood dyscrasias, request a medical consultation for blood studies and postpone treatment until normal values are reestablished.
- Medical consultation may be required to assess disease control and patient's ability to tolerate stress.

Teach patient/family:
- Importance of good oral hygiene to prevent soft tissue inflammation
- To prevent trauma when using oral hygiene aids
- Importance of updating health and drug history if physician makes any changes in evaluation or drug regimens
- To see physician immediately if rash develops because of drug

Appendixes

Appendix A

Abbreviations

ā before
aa of each
ab antibody
abd abdomen
ABGs arterial blood gases
ac before meals *(ante cibum)*
ACE angiotensin-converting enzyme
ACEI angiotensin-converting enzyme inhibitor
Ach acetylcholine
ACT activated clotting time
ACTH adrenocorticotropic hormone
ad lib as desired
ADH antidiuretic hormone
ADP adenosine diphosphate
ADR adverse drug reaction
AIDS acquired immunodeficiency syndrome
aka also known as
ALT alanine aminotransferase, serum
ama against medical advice
amb ambulation
amp ampule
ANA antinuclear antibody
ant anterior
ANUG acute necrotizing ulcerative gingivitis
AP anteroposterior
APAP acetaminophen
APB atrial premature beat
aPTT activated partial thromboplastin time
ARC AIDS-related complex
AROM active range of motion
ASA acetylsalicylic acid (aspirin)
asap as soon as possible
ASHD arteriosclerotic heart disease
AST aspartate aminotransferase, serum
AV atrioventricular
BAC blood alcohol concentration
bid twice a day *(bis in die)*
BM bowel movement
BMR basal metabolic rate
bol bolus
BP blood pressure
BPH benign prostatic hypertrophy
bpm beats per minute
BS blood sugar
BUN blood urea nitrogen
Bx biopsy
c̄ with
C Celsius (centigrade)
C section Cesarean section
CA cancer
Ca calcium
CAD coronary artery disease
cAMP cyclic adenosine monophosphate
cap capsule
cath catheterization or catheterize
CBC complete blood count
CCB calcium channel blocker

CC	chief complaint
cc	cubic centimeter
cGMP	cyclic guanosine monophosphate
CHD	coronary heart disease
CHF	congestive heart failure
cm	centimeter
CML	chronic myeloid leukemia
CMV	cytomegalovirus I
CNS	central nervous system
CO_2	carbon dioxide
CoA	coenzyme A
c/o	complains of
CO	cardiac output
COMT	catechol-*O*-methyltransferase
con rel	controlled release
conc	concentration
COPD	chronic obstructive pulmonary disease
COX2	cyclooxygenase 2
CPAP	continuous positive airway pressure
CPK	creatinine phosphokinase
CPR	cardiopulmonary resuscitation
CrCl	creatinine clearance
CRD	chronic respiratory disease
CRF	chronic renal failure
C&S	culture and sensitivity
CSF	cerebrospinal fluid
CTZ	chemoreceptor trigger zone
CV	cardiovascular
CVA	cerebrovascular accident
CVP	central venous pressure
$CysLT_1$	cysteinyl leukotriene receptor
D&C	dilation and curettage
del rel	delayed release
DIC	disseminated intravascular coagulation
DM	diabetes mellitus
DMARD	disease-modifying antirheumatic drugs
DNA	deoxyribonucleic acid
DOB	date of birth
dr	dram
dsg	dressing
DVT	deep vein thrombosis
D_5W	5% glucose in distilled water
dx	diagnosis
EBV	Epstein-Barr virus
ECG	electrocardiogram (EKG)
EEG	electroencephalogram
EENT	ear, eye, nose, and throat
elix	elixir, hydroalcoholic solution containing an active drug(s)
ENDO	endocrine systems
EPO	erythropoietin
EPS	extrapyramidal symptoms
ESR	erythrocyte sedimentation rate
ext rel	extended release
F	Fahrenheit
FBS	fasting blood sugar
FHT	fetal heart tones
FIO_2	inspired oxygen concentration
FSH	follicle-stimulating hormone
fx	fracture
g	gram
GABA	γ-aminobutyric acid
gal	gallon
GERD	gastroesophageal reflux disease
GGTP	γ-glutamyl transpeptidase
GHb	glycosylated hemoglobin
GI	gastrointestinal

G6PD glucose-6-phosphate dehydrogenase
gr grain
GR glucocorticoid receptor
gtt drop
GTT glucose tolerance test
GU genitourinary
Gyn gynecology
HbA_{1c} laboratory test for glycosylated hemoglobin
Hct hematocrit
HCG human chorionic gonadotropin
HDL high-density lipoprotein
HEMA hematologic system
Hgb hemoglobin
HIV human immunodeficiency virus
H&H hematocrit and hemoglobin
H&P history and physical examination
5-HIAA 5-hydroxyindoleacetic acid
HMG-CoA 3-hydroxy-3-methylglutaryl–coenzyme A reductase
5-HT 5-hydroxytryptamine (serotonin)
H_2O water
HPA hypothalamic-pituitary-adrenocortical axis
HR heart rate
HRT hormone replacement therapy
hr hour
hs at bedtime *(hora somni)*
HSV herpes simplex virus
HSV-2 herpes genitalis
hypo hypodermically
Hx history
IBS irritable bowel syndrome
ICP intracranial pressure
ICU intensive care unit
IDDM insulin-dependent diabetes mellitus
I&D incision and drainage
IgG immunoglobulin G
IL-2 interleukin-2
IM intramuscular
immed rel immediate release
inf infusion
inh inhalation
inj injection
INR international normalizing ratio
INTEG relating to integumentary structures
IOP intraocular pressure
IPPB intermittent positive-pressure breathing
ITP idiopathic thrombocytopenic purpura
IU international units
IUD intrauterine contraceptive device
IV intravenous
IVP intravenous piggyback
K potassium
kg kilogram
L or l left; liter
lat lateral
lb pound
LDH lactic dehydrogenase
LDL low-density lipoprotein
LDL-C low-density lipoprotein–cholesterol
LE lupus erythematosus
LFT liver function test

LH luteinizing hormone
LHRH luteinizing hormone–releasing hormone
liq liquid
LLQ left lower quadrant
LMP last menstrual period
LOC loss of consciousness
lot lotion
loz lozenge
LR lactated Ringer's solution
LRI lower respiratory infection
LVD left ventricular dysfunction
m meter
m^2 square meter
MAC *Mycobacterium avium* complex
MAO monoamine oxidase
MAOI monoamine oxidase inhibitor
max maximum
META metabolic
mEq milliequivalent
mg milligram
μg microgram
MI myocardial infarction
min minute
mixt mixture
ml milliliter
mm millimeter
mo month
MPA mycophenolic acid
MS musculoskeletal
MVA motor vehicle accident
ng nanogram
Na sodium
NC nasal cannula
neg negative
NIDDM non–insulin-dependent diabetes mellitus
NKA no known allergies
NMDA *N*-methyl-*D*-aspartate
NMI no middle initial
noc nocturnal (night)
NPH neutral protamine Hagedorn
NPO nothing by mouth *(nil per os)*
NS normal saline
NSAID nonsteroidal antiinflammatory drug
NV neurovascular
O_2 oxygen
OBS organic brain syndrome
OC oral contraceptive
OD right eye *(oculus dexter)*
oint ointment
OOB out of bed
ophth ophthalmic
OR operating room
ORIF open reduction, internal fixation
os left eye *(ocular sinister)*
OTC over the counter
ou each eye *(oculus uterque)*
oz ounce
p̄ after (post)
p pulse
PABA para-aminobenzoic acid
PAC premature atrial contraction
pCO_2 arterial carbon dioxide tension (pressure tore)
pO_2 arterial oxygen tension (pressure tore)
PAT paroxysmal atrial tachycardia
PBI protein-bound iodine
PBP penicillin binding protein
pc after meals *(post cibum)*

PCA patient-controlled analgesia
PCN penicillin
PE physical examination
PG prostaglandin
pH hydrogen ion concentration
PMDD premenstrual dysphoric disorder
PMS premenstrual syndrome
PNS peripheral nervous system
PO by mouth *(per os)*
postop postoperatively
PP postprandial
ppm parts per million
preop preoperatively
prep preparation
prn as needed *(pro re nata)*
PSA prostate-specific antigen
PT prothrombin time
PTSD posttraumatic stress disorder
PTT partial thromboplastin time
PVC premature ventricular contraction
PVD peripheral vascular disease
q every
qAM every morning
qd every day
qh every hour
qid four times a day
qod every other day
qPM every night
qt quart
q2h every 2 hours
q3h every 3 hours
q4h every 4 hours
q6h every 6 hours
q12h every 12 hours
qwk every week
r right
rap disintegr rapidly disintegrating
RAR retinoic acid receptor
RBC(s) red blood count or cell(s)
RDA recommended dietary allowance
rec rectal
REM rapid eye movement
RESP respiratory system
rhPDGF-BB recombinant human platelet–derived growth factor
RNA ribonucleic acid
R/O rule out
ROAD reversible obstructive airway disease
ROM range of motion
RTI respiratory tract infection
Rx therapy, treatment, or prescription
$\bar{s}$ without
SA sinoatrial
SAN sinoatrial node
SC subcutaneous
sec second
SERM selective estrogen receptor modulator
SGOT serum glutamic-oxaloacetic transaminase (now AST)
SGPT serum glutamic pyruvate transaminase (now ALT)

SIADH syndrome of inappropriate antidiuretic hormone
sig patient dosing instructions on prescription label
SL sublingual
SLE systemic lupus erythematosus
slow rel slow release
SMBG self-monitored blood glucose
SMZ sulfamethoxazole
SOB short of breath
sol solution
ss one half
SSRI selective serotonin reuptake inhibitor
stat at once
STD sexually transmitted disease
surg surgical
sus rel sustained release dose form
supp suppository
Sx symptoms
syr syrup, a highly concentrated sucrose solution containing a drug(s)
T temperature
$T_{1/2}$ drug half-life
T_3 triiodothyronine
T_4 thyroxine
tab tablet
TB tuberculosis
TBG thyroxine-binding globulin
tbsp tablespoon
TCA tricyclic antidepressant
TD transdermal
temp temperature
TG total triglycerides
TIA transient ischemic attack
tid three times daily *(ter in die)*
time rel time release dose form
tinc tincture, alcoholic solution of a drug
TMD temporomandibular dysfunction
TMJ temporomandibular joint
TMP trimethoprim
TNF tumor necrosis factor
top topical
tPA tissue plasminogen activator
TPN total parenteral nutrition
TPR temperature, pulse, respirations
TSH thyroid-stimulating hormone
tsp teaspoon
TT thrombin time
Tx treatment
U unit
UA urinalysis
ULDL ultra-low-density lipoprotein
URI upper respiratory infection
USP United States Pharmacopeia
UTI urinary tract infection
UV ultraviolet
vag vaginal
visc viscous
VD venereal disease
VHDL very-high-density lipoprotein
VLDL very-low-density lipoprotein
VO verbal order
vol volume
VPB ventricular premature beats
VS vital signs
WBC white blood cell; white blood cell count
WHO World Health Organization

wk	week
WNL	within normal limits
wt	weight
yr	year
>	greater than
<	less than
≠	not equal
↑	increase
↓	decrease
2°	secondary

Appendix B

Drugs Causing Dry Mouth

Drug category	Brand name	Generic name
ANOREXIANT	Adipex-P, Fastin, Ionamin	phentermine
	Anorex	phendimetrazine
	Mazanor, Sanorex	mazindol
	Tenuate, Tepanil	diethylpropion
ANTIACNE	Accutane	isotretinoin
ANTIANXIETY	Atarax, Vistaril	hydroxyzine
	Ativan	lorazepam
	BuSpar	buspirone
	Equanil, Miltown	meprobamate
	Librium	chlordiazepoxide
	Paxipam	halazepam
	Serax	oxazepam
	Sonata	zalephon
	Valium	diazepam
	Xanax	alprazolam
ANTIARTHRITIC	Arava	leflunomide
ANTICHOLINERGIC/ ANTISPASMODIC	Anaspaz	hyoscyamine
	Sal-Tropine	atropine
	Bellergal	belladonna alkaloids
	Bentyl	dicyclomine
	Ditropan	oxybutynin
	Donnatal, Kinesed	hyoscyamine atropine, phenobarbital, scopolamine
	Librax	chlordiazepoxide, clidinium
	Pro-Banthine	propantheline
	Transderm-Scop	scopolamine
ANTICONVULSANT	Felbatol	felbamate
	Lamictal	lamotrigine
	Neurontin	gabapentin
	Tegretol	carbamazepine
ANTIDEPRESSANT	Anafranil	clomipramine
	Asendin	amoxapine
	Celexa	citalopram
	Effexor	venlafaxine

	Elavil	amitriptyline
	Luvox	fluvoxamine
	Marplan	isocarboxazid
	Nardil	phenelzine
	Norpramin	desipramine
	Parnate	tranylcypromine
	Paxil	paroxetine
	Prozac	fluoxetine
	Replax	eletriptan
	Sinequan	doxepin
	Tofranil	imipramine
	Wellbutrin, Zyban	bupropion
	Zoloft	sertraline
ANTIDIARRHEAL	Imodium AD	loperamide
	Lomotil	diphenoxylate, atropine
	Motofen	difenoxin
ANTIHISTAMINE	Actifed	triprolidine with pseudoephedrine
	Atarax	hydroxyzine
	Benadryl	diphenhydramine
	Chlor-Trimeton	chlorpheniramine
	Claritin	loratadine
	Dimetapp	pseudoephedrine
	Phenergan	promethazine
ANTIHYPERTENSIVE	Capoten	captopril
	Catapres	clonidine
	Coreg	carvedilol
	Ismelin	guanethidine
	Aceon	perindopril
	Minipress	prazosin
	Serpasil	reserpine
	Wytensin	guanabenz
	Vasotec	enalapril
ANTIINFLAMMATORY ANALGESIC	Dolobid	diflunisal
	Celebrex	celecoxib
	Feldene	piroxicam
	Motrin	ibuprofen
	Nalfon	fenoprofen
	Naprosyn	naproxen
	Vioxx	rofecoxib
ANTIINFLAMMATORY GI	Colazal	balsalazide
ANTINAUSEANT	Antivert	meclizine
	Dramamine	dimenhydrinate
	Emend	aprepitant
	Marezine	cyclizine

ANTIPARKINSONIAN	Akineton	biperiden
	Artane	trihexyphenidyl
	Cogentin	benztropine mesylate
	Larodopa	levodopa
	Parsidol	ethopropazine
	Sinemet	carbidopa, levodopa
	Tasmar	tolcapone
ANTIPSYCHOTIC	Abilify	aripiprazole
	Clozaril	clozapine
	Compazine	prochlorperazine
	Eskalith	lithium
	Haldol	haloperidol
	Mellaril	thioridazine
	Navane	thiothixene
	Orap	pimozide
	Risperdal	resperidone
	Sparine	promazine
	Thorazine	chlorpromazine
	Triavil	amitriptyline, perphenazine
	Zyprexa	olanzapine
ANTISECRETORY	Aciphex	rabeprazole
	Nexium	esomeprazole
ANTISPASMODIC	Detrol	tolterodine
ANTIVIRAL	Sustiva	efavirenz
	Copegus	ribavirin
BRONCHODILATOR	(generic)	ephedrine
	Isuprel	isoproterenol
	Proventil, Ventolin	albuterol
	Xopenex	levalbuterol
CNS STIMULANT	Dexedrine	dextroamphetamine
	Desoxyn	methamphetamine
DECONGESTANT	Sudafed	pseudoephedrine
DIURETIC	Aldactone	spironolactone
	Diuril	chlorothiazide
	Dyazide, Maxzide, Dyrenium	triamterene
	Esidrix, HydroDIURIL	hydrochlorothiazide
	Lasix	furosemide
	Midamor	amiloride
MIGRAINE	Amerge	naratriptan
	Axert	almotriptan

	Frova	fovatriptan
	Maxalt	rizatriptan
	Replax	eletriptan
MUSCLE RELAXANT	Flexeril	cyclobenzaprine
	Lioresal	baclofen
	Norflex	orphenadrine
NARCOLEPSY	Provigil	modafinil
OPIOID ANALGESIC	Buprenex	buprenorphine
	Demerol	meperidine
	MS Contin	morphine
	Synalgos DC	dihyrocodeine combinations
OPHTHALMIC	Azopt	brinzolamide
SEDATIVE	Dalmane	flurazepam
	Halcion	triazolam
	Restoril	temazepam

Appendix C

Controlled Substances Chart

Drugs	United States	Canada
Heroin, LSD, peyote, marijuana, mescaline, phencyclidine	Schedule I (CI)	Schedule H
Opium, fentanyl, morphine, meperidine, methadone, oxycodone (and its combinations), hydromorphone, codeine (single-drug entity), and cocaine	Schedule II (CII)	Schedule N
Short-acting barbiturates	Schedule II	Schedule C
Amphetamine and methylphenidate	Schedule II	Schedule G
Codeine combinations, hydrocodone combinations, glutethimide, paregoric, phendimetrazine, thiopental, testosterone, and other androgens	Schedule III (CIII)	Schedule F
Benzodiazepines (diazepam, midazolam, etc.), chloral hydrate, meprobamate, phenobarbital, propoxyphene (and combinations), pentazocine (and combinations), and methohexital	Schedule IV (CIV)	Schedule F
Antidiarrheals and antitussives with opioid derivatives	Schedule V (CV)	

Appendix D

FDA Pregnancy Categories

A Studies have failed to demonstrate a risk to the fetus in any trimester

B Animal reproduction studies fail to demonstrate a risk to the fetus; no human studies available

C Given only after risks to the fetus are considered; animal reproduction studies have shown adverse effects on fetus; no human studies available

D Definite human fetal risks; may be given in spite of risks if needed in life-threatening conditions

X Absolute fetal abnormalities; not to be used anytime during pregnancy because risks outweigh benefits

Appendix E

Drugs That Affect Taste

ALCOHOL DETOXIFICATION
disulfiram (Antabuse)

ALZHEIMER'S
donepezil (Aricept)

ANALGESICS (NSAIDS)
diclofenac (Voltaren)
etodolac (Lodine)
ketoprofen (Orudis)
meclofenamate (Meclofen)
sulindac (Clinoril)

ANESTHETICS (GENERAL)
midazolam (Versed)
propofol (Diprivan)

ANESTHETICS (LOCAL)
lidocaine transoral delivery system (Dentipatch)

ANOREXIANTS
diethylpropion (Tenuate)
mazindol (Mazanor)
phendimetrazine (Adipost)
phentermine (Ionamin)

ANTACIDS
aluminum hydroxide (Amphojel)
calcium carbonate (Tums)
lansoprazole (Prevacid)
magaldrate (Riapan)
omeprazole (Prilosec)
sucralfate (Carafate)

ANTIANXIETY
buspirone (BuSpar)

ANTIARTHRITIC
leflunomide (Arava)

ANTICHOLINERGICS
clidinium (Quarzan)
mepenzolate (Cantil)
propantheline (Pro-Banthine)

ANTICONVULSANTS
fosphenytoin (Cerebyx)
phenytoin (Dilantin)
topiramate (Topamax)

ANTIDEPRESSANTS
amitriptyline (Elavil)
clomipramine (Anafranil)
desipramine (Norpramin)
doxepin (Sinequan)
fluoxetine (Prozac)
imipramine (Tofranil)
nefazodone (Serzone)
nortriptyline (Pamelor)
protriptyline (Vivactil)
sertraline (Zoloft)

ANTIDIABETICS
metformin (Glucophage)
tolbutamide (Orinase)

ANTIDIARRHEALS
bismuth subsalicylate (Pepto-Bismol)

ANTIEMETICS
aprepitant (Emend)
dolasetron mesylate (Anazemet)

ANTIFUNGALS
terbinafine (Lamisil)

ANTIGOUT
allopurinol (Zyloprim)
colchicine

ANTIHISTAMINE (H_1) ANTAGONISTS
azelastine (Astelin)
cetirizine (Zyrtec)

ANTIHISTAMINE (H_2) ANTAGONISTS
famotidine (Pepcid)

ANTIHYPERLIPIDEMICS
clofibrate (Atromid-S)
fluvastatin (Lescol)

ANTIINFECTIVES
ciprofloxacin (Ciloxan)
daptomycin (Cubicin)
ethionamide (Trecator-SC)
gatifloxacin (Zymar)
gemifloxacin (Factiv)
levofloxacin (Levoquin)
lincomycin (Lincocin)
metronidazole (Flagyl)
ofloxacin (Floxin)

ANTIINFLAMMATORY/ ANTIARTHRITIC
auranofin (Ridaura)
aurothioglucose (Solganal)
celecoxib (Celebrex)
rofecoxib (Vioxx)
sulfasalazine (Azulfidine)

ANTIMIGRAINE
almotriptan (Axert)
fovatriptan (Frova)

ANTIPARKINSON
entacapone (Comtan)
levodopa (Larodopa)
levodopa-carbidopa (Sinemet)
pergolide (Permax)
pramipexole dihydrochloride (Mirapex)

ANTIPSYCHOTICS
lithium (Eskalith)
pimozide (Orap)
prochlorperazine (Compazine)
quetiapine fumarate (Seroquel)
risperidone (Risperdal)

ANTITHYROID
methimazole (Tapazole)
propylthiouracil

ANTIVIRALS
acyclovir (Zovirax)
amprenavir (Agenerase)
atazanavir (Reyataz)
delavirdine mesylate (Rescriptor)
didanosine (Videx)
efavirenz (Sustiva)
foscarnet (Foscavir)
indinavir (Crixivan)
penciclovir (Denavir)
ribavirin (Copegus)
rimantadine (Flumadine)
ritonavir (Norvir)
saquinavir (Invirase)
valcyclovir (Valtrex)
zidovudine (Retrovir)

ANXIOLYTIC/SEDATIVES
chloral hydrate
estazolam (ProSom)
quazepam (Doral)
zolpidem (Ambien)

ASTHMA PREVENTIVES
cromolyn (Intal)
nedocromil (Tilade)

BRONCHODILATORS

albuterol (Proventil)
bitolterol (Tornalate)
formoterol fumarate (Foradil)
ipratropium (Atrovent)
isoproterenol (Isuprel)
metaproterenol (Alupent)
pirbuterol (Maxair)
terbutaline (Brethine)

CALCIUM-AFFECTING DRUGS

alendronate (Fosamax)
calcitonin (Calcimar)
etidronate (Didronel)

CANCER CHEMOTHERAPEUTICS

capecitabine (Xeloda)
fluorouracil (Efudex)
levamisole (Ergamisol)
tamoxifen (Nolvadex)

CARDIOVASCULAR

amiodarone (Cordarone)
amlodipine (Norvasc)
bepridil (Vascor)
captopril (Capoten)
clonidine (Catapres)
diltiazem (Cardizem)
enalapril (Vasotec)
flecainide (Tambocor)
fosinopril (Monopril)
guanfacine (Tenex)
labetalol (Trandate)
losartan (Cozaar)
mecamylamine (Inversine)
mexiletine (Mexitil)
moricizine (Ethmozine)
nadolol (Corgard)
nifedipine (Procardia XL)
penbutolol (Levabol)
perindopril (Aceon)
propafenone (Rythmol)
quinidine (Cardioquin)
valsartan (Diovan)

CNS STIMULANTS

dextroamphetamine (Dexedrine)
methamphetamine (Desoxyn)

DECONGESTANT

phenylephrine (Neo-Synephrine)

DIURETICS

acetazolamide (Diamox)
methazolamide (Naptazine)
polythiazide (Renese)

GLUCOCORTICOIDS

budesonide (Rhinocort)
flunisolide (Aerobid)
rimexolone (Vexol)

GALLSTONE SOLUBILIZATION

ursodiol (Actigall)

HEMORHEOLOGIC

pentoxifylline (Trental)

IMMUNOMODULATORS

interferon alfa (Roferon-A)
levamisole (Ergamisol)
tacrolimus (Protopic)

IMMUNOSUPPRESSANTS

azathioprine (Imuran)

IRRITABLE BOWEL SYNDROME

alosetron (Lotronex)

METHYLXANTHINES

aminophylline (Somophyllin)
dyphylline (Dilor)
oxtriphylline (Choledyl)
theophylline (Theo-Dur)

NICOTINE CESSATION

nicotine polacrilex (Nicorette)

OPHTHALMICS
apraclonidine (Iopidine)
brimonidine (Alphagan)
brinzolamide (Azopt)
dorzolamide (Truspot)
olopatadine (Pantanol)

PROTON PUMP INHIBITORS
esomeprazole (Nexium)
lansoprazole (Prevacid)
omeprazole (Prilosec)

RETINOID, SYSTEMIC
acitretin (Soriatane)

SALIVARY STIMULANT
pilocarpine (Salagen)

SKELETAL MUSCLE RELAXANTS
baclofen (Lioresal)
cyclobenzaprine (Flexeril)
methocarbamol (Robaxin)

VITAMINS
calcifediol (vitamin D)
calcitriol (vitamin D)
dihydrotachysterol (vitamin D)
phytonadione (vitamin K)

Appendix F

Combination Products

How to use this appendix: Drugs are frequently combined into a single dose unit (or product) for patient convenience, as well as for other reasons. Only selected products, both prescription and OTC, are shown in this appendix. The list is alphabetical by the brand name of the combination product. Brand names for identical drug combinations are listed together. When the patient's drug history includes one of these combination products, it can be easily accessed through the index. The active ingredients and dose amounts follow each brand name. The ingredients are listed in random order, because all ingredients should be therapeutically useful and important. Information for each ingredient can be found in the individual drug monograph in the main body of the book.

Accuretic: quinapril 10 mg with hydrochlorothiazide 12.5 mg, or quinapril 20 mg with hydrochlorothiazide 12.5 mg, or quinapril 20 mg with hydrochlorothiazide 25 mg

Aceta with Codeine, Tylenol with Codeine No. 3: acetaminophen 300 mg with codeine phosphate 30 mg

Actifed Cold and Allergy, Allerfrim, Aprodine, Cenafed Plus, Genac: pseudoephedrine HCl 60 mg with triprolidine HCl 2.5 mg

Activella: norethindrone acetate 0.5 mg with estradiol 1 mg

Adderall 5: amphetamine aspartate 1.25 mg, amphetamine sulfate 1.25 mg, dextroamphetamine saccharate 1.25 mg, and dextroamphetamine sulfate 1.25 mg

Adderall 7.5: amphetamine aspartate 1.875 mg, amphetamine sulfate 1.875 mg, dextroamphetamine saccharate 1.875 mg, and dextroamphetamine sulfate 1.875 mg

Adderall 10: amphetamine aspartate 2.5 mg, amphetamine sulfate 2.5 mg, dextroamphetamine saccharate 2.5 mg, and dextroamphetamine sulfate 2.5 mg

Adderall 12.5: amphetamine aspartate 3.125 mg, amphetamine sulfate 3.125 mg, dextroamphetamine saccharate 3.125 mg, and dextroamphetamine sulfate 3.125 mg

Adderall 15: amphetamine aspartate 3.75 mg, amphetamine sulfate 3.75 mg, dextroamphetamine saccharate 3.75 mg, and dextroamphetamine sulfate 3.75 mg

Adderall 20: amphetamine aspartate 5 mg, amphetamine sulfate 5 mg, dextroamphetamine sulfate 5 mg, and dextroamphetamine saccharate 5 mg

Adderall 30: amphetamine aspartate 7.5 mg, amphetamine sulfate 7.5 mg, dextroamphetamine sulfate 7.5 mg, and dextroamphetamine saccharate 7.5 mg

Adderall XR10 mg: amphetamine aspartate 2.5 mg, amphetamine sulfate 2.5 mg, dextroamphetamine sulfate 2.5 mg, and dextroamphetamine saccharate 2.5 mg
Adderall XR 20 mg: amphetamine aspartate 5 mg, amphetamine sulfate 5 mg, dextroamphetamine sulfate 5 mg, and dextroamphetamine saccharate 5 mg
Adderall XR 30 mg: amphetamine aspartate 7.5 mg, amphetamine sulfate 7.5 mg, dextroamphetamine sulfate 7.5 mg, and dextroamphetamine saccharate 7.5 mg
Advicor: niacin 500 mg and lovastatin 20 mg; niacin 750 mg and lovastatin 750 mg; niacin 1000 mg and lovastatin 20 mg
Advair Diskus: salmeterol 50 μg and fluticasone propionate 100, 250, or 500 μg
Aggrenox: aspirin 25 mg with dipyridamole 200 mg
Ak-Trol Ointment, Dexasporin Ointment, Dexacidin Ointment, Maxitrol Ointment: dexamethasone 1 mg, polymyxin B sulfate 10,000 U, and neomycin sulfate 3.5 mg/g
Ak-Trol, Maxitrol, Dexacidin Suspension: dexamethasone 1 mg, polymyxin B sulfate 10,000 U, and neomycin sulfate 3.5 mg/ml of supension
Aldactazide 25/25: spironolactone 25 mg with hydrochlorothiazide 25 mg
Aldactazide 50/50: spironolactone 50 mg with hydrochlorothiazide 50 mg
Aldoclor-150: methyldopa 250 mg with chlorothiazide 150 mg
Aldoclor-250: methyldopa 250 mg with chlorothiazide 250 mg
Aldoril-15: methyldopa 250 mg with hydrochlorothiazide 15 mg
Aldoril-25: methyldopa 250 mg with hydrochlorothiazide 25 mg
Aldoril D30: methyldopa 500 mg with hydrochlorothiazide 30 mg
Aldoril D50: methyldopa 500 mg with hydrochlorothiazide 50 mg
Aleve Sinus and Headache, Aleve Cold and Sinus: naproxen sodium 220 mg with pseudoephedrine HCl 120 mg
Alka-Seltzer Plus Cold and Sinus: acetaminophen 250 mg with phenylephrine HCl 5 mg
Alka-Seltzer Plus Cold and Sinus, Ornex No Drowsiness, Phenapap, Sinutab Without Drowsiness Regular Strength, Sudafed Cold and Sinus Non-Drowsy: acetaminophen 500 mg with pseudoephedrine HCl 30 mg
Allegra-D: fexofenadine 60 mg with pseudoephedrine HCl 120 mg
Anacin, P-A-C Analgesic: aspirin 400 mg with caffeine 32 mg
Anacin Maximum Strength: aspirin 500 mg with caffeine 32 mg
Anexsia 5/500, Bancap HC, Ceta-Plus, Co-Gesic, Dolacet, Duocet, Hydrocet, Hydrogesic, Hy-Phen, Lorcet-HD, Lortab 5/500, Margesic H, Panacet 5/500, Stagesic, T-Gesic, Vicodin: hydrocodone bitartrate 5.0 mg with acetaminophen 500 mg
Anexsia 7.5/650, Lorcet Plus: hydrocodone bitartrate 7.5 mg with acetaminophen 650 mg
Anexsia 10/660, Vicodin HP: hydrocodone bitartrate 10 mg with acetaminophen 660 mg
Apresazide 25/25: hydralazine HCl 25 mg with hydrochlorothiazide 25 mg
Apresazide 50/50: hydralazine

HCl 50 mg with hydrochlorothiazide 50 mg

Apresazide 100/50: hydralazine HCl 100 mg with hydrochlorothiazide 50 mg

Arthrotec: diclofenac 75 mg with misoprostol 200 μg; or diclofenac 50 mg with misoprostol 200 μg

Aspirin Free Excedrin, Premsyn PMS, Vitelle Lurline PMS, Pamprin Multi-Symptom Maximum Strength: acetaminophen 500 mg with caffeine 65 mg

Atacand HCT: candesartan cilexetil 16 mg with hydrochlorothiazide 12.5 mg; candesartan cilexetil 32 mg with hydrochlorothiazide 12.5 mg

Avandamet: rosiglitazone maleate 1 mg with metformin HCl 500 mg, rosiglitazone maleate 2 mg with metformin HCl 500 mg or rosiglitazone maleate 4 mg with metformin HCl 500 mg

Avalide: irbesartan 150 mg with hydrochlorothiazide 12.5 mg; irbesartan 300 mg with hydrochlorothiazide 12.5 mg

Azo-Sulfisoxazole: sulfisoxazole 500 mg with phenazopyridine HCl 50 mg

Barbidonna: belladonna alkaloids, atropine sulfate 0.025 mg, hyoscyamine sulfate 0.1286 mg, scopolamine hydrobromide 0.0074 mg, and phenobarbital 16 mg

Barbidonna No. 2: belladonna alkaloids, atropine sulfate 0.025 mg, hyoscyamine sulfate 0.1286 mg, scopolamine hydrobromide 0.0074 mg, and phenobarbital 32 mg

BC Powder Original Formula: aspirin 650 mg with caffeine 32 mg, salicylamide 195 mg

BC Powder Arthritis Strength: aspirin 742 mg with caffeine 36 mg, salicylamide 222 mg

Bellergal-S, Phenerbel-S, Folergot-DF: ergotamine tartrate 0.6 mg with levorotatory belladonna alkaloids maleates 0.2 mg and phenobarbital 40 mg tablets

Benylin Expectorant Liquid: dextromethorphan hydrobromide 5 mg with guaifenesin 100 mg/5 ml

Bromfed, Bromfenex, Ultrabrom: pseudoephedrine HCl 120 mg with brompheniramine maleate 12 mg

Bromfed Tablets: pseudoephedrine HCl 60 mg with brompheniramine maleate 4 mg

Bromfenex-PD, Bromfed-PD, Dallergy-JR, ULTRAbrom PD: pseudoephedrine HCl 60 mg with brompheniramine maleate 6 mg

Bromo-Seltzer: acetaminophen 325 mg, citric acid 2.224 g, sodium bicarbonate 2.781 g/capful measure

Butibel: belladonna extract 15 mg (0.187 mg of alkaloids of belladonna leaf) with butabarbital sodium 15 mg

Butibel Elixir: belladonna extract 15 mg with butabarbital sodium 15 mg in each 5 ml

Cafergot, Ercaf, and Wigraine: ergotamine tartrate 1 mg with caffeine 100 mg

Cafergot Suppositories, Cafatine, Cafetrate, Wigraine: ergotamine tartrate 2 mg, caffeine 100 mg

Cafergot-PB: levoalkaloids of belladonna 0.125 mg with pentobarbital sodium 30 mg

Caladryl Lotion: diphenhydramine HCl 1% with calamine 8%, camphor 0.1%, alcohol 2.2%

Capital with Codeine Suspension or **Tylenol with Codeine Elixir:** acetaminophen 120 mg/5 ml with codeine 12 mg/5 ml

Capozide 25/15: captopril 25 mg with hydrochlorothiazide 15 mg
Capozide 25/25: captopril 25 mg with hydrochlorothiazide 25 mg
Capozide 50/15: captopril 50 mg with hydrochlorothiazide 15 mg
Capozide 50/25: captopril 50 mg with hydrochlorothiazide 25 mg
Carisoprodol Compound, Sodol Compound, Soma Compound: carisoprodol 200 mg with aspirin 325 mg
Chardonna-2: belladonna extract 15 mg with phenobarbital 15 mg
Children's Advil Cold: ibuprofen 100 mg and pseudoephedrine HCl 15 mg/5 ml
Cheracol Cough Syrup, Gani-Tuss Liquid, Guiatuss AC Syrup, Halotussin AC Liquid, Mytussin AC Cough Syrup, Romilar AC Liquid, Tuss-Organidin NR Liquid, Tuss-Organidin-S NR Liquid: codeine phosphate 10 mg and guaifenesin 100 mg/5 ml
Ciprodex Otic: ciprofloxacin 0.3% with dexamethasone 0.1%
Claritin-D 12 Hour: loratadine 5 mg with pseudoephedrine sulfate 120 mg
Claritin-D 24 Hour: loratadine 10 mg with pseudoephedrine sulfate 240 mg
Clorpres: clonidine HCl 0.1 mg with chlorithalidone 15 mg; clonidine HCl 0.2 mg with chlorithalidone 15 mg; clonidine HCl 0.3 mg with chlorithalidone 15 mg
CombiPatch: estradiol 0.05 mg with norethindrone acetate 0.14 mg; estradiol 0.05 mg with norethindrone acetate 0.25 mg
Combipres 0.1: clonidine HCl 0.1 mg with chlorthalidone 15 mg
Combipres 0.2: clonidine HCl 0.2 mg with chlorthalidone 15 mg
Combipres 0.3: clonidine HCl 0.3 mg with chlorthalidone 15 mg
Combivent: albuterol sulfate 103 µg with ipratropium bromide 18 µg
Combivir: lamivudine 150 mg with zidovudine 300 mg
Comtrex Allergy-Sinus, Actifed Cold and Sinus Maximum, Good Sense Maximum Sinus, Sine-off Sinus Medicine, Sinutab Maximum Strength Sinus Allergy: pseudoephedrine HCl 30 mg with chlorpheniramine maleate 2 mg and acetaminophen 500 mg
Corzide 40/5: bendroflumethiazide 5 mg with nadolol 40 mg
Corzide 80/5: bendroflumethiazide 5 mg with nadolol 80 mg
Cosopt: dorzolamide HCl 2% with timolol maleate 0.5% in 5, 10 ml
Cystex: methenamine 162 mg, sodium salicylate 162.5 mg, benzoic acid 32 mg
Darvocet-N 50, Propoxyphene Napsylate with Acetaminophen Tablets: acetaminophen 325 mg with propoxyphene napsylate 50 mg
Darvocet-N 100, Propacet 100: propoxyphene napsylate 100 mg with acetaminophen 650 mg
DarvonA 500: propoxyphene napsylate 100 mg with acetaminophen 500 mg
Darvon Compound-65 Pulvules: aspirin 389 mg with caffeine 32.4 mg, propoxyphene HCl 65 mg
Deconamine SR, Brexin-LA, Colfed-A, Deconomed, Rinade B.I.D, Kronofed-A, N D Clear, Time-Hist: pseudoephedrine hydrochloride 120 mg with chlorpheniramine maleate 8 mg
Demi-Regroton: chlorthalidone 25 mg with reserpine 0.125 mg

Diovan HCT: valsartan 160 mg and hydrochlorothiazide 12.5 mg; valsartan 80 mg with hydrochlorothiazide 12.5 mg

Diutensin-R: methyclothiazide 2.5 mg with reserpine 0.1 mg

Drixoral Cold and Allergy: pseudoephedrine sulfate 120 mg with dexbrompheneramine 6 mg

Dristan Cold Non-Drowsy Maximum Strength, Mapap Sinus Maximum Strength, Nasal Decongestant Sinus Non-Drowsy, Ornex No Drowsiness Maximum Strength, Sine-off No Drowsiness Formula, Sinutab Sinus Without Drowsiness Formula, Sinus-Relief Maximum Strength, Sudafed Sinus Headache Non-Drowsy, SudoGest Sinus Maximum Relief, Tavist Sinus Maximum Strength, Tylenol Sinus Non-Drowsy Maximum Strength: pseudoephedrine HCl 30 mg, acetaminophen 500 mg

DuoNeb Inh Sol: ipratropium HBr 0.5 mg and albuterol sulfate 3 mg/3 ml

Duratuss, Entex PSE, Guai-Vent/PSE, Guaifenex PSE 120, Guaimax-D: pseudoephedrine HCl 120 mg with guaifenesin 600 mg

Duratuss HD Elixir, Hydro-Tussin HD, Su-Tuss HD: pseudoephedrine HCl 30 mg with hydrocodone bitartrate 2.5 mg and guaifenesin 100 mg per 5 ml

Dyazide: hydrochlorothiazide 25 mg with triamterene 37.5 mg

Empirin with Codeine 30 mg (No. 3): aspirin 325 mg with codeine phosphate 30 mg

Empirin with Codeine 60 mg (No. 4): aspirin 325 mg with codeine phosphate 60 mg

Enduronyl: deserpidine 0.25 mg with methylclothiazide 5 mg

Enduronyl-Forte: deserpidine 0.5 mg with methylclothiazide 5 mg

Entex LA: guaifenesin 400 mg with phenylephrine HCl 30 mg

E-Pilo and PE (products 1 through 6): epinephrine bitartrate 1% with pilocarpine HCl 1%, 2%, 3%, 4%, 6%

Esgic, Fioricet, Repan: acetaminophen 325 mg with butalbital 50 mg and caffeine 40 mg

Esgic-Plus: butalbital 50 mg with acetaminophen 500 mg and caffeine 40 mg

Esimil: guanethidine monosulfate 10 mg with hydrochlorothiazide 25 mg

Estratest, Syntest: methyltestosterone 2.5 mg with esterified estrogens 1.25 mg

Estratest HS, Syntest HS: methyltestosterone 1.25 mg with esterified estrogens 0.625 mg

Etrafon 2-10, Triavil 2-10: perphenazine 2 mg with amitriptyline HCl 10 mg

Etrafon, Triavil 2-25: perphenazine 2 mg with amitriptyline HCl 25 mg

Etrafon-A, Triavil 4-10: perphenazine 4 mg with amitriptyline HCl 10 mg

Etrafon-Forte, Triavil 4-25: perphenazine 4 mg with amitriptyline HCl 25 mg

Excedrin Migraine, Excedrin Extra Strength: aspirin 250 mg with acetaminophen 250 mg and caffeine 65 mg

Excedrin PM Liquid: acetaminophen 167 mg and diphenhydramine HCl 8.3 mg/5 ml or acetaminophen 1000 mg and diphenhydramine HCl 50 mg/30 ml

Excedrin PM (caplets), Bufferin AF Nighttime: acetaminophen 500 mg with diphenhydramine citrate 38 mg

Excedrin PM (liquigels), Bayer Select Maximum Strength Night Time Pain Relief, Sominex Pain Relief, Tycolene PM, Extra Strength Tylenol PM (gelcaps): acetaminophen 500 mg with diphenhydramine HCl 25 mg

Femhrt: norethindrone acetate 1 mg with ethinyl estradiol 5 μg

Fioricet with Codeine: acetaminophen 325 mg, butalbital 50 mg, caffeine 40 mg, and codeine phosphate 30 mg

Fiorinal, Butalbital Compound: aspirin 325 mg with butalbital 50 mg, caffeine 40 mg

Fiorinal with Codeine No. 3: aspirin 325 mg with butalbital 50 mg, caffeine 40 mg, codeine phosphate 30 mg

Flexaphen: chlorzoxazone 250 mg with acetaminophen 300 mg

Glucovance: glyburide 1.25 mg with metformin HCl 250 mg; glyburide 2.5 mg with metformin HCl 500 mg; glyburide 5 mg with metformin HCl 500 mg

Goody's Extra Strength Headache Powder: aspirin 520 mg with acetaminophen 260 mg and caffeine 32.5 mg per powder

Goody's Body Pain Powder: aspirin 500 mg with acetaminophen 325 mg

Helidac: bismuth subsalicylate 262.4 mg with metronidazole 250 mg (tabs) plus tetracycline 500 mg (caps)

Humibid DM, Fenesin DM, Guaifenex DM, Iobid DM, Muco-Fen-DM: dextromethorphan hydrobromide 30 mg with guaifenesin 600 mg

Hycodan, Hydromet, Hydromide, Hydropane, Tussigon: hydrocodone bitartrate 5 mg with homatropine methylbromide 1.5 mg

Hydrap-ES, Ser-Ap-Es, Tri-Hydroserpine, Marpres: hydrochlorothiazide 15 mg with hydralazine 25 mg and reserpine 0.1 mg

Hydropres-50, Hydro-Serp, Hydroserpine No. 2: reserpine 0.125 mg with hydrochlorothiazide 50 mg

Hydroserpine No. 1, Salutensin-Demi: reserpine 0.125 mg with hydrochlorothiazide 25 mg

Hyphed Syrup, Histinex PV, P-V-Tussin, Tussend Syrup: hydrocodone bitartrate 2.5 mg with pseudoephedrine HCl 30 mg and chlorpheniramine maleate 2 mg in each 5 ml

Hyzaar: losartan potassium 50 mg with hydrochlorothiazide 12.5 mg or losartan potassium 100 mg with hydrochlorothiazide 25 mg

Iberet-500 Filmtabs, Generet-500: iron 105 mg, vitamins B_1 6 mg, B_2 6 mg, B_3 30 mg, B_5 10 mg, B_6 5 mg, B_{12} 25 μg, and C 500 mg

Inderide 40/25, Propranolol HCl, Hydrochlorothiazide Tablets 40/25: propranolol HCl 40 mg with hydrochlorothiazide 25 mg

Inderide 80/25, Propranolol HCl, Hydrochlorothiazide Tablets 80/25: propranolol HCl 80 mg with hydrochlorothiazide 25 mg

Kaletra: lopinavir 133.3 mg with ritonavir 33.3 mg

Kaletra Oral Solution: lopinavir 80 mg with ritonavir 20 mg/ml

Legatrin PM: acetaminophen 500 mg with diphenhydramine hydrochloride 50 mg

Lexxel: enalapril maleate 5 mg with felodipine 5 mg; enalapril

maleate 5 mg with felodipine 2.5 mg
Librax: clidinium 2.5 mg with chlordiazepoxide HCl 5 mg
Lopressor HCT 50/25: metoprolol tartrate 50 mg with hydrochlorothiazide 25 mg
Lopressor HCT 100/25: metoprolol tartrate 100 mg with hydrochlorothiazide 25 mg
Lopressor HCT 100/50: metoprolol tartrate 100 mg with hydrochlorothiazide 50 mg
Lorcet-HD, Hydrogesic, Hy-Phen, Margesic H, Lortab 5/500, Anexsia 5/500, Panacet 5/500: hydrocodone bitartrate 5 mg with acetaminophen 500 mg
Lorcet Plus, Anexsia 7.5/650: hydrocodone bitartrate 7.5 mg with acetaminophen 650 mg
Lorcet 10/650: hydrocodone 10 mg with acetaminophen 650 mg
Lortab ASA, Alor 5/500, Azdone, Damason-P, Panasal 5/500: hydrocodone bitartrate 5 mg with aspirin 500 mg
Lortab 2.5/500: hydrocodone 2.5 mg with acetaminophen 500 mg
Lortab 7.5/500: hydrocodone bitartrate 7.5 with acetaminophen 500 mg
Lortab Elixir: 2.5 mg hydrocodone with 167 mg acetaminophen in 5 ml
Lotensin HCT 5/6.25: benazepril 5 mg and hydrochlorothiazide 6.25 mg
Lotensin HCT 10/12.5: benazepril 10 mg and hydrochlorothiazide 12.5 mg
Lotensin HCT 20/12.5: benazepril 20 mg with hydrochlorothiazide 12.5 mg
Lotensin HCT 20/25: benazepril 20 mg with hydrochlorothiazide 25 mg
Lotrel 2.5/10: amlidopine 2.5 mg with benazepril HCl 10 mg
Lotrel 5/10: amlidopine 5 mg with benazepril HCl 10 mg
Lotrel 5/20: amlidopine 5 mg with benazepril HCl 20 mg
Lotrel 10/20: amlidopine 10 mg with benazepril HCl 20 mg
Lotrisone: clotrimazole 1% and betamethasone dipropionate 0.05%
Lufyllin-EPG Elixir: ephedrine HCl 24 mg with dyphylline 150 mg and guaifenesin 300 mg and phenobarbital 24 mg/15 ml
Maxzide-25 MG: triamterene 37.5 mg with hydrochlorothiazide 25 mg
Maxzide: hydrochlorothiazide 50 mg with triamterene 75 mg
Melagesic PM: acetaminophen 500 mg with melatononin 1.5 mg
Metaglip: glipizide 2.5 mg with metformin HCl 250 mg; glipizide 2.5 mg with metformin HCl 500 mg; glipizide 5 mg with metformin HCl 500 mg
Metatensin No. 2: reserpine 0.1 mg with trichlormethiazide 2 mg
Metatensin No. 4: reserpine 0.1 mg with trichlormethiazide 4 mg
Micardis HCT: telmisartan 40 mg with hydrochlorothiazide 12.5 mg; telmisartan 80 mg with hydrochlorothiazide 12.5 mg
Micranin: meprobamate 200 mg with aspirin 325 mg
Midol Maximum Strength PMS Caplets: acetaminophen 500 mg with caffeine 60 mg, pamabrom 25 mg, and pyrilamine maleate 15 mg
Midol PM, Compoze NightTime Sleep Aid, 40 Winks, Maximum Strength Nytol, SnoozeFast, Sominex, Twilite: diphenhydramine 50 mg

Minizide 1: prazosin HCl 1 mg with polythiazide 0.5 mg
Minizide 2: prazosin HCl 2 mg with polythiazide 0.5 mg
Minizide 5: prazosin HCl 5 mg with polythiazide 0.5 mg
Moduretic: amiloride HCl 5 mg with hydrochlorothiazide 50 mg
Monopril HCT: fosinopril sodium 10 mg with hydrochlorothiazide 12.5 mg; fosinopril sodium 20 mg with hydrochlorothiazide 12.5 mg
Motrin Sinus Headache, Advil Cold and Sinus, Advil Flu and Body Ache, Dristan Sinus: ibuprofen 200 mg, pseudoephedrine HCl 30 mg
Murocoll-2: scopolamine hydrobromide 0.3%, phenylephrine hydrochloride 10% drops
MycoLog II, Mycogen II, Myco-Triacet II, Mytrex: triamcinolone acetonide 0.1% and nystatin 100,000 U/g (ointment or cream)
Mylanta Liquid: aluminum hydroxide 200 mg, magnesium hydroxide 200 mg, simethicone 20 mg
Naldecon-DX Senior, Diabetic Tussin Maximum Strength DM, Robitussin Cough and Congestion Formula: dextromethorphan hydrobromide 10 mg/5 ml with guaifenesin 200 mg/5 ml
Norco: hydrocodone bitartrate 10 mg with aspirin 325 mg
Norco 5/325: hydrocodone bitartrate 5 mg and acetaminophen 325 mg
Norgesic: orphenadrine citrate 25 mg with aspirin 385 mg, caffeine 30 mg
Norgesic Forte: orphenadrine citrate 50 mg with aspirin 770 mg, caffeine 60 mg
Ortho-Prefest: estradiol 1.0 mg and norgestimate 0.09 mg
Palgic-D, Coldec-D: pseudoephedrine HCl 90 mg with carbinoxamine maleate 8 mg
Pancof XP: hydrocodone bitartrate 3 mg with guaifenesin 100 mg and pseudoephedrine HCl 15 mg in each 5 ml
Parepectolin: attapulgite 600 mg/15 ml
Pediazole, Eryzole: erythromycin ethlysuccinate (equivalent to 200 mg of erythromycin) per 5 ml with sulfisoxazole acetyl (equivalent to 600 mg of sulfisoxazole) per 5 ml
Pepcid Complete: calcium carbonate 800 mg, magnesium hydroxide 165 mg, famotidine 10 mg
Percocet (note many available strengths)—**Percocet 2.5/325:** oxycodone hydrochloride 2.5 mg with acetaminophen 325 mg; **Percocet 5/325:** oxycodone hydrochloride 5 mg with acetaminophen 325 mg; **Percocet 7.5/500:** oxycodone hydrochloride 7. 5 mg with acetaminophen 500 mg; **Percocet 10/325:** oxycodone hydrochloride 10 mg with acetaminophen 325 mg; **Percocet 10/650:** oxycodone hydrochloride 10 mg with acetaminophen 650 mg
Percodan, Roxiprin: oxycodone hydrochloride 4.5 mg, oxycodone terephthalate 0.38 mg, and aspirin 325 mg
Percodan-Demi: aspirin 325 mg with oxycodone HCl 2.25 mg, oxycodone terephthalate 0.19 mg
Percogesic, Aceta-Gesic, Major-Gesic, Phenylgesic: acetaminophen 325 mg with phenyltoloxamine citrate 30 mg
Peri-Colace, D-S-S Plus 100, Genasoft Plus, Peri-Dos: docusate sodium 100 mg with casanthranol 30 mg

Pravigard PAC: pravastatin 20 mg with buffered aspirin 81 mg; pravastatin 40 mg with buffered aspirin 81 mg; pravastatin 80 mg with buffered aspirin 81 mg; pravastatin 20 mg with buffered aspirin 325 mg; pravastatin 40 mg with buffered aspirin 325 mg; pravastatin 80 mg with buffered aspirin 325 mg

Premphase: conjugated estrogens 0.625 mg with medroxyprogesterone acetate 5 mg

Prempro: conjugated estrogens 0.625 mg with medroxyprogesterone acetate 2.5 mg; conjugated estrogens 0.625 mg with medroxyprogesterone acetate 5 mg

Prevpac: lansoprazole 30 mg (2 caps), amoxicillin 500 mg (4 caps), and clarithromycin 500 mg (2 tabs)

Primatene Dual Action: ephedrine HCl 12.5 mg with theophylline 60 mg and guaifenesen 100 mg

Primatene: ephedrine HCl 24 mg with theophylline 130 mg and phenobarbital 7.5 mg

Primaxin IM: imipenem 500 mg with cilastatin 500 mg; imipenem 750 mg with cilastatin 750 mg for injection

Primaxin IV: imipenem 250 mg with cilastatin 250 mg; imipenem 500 mg with cilastatin 500 mg for injection

Profen II Tabs: pseudoephedrine HCl 45 mg with guaifenesin 800 mg

Pyridium Plus: phenazopyridine HCl 150 mg with hyoscyamine hydrobromide 0.3 mg and butabarbital 15 mg

Rauzide: bendroflumethiazide 4 mg with rauwolfia serpentina powdered 50 mg

Rebetron: ribavirin 200 mg and interferon alfa-2b 3 million IU

Regroton: reserpine 0.25 mg with chlorthalidone 50 mg

Renese-R: reserpine 0.25 mg with polythiazide 2 mg

Rifamate: isoniazid 150 mg with rifampin 300 mg

Rifater: isoniazid 50 mg with rifampin 120 mg and pyrazinamide 300 mg

Robitussin-DM, Robitussin Sugar Free Cough, Cheracol Plus, Cheracol-D, Genatuss DM, Mytussin DM, Tussin DM, Diabetic Tussin DM, Extra Action Cough Syrup, Guiatuss-DM, Gani-Tuss DMNR, Guiafenesin DMNR, Situssin DM, Phanatuss DM, Tolu-Sed DM: dextromethorphan hydrobromide 10 mg/5 ml with guaifenesin 100 mg/5 ml

Seasonale: ethinyl estradiol 0.03 mg with levonorgestrel 0.15 mg

Singlet for Adults Tablets, Simplet Tablets, TheraFlu Cough and Cold Medicine Powder, Triaminicin Cold-Allergy Sinus Medicine: pseudoephedrine HCl 60 mg, chlorpheniramine maleate 4 mg, and acetaminophen 650 mg

Stalveo 50: carbidopa 12.5 mg with levodopa 50 mg and entacapone 200 mg

Stalveo 100: carbidopa 25 mg with levodopa 100 mg and entacapone 200 mg

Stalveo 150: carbidopa 37.5 mg with levodopa 150 mg and entacapone 200 mg

Suboxone: buprenorphine 2 mg with naloxone 0.5 mg; buprenorphine 8 mg with naloxone 2 mg

Synalgos-DC, DHC Plus: aspirin 356.4 mg with caffeine 30 mg and dihydrocodeine bitartrate 16 mg

Talacen: pentazocine HCl 25 mg with acetaminophen 650 mg

Talwin Compound Caplets: pentazocine HCl 12.5 mg with aspirin 325 mg

Tarka 1:240: trandolapril 1 mg with verapamil 240 mg

Tarka 2:180: trandolapril 2 mg with verapamil 180 mg

Tarka 2:240: trandolapril 2 mg with verapamil 240 mg

Tarka 4:240: trandolapril 4 mg with verapamil 240 mg

Teczem: enalapril maleate 5 mg with diltiazem maleate 180 mg

Tenoretic 50: atenolol 50 mg with chlorthalidone 25 mg

Tenoretic 100: atenolol 100 mg with chlorthalidone 25 mg

Teveten HCT: eprosartan 600 mg with hydrochlorothiazide 12.5 mg; eprosartan 600 mg with hydrochlorothiazide 25 mg

Timentin Inj: ticarcillin disodium 3 g with clavulanate potassium 100 mg

Timolide 10/25: timolol maleate 10 mg with hydrochlorothiazide 25 mg

TracTabs 2X: methenamine 120 mg, methylene blue 6 mg, phenyl salicylate 30 mg, atropine 0.06 mg, hyoscyamine SO_4 0.03 mg, benzoic acid 7.5 mg

Triad, Esgic, Margesic, Medigesic: butalbital 50 mg with acetaminophen 325 mg and caffeine 40 mg

Triaminic Cough and Cold Soft Chews, Triaminic Cough Soft Chews: pseudoephedrine HCl 15 mg with dextromethorphan HBr 5 mg and chlorpheniramine maleate 1 mg

Triaminic Cold and Cough Liquid, Tri-Acting Cold and Cough, Thera-Hist Cold and Cough, PediaCare Multi-Symptom Cold, PediaCare Cough-Cold, Kid Care Children's Cough/Cold: pseudoephedrine HCl 15 mg with dextromethorphan HBr 5 mg and chlorpheniramine maleate 1 mg/5 ml

TriHemic 600: iron 115 mg, vitamin B_{12} 25 μg, vitamin C 600 mg, folic acid 1 mg, and intrinsic factor 75 mg

Trinalin Repetabs: pseudoephedrine HCl 120 mg with azatadine maleate 1 mg

Trinsicon, Feotrinsic, Foltin, Livitrinsic-F, Contrin: iron 110 mg, vitamin B_{12} 15 μg, vitamin C 7.5 mg, folic acid 0.5 mg, and intrinsic factor 240 mg

Trizivir: abacavir sulfate 300 mg, lamivudine 150 mg, and zidovudine 300 mg

Tussafed HC Syrup, Donatussin DC: hydrocodone bitartrate 2.5 mg with phenylephrine HCl 7.5 mg and guaifenesin 50 mg in each 5 ml

Tussionex Pennkinetic Suspension: chlorpheniramine (polistirnex) 8 mg and hydrocodone (polistirnex) 10 mg in 5 ml

Tylenol Flu Night Time Maximum Strength (powder): pseudoephedrine HCl 60 mg, diphenhydramine HCl 50 mg, and acetaminophen 1000 mg dissolved in 6 oz hot water

Tylenol Children's Sinus Suspension: acetaminophen 160 mg with pseudoephedrine HCl 15 mg

Tylenol PM Extra Strength: acetaminophen 500 mg with diphenhydramine 25 mg

Tylenol with Codeine No. 2: acetaminophen 300 mg with codeine phosphate 15 mg

Tylenol with Codeine No. 3: acetaminophen 300 mg with codeine phosphate 30 mg

Tylenol with Codeine No. 4: acetaminophen 300 mg with codeine phosphate 60 mg

Tylox, Roxicet 5/500, Roxilox: acetaminophen 500 mg with oxycodone HCl 5 mg

Ultracet: acetaminophen 325 mg and tramadol HCl 37.5 mg

Unasyn Inj: ampicillin sodium 1 g with sulbactam sodium 500 mg; ampicillin sodium 2 g with sulbactam sodium 1 g; ampicillin sodium 10 mg with sulbactam sodium 5 g

Uniretic 7.5: moexipril HCl 7.5 mg with hydrochlorothiazide 12.5 mg

Uniretic 15: moexipril HCl 15 mg with hydrochlorothiazide 25 mg

Uniretic: moexipril HCl 15 mg with hydrochlorothiazide 12.5 mg

Unisom Nighttime Sleep Aid: doxylamine succinate 25 mg

Unisom With Pain Relief: diphenhydramine HCl 50 mg with acetaminophen 650 mg

Urised, Uritin, Atrosept, Dolsed, UAA, Uridon Modified: methenamine 40.8 mg, phenyl salicylate 18.1 mg, atropine 0.03 mg, hyoscyamine 0.03 mg, and methylene blue 5.4 mg

Urisedamine: methenamine mandelate 500 mg with hyoscyamine 0.15 mg

Vanquish Caplets: aspirin 227 mg with acetaminophen 194 mg, caffeine 33 mg, and buffers

Vaseretic 5-12.5: enalapril maleate 5 mg with hydrochlorothiazide 12.5 mg

Vaseretic 10-25: enalapril maleate 10 mg with hydrochlorothiazide 25 mg

Vicks Children's NyQuil Cough/Cold Liquid, Vicks Pediatric Formula 44 Cough and Cold Liquid, All-Nite Children's Cough and Cold, Nitetime Children's: pseudoephedrine HCl 10 mg, chlorpheniramine maleate 0.67 mg, dextromethorphan hydrobromide 5 mg/5 ml

Vicks Chloraseptic Sore Throat Lozenges: benzocaine 6 mg with 10 mg menthol; **Children's Vicks Chloroseptic Spray:** phenol 0.5%; **Vicks Chloraseptic Mouthrinse:** phenol 1.4%

Vicks 44D Cough and Head Congestion, Robitussin Honey Cough and Cold: dextromethorphan hydrobromide 10 mg/5 ml with pseudoephedrine HCl 20 mg/5 ml

Vicodin Tuss Syrup, Vitussin Syrup, Codiclear HD Syrup, Hycosin Expectorant, Hycotuss Expectorant, Hydrocodone GF Syrup, Kwelcof Liquid: hydrocodone bitartrate 5 mg with guaifenesin 100 mg/5 ml

Vicodin: acetaminophen 500 mg with hydrocodone bitartrate 5.0 mg

Vicodin-ES: acetaminophen 750 mg with hydrocodone bitartrate 7.5 mg

Vicodin-HP: acetaminophen 660 mg with hydrocodone bitartrate 10 mg

Vicoprofen: hydrocodone bitartrate 7.5 mg with ibuprofen 200 mg

Wigraine, Cafergot, Ercaf: ergotamine tartrate 1 mg and caffeine 100 mg

Wigraine Suppositories, Cafatine, Cafetrate: ergotamine tartrate 2 mg, caffeine 100 mg

Zestoretic 10/12.5, Prinzide: lisinopril 10 mg with hydrochlorothiazide 12.5 mg

Zestoretic 20/12.5, Prinzide 12.5: lisinopril 20 mg with hydrochlorothiazide 12.5 mg

Zestoretic 20/25, Prinzide 25: lisinopril 20 mg with hydrochlorothiazide 25 mg

Ziac 2.5: bisoprolol fumarate 2.5 mg with hydrochlorothiazide 6.25 mg
Ziac 5: bisoprolol fumarate 5.0 mg with hydrochlorothiazide 6.25 mg
Ziac 10: bisoprolol fumarate 10 mg with hydrochlorothiazide 6.25 mg
Ziradyl Lotion: diphenhydramine HCl 1% with zinc oxide 2%, alcohol 2%, camphor, and parabens
Zosyn: piperacillin 2 g with tazobactam 0.25 g; piperacillin 3 g with tazobactam 0.375 g, piperacillin 4 g with tazobactam 0.5 g and piperacillin 36 g with tazobactam 4.5 g in vials for IV administration
Zydone: hydrocodone bitartrate 5 mg and acetaminophen 400 mg; or hydrocodone bitartrate 7.5 mg and acetaminophen 400 mg; or hydrocodone bitartrate 10 mg and acetaminophen 400 mg
Zyrtec-D 12 Hr: cetirizine HCl 5 mg with pseudoephedrine HCl 120 mg

Appendix G

Dose Calculations by Weight

Manufacturer-recommended doses are based on extensive clinical trials and are usually intended for the average, healthy adult male of average weight and age. Thus age, sex, weight, and chronic diseases of the major organs of metabolism (liver) and excretion (kidney) may affect the usual safe and effective FDA-approved dose recommendations.

Creatine clearance, peak and trough blood levels, and symptomatic patient response are often used to titrate doses for a given therapeutic effect.

Dentists seldom treat infants, but doses for pediatric and geriatric patients require an adjustment downward from the usual adult dose.

Geriatric patients may be particularly susceptible to effects produced by CNS depressants or drugs that affect renal function.

No reliable general rule for dose calculations can supplant clinically derived doses, and many drug monographs now list doses for children based on a mg/kg or mg/lb basis. Children's doses are also based on a reduction of adult doses as determined by body surface area and weight.

Clark's rule has been used for many years as a general guide for calculating children's doses.

Clark's Rule:

$$\frac{\text{Child's weight (lb)}}{150} \times \text{Adult dose} = \text{Child's dose}$$

weight lb/kg chart

1 kg = 2.2 lb

kilograms (kg)	pounds (lb)
10	22
20	44
25	55
30	66
35	77
40	88
45	99
50	110
55	121
60	132

Appendix H

Herbal and Nonherbal Remedies

Aloe vera
(Aloe vera, Aloe barbadensis)
Other names: Burn plant, curaçao aloes
Class: Herbal remedy
Major ingredients: The term *aloe vera* conventionally refers to the gel within the aloe leaf. (The glands in the leaf surface contain a different and unsafe substance called "drug aloe," and are not present, save in trace amounts, in aloe gel products.) The major active ingredients of aloe vera gel are thought to be its polysaccharides, especially one called *acemannan.* Other potentially important constituents include sitosterols and lignins.

Claimed actions: Aloe vera juice is widely credited with the ability to enhance skin regeneration after burns or wounds, but randomized controlled trials (RCTs) of aloe for speeding resolution of sunburn, skin damage caused by radiation therapy, and wounds have generally failed to find benefit. Based on the same putative tissue healing effect, aloe has been recommended for treatment of stomach ulcers and other gastrointestinal tract diseases, but there is no meaningful supporting evidence for these uses. Other claimed effects that lack supporting evidence from properly designed RCTs include immune stimulation and suppression of HIV infection. (Acemannan, however, is an FDA-approved treatment for fibrosarcoma in cats and dogs.) Two RCTs indicate that oral aloe gel might have a hypoglycemic effect in type 2 diabetes, but it has been suggested that these benefits were due to trace contamination of the aloe gel with parts of the leaf glands, supplying some drug aloe.
Uses: Preliminary RCTs of moderate-to-low quality suggest that aloe vera cream may offer benefit for seborrhea, psoriasis, and genital herpes, reducing symptoms and speeding resolution. Other uses based on the claimed actions noted previously lack RCT support.
Administration: In most of the studies that produced positive results for seborrhea, psoriasis, and genital herpes, aloe was applied as a cream containing 0.5% of aloe extract administered 3 times daily. One study used a cream containing 30% aloe gel. Whole aloe gel (rather than cream) applied topically has generally shown less benefit. A typical oral dose of aloe vera juice is 1 tablespoon twice daily. Maximum safe doses in pregnant or nursing women, young children, and individuals with severe hepatic or renal disease have not been established.
Side effects: Use of aloe gel, either internally or externally, has not been associated with any signifi-

cant side effects, other than nonspecific digestive distress or allergic reactions. Drug aloe (made from the leaf glands, and not generally available in the United States) is a strong laxative and should not be used.

Dental considerations:
Some people may swish or gargle with aloe preparation in hopes of treating periodontal disease. There is no evidence for or against this use.

Drug interactions: If aloe vera products can in fact reduce blood sugar in type 2 diabetes, potentiation interactions with oral hypoglycemics would be a possibility. However, no such interactions have as yet been reported.

Bilberry fruit
(Vaccinium myrtillus)

Other names: Blueberry, huckleberry, hurtleberry, myrtilli fructus

Class: Herbal remedy

Major ingredients: The fruit is the medicinal part under discussion in this article. (Bilberry leaf is an entirely different and much less common product, with different uses, often proposed for glucose control.) The proposed active ingredients of bilberry fruit are its anthocyanosides. Other constituents include flavone glycosides, iridoids, tannins, caffeic acid derivatives, and fruit acids.

Claimed actions: The anthocyanosides in bilberry have antioxidant properties. In vitro and other highly preliminary evidence suggests that they influence collagen metabolism by increasing cross-linkage of collagen fibers, inhibiting collagen degradation, promoting collagen biosynthesis, reducing inflammatory activity, and scavenging free radicals. The net effect may be decreased capillary permeability and hence reduced capillary leakage in venous insufficiency and ischemia reperfusion. Other in vitro studies hint that anthocyanosides may have an affinity for the retina, where they speed recovery of rhodopsin and alter enzymatic reactions in retinal tissues. At very high doses, anthocyanosides inhibit platelet aggregation.

Uses: Bilberry fruit is widely used in the belief that it enhances night vision, but the basis for this use rests largely on anecdotes and a few poorly controlled studies performed in the 1960s. More recent and better-designed RCTs have failed to find any benefit. However, weak evidence from small, poor-quality clinical trials hints at benefits in diabetic or hypertensive retinopathy, as well as venous insufficiency.

Administration: A typical dose of bilberry fruit is 160 mg twice a day of an extract standardized to contain 25% bilberry anthocyanosides. Maximum safe doses in pregnant or nursing women, young children, and individuals with severe hepatic or renal disease have not been established, but pregnant women have been given bilberry at the aforementioned dose in clinical trials.

Side effects: Animal and human trials indicate that bilberry fruit has a low order of toxicity. Reported side effects are limited to rare allergic reactions and nonspecific gastroinstestinal effects.

Dental considerations:
Ask why the product is being used.
Drug interactions: If taken in high doses, bilberry could conceivably potentiate anticoagulant or antiplatelet agents, but no such interactions have been reported.

Bistort
(Polygonum bistorta)
Other names: Adderwort, dragonwort, Easter mangiant, English serpentary, oderwort, osterick, passions, patience dock, snakeweed, sweet dock, twice writhen
Class: Herbal remedy
Major ingredients: Tannins.

Claimed actions: Astrigent, antidote for selected poisons or venoms, antidiarrheal and antiinflammatory.
Uses: Uses have included all forms of diarrhea and cholera. It has also been used in a mouth rinse for gum disease, canker sores, and stomatitis. Externally, uses include sores, wounds, and hemorrhage. It was used traditionally to treat insect bites, snake bites, gonorrhea, smallpox, measles, and intestinal worms.
Side effects: Increase in mucous production, irritation of the GI tract, and possible hepatic damage.
Administration: The leaves, roots, and rhizomes may be used to form a powder; also used as a tea, tincture, infusion, or ointment.
Dental considerations:
Awareness of patient use of product for sore throat or mouth rinse.
Drug interactions: Tinctures contain alcohol and should not be used with disulfiram.

Black cohosh
(Cimicifuga racemosa, Cimicifugae racemosae rhizoma)
Other names: Black snakeroot, baneberry
Class: Herbal remedy
Major ingredients: The active chemicals are described as triterpene glycosides (acetin, 27-deoxyacetin, cimigoside, cimicifugoside, and racemoside) along with phytosterin and flavone derivatives. Other constituents include ferulic acids, isoflavones, fatty acids, and a volatile oil. The fresh and dried rhizomes are the portion of the plant used.

Claimed actions: Black cohosh is not a typical phytoestrogen (plant-based substance with estrogenic actions), because none of its constituents bind to estrogen receptors. It has been hypothesized, though, that some unknown constituent(s) of black cohosh undergoes metabolic activation and acquires selective estrogen receptor modifier activity. Effects have been noted on estrogen receptors in bone (possibly reducing bone breakdown), the brain/hypothalamus (altering LH release and reducing vasomotor symptoms), and the vaginal cell wall (partially reversing atrophy). Uterus and breast estrogen receptors appear to be relatively unaffected.
Uses: Black cohosh is primarily used to treat menopausal syndrome. Limited evidence from placebo-controlled RCTs suggests that it can reduce hot flashes and vaginal dryness, without causing uterine hypertrophy. Black cohosh is also sometimes recommended for

treatment of premenstrual syndrome and dysmenorrhea disorders, but there is no meaningful evidence to support these uses.
Administration: The typical dosage of black cohosh is 1 or 2 tablets twice daily of a standardized extract manufactured to contain 1 mg of 27-deoxyaceteine per tablet. It has been suggested that black cohosh should not be used for more than 6 months except under the supervision of a physician.
Contraindications: The herb is not recommended for use by pregnant or nursing women.
Side effects: In clinical trials, use of black cohosh has not been associated with any significant side effects, other than occasional allergic reactions or nonspecific GI distress. However, there is one case report of autoimmune hepatitis apparently induced by the use of black cohosh. Overdosage may cause vomiting, headache, hypotension, and other symptoms.
Dental considerations:
Ask why the product is being used.
Drug interactions: Weak evidence hints that black cohosh can potentiate antihypertensive drugs.

Boswellia
(Boswellia serrata)
Other names: Frankincense, salai guggul
Class: Herbal remedy
Major ingredients: Boswellia is the dried oleo-resin made from the sap of the *Boswellia serrata* tree. Its major ingredients include boswellic acids and volatile oils.

Claimed actions: Whole boswellia as well as isolated boswellic acids have shown antiinflammatory effects in in vitro, animal, and preliminary human trials.
Uses: Preliminary RCTs suggest that boswellia might reduce symptoms of asthma, osteoarthritis, and inflammatory bowel disease, presumably through antiinflammatory effects. RCTs on boswellia for rheumatoid arthritis were of low quality and produced inconsistent results. Boswellic acids are undergoing study for palliative treatment of malignant glioma, in which they may reduce cerebral edema and possibly slow tumor growth.
Administration: In most clinical trials, boswellia was taken at a dose of 300 to 400 mg 3 times a day, in the form of an extract standardized to contain 37.5% boswellic acids. Higher doses have also been tried. Safety in pregnant or nursing women, young children, and individuals with severe hepatic or renal disease has not been established.
Side effects: No significant side effects, other than rare allergic reactions and nonspecific gastrointestinal distress, have been noted in clinical trials. However, these trials generally used a pharmaceutical grade extract of the herb boswellia, or simply purified boswellic acids. Preparations made from the whole herb, or under less careful supervision, might present additional risks.
Dental considerations:
Ask why the product is being used.
Drug interactions: No dental drug interactions are reported.

Butterbur
(Petasites hybridus, P. albus, P. vulgaris)

Other names: Petasin, blatterdock, butterfly dock, capdockin, flapperdock, umbrella leaves
Class: Herbal remedy
Major ingredients: The entire plant is used medically. The major active ingredients are thought to be the sesquiterpene alcohol esters petasin and isopetasin. Hepatotoxic pyrrolizidine alkaloids are present in the crude herb, but are removed during the manufacturing process for standardized products.

Claimed actions: Preliminary evidence suggests that butterbur, presumably through its petasin and isopetasin content, has antiinflammatory, antispasmodic, and antihistaminic properties. Its proposed antiinflammatory effect appears to be mediated through peptidoleukotrienes rather than prostaglandins.
Uses: Standardized butterbur extract is widely used for prophylaxis of migraine headaches, but only one RCT supports this use. A double-blind comparative study without a placebo group found weak evidence that butterbur extract might have utility in allergic rhinitis. Another RCT failed to find butterbur effective for allergic skin disease. Other proposed uses based on the apparent actions of butterbur, but that lack meaningful supporting evidence, include asthma, bladder spasms, gallbladder pain, irritable bowel syndrome, musculoskeletal pain, and tension headaches.
Administration: The typical dosage of butterbur is 50 mg twice daily of an extract standardized to contain 7.5 mg of petasin and isopetasin; only products that are certified free from pyrrolizidine alkaloids should be used. Until further safety studies are performed, butterbur extract is not recommended for pregnant or nursing women, young children, or those with liver disease.
Side effects: In clinical trials of pharmaceutical grade standardized butterbur extract, no significant side effects were seen, other than occasional allergic reactions and nonspecific gastrointestinal irritation. However, there is one case report of cholestatic hepatitis apparently linked to use of butterbur extract. Unprocessed butterbur contains toxic pyrrolizidine alkaloids and should not be used at all.
Dental considerations:
Ask why the product is being used.
Drug interactions: No dental drug interactions are reported.

Chamomile
(*Matricaria chamomilla, Matricaria recutita, Anthemis nobilis,* and *Matricariae flos*)
Other names: Roman chamomile, common chamomile, German chamomile
Class: Herbal remedy
Major ingredients: Volatile oil containing alpha-bisabolol and other bisabolol derivatives (chamazulene, apigenin), various flavonoids, umbelliferone (a coumarin-like ingredient), and many other components. The portion of the plant used is the dried flower.

Claimed actions: Antiinflammatory, antispasmodic, antibacterial, carminative, and to promote wound healing.
Uses: Chamomile cream is widely

used to treat eczema and minor wounds, but there is only scant preliminary evidence to support this use. One RCT failed to find chamomile cream helpful for the treatment of radiation-therapy–induced skin damage; another failed to find benefit for apthous ulcers caused by 5-FU chemotherapy. One RCT did find evidence that inhalation of chamomile essential oil can reduce common cold symptoms. Oral chamomile has been used to treat inflammation and spasm in the GI tract, but this indication has no reliable supporting evidence.
Administration: Available in a variety of dose forms, including teas, infusions (external use), a mouth rinse, and oral dose forms.
Side effects: Slight risk of contact dermatitis: possible cross allergies with ragweed.
Dental considerations:
Ask why the product is being used. In patients taking warfarin or other oral anticoagulant, inquire about bleeding history. Inquire about unusual bleeding episodes following dental treatment.
Drug interactions: Evidence is lacking, but theoretically patients taking oral anticoagulants could show increased bleeding times. Possible risk of increased sedation with CNS depressants. Black cohosh may also inhibit CYP 3A4 activity, potentially changing serum levels of numerous drugs, but case reports are lacking.

Chaste tree, chasteberry
(Vitex agnus-castus, angi casti fructrus)

Other names: Chaste tree fruit, monk's pepper, chaste tree
Class: Herbal remedy
Major ingredients: Iridoid glycosides (agnuide and aucubin), flavonoids, progestins, testosterone, and multiple essential oils. The portion of the plant used is the dried, ripe fruit.

Claimed actions: Chasteberry is thought to inhibit the release of prolactin through action on dopamine receptors, although the evidence for this effect remains incomplete. It does not have a direct estrogen-like or progesterone-like effect.
Uses: Chasteberry is primarily used for the treatment of cyclic breast pain, a use supported by several RCTs. It may also produce benefits in premenstrual syndrome, although the evidence for this indication is largely limited to one well-designed RCT. Other proposed uses, all based on its prolactin-related actions and lacking significant clinical trial support, include amenorrhea, luteal phase defect, and infertility. There is no evidence or rationale to indicate that chasteberry is helpful for menopausal syndrome, but it is sometimes recommended for that purpose. There is a possible risk of increased ovulation and pregnancy in some women. Avoid use in pregnancy and lactation.
Administration: The typical dosage of chasteberry extract is 20 to 40 mg daily, usually in one AM dose.
Contraindications: Because of its effect on prolactin, chasteberry should not be used by pregnant or lactating women.

Side effects: Chasteberry was well tolerated in clinical trials, producing no more than nonspecific reactions. There is one case report of ovarian hyperstimulation apparently caused by chasteberry.

Dental considerations:
Ask why the product is being used.

Drug interactions: Based on its presumed mechanism of action, chasteberry might potentiate the action of bromocriptine. Dopamine receptor antagonists could in theory block some herbal effects.

Chondroitin sulfate
Other names: Chondroitin
Class: Nonherbal remedy
Major ingredient: Chondroitin sulfate is a mucopolysaccharide, that is, a glycosaminoglycan (GAG). It is found in mammalian cartilaginous tissue and is believed to play a role in flexibility. It is highly viscous and related chemically to sodium hyaluronate.

Claimed actions: It has useful viscoelastic properties suitable for use in selected types of ocular surgery, usually in combination with sodium hyaluronate. Orally administered GAGs are believed to concentrate in cartilage. Chondrocytes use GAGs to form a new cartilage matrix. It may also inhibit leukocyte elastase where high concentrations are associated with rheumatoid arthritis. Other properties may include bringing synovial fluid into the joint. All of these may contribute to reduced inflammatory activity in joints. Serum lipid–lowering and antithrombogenic effects have also been suggested.

Uses: The primary use of chondroitin as a dietary supplement is for the treatment of osteoarthritis, often in combination with glucosamine. The results of several RCTs of varying quality indicate that chondroitin can reduce symptoms to approximately the same extent as NSAIDs; weaker evidence supports a possible disease-modifying effect (slowing progressive joint damage). Chondroitin in an ophthalmic solution has been used to treat dry eyes. In combination with sodium hyaluronate it is used to support ocular surgery during cataract removal and lens implantation surgery. Its use in cardiovascular diseases remains in doubt.

Administration: A variety of oral dose forms are available, many in combination with glucosamine. Professionally used ophthalmic preparations are also available.

Side effects: Long-term side effects are unknown. GI complaints may be reported on occasion.

Dental considerations:
Ask why the product is being used. Arthritic patients may also be taking aspirin, NSAIDs, or arthritic disease modifying drugs in addition to chondroitin. Question the patient about other antiarthritic drugs used, including OTC drugs.

Drug interactions: None reported with dental drugs.

Conjugated linoleic acids
Other names: CLAs
Class: Nonherbal remedy
Major ingredients: Conjugated linoleic acids are mixed isomers of the essential omega-6 fatty acid linoleic acid.

Claimed actions: The essential

fatty acids in CLAs are hypothesized to affect fat metabolism. Limited and inconsistent evidence suggests that CLA supplements might increase fat metabolism while retaining lean muscle mass. CLA also has functional similarities to thiazolidinedione, which led to investigation of potential hypoglycemic effects; however, the limited evidence that is available suggests a possible *hyper*glycemic effect instead. Chemopreventive and hypolipidemic effects have also been hypothesized.

Uses: The most common use of CLA is as an aid to enhancing body composition, said to "burn fat" while helping to increase muscle mass. However, the clinical evidence for this effect is limited to small RCTs with inconsistent results. CLA does not appear to aid weight loss per se.

Administration: A typical dose is 3 to 5 g daily.

Contraindications: At this time, CLA should not be used by nursing mothers, because one clinical trial found that CLA supplements reduced the fat content of breast milk.

Side effects: CLA generally causes no side effects other than nonspecific digestive distress. Safety for pregnant women, young children, and individuals with liver disease has not been established.

Dental considerations:
Ask why the product is being used.

Drug interactions: One study found potential hyperglycemic effects with CLA, suggesting antagonistic interactions with hypoglycemic agents. However, no such interactions have been reported.

Coenzyme Q_{10}
Other names: CoQ_{10}, ubiquinone
Class: Nonherbal remedy
Major ingredients: Coenzyme Q_{10} is a cofactor found in all animal and plant cells. No dietary intake is needed, because the body manufactures it from other, widely available precursors.

Claimed actions: CoQ_{10} is an essential cofactor in the Kreb's cycle, playing a role in the aerobic production of ATP. Because heart muscle depends entirely on aerobic energy production, CoQ_{10} supplementation has been suggested as a way to enhance myocardial function. Further support for this treatment approach comes from evidence of reduced myocardial CoQ_{10} in people with congestive heart failure. In addition, certain medications often taken by individuals with heart disease, most notably statins, are thought to either suppress the endogenous production of CoQ_{10} or interfere with its function. This suggests a need for repletion; however, there remains little evidence as yet that exogenous CoQ_{10} provides any objective or subjective benefit for people using such medications (other than restoring normal CoQ_{10} levels). Other proposed uses of CoQ_{10} are based on its antioxidant properties, or other unknown mechanisms.

Uses: Incomplete and somewhat inconsistent evidence from double-blind trials suggests that CoQ_{10} may offer benefit as adjuvant therapy for congestive heart failure, enhancing cardiac performance. Weaker and again inconsistent evidence suggests possible benefits in cardiomyopathy, hypertension, cardiac reperfusion injury, and diabetes. Weak evidence hints that CoQ_{10} might reduce doxorubicin cardiotoxicity, improve renal function in chronic renal failure, enhance antibody response to hepatitis B vaccine, aid recovery from periodontal disease, reduce symptoms of muscular dystrophy and neurogenic atrophy, and slow the progression of Parkinson's disease. CoQ_{10} does not appear to be helpful as a sports supplement. See Drug Interactions below for a list of the medications for which CoQ_{10} has been recommended as a repletion agent.

Administration: A typical dosage of CoQ_{10} is 30 to 150 mg taken two or three times daily. Maximum safe doses in pregnant or nursing women, young children, and individuals with severe hepatic or renal disease have not been established.

Side effects: CoQ_{10} appears to offer little to no toxic risk. Use of CoQ_{10} in human trials continuing for up to 6 years has shown no serious side effects. Mild nonspecific gastrointestinal distress may occur. There have been a few questionable case reports of a CoQ_{10} withdrawal syndrome in individuals using the supplement for CHF.

Dental considerations:
Patients who believe that CoQ_{10} offers benefit for periodontal disease may be advised that the evidence for benefit with this expensive supplement is exceedingly weak.

Drug interactions: CoQ_{10} has a molecular similarity to vitamin K, which has led to concerns that CoQ_{10} use might antagonize the effects of warfarin. However, one study designed to evaluate this possibility found that use of CoQ_{10} caused no change in INR or warfarin dosage. Drugs thought to interfere with the production or action of CoQ_{10}, and therefore to potentially benefit from repletion, include the following: beta-blocking agents (alprenolol, metoprolol, and propranolol to a greater extent than timolol), clonidine, hydrochlorothiazide, methyldopa, oral hypoglycemics (dymelor, glyburide, phenformin, and tolazamide to a greater extent than chlorpropamide, glipizide, and tolbutamide,) phenothiazines, statins, and tricyclic antidepressants. The best evidence for tangible benefit with exogenous CoQ_{10} supplementation exists for statins and tricyclics, but the evidence is not strong.

Cranberry
(Vaccinium macrocarpon)
Class: Herbal remedy
Major ingredients: The berries are the medicinal part used. Cranberries contain a variety of proanthocyanidins, and these are its presumed active ingredients. Other constituents include fructose and various plant acids, such as citric and malic acid.

Claimed actions: Proanthocyanidin complexes in cranberry are thought to reduce bacterial adhesion to uroepithelial cells by impairing the action of bacterial adhesins, thus interfering with the early stages of infection. This pro-

posed mechanism would not tend to suggest benefits for infections that are already underway.
Uses: Limited evidence from RCTs indicates that regular use of cranberry juice concentrate can reduce the incidence of acute urinary tract infections in women. There is no evidence of benefit once an acute infection has begun. Effectiveness for treatment of chronic bacteriuria/pyuria is unclear. One small study suggests that cranberry juice might increase insulin secretion in individuals with type 2 diabetes, but the clinical significance of this finding is unclear.
Administration: Dry cranberry juice extract is often taken at a dose of 500 to 2000 mg, three times daily, depending on the product's concentration. Cranberry juice itself is very bad tasting, and palatable cranberry beverages contain little cranberry. Maximum safe doses in pregnant or nursing women, young children, and individuals with severe hepatic or renal disease have not been established.
Side effects: Use of cranberry concentrate is not associated with side effects other than occasional allergic reactions and nonspecific, mild gastrointestinal distress. Some concerns have been expressed about possible lithogenic actions of cranberry, but it appears that on balance intake is more likely to reduce risk of urolithiasis than to increase it.
Dental considerations:
Weak evidence hints that the proanthocyanidins in cranberry might offer dental benefits by impairing aggregation of the bacteria involved in plaque formation. However, because it is difficult to tolerate the taste of pure cranberry unless sweetener is added, this finding will not have practical use unless an artificial sweetener can be used.
Drug interactions: Based on case reports, it appears that high intake of cranberry can increase the action of warfarin, leading to excess anticoagulation. In addition, because cranberries reduce urinary pH, excretion of various drugs might be increased, including opiates, antidepressants, antipsychotics, and some antibiotics. However, there are no actual case reports of such interactions.

Creatine
Other names: Creatine monohydrate
Class: Nonherbal remedy
Major ingredient: Creatine is manufactured in the body from arginine, glycine, and methionine. There is no dietary requirement for creatine.

Claimed actions: Exogenous creatine is thought to increase muscle supplies of phosphocreatine, enabling more rapid restoration of ATP levels after a short, high-intensity burst of exertion. Increased creatine levels may also enhance nerve function. These two effects combined are the basis for the use of creatine in neuromuscular disorders. In mitochondrial disorders, exogenous creatine is thought to stabilize mitochondrial creatine kinase, decreasing demand on the damaged mitochondria. Creatine may also reduce lipid levels, through an as yet unidentified mechanism.
Uses: Numerous small RCTs indi-

cate that creatine may slightly increase performance in high-intensity repetitive burst exercise, but the evidence is not entirely consistent and rather specific parameters of duration and rest appear to be necessary for benefit. Creatine is not helpful in endurance exercise, and may or may not enhance resistance exercise capacity. Other small RCTs suggest possible benefit in congestive heart failure (increasing exercise tolerance) and hyperlipidemia. Results have been mixed in studies of creatine as an aid to recovery of muscle strength after limb immobilization, or as a treatment for a variety of neuromuscular and mitochondrial disorders.

Administration: A typical daily dose of creatine is 2 to 5 g daily. Athletes typically begin with a loading dose of 15 to 30 g daily for several days, but there is no evidence that this offers additional value.

Side effects: Creatine has a low order of toxicity, but long-term safety studies have not been performed. Common side effects of creatine supplementation include weight gain, mostly from water retention, as well as mild gastrointestinal distress and possibly muscle cramping and dehydration. Contrary to some reports, there is no evidence that creatine diminishes the body's ability to tolerate increased environmental temperatures. Maximum safe doses in pregnant or nursing women, young children, and individuals with severe hepatic or renal disease have not been established.

Dental considerations:
Ask why the product is being used.

Drug interactions: No dental drug interactions are reported.

Dong quai
(Angelica sinensis)

Other names: Chinese angelica, dang-gui

Class: Herbal remedy

Major ingredients: Active constituents of dong quai may include butylidene phthalide, ferulic acid, beta-sitosterol, a variety of coumarins (oxypeucedanin, osthol, and others), an essential oil, polysaccharides, lactones, and vitamins E and B_{12}. The portion of the plant used is the root.

Claimed actions: Vasodilation, antispasmodic in blood vessels, CNS stimulation, and immunosuppressant and antiinflammatory properties. The mechanism of action of these effects is unclear. Contrary to some reports, dong quai does not appear to have phytoestrogen constituents.

Uses: It is used in Chinese herbal medicine in combination with other herbs. Uses include dysmenorrhea, other menstrual problems, and menopausal symptoms. Other uses include arthritis, hypertension, and ulcers. However, significant clinical studies are lacking. One RCT failed to find dong quai helpful for menopausal symptoms. The remedy does not appear in the German Commission E monographs.

Administration: Administered orally as in infusion, a tincture, or a chewable root.

Contraindications: Women who have had breast cancer should not use dong quai: despite a lack of

estrogenic action, dong quai may stimulate breast cancer cell growth (in vitro evidence only).
Side effects: In clinical trials, dong quai has been generally well tolerated. Photosensitization is possible on theoretic grounds. Safety for pregnant or nursing women, young children, and individuals with severe liver or kidney disease has not been established.
Dental considerations:
Ask why the product is being used. In patients taking warfarin or other oral anticoagulant, inquire about bleeding history. Inquire about unusual bleeding episodes following dental treatment. Caution suggested for combination treatment with photosensitizing drugs.
Drug interactions: Dong quai may interact adversely with anticoagulants or antiplatelet agents.

Echinacea
(Echinacea angustifolia, Echinacea purpurea, Echinacea pallida)
Other names: American cone flower, Kansas snakeroot, purple cone flower
Class: Herbal remedy
Major ingredients: Caffeic acid glycoside (echinacoside), alkylamides (echinacein and others), essential oils (humulene and others), a variety of flavonoids, and many other components. As with any plant, the contents vary with the species, the parts of the plant used, and whether the plant is dried or fresh. The portion of the plant used is the flower, other aboveground parts, and even the roots. Most studies finding benefit for the common cold involved preparations made from the aboveground portion of the *E. purpurea* species.

Claimed actions: Stimulation of the immune system (some laboratory data suggest an increase in macrophage phagocytic activity and numbers of neutrophils); possible antibacterial, antiviral, and antiinflammatory activity lack strong support.
Uses: Considerable (though not entirely consistent) evidence from RCTs indicates that acute use of echinacea may reduce the symptoms and duration of the common cold and influenza. Chronic use of echinacea does not appear to offer prophylactic benefits against colds. Other uses that have been proposed, but that lack meaningful supporting evidence, include wound healing, *Candida* infections, supportive therapy for lower urinary tract infections, rheumatoid arthritis, and supportive use in colon cancer.
Administration: Available in a variety of preparations for internal (oral administration) and external use.
Contraindications: On theoretic grounds, should not be used in patients with autoimmune diseases or progressive infectious diseases, including tuberculosis, multiple sclerosis, leukocytosis, and collagen diseases, or individuals taking immunosuppressive medications.
Side effects: Generally limited to parenteral doses only. Fatigue, headache, and dizziness were reported with oral doses. There is a possible risk of cross-allergic reaction with chamomile or ragweed.
Dental considerations:
Ask why it is being used. Avoid use

during immunosuppression. Use with caution in asthma, atopy, or allergic rhinitis, because of potential for allergic reactions.
Drug interactions: May decrease effectiveness of immunosuppressants. Discontinue before use of general anesthetics.

Eleutherococcus
(Eleutherococcus senticosus; Acanthopanax senticosus)
Other names: Siberian ginseng, Russian ginseng, eleutheroginseng
Class: Herbal remedy
Major ingredients: Major constituents include a variety of unrelated lignans, setoids, phenylacrylic acid derivatives, polysaccharides, steroid glycosides, and triterpene saponins all somewhat misleadingly named eleutherosides (eleutheroside A, B, etc.). The root and rhizome are the medicinal parts used. Note that despite the common name "Russian ginseng," eleutherococcus has no botanic or biochemical similarity to true ginseng, *Panax ginseng*.

Claimed actions: Eleutherococcus is said to act as an "adaptogen," a substance that enhances an organism's general ability to adapt to stress of all kinds. However, the supporting evidence that eleutherococcus (or any other substance) has adaptogenic properties is limited to human and animal trials of substandard methodology. Some evidence indicates that eleutherococcus may increase maximal oxygen intake during intense exercise. Immunomodulatory effects have been seen in some studies, specifically increases in helper/inducer T-lymphocytes.
Uses: One RCT found evidence that regular use of eleutherococcus by individuals with chronic recurrent genital herpes reduced the rate of flare-ups. One RCT failed to find eleutherococcus helpful for chronic fatigue syndrome. The majority of RCTs evaluating eleutherococcus for possible sports performance enhancement effects have failed to find benefit.
Administration: A typical dose of eleutherococcus is 2 to 3 g daily of the whole herb or 300 to 400 mg of a standardized extract. Maximum safe doses in pregnant or nursing women, young children, and individuals with severe hepatic or renal disease have not been established.
Side effects: Eleutherococcus is thought to have a low order of toxicity; however, most safety studies were performed in the former Soviet Union and it is not clear whether they may be fully relied on. In clinical trials, no significant side effects have been seen.
Dental considerations:
Ask why the product is being used.
Drug interactions: There is one case report in which it appears that use of eleutherococcus interfered with a laboratory test for serum digoxin levels, causing the test to falsely report an elevation that did not in fact exist. Based on its possible immunomodulatory actions, eleutherococcus could conceivably interfere with the action of immunosuppressive drugs, but no such interactions have been reported.

Evening primrose oil
(Oenothera biennis)
Other names: Evening primrose
Class: Herbal remedy
Major ingredients: The oil is a mixture of fatty acids, including linoleic acid (50%-80%), gamma-linolenic acid (GLA, 6%-11%), and smaller amounts of other fatty acids, including palmitic acid, oleic acid, and stearic acid. Other ingredients include tannins, sitosterol, and trace minerals. The portion of the plant used is the seed.

Claimed actions: Antiatherosclerotic, relief of premenstrual tension, relief of mastalgia, and antiinflammatory actions for arthritis and dermatologic conditions. The fatty acids contained in the oil may function like essential oils and act as precursors of prostaglandins that help regulate metabolic functions.
Uses: Evening primrose is primarily used as a source of GLA. Some RCT evidence suggests that evening primrose or GLA can reduce symptoms of diabetic neuropathy after many months of use. Weak RCT evidence hints that GLA from borage oil may help adult periodontitis. Other potential indications of GLA or evening primrose oil with weak supporting evidence at best include hyperlipidemia, PMS, rheumatoid arthritis, and weight loss. Claims are also made that GLA is effective in controlling symptoms of atopic dermatitis, but the most recent and best-designed RCTs failed to find benefit. The same can be said of GLA for cyclic mastitis. One RCT failed to find evening primrose oil effective for ADHD. This herb is not listed in the German Commission E monographs.
Administration: Available for oral administration in capsules.
Side effects: Few side effects are noted and occur only occasionally. They generally include GI complaints, including GI upset and nausea.
Dental considerations:
Ask why the product is being used. As noted previously, has shown some promise for periodontitis.
Drug interactions: No dental drug interactions are reported.

Feverfew
(Tanacetum parthenium, Chrysanthemum parthenium)
Other names: Featherfew, feverfew leaf, bachelor's button
Class: Herbal remedy
Major ingredients: Sesquiterpene lactones, especially parthenolide 85%, were once considered the active ingredient in feverfew. However, studies using parthenolide-rich extracts found no benefit, and attention has now focused elsewhere. One bioactive candidate is tanetin, a lipophilic avonol (6-hydroxykaempferol 3,7,4'-trimethyl ether) that inhibits proinflammatory eicosanoids). Other constituents include volatile oils (camphor, *trans*-chrysanthylacetate), flavonoids (luteolin, apigenin), and many other constituents. The portion of the plant used is the leaf.

Claimed actions: Inhibition of proinflammatory eicosanoids resulting in antiinflammatory actions. May decrease platelet aggregation and serotonin release (laboratory studies). It is not listed in the German Commission E monographs.

Uses: A few small RCTs have found that regular use of feverfew leaf can reduce the severity, duration, or incidence of migraines. Studies using feverfew extracts standardized to parthenolide content, however, have failed to find benefits. Other proposed uses, including osteoarthritis, rheumatoid arthritis, and stimulation of menstruation, lack RCT support.

Administration: Available in many oral dose forms or used to make an infusion. Safety in lactating women or individuals with severe hepatic or renal disease is not established.

Contraindications: Because of history of use as an abortifacient, should not be used during pregnancy.

Side effects: Oral products produce few complaints; chewing the leaves may lead to oral ulcerations and swelling of circumoral tissues. There is the potential risk of increased bleeding time.

Dental considerations:

Ask why the product is being used. In patients taking warfarin or other oral anticoagulant, inquire about bleeding history. Inquire about unusual bleeding episodes following dental treatment.

Drug interactions: On a theoretic basis, feverfew might potentiate the effects of antiplatelet agents and increase gastric side effects of NSAIDs. However, no such interactions have been reported. Advise patients not to take this herb for 2 to 3 weeks before surgery.

Garlic

(Allium sativum)

Other names: Allium, poor man's treacle

Class: Herbal remedy

Major ingredients: A volatile oil containing several sulfur compounds, a sulfur-containing amino acid identified as alliin. With grinding, alliin is converted to allicin, responsible for the typical odor of garlic, as well as much of its bioactivity. Ajoene and s-allylcysteine are also active compounds. The portion of the plant used is whole, fresh or dried, garlic clove, and oil of garlic.

Claimed actions: With oral use, actions claimed for garlic include hypolipidemic, antiplatelet aggregation, antihypertensive, antioxidant, antiatherosclerotic, and immune stimulant activity. In vitro studies have found topical antibiotic, antifungal, and antiviral actions. Antithrombotic effects have been documented in vitro and in vivo.

Uses: Despite widespread use for hyperlipidemia, current evidence from well-designed RCTs suggests that garlic does not improve lipid levels to more than a minimal extent. Some evidence from preliminary RCTs indicates that regular use of standardized garlic extracts may reduce incidence of the common cold in adults and children. Weak RCT evidence indicates possible antihypertensive and antiatherosclerotic actions. One RCT suggests that oral use of garlic can decrease insect (tick) bites. Topically, garlic has been used to treat a wide array of bacterial,

fungal, and viral infections, but there are no rigorous supporting data. Oral antibiotic effectiveness is unlikely. Use in GI fungal infections remains in doubt. Long-term effects are unknown.
Administration: Available in a variety of oral dose forms. The best-studied form of garlic is garlic powder specially stabilized to provide alliin, which can be converted to allicin. Raw garlic also provides alliin/allicin, but other forms of garlic such as cooked garlic, garlic oil, and aged garlic products do not provide alliin. (Nonetheless, some pharmacologic effects have been seen with them, presumably from other constituents.)
Side effects: The taste and odor of garlic is by far the most common complaint. Rarely GI symptoms may occur with larger doses. Halitosis and burning of the mouth have been reported. There is one case report of spontaneous spinal epidural hematoma attributed to use of garlic products. Note that standardized garlic is more similar to raw garlic than to cooked garlic, and therefore the common food use of cooked garlic cannot be taken as evidence of safety.
Dental considerations:
Ask why the product is being used. Inquire about unusual bleeding episodes following dental treatment.
Drug interactions: Garlic might potentiate antiplatelet or anticoagulant agents. Because of increased risk of bleeding, advise patients not to take this herb for 2 to 3 weeks before surgery. Garlic has been found to reduce plasma concentrations of saquinavir and possibly increase the gastrointestinal toxicity of ritonavir (drugs used for HIV).

Ginger
(Zingiber officinale, Zingiberis rhizoma)
Other names: Ginger root
Class: Herbal remedy
Major ingredients: The root contains a volatile oil and other chemicals termed *pungent principles.* These latter compounds are collectively known as gingerols, shogaols, and gingerdiols. The portion of the plant used is the root.

Claimed actions: Motion sickness prevention, promotion of salivary and gastric secretions, positive inotropic action, and antiplatelet and antiinflammatory effects have all been claimed for this herb. Gluonolactone, an active ingredient, has been reported to have serotonin (5-HT) antagonist activity, and gingerols may have a positive inotropic effect.
Uses: Incomplete and somewhat inconsistent evidence from multiple RCTs of varying quality suggests that ginger can reduce motion sickness symptoms. Other RCTs suggest benefits for nausea and vomiting of pregnancy (morning sickness). Results are contradictory on benefits for postsurgical anesthesia. Ginger has also been used for nausea of chemotherapy, but supporting evidence is weak. RCTs have shown equivocal results regarding efficacy in osteoarthritis.
Administration: Only the rhizome (rootlike stalk) of the plant is used. The German Commission E monographs list the dose at 2 to 4 g daily. Despite ginger's medical use in

nausea and vomiting of pregnancy, safety in pregnancy and lactation is not established.

Side effects: Generally not reported except for toxic doses that could include CNS depression and arrhythmia.

Dental considerations:

Ask why the product is being used.

Drug interactions: Although ginger has shown antiplatelet rather than anticoagulant effects, there is one case report in which use of ginger apparently potentiated phenprocoumon. Interactions with other anticoagulants or antiplatelet agents are possible.

Ginkgo

(Ginkgo biloba, Ginkgo folium)

Other names: Maidenhair tree, ginkyo

Class: Herbal remedy

Major ingredients: Common ingredients with claimed pharmacologic activity include multiple flavonoids (biobetin, ginkgetin), flavone glycosides (quercctin), bioflavones, terpenoids (ginkgolides A, B, and C), and bilobalide. The portion of the plant used is the leaf only, made in a specific 50:1 extract. Thus the commonly tested treatment is more properly called ginkgo biloba extract (GBE) rather than ginkgo. The seeds are toxic.

Claimed actions: Improvement in blood flow in the microcirculation, inhibition of development of trauma-induced or toxin-induced cerebral edema, improved hypoxic tolerance in cerebral tissues, reduction in retinal edema, increased memory performance, inhibition of age-related reduction in muscarinic receptors, and antagonism of platelet-activating factor (PAF). It may also have monoamine oxidase inhibition properties.

Uses: Significant, though not entirely consistent, evidence from multiple RCTs supports use in Alzheimer's dementia and other forms of dementia. Significant evidence also exists for benefit in intermittent claudication. Weaker evidence from RCTs supports use in normal age-related memory impairment, PMS, Raynaud's phenomenon, and vertiginous syndromes. Other potential uses with limited support include idiopathic sudden hearing loss, glaucoma, macular degeneration and diabetic microvascular disease. Contrary to earlier reports, ginkgo does not appear to be effective for sexual dysfunction (in men or women), tinnitus, or mountain sickness.

Administration: Capsules and tablets of leaf extracts are available for use. Doses range from 120 to 240 mg of 50:1 dry extract for 8 weeks for chronic diseases. Use for longer than 3 months requires reevaluation of benefits.

Contraindications: Pregnancy and lactation. Individuals with seizure disorders should not use ginkgo.

Side effects: In clinical trials, ginkgo has been well tolerated, producing no more than occasional mild allergies and nonspecific digestive distress. There are several reports of internal bleeding attributable to use of ginkgo, including bleeding episodes during surgery. Seizures have also been reported. In addition, one report of oral ulcerations is noted.

Dental considerations:
Ask why the product is being used. Inquire about unusual bleeding episodes following dental treatment.
Drug interactions: There is considerable evidence for anticoagulant and antiplatelet activity with ginkgo; do not combine with other anticoagulant or antiplatelet agents except under close supervision. Discontinue ginkgo use 2 weeks before surgery and general anesthesia. Ginkgo might also decrease effectiveness of calcium channel blockers and increase ototoxicity of aminoglycosides. Possible interaction between ginkgo and trazodone (Desyrel) may cause excess stimulation of GABA receptors leading to CNS depression and possible coma.

Ginseng
(*Panax quinquefolium,* American; *Panax ginseng,* Korean)
Class: Herbal remedy
Major ingredients: Constituents vary with the species of ginsing used. Contains steroid-like compounds called *ginsenosides* or *panaxosides.* Other ingredients include a volatile oil and flavonoids along with smaller quantities of other substances.

Claimed actions: Panax ginseng is said to act as an "adaptogen," a substance that enhances an organism's general ability to adapt to stress of all kinds. However, the supporting evidence that ginseng (or any other substance) has adaptogenic properties is limited to animal studies and a few human trials of substandard methodology. Despite earlier reports, ginseng itself does not appear to have estrogenic effects.
Uses: Preliminary RCTs suggest that American ginseng but not *Panax ginseng* may improve glucose control in type 2 diabetes. Other uses with limited and in some cases inconsistent RCT support include increasing immune response to influenza vaccine, enhancing mental function, improving blood sugar control in diabetes, correcting erectile dysfunction, and enhancing sports performance.
Administration: The root is used for teas and various other oral preparations.
Contraindications: Worrisome data from animal studies suggest possible teratogenic effects. Do not use during pregnancy.
Side effects: Ginseng appears to have a low level of toxicity. In clinical trials, few side effects were seen beyond occasional allergic reactions and nonspecific digestive distress. However, adulterants included with ginsing products may increase risk for other side effects.
Dental considerations:
Ask why the product is being used.
Drug interactions: No specific dental drug interactions are reported, but ginsing may interact with monoamine oxidase inhibitors. Interactions with warfarin are unclear. Discontinue 7 days before general anesthesia and general surgical procedures.

Glucosamine sulfate
Other names: Chitosamine, glucosamine
Class: Nonherbal remedy
Major ingredient: Glucosamine

sulfate, an aminomonosaccharide (2-amino-2-deoxyglucose), is a component of mucopolysaccharides and mucoproteins. Other salt forms may also be used.

Claimed actions: Glucosamine is used in the synthesis of glycoproteins and glycosaminoglycans (GAGs). It is formed in the body from glucose through intermediary metabolic steps to be incorporated into GAGs, which are essential for cartilage function in joints. Exogenous glucosamine is thought to enhance joint proteoglycan content, thereby improving function of the failing joint.

Uses: Most but not all published RCTs indicate that glucosamine is superior to placebo and equally effective (though slower acting) than standard NSAIDs for the treatment of osteoarthritis. Incomplete RCT evidence additionally points toward a possible disease-modifying effect (retarding progressive joint damage). Other proposed uses include prevention and treatment of tendon and other soft tissue injuries, but there is no meaningful evidence to support these indications.

Administration: The usual dose is 500 mg three times daily.

Side effects: Side effects are uncommon but can include GI effects such as nausea, heartburn, diarrhea, and epigastric pain. CNS side effects are also rarely observed; they may include headache, insomnia, and drowsiness. Contrary to earlier reports, glucosamine does not appear to be harmful for patients with diabetes. However, arthritic patients may be taking aspirin, NSAIDs, or disease-modifying osteoarthritis drugs in addition to glucosamine and chondroitin. Question the patient about other antiarthritic drugs used, including OTC drugs.

Dental considerations:

Ask why the product is being used.

Drug interactions: No dental drug interactions are documented.

Goldenseal

(Hydrastis canadensis)

Other names: Eye root, yellow root, turmeric root

Class: Herbal remedy

Major ingredients: Contains the isoquinoline alkaloids hydrastine and berberine, other related alkaloids, and a volatile oil.

Claimed actions: Astringent and antiseptic. May also stimulate the secretion of bile and may have laxative action. Hydrastine has been shown to cause vasoconstriction in peripheral vessels. Berberine may have some antibacterial actions. This herb is not included in the German Commission E monographs.

Uses: No proposed uses of goldenseal are supported by RCTs. Goldenseal is frequently added to preparations designed to treat the common cold, but there is no evidence (nor traditional history) to suggest that it is effective for this purpose. Goldenseal is also widely used topically for minor skin wounds and mucous membrane irritation, again without supporting evidence. Its constituent, berberine, may have some action against intestinal infections, but unrealistically high doses of goldenseal would be required to match the dose of berberine used in studies. Berberine (not goldenseal) has also been used in the treatment of eye infections. Numerous other proposed uses of goldenseal that lack evidence of efficacy include "masking" a positive drug screen, treating minor cardiac arrythmias, and reducing crampy intestinal pain and dyspepsia.

Administration: Typical dosages for oral use are 500 mg three times daily, often in combination with other herbs. Topical goldenseal preparations vary in concentration.

Contraindications: It is contraindicated for use in pregnancy and lactation, and by individuals with hepatic disease.

Side effects: Safe in usual doses; adverse effects are more often observed with toxic doses (may include hypertension, convulsions, and breathing difficulties). Photosensitivity is a theoretic possibility.

Dental considerations:
Ask why the product is being used.

Drug interactions: None reported.

Gotu kola
(Centella asiatica)

Other names: TECA (titrated extract of *Centella asiatica*), TTFCA (total triterpenic fraction of *Centella asiatica*), hydrocotyle, Indian pennywort

Class: Herbal remedy

Major ingredients: The aboveground parts of the plant are used. The major constituents are the triterpene acids and esters known as asiaticosides, asiatic acid, madecassic acid, and madecassoside. (Note: Gotu kola, unlike the unrelated kola nut, does not contain caffeine.)

Claimed actions: Gotu kola, or its triterpenic extract, is said to enhance the structure and function of connective tissues, an effect possibly mediated by actions on collagen cross-linking and fibronectin production. This is the basis for most of its proposed uses. However, the supporting evidence for such an effect is generally weak. Gotu kola extracts may also weaken the protective outer coating of *Mycobacterium leprae,* and on that basis it has been used for leprosy.

Uses: Several small RCTs found that gotu kola can decrease pain, edema, and leg fatigue in chronic venous insufficiency of the lower extremity. There is no evidence that it can alter the appearance of visible varicosities. Other small RCTs suggest benefit in the treatment of keloids, leprosy, and reducing the startle reflex to sudden loud noises. Oral and topical gotu kola have been additionally recommended for virtually all diseases of the skin or diseases that have skin manifestations, but there is no RCT evidence to support these uses.

Administration: The studied dose of gotu kola is 20 to 40 mg 3 times daily of a triterpenic extract standardized to contain 40% asiaticoside, 29% to 30% asiatic acid, 29% to 30% madecassic acid, and 1% to 2% madecassoside. Safety in pregnancy has not been established, but pregnant women have been in enrolled in clinical trials, and no harmful effects were seen.

Side effects: Gotu kola appears to have a low order of toxicity. In clinical trials, use of gotu kola has not been associated with significant side effects other than occasional allergic reactions and mild nonspecific digestive distress. However, based on a study in mice, there are some concerns that topical gotu kola might have cancer-promoting actions.

Dental considerations:
Ask why the product is being used.

Drug interactions: No dental drug interactions are reported.

Grape seed extract

(Vitis vinifera, Vitis coignetiae)

Other names: Grape seed extract, grape seed oil, muskat, de pepins de raisin

Class: Herbal remedy

Major ingredients: The oil of the grape seed is one of the two major sources of oligomeric proanthocyanidin complexes (OPCs), less commonly called procyanidolic oligomers (PCOs). (The other is the bark of maritime pine.) Other constituents include essential fatty acids and tocopherols (vitamin E). Pycnogenol, a trademarked and patented herbal product and dietary supplement, contains similar but not identical OPCs from the bark of the maritime pine (*Pinus maritime,* sometimes called *Pinus nigra* var. *maritime*). *V. coignetiae* also contains epsilon-viniferin, oligostilbenes and amyelopsins, and 51-nucleotidase inhibitors. Resveratrol (3,5,41-trihydroxystilbene) is present when herbal preparations are mixed with grape skin extract. The part used is the seed or sometimes the skin of the grape.

Claimed actions: OPCs have significant free-radical scavenging actions, and may also act to protect connective tissue by inhibiting hyaluronidase, elastase, and collagenase and increasing collagen cross-linking. These effects, and others, may lead to decreased capillary permeability. OPCs also inhibit platelet aggregation and alter prostaglandin metabolism.

Uses: The best-documented use of OPCs is treatment of chronic venous insufficiency, in which several RCTs suggest that OPC treatment can reduce lower extremity pain, edema, and fatigue. Effects on visible varicosities have not been documented. Weaker RCT evidence suggests possible benefit for reducing edema caused by surgery or minor injury. Other indications for OPCs from grape seed that have some support from small RCTs include reducing capillary fragility in liver cirrhosis and alleviating symptoms of allergic rhinitis. Related OPCs from pine bark have shown some potential benefit for periodontal disease, when used in the form of chewing gum. Grape seed OPCs have failed to prove effective for reducing lipid levels. Supposed benefits for cardiovascular disease are entirely theoretic, based on antioxidant and antiplatelet properties.

Administration: Administered orally in tablets or capsules. Doses range from 40 to 300 mg per day, with maintenance doses at 40 to 80 mg daily.

Contraindications: OPCs are thought to have antiplatelet activity, and on this basis they should not be taken by individuals using anticoagulant or antiplatelet agents.

Side effects: Grape seed OPCs

have undergone extensive safety testing and appear to have a low degree of toxicity.

Dental considerations:

Determine why the patient is taking botanic products. Patients should discontinue use 2 weeks before surgery. As noted previously, OPCs from pine bark have shown some promise for periodontitis.

Drug interactions: Although there are theoretic concerns that OPCs could potentiate antiplatelet or anticoagulant agents, there are no well-documented case reports to support this concern.

Green tea

(Camellia sinensis)

Other names: EGCG, *Camellia thea, Camellia theifera,* epigallocatechin gallate, green tea polyphenols, thea bohea, thea sinensis, thea viridis

Class: Herbal remedy

Major ingredients: The major constituents of green tea include catechin polyphenols (especially epigallocatechin gallate), as well as triterpene saponins, caffeine, theobromine, theophylline, flavonoids, caffeic acid derivatives, and volatile oil. The product is made by steaming the fresh-cut leaf of the plant.

Claimed actions: Observational studies have inconsistently suggested that green tea might reduce cancer and heart disease risk. The polyphenols in green tea have antioxidant properties. Other reported actions of green tea with weak supporting evidence include enhanced thermogenesis, hypolipidemic effects, antiinflammatory actions in periodontal disease, hepatoprotection, and protection of skin from sun damage.

Uses: Green tea, or extracts made from it, is widely used in the expectation that it will reduce risk of heart disease and cancer, but at present the supporting evidence for benefit is weak and there are no meaningful RCTs indicating benefit. One small double-blind placebo-controlled trial did provide evidence that sugarless green tea candy chews have a favorable effect in periodontal disease, as shown by relative improvements in approximal plaque index and sulcus bleeding index. More recently, green tea has become a common ingredient in weight loss products, based only on scant preliminary evidence; the one RCT on this proposed use failed to find benefit for preventing weight regain after weight loss. Neither topical nor oral green teas have proven to provide the same level of protection from the sun as standard sunblocks, though they may provide some protection.

Administration: Three cups of green tea daily, or 100 to 150 mg 3 times daily of a green tea extract standardized to contain 80% total polyphenols and 50% epigallocatechin gallate.

Side effects: Green tea contains less caffeine and related stimulants than does black tea, but caffeine-related side effects may occur, such as agitation and insomnia.

Dental considerations:

Ask why the product is being used. Those chewing green tea candies for putative anti–periodontal-disease actions should be cautioned not to consider it a substitute for standard care.

Drug interactions: Green tea contains high levels of vitamin K, and would therefore be expected to decrease the effectiveness of coumadin and related drugs. The caffeine in green tea could interact with MAO inhibitors.

Guggul

(Commiphora mukul)

Other names: False myrrh, gum guggul, gugulipid, mukul myrrh tree

Class: Herbal remedy

Major ingredients: Guggul is the oleo-gum-resin obtained by drying the sap of the *Commiphora mukul* tree. Its active ingredients are thought to be ketonic steroids known as guggulsterones.

Claimed actions: Guggulsterones are strong antagonists of two nuclear hormone receptors involved in cholesterol metabolism, which provides a plausible basis for the use of guggul in the treatment of hyperlipidemia, its major proposed use. It is widely claimed that guggul increases thyroid activity and thereby aids weight loss, but there is no meaningful supporting evidence for either part of this claim.

Uses: Although earlier RCTs performed by Indian researchers did report hypolipidemic actions, a more recent, larger, and better-designed RCT performed in the United States failed to find benefits; in fact, guggul appeared to *increase* levels of LDL-C. One RCT found guggul ineffective as a weight loss aid. Other proposed uses of guggul that lack reliable supporting evidence include improving glucose control in diabetes, aiding weight loss, and treating acne.

Administration: Guggul is typically used in a standardized extract form to provide 100 mg of guggulsterones daily (especially E- and Z-guggulsterone). Safety in pregnant or lactating women and in individuals with severe hepatic or renal disease is not known.

Side effects: Guggul appears to have a low order of toxicity. In clinical trials of standardized guggul extract, no significant side effects other than occasional allergic reactions (especially skin rash) and nonspecific gastrointestinal distress have been seen.

Dental considerations:

Ask why the product is being used.

Drug interactions: No dental drug interactions are reported.

Hawthorn

(Crataegus oxyancantha, Crataegi folim cum flore, C. monogyna, C. Laevigata)

Other names: English hawthorn, maybush

Class: Herbal remedy

Major ingredients: Flavonoids (hyperoside, vitexin-rhamnose, rutin, and proanthocyanidins) with vasodilating properties, as well as inhibition of vasoconstriction. Proanthocyanidins are reported to block angiotensin-converting enzyme (ACE). It also contains tyramine, a biogenic amine. The plant parts used include the flowers, leaves, fruits, and mixtures of other plant parts.

Claimed actions: Hawthorn appears to have inotropic actions; in addition, some evidence suggests that hawthorn has antiarrhythmic actions by blocking repolarizing potassium currents in ventricular myocardium, a mechanism similar to that of class III antiarrhythmics. Other reported effects include inhibition of angiotensin-converting enzyme and inhibition of cyclic AMP phosphodiesterase.
Uses: Moderately strong evidence from multiple RCTs indicates that hawthorn improves signs and symptoms of class I or II congestive heart failure. However, there is no evidence that hawthorn can reduce risk of morbidity and mortality (a benefit shown with ACE inhibitors). Weaker RCT support indicates benefits in angina. Other proposed indications that lack substantive support include atherosclerosis, hypertension, benign cardiac arrythmias, and prevention of postischemic arrythmias.
Administration: Available in oral dose forms as an extract and plant parts for brewing teas.
Side effects: No contraindications or side effects are listed.
Dental considerations:
Ask why the product is being used. Monitor vital signs in patients with cardiovascular disease.
Drug interactions: There are theoretic concerns of possible adverse interactions if herb is used with other drugs that may affect cardiac function.

Horse chestnut extract
(Aesculus hippocastanum)
Other names: HCE; raw form—buckeye, conkers
Class: Herbal remedy
Major ingredients: The major constituents of horse chestnut are triterpene saponins, especially escin (also spelled "aescin"). Other constituents include flavonoids, polysaccharides, and oligomoeric proanthocyanidins. Whole horse chestnut contains the toxic coumarin glycoside esculin (also spelled "aesculin"), but the standard horse chestnut extract product has had the esculin removed. Horse chestnut seed and leaf are both used medicinally.

Claimed actions: Horse chestnut extract (HCE) is thought to reduce capillary permeability. Proposed mechanisms include venotonic, antiinflammatory, antihydrolase, and anti–neutrophil-adherence properties.
Uses: Several moderate-size RCTs of varying quality have found evidence that HCE can reduce symptoms of venous insufficiency in the lower extremities, including edema, pain, and fatigue. Benefits (prevention or treatment) regarding visible varicosities have not been documented. One RCT suggests benefits for hemorrhoids. Weaker forms of evidence suggest potential benefits for aiding resolution of phlebitis and reducing edema after surgery or injury. Topical horse chestnut for bruising has similarly weak supporting evidence.
Administration: HCE is taken at a dose of 300 mg twice daily, in a form standardized to contain 50 mg escin per dose. Enteric-coated capsules are used to avoid otherwise predictable stomach discomfort. Safety in pregnant women has not been established, but animal data

are reassuring and pregnant women have been enrolled in RCTs of horse chestnut.

Side effects: Whole horse chestnut, as opposed to HCE, is a toxic herb and should not be used. HCE predictably causes gastric irritation if it is not delivered in an enteric-coated capsule; enteric-coated HCE is not associated with any significant side effects other than occasional allergic reactions.

Dental considerations:
Ask why the product is being used.

Drug interactions: Horse chestnut, because of its saponin content, might potentiate the effects of antiplatelet or anticoagulant agents.

Hydroxymethyl butyrate (HMB)
Other names: Beta-hydroxy beta-methylbutyric acid

Class: Nonherbal remedy

Major ingredients: Hydroxymethyl butyrate is a naturally occurring degradation product of the amino acid leucine.

Claimed actions: During intense exercise, muscle tissue degradation occurs, which leads to leakage of leucine and its subsequent transformation to HMB. It has been hypothesized that increased HMB levels from exogenous sources provides a downstream feedback signal that slows muscle protein degradation.

Uses: Several small RCTs, some published only in abstract form, indicate that use of HMB may enhance response to weight training, resulting in increased muscle mass. On this basis, HMB has become a popular supplement for bodybuilders. However, the supporting evidence must be regarded as weak, and the benefits, if any, are modest. Even weaker evidence hints that HMB might have an antihypertensive or hypolipidemic effect.

Administration: A typical dosage of HMB is 1 g three times daily. Maximum safe doses in young children, pregnant or nursing women, and individuals with severe hepatic or renal disease have not been established.

Side effects: HMB appears to have a low order of toxicity. No significant side effects have been seen in clinical trials, other than occasional nonspecific digestive distress. However, long-term safety studies have not been performed.

Dental considerations:
Ask why the product is being used.

Drug interactions: No dental drug interactions are reported.

Kava
(Piper methysticum, Piperis methystrici rhizoma)

Other names: Kava-kava, kew, tonga

Class: Herbal remedy

Major ingredients: Kava lactones (kava alpha-pyrones), including methysticin, kawain, and others. The plant parts used are the dried rhizomes.

Claimed actions: These lactones have demonstrable pharmacologic activity on the CNS. Reported actions include sedation, muscle relaxation, and anticonvulsive and antispasmodic effects. Suggested mechanisms of action range from GABA receptor modification to do-

pamine antagonist activity. A local anesthetic action is also claimed.
Uses: Meaningful evidence from multiple RCTs demonstrates significant improvement of symptoms in various anxiety disorders. Other proposed uses lack support, including relief of general tension, stress, and insomnia. An intoxicating effect has also been reported in very high doses.
Administration: Standardized products for oral administration are available; in some areas the kava-kava is chewed. Use should be limited to no more than 3 months. It should not be used in patients with endogenous depression or Parkinson's disease or during pregnancy and lactation.
WARNING: Kava has been taken off the market in numerous countries because of reports of severe liver injury, in some cases requiring transplantation; this appears to be a rare idiosyncratic or allergic reaction rather than ordinary liver toxicity, but it has been seen even with traditionally prepared kava, as well as pharmaceutical-grade standardized products. Until further is known, however, kava should be considered an unsafe herb.
Contraindications: Reports of dystonic reactions suggest that kava should not be used by patients taking antipsychotic medications. Also, apparent antidopaminergic actions contraindicate use in Parkinson's disease, and CNS effects and possible potentiation of alcohol toxicity contraindicate use in alcoholism. Whether or not the risk of liver damage (see WARNING) is increased in patients with preexisting liver disease remains unknown.
Side effects: Kava is generally well tolerated in normal doses. GI complaints may occasionally accompany use. Chewing kava-kava can result in circumoral numbness. Patients using kava-kava may have reduced alertness, and very high intake can cause inebriation. See WARNING concerning liver damage.
Dental considerations:
Caution against use of kava in all patients, especially those with existing liver disease.
Drug interactions: May potentiate CNS sedation if used in combination with other CNS depressants. May increase risk of dystonic reactions if given in combination with antipsychotics. Discontinue 24 hours before general anesthesia and surgical procedures.

Lemon balm
(Melissa officinalis)
Other names: Honey plant, Melissa, sweet Mary, balm mint
Class: Herbal remedy
Major ingredients: Volatile oil extract by distillation from leaves or whole plant, contains geranial, neral, citronellal, linalool, and others. Other constituents include glycosides, caffeic acids, flavonoids, and titerpene acids.

Claimed actions: Some evidence indicates that topical lemon balm extract blocks herpes virus receptors on host cells, and may also inhibit viral-related protein synthesis by action on elongation factor eEF-2. Taken internally, lemon balm may cause sedation through CNS nicotinic and muscarinic receptor-binding properties, although this mechanism is not well established.

Uses: Several RCTs of moderate to low quality found evidence that use of topical lemon balm preparations can reduce the severity of acute genital or oral herpes recurrences if applied at the beginning of symptoms. There are no meaningful data on possible prophylactic effect. For oral use, lemon balm alone or combined with valerian has shown some potential value for insomnia, but not all data are consistent. One RCT found that lemon balm extract reduced agitation in individuals with Alzheimer's disease. Other proposed uses of lemon balm lack supporting evidence. These include anxiety disorders, dry skin, headache, influenza, menstrual problems, and muscle spasms.

Administration: Topical lemon balm for herpes is used in the form of a 70:1 extract cream, applied twice daily, and standardized using bioassay for inhibition of viral cellular lysis. Typical oral doses are 1.5 to 4.5 g/day of dried herb daily, or the equivalent in a standardized extract form. Maximum safe dosages of oral lemon balm for young children, pregnant or nursing women, and individuals with severe hepatic or renal disease are not known.

Side effects: Use of topical lemon balm has not been associated with any significant side effects other than occasional allergic reactions. Oral lemon balm is generally regarded as safe. However, based on weak evidence that it may have a sedative effect, people taking oral lemon balm might be at increased risk if they drive or operate heavy machinery, or engage in any other activity that requires a high level of alertness.

Dental considerations:

Ask why the product is being used. Pregnant women should be cautioned not to regard topical lemon balm as effective prevention against transmission of herpes to the newborn. See also Drug Interactions.

Drug interactions: In animal studies, lemon balm extracts have produced dose-dependent potentiation of pentobarbital.

Licorice

(Glycyrrhiza glabra)

Other names: Licorice root, liquorice, licorice, deglycyrrhizinated licorice, DGL, sweet wood, Yasti Madhu, sweet wort, Reglisse, and Subholz

Class: Herbal remedy

Major ingredients: Whole licorice contains as its principle presumed active ingredient a terpenoid called glycyrrhizin glycoside (glycyrrhizinic acid). Deglycyrrhizinated licorice (DGL) is a popular form of licorice that has had this constituent removed. Other constituents include asparagine, biotin, choline, fat, gum, inositol, lecithin, glycosides, volatile oil, coumarins, estrogenic substances, sterols, saponins, manganese, PABA, pantothenic acid, various pentacyclic triterpenes, phosphorous, B vitamins (1, 2, 3, 6, and 9), vitamin E, and a yellow dye.

Claimed actions: Glycyrrhizin has mineralocorticoid effects in high doses or with prolonged use. Licorice, possibly because of its glycyrrhizin content, is thought to potentiate topical or oral corticosteroids and exert an estrogen-like effect. Other claimed actions with less substantiation include demulcent, diuretic, expectorant, antitussive, laxative, emetic, emollient, antiinflammatory, tissue healing, and antiarthritic effects.

Uses: There are no well-documented uses of licorice or DGL. DGL has shown some promise for peptic ulcer disease, but published studies involved combination products with other active ingredients such as antacids. Various additional claims of effectiveness have been made for whole licorice, including hypoglycemia, bronchitis, colitis, cystitis, stress, colds, high cholesterol, fever, nausea, inflammation, coughs, laryngitis, chronic fatigue syndrome, and general debility. Externally, licorice preparations have been used for eczema, psoriasis, burns, boils, sores, ulcers, and redness of the skin. DGL lozenges have been recommended for mouth ulcers. However, there is no reliable substantiation for any of these uses.

Side effects: Glycyrrhizin has direct mineralocorticoid effects and also increases corticosteroid activity by inhibiting metabolic inactivation of cortisol. Signs of pseudohyperaldosteronism have been seen within a few weeks of usage, including headache, muscle weakness, muscle cramps, hypertension, heart failure, arrhythmias, water retention, sodium retention, and potassium loss. The DGL form has not been associated with any significant side effects other than occasional allergic reactions or nonspecific gastrointestinal distress.

Administration: It is given by powder, liquid, or capsules. Topically a 2% licorice juice has been used as an antibacterial ointment. A mouthwash with 200 mg of deglycyrrhizinated licorice in 200 ml of warm water has also been used. Snuff often contains a great deal of licorice.

Contraindications: Licorice use should be avoided by pregnant women (it may cause reduced gestational age at birth), women with a history of breast cancer (because of potential estrogenic effects), or by men with a history of infertility or decreased libido (licorice may reduce testosterone levels). Licorice should not be used by patients taking thiazide or loop diuretics, digitalis, or potassium-sparing diuretics, because of its mineralocorticoid effects. However, DGL products should not interact with these medications.

Dental considerations:
Limit use of whole licorice to no more than 6 weeks. DGL lozenges have been proposed for apthous ulcers, but there is no supporting evidence for this use.

Drug interactions: Tobacco may alter metabolism leading to toxicity. May potentiate corticosteroid drugs, so use in combination only with caution. May potentiate or antagonize diuretics, and the increased potassium loss caused by licorice presents increased risks for individuals using digoxin or antiarrhythmic drugs.

Myrrh
(Commiphora myrrha)
Other names: Bola, gum myrrh tree, mu-yao

Class: Herbal remedy
Major ingredients: A volatile oil (primarily sesquiterpenes), triterpenes, and gum resin

---

Claimed actions: Analgesic, antifungal, antiseptic, astringent, carminative, emmenagogue, expectorant, antispasmodic, disinfectant, immune stimulant, circulatory stimulant, stomachic, tonic, and vulnerary.
Uses: It has been used as a disinfectant, as an astringent, and to treat disorders of the female reproductive system. It has long been used in the treatment of oral ulcers and gingivitis, halitosis, denture-irritated mouth, and sore teeth and gums. Other uses include nonspecified chest problems and diphtheria. In Chinese medicine it is used for rheumatism, arthritis, and circulatory problems.
Administration: Infusion, mouthwash, tincture, incense, capsules, and dental powder.
Contraindications: Diabetes, pregnancy.
Side effects: Because of its claimed uterine stimulant effects, avoid use in pregnancy. Because of resin content and difficult clearance from the body may cause minor renal damage if used over an extended period of time. Avoid high dose for chronic use.
Dental considerations:
Myrrh has been approved by Commission E (Germany) for treatment of inflammation of the mouth and pharynx, but topical uses are not substantiated. A tea, prepared by placing 1 to 2 teaspoonfuls in a cup of boiling water and steeping for 10 to 15 minutes, has been used for oral administration three times daily.
Drug interactions: Enhancement of oral hypoglycemic agents.

Nettle root
(Urtica dioica radix)
Other names: Stinging nettle
Class: Herbal remedy
Major ingredients: The presumed active constituents of nettle root are beta-sitosterol and other related sitosterols. Other possibly active constituents include lectins, lignans, polysaccharides, and hydroxycoumarins. Note that nettle leaf is an entirely different herbal product from the one discussed in this article.

Claimed actions: The sitosterols in nettle root, especially beta-sitosterol, have multiple actions of possible relevance to prostate disease, including reducing inflammation in the prostate and alteration of sex hormone binding properties.
Uses: Several small RCTs indicate that nettle root can improve symptoms of benign prostatic hyperplasia (BPH).
Administration: When taken for BPH, the typical dose is 120 mg of the dry extract twice daily, or 4 to 6 g daily of the whole root. Nettle root is often sold in combination with other herbs thought to be effective for BPH, including saw palmetto and pygeum, and there is some evidence of a potentiating effect with the latter. Maximum safe dosages in young children, lactating women, and individuals with severe hepatic or renal disease are not known.

Contraindications: Nettle should not be used by pregnant women, based on animal studies showing uterotonic action, as well as its traditional use as an abortifacient.
Side effects: Although extensive safety studies have not been reported, nettle root appears to be of a low order of toxicity. In drug monitoring studies, side effects were rare and nonspecific.
Dental considerations:
Ask why the product is being used.
Drug interactions: None known, but there are weak theoretic concerns regarding interactions with antihypertensive, hypoglycemic, or sedative pharmaceuticals.

Passionflower
(Passiflora incarnate)
Other names: Passion vine
Class: Herbal remedy
Major ingredients: Passionflower contains harman and harmaline, alkaloids that might possess MAOI activity. Other constituents include cyanogenic glycosides, flavonoids, and maltol. The aerial parts of the plant are used.

Claimed actions: Sedative and antispasmodic uses are claimed, based primarily on animal studies.
Uses: Scant preliminary evidence from small RCTs found suggestive evidence that passionflower might be helpful for the treatment of anxiety, as well as for withdrawal from opiate dependency. Its common use for "nervous stomach" has not been formally investigated.
Administration: A typical dosage of crude passionflower is 1 g three times daily. Concentrated extracts and tinctures are also available. Maximum safe doses in nursing women, young children, and individuals with severe hepatic or renal disease have not been established.
Contraindications: Use of passionflower during pregnancy is not advised, because of the uterotropic actions of harman and harmaline.
Side effects: Passionflower is generally well tolerated when taken in usual doses.
Dental considerations:
Ask why the product is being used.
Drug interactions: Passionflower might potentiate the action of sedative drugs, including those used for dental anesthesia. Interactions with MAOI drugs are also possible.

Peppermint
(Mentha piperita)
Other names: Peppermint oil, essential oil of peppermint, mint, brandy mint, menthol
Class: Herbal remedy
Major ingredients: The primary active constituent in peppermint is assumed to be menthol. Other constituents of the essential oil include menthone, menthofurane, menthyl acetate, neomenthol, and isomenthone. The whole leaf additionally contains caffeic acids and flavonids. The leaf and flowers are the parts used medicinally. Most tested uses of peppermint involved preparations of the essential oil rather than whole leaf.

Claimed actions: Some evidence indicates that menthol relaxes gastrointestinal smooth muscle. Peppermint oil has a cooling effect on the skin, and may have cholagogue properties.
Uses: Several preliminary RCTs

somewhat inconsistently suggest that peppermint oil can alleviate symptoms of irritable bowel syndrome; other RCTs suggest that peppermint oil can decrease intestinal spasm during a barium enema. Other uses of peppermint oil with only minimal supporting evidence include functional dyspepsia and dissolution of gallstones. Inhaled peppermint oil has shown some promise for upper respiratory infections; peppermint oil applied to the temples may produce a subjective decrease in headache sensation. There are no well-documented uses of peppermint leaf.
Administration: In clinical trials, peppermint oil was given in enteric-coated form at a dose of 0.2 to 0.4 ml 3 times a day. Whole peppermint leaf is taken in tea form.
Contraindications: Because of the potential toxicity of excessive peppermint oil, use in pregnant or nursing women and in individuals with severe hepatic or renal disease is not advised.
Side effects: Peppermint leaf has a low order of toxicity and is generally regarded as safe (GRAS). However, even at normal doses, peppermint oil can cause esophageal reflux, which is the reason for usage of enteric-coated capsules. Excessive intake of peppermint oil can cause CNS and renal damage. At normal doses, however, peppermint oil generally causes few side effects. Inhalation occasionally causes hypersensitivity reactions.
Dental considerations:
Ask why the product is being used.
Drug interactions: Animal studies suggest that oral peppermint oil can increase cyclosporine bioavailablity. This could cause cyclosporine levels to rise to toxic levels; conversely, if cyclosporine levels are adjusted while an individual is taking peppermint oil, discontinuation could cause a fall to subtherapeutic levels.

Probiotics
Other names: Friendly bacteria, acidophilus
Class: Nonherbal remedy
Major ingredients: Probiotics in common use include *Lactobacillus acidophilus, Lactobacillus GG,* and other lactobacilli; *Bifidobacterium bifidum; Saccharomyces boulardii* (a yeast); *Streptococcus thermophilus;* and *S. salivarius.*

Claimed actions: Probiotics are microorganisms (usually bacteria, but also yeasts) that colonize the digestive tract and other tissues and exist in healthy symbiosis with the body. They compete with and potentially inhibit pathogenic organisms, and may aid digestion and assist in the formation of vitamin K. Altered bowel flora may cause immunomodulatory effects as well.
Uses: Numerous RCTs have evaluated the use of probiotics for preventing or treating various forms of diarrhea, including acute viral diarrhea, traveler's diarrhea, antibiotic-associated diarrhea, and chemotherapy- or radiation-induced diarrhea. In general, the results have been supportive. Probiotics may also help prevent caries. One large RCT found that use of *Lactobacillus GG* in milk given to children ages 1 to 6 reduced incidence of caries as compared with unfortified milk. Other RCTs sug-

gest benefits for inflammatory bowel disease, irritable bowel syndrome, and eczema. Weaker or mixed evidence has been presented regarding usefulness for urinary tract infection prophylaxis, hyperlipidemia, and prevention of upper respiratory tract infections.

Administration: A typical dose of bacterial probiotics supplies about 5 billion live organisms daily. *S. boullardii* yeast is taken at a dose of 500 mg twice daily. Surveys of products on the market have shown wide variability in quality.

Side effects: Aside from a short-term increase in intestinal gas production, use of probiotics by healthy people has not been associated with any significant side effects. Immunocompromised individuals may be at risk from invasive infection by the probiotic, however.

Dental considerations:

Ask why the product is being used. As noted previously, some evidence indicates potential benefit for caries prophylaxis in children.

Drug interactions: No dental drug interactions are reported. Use of probiotics during and for a short while after antibiotic usage may prevent antibiotic-associated diarrhea and restore normal bowel flora.

Proteolytic enzymes

Other names: Pancreatic enzymes, digestive enzymes

Class: Nonherbal remedy

Major ingredients: Commercial products generally include one or more of the following proteolytic enzymes: bromelain, chymotrypsin, pancreatin, papain, or trypsin.

Claimed actions: Although the primary physiologic use of proteolytic enzymes is to digest protein, it appears that some portion of exogenously delivered proteolytic enzymes enters systemic circulation and exerts an antiinflammatory effect.

Uses: Proteolytic enzyme mixtures have been tried for reducing pain and edema following surgery, but the results of the numerous reported RCTs have been mixed. Other RCTs suggest possible benefits for sports injuries and other minor injuries, again reducing pain and edema. Proteolytic enzymes have also shown some promise for osteoarthritis and herpes zoster. Other claimed uses, but that lack RCT support, include food allergies and rheumatoid arthritis.

Administration: Proteolytic enzymes are delivered orally in a variety of enteric-coated or non–enteric-coated forms. Dosage depends on the particular product. Maximum safe doses for pregnant or nursing women, young children, and individuals with severe hepatic or renal disease have not been established.

Side effects: In clinical trials, use of proteolytic enzymes has not been associated with any significant side effects beyond occasional allergic reactions or nonspecific digestive distress.

Dental considerations:

Ask why the product is being used.

Drug interactions: Papain might potentiate anticoagulant and antiplatelet agents. Pancreatin could interfere with the absorption of folic acid supplements.

Pyruvate

Other names: Dihydroxyacetone pyruvate, DHAP

Class: Nonherbal remedy

Major ingredients: Pyruvate is a product of aerobic glycolysis. It enters the mitochondria to form acetyl CoA by oxidative decarboxylation. There is little pyruvate in the diet; it is synthesized endogenously.

Claimed actions: Some evidence suggests that exogenous pyruvate has a feedback-inhibition effect on lipid synthesis. Weaker evidence hints that increased supply of pyruvate might enable a higher rate of ATP synthesis during exercise.

Uses: Limited evidence from small RCTs indicates that pyruvate supplements may aid weight loss or body composition (fat/muscle proportion). In general, evidence from clinical trials does not support use of pyruvate as a sports performance enhancing agent.

Administration: Pyruvate is typically taken at a dose of 30 g daily, in divided doses. It is often sold in combination with dihydroxyacetone, under the name DHAP (dihydroxyacetone pyruvate). Maximum safe doses are not known for pregnant or nursing women, young children, and individuals with severe hepatic or renal disease.

Side effects: In clinical trials, use of pyruvate has not caused significant side effects other than occasional allergic reactions and nonspecific digestive distress.

Dental considerations:

Ask why the product is being used.

Drug interactions: No dental drug interactions are reported.

Quercetin

Other names: Quercetin chalcone

Class: Nonherbal remedy

Major ingredients: Quercetin is a bioflavonoid found in many foods, particularly apples, black tea, grapefruit, onions, and red wine.

Claimed actions: Some evidence suggests that exogenous quercetin has antiinflammatory effects and also inhibits nitric oxide and tyrosine kinase. Quercetin, like many bioflavanoids, has antioxidant and chemopreventive properties in vitro. It is also said to have the cromolyn-like effect of stabilizing mast cells, but the supporting evidence for this claim is weak, and there are no RCTs that show actual clinical effect in allergies.

Uses: One small RCT found limited evidence that quercetin may be effective for the treatment of chronic prostatitis. Another small RCT hints at benefits for interstitial cystitis. Other proposed uses that lack RCT substantiation include allergies (eczema, asthma, allergic rhinitis), viral infections, and prevention of cataracts, cancer, and heart disease.

Administration: Quercetin is usually taken orally at a dose of 500 mg two times daily. Quercetin chalcone is marketed as having better oral absorption than quercetin, but this has not been reliably substantiated. Maximum safe doses in young children and in individu-

als with severe hepatic or renal disease have not been established.
Contraindications: Weak evidence hints that use of quercetin by pregnant or nursing mothers might increase the risk of infant leukemia.
Side effects: Use of quercetin in clinical trials has not been associated with any significant side effects beyond occasional allergic reactions and nonspecific digestive distress. However, despite in vitro evidence of chemoprevention, there are some indications that quercetin could have a carcinogenic effect under certain circumstances that are not well defined as yet.
Dental considerations: Ask why the product is being used.
Drug interactions: No dental drug interactions are reported.

Sage
(Salvia officinalis)
Other names: Broad-leaf sage, common sage, Dalmatian sage, garden sage, true sage
Class: Herbal remedy
Major ingredients: volatile oils, phenolic acids, tannins, diterpene bitter principles, triterpenes, steroids, flavones, and flavonoid glycosides

---

Claimed actions: Antibacterial, fungistatic, virustatic, astringent, carminative, secretion promotion, and perspiration inhibition.
Uses: From the earliest of times, uses have included treatment of open sores and wounds, sore throat, and fertility problems. Sage is also used to treat gum disease, canker sores, and halitosis. Other uses include antioxidant effects, menstrual pain, menopausal symptoms, and muscle spasms. Orally ingested sage is reported to reduce perspiration and to encourage appetite. Other uses include stomatitis, gingivitis, pharyngitis, and hyperhidrosis. It has been used topically to treat itching associated with insect bites along with herpes lesions, shingles, and psoriasis.
Administration: Dried leaves, extract, tincture, and essential oil.
Contraindications: Pregnancy.
Side effects: Reported side effects include vertigo, tachycardia, and, for patients prone to seizures, a risk of seizure.
Dental considerations:
Efficacy for use of sage gargle for gum disease is not established.
Drug interactions: Insulin or oral hypoglycemics, seizure medications. Some sage products may contain alcohol (tincture) and should not be used with disulfiram.

SAMe
Other names: Ademethionine, adenosylmethionine, S-adenosylmethionine, S-adenosyl-l-methionine (pronounced "Sammy")
Class: Nonherbal remedy
Major ingredients: S-adenosylmethionine.

Claimed actions: A naturally occurring molecule found in most body tissues, SAMe is an active methyl carrier playing an essential role in transmethylation. It is involved in the synthesis, metabolism, and activation of hormones, neurotransmitters, phospholipids, proteins, nucleic acids, and some natural medications. SAMe is inti-

mately linked to vitamin B_{12} and folic acid metabolism. When these vitamins are absent, reduced levels of SAMe can result. As a result, SAMe affects serotonin and many body tissues, including cartilage and membranes. It functions as an antidepressant via an unknown mechanism, but is associated with increased levels of serotonin, dopamine, and norepinephrine.
Uses: A moderate level of evidence from placebo-controlled and comparative RCTs indicates that oral SAMe can reduce symptoms of osteoarthritis, to approximately the same extent as low doses of NSAIDs. Weaker RCT evidence supports efficacy in depression, fibromyalgia, and cholestasis, and in highly preliminary studies SAMe has shown promise for Gilbert's disease and other liver disorders.
Administration: Oral dose forms have variable bioavailability; doses used in clinical trials were generally 1200 to 1600 mg daily, taken in divided doses.
Contraindications: None reported; however, there is a possible risk of hypomania in patients with bipolar disorder.
Side effects: GI—diarrhea, nausea, vomiting. CNS—hypomania in bipolar disorder, anxiety.
Dental considerations:
Determine why the patient is taking the drug.
Drug interactions: SAMe might interfere with the effectiveness of L-dopa, used for Parkinson's disease. Based on a case report of a toxic interaction with clomipramine, combination use with standard antidepressants should be done only with caution.

Saw palmetto
(Serenoa repens, Sabal fructus)
Other names: Sabal, cabbage palm, saw palmetto berry
Class: Herbal remedy
Major ingredients: Contains various sitosterols (phytosterols) such as beta-sitosterol and other sitosterol compounds, flavonoids, polysaccharides, and free fatty acids. The portion of the plant used is the ripe, dried fruit.

Claimed actions: Reported to be antiandrogenic and antiinflammatory, and may have some low-level estrogenic activity. The antiandrogenic activity is suggested to occur by inhibition of the enzyme testosterone-5-alpha-reductase. This action prevents the conversion of testosterone to dihydrotestosterone, the active androgenic hormone. Some data support blockade of dihydrotestosterone to receptors in the cell nucleus. Limited data seem to support the estrogenic effects. The antiinflammatory effects remain doubtful. Use of saw palmetto does not affect PSA levels.
Uses: This herbal product has been used in the treatment of symptoms associated with benign prostatic hyperplasia, in particular urinary difficulties. Clinical trials show better results than placebo and apparent comparative results to finasteride (Proscar) and other pharmaceuticals for BPH. Saw palmetto appears to cause some reduction of the size of the prostate gland, though not to the same extent as finasteride. (Note: Several effective pharmaceuticals for BPH cause no change in prostate gland

size.) Use in prostatitis and baldness remains speculative.

Administration: Saw palmetto is taken at a dose of 160 mg twice a day of an extract standardized to contain 85% to 95% fatty acids and sterols.

Side effects: In clinical trials, side effects associated with saw palmetto have been few and nonspecific. There is one case report of saw palmetto apparently causing increased bleeding during surgery; for this reason, use of saw palmetto should be discontinued 2 weeks before surgery. Whether it can influence other androgens or even show estrogenic effects in women is not clear. Avoid use in pregnancy and in women of childbearing age.

Dental considerations:

Ask why the product is being used.

Drug interactions: No dental drug interactions are reported.

St. John's wort

(Hypericum perforatum, Hyperici herba)

Other names: Hypericum, kaimath weed, John's wort

Class: Herbal remedy

Major ingredients: Contains quinoids (hypericin, pseudohypericin), anthraquinones, flavonoids (hyperoside, quercitin, rutin), bioflavonoids, and a volatile oil. One of the pharmacologically active components is hyperforin; another, hypericin, has photosensitizing properties. Flavonoids including amentaflavone may contribute to the pharmacologic action of the herb. The portions of the plant used are the aboveground parts harvested during the flowering season.

Claimed actions: The primary actions are antidepressant, antiinflammatory, and antimicrobial. The constituent hyperforin appears to inihibit uptake of serotonin, dopamine, and norepinephrine.

Uses: It is used for the treatment of mild to moderate major depression; according to most but not all of the many RCTs performed it is more effective than placebo and, except in severe major depression, as effective as tricyclics or SSRIs. The volatile oil seems to increase the healing of burns. Hypericin has shown in vitro activity against the HIV virus, but human trials indicate that to produce any clinical effect, hypericin must be taken in toxic doses. One RCT failed to find St. John's wort helpful for polyneuropathy. Topical St. John's wort has shown some promise for eczema.

Administration: A variety of oral preparations are available, standardized to either hypericin or hyperforin.

Side effects: In the extensive clinical trial experience with St. John's wort, side effects have been limited and generally nonspecific. Photosensitization may occur at higher doses or with topical use. Like all antidepressants, St. John's wort can cause episodes of mania in people with bipolar disorder. There are some reports that use of St. John's wort by individuals with Alzheimer's disease may increase agitation. Its safety during pregnancy and lactation is unknown.

Dental considerations:

Ask why the product is being used.

Drug interactions: St. John's wort affects a variety of cytochromes, as well as the transport protein p-glycoprotein, and can reduce levels and thereby activity of numerous medications to an extent that is clinically significant. Interacting drugs include oral contraceptives (leading to unwanted pregnancy), protease inhibitors and nonnucleoside reverse transcriptase inhibitors (leading to reduced anti-HIV effectiveness), cyclosporine (leading to organ rejection), clozapine, digoxin, losartan, metronidazole, olanzapine, omeprazole, statins, warfarin, and various chemotherapy drugs. Note also that if blood levels of a drug are stabilized while a patient is on St. John's wort, discontinuation of the herb may cause a dangerous rise in levels. In addition, St. John's wort should be used only with caution if at all in patients taking other antidepressive medications, including MAO inhibitors, tricyclic antidepressants, and selective serotonin reuptake inhibitors, because case reports suggest a risk of serotonin syndrome. Combined use with tramadol might present a similar risk. Although St. John's wort does not appear to have MAO inhibitor actions at normal doses, one case report exists of an MAO-like interaction between St. John's wort and tyramine-containing foods. Discontinue use 2 weeks before general anesthesia. Avoid dental (or other) drugs with a potential for photosensitivity.

Stevia

(Stevia rebaudiana)

Other names: Caa'inhem, Paraguayan sweet herb, sweet herb, sweet leaf of Paraguay, sweetleaf

Class: Herbal remedy

Major ingredients: The leaves of this plant are used medicinally. Major active constituents include diterpene steviosides and rebaudioside. Flavonoids and volatile oil are present as well.

Claimed actions: Steviosides are sweeter than sucrose by weight, producing a taste said to be preferable to saccharine, though not entirely without aftertaste. At much higher doses than reasonable intake for use as a sugar substitute, steviosides have shown an antihypertensive effect.

Uses: Stevia enjoys wide use as a noncaloric sweetening agent in Japan and several other countries. However, in the United States stevia has not received approval for use under this designation; it is nonetheless used widely as a sweetener without claiming it as such. Concentrated steviosides at far higher doses are beginning to be used by people with hypertension; such use may be expected to increase in the future.

Administration: Approximately one-sixth teaspoon of ground stevia (or 2 to 4 drops of stevia liquid extract) equals the sweetness of one teaspoon of ordinary sugar. This supplies about 30 mg of steviosides. For hypertension, the dose used in clinical trials was 250 to 500 mg of concentrated steviosides three times daily. Maximum safe doses in pregnant or nursing women, young children, and individuals with severe hepatic or renal disease have not been established.

Side effects: Stevia is generally

regarded as a safe herb, but animal studies suggest that high doses may have antifertility actions in both males and females. The widespread use of stevia in Japan suggests reasonable safety in children and pregnant women.
Dental considerations: Patients may be using stevioside-sweetened products to avoid caries, a use that may be reasonable.
Drug interactions: If someone is used to taking 25 teaspoons of sugar a day, the equivalent in stevia might produce an antihypertensive effect. Certain more susceptible people might respond at a lower dose. This suggests the possibility of potentiation interactions with antihypertensives, but no such interactions have been reported as yet.

Valerian
(Valeriana officinalis, Valerianae radix)
Other names: Valerian root, Indian valerian
Class: Herbal remedy
Major ingredients: Valepotriates (isovaltrate and others), a volatile oil (bornyl isovalerenate and isovalerenic acid), sesquiterpenes, and multiple other substances. Pharmacologically active components are not identified with any certainty, but may be isovaleric acid and related derivatives. The portions of the plant used are the fresh underground parts and roots.

Claimed actions: Sedation, reduction in nervousness, sleep promoting, and antispasmodic. Laboratory data suggest that it may increase GABA levels at synapses.
Uses: Evidence from several RCTs suggests that valerian can improve sleep, especially with continued use. Other proposed uses of valerian lack meaningful supporting evidence. These include restlessness, reduction in nervousness (anxiolytic), agitation associated with menstruation, colic, stomach cramps, and uterine spasticity. Antispasmodic properties are not well defined. It has also been used externally by adding to bath water.
Administration: Available for oral use in a variety of oral products, including tinctures, infusions, and extracts.
Side effects: Generally not observed in usual doses. GI complaints, headache, sleeplessness, mydriasis, excitability, and cardiac disturbances may occur with long-term use.
Dental considerations:
Ask why the product is being used.
Drug interactions: Although no interactions are reported, monitor patients for increased sedation when using other CNS depressants. May potentiate CNS depressants.

Yohimbe bark
(Pausinystalia yohimbe)
Other names: Yohimbe cortex
Class: Herbal remedy
Major ingredients: The principal alkaloid is yohimbine (quebrachine) with lesser amounts of stereoisomers of yohimbine along with other indole alkaloids, including corynantheidine and allo-yohimbine. It also contains a variety of plant tannins. The portion of the

plant used is the dried bark of the trunk and branches of the tree.

Claimed actions: The major effects of this drug are due to yohimbine. Do not confuse the prescription drug yohimbine with yohimbe. Yohimbine has α_2-adrenergic antagonist activity. Presynaptic α_2-adrenergic receptors regulate norepinephrine release. In a feedback-type action, antagonism of these receptors is associated with greater norepinephrine release. It may also dilate blood vessels; claims are made for a calcium channel blocking action and inhibition of monoamine oxidase enzymes.
Uses: It has been used to treat erectile dysfunction, as an aphrodisiac, for exhaustion, and even for orthostatic hypotension. Limited data concern yohimbine and not yohimbe. Yohimbine has not been approved for this application. According to the German Commission E monographs, yohimbe's effectiveness is not documented and it is not recommended.
Administration: Limited products are available and usually in combination with other ingredients.
Side effects: Usual doses produce few side effects; however, in large doses significant adverse effects are reported. These include increased salivation, anxiety, hallucinations, exanthema, nervousness, irritability, tachycardia, and sweating. Other effects may also be observed. Cardiac failure, which could be fatal, is reported. Contraindicated in patients with hepatic or renal impairment and psychiatric disorders.
Dental considerations:
Ask why the product is being used.
Drug interactions: No specific dental drug interactions are reported, but it may have MAO inhibitory action. Avoid use of indirect-acting sympathomimetics and tricyclic antidepressants.

Xylitol

Class: Nonherbal remedy
Major ingredients: Xylitol is a polyol with the same intensity of sweetness as sucrose, but it cannot serve as a metabolic base for oral microbes.

Claimed actions: Xylitol inhibits the growth of *Streptococcus mutans,* and on this basis has been proposed as a prophylactic agent against dental caries. Xylitol may also inhibit growth of *S. pneumoniae* and thereby reduce risk of respiratory infections caused by this organism.
Uses: In several large randomized controlled trials, children who used gums, lozenges, syrups, toothpastes, or candies containing xylitol experienced a reduced incidence of caries as compared with control groups. Use of xylitol by nursing mothers may also confer some protection to the child, presumably because infants receive their initial *S. mutans* colonization from the mother. Other RCTs suggest that xylitol use by children may reduce incidence of otitis media. Xylitol has additionally been suggested as a prophylactic for periodontal disease, but this potential use has not yet undergone significant study.
Administration: A typical dose of xylitol used in clinical trials for caries prevention was 4.3 to 10 g

daily. Higher doses appear to be more effective than lower doses. **Side effects:** High consumption of xylitol can cause mild digestive distress and possibly diarrhea, especially in children.

Dental considerations:
Patients should be reminded that xylitol gum and related products should be used in addition to standard dental hygiene recommendations, not as a substitute for them.

Drug interactions: No dental drug interactions are reported.

BIBLIOGRAPHY

Blake S: *Alternative remedies CD-ROM,* St Louis, 2001, Mosby.

Blumenthal M et al: *The complete German Commission E monographs,* Austin, 1998, American Botanical Council.

Miller LG: Herbal medicinals: selected clinical considerations focusing on known or potential drug-herb interactions, *Arch Intern Med* 158(20):2200-2211, 1998.

Mosby's drug consult 2004: the comprehensive reference for generic and brand name drugs, ed 14, St Louis, 2004, Mosby.

Mosby's handbook of herbs and supplements and their therapeutic uses, St Louis, 2003, Mosby.

Natural medicines comprehensive database, Stockton, CA, 2004, Pharmacist's Letter/Prescriber's Letter, Therapeutic Research Faculty.

Nonherbal dietary supplements, *Pharmacist's Letter* 98(4), 1998.

O'Hara MA et al: A review of 12 commonly used medicinal herbs, *Arch Fam Med* 7:523-536, 1998.

PDR for herbal remedies, Montvale, NJ, 1998, Medical Economics.

Therapeutic use of herbs, continuing education booklets part 1 and part 2, Stockton, CA, 1998, Pharmacist's Letter.

Appendix I

Drugs Affecting the Cytochrome P-450 Isoenzymes

The cytochrome P-450 (CYP450) families of isoenzymes act as major enzyme systems for the oxidative metabolism of a large number of drugs. The highest concentrations of CYP450 enzymes are found in the liver and intestine, with lesser amounts in other tissues. They are distinguished from one another by family names using letters and numbers; for example, CYP1A2, CYP2D6, or CYP3A4. A number of drugs and foods can induce or inhibit specific isoenzymes, and in some instances this has resulted in serious drug interactions. It is also true that one drug may be a substrate for CYP450 and at the same time cause induction or inhibition of that same enzyme. Because enzymes are substrate specific, each CYP450 isoenzyme will catalyze the metabolism of only selected drugs. On the other hand, more than one CYP450 isoenzyme may participate in the metabolism of a drug.

An example of a drug interaction involving CYP3A4 is provided. Lovastatin (Mevacor, a drug that interferes with cholesterol synthesis) is a substrate for CYP3A4. Erythromycin (a macrolide antiinfective) is an inhibitor of CYP3A4. Thus erythromycin, by its effects on the CYP3A4 isoenzyme, inhibits the metabolism of lovastatin when the drugs are taken concurrently. This results in decreased clearance of the drug from the body and increased plasma levels of lovastatin. Significant increases in the plasma levels of lovastatin have been associated with the risk of a potentially serious adverse effect known as *rhabdomyolysis.* Thus erythromycin is contraindicated when a patient is also taking lovastatin. In some cases, inhibition of CYP450 in the intestines will result in altered drug absorption. This can mean either too little drug is absorbed or more drug is absorbed than expected. Either effect will modify the anticipated response. When a drug is both a substrate and an inducer of CYP450 enzymes, the anticipated response of a second dose will be less than expected. For some drugs, this can be overcome by giving higher than normal doses. Grapefruit juice is an example of a food that is an inhibitor of CYP3A4.

The following table lists a number of drugs that function either as substrates, inhibitors, or inducers of one or more of the CYP450 isoenzymes. It is almost impossible to list all of the potential or established drug interactions, but some involve commonly used dental drugs. When the notation of dental drug interaction appears, refer to the individual monograph for each drug to see the specific drug interactions as related to this family of enzymes only. (Hint: Select the generic name and use the colored tabs on the side of the book to quickly locate a drug.)

Isoenzyme	Drug	Substrate	Inducer	Inhibitor	Dental drug interaction
CYP1A2					
	acetaminophen	X			
	aprepitant (Emend)	X			
	atazanavir (Reyataz)		X		
	caffeine	X			
	ciprofloxacin (Cipro)			X	X
	clozapine (Clozaril)	X			
	cimetidine (Tagamet)			X	
	cyclobenzaprine (Flexeril)	X			
	erythromycin			X	
	estradiol	X			
	fluvoxamine (Luvox)			X	X
	naproxen (Naprosyn)	X			
	norfloxacin (Noroxin)			X	
	olanzapine (Zyprexa)	X			
	rifampin (Rifadin)		X		
	riluzole (Rilutrex)	X			
	theophylline	X			X
	tacrine (Cognex)	X		X	
	ticlopidine (Ticlid)			X	
	verapamil (Calan)	X			
	warfarin (Coumadin)	X			
	zileuton (Zyflo)	X			
Nondrug substance					
	Cigarette smoke		X		
CYP2B6					
	bupropion (Wellbutrin)	X			
	efivarenz (Sustiva)	X			

Isoenzyme	Drug	Substrate	Inducer	Inhibitor	Dental drug interaction
CYP2C8-10					
	cimetidine (Tagamet)			X	
	diazepam (Valium)	X			
	diclofenac (Cataflam)	X			
	fluvastatin (Lescol)	X			
	omeprazole (Prilosec)			X	
	paclitaxel (Taxol)	X			
	phenobarbital		X		
	rifampin (Rifadin)		X		
CYP2C9	amitriptyline (Elavil)	X			
	aprepitant (Emend)		X		
	atazanavir (Reyataz)			X	
	bosentan (Tracleer)	X			
	celecoxib (Celebrex)	X			
	clopidrogel (Plavix)			X	
	diclofenac	X			
	fluconazole (Diflucan)			X	
	fluvastatin (Lescol)	X			
	fluvoxamine (Luvox)			X	
	formoterol (Foradil)	X			
	glipizide (Glucotrol)	X			
	ibuprofen	X			
	imipramine (Tofranil)	X			
	ketoconazole (Nizoral)			X	
	metronidazole (Flagyl)			X	

Isoenzyme	Drug	Substrate	Inducer	Inhibitor	Dental drug interaction
	montelukast (Singulair)	X			
	naproxen	X			
	phenytoin (Dilantin)	X			
	piroxicam (Feldene)	X			
	rifampin (Rifacdin)				
	ritonavir (Norvir)			X	
	secobarbital		X		
	sildenafil (Viagra)	X			
	valdecoxib (Bextra)	X			
	warfarin (Coumadin)	X			
	zafirlukast (Accolate)	X		X	
	zileuton (Zyflo)	X			
CYP2C19					
	aprepitant (Emend)	X		X	
	citalopram (Celexa)	X			
	diazepam (Valium)	X			
	escitalopram (Lexapro)	X			
	felbamate (Felbatol)			X	
	fluoxetine (Prozac)			X	
	formoterol (Foradil)	X			
	lansoprazole (Prevacid)	X			
	nelfinavir (Viracept)	X			
	omeprazole (Prilosec)	X			
	oxcarbazepine (Trileptal)			X	
	propranolol (Inderal)	X			
	rifampin (Rifadin)		X		

Isoenzyme	Drug	Substrate	Inducer	Inhibitor	Dental drug interaction
CYP2D6					
	amitriptyline (Elavil)	X			
	bupropion (Wellbutrin)			X	
	cevimeline (Evoxac)	X			
	chlorphe-niramine			X	
	codeine	X			
	desipramine (Norpramin)	X			
	dextromethor-phan	X			
	diphenhydra-mine (Benadryl)			X	X
	donepezil (Aricept)	X			
	escitalopram (Lexapro)	X			
	fluoxetine (Prozac)			X	
	fluvoxamine (Luvox)			X	
	formoterol (Foradil)	X			
	haloperidol (Haldol)	X			
	mexiletine (Mexitil)	X			
	oxycodone	X			
	paroxetine (Paxil)			X	
	propoxyphene	X			
	ritonavir (Norvir)			X	
	sertraline (Zoloft)			X	X
	timolol (Blocadren)	X			
	tolterodine (Detrol)	X			
	tramadol (Ultram)	X			
	venlafaxine (Effexor)	X			

Isoenzyme	Drug	Substrate	Inducer	Inhibitor	Dental drug interaction
CYP2E1					
	acetaminophen	X			
	chlorzoxazone (Paraflex)	X			
	disulfiram			X	
	ethanol	X	X		
	isoniazid		X		
CYP3A3					
	alprazolam (Xanax)	X			
	cimetidine (Tagamet)			X	
	erythromycin	X			
	midazolam (Versed)	X			
	ranitidine (Zantac)			X	
	rifabutin (Mycobutin)		X		
	rifampin (Rifadin)		X		
CYP3A4					
	alfuzosin (Uroxatral)	X			
	alprazolam (Xanax)	X			X
	amprenavir (Agenerase)	X		X	X
	amiodarone (Cordarone)	X		X	
	apepitant (Emend)	X			
	atazanavir (Reyataz)	X			X
	atorvastatin (Lipitor)	X			X
	buspirone (BuSpar)	X			X
	bosentan (Tracleer)	X	X		
	carbamazepine (Tegretol)	X	X		X
	clorazepate (Tranxene)	X			X
	chlordiazepoxide (Librium)	X			X

Isoenzyme	Drug	Substrate	Inducer	Inhibitor	Dental drug interaction
	cimetidine (Tagamet)			X	
	citalopram (Celexa)	X			X
	clarithromycin (Biaxin)	X		X	X
	cyclosporine (Sandimmune)	X			
	delavirdine (Rescreptor)	X		X	
	dexamethasone (Decadron)	X		X	X
	diazepam (Valium)	X			X
	diltiazem (Cardizem)	X			
	dutasteride (Avodart)	X			
	efavirenz (Sustiva)		X		
	eletriptan (Replax)	X			
	eplerenone (Inspra)	X			
	erythromycin	X		X	X
	escitalopram (Lexapro)	X			
	estazolam (ProSom)	X			X
	felodipine (Plendil)	X			X
	fluconazole (Diflucan)			X	X
	fluvastatin (Lescol)	X			
	fluvoxamine (Luvox)			X	
	fomaterol (Foradil)	X			
	indinavir (Crixivan)	X		X	X
	itraconazole (Sporanox)			X	X
	ketoconazole (Nizoral)			X	X
	lovastatin (Mevacor)	X			X

Isoenzyme	Drug	Substrate	Inducer	Inhibitor	Dental drug interaction
	lidocaine	X			
	metronidazole (Flagyl)			X	X
	midazolam (Versed)	X			X
	montelukast (Singulair)	X			
	nefazodone (Serzone)			X	X
	nelfinavir (Viracept)	X		X	X
	nevirapine (Viramune)	X	X		
	nicardipine (Cardene)	X			
	nifedipine (Procardia)	X			
	nisoldipine (Sular)	X			
	omeprazole (Prilosec)			X	
	oxcarbamazepine (Trileptal)		X		
	paclitaxel (Taxol)	X			
	phenobarbital	X	X		X
	quazepam (Doral)	X			X
	ritonavir (Norvir)	X		X	X
	saquinavir (Fortovase)	X		X	X
	sertraline (Zoloft)			X	X
	sildenafil (Viagra)	X			X
	simvastatin (Zocor)	X			X
	tacrolimus (Prograf)	X			
	tadalafil (Cialis)	X			X
	tiagabine (Gabitril)	X			
	triazolam (Halcion)	X			X

Isoenzyme	Drug	Substrate	Inducer	Inhibitor	Dental drug interaction
	trimetrexate (Neutrexin)	X			
	valdecoxib (Bextra)	X			
	vardenafil (Levitra)	X			X
	verapamil (Calan)	X		X	
	warfarin (Coumadin)	X			X
	zafirlukast (Accolate)			X	
	zaleplon (Sonata)	X			
	zileuton (Zyflo)	X			
	zolpidem (Ambien)	X			X
NONDRUG PRODUCTS					
	Grapefruit juice			X	X
	St. John's wort		X		X
CYP3A5					
	levostatin (Mevacor)	X			
	midazolam (Versed)	X			
	nifedipine (Procardia)	X			

Appendix J

Prescription Examples

This appendix illustrates a number of prescriptions that can be used as a guide to help you write prescriptions for dental patients. They can be used as written or modified to address each patient's specific needs and your personal preferences. They are not a substitute for your clinical judgment. The process of selecting and prescribing a medication for a patient is usually straightforward, but it can be challenging in some cases. It is important for the prescribing dentist to be completely knowledgeable about any drug prescribed. Complete prescribing information should be consulted before selecting a drug. This means knowing how the drug acts, its intended use, the dose and dose forms, how frequently the drug should be taken, and adverse effects and drug interactions. These essential drug facts are tools for the profession. In the following examples, prescriptions for brand name drugs are for illustrative purposes only and do not constitute a recommendation for that particular product. In an era of expensive brand name products, generics are generally the less expensive way to prescribe medications, but in some cases (especially for new drugs or specialty products) only brand name products are available.

Before prescribing or recommending (in the case of OTC products) a medication for a patient, it is strongly suggested that the dentist adhere to the following protocol:

a. Examine and evaluate the patient, leading to a diagnosis.
b. Obtain the patient's medical and drug history (including the use of OTC drugs, illegal drugs, and herbal or nonherbal remedies).
c. Determine the duration of drug therapy and the required number of doses.
d. Assess the patient's prior experience with drugs, including drug allergy.
e. Research the potential side effects and drug interactions.
f. Adhere to all federal and state laws regulating drug use in practice.
g. Consider the cost to the patient if less expensive alternatives are available.
h. Consider the patient's ability to use more complex dose forms or to follow complex instructions for use.
i. Have an alternative selection in mind in the event a patient cannot tolerate the prescribed drug.

I. ANALGESICS

Controlled substances (requires state and DEA registration to prescribe with DEA number included on the prescription)

Prescription examples are for acute pain without regard to intensity of pain. Because acute pain is generally managed within 3-4 days, prescriptions should limit the number of doses to be dispensed. In given situations, more than 10 or 12 doses may be required. *If the analgesic product you are using is not illustrated, don't worry. These are merely examples provided for guidance in prescription writing and are not inclusive of all analgesic products, which number into the hundreds.* For illustrative purposes, both brand and generic names are used. Note that the directions for use indicate a specific time interval for optimum response; prn use is avoided to ensure more appropriate dosing intervals for the analgesic. By the clock dosing is much more effective than as needed doses. The cautions of sedation, hazard of operating an automobile, and avoidance of alcohol are appropriate for each product.

Rx
Darvocet-N 100*
Disp: 12 (twelve) tabs
Sig: Take 1 (one) tab PO q4h for pain relief.
*(The maximum recommended dose for propoxyphene napsylate is 600 mg/day. Do not take with alcohol, and reduce the dose or select another drug if significant liver or renal failure is present.)

Rx
Empirin with Codeine #4*
Disp: 12 (twelve) tabs
Sig: Take 1 (one) tab PO q4h for pain relief.
*(This product contains 60 mg of codeine phosphate, a preferable oral adult dose; the No. 3 product contains 30 mg of codeine phosphate.)

Rx
Fiorinal with Codeine 30 mg*
Disp: 12 (twelve) caps
Sig: Take 1 (one) cap PO q4-6h for pain relief.
*(This product contains a short-acting barbiturate. Fioricet with Codeine 30 mg contains acetaminophen instead of aspirin.)

Rx
Lortab 5/500
Disp: 12 (twelve) tabs
Sig: Take 1 (one) tab PO q6h for pain relief.

Rx
Percodan
Disp: 10 (ten) tabs
Sig: Take 1 (one) tab PO q6h for pain relief.

Rx
Tylenol with Codeine Elixir*
Disp: 90 ml (volume may vary with duration and patient's age)
Sig: Take 5 ml (one teaspoonful) q6-8h for pain relief.
*(This is an example for a child age 3-6 yr. For a child age 7-12 yr the dose is 10 ml, and for adults the dose is 15 ml. Be sure you know the quantities of acetaminophen and codeine phosphate contained

in each 5 ml dose. This product also contains alcohol. Your pharmacist can increase the amount of codeine in each 5 ml dose unit; consult your pharmacist for instructions.)

Rx
Tylenol with Codeine #4*
Disp: 12 (twelve) tabs
Sig: Take 1 (one) tab PO q4h for pain relief.
*(This product contains 60 mg of codeine phosphate, a preferable oral adult dose; the No. 3 product contains 30 mg of codeine phosphate.)

Rx
Vicodin
Disp: 10 (ten) tabs
Sig: Take 1 (one) tab PO q6h for pain relief.

Rx
Zydone 5/400*
Disp: 10 (ten) tabs
Sig: Take 1 (one) or 2 (two) tabs PO q4-6h for pain relief.
*(Because Zydone is available in several strengths, the prescription must be specific as shown in the example.)

Nonnarcotics or analgesics not classified as controlled substances

Doses for aspirin and acetaminophen for both adults and children are given in the respective monographs. For consistent dose levels and effects, it is important to prescribe NSAIDs by the clock rather than prn.

Rx
diclofenac sodium 50 mg tabs (immediate release type)
Disp: 9 (nine) tabs
Sig: Take 1 (one) tab PO q8h for pain relief.

Rx
diflunisal 500 mg tabs*
Disp: 7 (seven) tabs
Sig: Take 2 (two) tabs PO the first dose; then 1 (one) tab PO q12h for pain relief.
*(The 250 mg tabs may be sufficient for some patients. The initial dose is 500 mg; do not exceed doses of 1.5 g/day.)

Rx
etodolac 400 mg tabs*
Disp: 16 (sixteen) tabs
Sig: Take 1 (one) tab PO q6-8h for pain relief.
*(The 200 mg tabs may be sufficient for some patients. Dose limit is 1200 mg/day.)

Rx
ibuprofen* 400 mg tabs†
Disp: 24 (twenty-four) tabs
Sig: Take 1 tab PO q4h for pain relief.
*(Special preparations for children, such as Children's Motrin with specified doses, are available for toothaches; doses are printed on the package.)
†(If larger doses are preferred, the time interval between doses must be adjusted to reflect the larger dose; for example, 600 mg every 6 hours. Another option is to recommend OTC ibuprofen in 200 mg

tablets and tell the patient to take 2 tabs every 4 hours. For some patients, a prescription may be required to ensure a desirable patient benefit. Ibuprofen also can be used for chronic pain.)

Rx
ketoprofen 25 mg caps (or 50 mg caps)*
Disp: 12 (twelve) caps
Sig: Take 1 (one) cap PO q6-8h for pain relief.
*(The larger dose may be required for some patients. Select the smaller dose for the elderly and patients with severe renal or hepatic disease; also available OTC in 12.5 mg tabs.)

Rx
meclofenamate sodium* 50 mg caps
Disp: 18 (eighteen) caps
Sig: Take 1 (one) cap PO q4-6h for pain relief.
*(Total daily dose is limited to 400 mg.)

Rx
naproxen sodium tabs 550 mg tabs
Disp: 10 (ten) tabs
Sig: Take 1 (one) tab PO q12h for pain relief.
(Naproxen sodium also can be used for chronic pain.)

Rx
Ultram 50 mg tabs*
Disp: 12 (twelve) tabs
Sig: Take 1 (one) tab PO q4-6h for pain relief.
*(For more severe pain, the 100 mg tabs can be prescribed. Do not exceed the daily dose limit of 400 mg.)

Rx
Vioxx 50 mg tabs
Disp: 5 (five) tabs
Sig: Take 1 (one) tab PO daily for pain relief.

II. ANTIINFECTIVES

The primary considerations when selecting an antiinfective drug include potential causative organisms, the severity of the infection, the age of the infection (cellulitis vs. pus formation), the patient's prior history of antiinfective drug use, and the immunologic status of the patient. The duration of antiinfective drug therapy differs somewhat among clinicians, ranging from 5-10 days. Certainly surgical intervention or removal of a necrotic pulp makes a significant difference not only in resolution, but also the duration of the infection. The examples provided for illustration purposes show doses calculated to cover the patient for 7-10 days. Examples include both generic and brand name products. One or two examples of prescriptions for children are shown; doses were calculated using mg per kg of body weight and reflect manufacturers' or USP recommended doses. Antiinfectives should be prescribed to take at specific intervals, such as every 6 hours. Using symbols, such as qid for four times a day, may not allow for proper intervals between doses. However, for some drugs, such as rinses or lozenges, abbreviations such as qid or tid are satisfactory. *Note that these prescriptions are intended to help you develop your own prescription as dictated by the patient's need and circumstance.*

Rx
amoxicillin trihydrate 500 mg caps*
Disp: 21 (twenty-one) caps
Sig: Take 1 (one) cap PO q8h for infection until all are taken.
*(Some may prefer to give an initial loading dose of 1000 mg followed by the 500 mg doses.)

Rx
penicillin V potassium 500 mg tabs*
Disp: 28 (twenty-eight) tabs
Sig: Take 1 (one) tab PO q6h for infection until all are taken.
*(Some may prefer to give an initial loading dose of 1000 mg followed by the 500 mg doses.)

Rx for prophylaxis against bacterial endocarditis for three different appointments

---

Rx
amoxicillin trihydrate 500 mg caps
Disp: 12 (twelve) caps
Sig: Take 4 (four) caps PO 1 hour before each dental appointment.

Rx for a child weighing 30 kg (66 lb)

The package insert dose for children is 20 mg/kg/day (in equal doses given every 8 hours) for mild/moderate infections and 40 mg/kg/day (in equal doses given every 12 hours) for severe infections. The example chosen is 20 mg/kg/day; this means the total daily dose will be 600 mg, or 200 mg every 8 hours in individual doses.

Rx
amoxicillin for oral suspension 200 mg/5 ml
Disp: 150 ml*
Sig: Take 5 ml PO q8h for infection until all is taken.
*(This is enough volume to provide doses for 10 days.)

Rx
cefadroxil 500 mg caps
Disp: 14 (fourteen) caps
Sig: Take 1 (one) cap PO q12h for infection until all are taken.

Rx for prophylaxis against bacterial endocarditis for a single appointment

---

Rx
cefadroxil 1 g tabs*
Disp: 2 (two) tabs
Sig: Take 2 (two) tabs PO 1 hour before appointment.
*(Alternatively, 500 mg caps could also be used, noting that 4 caps are required for a single use.)

Rx
clindamycin hydrochloride 300 mg caps*
Disp: 28 (twenty-eight) caps
Sig: Take 1 (one) cap PO q6h for infection until all are taken.
*(Doses of 150 mg also are used depending on severity of the infection.)

Rx
azithromycin 250 mg caps
Disp: 6 caps
Sig: Take 2 (two) caps PO the first day, then 1 (one) cap daily for infection until all are taken. Take 1 hour ac or 2 hours pc.

Rx
Biaxin 250 mg tabs*
Disp: 20 (twenty) tabs
Sig: Take 1 (one) tab PO q12h for infection until all are taken.
*(The 500 mg dose may be required for some infections, such as maxillary sinusitis subsequent to loss of root tip in the sinus cavity.)

Rx for prophylaxis against bacterial endocarditis for six appointments

Rx
clindamycin hydrochloride 300 mg caps
Disp: 12 (twelve) caps
Sig: Take 2 (two) caps PO 1 hour before each appointment.

Rx
doxycycline 100 mg caps
Disp: 11 (eleven) caps
Sig: Take 1 (one) cap PO q12h the first day, then take 1 (one) cap PO daily for infection until all are taken.

Rx
Ery-Tab 250 mg tabs*
Disp: 40 (forty) tabs
Sig: Take 1 (one) tab PO q6h for infection until all are taken.
*(This is an erythromycin base; other dose options depending on the dose form selected include 333 mg q8h or 500 mg q12h.)

Rx
erythromycin ethyl succinate 400 mg tabs
Disp: 40 (forty) tabs
Sig: Take 1 (one) tab PO q6h for infection until all are taken.

Rx
metronidazole 250 mg tabs
Disp: 21 (twenty-one) tabs
Sig: Take 1 (one) tab PO q8h for infection until all are taken; avoid use of alcohol products.

III. ANTIFUNGAL ANTIINFECTIVES

These are examples (not all products are illustrated) of prescriptions for drugs for *Candida* infections of the oral cavity, which are usually prescribed for use over 14 days. Remember that patient evaluation, history, and diagnosis always precede drug selection.

Rx
clotrimazole 10 mg troches
Disp: 70 troches
Sig: Slowly dissolve 1 (one) troche in your mouth 5 times a day while awake until all are used.

Rx
fluconazole 50 mg tabs*
Disp: 15 (fifteen) tabs
Sig: Take 2 (two) tabs PO the first day, then take 1 (one) tab PO daily for infection until all are taken.
*(The 100 mg dose size may be required for more severe infections or for immunocompromised patients.)

Rx
nystatin ointment*
Disp: 15 (fifteen) g
Sig: Apply a small amount to affected areas after each meal and at bedtime.
*(Possible use in angular cheilitis associated with candidiasis.)

Rx
nystatin oral suspension (100,000 u/ml)
Disp: 320 ml
Sig: Rinse for 1 min with 5 ml of solution q6h while awake and then expectorate. One rinse should be used just before bedtime.*
*(Dentures also should be carefully cleaned and then soaked in the oral solution for approximately 15 min each day during treatment.)

Although some sugar is contained in the commercial preparation of nystatin oral suspension, it is still effective against candidiasis. An alternative choice for oral nystatin rinse when sugar is not desirable for the patient is shown in the following example. Be sure to check labels for sugar content in all locally acting oral products.

Rx
nystatin extemporaneous powder
Disp: 50 million units*
Sig: Add 1/8 tsp (500,000 U) to 1 cup water (8 oz) and rinse qid for 2 weeks.
*(This is the smallest container of powder available; it supplies enough powder for 25 days of use.)

IV. OTHER DENTAL PRESCRIPTIONS

The following prescriptions are examples for a variety of dental diseases. They are grouped according to their usual applications. *Again, there may be many choices for treatment that are not shown; these are examples for assistance in prescription writing.*

Recurrent aphthous stomatitis

Rx
Aphthasol Oral Paste 5%
Disp: 5 (five) g
Sig: Dab a small amount of paste on ulcer qid, pc, and hs.

Rx
Benadryl Elixir 40 ml*
Kaopectate 80 ml
Water q.s. ad. 240 ml
Sig: Rinse with 5 ml for 1-2 min prn for comfort and then expectorate.
*(A 50/50 mixture of Benadryl/Kaopectate also can be used. Benadryl Elixir alone also serves as a palliative rinse, but it contains alcohol; when alcohol is to be avoided use Children's Benadryl, which is alcohol free.)

Rx
chlorhexidine rinse 0.12% or write Peridex
Disp: 16 (sixteen) oz
Sig: Rinse with 15 ml twice daily after brushing.*
*(Optional application route: moisten a cotton-tipped applicator and dab on aphthous ulcer bid.)

Rx
fluocinonide gel 0.05% or write Lidex Gel
Disp: 15 (fifteen) g
Sig: Apply small amount (dab on or use cotton-tipped applicator) to ulcers bid.

Rx
Xylocaine Viscous 2%
Disp: 100 ml
Sig: Rinse with 5 ml for 1-2 min q4h.
(Optional choice: rinse before meals and at bedtime.)

Desquamative lesions (lichen planus, phemphigoid)

Rx
Diprolene gel 0.05%*
Disp: 15 (fifteen) g
Sig: Apply a small amount to lesions tid. Apply the last dose at bedtime.
*(This is a very-high-potency glucocorticoid; consider switching to a high-potency gel once severe lesions are under control.)

Rx
Lidex gel 0.05%*
Disp: 30 (thirty) g
Sig: Apply a small amount to lesions tid. Apply the last dose at bedtime.
*(This is a high-potency topical glucocorticoid. Alternatively, if the lesions are small, dab a small amount directly on the lesions.)

Rx
prednisone 5 mg tabs
Disp: 44 tabs
Sig: Take 2 (two) tabs PO AM and PM × 2 days, then reduce by 1 (one) tab each day until all are taken.

Drugs affecting salivary flow
Prescriptions to reduce salivary flow (using four appointments as an example, because the number of tablets to dispense depends on the number of appointments):

Rx
atropine sulfate 0.4 mg tabs
Disp: 4 (four) tabs
Sig: Take 1 tab PO 30-60 min before appointment.

Rx
Pro-Banthine 15 mg tabs
Disp: 4 (four) tabs
Sig: Take 1 (one) tab PO 45-60 min before appointment.
*(Many pharmacies may no longer stock this particular drug.)

Prescription to stimulate salivary flow in selected patients:

Rx
Evoxac 30 mg caps
Disp: 42 (forty-two) caps*
Sig: Take 1 (one) cap PO three times a day.
*(Larger doses increase risk of side effects; enough doses are ordered for a 2-week period to evaluate patient response.)

Drugs for herpes labialis

Rx
acyclovir 200 mg caps
Disp: 35 (thirty-five) caps
Sig: Take 1 (one) cap PO 5 times a day.

Rx
acyclovir cream 5%
Disp: 3 (three) g
Sig: At the first sign of lesion, apply a small amount to affected areas 6 × daily for 1 week.

Rx
Denavir Cream 1%
Disp: 2 (two) g
Sig: At first sign of lesion, apply a small amount to affected area q2h (while awake) × 4 days.

Mild allergic reactions

Rx
Benadryl 25 mg caps*
Disp: 15 (fifteen) caps
Sig: Take 1 (one) cap q4-8h for symptom relief.
Caution: sedation. *(Adults can take up to 50 mg per dose. Alternative long-acting, nonsedating antihistamines also are available, as well as other rapid-onset, short-acting, sedating antihistamines. However, for immediate hypersensitive reactions, rapid-acting drugs are preferred.)

Rx
Medrol Dosepak 4 mg tabs
Disp: 1 unit
Sig: Follow labeled directions on package for use.
(Note: A pack contains 21 tabs.)

Other dental prescriptions:

Fluoride toothpaste

Rx
1.1% neutral sodium fluoride toothpaste*
Disp: 2 (two) tubes
Sig: Apply thin ribbon to dry toothbrush and brush for 2 min. Spit out excess; do not eat, drink, or rinse for 30 min after use.
*(You may prefer to write PreviDent 5000 Plus.)

Appendix K

Selected References

Advisory Statement: Antibiotic prophylaxis for dental patients with total joint replacements, *JADA* 134:895-899, July 2003.

American Dental Association: Anesthesia color code revision, *ADA News* 24:12, July 2003.

Borea G et al: Tranexamic acid as a mouthwash in anticoagulant-treated patients undergoing oral surgery, *Oral Surg Oral Med Oral Pathol* 75:29-31, 1993.

Cohen DM, Bhattacharyya I, Lydiatt WM: Recalcitrant oral ulcers caused by calcium channel blockers: diagnosis and treatment considerations, *JADA* 130:1611-1618, Nov 1999.

Cupp MJ, Tracy TS: Role of the cytochrome P450 3A subfamily, *US Pharmacists* 22:HS9-HS21, 1997.

Dajani AS et al: Prevention of bacterial endocarditis: recommendations by the American Heart Association, *JAMA* 277:1794-1801, June 1997.

DePaola LG: Managing the care of patients infected with blood borne diseases, *JADA* 134:350-358, 2003.

Drug interaction facts, updated quarterly, St Louis, Facts and Comparisons.

Facts and comparisons, updated monthly, St Louis, Facts and Comparisons.

Fye KH et al: Celecoxib-induced Sweet's syndrome, *J Am Acad Dermatol* 45:300-302, Aug 2001.

Gahart BL: *2000 intravenous medications,* ed 16, St Louis, 1999, Mosby.

Halevy S, Shai A: Lichenoid drug eruptions, *J Am Acad Dermatol* 29:249-255, 1993.

Hardman JG et al: *Goodman and Gilman's the pharmacological basis of therapeutics,* ed 10, New York, 2002, McGraw-Hill.

Little JW, Falace DA: *Dental management of the medically compromised patient,* ed 6, St Louis, 2002, Mosby.

Mancano MA: Drug interactions with protease inhibitors: part I, *Pharmacy Times* 67:14-17, June 2001.

The medical letter, handbook of adverse drug interactions, New Rochelle, NY, 1999, The Medical Letter.

Mosby's drug consult 2004: the comprehensive reference for generic and brand name drugs, ed 14, St Louis, 2004, Mosby.

Pharmacist's Letter 18, 2002.

Pharmacist's Letter 19, 2003.

Physicians' desk reference, ed 58, Montvale, NJ, 2000, Medical Economics.

Rees TD: Oral effects of drug abuse, *Crit Rev Oral Biol Med* 3(3):163-184, 1992.

Rees TD: Systemic drugs as a risk factor for periodontal disease initiation and progression, *Compendium* 16:20-42, 1995.

Shulman JD, Wells LM: Acute fluoride toxicity from ingesting home-use dental products in children birth to 6 years of age, *J Public Health Dent* 57(3):150-158, 1997.

Skidmore-Roth L: *Mosby's 2002 nursing drug reference,* St Louis, 1999, Mosby.

Taylor SE: New drugs and product approval from 2002, *Texas Dental Journal* 120:1160-1169, 2003.

Taylor SE, Gage TW: New drugs and products approved from 2000, *Texas Dental Journal* 118:1070-1081, 2001.

United States Pharmacopeial Convention: *Drug information for the health care professionals USPDI,* ed 24, Englewood, CO, 2004, Micromedex.

United States Pharmacopeial Convention: *USP dictionary of USAN and international drug names 2001,* Rockville, MD, 2001, The Convention.

Valsecchi R, Cainelli T: Gingival hyperplasia induced by erythromycin, *Acta Derm Venereol (Stockh)* 72:157, 1992.

Westbrook P et al: Reversal of nifedipine-induced gingival hyperplasia by the calcium channel blocker, isradipine, *J Dent Res* 74(S1):208, 1995.

Westbrook SD, Paunovich ED, Freytes CO: Adult hemopoietic stem cell transplantation, *JADA* 134:1224-1230, Sep 2003.

Whal MJ: Altering anticoagulant therapy: a survey of physicians, *JADA* 127:625-638, 1996.

Whal MJ: Myths of dental surgery in patients receiving anticoagulant therapy, *JADA* 131:77-81, 2000.

Wright JM: Oral manifestations of drug reactions, *Dent Clin North Am* 28:529-543, 1984.

Zelickson BD, Rogers RS: Oral drug reactions, *Dermatol Clin* 5:695-708, 1987.

Generic and Trade Name Index

Index

Entries can be identified as follows: generic name, Trade Name, DRUG CATEGORY, *Combination Product.*

Entries can be identified as follows: generic name, Trade Name, DRUG CATEGORY, *Combination Product.*

Entries can be identified as follows: generic name, Trade Name, DRUG CATEGORY, *Combination Product.*

Entries can be identified as follows: generic name, Trade Name, DRUG CATEGORY, *Combination Product.*

Entries can be identified as follows: generic name, Trade Name, DRUG CATEGORY, *Combination Product.*

B

Entries can be identified as follows: generic name, Trade Name, DRUG CATEGORY, *Combination Product.*

Entries can be identified as follows: generic name, Trade Name, DRUG CATEGORY, *Combination Product.*

Entries can be identified as follows: generic name, Trade Name, DRUG CATEGORY, *Combination Product.*

Entries can be identified as follows: generic name, Trade Name, DRUG CATEGORY, *Combination Product.*

Entries can be identified as follows: generic name, Trade Name, DRUG CATEGORY, *Combination Product.*

Entries can be identified as follows: generic name, Trade Name, DRUG CATEGORY, *Combination Product.*

Entries can be identified as follows: generic name, Trade Name, DRUG CATEGORY, *Combination Product.*

E

Entries can be identified as follows: generic name, Trade Name, DRUG CATEGORY, *Combination Product.*

Entries can be identified as follows: generic name, Trade Name, DRUG CATEGORY, *Combination Product.*

Entries can be identified as follows: generic name, Trade Name, DRUG CATEGORY, *Combination Product.*

Entries can be identified as follows: generic name, Trade Name, DRUG CATEGORY, *Combination Product.*

Entries can be identified as follows: generic name, Trade Name, DRUG CATEGORY, *Combination Product.*

Entries can be identified as follows: generic name, Trade Name, DRUG CATEGORY, *Combination Product.*

I

Entries can be identified as follows: generic name, Trade Name, DRUG CATEGORY, *Combination Product.*

J

K

Entries can be identified as follows: generic name, Trade Name, DRUG CATEGORY, *Combination Product.*

Entries can be identified as follows: generic name, Trade Name, DRUG CATEGORY, *Combination Product.*

Entries can be identified as follows: generic name, Trade Name, DRUG CATEGORY, *Combination Product.*

Entries can be identified as follows: generic name, Trade Name, DRUG CATEGORY, *Combination Product.*

Entries can be identified as follows: generic name, Trade Name, DRUG CATEGORY, *Combination Product.*

Entries can be identified as follows: generic name, Trade Name, DRUG CATEGORY, *Combination Product.*

Entries can be identified as follows: generic name, Trade Name, DRUG CATEGORY, *Combination Product.*

Entries can be identified as follows: generic name, Trade Name, DRUG CATEGORY, *Combination Product.*

O

Entries can be identified as follows: generic name, Trade Name, DRUG CATEGORY, *Combination Product.*

Entries can be identified as follows: generic name, Trade Name, DRUG CATEGORY, *Combination Product.*

Entries can be identified as follows: generic name, Trade Name, DRUG CATEGORY, *Combination Product.*

Entries can be identified as follows: generic name, Trade Name, DRUG CATEGORY, *Combination Product.*

Entries can be identified as follows: generic name, Trade Name, DRUG CATEGORY, *Combination Product.*

Q

R

Entries can be identified as follows: generic name, Trade Name, DRUG CATEGORY, *Combination Product.*

Entries can be identified as follows: generic name, Trade Name, DRUG CATEGORY, *Combination Product.*

Entries can be identified as follows: generic name, Trade Name, DRUG CATEGORY, *Combination Product.*

T

Entries can be identified as follows: generic name, Trade Name, DRUG CATEGORY, *Combination Product.*

Entries can be identified as follows: generic name, Trade Name, DRUG CATEGORY, *Combination Product.*

Entries can be identified as follows: generic name, Trade Name, DRUG CATEGORY, *Combination Product.*

U

Entries can be identified as follows: generic name, Trade Name, DRUG CATEGORY, *Combination Product.*

Entries can be identified as follows: generic name, Trade Name, DRUG CATEGORY, *Combination Product.*

NEW DRUG UPDATES

Following are monographs for 13 new drugs that have received FDA approval since the publication of *Mosby's Dental Drug Reference,* seventh edition. These monographs follow the same format as those in the book. They are arranged in alphabetical order by generic name, and trade names are given for all medications in common use. Each monograph contains the same subsections as those listed and described on pages ix through xi.

Drug monographs included in this insert

Generic	Trade
acamprosate calcium	Campral
cinacalcet HCl	Sensipar
darifenacin HBr	Enablex
duloxetine HCl	Cymbalta
eszopiclone	Lunesta
omega-3-acid ethyl esters	Omacor
palifermin	Kepivance
rifaximin	Xifaxan
solifenacin succinate	Vesicare
telithromycin	Ketek
tinidazole	Tindamax
trospium chloride	Sanctura
voriconazole	Vfend, Vfend IV

acamprosate calcium

(a-kam-proe'sate)

Campral

Drug class.: Amino acid neurotransmitter analog

Action: Action not established, but it is suggested to involve interaction with glutamate and GABA neurotransmitter systems in the CNS restoring the balance between the systems.

Uses: Maintenance of alcohol abstinence in patients with alcohol dependence as part of a comprehensive treatment program.

Dosage and routes:

• *Adult:* PO patient must have achieved alcohol abstinence, 2 tabs (666 mg) tid with meals; moderate renal impairment: use starting dose of 333 mg tid

Available forms include: Del rel tab 333 mg

Side effects/adverse reactions:

▼ *ORAL:* Dry mouth, taste perversion

CNS: Depression, anxiety, dizziness, anorexia, tremor, diarrhea, insomnia, paresthesia, headache, alcohol craving, somnolence

CV: Palpitation, syncope, peripheral edema, hypertension

GI: Constipation, nausea, abdominal pain, vomiting, dyspepsia, flatulence

RESP: Cough, bronchitis

HEMA: Anemia, ecchymosis

GU: Impotence, UTI

EENT: Rhinitis, *abnormal vision*

INTEG: Rash, pruritus, sweating

ENDO: Hypothyroidism (rare)

META: ↑ AST, ↑ ALT

MS: Back pain, myalgia, arthralgia

MISC: Accidental injury, asthenia, weight gain, pain, flu syndrome

Contraindications: Hypersensitivity, severe renal impairment

Precautions: Reduce dose in moderate renal impairment, monitor for depression and suicidal tendencies, risk of impairment of motor skills or judgment; pregnancy category C, lactation, safety and efficacy in pediatric patients has not been established

Pharmacokinetics:

PO: absolute bioavailability ~11%, steady-state plasma levels 3-8 hrs; negligible plasma protein binding, excreted via urine; drug not metabolized.

Drug interactions of concern to dentistry:

• None reported.

DENTAL CONSIDERATIONS

General:

• The dental professional must be aware of the patient's disease, and the patient must be in active treatment for alcohol abuse.

• Avoid prescribing other addictive drugs, including opioids and benzodiazepines.

• Examine for oral manifestation of opportunistic infection.

• Assess salivary flow as a factor in caries, periodontal disease, and candidiasis.

• Consider semisupine chair position for patient comfort if GI side effects occur.

Consultations:

• Medical consultation may be required to assess disease control.

• Inform abuse counselor or provider if sedative medications are required for proper patient management.

Teach patient/family:

When chronic dry mouth occurs, advise patient:

- To avoid mouth rinses with high alcohol content due to drying effects
- To use daily home fluoride products for anticaries effect
- To use sugarless gum, frequent sips of water or saliva substitutes
- Place on frequent recall due to oral side effects.
- Importance of good oral hygiene to prevent soft tissue inflammation/infection.

---

cinacalcet HCl

(sin-a-kal'set)

Sensipar

Drug class.: Calcimimetic

Action: Directly lowers PTA levels by increasing the sensitivity of the calcium-sensitive receptor on parathyroid chief cells to extracellular calcium causing a decrease in serum calcium levels.

Uses: Secondary hyperparathyroidism in patients on dialysis for chronic kidney disease; hypercalcemia in patients with parathyroid carcinoma

Dosage and routes:

Chronic kidney disease on dialysis:

- *Adult:* PO 30 mg/d; depending on serum Ca^{++}, phosphorus and iPTH levels, adjust dose q2-4 wks to 60, 90, 120 and 180 mg/d. Take with food.

Parathyroid carcinoma:

- *Adult:* PO 30 mg bid; with monitoring of serum Ca^{++}, adjust dose q2-4 wks to 60 mg and 90 mg bid and 90 mg 3-4 times/day.

Available forms include: Tabs 30, 60, 90 mg

Side effects/adverse reactions:

CNS: Dizziness, anorexia

CV: Hypertension

GI: Nausea, vomiting, diarrhea

MS: Myalgia

MISC: Non-cardiac chest pain, asthenia, infection

Contraindications: Hypersensitivity

Precautions: Monitor serum calcium levels (risk of seizures), risk of hypocalcemia (paraesthesias, myalgia, cramps, tetany and seizures), moderate/severe hepatic impairment, pregnancy category C, lactation, safety and efficacy not established for pediatric patients

Pharmacokinetics:

PO: Peak plasma levels 2-6 hrs; plasma protein binding 93-97%; metabolized by CYP3A4, CYP2D6 and CYP1A2 isoenzymes, excreted mainly in urine (80%) and feces (15%).

Drug interactions of concern to dentistry:

- Increased plasma levels of drugs metabolized by CYP2D6 isoenzymes: amitriptyline (see Appendix I)
- Increased plasma levels: ketoconazole, erythromycin and other strong inhibitors of CYP3A4 isoenzymes (see Appendix I)

DENTAL CONSIDERATIONS

General:

- Determine why patient is taking the drug.
- Be aware of patient's disease, its progress and dialysis treatment
- Short appointments and a stress reduction protocol may be required for anxious patients.

• Monitor vital signs every appointment due to cardiovascular side effects.
• Patients taking opioids for acute or chronic pain should be given alternative analgesics for dental pain.
• Product may be used in outpatient therapy.
• Consider semisupine chair position for patient comfort if GI side effects occur.

Consultations:
• Consultation with physician may be needed if sedation or general anesthesia is required, including serum calcium, phosphorus and iPTH values.
• Precaution if dental surgery is anticipated, general anesthesia required
• Antibiotic prophylaxis may be indicated for patient on dialysis; complete physician consult.

Teach patient/family:
• Importance of good oral hygiene to prevent soft tissue inflammation/infection.
• Importance of updating health and drug history, reporting changes in health status, drug regimen changes or disease/treatment status.
• To prevent trauma when using oral hygiene aids.

darifenacin HBr

(dar-ee-fen'a-sin)
Enablex
Drug class.: Anticholinergic

Action: Competitive muscarinic receptor antagonist
Uses: Overactive bladder with symptoms of urge urinary incontinence, urgency and frequency

Dosage and routes:
• *Adult:* PO 7.5 mg/d; after 2 wks dose can be increased to 15 mg/d depending on response. NOTE: Daily dose should not exceed 7.5 mg/d in patients taking strong CYP3A4 inhibitors.
Available forms include: Ext rel tab 7.5, 15 mg

Side effects/adverse reactions:
▼ *ORAL: Dry mouth*
CNS: Dizziness
CV: Hypertension, peripheral edema
GI: Constipation, dyspepsia, abdominal pain, nausea, diarrhea.
RESP: Bronchitis
GU: UTI, acute urinary retention, vaginitis
EENT: ***Blurred vision, dry eyes, abnormal vision, sinusitis***
INTEG: Dry skin, rash, pruritis
META: Weight gain
MS: Back pain, arthralgia
MISC: Asthenia, flu-syndrome

Contraindications: Hypersensitivity, urinary retention, gastric retention, uncontrolled narrow angle glaucoma.

Precautions: Bladder outflow obstruction, gastric obstructive disorders, severe constipation, ulcerative colitis, myasthenia gravis, treated narrow-angle glaucoma, severe hepatic impairment, risk of heat prostration (due to decreased sweating), pregnancy category C, lactation, safety and efficacy in pediatric patients has not been established

Pharmacokinetics:
PO: Peak plasma levels ~7 hrs; mean oral bioavailability 15-19%; plasma protein binding 98%, extensive metabolism by CYP2D6

and CYP3A4 isoenzymes; renal excretion of metabolites (60%) and feces (40%)

Drug interactions of concern to dentistry:

• Increased anticholinergic effect: anticholinergic drugs

• Drugs metabolized by CYP2D6: use with caution

• Increased plasma levels: potent CYP3A4 inhibitors such as ketoconazole, itraconazole, clarithromycin (see Appendix I)

• Caution in use with other drugs that are CYP2D6 substrates such as tricyclic antidepressants.

DENTAL CONSIDERATIONS

General:

• Assess salivary flow as a factor in caries, periodontal disease, and candidiasis.

• To be aware of oral side effects and potential sequella.

• Consider semisupine chair position for patient comfort if GI side effects occur.

• Protect patient's eyes from accidental spatter during dental treatment.

Consultations:

• Physician should be informed if significant xerostomic side effects occur (e.g., increased caries, sore tongue, problems eating or swallowing, difficulty wearing prosthesis) so a medication change can be considered.

Teach patient/family:

When chronic dry mouth occurs, advise patient:

• To avoid mouth rinses with high alcohol content due to drying effects

• To use daily home fluoride products for anticaries effect

• To use sugarless gum, frequent sips of water or saliva substitutes

• Importance of updating health and drug history, reporting changes in health status, drug regimen changes or disease/treatment status.

---

duloxetine HCl

(doo-lox′e-teen)

Cymbalta

Drug class.: Antidepressant

Action: Selective inhibitor of neuronal uptake of serotonin and norepinephrine (SNRI)

Uses: Major depressive disorder (MDD)

Dosage and routes:

• *Adult:* PO 40 mg (20 mg bid) to 60 mg (30 mg bid)

Available forms include: Caps 20, 30, 60 mg

Side effects/adverse reactions:

▼ *ORAL: Dry mouth*

CNS: Decreased appetite, somnolence, dizziness, insomnia, tremor, anxiety, headache

CV: Hot flushes, palpitation, increased blood pressure

GI: Nausea, constipation, diarrhea, vomiting, abdominal pain, gastritis

RESP: URI, cough

HEMA: Anemia

GU: Decreased libido, abnormal orgasm, erectile dysfunction, delayed ejaculation, dysuria

EENT: Blurred vision, pharyngitis

INTEG: Pruritus, rash

META: Increases in ALT, AST, CPK and alkaline phosphatase

MS: Back pain, arthralgia

MISC: Fatigue, increased sweating, decreased weight

Contraindications: Hypersensitivity, MAO inhibitors, uncontrolled narrow-angle glaucoma, end stage renal disease

Precautions: Risk of hepatotoxicity, risk of increase in blood pressure, observe for suicide risk; activation of mania or hypomania, seizure disorders, abrupt discontinuation symptoms; patients with delayed gastric emptying, hepatic impairment, impaired motor skills; pregnancy category C; lactation, use in children is not established

Pharmacokinetics:

PO: Peak plasma levels ~6 hrs; food delays peak concentration time, plasma protein binding >90%; extensive metabolism involving CYP2D6 and CYP1A2; metabolites excreted in urine (70%); 20% in feces

Drug interactions of concern to dentistry:

• Increased plasma levels: inhibitors of CYP1A2 or CYP2D6 (see Appendix I)

• Drugs metabolized by CYP2D6: increased plasma levels (see Appendix I)

• Limited information available: use CNS depressants with caution, avoid alcohol-containing products

DENTAL CONSIDERATIONS

General:

• Prescribe CNS depressants in small quantities for limited use to prevent their use as a suicide tool.

• Determine why patient is taking the drug.

• Short appointments and a stress reduction protocol may be required for anxious patients.

• Examine for oral manifestation of opportunistic infection.

• Assess salivary flow as a factor in caries, periodontal disease, and candidiasis.

• Consider semisupine chair position for patient comfort if GI side effects occur.

Consultations:

• Consultation with physician may be needed if sedation or general anesthesia is required.

• Medical consult may be required to assess disease control and patient's ability to tolerate stress.

• Physician should be informed if significant xerostomic side effects occur (e.g., increased caries, sore tongue, problems eating or swallowing, difficulty wearing prosthesis) so a medication change can be considered.

Teach patient/family:

• Caution patients about driving or performing other tasks requiring alertness.

• Importance of updating health and drug history, reporting changes in health status, drug regimen changes or disease/treatment status.

• Place on frequent recall due to oral side effects.

When chronic dry mouth occurs, advise patient:

• To avoid mouth rinses with high alcohol content due to drying effects

• To use daily home fluoride products for anticaries effect

• To use sugarless gum, frequent sips of water or saliva substitutes

---

eszopiclone

(es-zoe'pik-lone)

Lunesta

Drug class.: Nonbenzodiazepine hypnotic

Controlled Substance Schedule IV

Action: Mechanism of action unclear; may interact with GABA-receptor complexes located near benzodiazepine receptors

Uses: Treatment of insomnia

Dosage and routes:

• *Adult:* PO 2 mg hs, adjust doses to individual's response; can be increased to 3 mg if required (take immediately before going to bed)

• *Elderly Adult:* PO 1 mg hs, adjust doses to individual's response; can be increased to 2 mg if required

Available forms include: Tabs 1, 2, 3 mg

Side effects/adverse reactions:

▼ *ORAL: Dry mouth, unpleasant taste,* mouth ulceration

CNS: Drowsiness, dizziness, light-headedness, headache, nervousness, somnolence, difficulty with coordination, anxiety, confusion, depression, hallucinations

CV: Chest pain, migraine, hypotension (rare), peripheral edema

GI: Dyspepsia, nausea, vomiting, diarrhea

RESP: Infection (unspecified)

GU: ***Dysmenorrhea, UTI, decreased libido, gynecomastia***

INTEG: Pruritus, urticaria, rash

MS: Leg cramps, joint pain

MISC: Accidental injury, viral infection

Contraindications: None reported.

Precautions: Reduce dose in elderly, take dose immediately before bedtime; treatment emergent reactions: risk of altered motor coordination, short term memory, alertness; use with caution in patients with altered metabolism, compromised respiratory function, severe hepatic impairment, patients with depression or suicidal tendencies; pregnancy category C, lactation, safety and efficacy in children <18 yrs is not established

Pharmacokinetics:

PO: Rapidly absorbed, peak levels <1 hr; plasma protein binding 52-59%, extensively metabolized, active metabolite, metabolized by CYP3A4 and CYP2E1 enzymes, elimination time 6 hrs, excreted in urine (75%), fatty meals delay absorption.

Drug interactions of concern to dentistry:

• Increased CNS depression: all CNS depressants, avoid alcohol use

• Avoid the use of potent CYP3A4 inhibitors: ketoconazole (see Appendix I)

DENTAL CONSIDERATIONS

General:

• Determine why patient is taking the drug.

• Short appointments and a stress reduction protocol may be required for anxious patients.

• To be aware of oral side effects and potential sequella.

• Assess salivary flow as a factor in caries, periodontal disease, and candidiasis.

• Consider semisupine chair position for patient comfort if GI side effects occur.

• Psychological and physical dependence may occur with chronic administration.

Consultations:

• Consultation with physician may be needed if sedation or general anesthesia is required.

• Medical consult may be required to assess disease control and patient's ability to tolerate stress.

Teach patient/family:

• Importance of good oral hygiene to prevent soft tissue inflammation/infection.

• Caution patients about driving or performing other tasks requiring alertness.
• Place on frequent recall due to oral side effects.
• Importance of updating health and drug history, reporting changes in health status, drug regimen changes or disease/treatment status.

When chronic dry mouth occurs, advise patient:
• To avoid mouth rinses with high alcohol content due to drying effects
• To use daily home fluoride products for anticaries effect
• To use sugarless gum, frequent sips of water or saliva substitutes

omega-3-acid ethyl esters

Omacor

Drug class.: Lipid regulating drug

Action: Not known, may interfere with selected enzymes that may reduce the synthesis of triglycerides

Uses: Adjunct to diet to reduce very high ≥500 mg/dl triglyceride levels in adults

Dosage and routes:
• *Adult:* PO 4 gm/d, as a single dose or in 2 equal doses (discontinue after 2 months if no response)

Available forms include: Caps 1 g

Side effects/adverse reactions:

▼ *ORAL: Taste perversion,* dry mouth

CV: Angina pectoris

GI: Dyspepsia, eructation

INTEG: Skin rash

META: ↑ AST, ↑ ALT

MS: Back pain

MISC: Flu-like syndrome, infection (nonspecified)

Contraindications: Hypersensitivity

Precautions: Ascertain triglyceride levels before use, couple with diet alteration, exercise and weight loss programs, including review of drugs that may increase triglyceride levels, reassess after 2 months and discontinue if results are unsatisfactory; pregnancy category C, lactation, safety and efficacy in pediatric patients <18 yrs is not established

Pharmacokinetics:

PO: Absorbed orally but kinetic data not provided or not known. Free forms of EPA and DHA are undetectable in the circulation.

Drug interactions of concern to dentistry:
• None reported, although testing has not been performed

DENTAL CONSIDERATIONS

General:
• Reassure patient that taste alteration is not due to a disease problem.
• Be aware that patients with high serum triglyceride levels may also have cardiovascular disease.
• Question patient about other drugs/herbals they may also be taking.
• Assess salivary flow as a factor in caries, periodontal disease, and candidiasis.
• Consider semisupine chair position for patient comfort if GI side effects occur.

Consultations:
• Medical consult as needed if cardiovascular disease is present.

• Medical consult may be required to assess disease control in the patient.

Teach patient/family:

• Importance of good oral hygiene to prevent soft tissue inflammation/ infection.

• To prevent trauma when using oral hygiene aids.

• Importance of updating health and drug history, reporting changes in health status, drug regimen changes or disease/treatment status.

• Ensure that patient is following prescribed diet and regularly takes medication.

When chronic dry mouth occurs, advise patient:

• To avoid mouth rinses with high alcohol content due to drying effects

• To use daily home fluoride products for anticaries effect

• To use sugarless gum, frequent sips of water or saliva substitutes

palifermin

(pal-ee-fer′min)

Kepivance

Drug class.: Human keratinocyte growth factor (KGF)

Action: KFG binds to KFG receptors present on epithelial cells including the tongue, salivary gland and buccal mucosa, as well as many other tissues. It is reported to produce proliferation, differentiation and migration of epithelial cells.

Uses: Decreases the incidence and duration of severe oral mucositis in patients with hematologic malignancies receiving myelotoxic therapy with hematopoietic stem cell support

Dosage and routes:

• *Adult:* IV 60 mcg/kg/d as an IV bolus 3 consecutive days before myelotoxic therapy and 3 consecutive days after myelotoxic therapy

Available forms include: Vials 6.25 mg

Side effects/adverse reactions:

▼ *ORAL: Dysesthesia, discoloration of tongue, altered taste, tongue thickening*

CNS: Paresthesia

CV: Hypertensiion

INTEG: Skin rash, erythemia, edema, pruritus

META: ↑ serum lipase, ↑ serum amylase

MS: Arthralgia

MISC: Fever, pain

Contraindications: Hypersensitivity to *E. coli* derived proteins

Precautions: Potential for stimulation of tumor growth, use in nonhematologic malignancies not established, pregnancy category C, lactation, safety and efficacy for pediatric patients is not established

Pharmacokinetics:

IV: After IV bolus levels decrease rapidly in first 30 minutes; plateau concentration 1-4 hrs, other data not available

Drug interactions of concern to dentistry:

• Has not been studied

DENTAL CONSIDERATIONS

General:

• Administered in the cancer center treatment facility at the time of myelotoxic therapy and hematopoietic transplantation.

• Hospital dentists in cancer centers will be involved in treatment of oral mucositis in cancer patients following established protocols.

rifaximin

(rif-ax'i-min)

Xifaxan

Drug class.: Semisynthetic, nonsystemic antiinfective

Action: Inhibits bacterial RNA synthesis through binding to the beta-subunit of bacterial DNA-dependent RNA polymerase

Uses: Traveler's diarrhea caused by noninvasive strains of *E. coli*

Dosage and routes:

• *Adult and child:* >12 yrs: PO 200 mg tid × 3 days

Available forms include: Tab 200 mg

Side effects/adverse reactions:

▼ *ORAL:* Dry lips

CNS: Headache, dizziness

GI: Flatulence, abdominal pain, rectal tenesmus, nausea, constipation, vomiting, bowel movements

RESP: URTI

HEMA: Lymphocytosis

GU: Urinary frequency

EENT: Ear pain, motion sickness, tinnitus

INTEG: Rash, hives, allergic dermatitis, urticaria

META: Dehydration, ↑ asparate aminotransferase

MS: Muscle pain, arthralgia

MISC: Fever, ***angioedema,*** fatigue, malaise

Contraindications: Hypersensitivity to this drug or any rifamycin antiinfective

Precautions: Effective in *E. coli* associated diarrhea only, discontinue if diarrhea becomes worse in 24-48 hrs, pregnancy category C, lactation, children <12 yrs of age

Pharmacokinetics:

PO: Low systemic absorption from GI mucosa, excreted as unchanged drug in feces (96%), small amounts appear in urine, measurable plasma levels indicate less than 0.4% is absorbed.

Drug interactions of concern to dentistry:

• None reported

DENTAL CONSIDERATIONS

General:

• This drug is not substantially absorbed and for acute use only. Patients are not likely to appear in the dental office.

solifenacin succinate

(sol-i-fen'a-sin)

Vesicare

Drug class.: Anticholinergic

Action: Competitive muscarinic receptor antagonist

Uses: Overactive bladder with symptoms of urge urinary incontinence, urgency and urinary frequency

Dosage and routes:

• *Adult:* PO 5 mg/d; dose may be increased to 10 mg/d depending on patient's response (Patients taking ketoconazole or other potent CYP3A4 isoenzyme inhibitors: limit 5 mg/d)

Moderate hepatic impairment or severe renal impairment

• *Adult:* PO Maximum dose 5 mg/d

Available forms include: Tabs 5, 10 mg

Side effects/adverse reactions:

▼ *ORAL: Dry mouth*

CNS: Dizziness, depression

CV: Hypertension, prolonged QT interval
GI: Constipation, nausea, dyspepsia, abdominal pain, vomiting
RESP: Cough
GU: Urinary retention, UTI
EENT: Blurred vision, dry eyes, pharyngitis
*MISC: **Angioedema,*** flu-like syndrome, fatigue

Contraindications: Hypersensitivity, urinary retention, gastric retention, uncontrolled narrow-angle glaucoma

Precautions: Bladder outflow obstruction, decreased GI motility, treated narrow angle glaucoma, renal impairment, reduced hepatic function; pregnancy category C, lactation, safety and efficacy not established in pediatric patients

Pharmacokinetics:
PO: Absolute bioavailability 90%, peak plasma levels 3 to 8 hrs, plasma protein binding 98%, extensive hepatic metabolism by CYP3A4 isoenzymes; metabolites excreted in urine (69%), some fecal elimination

Drug interactions of concern to dentistry:
- Increased anticholinergic effects: anticholinergic drugs
- Dose limit with: ketoconazole and other potent CYP3A4 isoenzyme inhibitors (see Appendix I)
- Use with caution: CYP3A4 isoenzyme inducers

DENTAL CONSIDERATIONS

General:
- Assess salivary flow as a factor in caries, periodontal disease, and candidiasis.
- Consider semisupine chair position for patient comfort if GI side effects occur.
- Protect patient's eyes from accidental spatter during dental treatment.

Consultations:
- Medical consult may be required to assess disease control in the patient.
- Physician should be informed if significant xerostomic side effects occur (e.g., increased caries, sore tongue, problems eating or swallowing, difficulty wearing prosthesis) so a medication change can be considered.

Teach patient/family:
- Place on frequent recall due to oral side effects.
- Importance of good oral hygiene to prevent soft tissue inflammation/infection.
- Importance of updating health and drug history, reporting changes in health status, drug regimen changes or disease/treatment status.

When chronic dry mouth occurs, advise patient:
- To avoid mouth rinses with high alcohol content due to drying effects
- To use daily home fluoride products for anticaries effect
- To use sugarless gum, frequent sips of water or saliva substitutes

---

telithromycin

(tel-ith-roe-mye'sin)

Ketek

Drug class.: Semisynthetic antiinfective ketolide

Action: Blocks bacterial protein synthesis by binding to the 50S ribosomal subunit

Uses: Acute bacterial exacerbation of chronic bronchitis (*S. pneumo-*

niae, H. influenzae, M. catarrhalis); acute bacterial sinusitis (*S. pneumoniae, H. influenzae, M. catarrhalis, S. aureus);* community acquired pneumonia *(S. pneumoniae, H. influenzae, M. catarrhalis, C. pneumoniae, M. pneumoniae)*
Dosage and routes:
Acute exacerbation of chronic bronchitis, acute bacterial sinusitis
• *Adult:* ≥18 yrs: PO 800 mg/d × 5 days
Community acquired pneumonia
• *Adult:* ≥18 yrs: PO 800 mg/d × 7-10 days
Available forms include: Tab 400 mg
Side effects/adverse reactions:
▼ *ORAL: Taste alteration,* candidiasis, stomatitis, glossitis, dry mouth, facial edema
CNS: Headache, dizziness, vertigo, insomnia, somnolence, anxiety, paresthesia
CV: Bradycardia, flushing, hypotension (rare), ***atrial arrhythmias, prolonged QT interval***
GI: Diarrhea, nausea, vomiting, ***pseudomembranous colitis, hepatic dysfunction,*** abdominal pain
HEMA: Increased platelet count
GU: Vaginal candidiasis, vaginitis
EENT: Blurred vision, difficulty in focusing, diplopia
INTEG: Rash, ***erythema multiforme*** (rare), urticaria
META: ↑ ALT, ↑ AST, ↑ bilirubin
MS: Cramps
MISC: Fatigue, severe allergic reactions (***angioedema, anaphylaxis***)
Contraindications: Hypersensitivity to this drug or any macrolide antibiotic, pimozide, patients with proarrhythmic conditions, quinidine, procainamide, dofetilide, simvastatin, lovastatin, atorvastatin, ergot alkaloids, hypokalemia
Precautions: Renal impairment, may prolong QT interval, exacerbation of myasthenia gravis, not for prophylactic use, use only for patients 18 yrs of age or older; pregnancy category C, caution in lactation
Pharmacokinetics:
PO: Absolute bioavailability 57%, peak levels 0.5-4 hrs, protein binding 60% to 70%, partially metabolized by CYP3A4, excretion 37% by metabolism, 13% excreted in urine and 7% in feces.
Drug interactions of concern to dentistry:
• Increased plasma levels: itraconazole, ketoconazole
• Increased plasma levels of midazolam, theophylline
• Inhibits the enzyme CYP3A4 (see Appendix I): do not use with CYP3A4 enzyme inducers

DENTAL CONSIDERATIONS
General:
• Determine why patient is taking the drug.
• This drug is used for URTI. Evaluate respiration characteristics for absence of disease.
• Consider semisupine chair position for patients with respiratory disease.
• Monitor vital signs every appointment due to cardiovascular side effects.
• Examine for oral manifestation of opportunistic infection.
• To be aware of oral side effects and potential sequella.
• Consider semisupine chair position for patient comfort if GI side effects occur.

Consultations:

• Consultation with physician may be needed if sedation or general anesthesia is required.

• Consult with patient's physician if an acute dental infection occurs and another antiinfective is required.

• Medical consult may be required to assess disease control and patient's ability to tolerate stress.

Teach patient/family:

• Alert the patient to the possibility of secondary oral infection and the need to see dentist immediately if signs of infection occur.

• Importance of updating health and drug history, reporting changes in health status, drug regimen changes or disease/treatment status.

---

tinidazole

(tye-ni'da-zole)

Tindamax

Drug class.: Antiprotozoal

Action: Unknown; free nitro radicals may be responsible for action against *Trichomonas*

Uses: Trichomoniasis, giardiasis, amebiasis

Dosage and routes:

Trichomoniasis (both male and female)

• *Adult:* PO 2 gm as a single dose with food

Giardiasis

• *Adult:* PO 2 gm as a single dose with food

• *Child >3 yrs:* PO 50 mg/kg as a single dose, (2 gm limit) with food

Intestinal amebiasis

• *Adult:* PO 2 gm/d × 3 days taken with food

• *Child >3 yrs:* PO 50 mg/kg/d (limit 2 gm/d) × 3 days with food

Amebic liver abscess

• *Adult:* PO 2 gm/d × 3-5 days taken with food

• *Child >3 yrs:* PO 50 mg/kg/d (limit 2 gm/d) × 3-5 days with food

Available forms include: Tabs 250, 500 mg

Side effects/adverse reactions:

▼ *ORAL: Metallic/bitter taste,* dry mouth, candidiasis, discolored tongue, stomatitis

CNS: Weakness, fatigue, anorexia, malaise, headache, dizziness, seizures, transient peripheral neuropathy

CV: Palpitation, flushing

GI: Nausea, vomiting, dyspepsia, cramps, constipation, diarrhea

RESP: Bronchospasm (rare)

HEMA: Transient neutropenia, transient leukopenia

GU: ***Discolored urine, vaginal discharge***

EENT: Pharyngitis

INTEG: Rash, urticaria, pruritis

META: ↑ transaminase levels

MS: Myalgia

MISC: ***Angioedema,*** fever

Contraindications: Hypersensitivity to this drug or other nitroimidazole derivatives; first trimester of pregnancy

Precautions: CNS disease (risk of seizures and peripheral neuropathy), history of blood dyscrasia, severe hepatic impairment, candidiasis may also be present, take tablets with food, differential and total leukocyte test recommended during therapy, pregnancy category C, lactation, pediatric use limited to giardiasis and amebiasis

Pharmacokinetics:

PO: Rapidly and completely absorbed, peak plasma levels ~1.6

hrs; plasma protein binding 12%; significant metabolism mainly by CYP3A4 isoenzymes; excreted mainly in urine, small fraction in feces

Drug interactions of concern to dentistry:

• Avoid alcohol or alcohol containing products.

• Enhanced effect of warfarin, lithium, cyclosporine.

• Reduced plasma levels: inducers of CYP3A4 isoenzymes (see Appendix I)

• Do not use with oxytetracycline.

DENTAL CONSIDERATIONS

General:

• NOTE: This is a short duration use drug; side effects usually should be of a short duration

• Examine for oral manifestation of opportunistic infection.

• Consider semisupine chair position for patient comfort if GI side effects occur.

Consultations:

• Consultation with physician may be needed if sedation or general anesthesia is required.

• Consult with patient's physician if an acute dental infection occurs and another antiinfective is required.

Teach patient/family:

• Taste alteration should rapidly return to normal after drug regimen is completed.

• Avoid alcohol containing mouth rinses while drug effects persist.

• Alert the patient to the possibility of secondary oral infection and the need to see dentist immediately if signs of infection occur.

• Importance of good oral hygiene to prevent soft tissue inflammation/infection.

• To prevent trauma when using oral hygiene aids.

---

trospium chloride

(trose'pee-um)

Sanctura

Drug class.: Anticholinergic

Action: Competitive muscarinic receptor antagonist

Uses: Overactive bladder with symptoms of urge urinary incontinence, urgency and urinary frequency

Dosage and routes:

• *Adult:* PO 20 mg bid at least 1 hr before meals

• *Elderly Adult:* PO 20 mg/d (to lessen frequency of side effects)

Available forms include: Tab 20 mg

Side effects/adverse reactions:

▼ *ORAL: Dry mouth,* dysgeusia

CNS: Headache, hallucinations

CV: Tachycardia, palpitation, syncope, hypertension

GI: Constipation, abdominal pain, dyspepsia, flatulence, abdominal distention, vomiting

GU: Urinary retention

EENT: Dry eyes, blurred vision, dry throat

INTEG: ***Stevens-Johnson Syndrome,*** dry skin

MS: Rhabdomyolysis

MISC: Fatigue, ***anaphylaxis, angioedema***

Contraindications: Urinary retention, gastric retention or uncontrolled narrow-angle glaucoma, hypersensitivity

Precautions: Bladder outflow obstruction, gastrointestinal obstructive disorders, ulcerative colitis, intestinal atony, myasthenia gravis,

controlled-angle glaucoma, severe renal impairment, moderate to severe hepatic impairment, risk of heat prostration (due to decrease in sweating); pregnancy category C, lactation, safety and efficacy in pediatric patients is not established.
Pharmacokinetics: Absolute bioavailability 9.6%, peak plasma levels 5-6 hrs; fatty meal reduces absorption; plasma protein binding 50-85%, metabolism not fully described; excretion mainly in feces (80%) with lesser amount in urine (5.8%).

Drug interactions of concern to dentistry:

- Drug interactions have not been studied, but expect increased anticholinergic effects when other anticholinergics are given.

DENTAL CONSIDERATIONS

General:

- Examine for oral manifestation of opportunistic infection.
- Consider semisupine chair position for patient comfort if GI side effects occur.
- Protect patient's eyes from accidental spatter during dental treatment.
- Assess salivary flow as a factor in caries, periodontal disease, and candidiasis.
- Monitor vital signs every appointment due to cardiovascular side effects.

Consultations:

- Physician should be informed if significant xerostomic side effects occur (e.g., increased caries, sore tongue, problems eating or swallowing, difficulty wearing prosthesis) so a medication change can be considered.

Teach patient/family:

When chronic dry mouth occurs, advise patient:

- To avoid mouth rinses with high alcohol content due to drying effects
- To use daily home fluoride products for anticaries effect
- To use sugarless gum, frequent sips of water or saliva substitutes
- Place on frequent recall due to oral side effects.
- Importance of good oral hygiene to prevent soft tissue inflammation/infection.
- Importance of updating health and drug history, reporting changes in health status, drug regimen changes or disease/treatment status.

---

voriconazole

(voe-ri-cone'a-zole)
VFEND, VFEND IV
Drug class.: Triazole antifungal

Action: Inhibits cytochrome P450 mediated ergosterol synthesis leading to loss of cell wall integrity
Uses: Treatment of infections due to *Aspergillus fumigatus, Scedosporium apiospermum, Fusarium* species and esophageal candidiasis, candidemia in non-neutropenic patients, disseminated candida infections in skin, abdomen, bladder wall and wounds
Dosage and routes:
Invasive aspergillous or serious infections due to Scedosporium or Fusarium

- *Adult:* IV loading dose 6 mg/kg q12h first day; then IV 4 mg/kg q12h or PO 200 mg q12h; IV not for bolus injection.

NEW DRUG UPDATES

Candidemia in neutropenic patients and other deep tissue candida infections

• *Adult:* IV loading dose 6 mg/kg q12h first day; then IV 3-4 mg/kg q12h or PO 200 mg q12h; IV not for bolus injection.

Esophageal candidiasis

• *Adult:* PO 200 mg q12h; oral doses must be taken at least 1 hr before or 1 hr after meals

Adjustment: Mild to moderate hepatic cirrhosis: reduce dose by 50%

Available forms include: Tabs 50, 200 mg; powder for oral susp 45 g (providing 40 mg/ml); vials 200 mg

Side effects/adverse reactions:

▼ *ORAL:* Dry mouth, glossitis, possible gingival overgrowth

CNS: Headache, hallucinations

CV: Peripheral edema, tachycardia, arrhythmias

GI: Nausea, diarrhea, abdominal pain, vomiting, cholestatic jaundice

RESP: Respiratory disorder (not specified)

HEMA: ***Agranulocytosis,*** anemia

GU: ***Acute renal failure,*** abnormal renal function

EENT: Visual disturbances, photophobia, chromatopsia, photosensitivity

INTEG: Rash, ***Stevens-Johnson Syndrome, toxic epidermal necrosis, erythema multiforme***

META: ↑ liver function tests, ↑ alkaline phosphatase, ↑ hepatic enzymes, hypokalemia, bilirubinemia, ↑ creatinine

MS: Arthralgia

MISC: Fever, sepsis, chills, ***anaphylaxis***

Contraindications: Hypersensitivity, allergy to other azole antifungals, pimozide, quinidine (prolonged QT interval), sirolimus, rifampin, long-acting barbiturates, ritonavir, efavirenz, rifabutin, ergot alkaloids, carbamazepine

Precautions: Visual function tests after 28 days of use; risk of serious hepatic reactions, monitor liver function, pregnancy category D, may be associated with prolonged QT interval and arrhythmias, infusion reactions, no night driving, risk of operating car or machinery, avoid strong sunlight, safety and efficacy in pediatric patients <12 yrs of age has not been established, lactation

Pharmacokinetics:

PO/IV: Steady state peak plasma levels in 24 hrs; oral bioavailability 96%, maximum plasma levels 1-2 hrs; plasma protein binding (58%), metabolized by CYP2C19, CYP2C9, CYP3A4 isoenzymes; metabolites excreted in urine (80-83%).

Drug interactions of concern to dentistry:

• A large number of drugs may interact with this drug. See contraindications. Other drugs that induce or inhibit CYP2C9 or CYP3A4 should be used with caution.

• Increased plasma levels of cyclosporine, tacrolimus, benzodiazepines

• Voriconazole may inhibit CYP2CP, CYP3A4 (see Appendix I)

DENTAL CONSIDERATIONS

General:

• Patient on chronic drug therapy may rarely present with symptoms of blood dyscrasias which can include infection, bleeding and poor healing.

• Avoid dental light in patient's eyes; offer dark glasses for patient comfort.

• Protect patient's eyes from accidental spatter during dental treatment.

• Examine for oral manifestation of opportunistic infection.

• Assess salivary flow as a factor in caries, periodontal disease, and candidiasis.

• Advise patient if dental drugs prescribed have a potential for photosensitivity.

• Monitor vital signs every appointment due to cardiovascular side effects.

Consultations:

• Consult with patient's physician if an acute dental infection occurs and another antiinfective is required.

• Medical consult may be required to assess disease control and patient's ability to tolerate stress.

• In a patient with symptoms of blood dyscrasias, request a medical consult for blood studies and postpone treatment until normal values are re-established.

Teach patient/family:

• Importance of good oral hygiene to prevent soft tissue inflammation/infection.

• To prevent trauma when using oral hygiene aids.

• Importance of updating health and drug history, reporting changes in health status, drug regimen changes or disease/treatment status.

When chronic dry mouth occurs, advise patient:

• To avoid mouth rinses with high alcohol content due to drying effects

• To use daily home fluoride products for anticaries effect

• To use sugarless gum, frequent sips of water or saliva substitutes

NEW COMBINATION PRODUCTS

Following are six new combination products that have been added since the publication of *Mosby's Dental Drug Reference,* seventh edition. These products follow the same format as those in found in Appendix F.

Caduet: amlodipine besylate 2.5 mg with atorvastatin calcium 10 mg, amlodipine besylate 2.5 mg with atorvastatin calcium 20 mg, amlodipine besylate 2.5 mg with atorvastatin calcium 40 mg, amlodipine besylate 5 mg with atorvastatin calcium 10 mg; amlodipine besylate 5 mg with atorvastatin calcium 20 mg, amlodipine besylate 5 mg with atorvastatin calcium 40 mg, amlodipine besylate 5 mg with atorvastatin calcium 80 mg; amlodipine besylate 10 mg with atorvastatin calcium 10 mg; amlodipine besylate 10 mg with atorvastatin calcium 20 mg; amlodipine besylate 10 mg with atorvastatin calcium 40 mg; amlodipine besylate 10 mg with atorvastatin calcium 80 mg
Combunox: oxycodone HCl 5 mg with ibuprofen 400 mg
Epzicom: abacavir 600 mg with lamivudine 300 mg
Parcopa: carbidopa 10 mg with levodopa 100 mg; carbidopa 25 mg with levodopa 100 mg; carbidopa 25 mg with levodopa 250 mg.
Truvada: tenofovir disoproxil fumarate 300 mg with emtricitabine 200 mg
Vytorin: ezetimibe 10 mg with simvastatin 10 mg; ezetimibe 10 mg with simvastatin 20 mg; ezetimibe 10 mg with simvastatin 40 mg; ezetimibe 10 mg with simvastatin 80 mg

RECENTLY APPROVED DRUGS – THOSE NOT LIKELY TO BE ENCOUNTERED IN THE DENTAL OFFICE

generic name (TRADE NAME-[Manufacturer]) Indication

apomorphine HCl (APOKYN-[Mylan Bertek Pharmaceuticals]) This is an injectable drug used to treat acute episodes of hypomobility or "off" episodes in advanced Parkinson's disease.

azacitidine (VIDAZA-[Pharmion]) This new injectable drug is a pyrimidine nucleoside analog of cytidine for use in 5 subtypes of myelodysplastic syndrome.

bevacizumab (AVASTIN-[Genentech]) is a recombinant monoclonal Ig G1 antibody that inhibits the activity of human vascular endothelial growth factor (VEGF). It is an injectable antineoplastic drug designed to hinder tumor growth by neutralizing vascular endothelial growth factor protein and inhibiting blood vessel growth. It is used in combination with 5-fluorouracil for treatment of patients with metastatic carcinoma of the colon or rectum.

cetuximab (ERBITUX-[Bristol, Myers, Squibb]) This is a monoclonal antibody that binds to human epidermal growth factor (EGFR). It is used in combination with irinotecan for the treatment of patients with metastatic colorectal carcinoma in patient's refractory to irinotecan alone. It is used alone to treat patients with metastatic colorectal cancer intolerant to irinotecan.

clofarabine (CLOLAR-[Genzyme]) A new antineoplastic drug (a purine nucleoside) used to treat pediatric patients with relapsed or refractory acute lymphoblastic leukemia.

erlotinib (TARCEVA-[Genentech]) An oral tablet form of human epidermal growth factor receptor type 1/ epidermal growth factor receptor (HER1/EGFR) tyrosine kinase inhibitor. It is approved for used in the treatment of patients with locally advanced or metastatic non-small cell lung cancer after failure of at least one prior chemotherapy regimen. Ketoconazole interacts with erlotinib to increase plasma levels and caution should be used when administering Tarceva with ketoconazole and other strong inhibitors of CYP3A4.

iloprost (VENTAVIS-[CoTherix]) This is an inhalational drug is indicated for the treatment of patients with pulmonary arterial hypertension with New York Heart Association class III or IV symptoms.

lanthanum carbonate (FOSRENOL-[Shire]) An orally administered drug that binds dietary phosphate in the GI tract and reduces serum phosphate in dialysis patients with end stage kidney disease.

pegaptanib sodium (MACUGEN-[Pfizer]) This drug is a selective vascular endothelial growth factor (VEGF) antagonist (injected directly into the eye) for use in the treatment of patients with neovascular (wet) age-related macular degeneration.

premetrexed disodium (ALIMATA-[Lilly]) A new anti-antifolate chemotherapeutic agent indicated for treatment patients with malignant pleural mesothelioma when surgery cannot be used.

ziconotide (PRIALT-[Elan Pharmaceuticals]) This new drug is a synthetic peptide for intrathecal administration. It is indicated for the management of severe chronic pain in patients for whom intrathecal therapy is warranted and who are intolerant of or refractory to other treatment, such as systemic analgesics, adjunctive therapies or intrathecal morphine. Drug interactions an increased incidence of CNS adverse reactions when used with other CNS depressants.